Principles and Practice of Psychopharmacotherapy

Third Edition

Principles and Practice of Psychopharmacotherapy

Third Edition

Philip G. Janicak, M.D.
Professor of Psychiatry
Medical Director, Psychiatric Clinical Research Center
Department of Psychiatry
University of Illinois at Chicago
Chicago, Illinois

John M. Davis, M.D.
Gilman Professor of Psychiatry
Psychiatric Institute
Department of Psychiatry
University of Illinois at Chicago
Chicago, Illinois

Sheldon H. Preskorn, M.D.
Professor and Vice-Chairman of Psychiatry
University of Kansas-Wichita
Wichita, Kansas

Frank J. Ayd, Jr., M.D.
Emeritus Director
Taylor Manor Hospital
Ellicott City, Maryland

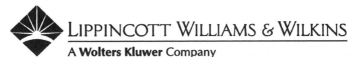
LIPPINCOTT WILLIAMS & WILKINS
A **Wolters Kluwer** Company
Philadelphia • Baltimore • New York • London
Buenos Aires • Hong Kong • Sydney • Tokyo

Acquisitions Editor: Charles W. Mitchell
Developmental Editor: Joyce A. Murphy
Production Editor: Frank Aversa
Manufacturing Manager: Colin J. Warnock
Cover Designer: Matthew Cray Janicak
Compositor: Techbooks
Printer: RR Donnelley/Crawfordsville

Library of Congress Cataloging-in-Publication Data

Principles and practice of psychopharmacotherapy / Philip G. Janicak...[et al.].—3rd ed.
    p. ; cm.
  Includes bibliographical references and index.
  ISBN 0-7817-2794-4
    1. Mental illness—Chemotherapy. 2. Psychopharmacology. I. Janicak, Philip G.
    [DNLM: 1. Mental Disorders—drug therapy. 2. Psychotropic Drugs—metabolism.
  3. Psychotropic Drugs—therapeutic use. WM 402 P957 2001]
  RC483 .P74 2001
  616.89′18—dc21   2001018654

10 9 8 7 6 5 4 3 2 1

Josephine, Edward, Mary, and Matthew,
For the gift of a life filled with love.

Our patients and their families.
If this endeavor alleviates your suffering in any way,
our efforts will have been rewarded
a thousand-fold.

PHILIP G. JANICAK

To my family with love and thanks:
Deborah, Richard, Kathy, Markey, Jody, and Rob.

To the international community of physicians and scientists
dedicated to developing better ways
of treating mental illness.

JOHN M. DAVIS

To Belinda and Erika,
with love and gratitude for your support, encouragement, and understanding.

In loving memory of my parents, Harrison and Marie.

SHELDON H. PRESKORN

My wife and my family,
For their love, support, and understanding.

My patients, who have taught me so much.
My colleagues, who have shared their knowledge with me.

FRANK J. AYD, JR.

Contents

Foreword

Prior to the fall of 2000, I had known three of the authors of this remarkable textbook reasonably well. However, only recently had I reason to talk at length with Dr. Janicak and, immediately thereafter, to read in detail the second edition of the present book. I found it excellently organized, full of useful information that is well presented and encyclopedic in scope. I therefore accepted with pleasure the invitation to write the foreword to the third edition, in its final stages of composition when Dr. Janicak and I met while he was visiting the Boston area. I'm ashamed to say that I had personally been guilty of regional ethnocentricity, having read and used books on psychopharmacology mainly by Bostonians or, in the past, by Klein and Davis when they were in New York and Bethesda, respectively.

The third edition is truly remarkable in its scope, depth, and readability. It is both comprehensive and remarkably up-to-date. The field (and the practice) of clinical psychopharmacology has expanded radically over the past few years, in the number and types of drugs available to treat psychiatric disorders, the types of formulations being used (or in testing), and the depth of knowledge of their pharmacodynamics and pharmacokinetics. This parallels the growth in psychiatry and brain science.

One wonders whether the apparent expansion of polypharmacy, seen in psychiatric inpatients and outpatients, is not a result of many more kinds of drugs to use. Also, many newer drugs—gabapentin, olanzapine, quetiapine, mirtazapine, nefazodone, the several SSRIs–are not only reasonably safe in overdose but have a confusing (or encouraging, take your choice) range of probable efficacies that can lead competent psychiatrists to place patients who are not improving on monotherapy or duotherapy onto a larger group of medications. A depressed psychotic with chronic probable schizoaffective disorder is not uncommonly found on an atypical antipsychotic in its full regular dose, plus an older neuroleptic because psychotic symptoms persist; plus two mood stabilizers; one antidepressant; trazodone and zopiclone for insomnia; a benzodiazepine for daytime anxiety; and buspirone to potentiate the antidepressant. When such a patient is admitted to a psychiatric unit, the allowed stay is likely to be too short to permit any major withdrawal of the multiple medications. The sort of problem presented above is not solved simply, but the third edition does give a great deal of information on each of the drugs involved, their demonstrated efficacies, their potential side effects, and their likely interactions with other drugs. The clinician can use this book to understand possible complications, and can use this knowledge to intelligently begin unscrambling to polydrug regimens systematically, to retain contributions that seem both useful and benign, and to use theraputic drug monitoring (the authors' term) to assess levels of the various drugs in biological fluids as a method to assess possible interactions that may have toxic potential.

This book gives the studious reader a broad education in clinical research design, statistics, and especially pharmacokinetics, drug metabolism, and pharmacodynamics. All this plus useful guides to the selection of clinical treatments and algorithms to follow if the first option fails after an adequate trial. This book also gives the best up-to-date coverage of the newer atypical antipsychotics, including ziprasidone, which, as of this writing, is teetering on the edge of becoming available in U.S. drug stores. It covers not only mirtazapine and newer MAOIs, but also reboxetine, a noradrenergic antidepressant available only in Europe; as well as newer biological therapeutics such as transcranial magnetic stimulation and vagal nerve stimulation used as treatments (so far) mainly for affective disorders. Its coverage of electroconvulsive therapy is accurate and up-to-date.

This book manages to review, in adequate detail, a vast number of studies that form the basis for its meta-analyses and many of its recommendations. The contents outline, figures, and tables enable the reader to easily find the information he needs at the level he is prepared to digest it.

The book is written cohesively and provides the kind of compendium that Goodman and Gilman provided to pharmacology when they first wrote their textbook in the 1940's, now multiauthored and vastly larger.

Each chapter begins with a review of the status of knowledge about the etiology, course, biology, and genetics of the disorders to be treated. These sections alone would make the book useful to residents or past-residents reviewing material before taking their psychiatric boards.

As a practicing clinician with my own experiences and prejudices, I may not agree absolutely with every recommendation or warning in this book but I strongly believe this is the best, most comprehensive, most timely, and most usable textbook about our field to date.

Jonathan Cole, M.D.

Preface to the First Edition

Over the last three decades there has been an explosion of information about drug therapies for the management of mental disorders. This phenomenon closely parallels the expansion of ever more sophisticated technologies that subserve the field of neuroscience. As a result, pathophysiology has become an increasingly more appropriate foundation upon which to diagnose disorders, as well as to develop more effective biological remedies. A further development has been the growing number of well-conceived and carefully executed clinical drug trials, making assimilation of this expansive literature a daunting task.

The goal of *Principles and Practice of Psychopharmacotherapy* is to provide a clinical logic that incorporates contemporary knowledge about drug therapies into the overall management of the mentally ill. The intended audience includes: residents in psychiatry and family practice, as well as the general practitioners of these medical specialties; psychiatric nurses, psychologists, and social workers; and other mental health professionals who are involved with patients taking psychotropic medications.

We have highlighted what we believe to be the unique strengths of this work. First, this book has been conceived and written by four authors only. Each is a professor of psychiatry, and combined, we bring to this effort over 100 years of research and clinical experience. This work has truly been a team effort, with extensive meetings and phone discussions, and careful reviews and critiques of original and subsequent drafts by each author over the last two years. Further, expert opinion has also been sought and graciously given in the form of detailed critiques by such recognized leaders as Max Fink, M.D., Ghanshyam Pandey, Ph.D., and Donald Klein, M.D. The results are:

A work characterized by a comprehensive summarization of the literature (e.g., about 2000 references, most since 1985);

A uniformity and succinctness of style and organization throughout the text; and

The development of treatment strategies based on the best scientific data available and tempered by our combined clinical experience.

In Chapter 1 we formulate seven guiding principles that clearly demarcate the role of drug therapy within the context of a comprehensive, often lifelong, treatment approach. Next, to help guide therapeutic choices, we provide statistical summarizations, by means of meta-analyses, of the extensive, ever more methodologically rigorous, literature comparing various drug and somatic therapies to placebo or to each other.

To set the stage for such an exercise, we discuss in Chapter 2 the qualities that characterize a well-designed study and the issues critical to appreciating the strengths and the weaknesses of combining the outcomes of multiple trials to derive a "bottom-line" conclusion on relative efficacy.

In Chapter 2 we also explore the role of drug therapy from the patient-consumer's perspective. Thus, such issues as informed consent, the cost of treatment, and labelled versus nonlabelled uses for FDA-approved medications are carefully considered.

In Chapter 3 we discuss the relevant pharmacokinetic principles, particularly as they apply to the treatment recommendations rendered throughout the text.

In Chapters 4 through 12 we deal with the major classes of psychotropics as well as the pertinent diagnostic issues related to various drug therapies. This constitutes the core of our work, and includes the:

Antipsychotics
Antidepressants
Somatic therapies
Mood stabilizers
Anxiolytics/sedative-hypnotics

Our approach to each of these drug groups and related somatic therapies begins with a consideration of the possible mechanisms of action, followed by a comprehensive literature review on efficacy and adverse effects. These discussions then serve as the basis for the development of a clinical therapeutic strategy. Knowing that many patients fail standard treatment recommendations, because of either insufficient efficacy or intolerance to adverse effects, led us to emphasize the latter's importance.

The book concludes with Chapters 13 and 14 on disorders that require separate consideration. The first group includes Panic, Obsessive-Compulsive, Post-Traumatic Stress, Somatoform, and Dissociative disorders. Although traditionally these are classified as anxiety disorders, their symptoms and varied treatment responsivity require a separate series of discussions. Finally, certain groups of patients are considered in light of their specialized needs when contemplating psychotropic drug therapy. They include the pregnant patient, children and adolescents, the elderly, the personality disordered, as well as patients whose conditions are complicated by medical problems (e.g., the alcoholic patient; the HIV-infected patient).

Throughout the book an attempt is made to create a "reader-friendly" compendium. Thus, for any given topic one can quickly peruse the introductory and conclusionary statements; the critical points in the text as indicated by italics, boldface, or bulleted lists; the tabular data (e.g., statistical summaries of the comparative efficacy of a new agent versus placebo and a standard drug therapy); and the treatment strategy diagrams, all of which succinctly outline our suggested approach to a given disorder. This allows the reader to quickly assimilate the most important information, while also providing a more in-depth discussion to be reviewed as time permits. Illustrative case examples are also provided to underscore a particular clinical issue.

As "no man is an island," no author (or group of authors) could presume to take sole credit for such an endeavor as we now put forth. Therefore, it is with gratitude that we acknowledge the editorial assistance of Nijole Beleska Grazulis, M.S., who also indexed this work. We thank Dave Retford, Barbara Felton, Molly Mullen, Jonathan Pine, Gillian Casey, and Wayne Hubbel of Williams & Wilkins for their guidance and expertise. Further, Drs. Janicak and Davis sincerely thank Rajiv P. Sharma, M.D., Javaid I. Javaid, Ph.D., Subhash Pandey, Ph.D., Mark Watanabe, Ph.D., Sheila Dowd, Alan Newman, and Jane Retallack for their efforts on behalf of this enterprise. Dr. Preskorn thanks Sharon Hickok for her assistance in making this textbook a reality, and his mentors, colleagues, residents, medical students, and patients, who have provided insights and intellectual stimulation throughout the years. Dr. Ayd thanks Mary Ann Ayd and Ann Lovelace.

Finally, good night, Michael Fisher, wherever you are.

Philip G. Janicak, M.D.
John M. Davis, M.D.
Sheldon H. Preskorn, M.D.
Frank J. Ayd, Jr., M.D.

Preface

In the decade since this textbook was first conceived and created, nothing short of a revolution has occurred in the practice of psychopharmacotherapy. In addition to the growing population of antidepressants, antipsychotics, and mood stabilizers, we have witnessed the ascendancy of:

- *Genetics* as a promising approach for future drug development
- *Natural remedies* as potential partners with standard drug development
- *Novel somatic approaches* that may supplement or complement existing treatments
- Treatment *guidelines* and *strategies* that are increasingly based on the principles of sound clinical practice.

The pace of these developments continues to accelerate (along with the ongoing expansion of the universe). One obvious result is the sheer mass of research data and associated clinical experience that must be considered and then mastered if optimal drug therapeutic strategies are to be implemented. The third edition of this textbook is an attempt to accomplish these goals by reviewing, synthesizing, and then organizing this material into clinical therapeutic strategies. Our combined contribution represents a wealth of research and clinical experience that makes such an endeavor possible.

In addition, the dedicated work of several colleagues has been invaluable. They include Charles Mitchell and Joyce Murphy at Lippincott Williams & Wilkins. Barbara Felton has now been taken off the endangered species list and once again has brought editorial expertise and patient guidance to this iteration of our text. Others who have generously given of their time and expertise include Elizabeth Winans, Pharm.D., Brian Martis, M.D., Sylvia Dennison, M.D., Mary Kay Sheehan, MSN, Laura Miller, M.D., Mani Pavuluri, M.D., and Mary Zayas. Dr. Davis thanks Michael Bennett and Nancy Chen, M.S. Dr. Preskorn acknowledges Jane Loux, Jalen Fitzpatrick, and Cheryl Carmichael. Dr. Ayd thanks Loretta Ayd Simpson, Virginia McClellan, and Ann Lovelace.

And, oh yes, one more bit of progress has been the increasing number of Michael Fisher sightings in the Boston area.

Philip G. Janicak, M.D.
John M. Davis, M.D.
Sheldon H. Preskorn, M.D.
Frank J. Ayd, Jr., M.D.

Principles and Practice
of Psychopharmacotherapy

Third Edition

1

General Principles

The art and the science of psychopharmacotherapy have expanded rapidly in the past decade, creating both an opportunity and a challenge. The contributions made by neuroscience have facilitated a more rapid approach to the development of new psychotropics. For example, since the first edition was published in 1993, the novel antipsychotics have been widely used clinically; and even while these agents are positively affecting the lives of countless patients, newer compounds such as ziprasidone, iloperidone and aripiprazole are poised to prove their worth in the broader clinical arena. In addition, the novel antipsychotics are showing promise for other disorders such as the life-threatening water imbalance problem in some schizophrenic patients and as an effective intervention for more severe, treatment-refractory mood disorders. Finally, a variety of subgroups, such as the dual-diagnosed (mental disorder plus alcohol/substance abuse) and female patients of childbearing potential, are now being more carefully considered in clinical drug trials. In general, the need to know more about the differences in physiological processes, clinical presentation, and treatment response has generated an increased appreciation of the specific needs related to gender and those patients with comorbid substance abuse or dependence.

As a result, while improved therapies to ease a patient's suffering are constantly emerging, the practitioner is required to continually assimilate new information about recent advances, including *novel agents* targeted to affect specific components of various neurotransmitter systems, *combination strategies*, *alternative uses* of existing agents, and the *specialized requirements* of a growing number of identified diagnostic subtypes. Throughout this book, we provide a **decision-making method** that incorporates this growing database for the optimal use of drug therapies in clinical practice.

Our model of pharmacotherapy is grounded on a scholarly review and summation of the critical supporting research. Beginning with a discussion of the major principles underlying our approach, we follow with chapters on specific psychiatric disorders and their related drug therapies. There is an emphasis on the historical development of our present diagnostic system to underscore the fluid nature and increasing sophistication in defining various psychiatric disorders. **The goal is to provide a logical treatment strategy that can be readily applied and easily adapted to an ever-increasing body of relevant scientific data.**

This approach is based on several underlying assumptions:

- The *medical model* serves as the foundation for the treatment of psychiatric disorders.
- A *nontheoretical approach* is advocated in considering etiology/pathogenesis.
- An *empirically based foundation,* derived from scientific investigation, is used to guide treatment decisions.

All modalities, from electroconvulsive therapy (ECT) to psychotherapy, can be incorporated into our approach when empirical data support their utility. When sufficient data are lacking, we offer suggestions based on our cumulative clinical and research experience.

PRINCIPLES OF PSYCHOPHARMACOTHERAPY

Principle 1

The diagnostic assessment, subject to revisions, is fundamental to our model (Table 1-1).

Patients present with symptoms. The clinician's goal is to formulate these problems within the context of the highest level of diagnostic sophistication (Table 1-2) based on both the

TABLE 1-1. *Principles of psychopharmacotherapy*

Principle 1	The diagnostic assessment, subject to revisions, is fundamental to our model.
Principle 2	Pharmacotherapy alone is generally insufficient for complete recovery.
Principle 3	The phase of an illness (e.g., acute, relapse, recurrence) is of critical importance in terms of the specific intervention and the duration of treatment.
Principle 4	The risk-to-benefit ratio must always be considered when developing a treatment strategy.
Principle 5	Prior personal (and possibly family) history of a good or a poor response to a specific agent usually dictates the first-line choice for a subsequent episode.
Principle 6	It is important to target specific symptoms that serve as markers for the underlying psychopathology and to monitor their presence or absence over an entire course of treatment.
Principle 7	It is necessary to observe for the development of adverse effects throughout the entire course of treatment. Such monitoring often involves the use of the laboratory to ensure safety, as well as optimal efficacy.

subjective and the objective components of the evaluation (1, 2). To accomplish this task, the clinician must realize that behavioral symptoms in psychiatry are analogous to localizing signs in neurology. Such symptoms as depressed mood or auditory hallucinations are mediated through the function or dysfunction of specific brain regions. Different etiologically determined disorders can cause dysfunction in the same brain region, leading to similar phenomenological presentations. For example, a brain tumor, a stroke, or demyelinating plaque can all affect the frontal lobe, culminating in similar behavioral symptoms.

The increased specificity of a syndromic, as compared with a symptomatic, diagnosis comes from the use of both inclusion criteria (i.e., a constellation of symptoms and signs present for a set interval of time) and exclusion criteria (i.e., conditions that may mimic the syndrome under consideration but have a known pathophysiological or etiological basis) (3). Currently, most psychiatric diagnoses are at the syndromic level, with similar presentations often representing substantially different underlying disorders. Therefore, considerable variability is found in the treatment outcome of patients diagnosed with the same syndrome. Further, patients with the same pathophysiology may be erroneously differentially categorized because of alternate syndromic presentations. A classic example is multiple sclerosis, which typically presents with signs and symptoms separated in time and space. Another example is tertiary syphilis, known as the "great mimic" due to its myriad clinical presentations. For this reason, clinicians must be ready to

TABLE 1-2. *Levels of diagnostic sophistication*

Diagnostic level	Description	Example	Diagnostic impression
Symptomatic	Isolated symptoms	Auditory hallucinations	Psychosis, NOS
Syndromic	Constellation of signs and symptoms Inclusion/exclusion criteria	Irritability Pressured, irrelevant speech Insomnia Poor judgment	Bipolar disorder, manic phase, with mood congruent psychotic features
Pathophysiologic	Demonstrable structural or biochemical changes	Elevated TFTs Lowered TSH	Hyperthyroidism
Etiologic	Known causative factors	Positive for thyroid antibodies Diffuse toxic goiter on ultrasonogram	Thyrotoxicosis secondary to Graves' hyperthyroidism

NOS, not otherwise specified; TFTs, thyroid function tests; TSH, thyroid-stimulating hormone.

alter their diagnosis, as well as treatment plans, if dictated by changes in the course of illness.

Although criteria-based syndromes have certain limitations, we emphasize their usefulness as a first step in developing an empirical approach to psychopharmacological and somatic therapies. Systematic studies of the effects of psychotropics on such syndromes permit investigators to:

- Conduct *sequential investigations* in different groups of patients with the same signs and symptoms with reasonable confidence that they are treating patients with similar syndromes.
- *Clarify the effectiveness* of a specific treatment.
- Compare the *relative effectiveness* of one treatment with another when assessing the outcome in patients with similar syndromic diagnoses.
- Clarify which particular symptoms may be *critical in predicting a drug versus placebo difference* (e.g., neurovegetative symptoms of depression).
- Clarify *atypical or specific subtypes of presentations that may not benefit from standard treatments* (e.g., atypical or psychotic depressive disorders).
- Perform *replication studies*, as well as *multisite clinical trials*.

Finally, diagnoses based on etiology or pathophysiology are superior to symptomatic or syndromic diagnoses in terms of their specificity and usefulness (4). With the completion of the first phase of the Human Genome Project, the promise of greater homogeneity in diagnostic categories based on genetic information will increasingly guide treatment strategies (5). As in other areas of medicine, the likelihood of a successful outcome increases based on the level of diagnostic specificity, because treatment can then be targeted to the underlying causative factors.

Principle 2

Pharmacotherapy alone is generally insufficient for complete recovery.

Although drug therapy may be the cornerstone of recovery, some type of educational and psychosocial intervention is almost always needed, as well as more specialized forms of psychotherapy when indicated. Examples of the latter include the use of anxiolytic agents in combination with behavior modification for phobic disorders or the use of interpersonal psychotherapy plus antidepressants for depressive disorders. Further, because many of the psychotropics often have a delayed onset of action, early counseling may avoid premature discontinuation by a patient, as well as providing hope and reassurance during this lag phase. In addition to communicating in an understandable fashion the nature of the symptoms and the disorder, and incorporating the patient and the family as active participants in the treatment plan, the clinician must generally be prepared to respond to these questions:

- What is happening to me?
- Will I get better?
- What will it take?
- What are the limitations of my condition and of the proposed treatment?
- What will it cost?

Simple, straightforward explanations of a patient's condition and the rationale for a specific course of action are generally well received. For those unable to benefit because of cognitive disruption, reassurance and expressions of empathy and concern are often therapeutic. A thorough, brief review of what is known about the patient's disorder should be communicated while dispelling common myths about his or her condition (e.g., the problem is related to a lack of moral strength). A patient's prognosis should be realistically and, to the extent possible, optimistically explained. Various treatment options should also be discussed, as noted in the section "Informed Consent" of Chapter 2.

Whereas the clinician should always take the role of counselor and advisor, the ultimate course of action should be left to the patient, except in those few instances in which the patient cannot make a rational, prudent, and informed decision on his or her own behalf. Bringing the patient into the process as an active, informed participant is beneficial to self-esteem and improves compliance. There are, however, two instances in which the clinician should not defer to the patient's wishes: if the illness significantly affects the ability to make an informed decision and when a treatment is requested (e.g., a drug of abuse) that cannot be provided in good faith.

The educational process should continue throughout the entire treatment relationship and often involves clarifying issues as they arise. When a patient does not respond to the first line of treatment, the next step is to address the possible reasons this lack of response has occurred, as well as the rationale for attempting second and subsequent treatment strategies. Finally, because many psychiatric disorders are recurrent, educating the patient and the family as to the early warning signs of a relapse may allow for earlier intervention and perhaps even prevention. In this way, a patient may suffer fewer adverse sequelae, often avoiding unnecessary hospitalizations and prolonged recovery phases from subsequent, repeated exacerbations.

In addition to adequate pharmacotherapy, specific forms of psychotherapy may also be indicated. These may include cognitive or interpersonal psychotherapy or various behavior desensitization and biofeedback techniques. Some patients may benefit from insight-oriented psychotherapy; group, family, or marital counseling; or both. Finally, in more chronic disorders, patients often benefit from vocational rehabilitation. A knowledgeable clinician realizes that these disorders do not occur in a vacuum, and, regardless of diagnosis, each patient requires an individualized treatment plan to optimize outcome.

Principle 3

The phase of an illness (e.g., acute, relapse, recurrence) is of critical importance in terms of the initial intervention and the duration of treatment.

Once an acute episode has been adequately controlled, ongoing treatment is often necessary for several months to prevent relapsing back into the acute phase. Some patients should also receive indefinite prophylaxis due to the high likelihood of recurrence. Because it is difficult to accurately predict which patients will have subsequent episodes, however, clinicians may be reluctant to expose those who will not experience a recurrence to the adverse effects of long-term therapy.

The course of an illness also dictates the need for and the duration of maintenance and prophylactic therapy. In particular, prophylaxis may not be indicated for an uncomplicated first episode depending on the specific disorder and the patient's response to standard interventions. Conversely, patients with histories of multiple recurrences, with family histories of a psychiatric disorder, with prolonged durations of, or particularly severe, acute episodes, and with delayed rate of response to treatment intervention are indications for ongoing prophylaxis.

Some medications are clearly appropriate during an acute phase of treatment but not for maintenance or prophylactic purposes. Conversely, certain drugs may not be very useful for acute management but are exceptionally beneficial for maintenance or prophylaxis. For example, in an acute manic episode, adjunctive benzodiazepines may rapidly sedate patients; however, these drugs are not ideal as maintenance strategies once the acute symptoms are under control. With early signs of breakthrough and possible relapse, however, they may again play a role in preventing a relapse of the full manic phase. The converse example is lithium, which is relatively ineffective with more severe, manic exacerbations such as stage 2 or stage 3 mania, but can be very effective for maintenance and prophylaxis once the acute symptoms have been controlled with other drug or somatic interventions.

Principle 4

The risk-to-benefit ratio must always be considered when developing a treatment strategy.

Specific factors to consider are both psychiatric and physical contraindications. For example, bupropion is contraindicated in a depressed patient with a history of seizures due to the increased risk of recurrence while on this agent. Conversely, it may be an appropriate choice for a bipolar disorder with intermittent depressive episodes that is otherwise under good control with standard mood stabilizers. This consideration is based on the limited data suggesting that bupropion is less likely to induce a manic switch in comparison with standard heterocyclic antidepressants. Another example is the avoidance of benzodiazepines for the treatment of panic disorder in a patient with a history of alcohol or sedative-hypnotic abuse due to the increased risk of misuse or dependency. In this situation, a selective serotonin reuptake inhibitor (SSRI) may be more appropriate.

Assessment of physical, as well as psychiatric status, is also critically important. The presence of intercurrent medical disorders, as well as any medication used to manage them, increases the likelihood of an adverse outcome with an otherwise appropriate medication. With a recent history of myocardial infarction, certain tricyclic antidepressants (TCAs) or low-potency antipsychotics might be contraindicated due to potential adverse effects on cardiac function. Another example is the avoidance of carbamazepine in a bipolar patient with a persistently low white blood cell count. Finally, β-blockers are typically contraindicated in a patient with asthma.

A related issue is the patient's ability to metabolize and eliminate drugs adequately. For example, lithium is excreted entirely by the kidneys, and if a patient suffers from significantly impaired renal function, high, potentially toxic levels could develop on standard doses. Although the dose could be adjusted to compensate for the decrease in drug clearance, it might be more appropriate to choose another mood stabilizer such as valproate or carbamazepine, because they are primarily metabolized through the liver.

A final consideration is that of economics, which includes the procurement costs and myriad other factors that can increase the overall expense of treatment (see section "Cost of Treatment" in Chapter 2).

Principle 5

Prior personal (and possibly family) history of a good or a poor response to a specific agent usually dictates the first-line choice for a subsequent episode.

Given the development of new drugs with more refined mechanisms of action, patients' responses to therapeutic interventions increasingly become critical sources of data. Poor or inadequate response to a previous trial of a specific class of medication (e.g., an SSRI) would suggest the need to try a different pharmacological class (e.g., bupropion). Response (whether improvement or deterioration) also provides insights into the underlying pathophysiology. Therefore, the careful monitoring of outcome can generate in-

formation for modifying previously suboptimal therapies. If prior or initial response is inadequate, common issues to consider include:

- Appropriate *diagnosis,* including specific subtypes (e.g., delusional depression)
- Adequacy of *treatment* (e.g., sufficient dose, blood concentration, or duration)
- *Noncompliance*
- Intercurrent *substance* or *alcohol abuse, medical problems,* the concomitant use of *prescription* or *over-the-counter medications*
- Lack of adequate or appropriate *social support*
- The presence of an *Axis II* diagnosis

Principle 6

It is important to target specific symptoms that serve as markers for the underlying psychopathology and to monitor their presence or absence over an entire course of treatment.

For example, in a bipolar patient, reduction of the amplitude of mood swings may be the focus of acute therapy. During the maintenance phase, however, the most sensitive predictor of an impending relapse might be a decreased need for sleep. Careful attention to the onset of such a symptom might lead to early treatment, preventing a full-blown recurrence.

It is also important to recognize that certain symptoms may respond before others. In a depressive episode, vegetative symptoms such as sleep and appetite disturbances will often respond early in the course of treatment, whereas mood may take several weeks to improve. Cognizant of these different temporal patterns of response, the clinician may be encouraged to continue with a certain approach. Also, educating the patient regarding the differential time course to response for various symptoms may facilitate compliance. Subsequently, during the maintenance/prophylactic phase, the clinician should monitor how effectively a treatment prevents the reemergence of the acute symptoms.

Principle 7

It is necessary to watch for the development of adverse effects throughout the entire course of treatment. Such monitoring often involves

the use of the laboratory to ensure safety, as well as optimal efficacy (6).

It is important to confirm that the adverse effects are actually caused by a specific treatment. Because patients in clinical studies often experience a wide range of adverse effects while on placebo, one should not prematurely conclude that such events are due to active medication.

With the development of new, more specific agents, it is increasingly important to note and report undesirable behavioral effects, as well as physical reactions. For example, if a patient becomes excessively passive, there is a chance that the behavior will be missed or attributed to the underlying psychiatric condition. In fact, it might be a previously unrecognized effect of a new medication. The identification of previously unknown adverse effects (while undesirable in themselves) can be the basis for the next round of serendipitous discoveries about the underlying pathophysiology of a given disorder.

In this context, the first role of the laboratory is to detect specific adverse effects to target organs (see "Role of the Laboratory" later in this chapter). Monitoring will generally be tailored to the specific therapy used because of its known potential for causing certain problems. Examples include *periodic blood counts with carbamazepine or clozapine and thyroid and renal function studies with long-term maintenance lithium.*

Another use of the laboratory is for therapeutic drug monitoring (TDM) of psychotropics with defined optimal ranges, narrow therapeutic indices, or both. Although TDM is not essential for many psychotropics, it is for others, including lithium, several TCAs, valproate, and carbamazepine. It may also be helpful to optimize the use of certain antipsychotics (e.g., haloperidol, clozapine) (7).

The same dose of many of these drugs produces substantially different concentrations among different patients due to multiple factors. Elimination rates can vary to a clinically significant degree among different patients on the same dose, such that some will develop subtherapeutic concentrations, others concentrations in the therapeutic range, and still others toxic concentrations. TDM can provide the necessary information on how rapidly a patient eliminates the drug, so the dose can be adjusted to maximize safety and efficacy.

ROLE OF NEUROSCIENCE

Psychopharmacotherapy is still an empirically based approach. Advances in the neurosciences, however, are occurring at an increasingly rapid pace and will ultimately provide a much more complete understanding of cerebral structure and function, as well as guide clinical drug therapies in the future.

One important example is the use of *brain imaging* such as positron emission tomography (PET), single photon emission computerized tomography (SPECT), and magnetic resonance imaging (MRI). These techniques are allowing us to localize brain regions underlying many behavioral symptoms (e.g., anxiety, vigilance, sadness), while at the same time enabling us to attain greater levels of diagnostic sophistication.

Perhaps most critical to a discussion on psychotropics is the explosion of knowledge about the fundamental subcellular processes that contribute to psychiatric disorders. We have been able to isolate and study many biologically important substances (e.g., neurotransmitters, receptor subtypes, various components of the postligand—receptor interface, including various subsequent messenger systems). The goal is to characterize the cascade of subsequent intraneuronal events, culminating in genetically determined cell protein alterations. Once these processes are characterized, they can provide insights into pathoetiology, as well as become the targets for specific drug development. Concurrently, observing how new drugs interact with these cellular components enhances our knowledge of their functional role in mediating specific behavioral symptoms. Newer agents can then serve as probes to test whether these components are relevant to a given psychiatric disorder.

Mechanism of Action

Psychotropic drugs affect specific biochemical processes, most often involving enzymes, receptors, or ion channels. A given drug's action that produces a physiological response (whether intended or otherwise) is termed the "mechanism of action." **It is axiomatic that central effects mediate the clinical actions of psychotropic medications. But, for any given drug, the effects on known processes may not be the mechanism mediating clinical response. Instead, the clinical outcome may be the result of some as yet unrecognized central action, due in part to the limited understanding of the pathophysiology underlying specific psychiatric disorders.** When the fundamental biology underlying a disorder is unknown, it is impossible to state how a drug is correcting a given syndrome. Typically, proposed mechanisms of action for behavioral effects are simply the actions of the particular drug on known central biochemical processes. Whether these actions are truly the mechanisms underlying the behavioral effect (e.g., amelioration of depression) must be viewed with healthy skepticism.

With the rapid ongoing developments in neuroscience, we are likely to see further reliance on drug probes to test the functional integrity of neurotransmitter systems in specific disorders. An ever-increasing number of biochemical processes are being elucidated that may mediate a specific psychotropic's effects, including:

- *Enzymes* responsible for the synthesis and degradation of an expanding list that includes neurotransmitters, neuropeptides, and neurohormones
- *Storage of neurotransmitters in vesicles* within the cytoplasm
- *Release mechanisms*
- *Presynaptic membrane uptake pumps*
- *Subtypes of pre- and postsynaptic receptors*
- *Receptor subcomponents* (e.g., G-proteins)
- *Subsequent messenger systems* (cAMP, PKC)
- *Ion channels*

As these various processes are better characterized, they will increasingly become the targets for future drug development.

Drug Development and Its Implications

The first psychotropics of the modern era (e.g., lithium, neuroleptic antipsychotics, tricyclic and monoamine oxidase inhibitor antidepressants) were discovered serendipitously. These agents were not engineered to have selective actions, but instead produce a wide range of central biochemical effects and generally affect more than one neurotransmitter system simultaneously, resulting in multiple repercussions:

- *Such drugs can be helpful in more than one condition* because they act by more than one mechanism.
- *Any number of these drugs' actions could be responsible for the clinical effect;* therefore, such drugs provide limited insight into the pathophysiology of a given condition.
- Generally, due to their multiplicity of effects (positive as well as negative), *these "broad-spectrum" medications are more poorly tolerated* than agents with fewer biochemical interactions.

Future attempts to focus the actions of newer agents can greatly reduce the "signal-to-noise ratio" and enhance the development of more specific treatments (8).

Although there are many problems with the first generation of modern psychotropics, they have been extremely effective and have provided insights into the underlying pathophysiology. Studying the effects of these agents on specific biochemical functions has had great heuristic value, generating numerous hypotheses that have guided subsequent drug development. One set of hypotheses deals with the possible mechanisms underlying the clinical efficacy of these agents, and includes:

- The *dopamine hypothesis,* based on the actions of neuroleptics
- The *catecholamine* and the *indolamine hypotheses,* based on the actions of various antidepressants
- The *permissive, adrenergic-cholinergic balance,* and *bidimensional hypotheses,* based on both the effects of antidepressants and on the modulating interactions among various neurotransmitter systems

Concurrently, hypotheses were also developed regarding the undesirable or toxic effects associated with the various biochemical actions of these agents. Examples include the following:

- *Orthostatic hypotension* secondary to α_1-adrenergic receptor blockade
- *Cardiotoxicity* secondary to membrane stabilization
- *Central anticholinergic syndrome* due to the potent muscarinic-cholinergic effects of many psychotropics

Chemists can now better define the structure-activity relationship of these early psychotropics to guide the development of newer drugs. Such relationships are refined by *in vitro* testing to determine whether newly synthesized compounds have the desired biochemical effect on specific targets, such as enzyme inhibition or receptor blockade. Simultaneously, these agents are tested for any undesirable effects. Where such effects exist, modifications can be made to the chemical structure to eliminate or reduce such unwanted qualities. When a new psychotropic drug meets the desired inclusion and exclusion criteria, it is then tested in the clinic to determine whether it possesses the desired therapeutic effect. Results from these clinical studies provide critical feedback regarding the mechanisms of action, which will guide the development of future generations of agents.

SSRIs (e.g., fluoxetine, sertraline, paroxetine, fluvoxamine, citalopram), bupropion, venlafaxine, nefazodone, and mirtazapine represent agents engineered to eliminate many of the earlier generation antidepressant side effects (9, 10). Beginning in the late 1980's, the introduction of these agents had important research and clinical implications. From the research standpoint, they advance our understanding of the pathophysiology of various disorders, while providing a way to test for the existence of putative biochemically distinct subtypes. Such attempts were unsuccessful with earlier generation psychotropics, in part due to their lack of specific action. For example, the TCAs are effective in depressive disorders, enuresis, and panic attacks, but different mechanisms are believed to be responsible for these varied efficacies. In a similar way, all TCAs have effects on both the norepinephrine and the serotonin reuptake systems within the clinically relevant concentration range. Attempts in the past to distinguish between "serotonergic" and "adrenergic" depressive disorders with such agents were unsuccessful because of the nonspecific nature of these drugs' effects, even if two such forms of depressive disorders exist. Newer agents, however, are orders of magnitude different in their affinity for one neurotransmitter system versus another and can be used as probes to expand our understanding of the relevant neurobiology.

Clinically, these newer agents also have several advantages because they:

- Are generally *safer* and *better tolerated*
- Have *more specific pharmacological actions*
- *Can test the functional integrity* of a given neurotransmitter system in a specific syndrome or patient

Thus, the first era of modern psychopharmacotherapy (i.e., serendipitous discovery) is giving way to the second era, which is the refinement of drugs based on known biochemical effects. This process will eventually lead to the next era, which will be the synthesis of compounds with specific interactions at newly discovered subcomponents of the neuron. The existence of such agents will also permit the development of an empirically based hierarchical treatment plan that will define the agent of first choice and then which agent is most likely to help when the first choice is unsuccessful or poorly tolerated. The approach used in this book will allow the reader to both anticipate such developments and incorporate them as they occur.

DIAGNOSTIC ASSESSMENT

Diagnosis is critical to understanding a patient's presenting complaints, as well as serving as the basis for developing treatment strategies. For this reason, each treatment section of this textbook is preceded by introductory discussions of the major psychiatric disorders, including an historical perspective to underscore the evolving nature of our nomenclature and the criteria used to define specific categories (see Appendix A). We further refine this organization by incorporating factors that often affect presentation and response to treatment. Such variables include:

- *Phase of the illness* being treated (i.e., acute, prevention of relapse, prevention of recurrence)
- *Confounding issues* such as other psychiatric or medical conditions
- *Psychosocial stressors*, to the extent that they affect symptom presentation and effectiveness of treatment

Our model of pharmacotherapy recognizes that the current understanding of pathophysiology and etiology is advancing but still at a rudimentary stage. **Therefore, diagnostic assessment of any patient is an ongoing process that must be continuously updated throughout treatment.** Such revisions are based on information acquired from the patient during follow-up, including response, partial response, or lack of response to specific interventions, as well as the emergence of new knowledge from subsequent scientific investigations.

The diagnostic assessment consists of several stages, including the following:

- A *subjective account* by the patient of the pertinent information, including personal and family histories
- *Objective parameters,* including the mental status exam
- The clinician's *initial impression,* culminating in a preliminary diagnosis
- *Treatment planning,* including further diagnostic workup, first-line treatment strategies, and education of the patient and the family

Subjective Component

This aspect of a psychiatric evaluation incorporates several sources of information, including the individual's own account, family and friends' reports, the referral source, and any earlier database (e.g., the chart from a previous hospitalization). Basic identifying information such as age, sex, race, marital status, present family situation, living circumstances, work skills, present work situation, and sources of income is essential. The individual's communication of the basic problems, or the "chief complaint," will set the stage for an elucidation of the chronology of precipitating events that culminated in seeking help.

Next is an exploration of any prior psychiatric history, or treatment, or both, either personally or in other family members; serious past or ongoing medical problems, either personally or in family members; and the use or abuse of medications, illicit drugs, or alcohol.

Objective Component

Objective data include a thorough physical evaluation (including a thorough neurological exam), supplemented by laboratory data such as routine blood work, urinalysis, chest x-ray, ECG, and drug screen (see "Role of the Laboratory" later in this chapter). All this information is routinely collected when a person first enters the hospital; on an outpatient basis, however, the clinician may select only those tests deemed appropriate at the time.

The mental status examination is the most important aspect of this phase and scrutinizes how an individual is feeling, acting, and thinking at the time of the interview (i.e., a cross-sectional versus longitudinal evaluation). The clinician begins with a basic observation of *overt appearance* and *motoric behavior*, including *affect* (i.e., overt emotional reactions in terms of intensity, quality, appropriateness, and continuity) and *mood* (i.e., underlying feeling tone). It is important to note that affect and mood may not always be synonymous, and this discrepancy can complicate the diagnostic assessment.

Thought processes, including memory and orientation, reflect one's ability or inability to assimilate and communicate ideas in a logical and coherent fashion. *Thought content* explores the substance of one's ideation, and typical aberrations such as obsessions, phobias, illusions, delusions, or hallucinations may be elicited. Evaluation of *memory* and *orientation* is critical to the differentiation of a psychiatric versus a nonpsychiatric medical disorder. Memory for immediate, recent, and remote events can be readily tested, as well as orientation to time, place, person, space, and situation. Assuming the level of anxiety is not sufficient to impair responses to questions in these areas, deficits usually imply some impairment of brain functioning, which may or may not be reversible.

Intellectual capacity is considered in the context of an individual's social, cultural, and educational opportunities. The presentation of problem-solving situations congruent with one's life circumstances is an excellent way to determine intellect and capacity to make sound *judgments. Insight* has many levels of meaning. It may simply refer to a basic appreciation of how and why individuals finds themselves in their present situations, or it can refer to a person's appreciation of a more complex set of causal relationships that have culminated in the present problem. One's *abstractive ability* is the capacity to perceive a conceptual commonality in otherwise apparently distinct or separate entities. This ability can be tested by the patient's understanding of proverbs and appreciation of humor.

To summarize, the mental status exam highlights several aspects of functioning. Each succeeding component requires that earlier aspects be intact for adequate reality testing, as well as the optimal expression of one's personality, as subjectively perceived and objectively observed, in terms of emotions, thoughts, and behavior.

Initial Impression

Having obtained the necessary information from subjective and objective sources, the next step is the development of a preliminary diagnostic assessment, including commentary when possible on the five major axes (*Diagnostic and Statistical Manual of Mental Disorders, 4th ed., revised* (DSM-IV) [11]), as well as other differential diagnostic considerations (see Appendix A). The diagnostic assessment serves many purposes:

- It is a *shorthand way of labeling and referring* to patients' complaints.
- It *provides a way of conceptualizing complaints* within the framework of our current knowledge, so that appropriate treatment can be instituted.
- It *facilitates research* by allowing data to be systematically collected from different patients with the same condition.
- It is important for *billing*.

The most basic assessment is a *description of the phenomena* (e.g., anxiety, etiology undetermined). An assessment also takes the additional form of an *"initial impression"* (e.g., phobic disorder) and a *differential diagnosis* of other possible categories that need further exploration (e.g., rule out hyperthyroidism, rule out an agitated depression). As such, diagnosis serves an analogous function in medicine as does hypothesis formulation in science. The value of a given diagnosis (or hypothesis) is determined by the degree to which it explains the facts of the case (i.e., the presentation, the course, and the response to treatment). If the diagnosis does not lead to an acceptable treatment outcome based on these criteria, it must be revised, just as a hypothesis may need to be revised in the course of a scientific experiment.

Treatment Planning

The last step (and obvious culmination) of the diagnostic assessment is formulation of the initial treatment plan, including the potential role of pharmacotherapy. The first consideration is to decide what *other diagnostic workup* is necessary. Typical procedures include the obtaining of corroborative history from spouse and family, psychological testing, and other physical and neurological evaluations as dictated by the initial findings. These steps should further refine the working diagnostic impression. Often there is also the need to consider and treat more than one problem. The course of *treatment* in a hospitalization may simply consist of separating the individual from recent environmental stresses and allowing the patient's own restorative resources to stabilize in the protective and supportive milieu of an inpatient setting.

Other treatments are often necessary, however, and may include:

- *Psychotherapy* (e.g., individual, family)
- *Sociotherapy* (e.g., recreational, occupational, and activities therapy)
- *Pharmacotherapy* (e.g., anxiolytics, antidepressants, antipsychotics)
- *Somatic therapy* (e.g., electroconvulsive treatment)

Although the focus of this text is pharmacotherapy, incorporating these other modalities is often critical to a successful outcome and is also discussed.

Diagnostic Approaches

Although the ideal course would be to consider the symptoms as the behavioral manifestations of an underlying cerebral pathology and to formulate subsequent treatment plans on this assumption, currently most treatments are dictated by a specific diagnosis.

This text develops a hierarchical framework for considering first-line treatment choices and subsequent options if initial interventions fail. We begin with treatment recommendations from the standpoint of our current diagnostic nosology. We also consider patients who do not easily fit into a single major diagnostic category, or in whom treatment based on syndromic constellations proves unsuccessful. When possible, we suggest a strategy based on data about the underlying pathophysiology. These working strategies are drawn from the presenting behavioral symptoms and quality of response to earlier therapeutic trials.

A hypothetical vignette may serve to illustrate such a paradigm shift from a syndromic to a pathophysiological approach in patients who do not respond adequately to standard therapeutic trials.

Case Example: The patient's presenting problems are anger and impulse control, symptoms that may not fit well into an Axis I or II diagnostic category. The clinician may conceptualize these symptoms as cyclothymia and begin treatment with a mood stabilizer such as lithium. If this is unsuccessful, a reasonable second approach might be a trial with valproate or carbamazepine. If symptoms persist, one might consider dysthymia because of the presence of persistent dysphoric symptoms, and initiate treatment with a SSRI. In this scenario, however, the patient not only remains symptomatic but also evidences some worsening of impulsivity and anger.

At this point, having exhausted therapeutic approaches based on empirical data, it may be useful to shift paradigms. Whereas previously trial and error may have been the only recourse, we are now approaching the point at which a pathophysiological paradigm may help guide the selection of subsequent drug therapies. Considerable evidence indicates that impulsivity in various mammalian species is mediated in part through serotonin mechanisms. More specifically, serotonin may influence the function of the amygdaloid and septal-hippocampal formations, perhaps through 5-HT_{1A} receptors located in these regions.

There is also evidence of low levels of 5-hydroxyindoleacetic acid (5-HIAA) in the cerebrospinal fluid (CSF) of impulsive individuals. We might hypothesize that, in a nonresponsive, impulsive patient, diminished serotonin plays a role in the pathophysiology. This hypothesis could now be tested and simultaneously serve as the foundation for a pathophysiologically based treatment by choosing therapies specific for various components of this system. For example, the 5-HT_{1A} agonist buspirone might be tried, because there is limited evidence from open trials that it has antiaggressive properties.

Education

Educating a patient, as well as the family, is of the utmost importance for any treatment plan to succeed. Good clinicians, like good teachers:

- *Communicate* at a level appropriate to the individual's ability to comprehend.
- Convey their suggestions in the context of a working *theoretical framework* (be it right or wrong!)
- Encourage the patient and the family to become *active participants* in treatment.

ROLE OF THE LABORATORY

Interest in the neurobiological substrates of psychiatric disorders has paralleled the increase in effective somatic therapies, which, in turn, have extended the laboratory's role in evaluating patients. Although the laboratory can never replace clinical acumen in psychiatry, or in any other medical specialty, it can play a significant role in:

- Elucidating and quantifying *biological factors* associated with various psychiatric disorders
- Determining the *choice of treatment*
- Monitoring *clinical response*

This section reviews the standard medical assessment for the psychiatric patient, summarizes specific tests frequently used in the clinical and research setting, and discusses the laboratory's role in treatment evaluation (e.g., therapeutic drug monitoring) (6, 12–14).

Medical Assessment

General principles for assessment include the following:

- A *detailed physical examination,* which may reveal medical problems previously missed; new, unrelated medical problems; incorrect diagnoses; or adverse effects associated with various treatments
- The *avoidance of wasteful screening batteries with limited clinical utility.* Instead, specific lab tests based on a careful assessment and integration of the history and the physical examination are the ideal
- Recognition of *presenting signs and/or symptoms that dictate the need for further medical evaluation* (e.g., a known history of recurring or chronic medical illness, prominent physical symptoms, evidence of an organic mental disorder on the Mini-Mental State Examination, substance abuse disorder)
- In specific cases, the use of *treatment options that require lab testing* (e.g., lithium, clozapine, ECT)

Admission Assessment for Inpatients

A screening battery to evaluate the general physical condition of the patient is outlined in Table 1-3. Supplementary lab and diagnostic tests may be required when specific clues from the history, physical examination, or initial lab screen suggest a physical disturbance (Table 1-4). Finally, Table 1-5 lists tests often used for specific clinical circumstances.

Laboratory Tests

Demonstrable lab abnormalities in psychiatric disorders are not sufficiently specific or sensitive to identify with certainty the correct diagnosis or appropriate treatment. They can, however, indi-

TABLE 1-3. *General laboratory evaluation*

Complete blood count (CBC) and differential
General chemistries
Thyroid function tests (e.g., TSH, T_3, T_4)
Screening for syphilis (e.g., VDRL or RPR)
Urinalysis
Chest x-ray
Electrocardiogram (when indicated)
Pregnancy test (in all eligible females)

Adapted from Israni TH, Janicak PG. Laboratory assessment in psychiatry. In: Flaherty J, Davis JM, Janicak PG, eds. *Psychiatry: diagnosis and therapy.* 2d ed. Norwalk, CT: Appleton and Lange, 1993:30–39.

cate an association between a given disorder and a specific measure, which may or may not be relevant to its pathogenesis or etiology. Biological markers may be "*state-dependent,*" serving as aids in the diagnosis of a specific psychiatric illness with which they are associated, as well as useful for following treatment response. On the other hand, "*trait*" markers may help in identifying vulnerable individuals.

Neuroendocrine Tests

Given that the seat of hormonal modulation is in the limbic-hypothalamic-pituitary axis, endocrine changes serve as important correlates

TABLE 1-4. *Supplemental assessments*

Skull films; CT scan; MRI
EEG; evoked potentials
Polysomnography; nocturnal penile tumescence
Urinary toxicology screen
Blood and/or breath alcohol levels
Serum concentrations of medications
B_{12} and folate levels
Heavy metal screens
Serum ceruloplasmin
Erythocyte sedimentation rate (ESR)
HIV testing
Antinuclear antibodies
Monospot test
TB skin test
Blood cultures
Urine porphyrins; osmolality
Stool for occult blood
Arterial blood gases
Lumbar puncture with CSF studies

Adapted from Israni TH, Janicak PG. Laboratory assessment in psychiatry. In: Flaherty J, Davis JM, Janicak PG, eds. *Psychiatry: diagnosis and therapy.* 2d ed. Norwalk, CT: Appleton and Lange, 1993:30–39.

TABLE 1-5. *Batteries for specific clinical circumstances*

Elderly psychiatric patients
  CBC with differential
  ESR
  Serum B$_{12}$ and folate levels
  SMA-20
  Liver function tests
  Serological test for syphilis
  Urinalysis
  Lumbar puncture
  Chest x-ray
  ECG
  Skull x-ray; EEG if necessary
  CT scan; MRI if indicated
Suspected substance abuse
  Breath and blood alcohol levels
  Urine drug screen
  Serum toxicological screen with gas
    chromatography–mass spectroscopy
    (GG-MS)
Lithium workup
  CBC
  Serum electrolytes
  Blood urea nitrogen, serum creatinine
  Thyroid function tests
  ECG (if age >45 years or clinically indicated)
  Urinalysis
  Pregnancy test
Valproate Workup
  CBC with differential
  Liver function tests
  Serum electrolytes
  Pregnancy test
Carbamazephine workup
  CBS with differential
  Liver function tests
  Serum electrolytes
  Blood urea nitrogen, serum creatinine
  Pregnancy test
Clozapine
  CBC with differential (baseline; weekly for
    6 months, then biweekly)
Electroconvulsive therapy
  CBC
  Blood chemistries
  Chest x-ray; spinal x-ray (if indicated)
  Urinalysis
  ECG

Adapted from Israni TH, Janicak PG. Laboratory assessment in psychiatry. In: Flaherty J, Davis JM, Janicak PG, eds. *Psychiatry: diagnosis and therapy.* 2d ed. Norwalk, CT: Appleton and Lange, 1993:30–39.

to major psychiatric disorders. These changes include basal hormone concentrations, as well as responses to pharmacological challenges. Equally important, endocrine disorders may present with psychiatric symptoms (e.g., manic symptoms in hyperthyroidism, severe depression in hypercortisolism, psychotic symptoms associated with Cushing's syndrome). Commonly used neuroendocrine tests include the following.

Dexamethasone Suppression Test

The dexamethasone suppression test (DST) procedure typically involves an oral dose of 1.0 mg of dexamethasone, taken at 11:00 pm. For inpatients, blood samples are typically drawn the next day at 8:00 am, 4:00 pm, and 11:00 pm, whereas for outpatients a single 4:00 pm sample is usually collected. These samples are then analyzed for plasma cortisol concentrations. *Normally, the single 1.0-mg dose of dexamethasone at 11:00 pm will suppress plasma cortisol secretion, resulting in concentrations below 5 μg/dL for the next 24 hours. Levels higher than this indicate nonsuppression or a positive test result.* Due to variation in assay methods, however, any concentration in the 4 to 7 μg/dL range must be interpreted with caution. An abnormal DST (nonsuppression) increases the probability of a major depressive episode or at least an affective component to the illness. It cannot, however, be used as a diagnostic test because of its low specificity (i.e., identifies only about 45% to 50% of patients with major depression); nor can it serve as an adequate screening device because almost 7% of normal control subjects and approximately 19% of acute schizophrenic patients may be nonsuppressors (15, 16). Some studies have indicated that failure of the DST to normalize after somatic treatment for depression might indicate a higher likelihood of relapse (17). If confirmed, this may have greater application in clinical psychiatry. Table 1-6 lists causes of false-positive and false-negative results on the DST.

Thyrotropin-Releasing Hormone Stimulation Test

After an overnight fast, an intravenous line is started at 8:30 am. At 8:59 am, blood samples are collected for baseline thyroid indices, including thyroid-stimulating hormone (TSH). At 9:00 am, synthetic thyrotropin-releasing hormone (TRH) is administered intravenously (usually a dose of

TABLE 1-6. *Causes of false positives or negatives on DST*

False positives	False negatives
Pregnancy	Addison's disease
Obesity	Hypopituitarism
Weight loss or malnutrition	Slow metabolism
Alcohol abuse/withdrawal	of dexamethasone
Infection	Drugs
Trauma	Exogenous
Diabetes mellitus	corticosteroids
Carcinoma	Indomethacin
Cushing's syndrome	High doses of
Anorexia nervosa	benzodiazepines
Renal/cardiac disease	High doses of
Cerebrovascular disease	cyproheptadine
Antipyschotic withdrawal	
Temporal lobe epilepsy	
Drugs	
Estrogens	
Narcotics	
Sedative-hypnotics	
Anticonvulsants	

Adapted from Roose RB, et al. Medical assessment and laboratory testing in psychiatry. In: Kaplan HI, Sadock BJ, eds. *Comprehensive textbook of psychiatry.* 7th ed. Philadelphia: Lippincott Williams & Wilkins, 2000:732–754.

500 μg given over 30 s). Transient side effects include gastrointestinal or genitourinary symptoms, a sensation of warmth, dryness of mouth or metallic taste, and tightness in the chest.

Plasma samples for TSH concentrations are then collected 15, 30, 60, and 90 min after the TRH infusion.

A normal response is an increase in plasma TSH of 5 to 15 μU/mL above baseline. A response of less than 5 μU/mL above baseline is generally considered to be blunted (some laboratories consider a response below 7 μU/mL to be blunted) and may be consistent with a major depression. An abnormal test is found in approximately 25% of patients with depression. A blunted TSH response (especially in conjunction with an abnormal DST) may help in confirming the differential diagnosis of a major depressive episode and support continued antidepressant treatment. An increased baseline TSH or an "augmented" TSH response (higher than 30 μU/mL), in conjunction with other thyroid indices, might identify patients with hypothyroidism, mimicking a depres-

sive disorder. These patients may benefit most from thyroid replacement therapy.

Other Neuroendocrine Tests

Other neuroendocrine tests include the following:

- *Blunted growth hormone response* to various stimuli, such as insulin-induced hypoglycemia, L-dopa, 5-hydroxytryptamine, apomorphine, D-amphetamine, clonidine, growth hormone-releasing hormone, and TRH. The growth hormone response to clonidine is one challenge test that has been consistently reported to be blunted by several different research groups. This test measures the responsiveness of postsynaptic α_2-adrenergic receptors and may be a "trait" marker for depression (18).
- *Blunted prolactin response* to such agents as fenfluramine, methadone, and l-tryptophan may be secondary to a possible serotonin deficiency in depression.
- *Plasma melatonin* levels and urinary levels of its primary metabolite, *6-hydroxymelatonin,* have been used in research as indices of noradrenergic functioning before and after treatment with antidepressants.

Biochemical Markers

Although research on neurotransmitters and their metabolites has found numerous abnormalities, no routine lab test has been developed to reliably enhance diagnosis or treatment (see section "Mechanism of Action" in Chapter 7). Some consistent findings include the following:

- An association between impulsive aggression, suicidal behavior, or both with decreased CSF levels of the serotonin metabolite *5-HIAA*
- Low 24-hour urinary *3-methoxy-4-hydroxyphenylglycol* (metabolite of norepinephrine), primarily in bipolar disorders (i.e., depressed phase)

Peripheral tissue markers include high-molecular-weight complex biomolecules (receptors) and enzyme systems that can be obtained from outside the CNS (e.g., in platelets, lymphocytes, skin fibroblasts, and erythrocytes) and are thought to reflect or parallel central neuronal activity.

Some noteworthy findings are as follows:

- *Increased platelet α_2-adrenergic receptors* in depression
- *Decreased β-adrenergic receptor binding sites* on lymphocytes in affective disorders
- Significantly *decreased ^{3}H-labeled imipramine binding sites in platelets* from depressed and obsessive-compulsive patients
- *Increased platelet 5-HT$_{2A}$ receptors in suicidal patients* independent of diagnosis (19, 20)

Genetic Markers

Gross *chromosomal abnormalities* can be used to identify various types of mental retardation, as in the case of Down's syndrome (i.e., trisomy 21) or fragile X syndrome. *Molecular genetics* examines specific DNA sequences or restriction fragment length polymorphisms (RFLPs) in the genes of patients with psychiatric disorders and normal control subjects, as well as specific HLA subtypes. Genetic *linkage studies* attempt to establish the chromosomal locus of certain disorders (e.g., chromosome 4 in Huntington's disease; chromosomes 14, 19, and 21 in Alzheimer's disease). Further, there have been conflicting results from studies of both the X-chromosome and chromosome 11 in bipolar disorder. High lithium erythrocyte-plasma ratios and high muscarinic acetylcholine receptor density, both of which have been reported in mood disorders, may be potential markers for candidate genes, particularly when the gene's locus on its chromosome is known.

Brain Imaging Techniques

In clinical psychiatry, brain imaging offers a modest amount of information, chiefly useful in differential diagnosis (21). In research, however, imaging has proved invaluable in clarifying the relationship between neuroanatomic regions and pathophysiology.

Questions that clinical psychiatrists pose and want such technology to answer include:

- Can a *diagnosis* be made solely from a functional image, and can repeated scans monitor the *progress* of the disorder with or without therapy?
- Can functional imaging *localize* those areas of the brain that subserve certain symptoms (e.g., hallucinations)?
- Can functional imaging define *biochemical characteristics* of a psychiatric disorder in a reproducible, generalizable, and predictive manner?
- Can functional imaging provide a rational *basis for selecting psychopharmacotherapy* (including type of drug and dose), as well as *predict the likely outcome*?

For example, Silbersweig et al. (22) used PET to identify increased activity in brain areas while schizophrenic patients were experiencing auditory hallucinations. Using a group (versus individual) analysis approach, a highly significant pattern of deep activation was observed (i.e., bilateral thalamus, left hippocampus-parahippocampal gyrus, and right ventral tegmentum). Autonomous activity in these areas is consistent with other reports and may account for the bizarre, involuntary experiences of these patients. Another example is a series of PET studies that demonstrated up to 80% striatal dopamine-2 receptor occupancy in acutely ill patients receiving antipsychotic treatment (23). Klemm et al. (24) have reported a similar result using a raclopride derivative (benzamide-123) developed for SPECT. The implication is that this more readily available (and less expensive) non-PET radiopharmaceutical procedure may be a potential tool for the clinical monitoring of patients on antipsychotics, and perhaps other psychotropics.

Some issues, however, presently preclude the routine use of most techniques, including the following:

- *Many steps* are required (e.g., data acquisition, tracer kinetic modeling, image processing, reconstruction, and analysis).
- Analysis involves *statistical techniques that may oversimplify* while producing compelling visual images.

- Data may be generated in a *resting* (or reference) state, in *response to a challenge* to a putative deficiency characteristic of a clinical syndrome, or in *both*.

Computerized Tomography

Computerized tomography (CT) is used in the clinical setting primarily to rule out organic lesions that might underlie or contribute to a psychiatric disorder. Specific indications may include:

- *First episode after age 40* of a psychotic, mood, or personality disorder
- *Abnormal motor movements*
- Delirium or *dementia* of unknown etiology
- Persistent *catatonia*
- *Anorexia nervosa*

Indications for using contrast include the presence of focal signs and symptoms or of any lesion noted on a noncontrast scan. Findings include the following:

- *Reversed cerebral asymmetry* in schizophrenics
- *Cerebellar atrophy, third ventricle enlargement,* and *high ventricle-to-brain ratios* in chronic schizophrenic patients
- A negative correlation between *ventricular enlargement* and *antipsychotic treatment-response* in chronic schizophrenics
- *Cortical atrophy,* as evidenced by sulcal widening, in chronic schizophrenia

In addition, abnormalities have been reported in depression, alcoholism, Alzheimer's disease, and multi-infarct dementia. It is important to note that these are statistical findings in the psychiatric research setting, and CT is not sufficiently sensitive or specific to be used as a routine diagnostic test.

Magnetic Resonance Imaging

Magnetic resonance imaging (MRI) uses a magnetic field to detect the frequencies at which substructures of chemical elements in body tissue resonate. The characteristic frequencies of various brain tissues are recorded to create an exquisitely detailed picture of brain structures.

The established clinical utility of MRI is in the diagnosis of primary degenerative dementias (e.g., Alzheimer's and Pick's diseases). In addition, recent studies of schizophrenia have demonstrated smaller frontal lobe size, ventricular enlargement (especially in the frontal horns), and temporal-limbic abnormalities, including complete or partial agenesis of the corpus callosum.

Possible advantages of MRI over CT include the following:

- *Imaging in all planes,* including sagittal and coronal, in addition to transverse
- *Higher resolution* of tissue structures
- *Better differentiation* of *gray matter* from white matter
- *Better definition of lesions* in *demyelinating disorders* (e.g., multiple sclerosis) and, therefore, early identification
- Excellent *visualization of the posterior fossa and pituitary regions*
- Potential for measuring *physiological variables*

In clinical practice, however, the CT scan is still frequently used, as it is convenient, safe, relatively comfortable, less expensive, and especially helpful as a diagnostic tool in patients with a history of cerebral concussion or subarachnoid hemorrhage.

Functional Magnetic Resonance Imaging. Functional magnetic resonance imaging (fMRI) is a potential tool to study the neuronal basis of behavior (25). The general principles behind this technique are closely related to neuronal metabolic activity and blood flow. Thus, fMRI can measure CNS hemodynamic changes that occur during activation paradigms, allowing functional evaluation of those regions that subserve sensory, motor, cognitive, and emotional processes. Because of the high spatial resolution, functional and structural aspects of the brain can also be correlated. In addition, fMRI is noninvasive and does not require exposure to radiation (26). Limitations include inadequate temporal resolution, high susceptibility to movement artifacts, and inadequate statistical models to analyze the large data sets generated.

Magnetic Resonance Spectroscopy. Magnetic resonance spectroscopy (MRS) has made it possible to measure various neurotransmitter systems, including choline-containing compounds in the CNS, *in vivo*, noninvasively, and without exposure to radioactivity. For example, preliminary reports used MRS to evaluate choline concentrations in the subcortical nuclei of elderly depressed patients before and after treatment, as well as in younger unmedicated depressed patients (27–29). One report found evidence for elevated choline levels, which resolved with treatment, and another found evidence of increased choline response in depressed patients relative to control subjects. Other studies have found decreased levels of *N*-acetylaspartate (NAA) moieties in the hippocampus and frontal cortex of patients with schizophrenia, consistent with postmortem studies indicating a loss of neurons in these areas (30). A decrease in dorsolateral prefrontal cortex (DLPC) NAA has also been reported in bipolar patients (31).

In summary, MRI, fMRI, and MRS provide the promise of powerful noninvasive techniques for studying both anatomical and biological activity in a variety of conditions, as well as the impact of treatment.

Other Imaging Techniques

Thus far, these techniques lack general applicability for routine psychiatric diagnosis or treatment.

Positron emission tomography. (PET) provides functional images of the brain and is particularly promising in the study of neurotransmitter systems and their interactions (32). A positron-emitting element (e.g., fluorine-18, carbon-11, carbon-14) is incorporated into a biologically significant compound (e.g., d-glucose), which is then administered intravenously. The distribution of the compound in different regions of the brain when the patient is at rest or engaged in a specific task is then mapped. This technique can also be used to measure receptor density or receptor-ligand activity in a given location.

Important PET scan findings include the following:

- Reduced *prefrontal metabolism* in schizophrenia
- High *metabolic rates* in the orbital frontal cortex and basal ganglia of patients with obsessive-compulsive disorder
- Neuroleptic *blockade of D_2 receptors* in schizophrenia (33, 34)
- Association of the personality dimension of introversion with increased activity in frontal lobe regions (35)

Single photon emission computed tomography (SPECT) is a method that allows the measurement of cerebral blood flow when certain designated brain areas are activated by having the subjects perform specific experimental tasks (e.g., cognitive challenge tests like Wisconsin Card-Sorting). As in PET, SPECT can visualize both cortical and subcortical structures. Although the pictures are not as clear as those produced by PET scanning, with increasing improvements in hardware and software SPECT may offer a reasonable and less expensive alternative to study brain activity (36).

Both SPECT and PET studies have revealed a characteristic pattern of hypoperfusion in posterior temporoparietal regions in Alzheimer's disease.

Regional Cerebral Blood Flow Mapping. Such mapping techniques use radioactive probes (e.g., xenon-13) to delineate perfusion of cortical structures. For example, they have generally confirmed prefrontal cortex dysfunction in schizophrenia (37).

Neurophysiological Testing

Electroencephalogram

The electroencephalogram (EEG) procedure is useful in differentiating some organic conditions from idiopathic psychiatric syndromes, as well as in helping to identify focal structural lesions in the cortex (38, 39). In some patients with episodic, paroxysmal behavioral disturbances and a presumptive diagnosis of schizophrenia, a sleep-deprived EEG with nasopharyngeal leads may help rule out an epileptiform disorder contributing to or underlying psychotic behavior. In general, an EEG is indicated in patients who are younger (especially under age 25) and presenting with their first psychotic episode, or in patients with a history of possible cerebral injury or neurological disturbance (e.g., accidents, unconsciousness, infections, perinatal complications, seizures). This procedure has the advantages of being safe, being relatively inexpensive, and allowing the patient to be relatively free from discomfort.

Limitations of the EEG are numerous, however, and include the following:

- An apparently *normal EEG does not exclude organic disease* or epilepsy.
- *ECT* and *psychotropics* affect the EEG making interpretation difficult at times.
- *Sampling error* is possible because the paroxysmal electrical activity may not have occurred during the time of recording. In such cases, a sleep-deprived EEG or a 24-hour ambulatory recording might be helpful.

Sometimes, videotaping a seizure can help define its type (e.g., epileptic or psychogenic) and quantify the abnormal behavior that accompanies the aberrant electrical activity.

In the search for specific neurophysiological markers of idiopathic psychiatric syndromes (e.g., schizophrenia, major mood disorders), studies have reported various nonspecific EEG abnormalities. In addition, psychiatric patients appear more sensitive to activation procedures such as the following:

- Sleep deprivation
- Provocative stimuli (e.g., photic stimulation with flashing strobe light)
- Hyperventilation

Thus far, however, no specific EEG patterns have been identified that can accurately aid in the diagnosis of a particular psychiatric condition.

Computed Topographic Mapping of the Electroencephalogram

Topographic mapping of the EEG, also referred to as brain electrical activity mapping, involves the recording of cortical electrical activity in certain specified frequencies, which a computer then graphically visualizes in two-dimensional, color-coded maps. This procedure is chiefly used in psychopharmacological and neuropsychological research.

Polysomnography

Polysomnography refers to sleep recordings that simultaneously monitor various physiological parameters (usually at night). The tests that may be carried out include EEG, electromyogram (EMG), electro-oculogram, ECG, rapid eye movement (REM), nocturnal penile tumescence (NPT), respiratory air flow, and vital signs. In a typical sleep laboratory, a 12- to 16-channel polygraph recording is made. Uses include the following:

- Investigation and diagnosis of *sleep disorders,* especially sleep apnea and narcolepsy
- Research in *depression* (e.g., REM density and latency; total sleep time)
- *Drug* and *alcohol withdrawal* studies
- NPT in the differentiation of functional from organic causes of *impotence*

Evoked Potentials

Evoked potentials are electrophysiological recordings (on the order of milliseconds, as opposed to minutes in other brain-imaging techniques like PET) evoked from specific cortical areas (e.g., visual, auditory, somatosensory) using discrete types of sensory stimulation (e.g., flashes of light). They can differentiate between certain organic and functional disorders (e.g., visual evoked potentials in suspected hysterical blindness), as well as evaluate demyelinating disorders such as multiple sclerosis. At this time, however, evoked potentials are mainly used in the study of biological markers. For example, several investigations have found low-amplitude, late (greater than 250 ms) brainstem auditory evoked potentials in schizophrenic patients, which suggest attentional and information-processing impairment (40, 41).

Other Techniques

The *electroretinogram* reflects central dopaminergic function. Eye tracking dysfunction, such as aberrant *smooth pursuit eye tracking movements,* may represent genetic vulnerability markers for schizophrenia (42–44). *EMG* and *nerve conduction studies* may help in cases where myopathies or peripheral neuropathies are suspected. *Magnetoencephalography* is a noninvasive technique that measures the weak magnetic fields generated by the electrical activity of the brain (including the deeper subcortical areas) and converts them back into electric signals, which are then recorded. It holds great promise for neuroscience research.

Therapeutic Drug Monitoring. The ideal drug treatment strategy achieves maximal therapeutic response with a minimum of side effects. In many branches of medicine, monitoring plasma levels, rather than dose of a drug, is often the optimal way to reach this goal (45). Although not a routine procedure in psychiatry, this approach is used for lithium, valproate, and carbamazepine, as well as for some antidepressants and antipsychotics. For many other psychoactive drugs, however, this approach is used on a case-by-case basis. The best use of this technique remains for those circumstances when response is not adequate or unexpected adverse events occur. Chapter 3 covers the pharmacokinetic principles relevant to the optimal dosing of medication and to the use of TDM. In this section, we review the clinical use of TDM as follows:

- State the *theoretical basis* of the blood level/clinical response relationship.
- Note the *methodological issues* that complicate the interpretation of results from plasma level/clinical response studies.
- Integrate results from existing valid studies to emphasize the *clinical applicability* of TDM.

Theoretical Basis

If a drug produced immediate pharmacological effects, then the monitoring of plasma levels would be less necessary. For example, one can directly observe the clinical stages of anesthesia and adjust the anesthetic dosage by monitoring its effects. On the other hand, there is often a long interval (e.g., weeks) between response and drug administration in clinical psychopharmacology. In such situations, if the plasma concentrations required for clinical response are known, doses can be adjusted more rapidly to achieve

the proper levels. Such monitoring is also useful when there are large interindividual differences among patients in the metabolism of a drug. In such instances, knowledge of the potential therapeutic range for a given agent could provide more precise guidelines for individualized dose adjustment.

For example, response to a given dose or plasma concentration of an antipsychotic can take weeks, so increasing the dose every few days can overrun this lag period, often leading to much higher than ideal concentrations. Although dose is usually adjusted based on clinical response, knowing the minimally effective level may avoid unnecessary medication exposure. The primary data in determining the minimally effective dose come from fixed dose-response trials. Plasma level studies can also supplement these data because there is a positive correlation between levels achieved and the dose required. Thus, one can estimate the average dose needed to produce a certain concentration. In another sense, plasma levels can be thought of as a fine-tuning of the dose.

The basic assumptions that underlie the relationship between plasma levels and clinical response are:

- An *optimal concentration* range exists at which maximal pharmacological response will occur.
- A relationship exists between the drug *concentration in plasma* and *at the site of action*.
- *Pharmacogenetic* and *environmental factors* vary the quantity of drug that reaches the receptor site in different individuals.

At too low concentrations there will be no response, followed by a rapidly increasing response once the threshold level is reached. After the maximal pharmacological response is achieved, further increases in concentration will not enhance response. Thus, a plasma level-response relationship often shows the typical sigmoidal shape. Further, at higher concentrations, various adverse effects of a drug may be more prominent. Thus, a composite plot of the clinical benefit versus drug plasma level will result in an inverted U-shaped relationship that defines the range (or "therapeutic window") to achieve optimal benefit in most patients. For most drugs, the upper end of the therapeutic window represents toxicity. Hypothetically, however, some drugs at higher concentrations could actually lose their clinical effectiveness as a result of altered pharmacodynamic actions. The only agent for which evidence exists to support this contention is the antidepressant nortriptyline, but even here, the data are limited. For a drug that does not have serious toxic effects at higher concentrations, the blood level/clinical benefit relationship will eventually plateau.

Methodological Issues

A number of methodological issues have confounded the interpretation of results, thus minimizing the clinical utility of the plasma level-therapeutic response relationship (46). These issues can be grouped as follows:

- *Dose* strategy
- *Assay* methods
- Patient *population*
- Study *design*

Dose Strategy. **The most insidious potential methodological error in plasma level/clinical response studies is the possible confound due to increasing the dose too soon when a patient fails to respond.** This error frequently results in missing the therapeutic threshold level because patients are not kept on the lower dose for a sufficient time to document ineffectiveness. Additionally, because patients may be responding at a slower rate than the rate of dose increases, responders at a higher dose may have actually improved at a lower dose had it been maintained for a longer period of time.

To illustrate, consider two examples of patients with inadequate clinical response. In the first, poor response is due to a low plasma level. When the clinician increases the dose, the plasma level also rises, and although there may be a response at the higher plasma level, frequently repeated dose increases can obscure the threshold level for response. In the second example, there is an adequate plasma level but a drug-refractory patient. When the dose is increased, the plasma level rises; the patient, however, will remain nonresponsive at any concentration if the patient's disorder is not responsive to a given drug's mechanism of action.

In research trials, one experimental design to solve this confound is to nonrandomly assign a fixed dose based on the patient's clinical condition at admission and then hold it constant throughout the rest of the study. The investigator may initially preassign patients to high, medium, or low doses based on the investigator's clinical judgment; this assignment, however, is done before treatment starts and is usually based on the severity of the symptoms present. In the absence of a large number of well-designed studies, this method is less rigorous but usable in the interpretation of dose-response studies.

A more rigorous method to define the plasma level/clinical response relationship is to use a constant (or fixed) dose design, regardless of clinical status. It can be a single fixed dose or random assignment to several different fixed doses (e.g., low, medium, and high) to investigate the low and the high end of a potential therapeutic window. When data from several fixed-dose studies indicate a possible therapeutic range for a specific drug, prospectively targeting patients to various plasma levels can then be a useful confirmatory study design. In this design, patients are maintained in a predetermined fixed plasma level range during the trial period.

Assay Methods. Analytic techniques can be broadly divided into *chemical* or *biological* assays. Chemical methods primarily use physicochemical characteristics of a drug in conjunction with analytic instrumentation, and are generally individualized for each compound or a group of similar compounds. **Currently, gas liquid chromatographic and high-pressure liquid chromatographic methods are the most commonly used for such analyses.** Biological methods, on the other hand, are based on some biological activity of the drug. In general, they do not quantitate the specific drug concentration, but rather the activity of the drug is transformed into a concentration equivalent. As a result, these methods cannot distinguish between compounds that have similar biological activities. This problem is highlighted by studies involving antipsychotics, because many laboratories used radioreceptor assay (RRA) for drug measurements. For example,

TABLE 1-7. *Antipsychotic levels by gas-liquid chromatography and radioreceptor assay[a]*

Drug	Number of subjects	Gas-liquid chromatography (ng/mL)	Radioreceptor assay (ng/mL)
Haloperidol	20	7.2	10.1
Butaperazine	10	152.0	201.0
Fluphenazine	20	0.97	7.1
Trifluoperazine	35	0.7	5.7

[a] Same plasma sample was analyzed by the two methods.
From Javaid JI, Pandey GN, Duslak B, et al. Measurement of neuroleptic concentrations by GLC and radioreceptor assay. *Commun Psychopharmacol* 1980;4:467–475, with permission.

Javaid et al. (47) have shown that in the same plasma sample, chemical assay and RRA resulted in substantially different levels for various antipsychotics (Table 1-7). Because RRA also measures pharmacologically active metabolites, this outcome is not surprising. A brief description of the principles of these methods, along with their utility, is given in Table 1-8.

In earlier studies, the method of blood collection and sample handling before analysis could also have resulted in variable plasma level measurements. For example, it has been reported that during blood collection of TCAs and phenothiazines, contact with rubber stoppers for extended periods of time could result in spuriously low plasma levels (47, 48).

Patient Population. When analyzing the results of studies that attempt to relate the plasma drug concentration to response, there are a number of patient variables that should be considered:

- *Refractory* patients
- *Nonhomogeneous* patient samples
- Patient *noncompliance,* particularly in outpatient studies
- Small patient *sample sizes*

Study Design. Important issues relating to study design are these:

- *Inadequate evaluation* of clinical response
- Concurrent *multiple-drug treatments*
- Too brief an *observation period*
- Variable time of *blood sampling*

As noted earlier, the interpretation of plasma level versus clinical response data even in well-designed studies is further complicated by the presence of multiple *active metabolites*

formed by biotransformation, which is a necessary step in the elimination process for most psychotropics.

Clinical Applicability

Substantial data indicating large differences in plasma levels among patients treated with the same dose of a psychotropic provide one rationale for adjusting the dose based on blood levels to achieve the optimal clinical effect; the putative therapeutic range, however, must be established for each individual drug. Valid studies must also define clinically meaningful limits. Thus, a large body of information is required before even an approximation of the therapeutic range can be determined.

Plasma levels of various psychotropics differ widely among individuals on the same dose due to differences in their rates of metabolism. Therefore, the clinician must adjust each patient's dosage to achieve maximal benefit with minimal side effects. Therapeutic drug monitoring can be used to address these issues:

- To determine *compliance*
- To establish *adequacy* of the pharmacotherapy in nonresponders
- To *maximize the clinical response* where the drug plasma level-response relationship has been established based on well-designed and executed studies
- To help define the *dose-response relationship*
- To clarify when potential *drug interactions* may alter steady-state concentration levels
- To avoid *toxicity* due to unnecessarily high plasma levels

TABLE 1-8. *Various techniques used for therapeutic drug monitoring*

Method	Principle	Comments
Chemical assays		
Spectrometric	Drug is extracted into organic solvent and subsequently measured by colorimetric reaction or fluorescence.	At therapeutic concentrations, sensitivity fair to poor for potent antipsychotics; specificity–poor to fair; rarely used at present.
GLC	Compounds are separated between moving gas phase and stationary liquid phase and detected by different detectors; the method is individualized for each compound or a group of similar compounds after extraction.	The ues of specific detectors, such as electron capture (ECD) and nitrogen/phosphorus (NPD), gives good-to-excellent sensitivity and specificity; commonly used in many labs for routine measurements.
HPLC	Compounds are separated between moving liquid phase and a stationary phase and detected by different detectors; the method is individualized for each compound or a group of similar compounds after extraction.	The use of special detectors, such as fluorescence or electrochemical detectors, results in good-to-excellent sensitivity and specificity; commonly used in many labs for routine measurements.
GC-MS	After extraction, the compounds are separated by GC and fragmented by MS; each compound gives specific mass fragments.	Very specific, with good-to-excellent sensitivity; not economical for routine analysis; generally used to establish specificities for other techniques.
Biological assays		
RRA	Radiolabeled drug bound to receptors can be displaced by unlabeled compounds with similar binding characteristics; the plasma can be used without extraction.	This method measures the inhibitory activity of the sample; although simple, with fair sensitivity, the method has poor specificity; some labs use in clinical studies.
RIA	Antibodies are prepared against the drug linked to a protein; the displacement by the sample of radiolabeled drug from antibody-antigen complex is determined; the sample can be used without extraction.	The method is sensitive and simple; however, the specificity is poor to fair and depends on the cross-reactivity of structurally related compounds; generally restricted to the labs that have specific antibodies because currently they are not commercially available.

From Javaid JI, Janicak PG, Holland D. Blood level monitoring of antipsychotics and antidepressants. *Psychiatr Med* 1991;9:163–187, with permission.

- To be used as a safeguard for the clinician in potential *medicolegal* situations (e.g., when a patient responds to either an unusually low or high dose of a drug)

Lithium. For most psychiatrists, lithium testing is the area of laboratory testing with which they are most familiar. Lithium has a well-defined, narrow serum concentration range (49). For acute mania, therapeutic lithium levels range between 0.5 mEq/L at the low end and about 1.5 mEq/L at the high end. Individual patients, however, may have idiosyncratic responses outside this range. Samples for blood levels should be drawn about four to five half-lives (i.e., 4 to 6 days) after an adjustment in dose, or more frequently if unexpected reactions occur. Blood samples should be collected 10 to 12 hour after the last dose.

After resolution of the acute phase, maintenance levels of at least 0.8 mEq/L are necessary for optimal efficacy and should be checked once every 6 to 12 months, or more often if clinically indicated. Other follow-up tests include periodic thyroid function tests, blood urea nitrogen, serum creatinine, serum calcium (because lithium may cause hypoparathyroidism), and an ECG. Thyroid function tests and renal function should be monitored approximately every 6 to 12 months (see the section "Maintenance/Prophylaxis Treatment" in Chapter 10).

Anticonvulsants. The plasma levels of anticonvulsants that are optimally therapeutic for psychiatric disorders have not been clearly established. Because there are data on their usefulness to treat seizure disorders, monitoring of blood levels has increased the safety of anticonvulsants (and indirectly their efficacy), while also verifying compliance and determining the cause of toxicity when more than one medication is concurrently administered (see the section "Alternative Treatment Strategies" in Chapter 10).

The anticonvulsant therapeutic range for plasma concentrations of *carbamazepine* is 4 to 12 μg/mL. Hematological assessment in patients on carbamazepine therapy is appropriate because aplastic anemia and agranulocytosis have been reported in association with its use.

Some data indicate that therapeutic serum levels of *valproate* for most patients will range from 45 to 125 μg/mL (50). Patients should be monitored closely for nonspecific symptoms like malaise, weakness, lethargy, facial edema, anorexia, and vomiting—all of which are indicative of hepatotoxicity. Liver function tests should be obtained before therapy and repeated if indicated, especially during the first 6 months.

Antidepressants. TDM is a standard of care issue when prescribing TCAs due to their narrow therapeutic index; the wide interindividual variability in their elimination rate, and the serious but often insidious nature of their toxicity. TDM generally only needs to be performed once in a patient on a TCA, because the goal is to characterize the patient's ability to clear the drug. TDM is only repeated if a problem with compliance is suspected or if something occurs that may change the patient's ability to clear the drug (e.g., an intercurrent disease or change of drug that induces or inhibits the CYP 450 enzyme system responsible for the metabolism of TCAs). For all other antidepressants, TDM may be done for the following reasons:

- Questionable patient *compliance*
- *Poor response* to an "adequate" dose, raising doubts about unusual pharmacokinetics, such as excessively slow or fast metabolism, leading to unusually low or high blood levels
- *Side effects* at a low dose
- *Medical illness; children* and *adolescents; elderly* patients
- Patients for whom *treatment is urgent* and it is imperative to achieve therapeutic levels as soon as possible

For example, a test dose may identify a fast metabolizer, who may require a higher dose; there is no evidence, however, that this approach could accelerate response, an issue that needs to be tested in controlled trials. Further, only limited evidence exists that high doses will shorten the lag period for any psychotropic agent (e.g., divalproex sodium loading dose strategy).

These issues are discussed in greater detail in the "Pharmacokinetics" section in Chapter 7.

Antipsychotics. Clear guidelines for measuring therapeutic serum concentrations of antipsychotics have not yet been established. There may, however, be specific situations in which they may be of value (e.g., monitoring of haloperidol [HPDL] levels might be useful in patients on concurrent carbamazepine therapy because the latter agent can substantially reduce serum HPDL concentrations). These issues are discussed in greater detail in the "Pharmacokinetics/ Plasma Level" section in Chapter 5.

Anxiolytics and Sedative-Hypnotics. Because of their large therapeutic index, measurement of anxiolytic or sedative-hypnotic serum concentrations is not usually necessary in clinical practice, unless abuse, overdose, or inadvertent toxicity are suspected. Some data indicate that plasma alprazolam levels of 40 ng/mL may be required to manage panic disorder (51) (see the sections "Adverse Effects of Anxiolytics" and "Adverse Effects of Sedative-Hypnotics" in Chapter 12).

Summary

Historically, many of the pioneers in psychiatry attempted to correlate "mental" symptoms with identifiable brain pathology. This tradition continues by using state-of-the-art techniques to search for biological correlates of psychopathology. This search, in turn, may lead to a better understanding of pathogenesis and causation, culminating in more specific treatment strategies.

The laboratory will play an increasingly important role in clinical psychiatry and presently is most helpful in:

- *Identification of medical disorders* that present with cognitive, affective, and behavioral changes, or when psychiatric disorders mimic medical-neurological syndromes
- Medical workup before *specialized treatment options*
- The selective use of *drug concentrations* to enhance efficacy and minimize toxicity

It is important that clinicians appreciate the need for the judicious use of the laboratory for a particular individual, while being sensitive to economic realities, degree of discomfort, and risk of adverse effects. Clinicians must also be cognizant of the nuances in interpreting laboratory data (i.e., their specificity, sensitivity, and predictive value). Finally, they need to integrate laboratory data with the patient's history, interview, and physical examination to formulate the most accurate diagnosis and appropriate treatment plan.

CONCLUSION

Clinicians should be prepared to take advantage of an ever-increasing number of newer, more specific agents. They can accomplish this by:

- Adopting a *medical model* when evaluating the patient's complaints
- Taking a *stepwise, empirically based approach to treatment* selection
- Adopting the stance of a *behavior psychopharmacologist* when evaluating a patient's response, recognizing that any reaction to medication (intended or otherwise) could provide useful information
- *Keeping current with recent, relevant developments* in the neurosciences

The application of our principles should help clinicians to incorporate new developments in psychopharmacology into their practice. The result will be improved patient care and further insights into pathophysiology, which can serve as the basis for our next generation of therapies.

REFERENCES

1. Kendell RE. *The role of diagnosis in psychiatry.* Oxford: Blackwell Scientific, 1975.
2. Lee S, Chow CC, Wang YK, et al. Mania secondary to thyrotoxicosis. *Br J Psychiatry* 1991;159:712–713.
3. Preskorn SH. Beyond DSM-IV: what is the cart and what is the horse? *Psychiatr Ann* 1995;25:53–62.
4. Preskorn S. The future of psychopharmacology: potentials and needs. *Psychiatr Ann* 1990;20:625–633.
5. Preisig M, Bellivier F, Fenton BT. Association between bipolar disorder and monoamine oxidase A gene polymorphism: results of a multicenter study. *Am J Psychiatry* 2000;157:948–955.
6. Janicak PG, Winans E. The laboratory in clinical psychiatry. In: Dickstein LJ, Riba MB, Oldham JM, eds. *American Psychiatric Press review of psychiatry. Vol. 16.* Washington, DC: American Psychiatric Press, 1997:V7–V29.
7. Preskorn SH, Burke M, Fast GA. Therapeutic drug monitoring. Principles and practices. *Psychiatr Clin North Am* 1993;16:611–646.
8. Preskorn SH. Should rational drug development in psychiatry target more than one mechanism of action in a single molecule? *Int Rev Psychiatry* 1995;7:17–28.
9. Preskorn SH. The relative adverse effect profile of non-SSRI antidepressants: relationship to *in vitro* pharmacology. *J Pract Psychiatry Behav Health* 2000;6:218–223.
10. Preskorn SH. The adverse effect profiles of the selective serotonin reuptake inhibitors: relationship to *in vitro* pharmacology. *J Psychiatr Pract* 2000;6:153–157.
11. American Psychiatric Association. *Diagnostic and statistical manual of mental disorders,* 4th ed. Washington, DC: American Psychiatric Press, 1994.
12. Israni TH, Janicak PG. Laboratory assessment in psychiatry. In: Flaherty J, Davis JM, Janicak PG, eds. *Psychiatry: diagnosis and therapy,* 2nd ed. Norwalk, CT: Appleton and Lange, 1993:30–39.
13. Stanga C, Preskorn SH. Use of the laboratory in psychiatry. In: Dunner DL, ed. *Current Psychiatric Therapy II.* Philadelphia: Saunders, 1997:2:59–74.
14. Roose RB, Deutsch LH, Deutsch SI. Medical assessment and laboratory testing in psychiatry. In: Sadock BJ, Sadock VA, eds. *Kaplan & Sadock's comprehensive textbook of psychiatry,* 7th ed. Baltimore: Lippincott Williams & Wilkins, 2000:732–754.
15. The APA Task Force on Lab Tests in Psychiatry. The DST: an overview of its current status in psychiatry. *Am J Psychiatry* 1987;144:1253–1262.
16. Sharma RP, Pandey GN, Janicak PG, et al. The effect of diagnosis and age on the DST: a meta-analytic approach. *Biol Psychiatry* 1988;24:555–568.
17. Arana GW, Baldessarini RJ, Ornstein M. The DST for diagnosis and prognosis in psychiatry. *Arch Gen Psychiatry* 1985;42:1193–1204.

18. Mokrani MC, Dual F, Crocq MA, et al. HPA axis dysfunction in depression: correlation with monoamine system abnormalities. *Psychoneuroendocrinology* 1997;22(suppl 1):S63–S68.
19. Pandey GN, Pandey SC, Dwivedi Y, et al. Platelet serotonin-2A receptors: a potential biological marker for suicidal behavior. *Am J Psychiatry* 1995;156:850–855.
20. Pandey GN. Altered serotonin function in suicide. Evidence from platelet and neuroendocrine studies. *Ann NY Acad Sci* 1997;836:182–200.
21. Drevets WC, Gadde KM, Ranga K, et al. Neuroimaging studies of mood disorders. In: Charney DS, Nestler EJ, Bunney BS, eds. *Neurobiology of mental illness.* Vol. 30. New York: Oxford University Press, 1999:394–418.
22. Silbersweig DA, Stern E, Frith C, et al. A functional neuroanatomy of hallucinations in schizophrenia. *Nature* 1995;378:176–179.
23. Farde L, Nordstrom AL, Wiesel FA, et al. Positron emission tomographic analysis of central D_1 and D_2 dopamine receptor occupancy in patients treated with classical neuroleptics and clozapine. *Arch Gen Psychiatry* 1992;49:538–544.
24. Klemm E, Grunwald F, Kasper S, et al. [1231] 1BZM SPECT for imaging of striatal D_2 dopamine receptors in 56 schizophrenic patients taking various neuroleptics. *Am J Psychiatry* 1996;153:183–190.
25. Doval O, Bello E, Singh J, et al. *The brain in motion: functional magnetic resonance imaging for clinicians.* Chicago: University of Illinois at Chicago Department of Psychiatry, 1999.
26. Burton MW, Small SL. An introduction to functional magnetic resonance imaging. *Neurologist* 1999;5:145–158.
27. Charles HC, Layers F, Boyko O, et al. Elevated choline concentrations in basal ganglia of depressed patients. *Biol Psychiatry* 1992;31:99A.
28. Charles HC, Lazeyras, AQ Krishnan KRR, et al. Brain choline in depression: *in vivo* detection of potential pharmacodynamic effects of antidepressant therapy using hydrogen localized spectroscopy. *Prog Neuropsychopharmacol Biol Psychiatry* 1994;18:1121–1127.
29. Renshaw PF, Stoll AL, Rothschild A, et al. Multiple brain ^{1}H-MRS abnormalities in depressed patients suggest impaired second messenger cycling. *Biol Psychiatry* 1993;33:44A.
30. Soares JC, Innis RB. Neurochemical brain imaging investigations of schizophrenia. *Biol Psychiatry* 1999;46:600–615.
31. Winsberg ME, Sachs N, Tate DL, et al. Decreased dorsolateral prefrontal *N*-acetyl aspartate in bipolar disorder. *Biol Psychiatry* 2000;47:475–481.
32. Smith GS, Dewey SL, Brodie JD, et al. Serotonergic modulation of dopamine measured with [^{11}C]raclopride and PET in normal human subjects. *Am J Psychiatry* 1997;154:490–496.
33. Kapur S, Remington G, Jones C, et al. High levels of dopamine D_2 receptor occupancy with low-dose haloperidol treatment: a PET study. *Am J Psychiatry* 1996;153:948–950.
34. Nyberg S, Eriksson B, Oxenstierna G, et al. Suggested minimal effective dose of risperidone based on PET-measured D_2 and 5-HT$_{2a}$ receptor occupancy in schizophrenic patients. *Am J Psychiatry* 1999;156:869–875.
35. Johnson DL, Wieber JS, Gold SM, et al. Cerebral blood flow and personality: a positron emission tomography study. *Am J Psychiatry* 1999;156:252–257.
36. Holman BL, Tumeh SS. Single-photon emission computed tomography (SPECT). *JAMA* 1990;263:561–564.
37. Sharif Z, Gewirtz G, Iqbal N. Brain imaging in schizophrenia: a review. *Psychiatr Ann* 1993;23:123–134.
38. Lishman WA. *Organic psychiatry. The psychological consequences of cerebral disorder,* 2nd ed. London: Blackwell Scientific, 1987.
39. Cummings JL. *Clinical neuropsychiatry.* Orlando: Grune & Stratton, 1985.
40. Kayser J, Bruder GE, Friedman D, et al. Brain event-related potentials (ERPs) in schizophrenia during a word recognition memory task. *Int J Psychophysiol* 1999;34:249–265.
41. Iwanami A, Okajima Y, Kuwakado D, et al. Event-related potentials and thought disorder in schizophrenia. *Schizophr Res* 2000;42:187–191.
42. Levy DL, Holzman PS, Matthysse S, et al. Eye tracking dysfunction and schizophrenia: a critical perspective. *Schizophr Bull* 1993;19:461–536.
43. Chen Y, Levy DL, Nakayama K, et al. Dependence of impaired eye tracking on deficient velocity discrimination in schizophrenia. *Arch Gen Psychiatry* 1999;56:155–161.
44. Holzman PS, Levy DL, Proctor LR. Smooth pursuit eye movements, attention, and schizophrenia. *Arch Gen Psychiatry* 1976;33:1415–1420.
45. Burke MJ, Preskorn SH. Therapeutic drug monitoring of antidepressants: cost implications and relevance to clinical practice. *Clin Pharmacokinet* 1999;37:147–165.
46. Javaid JI, Janicak PG, Holland D. Blood level monitoring of antipsychotics and antidepressants. *Psychiatr Med* 1991;9:163–187.
47. Javaid JI, Pandey GN, Duslak B, et al. Measurement of neuroleptic concentrations by GLC and radioreceptor assay. *Commun Psychopharmacol* 1980;4:467–475.
48. Cochran E, Carl J, Hanin I, et al. Effect of vacutainer stoppers on plasma tricyclic levels: a reevaluation. *Commun Psychopharmacol* 1978;2:495–503.
49. Janicak PG, Davis JM. Clinical usage of lithium in mania. In: Burrows GD, Norman TR, Davies B, eds. *Antimanics, anticonvulsants and other drugs in psychiatry.* New York: Elsevier, 1987:21–34.
50. Bowden CL, Janicak PG, Orsulak P, et al. Relationship of serum valproate concentrations to response in mania. *Am J Psychiatry* 1996;153:765–770.
51. Shader RI, Greenblatt DJ. Use of benzodiazepines in anxiety disorders. *N Engl J Med* 1993;328:1398–1405.

2

Assessment of Drug Efficacy and Relevant Clinical Issues

A series of related issues is pertinent to the decision-making process a clinician uses in the application of drug therapy. The *first section* of this chapter considers the quality of the research data on drug efficacy by classifying studies based on predetermined criteria for methodological rigor. The companion section on meta-analysis reviews the rationale and the potential complications inherent in statistically summarizing the data across several studies that assess drug efficacy. While mindful of the inherent shortcomings in this statistical approach, we believe such summarizations can provide the clinician with a meaningful quantitative statement about a specific drug's clinical value.

The *next section* addresses issues relevant to the clinician—patient relationship during the assessment, initial treatment, and maintenance/ prophylactic phases of psychopharmacotherapy.

The *final two sections* discuss the Food and Drug Administration (FDA) regulatory process and the cost of treatment. Expenses associated with assessment and treatment and, more importantly, the total economic impact on patients, their families, and society are considered.

EVALUATION OF DRUG STUDY DESIGNS

To accurately understand the literature, we have provided two perspectives so that practitioners can make the best decision about specific drug choices for their patients:

- We have *classified studies* (i.e., class I, II, III) based on their methodological rigor so that the reader can judge the quality of the data (Table 2-1).
- We *statistically summarize* drug outcome studies, producing a "bottom-line" quantitative assessment of the difference between an exper-

imental drug and placebo or other standard agent (see "Drug Management" later in this chapter).

We first consider the classification of studies by rigor (i.e., the extent to which the design allows the investigator to adequately test the hypothesis in question). There are several important elements in a well-controlled study, including:

- Placebo *control* (1)
- A proper *blind*
- *Random assignment*
- *Parallel* or *crossover* design
- No "active" *concomitant medications*
- An *adequate sample*
- The use of *valid measures* of outcome
- Proper presentation of the experimental *data*

Without adequate controls and appropriate methodology, the ability to generalize is compromised, bringing into question a study's validity, the interpretation of its results, or both.

Double-Blind Techniques

In a double-blind study, neither the patient nor the evaluator knows who is receiving active experimental medication or placebo. If enough patients are available for three or more groups, one or more active control medication groups can also be used. A standard active drug control serves two important purposes. First, it validates the experiment by demonstrating that the standard drug is clearly superior to placebo in this population. Second, it serves as a benchmark (because it has a known efficacy) by which to compare a new treatment. For example, a new drug could be equal to or better than a standard drug, and both should be better than placebo. Alternatively, the new drug could be less effective than the standard drug but more efficacious than placebo.

TABLE 2-1. *Classification of study designs*

Classification	Criteria
Class I: At least the first nine criteria	Random assignment (prospective)
	No concomitant active medication
	Parallel (or appropriate crossover) design
	Double-blind, placebo control
	Adequate handling of dropouts
Class II: Six of the eleven criteria	Adequate sample
	Appropriate population
	Standardized assessments
	Either clear presentation of data or appropriate statistics
Class III: Five of the eleven criteria	Adequate dose of medication
	Active controls[a]

[a] Desirable in all classes.

Random Assignment

Random assignment is the most important element of a controlled trial. Without it, patients most likely to respond could be preferentially assigned to one treatment arm, and any difference in efficacy would be secondary to this bias. When random assignment is used, a variety of confounding variables are equalized across the groups, including those of which the investigators are unaware (2).

Study Design

Parallel groups involve the assignment of patients to two or more treatments (e.g., new agent versus placebo, a standard agent, or both) that proceed concurrently. Unlike crossover designs, the carryover effects of the first treatment are then avoided.

In *crossover studies,* patients are randomly assigned to one of the two arms, so that generally a placebo is given first and then the active drug, or vice versa. The usual design is a placebo lead-in period, then active drug A or B, succeeded by a placebo period again, and then the "crossover" from A to B or B to A. This design can include a washout period during which placebo is administered between the first and second active drug phases, unless B is a placebo. If patients are maintained on placebo and the crossover to active treatment is not randomized (or in some other way controlled), they may be (and often are) switched concurrent with a spontaneous change in clinical state. Any coincidental

improvement or deterioration is in part due to this clinical change. In addition, change can be due to the cyclic nature of the disorder and not the drug's effect. Other, nonpharmacological interventions may also be introduced. For example, if staff become concerned about a patient, they may intervene with more intensive milieu, family, or individual therapy, while the clinician may feel compelled to switch from placebo to drug.

Concomitant Medications

Avoidance of active concomitant medication is the next important requirement. Such medication constitutes a major artifact because it can markedly weaken the drug—placebo difference. Thus, compared treatments may appear equally efficacious due to the concomitant medication and not any inherent efficacy of the experimental agent. Some studies have used multiple agents, in different doses, with some known to be specifically effective for the disorder under investigation. For example, in some studies, comparing carbamazepine or valproate with placebo or lithium, patients have also received adjunctive antipsychotics, making firm conclusions difficult (see the section "Alternative Treatment Strategies" in Chapter 10).

Concomitant medication should not be confused with rescue medications. The latter are nonspecific agents (or potentially effective drugs used in subtherapeutic doses) used so that patients can remain in the study for an adequate time, allowing for a valid comparison between the experimental agent and placebo (or standard drug). Often, rescue medications are used in the early phases and are decreased or eliminated before the critical evaluation at the end of the study. This enables more patients to complete the study (fewer dropouts), with the early impact of the rescue medication having at best only minimal effects on the final evaluations.

Augmentation or Combination Drug Studies

When it is likely that a second drug used in a copharmacy strategy can produce a better effect than a single drug, all patients can receive the standard drug and also be randomized to a second drug, placebo, or other comparator. Alternatively, designs can use placebo plus placebo, drug A plus placebo, drug B plus placebo, or both drugs combined.

Sample Adequacy

Equally critical to a properly designed study is sample adequacy (i.e., size and appropriateness). It is hard to make definitive conclusions with very small sample sizes (e.g., five per group) because variation is too great. The minimal sample size needed to make inferences also depends on how large the experimental drug-placebo effect size is (i.e., the larger the effect size, the smaller the sample needed).

The population studied should also be appropriate to the disorder. For example, in a study of antibiotics for pneumococcal pneumonia, the subject population should have this disease and not a viral pneumonitis. The same applies for an antipsychotic, which should not be studied in populations such as chronic, treatment-resistant or agitated, developmentally disabled patients. If studying an agent thought to benefit treatment resistance, however, one might deliberately select a patient population that satisfied such criteria.

Overly complicated entrance criteria may be counterproductive, in that patients who have a classic presentation may be excluded for trivial reasons because they fail to meet one or more less- important criteria. This may result in too small a sample size and can lead to the inclusion of patients who technically fit the criteria but are clearly inappropriate. This problem is particularly true with an uncommon disorder and with patients who are difficult to enroll in clinical trials (e.g., acutely manic).

Another issue is subjects who volunteer for an advertised study. Undoubtedly, some will have the true disorder, but others, although responding to an advertisement, may only minimally meet symptom criteria and may not have spontaneously sought help otherwise. This situation is particularly apparent when the disorder approximates normal emotions or problems. Some symptomatic volunteers may include newly recognized classic cases, whereas patients referred to a tertiary referral center may be an atypical, treatment-resistant population.

Rating Scales

Reliable and valid rating instruments are important. While a global assessment of clinical improvement is important, a valid rating scales can also qualitatively rate *symptom change*. In an open study, patients are often evaluated by the investigator's global impression, an approach obviously subject to bias. The use of adequately normed and standardized quantitative scales to assess patients at baseline and during treatment provides an element of objectivity. A reliably trained rater using valid instruments anchored by clear operational definitions makes it much harder for bias to enter, even if the study is not double-blind.

Data Analysis

The presentation of data and the statistical analysis are two critical factors. The inclusion of baseline and final ratings on each patient from a standardized (or even a simple global, semiquantitative) scale, allows for useful comparisons between those on active treatment or placebo. Even if formal analyses are not done, findings from such studies are often useful, and skeptical readers can always perform their own statistics.

Raw numbers provide the clinician with a "feel" for what actually happened, whereas the mean change scores on some abstract scale may have little intuitive meaning to the clinician. It is best to have the data speak directly to the reader in an uncomplicated fashion, and such information should always be included.

Equally important is the use of suitable quantitative statistical analyses, including more complicated models, because they can hold certain variables constant, control for artifacts, and provide supplementary information. Whatever statistics are used, they should be explicitly described in sufficient detail so the reader knows exactly what was done and can make a judgment about their appropriateness. For example, there are many different types of analyses of variance (ANOVA), analyses of covariance (ANCOVA), or multivariate analyses of variance (MANOVA), and some are not appropriate to the task at hand. If only the results of an ANOVA with a $p < 0.001$ are provided, the reader should be justifiably dubious, because this model may not be proper (p is an estimate of the probability that the results occurred by chance). Sufficient details are required to clarify which model was used, because the p value may be invalid with an inappropriate model.

Overly complicated statistics can introduce considerable bias into a study. When such models are used, they should be supplemented with raw data or simple, easily understood statistics. Usually, many patients drop out before studies are completed. *Observed data analysis* uses only the data actually observed at that time point. *Endpoint analysis* uses the last observation made on a subject. Patients often gradually improve or worsen. Some drop from the study when they get so much better that they are discharged or it seems pointless to continue in the study. Some can deteriorate to a dangerous state, so that they must be dropped for clinical reasons. In either case, reaching this point indicates that the drug is beneficial or not and is at least a qualitative endpoint. *Last observation carried forward* (LOCF), a standard method of data analysis, carries the last data point forward week by week. *Random regression models* can estimate what would happen at a later time point, assuming that patients change in a linear fashion. Improvement, however, often levels off. Thus, "creating" data points based on questionable assumptions can potentially introduce substantial bias.

Classifying Study Designs

Several features should be considered when classifying study designs by their quality. Although our classification is arbitrary, it is intended as a device to focus on all of the important criteria, not just one (e.g., "blinding").

A *class I* controlled study satisfies at least the first 10 of these criteria:

1. *Random* assignment
2. No *concomitant active medications*
3. *Parallel* (or appropriate crossover) design
4. Double-*blind, placebo* control
5. Adequate handling of *dropouts* (e.g., intent-to-treat analysis)
6. *Sample size* adequacy
7. Appropriate *population*
8. Standardized treatment *assessments*
9. Clear, descriptive *presentation of experimental data* or use of suitable quantitative *statistical analyses*
10. Adequate *dose* of medication
11. *Active control* (e.g., active standard drug)

The last criterion is a plus factor that enhances the value of any given study.

Class II studies are those that satisfy at least six of the 11 criteria. For example, a *single-blind study* introduces more bias, but if the other criteria (e.g., random assignment, parallel groups, etc.) are met, then the data may still be valid. An AB design with no randomization or statistical analyses may still have many excellent features. A mirror-image design, such as Baastrup and Schou's study (3) of lithium's prophylactic effects would be a good example (see the section "Maintenance/Prophylaxis" in Chapter 10). Such studies may have many elements of a better controlled design, including the following:

- Patients have a *classic presentation*.
- *Objective, quantifiable,* and *meaningful* measures are used to evaluate important clinical factors.
- An *adequate sample* is used.
- There is a *longer period of observation*.

A *class III* study is one that meets at least five of the 11 criteria. Whereas these studies have some important elements of a controlled trial, many aspects are uncontrolled. Because a bias can exist, however, does not mean it invalidates the result, only that it may. Because every question cannot be answered by a class I design for reasons of practicality or cost, class II and class III studies are very useful to at least partially resolve questions that would not otherwise be addressed.

An example of a class III study is the ABA design. A variable-length placebo lead-in period, drug period, and postdrug placebo period are suspect, however, because many nonrandom variables can influence their length. The choice of when to start an active drug may correspond to a worsening of the patient's condition, whereas the choice to stop treatment may foreshadow discharge with its own stresses. Such nonrandom events constitute major artifacts. With such a design, the staff can guess early and late in the hospitalization that patients are on placebo, and that they are on active treatment in the middle of the study, making the blind more illusionary than real.

Although there are many confounds with such a design, it does provide important information about whether a patient relapses when switched to placebo after an active drug. It is not possible to do a meaningful statistical analysis on an ABA design because there is no control group for comparison. The fact that some patients improve more on a drug in period B than in the placebo period A may be a factor of time or rater bias. Because there is no control group, one cannot say that this improvement is better than what would have occurred in the natural course of the illness. Relapse in the second placebo period, however, can provide some information.

Although ABA designs are only marginally better than open trials, they may be somewhat relevant to another scientific question (i.e., once the disease process is "turned off," will patients relapse when placebo is substituted?). For most psychotropics, we do not know whether relapse will occur immediately after a drug is stopped within a few days of achieving remission. The active disease may only have been suppressed, with relapse likely after discontinuation.

A *mirror-image study* (i.e., a design in which the time period on a new treatment is compared retrospectively with a similar time period without the new therapy) is often more like the "real world" of clinical practice, and hence its results may be easier to generalize. The bias in mirror-image studies, however, comes from nonrandom assignment and the absence of a blind. Because the control period occurred in a prior time segment, other variables could have changed in the interim. Without blinding, there is no way to avoid the possible bias of an evaluator's enthusiasm for a given treatment. Careful assessment by objective measurements can attenuate this bias.

Less Definitive Designs

Uncontrolled open studies are the most biased, with concomitant medication the source of greatest error. For example, a patient started on drug A who fails to immediately respond then has drug B added, but drug A could have a delayed effect on the patient, which is falsely attributed to the addition of drug B. Some case reports may attribute coincidental events to a specific drug. Thus, the critical reader should always clarify the role of concomitant medication as an artifact. Sometimes clinical myths can develop from several case reports on the efficacy of a specific drug when all patients were also on concomitant medication. Rare side effects can be defined by case reports, but the writer should always warn of coincidence, thus providing an honesty of purpose to the report.

Open designs can differ dramatically in their quality. Reports are often published on a variety of patients given different concomitant medications, diagnosed without the use of inclusion or exclusion criteria, and with outcome determined by the clinical investigator's opinion, based only on memory. By contrast, others include specified diagnostic criteria, include patients who are excellent examples of the disorder under study, use only one treatment, and are evaluated quantitatively and concurrently. Often the most important ingredient in an open study is the investigator's clinical judgment, which is, in fact, the measuring instrument. Whereas a more clinically experienced investigator may remain unbiased, those with less experience may unknowingly err in this regard. Open designs that incorporate quantitative evaluation of the medical record are superior to those that rely on clinician recall. We feel that a good open study can be better than a small-sample ABA study.

Systematic case-control studies (e.g., a nonrandomized control group) can also provide useful information, but unfortunately, they are rarely used in psychopharmacology research. In situations when uncommon conditions or those that pose an imminent danger to the patient (e.g., neuroleptic malignant syndrome) make it impossible to conduct prospective, controlled trials, case-control methodology can provide some degree of rigor. Because these studies are not random-assignment, however, the outcome can be substantially biased.

Good observational case-controlled or cohort studies can make reasonably accurate estimates. Comparisons of observational and randomized studies by Benson and Hartz (4) and Concato et al. (5) found similar results were obtained by both methods. It is unusual to have the same treatment investigated by both methodologies, however, and these comparisons may not have been representative of either design.

Finally, early in the investigation of a drug's effects, it is important to clarify which conditions are benefitted and which are not. For example, imipramine's efficacy for depression was discovered after it had been initially developed for the treatment of schizophrenia. Other examples include discovery that imipramine helped in panic attacks and that clomipramine was effective for obsessive-compulsive disorder. Because we cannot conduct class I, II, or III studies addressing all possible variables, good open studies can lead to the discovery of valuable information.

Conclusion

We apply our classification of study designs throughout the text to help the clinician interpret the quality of results from clinical trials. Further, we give the critical reader a perspective on the depth and validity of the available data. Most studies in our analyses of drug efficacy are class I or II, and if not, we discuss the studies accordingly.

STATISTICAL SUMMARIZATION OF DRUG STUDIES

Meta-analysis is a statistical method that combines data from individual drug studies to obtain a quantitative summary of their results. This statistical approach includes the following:

- The *overall effect* (i.e., how effective is a drug)
- The probability that this overall effect is *statistically significant*
- The *statistical confidence limits* on the overall effect
- The extent of *variability among all studies,* as well as the degree to which it is accounted for by discrepant results from a small fraction of the total number of studies
- The possible effects of methodological or substantive *variables that could alter the outcome*

When possible, meta-analyses were computed to summarize the overall effects from controlled clinical trials. These summarized data are used to compute an effect size and to calculate the probability that a given drug is different from placebo and equivalent to or more effective than standard drug treatments. The goal is to estimate the extent of clinical improvement with a specific treatment as an aid to therapeutic decision-making. In one sense, a meta-analysis can be seen as a quantitative literature review using a more explicit and structured approach. Thus, it can complement a narrative review and often accompanies a literature summary (6).

Unfortunately, efficacy is often assumed on the basis of clinical lore or by uncritically accepting the results of a few studies. An article may review several highly publicized references to support a certain position, but the careful reader may find that many of the studies quoted are poorly controlled or report duplicate data. A good example is the literature on clonazepam as a treatment for acute mania. Many review articles quote numerous references to support its efficacy, but a careful scrutiny of the literature reveals only one small, controlled study, the interpretation of which is limited by the use of active concomitant medication (see the section "Lithium Plus Benzodiazepines" in Chapter 10). Ideally, to make an informed judgment about a new drug, one should critically consider each individual study before drawing any conclusions. Although the number of uncontrolled trials vastly exceed those of their better-designed counterparts, a surprisingly large number of controlled reports are published. *Meta-analysis can provide a systematic estimate of the merit of these data.*

Omnibus Methods Versus Meta-Analysis

Meta-analysis is not simply counting the number of studies that find a significant difference or taking an average of their mean improvement. Hedges and Olkin (7) refer to such statistical models as omnibus or "vote-counting methods," noting that they have a number of methodological problems. They do not weigh studies according to the sample size. Furthermore, such methods only calculate one statistical parameter, indicating the probability that the studies considered together show a statistically significant difference. As a result, they can be overly influenced by one or a few disparate studies.

An important difference between such methods and meta-analysis is the ability to clarify whether all studies included show a consistent effect size (i.e., estimate homogeneity). For example, if a few studies find a large difference and the majority none, an omnibus method might still conclude a statistically significant difference. The appropriate conclusion, however, is that the results across studies are highly inconsistent. Thus, with omnibus methods, errors in a few small studies can disproportionately contribute to the final results, a phenomenon that Gibbons et al. (8) have illustrated with simulations. The meta-analytic methods in this text compare experimental with control groups, using estimates of homogeneity.

One of the major purposes of meta-analysis is to demonstrate whether findings are consistently and overwhelmingly statistically significant when studies are combined. When there is a consistent finding, with some studies clearly significant and others having strong trends, a box score method may misleadingly show some positive and some negative outcomes. Frequently, large studies are clearly positive, but some of the smaller, ostensibly negative studies may actually

show a strong trend that does not reach statistical significance due to their limited sample size.

With meta-analysis the statistical significance of the combined results can be overwhelming when all the differences are in the same direction. For example, when the authors performed a meta-analysis on the probability that maintenance antipsychotics produced a lower relapse rate in schizophrenics than placebo (53% relapsed on placebo and 20% on maintenance antipsychotics), the difference was significant to 10^{-100}! Typically, when multiple studies have the same outcome, the results of a meta-analysis will be markedly statistically significant. By contrast, p values of 0.05 or 0.01 are very difficult to interpret because an artifact from a single study could produce such "nonsignificant" significant levels.

Meta-Analytic Statistical Method

In preparing this book, we used a computer-assisted literature search for all studies on a given psychotropic, reviewed the bibliography of each report to identify other pertinent articles, and also obtained translations of the relevant non-English language articles whenever possible. All double-blind, random-assignment studies in the world literature that tested a given drug against placebo or other standard agents were systematically identified. Next, the standard techniques recommended by Hedges and Olkin (7) for continuous data or the Mantel-Haenszel model for discontinuous data were used (9). Because continuous data are more statistically powerful than discrete data, continuous data were preferentially used, when available, to derive the effect size. The sample size (N), mean (x), and standard deviations (SDs) were extracted, as well as how many patients had a good or poor response by deriving a standard cutoff point to separate responders from nonresponders. When a semiquantitative scale was provided, patients with moderate improvement or more were classified as "responders" and those with minimal improvement, no change, or worse as "nonresponders." For most medication studies, the majority of patients on placebo were usually rated only minimally improved. Thus, this level of change is an appropriate choice for a cutoff point to distinguish drug versus placebo differences. We note here the importance of having an a priori working definition of response threshold because choosing the best cutoff point in each individual study would bias the outcome (9).

Graphic Inspection of Results

The essence of meta-analysis is inspection of the data. Thus, this approach produces a visual or numeric representation of each study in the context of all the others. A review of the actual data gives the critical reader a feel for the data, as well as an index of suspicion if there is undue variability, which is far more important than any statistical parameter.

Studies in the literature often present a wide variety of data obtained with different rating scales, measuring instruments, and statistical techniques, which makes it difficult to compare results expressed in a wide variety of units. In statistics, actual scores are often converted to standardized scores by subtracting a given value for each subject from the mean and dividing the result by the standard deviation. This creates a new value in Z score units, with a mean of zero and a standard deviation of 1 (i.e., standard scores). In meta-analysis, the mean of the control group is subtracted from the mean of the experimental group and divided by the pooled group standard deviation, a process similar to the concept of percent change score. Thus, data are expressed in uniform units rather than in actual raw score means and standard deviations, which often vary substantially between studies. With meta-analysis, if a given study is discrepant (e.g., has a high placebo response rate or an unusually high drug efficacy rate), it will stand out. This information can be expressed graphically, using Z units derived from effect sizes, or percent response versus percent nonresponse, or the odds ratio (a statistical term used as an alternate to chi square). The reader can then note whether the finding is similar in all studies, or, conversely, whether there is a big effect in some but not others.

Therefore, meta-analysis abstracts results from each study and expresses them in a common unit, so one can easily compare, which allows us to focus on the hypothesis under ex-

amination rather than be distracted by the myriad differences among studies.

When the results from several studies are converted into similar units, a simple inspection of a graph or table readily reveals which studies have different outcomes from the majority. Such discrepancies can also be examined by a variety of statistical indices. For example, one can calculate a statistical index of homogeneity, remove the most discrepant study, and recalculate, revealing that all but one study is homogenous. If two studies are discrepant, one could remove both and again reexamine the indices of homogeneity, and so on. For an example, we summarize the relative efficacy of unilateral nondominant versus bilateral electrode placement for the administration of electroconvulsive therapy (ECT). Here, 10 studies had one result, and two others a different outcome (see Tables 8-10 and 8-11, in Chapter 8).

Effect Size

Effect size defines the magnitude of the difference between the experimental and the control groups regardless of sample size. This is quite different from the statistical significance, which is the probability that such a finding may occur by chance, leading to rejection of the null hypothesis. Statistical significance is determined in part by the sample size, so studies with a large number of subjects may find a highly significant result. In contrast, effect size is independent of sample size. Thus, in a six-person study, if two of three patients are benefitted by an antipsychotic and one of three improve on placebo, this result would not be statistically significant. But, if 200 of 300 patients benefit from an antipsychotic, while only 100 of 300 benefit from placebo, this would be highly statistically significant. Although the effect size (i.e., 67% on drug and 33% on placebo improving) is the same in both studies, only the results of the second study are clearly statistically significant because of its larger sample size.

The effect size of a *continuous variable* is frequently expressed as the difference between the mean of the experimental minus the mean of the control group divided by the pooled standard deviation. For example, in Chapter 5, data from the National Institute of Mental Health collaborative study demonstrated that antipsychotic-treated patients averaged a 4.2-point increase on a 6-point improvement scale, whereas the placebo patients averaged only a 2.2-point increase (i.e., an average difference of 2 points). The standard deviation of these data was approximately 1.7, so in effect size units, the improvement was approximately 1.2 (i.e., 2.0 ± 1.7) SD units. For *discontinuous data,* the effect size for a drug-placebo comparison is usually expressed as the difference between the percent improvement with the experimental drug and the percent improvement with placebo.

Interpretation of Effect Size

When there are a number of double-blind studies, the question of efficacy is usually readily determined. If the probability of a drug's superiority over placebo is massively significant (e.g., 10^{100} to 10^{20}), and the effect size is consistent from study to study, the possibility of a false-positive outcome is nil. The only possible exception is a major qualitative defect in the methodology.

Effect Size of Medical Drug Therapies

To provide a more general context in which to evaluate the effect sizes for various psychotropics, it is helpful to consider the data on the efficacy of various medical treatments, such as penicillin and streptomycin for pneumococcal pneumonia or tuberculosis, respectively. At the time penicillin was discovered, double-blind methodology was not used, and the standard therapy was sulfa drugs. In open studies, penicillin reduced the death rate from pneumonia by about 50%. When streptomycin was introduced, double-blind, random-assignment designs were being used, and the British conducted a multi-sanatorium study. They established an effect size for streptomycin, which can be expressed as a continuous variable (i.e., 0.8 effect size units) or as a discontinuous variable (i.e., 69% of patients improved with streptomycin versus 36% with placebo). We have tabulated drug therapies used as adjuncts to surgery to determine relative efficacies (Table 2-2). Because the results ranged from completely ineffective to substantially beneficial, this represents an unbiased sample of effect sizes chosen from this time period.

These examples quantitate the beneficial effects of an unbiased selection of standard antibiotics used as adjunctive treatments. The purpose is to give the clinician an appreciation for the magnitude of improvement, while also allowing us to place recent psychotropics in the context of other drugs' efficacy for common medical and surgical disorders. In general, psychotropics meet or exceed the effect of these medical drug treatments.

TABLE 2-2. *Effectiveness of new drug adjunctive therapies after surgery in comparison to standard nondrug treatments (1964–72)*

Treatment	Patients who developed complication or died (%)		Decrease in morbidity or mortality (%)
	Standard treatment	Standard plus adjunct	
Ampicillin for colon surgery	41	3	38
Neomycin-erythromycin for colon surgery	30	0	30
Antibiotics before heart surgery	33	26	7
Antibiotics after heart surgery	30	15	15
Heparin to prevent venous thrombosis	22	4	18
Chlorohexidine in contaminated wounds	13	13	0
Antibiotics after appendectomy	50	43	7
Vinblastine for cancer of lung	94	92	2
HATG with kidney transplant	34	31	3
Prednisone for cirrdosis	42	41	1
TSPA for cancer of colon	48	55	−7
Chemotherapy for cancer of breast	38	32	6
Average	*40%*	*30%*	*10%*

Confidence Interval

An important question in meta-analysis is the consistency of the results (i.e., its confidence interval). Thus, we not only want to know how much more effective a drug is but whether all the clinical trials agree on the size of the therapeutic effect.

Presentation of the confidence interval facilitates evaluation of the reported data in original measurement units, which simultaneously incorporates the statistical changes observed and the precision of the measurements in the units in which the data were measured. **The confidence interval provides a bridge to clinical importance, in that the reader can see the observed experimental change in the context of a range of uncertainty in the same units. Indeed, for this reason, the reporting of confidence intervals is required by many periodicals.**

Critical Issues in Meta-Analysis

There are several issues that must be considered when interpreting the results of a meta-analysis, including:

- *Choice of studies*
- *Selection of patients* who enter clinical trials
- The *"file drawer"* problem
- *Pattern of results*
- *Continuous versus catagorical* data
- Reporting of *standard deviations*
- *Crossover* designs
- *Redundant* data

Choice of Studies: The Need for a Valid Control Group

A critical methodological issue for a proper meta-analysis is the choice of studies. It is important that all studies meet reasonable criteria; otherwise, a potential bias is introduced. We chose only those studies that had an appropriate control group, which provided a standard by which a drug's effects could be measured. By contrast, there have been meta-analyses of multiple studies on psychotherapy, all done without comparison groups or with invalid comparison groups. Combining the effect size of these studies only reflects the enthusiasm of the investigator rather than any true effect, because there is no valid comparison.

Patients Who Enter Clinical Trials

Most clinical trials study "voluntary" patients who enter a research setting and are kept drug-free for 1 or more weeks. Severely disturbed patients, however, are usually not candidates for research. Because psychiatry lacks valid and reliable biological diagnostic tests, we do not know whether a given patient really has the disease under study. Further, some of the symptomatic volunteers who are often used in outpatient studies may not actually have the disease.

File Drawer Problem

One of the most important pitfalls in meta-analysis was labeled the "file drawer" problem by Easterbrook et al. (10). In a survey, these authors indicated that studies with positive outcomes were twice as likely to be published (and usually in more prestigious and therefore higher profile journals). Thus, there is a systematic tendency for positive results to be reported and negative results to be "filed away" and go unreported.

To minimize bias consequent to the tendency not to publish negative data, we attempted to include all double-blind, random-assignment trials from meeting presentations, reports of symposia, exhibits, or available unpublished data from the individual authors, the pharmaceutical industry, or the government.

Some investigators perform multiple statistical analyses and emphasize the most favorable outcome. Indeed, we have found reports of detailed statistical evaluations of the positive aspect of a study, with only passing reference to a negative finding that was not statistically significant. An example of this is a report on the benefit of lithium in treating alcohol dependence (11). Here, the negative result in nonaffectively disordered alcoholics is not adequately presented for comparison with their mood-disordered counterparts (see the section "The Alcoholic Patient" in Chapter 14).

The methodological rigor of a good meta-analysis guards against biases, fortuitous results, and, most important, being overly influenced by a few positive reports.

Certain meta-analytic techniques, particularly the vote-counting or omnibus methods, carry forward any positive result to the final summary statistics. Also, with a vote-counting method, one often tabulates the most positive rating outcome because it is emphasized by the study's author.

One safeguard is to calculate the number of patients whose negative results (hypothetically hidden in the file drawer) would result in converting a positive to a negative meta-analysis.

We believe the file drawer issue is less of a problem in meta-analysis than in the narrative review, which often lists only those publications that support a particular conclusion. Too often, narrative reviewers emphasize the results of other positive reviews. Thus, the reference list gives a false impression of more studies than were actually done, because duplicate publications and review articles are quoted as if they were independent studies. Other problems include:

- Studies listed as *"controlled"* do not include random-assignment or a valid control group.
- Studies are *misquoted.*
- A conclusion or abstract is quoted but is *not consistent* with the data in the article.
- The same data appear in *multiple publications.*

Interpretation of the Pattern of Results

The pattern and consistency of results across all studies are very important. For example, if there are a few small-sample positive studies and many large-sample negative studies, it is likely that the smaller studies were aberrations or wishful thinking. If the results between individual studies are highly discordant, it is a mistake to conclude that the overall effect is significant. Rather, the conclusion is that some studies show a drug effect and others do not, requiring one to explain the discrepancy. It is preferable to evaluate studies by some *a priori* criteria for methodological rigor and then examine whether there is a similar effect size in the more versus less rigorous studies.

Continuous Versus Categorical Data

For the most part, the meta-analyses used in this text are based on fourfold contingency tables, which include the number of responders or nonresponders to a given treatment. An advantage of dichotomous data is that information from each individual subject can be abstracted (i.e., the results come from actual patients). In one sense, this is not strictly a meta-analysis, because calculations are not done on summary statistical parameters but on observations of individual subjects. Such an approach has the advantage of directness, however, because the percentage of patients who respond or do not respond to a new treatment, standard treatment, or placebo is intuitively meaningful to clinicians, whereas a change of 0.8 SD units may not be.

Reporting of Standard Deviations

A meta-analysis for continuous data cannot be calculated unless the pertinent standard deviations are known. Unfortunately, clinical reports often give the sample size and mean ratings for the various groups but do not report the standard deviations (or standard error of the mean), which are necessary for effect size calculations. Thus, investigators should always report the indices of variability (e.g., confidence intervals, SDs) for the critical variables related to their primary hypothesis.

Crossover Designs

Because there was no method for doing a meta-analysis with crossover designs, we developed a method (a variation on Hedges' method for uncrossed designs) with suitable modification for paired data (12).

Redundant Data

It is inappropriate to statistically evaluate a patient studied with two different measures as if that patient were two different subjects (i.e., each patient can only be counted once). For example, investigators may initially report on the first 20 subjects, and in a second paper, report on a total of

60, including the original 20 subjects. The same patient counted twice (or more) will magnify any finding. Additionally, a bias is introduced by giving undue weight to the findings of groups who report their data in multiple publications, as opposed to those reporting their findings only once. Meta-analysis should eliminate duplicate publications of the same data.

Conclusion

The information presented in this section provides the background for later sections, which will quantitatively summarize the controlled literature for the various classes of psychotropics. In all cases, the data were obtained from controlled, clinical trials comparing a new (or experimental) treatment with placebo or a standard agent. The goal of these summations is to give a reader the critical "bottom line," devoid of our subjective bias, as well as the bias from isolated publications inconsistent with the trend seen when the controlled data are combined.

PATIENT ISSUES

Effects of Gender

In a 1996 editorial in the *American Journal of Psychiatry,* Dr. Leibenluft (13) articulates the ways in which gender matters in understanding psychiatric disorders. These include:

- When an illness is *more prevalent in one gender* (e.g., major depression)
- When an illness is *unique to one gender*
- When an illness is *more severe in one gender*
- When *risk factors differ by gender*
- When *treatment response differs* by gender.

In this text, the focus of our discussion is on the last issue. To illustrate the problem, we consider the effect of gender on drug pharmacokinetics (see Chapters 3, 5, 7, 10, and 12) and then address two important gender-related questions: the use of medications during pregnancy and the drug treatment of premenstrual dysphoric disorder (see Chapter 14).

Informed Consent

Assessment of Capacity to Consent

Treatment always implies a contract between the patient (consumer) and clinician (provider). Any contract assumes a patient has both the capacity to give consent and the willingness to do so. Clinicians who treat patients decide a question of capacity (either explicitly or implicitly) each time they hospitalize, perform surgery, or treat with drugs (14). There is an imperative embodied in the law which states that, with only certain exceptions, a valid consent is a necessary prerequisite in any clinical decision to provide treatment. There is an analogy to be drawn between capacity and mental illness. Clinicians often do not agree on the definition of a mental disorder, but it is a concept that is of constant practical significance. Persons are committed as a result of a mental disorder that significantly impairs their judgment, or are released if found not to have one. When insanity is an issue, persons will or will not be held responsible for their actions because of a mental disorder. With great difficulty and appreciable limitations, psychiatrists have developed standards for recognizing and categorizing these disorders. Although acceptance of the standards is not unanimous, they are at least consensual.

With psychiatric outpatients who are legally competent, issues of consent are not pertinent. These patients can simply take or not take their medication. In contrast, in the hospital setting (especially the public sector) there are a number of involuntary patients for whom legal issues are very relevant. Whereas voluntary patients can simply leave the hospital, involuntarily committed patients cannot. Further, although they can refuse oral medication, it can be given by injection when warranted.

We advocate a consumer-oriented approach to the clinician—patient relationship. Thus, a therapist should be an educator and advisor, rather than dictating treatment. Because patients must live with their disease, as well as tolerate the prescribed treatments, they should play an active part in related decisions. Ideally, different options are examined for their relative merits, and then the clinician recommends a treatment plan. In the typical outpatient practice, the two parties agree with the assessment and the treatment plan, with the patient always having the final say. If there is disagreement, a compromise can often be reached that is satisfactory to both. A third scenario occurs when a compromise cannot be reached. In most instances, the patient seeks care elsewhere, because clinicians, in good conscience, cannot comply with a treatment plan inconsistent with their professional judgment or solely dictated by the patient. Examples include the paranoid individual who declines medication based on delusional ideation but who is not committable, and the drug-seeking patient who demands medication that the physician cannot ethically prescribe.

The one exception to this approach involves patients who are unable to make an informed decision on their own behalf or who pose an immediate danger by virtue of their mental disorder. In this instance, the patient is protected by both the legal and medical systems. The laws of most states allow commitment when patients are an imminent danger to self or others due to their mental disorder. When no active treatment was available, confinement was the only option. With the availability of very effective drug therapies, hospitalization now typically lasts no more than a few weeks. Thus, treatment should be the focus of the medicolegal dialogue, with confinement only a vehicle to ensure its adequacy. Hospitalization without drug treatment is preventive detention. Medications treat the illness and, as a consequence, patients can return home with full rights not to take medication.

We suggest specific procedures for the clinical assessment of capacity to consent, as well as permissible courses of action that logically follow such assessments (15) (Fig. 2-1).

Mental Status Exam

Ability to Communicate. **The mental status exam is critical to the determination of a patient's capacity to consent, and the ability to communicate is an absolute prerequisite** (see the section "Diagnostic Assessment" in Chapter 1). Psychomotor impairments such as *mutism* or *catatonia* (withdrawn type) would severely affect an individual's fundamental ability to communicate any appreciation of the issues involved and their ramifications. Although an individual may actually be well oriented and may intellectually appreciate and even later remember events that occurred and the issues involved, that person is not capable of consenting if unable to demonstrate these faculties.

Memory. If a patient is able to communicate, the next factor to consider is *memory.* Most commonly recent recall is impaired, but in an acute situation (e.g., drug-induced delirium), immediate memory may also be disrupted. Frequently, immediate and recent memory impairment are superimposed on a more chronic organic state (e.g., degenerative dementia), with additional problems in remote memory. The more memory components involved, and the greater the severity of impairment in any one of them, the less able an individual will be to adequately register, retain, and recall information necessary to give consent. The most critical memory components involve the immediate-recent spectrum of functioning. Gross dysfunction can usually be tested by the standard mental status examination. **Intact immediate—recent memory components are also a prerequisite to giving informed consent.**

Orientation. In acute biological derangements such as phencyclidine intoxication or an electrolyte imbalance, *disorientation* can occur to all spheres (e.g., person, place, time, situation, and even spatial relationships). A person severely disoriented to a situation clearly lacks capacity, being unable to appreciate the nature of the interaction. One may be disoriented to other spheres, however, and still be capable of consenting. The clinician should ascertain which spheres are affected, as well as the severity of dysfunction in each. If there is a significant impairment of both memory and orientation, capacity should be regarded as at least diminished, if not entirely lacking. Because these problems may have a fluctuating course, intermittently improving and deteriorating, repeated assessment over time is necessary to reach a valid conclusion. **In summary, both memory and orientation must be substantially intact to support a conclusion that the patient can give consent.**

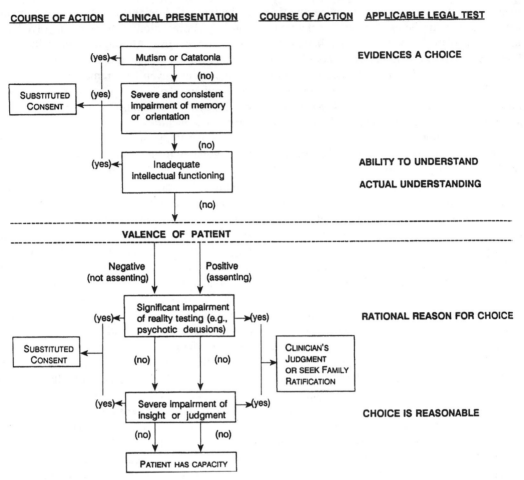

FIG. 2-1. Assessment of capacity to consent. Adapted from Janicak PG, Bonavich PR. The borderland of autonomy: medical-legal criteria for capacity to consent. *J Psychiatry Law* 1980;8:379.

Intellectual Functioning. The quality of a patient's *intellectual functioning* in the context of that person's educational, social, and cultural experiences must also be considered. Minimally, a patient should demonstrate the ability to express an understanding of basic issues at an appropriate level. This cognitive process can be tested by asking the patient to summarize or to reformulate and express a concept, question, or situation posed by the examiner. This exercise obviously calls for clinical judgment in choosing the items to which the patient responds, as well as in evaluating the intellectual level shown by the responses. The likelihood of clinical bias is generally greater the "higher" the cognitive process under examination. In a sense, one may be able to do no better than conscientiously apply one's own "reasonable person" standard. **The threshold for adequate intellectual function is a response that provides evidence of intact abstract and logical processing.**

Reality Testing. Next to be evaluated are *perception of reality* and the *quality of thought content.* An example would be a severely depressed patient who expresses feelings of guilt and worthlessness, at times to the extent of misperceiving the explanation of a treatment that is prescribed. For instance, from the clinician's viewpoint, the presented treatment recommendation is a means of alleviating the vegetative signs of depression; however, from the distorted viewpoint of a severely depressed patient, this may be interpreted as a justifiable punishment. A careful explanation of the mode and purpose of a proposed treatment should be followed by attempts to elicit feedback from patients that will reveal the extent of their reality testing.

Insight and Judgment. Issues of insight and judgment are more difficult to assess and can be conceptualized as the culmination of the previously discussed factors. At the very least, patients should manifest a basic awareness of the relationship between specific events in their life and the condition for which treatment is proposed. This would define the minimal insight necessary to give consent.

Although generally assessed together, intact insight does not imply sound judgment, which also involves an awareness of the current condition (i.e., a comprehension of both the problem and the process by which its alleviation may be accomplished). This assessment should be made in light of the patient's own expressed values, a process best accomplished by eliciting the premises that underlie the patient's decisions. If these premises have the quality of "reasonableness" (though perhaps, in the clinician's opinion, erroneous), it should be concluded that the patient has capacity. If they are not "reasonable," the inquiry should continue, with one possibility being that the premises are the product of the patient's illness. This conclusion would mitigate against a finding of capacity, though it should not be conclusive. It is only when the basis for a decision is clearly the result of the illness that the unreasonableness of the decision may indicate a lack of capacity. Thus, if the decision is unreasonable but is not the product of the illness, there should be a finding of capacity.

Age Factor. A final question is the issue of age, which may also play a significant role. In addressing this factor, Stanley et al. (16) compared elderly (mean age $= 69.2 \pm 5.3$) with younger (mean age $= 33.7 \pm 6.6$) medical patients for capacity to consent. Although both groups tended to make reasonable decisions, the elderly patients demonstrated poorer comprehension for various elements of the informed consent process. Thus, special care must be taken to ensure that older patients comprehend sufficiently to give a valid consent.

Tests of Capacity

In a review of the literature, Roth et al. (17) concluded that there are five categories for tests of competency (i.e., capacity):

- *"Evidencing a choice,"* which verifies the presence or absence of a decision by a patient for or against treatment
- The *"reasonable outcome of choice"* test, which evaluates the patient's ability to reach the "reasonable," the "right," or the "responsible" decision
- The *"choice based on rational reasons"* test, which attempts to ascertain the quality of a patient's thinking and whether it is a product of mental illness
- The *"ability of the patient to understand"* the risks, benefits, and alternatives to treatment (including no treatment)
- The *"actual understanding,"* which defines competence based on the accuracy of the patient's perceptions.

These authors (17) then assert that, in practice, competency is usually determined by the interplay of one or more of these tests and two other variables: *the risk-benefit ratio of treatment* and *the valence of the patient's decision* (i.e., consent to or refusal of treatment). We include valence as a factor in our guidelines, because agreement or lack of agreement between the patient and the clinician may dictate different courses of action, given the overriding preference to be in accord with the expressed wishes of the patient. We exclude the risk—benefit ratio as a factor, however, because ideally this consideration should occur before or after an assessment of capacity, but not as part of the actual determination.

Algorithm for Assessing the Capacity to Consent

We relate the major components of a psychiatric evaluation to various tests formulated by the courts. This schema assumes an adult patient not under legal guardianship with a nonemergent disorder. Components of the psychiatric evaluation are listed in the order they should be considered. We indicate the various courses of action the clinician may take (e.g., seek court determination of capacity to consent), relating the various tests of capacity to the most pertinent clinical factors (Fig. 2-1).

Obtaining Informed Consent

Once capacity has been assured, a patient's decision to accept or to refuse treatment must be ascertained as being informed and freely given. The information conveyed in a one-to-one, personal interaction with the patient should have these characteristics:

- *Accurate.*
- *Adequate* (complete in necessary detail, such as name, nature, and purpose of treatment).
- *Comprehensible* to the patient, and include the opportunity for the patient to ask questions.
- Appropriate.
- Describe potential *benefits,* including the likelihood of success.
- Indicate potential *risks* (e.g., side effects and complications).
- Present *alternatives,* if reasonable ones exist.
- Explain *anticipated results without treatment.*

Booklets, videocassettes, or audiotapes should never take the place of a personal encounter. A dated and signed progress note, including these details, is usually considered sufficient documentation.

Right to Treatment

One of the more controversial, if not paradoxical, developments in mental health law has been the establishment of a patient's right to treatment, followed by its legal counterpoint—the right to refuse treatment (18). Although some contend that there is no conflict between these two rights, the reality is that they are often at odds. The problem is most obvious with involuntarily committed patients, where the right to refuse treatment contradicts the reason for their hospitalization.

Although the principle of personal inviolability requires us to respect a patient's decisions about treatment in all ordinary situations, exceptions are necessary in extraordinary circumstances. The possibility of serious harm is the determining factor here, precluding an absolute right to make one's own health choices.

We would propose that all mentally ill persons, whether adjudicated or presumed incompetent, retain the right to articulate their objection to or refusal of treatment and that any such concerns must be heard. The critical factor regarding treatment refusals by the mentally ill is whether, when, how, and by whom such a refusal can be overridden. In our opinion, the decision to override a treatment refusal is best made by medical personnel rather than the legal system; the override decision should be allowed in all circumstances, not just emergencies; and it can and should be made expeditiously (19).

Consequences of Refusal of Treatment. The translation of the abstract right-to-refuse issue into real-world outcomes reveals serious consequences that are more complicated than may be assumed. For example, there is reliable research showing that psychotherapy without medication is not effective in treating such severe disorders as schizophrenia (20,21). Therefore, when medication is refused, often no effective, alternate, less restrictive treatment is available, and the only other real option is no treatment.

Judicial override has proven to be very harmful to the patients because this process often can take many months. During this medication-free period, serious harm may befall a patient, other patients, and their caregivers, as well as markedly lengthening the hospitalization. When the law requires that a patient's refusal be overridden only by judicial process, critical treatment time is lost, and it is important to consider whether this delay has any effect on recovery.

Although most controlled trials lasted only weeks, the longitudinal study of the effect of psychotherapy versus drugs by May et al. (20, 21) is particularly germane. Schizophrenic patients were randomly assigned to either antipsychotics or no medication. After 6 months or more, the initial nonmedication group was then given active drugs. Those patients who did not receive medication for the first 6 months did substantially worse during the following 3 to 5 years, spending twice as much time in the hospital as the initially medicated group. **This study documents the**

potential harmful consequences that may occur when patients do not receive early effective treatment.

Need for Periodic Review. Protected both as to the need for and the right to treatment, how can a patient be safeguarded subsequently? First, the course of treatment should be periodically reviewed, as already mandated by law or administrative regulation in the majority of states and their institutions. Second, a patient-initiated review mechanism should be formalized in the hospital setting, so that questions and concerns about the course of treatment can be voiced.

Compliance

Once capacity has been assured and informed consent given to a treatment plan, compliance becomes the next crucial issue.

Compliance is defined as adherence to the recommended treatment plan of a healthcare professional. Typically, it is partial at best, in that medications prescribed are taken less often than recommended, irregularly, and, at times, excessively. There are various reasons for noncompliance, which can be categorized as follows:

- Rational
- Capricious
- Absolute refusal
- Confusion
- Iatrogenic

Thus, no matter how astute a diagnostician or how brilliant the treatment recommendations, frequently these efforts are merely academic exercises and never actualized due to noncompliance.

Factors Decreasing Compliance

Patient compliance can be decreased significantly by several factors, including:

- The *stigma* of a mental disorder
- The frequent *denial* of illness
- The *disruption in cognitive processes* that is often a part of the illness
- Most importantly, *forgetfulness*

Side effects of medications, often not recognized as such by patients or inadequately inquired about by the clinician, also complicate adherence to therapy. The delay or time lag in the onset of action of many psychotropics, as well as a delayed time course for a recurrence triggered after stopping medication, also contribute. In this regard, the concept of prevention and prophylaxis must be carefully reviewed with the patient. Finally, the implications for various treatment "costs" related to compliance need to be explored and the means to circumvent impediments to a patient's cooperation sought (see "Cost of Treatment" later in this chapter).

Strategies to Increase Compliance

Because noncompliance occurs frequently, it is best to inquire directly about the issue and sometimes to evaluate it indirectly by using medication diaries, counting medications, or therapeutic drug monitoring.

The most critical factor in enhancing compliance is to encourage *active patient participation*, to the extent possible, in treatment planning and implementation. This includes *adequate communication* of the rationale for a given treatment in the context of an *empathic approach* and a *trusting relationship. Family and community involvement and support* is often a critical determining factor. Finally, *emphasis needs to be placed on the positive effects of medication* for the patient's quality of life. When possible, the most simplified drug regimen should be used. The patients and the family should know the prodromal symptoms that would alert them to return for a reevaluation of status, leading to appropriate actions to preclude a full episode (e.g., decreased sleep as a prodrome to a manic phase).

Treatment Termination

Termination of treatment may be initiated by the patient, by the clinician, or by mutual agreement. At this juncture, the potential for recurrence should be clearly discussed in the context of the risk-benefit ratio (e.g., diminished side effects or toxicity from drug discontinuation versus a recurrence of the disorder). Part of this process should be the identification of possible prodromal symptoms, which should alert the patient to return for a reevaluation of status and the possible resumption of medication to preclude a full episode (e.g., decreased sleep as a prodrome to a manic phase). After drug therapy is stopped, however, prediction of an impending episode may not be a useful strategy for certain disorders, making the decision to discontinue drug treatment more perilous (see discussion on intermittent antipsychotic maintenance strategy in Chapter 5).

Conclusion

Adequate compliance with treatment is a major issue affecting the potential for a successful outcome. As noted in this section, several factors may contribute to a patient's willingness to persist with treatment as prescribed. Perhaps foremost is the clinicians' ability to communicate their approach in an empathic and understandable manner.

DRUG MANAGEMENT

Acute, Maintenance, and Prophylactic Therapy

Because most psychiatric disorders are recurrent and chronic in nature, appropriate management always requires the consideration of three phases of treatment:

- *Acute*, or the control of a current episode
- *Maintenance,* or the prevention of relapse once an acute episode has been alleviated and it is assumed that the acute disease process has been suppressed but is still present
- *Prophylactic,* or the prevention of future episodic exacerbations

Acute interventions may produce a full response, partial response, or no response. The last outcome is usually due to problems such as:

- *Intolerance* due to side effects
- *Refractoriness*
- *Discontinuation* (i.e., cessation of treatment for any reason other than intolerance or refractoriness)

As emphasized earlier, adequacy and appropriateness of drug therapy should always be reviewed in the event of unsatisfactory results. If a patient has been properly diagnosed but only responds partially to an adequate drug trial, a more difficult clinical decision-making process then ensues. The two major options are to switch to a different subgroup of drug (e.g., from a conventional neuroleptic to a novel antipsychotic), or, alternatively, to augment the initial medication (e.g., adding lithium to an antidepressant regimen). In patients who are not helped by one drug treatment, switching to a different class within the same family is usually the approach that is most successful, for example, from a heterocyclic antidepressant (HCA) to a selective serotonin reuptake inhibitor (SSRI) or monoamine oxidase inhibitor. Regardless of the outcome with subsequent drug treatment trials, the same sequential logic can be applied.

The patient who manifests full remission should be continued on adequate maintenance therapy, usually for a period of several weeks to months, and often indefinitely. The exact duration is determined by such issues as the particular disorder, as well as the prior history of episode severity and frequency of relapses.

Prophylactic therapy beyond the first several months should be dictated by:

- *Chronicity* of illness
- Frequency and severity of *relapses*
- Associated *"comorbidity,"* such as other medical conditions or concurrent substance or alcohol abuse

During all phases of treatment, education, supportive therapy, and, at times, more specific types of psychotherapy are essential for a satisfactory outcome. For example, interpersonal therapy can complement adequate maintenance antidepressant treatment, possibly diminishing the frequency of episodes (see the section "Role of Psychosocial Therapies" in Chapter 7), and cognitive-behavioral techniques in combination with antiobsessive agents (e.g., clomipramine) can improve the quality of life for patients with obsessive-compulsive disorder, minimizing time spent on disabling rituals (see the section "Obsessive-Compulsive Disorder" in Chapter 13).

Monotherapy, Copharmacy, and Polypharmacy

As emphasized in Chapter 1, a major principle of drug therapy is the value of *monotherapy* (i.e., using only one medication). The rationale includes:

- Ease of *administration*
- Enhanced *compliance*
- Minimization of *side effects*
- Avoidance of *drug interactions*
- Easier assessment of the *benefit* or *lack of benefit* with a particular drug
- Lower *cost*

Copharmacy is the concurrent use of at least two agents to improve results. At times, it is necessary (e.g., an antiparkinsonian agent plus an antipsychotic to control extrapyramidal side effects [EPS]) or desirable (e.g., an antipsychotic plus an antidepressant to alleviate a psychotic depressive episode). The rational combination of medications is widely used in medicine when there is a sound pharmacological principle, empirical data to support a greater efficacy, reduced side effects, or enhanced safety. Examples include lithium potentiation of antidepressants, oral antipsychotics to supplement depot intramuscular preparations while establishing a new steady state plasma level or managing a sudden relapse, and drug combinations in the management of HIV/AIDS-related disorders.

If this strategy is required, we would discourage the use of fixed-ratio combinations (e.g., amitriptyline plus perphenazine) and instead recommend the use of these or other similar agents independently. The primary reason is to afford more flexibility in the choice of specific agents and relative dosing of each drug, thus enhancing efficacy and minimizing adverse effects.

When using more than one agent, it is important to make adjustments with a single drug at any given time. If more than one drug is increased, reduced, or switched concurrently, it will be difficult to identify which alteration was responsible for any significant change in status (whether good or bad).

The use of two or more agents concurrently has the potential for possibly deleterious *drug interactions*. Thus, as noted in subsequent chapters, the addition or elimination of an agent may significantly alter the activity of the concurrent drug treatment (e.g., carbamazepine lowering haloperidol plasma levels; nefazodone increasing the levels of triazolam).

Generally, one drug should be started at a time so that its results can be evaluated. Occasionally, emergency or practical considerations dictate starting more than one drug simultaneously, but later one can undergo a therapeutic discontinuation (e.g., antipsychotic plus mood stabilizer in a severe manic episode). While the addition of several medications does occur, we emphasize that the clinician should evaluate and document the patient's response to each newly added medication.

Polypharmacy is the irrational, simultaneous use of more than one agent from the same or different classes. Although there are some exceptions (e.g., low doses of trazodone given at bedtime for its sedative hypnotic effects during the early phases of treatment with fluoxetine, or the concurrent use of an SSRI and a $5-HT_{1A}$ agonist or HCA), this practice increases the risk of toxicity (via additive or synergistic effects) and adverse drug interactions, or both, while adding little to enhance clinical efficacy.

ROLE OF THE FOOD AND DRUG ADMINISTRATION

The Food and Drug Administration (FDA) was established in the 1930's by federal law to ensure the relative safety of food, cosmetics, and medicinals, as well as to regulate the marketing of such products, due to ongoing abuses in promotional claims. Since then, its scope of responsibilities has been revised, often in response to specific incidents such as the tragedy of thalidomide in the 1960's. In terms of medicinals, the FDA oversees drug development, including the extensive clinical trials that must be conducted to establish efficacy and safety for a defined indication. The focus of its activity is to ensure that a medication is not marketed in which the risk outweighs the benefit likely to be derived, and that a medication is not promoted by the manufacturer for unapproved uses.

Confusion can arise when a medication is generally deemed useful by the medical profession in a condition for which its use has not been FDA approved. Marketed drugs are frequently found helpful for disorders beyond the formal labeled indications. Part of the reason for this situation is the long and expensive process needed to produce sufficient data to obtain FDA labeling approval, which are estimated to cost as much as $300,000,000 to $1 billion. Frequently, there is not sufficient monetary incentive to warrant such expenditure, yet a compound is often found to be effective by researchers and clinicians in a given medical discipline.

The FDA has taken the position that the individual physician is in the best position to determine whether a medication may be helpful for a specific patient based upon that physician's reading of the literature as well as clinical experience. Otherwise, many patients would be denied effective treatment because of insufficient commercial incentive to carry out the costly process needed to receive marketing approval. A case in point is lithium, which languished in the United States for years, despite extensive use in the rest of the world for bipolar disorder. The reasons were twofold: (a) there had been several deaths earlier when lithium was used as a salt-substitute by individuals on a fluid-restricted diet; and (b) because lithium is a naturally occurring substance, no company could receive a patent for exclusive marketing rights. As a result, there was no way to recoup a sponsor's expenditure to receive marketing approval. Thus, for almost two decades, bipolar patients in the United States were denied the single most effective form of treatment. This situation could not be allowed to continue, given the personal, family, and societal cost of untreated bipolar disorder, so ultimately the federal government itself sponsored the research needed to achieve the appropriate labeling of lithium. A 5-year comparison with other countries shows that the United States and the United Kingdom exhibited similar patterns of drug availability, but the United States outpaced other countries (22).

For registration, the marketing company has to make a formal submission to the FDA, documenting a compound's efficacy and safety for a specific condition. The submission is referred to as a new drug application. To support labeling as an antidepressant, for example, a company must submit at least two unequivocal studies demonstrating the superiority of their drug over placebo (or appropriate control condition). Typically, a new drug application is considerably more extensive than just two pivotal studies. The extent of the application also depends on whether the drug is new to the market or whether the company is seeking an additional indication for which it can promote the sale of an existing approved drug. The FDA provides considerable protection for the patients by inspecting the studies to ensure safeguards against fraud. Also, an adequate sample size is required to ensure valid data.

Approved Versus Labeled

The words "approved" and "labeled" have different definitions. A medication is "approved" for marketing if its database supports its benefit for a recognized condition and its risks are sufficiently offset by its efficacy for a particular indication. The term "labeling" refers to the indications for which a medication can be promoted by the company marketing the compound. When a physician uses a drug for indications beyond those stated in the package insert, then an "approved" drug is being prescribed for an "unlabeled" indication. The physician must critically and carefully weigh the evidence supporting the drug's efficacy and balance the potential benefit against the potential risks for the indication in question. In all such circumstances, the patient also needs to be fully informed.

Even a modest new drug application will require a substantial investment of money and time. The financial expenditure includes the outlay for clinical trials to collect the data and to assemble the application. Time is also a crucial variable, because the only way to justify the expenditure is through sales of the product, making the remaining patent life an important variable in such a decision. If it is short, then the patent may expire before the new drug application can be assembled, submitted, and reviewed to receive "labeling" for that indication.

There are many worthwhile uses for medications that have not received formal "labeling" due to an economic decision. The data supporting such uses typically come from clinical experience in individual patients, then a series of case reports, and, finally, controlled studies, some of which may be funded by government grants to university-based researchers who have no commercial interest in the medication. At times, an individual clinician may have a personal interest in promoting a psychotropic drug, and sometimes off-label indications are not supported by adequate or unbiased data. This said, many off-labeled indications have been proven beyond a reasonable doubt. Results from such studies are published in medical journals but are generally not assembled into a formal new drug application to the FDA. Therefore, such an indication cannot be promoted by the marketing company, although physicians are free to prescribe the drug if they are convinced that the medical literature and their clinical experience support such a use.

A related issue is the wide availability of "natural" remedies, which bypass strict FDA regulations because they are not considered medicinals. As a result, patients often take these compounds unaware of their potential for deleterious effects and possible adverse drug interactions with concurrently prescribed agents. Thus, clinicians should always inquire about their use to minimize the potential for an adverse effect.

Research Studies Versus Clinical Application

To put this matter in perspective, the use of most FDA-approved drugs in clinical practice usually goes beyond the clinical database, even when the drug is being prescribed for the "labeled" indication. A major reason is the difference between patients who enter clinical trials and those whom most clinicians treat. To enter a clinical trial, a patient must meet rigorous inclusion and exclusion criteria, creating a narrow subgroup for whom the new drug will be indicated once marketed. Some of the most important differences include the following:

- The absence of patients on *concomitant psychotropics*
- The absence of patients with *serious medical conditions*

- The absence of patients with *concomitant substance abuse*
- The absence of patients with *central nervous system disease or trauma* (e.g., previous history of seizures, closed head trauma, or dementia)
- The limited, if any, experience with *hospitalized patients*
- The *underrepresentation of patients younger than 18* and *older than 65 or women of childbearing potential*

In reality, patients whose conditions are complicated by these issues are the most frequent recipients of medications, yet until recently they have usually been excluded from the clinical trials used for the approval process.

Furthermore, most psychiatric disorders are chronic, although some may go through intervals of apparent remission (e.g., major depressive disorder), whereas others are persistent but relatively asymptomatic (e.g., schizophrenia) with effective treatment. Hence, treatment with psychotropics is best considered in terms of months or years of continuous or intermittent therapy, rather than a few days or weeks. By contrast, the vast majority of the clinical trials involve short-term use. Thus, a typical database for the approval of a new antidepressant is usually based on experience with 2,000 to 8,000 patients (carefully selected as described earlier), with the majority exposed to the medication for less than 2 months. Often less than 25% will have received medication for more than 4 months, and less than 10% for more than 6 months. When a drug is marketed, most patients will be exposed to it for a minimum of 4 to 6 months. Yet, when treatment goes beyond 2 months, the database on the safety and continued efficacy of a medication is modest at best. Thus, although clinicians commonly use psychotropics for both maintenance and prophylactic purposes, an approved drug only has to be shown effective in the acute phase.

Only after a drug has been on the market for several years has sufficient experience been achieved so that many of these issues can be addressed with confidence. Even then most of that experience is nonsystematic. Problems may be detected in several ways:

- Clinicians are encouraged to send to the FDA *adverse experience reporting forms* when a patient develops a problem during treatment.
- The FDA may mandate specific *postmarketing surveillance programs* when a concern about the safety or efficacy of a new medication is suggested by either the preclinical or clinical database used for marketing approval.
- A *researcher may detect a problem* when studying patients treated with a medication, whether or not the primary focus is safety or efficacy.

The reality is that the application of many medications in clinical practice goes beyond the approved labeling in the package insert. To produce the data needed to address these clinical uses would simply be too costly and not practically feasible. Even now patients under HMO and managed care plans are often excluded from receiving the latest developments unless empirical trials with older treatments have failed. Thus, these patients may be treated with agents that are less effective and more toxic than their successors. In the long run, such policies are not cost-effective, in addition to being potentially harmful to patients.

Investigational Drugs

An investigational drug is typically one that has not been approved for marketing by the FDA for human use (23). This designation may also refer to agents approved by the FDA for a specific indication but being investigated for a nonlabeled use. Examples of the latter may include:

- A different *preparation* or *formulation*
- A higher than approved *dosage*
- Use by a different *patient population*

The Belmont Report (24), in considering differences between the research and the clinical setting, noted that departure from commonly accepted drug practice for individual patients should not be considered research. Innovative strategies, however, should be developed in research protocols as quickly as possible to assure safety and efficacy of such a practice.

A general rule is that if the intent of the activity is to contribute to the general knowledge base (e.g., large number of subjects, systematic data collection, intent to publish), the entire proposal should be submitted in writing and reviewed by the local institutional review board (IRB). These entities are committees formally designated by a research institution to review, approve, and monitor research on human subjects (25).

Investigational drugs may also be used on an emergency (i.e., life-threatening) basis, but should be reported to an IRB within 5 days. Subsequent use in other patients should be approved by the institution's IRB.

Compassionate use provisions have allowed the limited use of investigational drugs in the past. For example, the controversy surrounding AIDS and other life-threatening diseases has increased the pressure on the FDA to expand this program. Clozapine was also initially administered under such a program. Patients under the care of a responsible physician may now bring unapproved drugs into the United States or have them sent under specified conditions.

As required when using a marketed drug for FDA-labeled or nonlabeled indications, an important responsibility in the use of an investigational drug is the reporting of adverse effects to the FDA.

COST OF TREATMENT

Cost, in this context, implies more than just the price of the medication and the services of the treating clinician. Because most psychiatric disorders are chronic conditions, the cost of treatment must take into consideration the acute, maintenance, and prophylactic phases.

When calculating the total cost incurred by initiating therapy, one should consider:

- The *medication itself*
- *Ancillary procedures* to start and monitor therapy (e.g., preliminary and follow-up laboratory tests)
- Managing *adverse outcomes* (e.g., drug interactions that may require medical attention)
- Cost of *outpatient versus inpatient* treatment
- The comparative cost of *alternative therapies* (e.g., ECT versus medication for psychotic depression)

If such costs are prohibitive, it may be appropriate to select an alternative option so that compliance and overall outcome can be better assured.

Fortunately, for most psychotropics, side effects are minimal, usually involving nuisance complaints. With some agents, such as clozapine, however, the potential for more serious adverse effects does exist and must be carefully explained to the patient and family. Although managed care has successfully controlled overall financial costs, it is our responsibility to advocate for the optimal delivery of treatment, which necessarily takes into consideration not only the immediate expense of treatment but the impact of appropriate care in the long-term. As importantly, one should always factor in the cost of not providing adequate treatment, including:

- The *mortality* risk
- The *morbidity* risk and related costs such as:
  - *Adverse sequelae*
  - *Lost productivity*
  - *Disruption in socioeconomic relationships*

Price of Psychotropics

In general, the price on a per-milligram basis decreases as the dosage of the capsule or tablet increases or as the lot size increases (e.g., 1,000 vs. 100). The cost of generic substitutes is usually considerably less than that for the trade name psychotropic drugs, but issues of bioequivalence must also be considered (see the section "The Four Primary Pharmacokinetic Phases" in Chapter 3). Using the fewest tablets to achieve a targeted dose level is always less expensive. Unit dose systems, sustained release preparations, and concentrate forms all increase the cost (26).

The cost of medication can range from pennies to several dollars per week. The cost of providing outpatient treatment can amount to several hundred dollars a week, depending on the frequency of visits and therapist charges. The cost of hospitalization can range from $500 to $1,000 per day. The cost to the patient in terms of the social consequences can be incalculable. The use of a slightly more effective medication that prevents even one hospitalization could pay for several years of drug treatment. One side effect avoided, particularly if it would result in an emergency room visit or hospitalization, will quickly pay for any increased difference in medication expense. Thus, the cost to society for not providing the best medication can be quite substantial. More expensive but safer medications are preferable because of the high cost of treating adverse effects and of rehospitalization associated with earlier, less effective or less safe agents. A drug that causes fewer side effects also results in better compliance. Most importantly, when one provides optimal total care (i.e., inpatient, outpatient, drug management), one also helps to improve the patient's quality of life and contribution to society.

CONCLUSION

In this book, we critically review both the formal FDA "labeled" indications, as well as those indications accepted by experts in the field of psychopharmacotherapy. In terms of the latter, meta-analysis is used when possible to formally assess the size and quality of the database that supports the usefulness of a drug for a clinically accepted, but not formally "labeled," indication. These analyses can then aid the clinician in the decision to use a given drug for an "unlabeled" indication in a specific patient. Cost is considered in terms of price of medicine, as well as to the individual and society.

REFERENCES

1. Straus JL, von Ammon Cavanaugh S. Placebo effects. Issues for clinical practice in psychiatry and medicine. *Psychosomatics* 1996;37:315–326.
2. Jadad A, Moore RA, Carroll D, et al. Assessing the quality of reports of randomized clinical trials: is blinding necessary. *Control Clin Trials* 1996;51:1235–1241.
3. Baastrup P, Schou M. Lithium as a prophylactic agent. *Arch Gen Psychiatry* 1967;16:162–172.
4. Benson K, Hartz A. A comparison of observational studies and randomized controlled trials. *N Engl J Med* 2000;342:1878–1886.
5. Concato J, Shah N, Horwitz RI. Randomized, controlled trials, observational studies and the hierarchy of research designs. *N Engl J Med* 2000;342:1887–1892.
6. D'Agostino RB, Weintraub M. Meta-analysis: a method for synthesizing research. *Clin Pharmacol Ther* 1995;58:605–616.
7. Hedges LV, Olkin I. *Statistical methods for meta-analysis*. Orlando, FL: Academic Press, 1985.
8. Gibbons RD, Janicak PG, Davis JM. A response to Overall and Rhoades regarding their comment on the efficacy

of unilateral vs. bilateral ECT [Letter]. *Convuls Ther* 1987;3:228–237.

9. Fleiss JL. *Statistical methods for rates and proportions,* 2nd ed. New York: John Wiley & Sons,1981.

10. Easterbrook P, Berlin JA, Gopalan R, et al. Publication bias in clinical research. *Lancet* 1991;337:867–872.

11. Reynolds RN, Mercy J, Coppen A. Prophylactic treatment of alcoholism by lithium carbonate: an initial report. *Alcohol Clin Exp Res* 1977;1:109–111.

12. Gibbons R, Hedeker DR, Davis JM. Estimation of effect size from a series of experiments involving paired comparisons. *J Educ Stat* 1993;18:271–279.

13. Leibenluft E. Sex is complex. *Am J Psychiatry* 1996; 153:969–972.

14. Appelbaum PS, Grisso T. Assessing patients' capacities to consent to treatment. *N Engl J Med* 1988;319:1635–1638.

15. Janicak PG, Bonavich PR. The borderland of autonomy: medical-legal criteria for capacity to consent. *J Psychiatry Law* 1980:8;361–387.

16. Stanley B, Guido J, Stanley M, et al. The elderly patient and informed consent: empirical findings. *JAMA* 1984;252:1302–1306.

17. Roth LH, Meisel A, Lidz CW. Tests of competency to consent to treatment. *Am J Psychiatry* 1977;134:279–284.

18. Appelbaum PS. The right to refuse treatment with antipsychotic medications: retrospect and prospect. *Am J Psychiatry* 1988;145:413–419.

19. Brakel J, Davis JM. Taking harms seriously: involuntary mental patients and the right to refuse treatment. *Ind L Rev* 1991;25:429–473.

20. May PRA. *Treatment of schizophrenia: a comparative study of five treatment methods.* New York: Science House, 1968.

21. May PRA. Rational treatment for an irrational disorder: what does the schizophrenic patient need? *Am J Psychiatry* 1976;133:1008–1012.

22. Kessler DA, Hass AE, Feiden KL, et al. Approval of new drugs in the United States. Comparison with the United Kingdom, Germany, and Japan. *JAMA* 1996;276:1826–1831.

23. Teuting P. Investigational drugs and research. *Psychiatr Med* 1991;9:333–347.

24. The Belmont Report: ethical principles and guidelines for the protection of human subjects of research. [Report of the National Commission for the Protection of Human Subjects of Biomedical and Behavioral Research]. *OPRR Reports* April 18, 1979.

25. Kessler DA. The regulation of investigational drugs. *N Engl J Med* 1989;320:281–288.

26. Jurman RJ, Davis JM. Comparison of the cost of psychotropic medications: an update. *Psychiatr Med* 1991; 9:349–359.

3

Pharmacokinetics

GENERAL PRINCIPLES

The fundamental relationship between the pharmacodynamics of a drug (i.e., what the drug does to the body) and its pharmacokinetics (i.e., what the body does to the drug) is expressed by Equation 1:

$$\text{Effect} = \text{Affinity for site of action} \times \text{Drug level}$$
$$\times \text{Biological variance}$$

Pharmacodynamics (i.e., a drug's affinity for its sites of action) defines what the drug is theoretically capable of doing. For example, any drug that can block the dopamine-2 receptor is theoretically capable of causing extrapyramidal adverse effects (e.g., dystonia) (1–3). However, a sufficient amount of the drug must reach that target under clinically relevant dosing conditions to have a physiologically meaningful effect (4–7). The **pharmacokinetics** of a drug determine whether that amount is achieved under clinically relevant dosing conditions. **Equation 1 expresses the fundamental relationship between pharmacodynamics and pharmacokinetics.**

For most drugs, there is an optimal occupation of the target needed for an optimal response. Below a critical level, the target will not be sufficiently engaged to have a physiologically meaningful effect. Conversely, occupation above a critical upper limit will be associated with an increased likelihood of adverse effects (2, 3). This fact is fundamental to understanding the potential benefit of therapeutic drug monitoring (TDM), which is a means to determine the second variable in Eq. 1.

Drug level is determined by two variables—dosing rate and clearance, as expressed in Equation 2:

$$\text{Drug level} = \text{Dosing rate/Clearance}$$

Viewed from this perspective, clinical trials are in essence population pharmacokinetic studies in which the goal is to determine the dose of the drug needed to achieve the optimal drug level (i.e., concentration) in the average person enrolled in the study. The concept of the "average person" is critical because humans are not all the same including how they respond to a drug. That is the reason for the third variable in Eq. 1.

Biological differences among patients can shift their individual dose–response curves, either reducing or enhancing the magnitude of the drug response and sometimes even altering its fundamental nature. This biological heterogeneity results from differences in diagnosis, genetics, gender, age, organ function, and the internal environment of the body (8–11). The last variable includes the presence of other drugs, which can interact pharmacodynamically or pharmacokinetically, with the drug of interest.

Given this introductory background, the remainder of this chapter will focus on the clinically relevant aspects of pharmacokinetics (i.e., the second variable in Eq. 1). For ease of reference, a glossary of pharmacokinetic terms is provided at the end of this chapter.

FOUR PRIMARY PHARMACOKINETIC PHASES

The pharmacokinetics of a drug can be divided into four primary phases:

- Absorption
- Distribution
- Metabolism
- Elimination

Before discussing each of these four phases, a clinical vignette will be given to illustrate its clinical relevance.

Absorption

Case Example: A 37-year-old schizoaffective patient was treated with thioridazine (100 mg

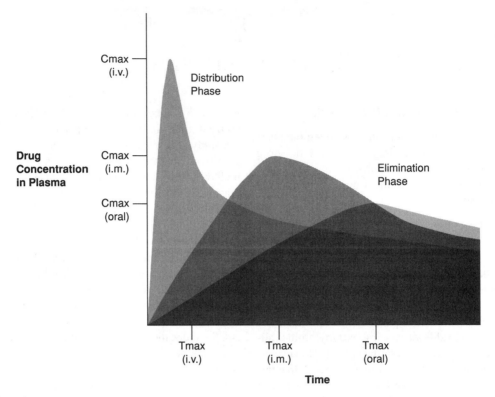

FIG. 3-1. Single-dose plasma drug concentration versus time curves for the same dose of the same drug given to the same individual by three different routes. (From Janicak PG, Davis JM. Pharmacokinetics and drug interactions. In: Sadock BJ, Sadock V, eds. *Kaplan & Sadock's comprehensive textbook of psychiatry, Vol. 2,* 7th ed. Philadelphia: Lippincott Williams & Wilkins, 2000:2251, with permission. Artwork created by Matthew Janicak.)

by mouth q.i.d.), phenytoin (100 mg by mouth q.i.d.), and amitriptyline (50 mg by mouth q.i.d.). The patient had been stabilized on this regimen for several weeks, but then complained of daytime sedation. The treating physician therefore combined all three into a single bedtime regimen. The patient expired the first night of the new schedule from an acute cardiac arrest.

In this case, each of the drugs the patient was taking was individually capable of slowing intracardiac conduction in a concentration-dependent manner. Death occurred as a result of their additive effect amplified by the decision to give each one as a single nighttime dose. That decision substantially increased the peak concentration of each drug and consequently resulted in a fatal arrhythmia.

The principal route of administration for psychoactive drugs is oral, with absorption generally occurring in the small bowel. The drug is then absorbed into the portal circulation and enters the liver. Drugs can be metabolized both by cytochrome P450 (CYP) enzymes in the bowel wall and in the liver before reaching the systemic circulation (i.e., first-pass metabolism). Most psychiatric medications are highly lipophilic, so they readily pass the blood–brain barrier and enter the CNS (12–15). In addition, because of their high lipophilicity, they generally share several other features:

- *Rapid* absorption
- *Complete* absorption
- Rapid and *extensive distribution* in tissue compartments

- High first-pass *effect*
- Large *volume of distribution*

Bioavailability refers to the portion of a drug absorbed from the site of administration. The reference site of administration is intravenous, because this route produces 100% *absorption.* Figure 3-1 illustrates three sample drug concentration curves in plasma as a function of time. The area under the curve (AUC) is the total amount of drug in the systemic circulation available for distribution to the sites of action. The same dose completely absorbed from any of these routes would produce an identical area under the curve (i.e., 100% bioavailability), although the shape would differ.

Any decrease in the total area under the curve for intramuscular or oral versus intravenous administration would represent a decrease in bioavailability based on that route of administration (16). Common factors that influence bioavailability include:

- *Physicochemical properties* of the drug
- *Formulation* of the product
- *Disease states* that influence gastrointestinal function or first pass-effect
- *Precipitation* of a drug at the injection site
- *Drug interactions* mediated by CYP enzymes in the bowel wall, liver, or transporters in the bowel wall

There are other clinically important parameters beyond the extent of absorption that are apparent on the single-dose plasma curve. These include the following:

- *Peak concentration* (C_{max})
- *Time to the peak concentration* (T_{max})

Generally, C_{max} will be inversely correlated to T_{max} (i.e., the shorter the time for a drug to be absorbed, the higher the peak concentration). A higher C_{max} and shorter C_{max} typically mean a more rapid appearance of clinical activity after administration. These parameters can also determine whether a drug should be developed for a specific indication, because T_{max} and C_{max} are generally a function of a compound's physicochemical properties.

In terms of physicochemical properties, the more polar a compound the slower the absorption from the gastrointestinal tract and the slower the penetration into the brain from the systemic circulation. These two phases (i.e., into the systemic circulation and into the brain) are usually correlated. Oxazepam, the most polar benzodiazepine (BZD), is slowly absorbed into the systemic circulation as well as into the brain (17, 18). Such pharmacokinetics are not the profile desired for use as a sedative-hypnotic. In contrast, lorazepam rapidly penetrates both compartments, inducing sleep in a relatively rapid time frame (14). Although rate of penetration into the brain generally parallels rate of penetration into the systemic circulation, this is not always true. An example is the original formulation of temazepam, which consisted of a hard gelatin capsule resistant to gastric breakdown (17). This formulation resulted in a slow absorption rate, diminishing its effectiveness as a sedative even though it penetrated the brain rapidly from the systemic circulation. A change in the formulation led to more rapid absorption, increasing its usefulness as a sedative-hypnotic.

Fast absorption may not always be desirable, because adverse effects may be a function of C_{max}. In the case example that began the discussion on absorption, failure to appreciate this fact led to a fatal outcome. **Cardiac toxicity, due to the stabilization of excitable membranes, is as much a function of the peak plasma concentration as it is of the steady-state tissue concentration.** Thus, changing a formulation to delay T_{max} and reduce C_{max} may significantly increase safety (e.g., reduce seizure risk with sustained release formulation of bupropion). Dividing the dose into smaller amounts and administering it more frequently can also accomplish the same result. In such a case, the average plasma concentration over the dosing interval and the amount absorbed will usually remain the same, but the peak concentration will be lower and the trough concentration higher.

Differences in bioavailability, particularly as they affect the rate of absorption, can vary significantly among formulations (i.e., products) of the same drug. The Food and Drug Administration considers a generic product to be comparable to a brand name if there is no more than a 20% difference (more or less) in bioavailability (i.e., T_{max} and C_{max}) (19). Hence, theoretically, there could be as much as a 40% difference between two generic preparations of the same drug. This possibility may explain why a patient who previously tolerated and benefitted from one generic preparation of a medication begins to develop side effects or suffers a relapse when another preparation is substituted.

Route of Administration

Different routes of administration can affect the rate of absorption, as well as the ratio of parent compound to its various metabolites. For example, the concentration versus time curve is usually shifted to the left with the intramuscular route, due to more rapid absorption (Fig. 3-1). Hence, T_{max} is shifted to the left (i.e., shortened) and C_{max} is higher, contracting the curve, even though the area under the curve (AUC) may be unchanged.

This pattern is not true for all drugs, however. For example, diazepam and chlordiazepoxide are unstable at a pH of 7.4 and tend to crystallize in tissue when given intramuscularly (14, 17, 18). Therefore, they are less bioavailable when given intramuscularly versus orally. Their absorption also tends to be erratic and variable, depending on where the injection was given (i.e., near blood vessels, in fat, or in muscle), as well as slower and less complete.

First-Pass Effect

When drugs are administered orally, they typically are absorbed in the small bowel, enter the portal circulation, and pass through the liver. Both CYP enzymes in the bowel wall and in the hepatocytes can metabolize a fraction of the drug before it reaches the systematic circulation (i.e., first-pass metabolism or first-pass effect). The extent of this effect can be broadly altered by diseases (e.g., cirrhosis, portacaval shunting, persistent hepatitis, congestive heart failure), and by some drugs (e.g., alcohol, ketaconazole, fluoxetine) influencing the peak concentrations achieved and the ratio of the parent compound to metabolites (11, 19, 20).

Transporters in the bowel wall can either actively take up or extrude drugs, thus increasing or decreasing absorption, respectively. Conversely, administered drugs or dietary factors can increase or decrease the activity of the transporters, altering the degree of absorption of another drug.

Once first-pass metabolism has occurred, metabolites are excreted into the bile and then the small bowel. Those that are lipid soluble are reabsorbed into the portal circulation, eventually entering the systemic circulation. These metabolites may have a similar or substantially different pharmacological profile from their parent drug. For example, chlorpromazine undergoes extensive hepatic biotransformation and has 168 theoretical metabolites, 70 of which have been identified in plasma and tissue. Some have dopamine receptor-blocking activity, although they are weaker than the parent compound, making it difficult to separate the effects (good or bad) of the parent compound from its numerous active metabolites.

In contrast to oral administration, drugs administered intravenously or intramuscularly directly enter the systemic circulation, avoiding the first-pass effect. This is why many drugs (e.g., fluphenazine) are more potent (i.e. greater effect per milligram dose taken) when administered intramuscularly. Hence, the intramuscular dose should be adjusted to compensate for this difference in absorption. Medical conditions such as cirrhosis can cause portacaval shunting, allowing drugs to avoid the first-pass effect and directly enter the systemic circulation, enhancing a psychotropic's effect. Coadministered drugs can affect first-pass metabolism or transport of another drug, thus altering its bioavailability (7, 10, 15). For example, acute alcohol intoxication can substantially reduce the first-pass effect on tricyclic antidepressants (TCAs), leading to a doubling of the C_{max} after the same dose (21). This effect contributes to the increased toxicity that occurs when an overdose of TCAs is taken with alcohol.

Distribution

Case Example: A 44-year-old chronic alcoholic man presented in the emergency room with

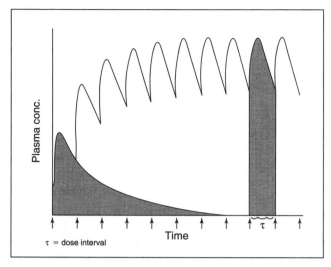

FIG. 3-2. Plasma drug concentration versus time curve following administration of a single oral dose and following repeated administrations of the same oral dose.

disorientation and combativeness after 2 days of abstinence. He complained of visual and tactile hallucinations and was found to have elevated heart rate, blood pressure, and temperature. *Lorazepam* was slowly administered intravenously, and after 15 minutes, the patient was mildly sedated. He was then transferred to an inpatient unit. During this 30-minute interval, he received no additional lorazepam, and when he arrived on the floor, his symptoms had returned. He became agitated, struck one of the nursing staff, and had to be physically restrained.

In this case, failure to account for the phenomenon of drug redistribution resulted in a potentially avoidable adverse outcome, as explained in the following discussion. Once in the systemic circulation, the drug distributes to organs in direct proportion to their fat and protein content (8). The rate of accumulation is a function of an organ's vascularity. Although highly lipid-soluble drugs accumulate in adipose tissue to the same extent that they accumulate in the brain, *the rate of accumulation is much faster in the brain than in adipose tissue.*

Figure 3-2 illustrates single and multiple dose pharmacokinetics, with the *Y* axis representing plasma drug concentration and the *X* axis the time elapsed since drug administration. When a single oral dose is administered, the drug reaches C_{max} and then undergoes a relatively rapid decline. **This initial decline is due primarily to drug distribution, rather than to elimination. Thus, the initial drug concentration drop is a function of the rate of uptake into other bodily compartments rather than elimination from the body.** This fact is particularly important with the first dose of an i.v.-administered psychotropic because:

- They are quite *lipophilic.*
- They have *large volumes of distribution.*
- Their *tissue concentrations are typically 10 to 100 times greater than their plasma concentrations.*

The acute effects of a single dose of most psychotropics are terminated by redistribution. An example would be the acute sedative effects of intravenously administered lorazepam, which rapidly enters the brain from the blood. A disproportionate amount of the dose enters the CNS because of its greater vascularity in comparison with peripheral adipose tissue. Brain concentration subsequently falls as the drug redistributes out of the brain into the plasma and then into other peripheral compartments. This fall in brain concentration terminates acute psychoactive effects of a single dose of a drug such as lorazepam.

Distribution of the drug is conceptualized as accumulation into various body compartments (e.g., fat, aqueous, bone, brain, etc.). The extent to which drugs differ in their rate and degree of accumulation into various organs is related to the number of compartments into which they equilibrate. Even within one apparent *compartment, such as blood, there may be more than one subcomponent for distribution, including the following*:

- Plasma *water*
- Plasma *protein*
- Circulating *cells* (particularly red blood cells)

Most psychotropics are highly protein-bound (22–25). Such bound drug often accounts for more than 90% of the total plasma concentration. The clinical significance is that even though the free-drug fraction is the smallest absolute amount, it is the most important, because its concentration determines the final equilibration with the site of action. Although a change in the bound amount from 95% to 90% may seem small, the corresponding change in the free fraction would be from 5% to 10%, doubling the effective drug concentration in equilibrium with the site of action. Thus, any condition that shifts the ratio of bound to free drug can change the concentration of the drug at its sites of action and thus the magnitude of its effect. Conditions that lead to a functional decrease in the amount of circulating protein include:

- *Malnutrition*, as with severe anorexia
- *Wasting*, as in the nephrotic syndrome
- *Aging* (25, 26)
- *Concomitant drugs* that compete for protein binding sites (27, 28)

Increasing the relative amount of the free fraction can increase toxicity. Most assays used in routine TDM do not distinguish between bound and free-drug fractions, and, hence, will not detect such changes unless specialized techniques are used.

Acute and chronic inflammatory processes can increase the amount of circulating α1-acid glycoprotein (which avidly binds a variety of psychotropics), increasing the absolute amount of bound drug, whereas the free fraction remains unchanged. In such circumstances, the circu-lating total concentrations may seem excessive, but actually simply represent an increase in the bound (but biologically inert) circulating fraction (29).

The absolute and the relative size of the body's fat compartment can change with normal aging and morbid obesity (8, 20, 30–32). As noted earlier, the percentage of total body water and protein content decreases in the elderly, whereas the percentage of fat content increases, providing a relatively larger reservoir in which to store psychotropics. These changes explain why many psychotropic drugs have a more persistent effect in the elderly. The morbidly obese patient also has an increased reservoir, and a drug's effect can persist in relation to the size of the adipose compartment.

Under steady-state conditions, there is a proportional relationship between the tissue and the plasma compartments (4, 16, 33). This fact underlies the usefulness of TDM, which utilizes drug concentration in plasma to assure adequacy of drug dose while helping to avoid toxicity. Although psychotropics do not exert their psychoactive effects in plasma, their plasma concentration is, nonetheless, in equilibrium with tissue levels. **Although tissue concentrations (depending on the organ) are 10 to 100 times greater than plasma concentrations, the latter provide an indirect measurement of the former** (2, 33).

Metabolism

Case Example: A 62-year-old man presented to his internist with a major depressive disorder. His past medical history was significant for two previous myocardial infarctions and related congestive heart failure, well-controlled by digoxin. There was also a past history of significant alcohol abuse, in remission for the past 4 years. The internist prescribed amitriptyline 75 mg p.o. at bedtime. One week later, the patient returned with a worsening of his depressive state, and the internist increased the dose to 100 mg. The patient continued to deteriorate and was referred to a psychiatrist, who hospitalized him. The patient was now suspicious, guarded, and irritable and was given the diagnosis of a psychotic depression. Haloperidol 10 mg p.o. at bedtime was added. Five days later, the patient was found unconscious in his room after complaining of faintness and heart palpitations. He was rushed to the coronary intensive care unit, where a 2:1 atrioventricular block and periodic runs of premature ventricular contractions were found on the ECG. Drug level monitoring revealed a total TCA plasma level of 950 ng/mL. All psychoactive drugs were stopped. As the plasma level fell, the cardiac and the psychotic symptoms resolved. This patient had several risk factors for the development of toxic TCA concentrations even while on a relatively low dose of amitriptyline. The following discussion elaborates on these factors.

Biotransformation

Most psychotropics undergo extensive *oxidative biotransformation* leading to the formation of more polar metabolites, which are then excreted in the urine. The necessary biotransformation steps may involve one or several of the following steps:

- Hydroxylation
- Demethylation
- Oxidation
- Sulfoxide formation

Whereas most drugs undergo extensive oxidative biotransformation (i.e., phase I metabolism) before elimination, some undergo simple conjugation with moieties such as glucuronic acid (i.e., phase II metabolism), and others are excreted unmetabolized (e.g., lithium) (35). Because conjugation can occur in most organs, phase II metabolism is not dependent on liver function. Thus, the clearance of drugs that undergo only glucuronidation is generally not affected by even significant liver impairment. These include all of the 3-hydroxybenzodiazepines (e.g., lorazepam, oxazepam, temazepam), which are as readily cleared by the old as by the young, as long as their renal function is normal. The same is true for patients with severely compromised liver function, which is another reason to use 3-

hydroxybenzodiazepines (e.g., lorazepam) early in the treatment of delirium tremens. Should such patients subsequently develop hepatic failure, they can still readily clear such drugs and thus avoid having them persist in the body to worsen cognitive function and level of arousal. By contrast, a drug like diazepam, which requires extensive biotransformation as a necessary step in its elimination, can persist in the body for a prolonged period should the patient develop hepatic failure (18). Further, the metabolites of diazepam have similar pharmacological properties, accumulate in the body, and ultimately contribute to the pharmacological effect.

Oxidative biotransformation results in the formation of metabolites whose pharmacological effects may be similar or dissimilar to the parent compound. Either way, active metabolites contribute to the final overall clinical effects. For example, norfluoxetine has essentially the same activity as fluoxetine in terms of both serotonin uptake blockade and inhibition of several CYP enzymes, but is cleared more slowly (11, 36, 37). As a result, norfluoxetine accumulates extensively in the body following chronic administration of fluoxetine, making it, rather than the parent compound, the principal determinant of the clinical effect.

In contrast, clomipramine's major metabolite, desmethylclomipramine, has a markedly different pharmacological profile from the parent drug (35). While clomipramine is a potent inhibitor of serotonin uptake, desmethylclomipramine is a more potent inhibitor of norepinephrine uptake. If clomipramine's value in obsessive-compulsive disorder (OCD) depends on its ability to block 5-HT uptake (and not of norepinephrine), then this effect should be a function of the relative ratio between clomipramine and desmethylclomipramine. Thus, clomipramine could lose its effectiveness for OCD if a patient were an efficient demethylator of this drug.

Another important situation occurs when the parent drug is biotransformed into a less efficacious and possibly more toxic metabolite. For example, if the concentration of the hydroxylated metabolite of imipramine (2-hydroxyimipramine) were increased, this TCA could lose its effectiveness while simultaneously increasing in toxicity (38).

Cytochrome P450 Enzyme Induction

Alcohol, nicotine, and most anticonvulsants induce a number of CYP enzymes (39, 40). This mechanism explains why barbiturates and carbamazepine induce the metabolism of other drugs as well as their own (i.e., **autoinduction**). Blood levels obtained 3 or 4 days after starting these drugs reflect the rate of elimination at that time; however, levels will subsequently fall on the same dose because autoinduction results in faster elimination (i.e., a shorter half-life) as a function of continued drug administration. Therefore, early TDM of carbamazepine will overestimate the eventual concentration reached after several weeks on the drug (see the section "Alternative Treatment Strategies" in Chapter 10).

Alcohol has a triphasic effect on the elimination rates of drugs that require extensive biotransformation (21). For example, *acute* alcohol ingestion in combination with a TCA in a teetotaler who attempts suicide will significantly block the first-pass metabolism of the TCA. This chemical inhibition can triple the peak concentration of a TCA by increasing its bioavailability. This is why the consumption of alcohol in association with a TCA overdose increases lethality.

Drinking on a regular basis for several weeks to months can induce CYP enzymes, resulting in a lower TCA plasma concentration. Thus, *subacute* and *subchronic* alcohol consumption induces liver enzymes and causes lower plasma levels of drugs that undergo oxidative biotransformation as a necessary step in their elimination.

Chronic alcohol ingestion can cause cirrhosis, reducing hepatic CYP enzyme concentration and liver mass, and causing portacaval shunting. These effects will result in increased plasma drug levels due to both greater bioavailability (due to reduced first pass metabolism) and due to decreased clearance. Thus, dose adjustment is necessary and should be guided by TDM when possible.

Cytochrome P450 Enzyme Inhibition

In contrast to anticonvulsants and alcohol, drugs such as bupropion, fluoxetine, flu- voxamine, nefazodone, quinidine, paroxetine, **and some antipsychotics can inhibit specific CYP enzymes** (7, 11, 36, 37, 41–44). Thus, TCAs, certain BZDs, bupropion, some steroids, and antipsychotics can all have their metabolism inhibited by drugs such as fluoxetine. For example, fluoxetine at 20 mg/day produces on average a 500% increase in the levels of coprescribed drugs which are principally dependent on CYP 2D6 for their clearance. That can lead to serious or even life-threatening toxicity if the drug has a narrow therapeutic index and the dose is not adjusted for the change in clearance caused by the coadministration of fluoxetine.

Hepatic Arterial Flow

After a drug enters the systemic circulation, the delivery back to the liver depends on left ventricular function. Hence, drugs may also affect the clearance of other drugs indirectly, through *an effect on hepatic arterial blood flow* (20, 31, 32). The rate of drug conversion is dependent on the rate of delivery to the liver, which is determined by arterial flow. *Cimetidine and β-blockers such as propranolol decrease arterial flow*, slowing the clearance of various drugs that undergo extensive oxidative biotransformation.

Effects of Disease on Hepatic Function

Diseases that *directly affect* hepatic integrity include cirrhosis, viral infections, and collagen vascular diseases. Diseases that *indirectly affect* function include metabolic disorders (e.g., azotemia secondary to renal insufficiency) and cardiac disease. Although decreased left ventricular output can result in a decrease in hepatic arterial flow, right ventricular failure causes hepatic congestion, reducing the first-pass effect and delaying biotransformation.

Thus, the patient with a toxic TCA concentration (see the case at the start of the "Metabolism" section) developed excessively high amitriptyline plasma levels due to the additive effects of diminished left ventricular function leading to decreased hepatic arterial blood flow; alcohol- and age-related decline in liver function; and, finally, haloperidol's inhibition of amitriptyline's metabolism (41).

Elimination

Case Example: A 48-year-old bipolar woman, stabilized on lithium 1,200 mg/day for the past 6 months, had a plasma level that varied between 0.8 and 1.0 mEq/L. She developed a recurrence of her rheumatoid arthritis, for which her internist prescribed ibuprofen (800 mg t.i.d.). A week later, she was brought to the emergency room in a confused, disoriented, and lethargic state. She was also ataxic and had periodic generalized myoclonic jerks. TDM revealed a lithium level of 4.0 mEq/L, and despite a rapid fall to under 0.5 mEq/L with plasma dialysis, her neurological status continued to deteriorate. After 5 days, she died.

Failure to account for a critical drug interaction, affecting the renal clearance of lithium, resulted in an otherwise avoidable fatality (45).

The last step in a drug's clearance from the body is elimination, which for most psychotropics occurs via the kidneys. At this point, most compounds have been converted into polar metabolites, which are more water- and less lipid-soluble than the parent compound, thus facilitating their clearance in urine. On the plasma drug concentration versus time curve, following a single dose, this step is reflected by the terminal elimination phase, which is typically a gradual and steady decline in the plasma drug level over time. The slope of this clearance curve is a function of the rates of biotransformation and elimination. Thus, the slope (the K_e or kinetic constant of elimination) represents a summation of the CYP enzymatic activity required for the biotransformation necessary for subsequent elimination and the glomerular filtration rate that clears polar metabolites from the blood (Fig. 3.1).

Obviously, *renal insufficiency* can delay clearance (8, 20). More specifically, it will result in the accumulation of higher concentrations of polar metabolites. Depending on the pharmacological profile of these metabolites, patients may accumulate compounds that are less effi-cacious, or more toxic, or both, than the parent compound. *Dehydration* can result in the same outcome because it diminishes glomerular filtration rate. Changing the *plasma pH* (e.g., giving cranberry juice to acidify, sodium bicarbonate to make more basic) can also hasten or retard the clearance of certain drugs (e.g., amphetamines) via the kidneys. Concurrent drugs may also affect the ability of the renal tubules to excrete a drug. Two examples are the effect of loop diuretics and nonsteroidal anti-inflammatory agents on renal clearance of lithium (45, 46).

Half-Life

Half-life is the time needed to clear 50% of a drug from the plasma. It also determines the length of time necessary to reach steady state. The general rule is that the time to reach steady-state concentration (C_{SS}) of a drug is five times the drug's half-life, not five times the dosing interval. The reason is that during every half-life period, a patient either clears or accumulates 50% of the eventual C_{SS} produced by that dosing rate. Therefore, in one half-life a patient will have reached 50% of the concentration that will eventually be achieved. In two half-lives, a patient achieves the initial 50% plus half of the remaining 50%, for a total of 75%. After three half-lives, a patient achieves the initial 50% and the next 25% plus half of the remaining 25%, for a total of 87.5%. At 97% (i.e., five half-lives), the patient is essentially at steady-state, which is the rationale behind the general rule. Parenthetically, washout or clearance of the drug from the body is the mirror image of drug accumulation.

Steady-State

C_{SS} is that total concentration of a drug in plasma that will not change as long as the dosing rate (i.e., dose per interval of time) remains unchanged or other factors do not alter the rate of metabolism or elimination. Dosing rate is most often thought of as the total amount of drug ingested in 24 hour (i.e., daily dosing rate). Once plasma steady-state is reached, the drug concentration in various body compartments (e.g., adipose tissue, the brain) is

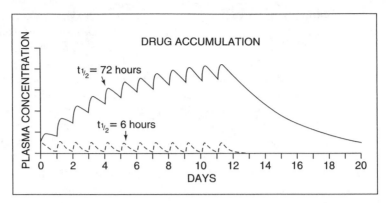

FIG. 3-3. Plasma drug concentration versus time curve for two model drugs: one with a half-life of 6 hours and one with a half-life of 72 hours.

at equilibrium. In this instance, the amount excreted every 24 hours will equal the amount taken every 24 hours, as long as other medical illnesses, personal habits, the physician, or the patient do not alter the elimination rate.

Another general rule is that the longer the half-life, the longer the interval between starting the drug and seeing its full effects, whether beneficial or adverse. Figure 3-3 demonstrates two different curves resulting from drugs with half-lives of 72 and 6 hours, respectively. Assuming a once-a-day dosing schedule, such as with a sedative-hypnotic at bedtime, drugs with these respective half-lives will accumulate in various tissues at two different rates and each to a different extent. In the case of the drug with a 72-hour half-life, the trough concentration before the next dose will be substantial relative to the peak concentration produced by the next dose. In the case of the drug with a 6-hour half-life, trough concentration will be trivial relative to the peak concentration produced by the next dose.

The length of the half-life determines the time needed to assess response, as well as to clear a drug. For example, flurazepam, a BZD sedative-hypnotic, may not achieve C_{SS} for several weeks after it is started (18, 19). Therefore, if a patient has been taking a p.r.n. sedative daily, declining cognitive function may actually be the result of a drug started 2 to 3 weeks previously! Conversely, it will take five times the half-life to clear 97% of the drug after its discontinuation. That can be of relevance when the desire is to quickly terminate an adverse effect or the potential for an

adverse effect (e.g., risk of a drug–drug interaction or tetratogenicity in the case of pregnancy). In other situations, the clinician may want delayed clearance to minimize the risk of a drug discontinuation syndrome (47).

To put this in perspective, the mean half-live of norfluoxetine is 20 days in a physically healthy older patient. That means it will take 100 days to achieve C_{SS} once fluoxetine has been started and 100 days to clear 97% of this active metabolite once the parent compound has been stopped. These times may be even longer at higher doses because fluoxetine has nonlinear pharmacokinetics over its recommended dosing range (i.e., autoinhibition).

Zero and First Order Kinetics

When only a fixed amount of drug is eliminated in a given interval of time, because enzymes for biotransformation and elimination are saturated, the kinetics of drug elimination are *zero order* (16). Alcohol is the classic example, where blood levels rise exponentially with increased amounts ingested, because elimination mechanisms are saturated and only a certain fraction of the total dose taken can be eliminated before the next dose is ingested.

First order kinetics means that the amount eliminated per unit of time is directly proportional to the amount ingested, so there is a linear relationship between dose change and plasma level change (i.e., 1 : 1). In contrast, with zero order kinetics there is a larger than proportional increase in the plasma concentration for each dose increment because the elimination mechanism is saturated.

Few drugs or substances exhibit zero order kinetics over their usual concentration ranges, but a number of psychotropics demonstrate nonlinear pharmacokinetics (a phenomenon between pure first order and pure zero order pharmacokinetics) meaning that the drug concentration increases disproportionately as its dose increases over its clinically relevant dosing range. The mechanism underlying this phenomenon is generally that different CYP enzymes (see the section "Drug–Drug Interactions") with different affinities and capacities mediate the biotransformation of the drug at different concentrations. At low concentration, the biotransformation is principally mediated by a CYP enzyme with higher affinity but lower capacity, which the drug saturates as its concentration increases (i.e., autoinhibits its own metabolism), and levels of the drug rise disproportionately with increasing dose until they reach a point at which a lower affinity but higher capacity CYP enzyme begins to mediate the drug's biotransformation (e.g., fluoxetine, nefazodone, paroxetine) (7, 11, 48). As an example, one third of patients on TCAs demonstrate nonlinear kinetics when concentrations exceed about 200 ng/mL (49, 50). Thus, they experience proportionally greater increases in drug plasma levels at the high end of the curve because of enzyme saturation.

ALTERATIONS IN PHARMACOKINETICS

Drug–Drug Interactions

Knowledge about pharmacokinetic interactions (i.e., the effects of one drug on the absorption, distribution, metabolism, or elimination of another coadministered drug) is critical for the safe and effective use of drug combinations. For most drugs, there are two phases of biotransformation prior to elimination: phase I, or oxidative metabolism, followed by phase II, or conjugation reactions (16). Knowledge of phase I metabolism has expanded substantially as a result of improved understanding of CYP enzymes. These advances came as a result of molecular biology, which per-

TABLE 3-1. *Human CYP enzymes as classified by family, subfamily, and gene* [a]

1A1	2A6	3A-3/4	4A9	7	11A1	17	19	21	27
1A2	2A7	3A5	4B1		11B1				
	2B6	3A7	4F2		11B2				
	2C8		4F3						
	2C9								
	2C18								
	2C19								
	2D6								
	2E1								
	2F1								

[a] Key to classification: (a) the first Arabic numeral represents the family; (b) the alphabetic letter represents the subfamily; and (c) the second Arabic numeral represents the individual gene within the subfamily.
From Preskorn S. *Clinical pharmacology of selective serotonin reuptake inhibitors.* Caddo, OK: Professional Communications, 1996.

mitted identification and cloning of the genes that encode specific CYP enzymes (Table 3-1).

The nosology for CYP enzymes involves grouping into families and subfamilies according to structural similarity. All CYP enzymes in the same family have at least 40% structural similarity, and those in the same subfamily have at least 60% structural similarity. The *family* is designated by the first Arabic number, the *subfamily* by an alphabetic letter, and the trailing Arabic number designates *the gene* that codes for a specific CYP enzyme (10, 35, 51).

Studies are now directed at identifying which CYP enzymes are involved in the biotransformation of specific drugs and also determining whether specific drugs can induce or inhibit specific CYP enzymes (Table 3-2) (52). The former can be determined by incubating a drug with a specific CYP enzyme and determining the affinity and capacity of that enzyme for biotransforming the drug. That information coupled with knowledge of the relative abundance of a specific CYP enzyme can be used to determine whether that CYP enzyme is primarily responsible for a drug's biotransformation.

In addition to such *in vitro* studies, the metabolism of the drug can be assessed in individuals who are genetically deficient in a specific CYP enzyme, but this approach is obviously limited to those CYP enzymes that have a genetic polymorphism, such as CYP 2D6 and CYP 2C19

TABLE 3-2. *How knowledge of drug-metabolizing enzymes will simplify understanding of pharmacokinetic interactions*

Drug A	$\longrightarrow$	Affects[a]	$\longrightarrow$	Enzyme X
Enzyme X	$\longrightarrow$	Metabolizes	$\longrightarrow$	Drugs B, C, D, E, F
Therefore, drug A	$\longrightarrow$	Affects[a]	$\longrightarrow$	Drugs B, C, D, E, F

[a] Could be inhibition or induction.

From Preskorn S. *Clinical pharmacology of selective serotonin reuptake inhibitors.* Caddo, OK: Professional Communications, 1996.

(35). Further confirmation can be obtained by coadministering a drug that is a known inhibitor of a specific CYP enzyme to determine whether such coadministration alters the clearance of the drug in question.

In vitro studies can also be used to determine if a drug is capable of inducing or inhibiting a specific CYP enzyme (53). Induction studies require the use of intact cells, because induction involves increasing the production of the CYP enzyme by increasing the translation of the gene. In contrast, inhibition studies can be done with microsome preparations or cells transfected with cDNA containing the gene coding for a specific CYP enzyme. In these studies, a potential inhibitor is added at varying concentrations to a bioassay containing the CYP enzyme in question and a drug that is a substrate for the enzyme. In this way, the kinetic inhibition constant (K_i) can be determined for the potential inhibitor relative to that specific CYP enzyme and substrate.

The K_i coupled with knowledge of the concentration of the potential inhibitor that should be expected under clinically relevant dosing can be used to estimate whether it is likely to inhibit the CYP enzyme to a clinically meaningful extent under usual dosing conditions (54–57). The concentration in question is that at the enzyme and is estimated by knowing the expected plasma concentration of the potential inhibitor under clinically relevant conditions and the partition coefficient of the inhibitor between the plasma compartment and the tissue site where biotransformation principally takes place. *That site is usually the liver, although some drugs are extensively metabolized by CYP enzymes in the bowel wall during the absorption phase (i.e., the first-pass metabolism).*

Such *in vivo* modelling is used to screen for potentially important pharmacokinetic drug–drug interactions. By knowing what CYP enzyme is principally responsible for the biotransformation of a specific drug and whether a second drug is capable of inducing or inhibiting that CYP enzyme, one can deduce whether coadministration of the second drug is likely to cause a clinically meaningful change in the clearance of the first drug (Table 3-2). Such screening is a cost- and time-effective way to determine which *in vivo* studies are most likely to yield clinically important information.

There are several ways of doing confirmatory *in vivo* studies. The most common involves measuring the clearance of a model substrate that is principally dependent on one CYP enzyme for its biotransformation before and after the addition of the potential inhibitor (37). The substrate may be given as a single test dose or dosed to steady state. Steady-state dosing is preferable because it more closely corresponds to the clinical situation. The inhibitor should be given at the clinically relevant dose and administered for a sufficient interval to assure that steady-state has been achieved, because the degree of inhibition is a function of the concentration of the inhibitor and any of its relevant metabolites, as well as their *in vitro* potency for inhibition.

This knowledge will allow the physician to determine whether a dose adjustment is needed when adding or stopping a drug that is capable of inducing or inhibiting the biotransformation of a concomitantly administered drug. Knowledge in this area is rapidly expanding as more of these studies are done. The results of specific studies are presented in the individual chapters dealing with the various classes of drugs.

One example is that certain anticonvulsants (e.g., CBZ, phenobarbital) potently *induce* specific CYP enzymes, principally CYP1A2 and 3A, causing plasma levels of antipsychotics to fall because of an acceleration in their metabolism (39, 40, 58, 59). Thus, the addition of carbamazepine to control mood swings in a psychotic patient previously stabilized may precipitate a psychotic exacerbation or relapse unless the antipsychotic dose is adjusted to compensate. Conversely, psychotropic drugs can inhibit specific CYP enzymes and thus increase the levels and the potential toxicity of concomitantly prescribed drugs dependent on that isoenzyme for their clearance. For example, fluoxetine and paroxetine substantially *inhibit* the CYP 2D6, important in the oxidative metabolism of drugs such as the TCAs (36, 41, 42, 51, 60). This effect can result in a quadrupling of the plasma concentration of TCAs and other CYP2D6 substrates/drugs and cause serious toxicity unless the dose is reduced (61, 62).

Effect of Gender

Gender differences in drug pharmacokinetics for females can be summarized as follows:

- **Absorption—bioavailability**
  - *Lower acidic environment* increases absorption of weak bases (e.g., TCAs, BZDs, some antipsychotics).
  - *Exogenous estrogen* may also increase absorption through this same mechanism.
  - *Slower transit time* in small intestine delays drug absorption and peak levels; lowers peak blood concentration.
- **Volume of distribution (VD)**
  - Drug *concentration and distribution are greater* in young women than in men.
  - *Protein binding is lower* in women than in men.
  - *Exogenous hormones* and *pregnancy* can alter protein binding.
- **Metabolism and elimination**
  - *Estradiol* and *progesterone* (used in oral contraceptives) reduce specific CYP enzyme activity (e.g., levels of APs such as HPDL, clozapine, and risperidone may rise).
- **Effects of pregnancy**
  - *Increased endogenous hormones of the luteal phase* cause decreased gastrointestinal motility and promote drug absorption.

- *Increased plasma* and *extracellular volumes* may lead to an increased VD and decreased drug levels.
- *Increased cardiac output* and *decreased albumin and α1-acid glycoproteins* can also lower drug levels (9, 63).

Effects of Aging and Disease

The pharmacokinetics of a drug can also change with aging and disease (8, 20, 26, 29, 32, 64–70). Several factors can alter the pharmacokinetic phases in the elderly, making them more prone to psychotropics' effects, including the following:

- A decrease in *intracellular water*
- A decrease in *protein binding*
- A decrease in *tissue mass*
- An increase in *total body fat*

These changes act synergistically to increase the effect of most psychotropic drugs in the elderly. An increase in the total body fat constitutes an enlarged reservoir for drug accumulation. The end result is that drugs tend to persist longer in the elderly.

The free-drug fraction also increases due to decreased protein binding so that for every milligram given, as well as for every drug concentration, there is a greater free drug concentration. In addition, *drug metabolism tends to decrease* in the elderly (related to diminished hepatic blood flow, liver mass, and CYP enzyme content and activity) (71). *Age-related decreases in renal excretion* also means that potentially active metabolites tend to accumulate more, and may be active in an undesirable way. All of these factors generally increase the effects of psychotropic drugs in the elderly; however, two age-related changes decrease drug accumulation and, hence, drug effect: decreased intestinal absorption and increased gastric pH.

In summary, for drugs that undergo extensive biotransformation before elimination, aging often produces a substantial lengthening of the time required to eliminate the drug (i.e., its half-life). **Thus, older patients frequently clear these agents much more slowly than their younger counterparts, making the elderly more susceptible to dose (i.e.,** concentration)–dependent adverse effects on the same amount of the same drug (72–82).

This phenomenon can also occur with diseases that alter the physiological mechanisms subserving the various pharmacokinetic phases.

THERAPEUTIC DRUG MONITORING

Therapeutic drug monitoring has four major clinical applications:

- To monitor *compliance*
- To increase *efficacy*
- To increase *safety*
- To protect against *medicolegal actions*

The characteristics of a drug that make TDM useful are listed in Table 3-3.

TDM can detect interindividual variability in pharmacokinetics that can determine clinical outcome (83–89). It is essentially a refinement of the traditional approach of adjusting dose based on clinical response. Using this strategy, the clinician titrates the dose based on an assessment of efficacy versus the development of nuisance or toxic effects. The discussion in this chapter has enumerated those pharmacokinetic factors that may produce variable clinical outcomes in different patients taking the same medication. TDM can be used to detect those differences among patients to guide rational dose adjustment.

Role of Therapeutic Drug Monitoring

One role for TDM is to guard against toxicity. This fact is particularly true for drugs that have narrow therapeutic indices, serious toxic effects, and substantial interindividual variabil-

TABLE 3-3. *Pharmacodynamic and pharmacokinetic characteristics of a drug that predict clinical usefulness of therapeutic drug monitoring*

Multiple mechanisms of action
Large interindividual variability in metabolism
Narrow therapeutic index
Delayed onset of action
Difficulty detecting early development of toxicity

ity in metabolism (85, 89). Such drugs include bupropion, clozapine, lithium, TCAs, some anticonvulsants, and low-potency antipsychotics. This role is especially crucial when early signs of toxicity are difficult to detect (90–92). For example, the early phases of a delirium due to toxic clozapine concentrations may mimic the worsening the underlying psychotic illness. Without guidance from TDM, the clinician might increase the clozapine dose due to presumed worsening of the psychotic disorder and inadvertently cause more toxicity.

TDM may provide objective data when there is a paucity of hard information. For example, TDM can provide additional information to determine the optimal dose of an antipsychotic for a given patient. In this instance, the patient is his own control, with an antipsychotic plasma level obtained after the dose has been stabilized. Then, TDM can be repeated when relapses occur to clarify whether noncompliance or drug refractoriness was responsible. Finally, this issue can be further clarified by repeating TDM when the patient is again stable. This approach avoids the initial impulse to increase the dose or to switch drugs, if the problem was at least partially attributable to noncompliance. It can also avoid a vicious cycle of increasing noncompliance due to adverse effects resulting from higher than necessary doses (and blood levels).

On occasion, TDM may also be used to aid in determining whether:

- There has been an *adequate trial*.
- A patient responded to the active drug or had a *placebo response*.
- The *likelihood of increased efficacy outweighs* the potential for *adverse effects*.

A sufficient dose for a sufficient interval constitutes an adequate trial. The question is whether the dose was sufficient. In drug-resistant cases, TDM can define dose adequacy by guiding its adjustment to eliminate differences introduced by pharmacokinetic variations among patients. Many clinicians assume a patient has experienced a placebo response if improvement occurs more rapidly than the typical time course. This assumption can be further substantiated by documenting a concentration well below that which is typically effective. Effective and safe levels in a patient responding to unusually low doses can help the clinician determine that the patient is likely to be a true drug, rather than a placebo, responder. This information can guide decisions about duration of drug therapy and whether other interventions may be indicated.

Rapid metabolizers may respond only to unusually high doses. TDM can alleviate concerns by providing a pharmacokinetic explanation for the necessity to use such high doses. Alternatively, some patients who only respond to high doses may also have high plasma drug levels and thus be at increased risk for serious toxicity. In such instances, prudence may dictate an alternative therapy, or at least following the patient's status more closely. An example would be a depressed patient requiring TCA plasma levels above 450 ng/mL (90) or a patient with schizophrenia requiring a clozapine level in excess of 750 ng/mL (85, 87). Although some patients may tolerate such levels, it would be prudent to obtain an ECG and an electroencephalogram (EEG) to assess for physiological evidence of toxicity even though it may not be clinically evident.

Timing of Samples for Therapeutic Drug Monitoring

Blood samples for TDM should be obtained in the elimination phase of drug dosing, because these levels are more reliable than those drawn during the absorption or distribution phases. Determining the elimination phase requires knowing when the C_{max} occurs, as well as the rapid fall off due to redistribution. Errors in the timing of samples (e.g., before steady-state has been reached or too early in a dosing interval) can produce misleading results and inappropriate dosing decisions.

Frequency of Therapeutic Drug Monitoring

The pharmacokinetics of a drug can also determine the frequency of monitoring. Many believe that TDM requires frequent blood drawings, primarily based on the experience with lithium. However, this drug is relatively unique in that its levels are determined by multiple independent factors. Thus, the plasma level of lithium is not solely a function of the dose and of renal status, but also of fluid and salt intake and output, which can vary independent of dose.

For most drugs, their concentration is a function of dose, as well as of the individual's rates of metabolism and elimination, which are relatively stable unless a moderating variable intervenes. Examples of such moderating variables include diseases that affect organs important for metabolism or elimination (e.g., liver or heart), or if the patient is exposed to a concurrent agent that induces or inhibits the CYP enzyme responsible for the biotransformation of the drug of interest.

Therapeutic drug monitoring is recommended as a standard aspect of care when the drug has a narrow therapeutic index and wide interindividual variability in clearance. For most drugs, such monitoring is recommended after the patient has been on a stable dose for 5 to 7 half-lives. After that, repeat monitoring is typically done only for cause. Reasons for repeat monitoring include an intervening factor in drug effectiveness or tolerability, or a change that might be reasonably expected to change the clearance of the drug (e.g., the addition or discontinuation of a second drug that would be expected to induce or inhibit the metabolism of the first drug, or the development of diseases that could adversely affect left cardiac ventricular, hepatic, or renal function).

Except in these situations, TDM does not need to be repeated because it is a measurement of the patient's ability to metabolize and eliminate a drug, which is generally a reproducible biological phenomenon and only changes for cause. This is also why TDM can be used to detect noncompliance. We note that for many agents, assays are not yet available or insufficient pharmacokinetic data exist to interpret plasma drug level results. Nonetheless, it is surprising how many drugs can be monitored, including most newer antidepressants, antipsychotics, and mood stabilizers.

CLINICAL APPLICATION OF PHARMACOKINETIC PRINCIPLES

Knowing the differential pharmacokinetics for a class of drugs allows the clinician to

choose specific members to either achieve a faster onset or a delayed offset of action (13, 14, 17, 18). For example, lorazepam is rapidly absorbed from the gastrointestinal tract into the systemic circulation and from there distributed into the brain. In contrast, oxazepam, the most polar BZD, is slowly absorbed from the gastrointestinal tract. Even after oxazepam is in the systemic circulation, it slowly enters tissue compartments, including the brain, during the distribution phase. Unlike lorazepam, oxazepam is not available in either the intramuscular or intravenous formulations. Thus, lorazepam would be preferable to achieve acute control of alcohol withdrawal (e.g., delirium tremens), whereas oxazepam would better stabilize a dependency-prone patient on sedative-hypnotics, because it does not cause the euphoria seen with the more rapidly absorbed members of this class.

Pharmacokinetics determines how long a drug's action will persist. For drugs that induce *tolerance*, knowledge of their elimination half-life can be used to predict the timing of a withdrawal syndrome after discontinuation. Again, a good example is the BZDs, because the principal difference among them is their pharmacokinetics rather than pharmacodynamics (17, 18). Thus, all these agents produce sedative-hypnotic tolerance, which may cause a minor (e.g., sleeplessness, increased anxiety) or a major (e.g., withdrawal delirium) abstinence syndrome when discontinued. When drugs are given in bioequivalent doses (i.e., adjusting the dose to compensate for differences in potency), the major determinant of the likelihood and the severity of an abstinence syndrome is their half-life. Longer acting BZDs (e.g., clonazepam) have their own *built-in taper* due to slow clearance, allowing time for readjustment of compensatory changes in the brain that eliminate or blunt withdrawal symptoms. In contrast, BZDs with very short half-lives (e.g., alprazolam) are more likely to produce withdrawal syndromes (93–96). This pharmacokinetic fact is the rationale for switching short-half-life BZD-dependent patients to an equipotent dose of a long-lived BZD, which can then be tapered more safely. The same is true for the withdrawal syndrome that can occur with selective serotonin reuptake inhibitors, being more common with short- (e.g., fluvoxamine, paroxetine) than with long-half-life (e.g., fluoxetine) members of this class (47, 48).

Differences in the half-life ($t_{1/2}$) determine how frequently drugs must be taken to maintain the desired effect. The knowledgeable practitioner will choose an agent from a class of similar compounds based in part on how well its pharmacokinetics meet the needs for which it is prescribed. When a clinician wants an immediate, but short-lived effect, the ideal agent would be rapidly absorbed into the systemic circulation and distributed into the brain, and then rapidly redistributed to other body compartments for eventual clearance. *Termination of the acute effects of a single dose of a psychotropic is primarily the result of redistribution from the brain to other body fat compartments, rather than final elimination* (13, 14, 17, 18). Sleep induction is a situation in which a rapid onset and reasonably rapid offset are desirable. In other situations, rapidity of onset might be less important than a sustained effect. Examples of the latter include maintenance and prophylactic strategies to prevent the recurrence of seizures, panic attacks, psychosis, or manic episodes. A short-lived agent, which requires multiple daily dosing to maintain effective concentrations, increases the likelihood of noncompliance, thus increasing the risk of relapse. Conversely, drugs such as fluoxetine have such long half-lives that the full effect can take weeks to develop and will persist for weeks after discontinuation. Such drugs can be considered depot preparations and may be best reserved for situations in which the benefits outweigh the disadvantages of such pharmacokinetics.

Single-Dose Prediction Test

The slope of the terminal elimination phase of the plasma drug concentration versus time curve can be used to predict the C_{SS} that will be achieved on a given drug dose (97). This strategy usually involves measuring the blood level 24 to 36 hours after a test dose. That level is a function of an individual's ability to eliminate the drug and hence is a measure of the individual's K_e. Because the K_e that determines the 24-hour single dose level is the same K_e that determines the C_{SS}, it can be used to predict the eventual C_{SS} on a given dose. Assuming linear pharmacokinetics, a change in dose will produce a proportional change in blood level, allowing the clinician to predict the dose required to achieve a desired concentration (e.g., see the section "Pharmacokinetics/Plasma Levels" in Chapter 5).

With repeated administration there is an ascending concentration until steady-state is reached. At that point, the concentration remains in a narrow range with continued drug administration, assuming that it does not influence its own metabolism (i.e., autoinduction or autoinhibition discussed earlier in this chapter).

Limitations Of Pharmacokinetics

This chapter has emphasized the clinical relevance of pharmacokinetics. However, there are limitations which are particularly important to consider when interpreting TDM results.

As pointed out in at the beginning of the chapter in Eq. 1, pharmacokinetics is only one of three variables that determine drug effect. Although a drug cannot exert its action without reaching a critical concentration at its *site of action,* achieving that concentration will not result in a clinically meaningful response if the site of action of the drug is not relevant to the disease the patient has. Also, there can be mutations in the site of action just as there are in cytochrome P450 enzymes. Such mutations in receptors can alter the binding affinity of the drug such that a different concentration is needed to occupy the target to a clinically meaningful degree. That phenomenon can explain why some patients may need a different concentration of the drug to achieve clinical benefit even though the drug is working through the same site of action (e.g., in a patient needing a lower concentration).

Another limitation is that the concentration most often measured is not the concentration of the drug at the site of action (Eq. 1). For convenience, most pharmacokinetics and most TDM is based on measuring the concentration of the drug in plasma, used as a surrogate for the concentration at the site of action. Although plasma drug concentration is reliably correlated with brain concentration, and even specific brain receptor occupancy as measured by positron emission tomography, there is still the possibility for differences in this relationship among individuals (1–3).

Other limitations stem from the fact that blood is actually composed of multiple compartments: cells, platelets, proteins, and plasma water (16). The cells, platelets, and proteins are analogous to peripheral compartments whereas water is the central compartment. It is the "free" concentration of drug in plasma water that is in equilibrium with the site of action. However, the concentration measured in plasma is generally the total concentration (free plus drug bound to plasma protein). Thus, changes in distribution can affect TDM results without reflecting a change in free drug concentration, site occupancy, and hence drug effect.

One such distribution phenomenon can occur as a result of *hemolysis* of the sample. Preparation of the TDM sample involves centrifugation to separate the cells and platelets from the plasma. If the sample is hemolyzed, then the centrifugation may not adequately separate cell fragments from the plasma. That can result in an increase in the apparent concentration of drug in plasma.

Protein binding is another distribution phenomenon that can affect TDM results (16). Most, but not all, psychiatric medications are highly protein bound such that modest changes in protein binding can theoretically result in large differences in the free fraction which is the concentration in equilbrium with the receptor. Theoretically, the displacement of the drug from its protein binding site by another drug could increase the free fraction of drug and thus receptor occupancy even though that change would not be reflected in the total drug concentration. Although this issue is commonly raised as a potential clinically important drug–drug interaction, that is rarely the case. *A more common problem is increased levels of circulating reactive protein* which can lead to increased total drug concentration (bound plus free) without changing the free concentration. A1-Acid glycoprotein is an example of a reactive protein which can be increased as a result of acute or chronic inflammatory processes (29). In such cases, the apparent drug concentration can increase in a given patient as a result of an acute infection, for example, without a change in the magnitude of drug effect because the free fraction remains the same.

There can also be *assay problems*. Common analytic approaches used in routine TDM involve either gas or liquid chromatography or antibody assays. These assays depend on the physiochemical properties of the drug to separate it from other elements in the plasma, typically by passing the sample through a separation column and then using a detector to measure the concentration. If the patient is on other drugs that are structurally similar to the drug of interest, the assay may not separate these two entities. In such a case, the concentration reported can be a combination of the concentrations of one or more drugs. **Thus, the patient's TDM results may change if the patient is taking a coprescribed drug not because of an interaction but because of a limitation in the assay.**

Another factor to be considered is the possibility of a *temporal dissociation* between changes in drug concentration and changes in drug effect (6, 98). Whereas a drug cannot exert an effect until it has reached its site of action, occupancy of the site does not necessarily coincide with the onset of a clinical effect. The clinically desired effect may result from an adaptational response of the brain to the occupancy of the site of action (e.g., receptor down-regulation). In such an instance, the drug concentration must be achieved and sustained for a period of time before the desired clinical action is realized. The reverse of such a temporal dissociation can occur when the drug is stopped (i.e., drug effect persists for a period of time after the drug has cleared from the body). Both of types of temporal dissociation must be considered when interpreting TDM results.

CONCLUSION

This chapter reviewed important pharmacokinetic principles of fundamental relevance to understanding much of what will be discussed subsequently. Understanding the pharmacokinetics of a drug is essential to the safe and effective prescribing of medications. Through the use of these principles, the clinician can frequently correct less than optimal outcomes. Knowledge of these principles is essential to understanding both the advantages and limitations of TDM. Reference to the principles reviewed in this chapter will frequently occur in subsequent chapters on specific drug therapies.

GLOSSARY

Absorption   Process by which a drug passes from the site of administration to the systemic circulation.

Area under curve (AUC)   The total area under the plot-of-drug concentration versus time following either a single dose or multiple doses of a specific drug product (e.g., formulation) in a specific patient by a specific route of administration.

Autoinduction   The induction of enzymes responsible for the biotransformation of a drug by the drug itself, such that the half-life decreases with chronic exposure to the drug (e.g., carbamazepine).

Autoinhibition   The inhibition or saturation of the highest affinity enzymes responsible for the biotransformation of a drug by the drug itself, such that lower affinity enzymes become important in elimination and the half-life increases with chronic exposure to the drug (e.g., fluoxetine, paroxetine).

Bioavailability   Fraction of the dose administered that is absorbed and reaches the systemic circulation as active drug. This fraction will range between 0 and 1.0.

Biotransformation   The process by which a drug is converted to more polar substances (i.e., metabolites), which are then eliminated from the body either in the urine or in the stool (e.g., demethylated and hydroxylated metabolites of tricyclic antidepressants; the three metabolites of bupropion).

Clearance (Cl)   The volume of plasma completely cleared of drug per unit of time, generally per minute.

Concentration maximum (C_{max}) The highest or peak plasma drug concentration occurring after a dose.

Concentration minimum (C_{min}) The lowest or trough plasma drug concentration occurring before the next dose.

Distribution Process by which a drug moves from the systemic circulation to the target site (e.g., brain) and to other tissue compartments (e.g., heart, adipose tissue).

Dosing rate The amount of drug delivered to the body per interval of time by a specific route of administration (i.e., oral [p.o.], intramuscular [i.m.], or intravenous [i.v.]).

Elimination half-life ($t_{1/2}$, plasma half-life) the time necessary for the concentration of drug in a bodily compartment (usually plasma) to decrease by one half as a result of clearance. Half-life is generally measured in hours. For psychotropic medications, half-life can be as short as 2 to 4 hours (e.g., triazolam to as long as 20 days (e.g., norfluoxetine, the demethylated metabolite of fluoxetine).

Elimination rate constant (K_e) Rate of decrease in drug concentration per unit of time as a result of elimination from the body.

Enterohepatic recirculation The reabsorption of drug and/or metabolites from the small bowel into the portal circulation after first pass metabolism has occurred. Such recirculation contributes to the total amount of drug and/or metabolites, which eventually enters the systemic circulation (e.g., demethylated and hydroxylated metabolites of tricyclic antidepressants).

First-order kinetics The amount of drug eliminated per unit of time is directly proportional to its concentration. In this state, the mechanisms for biotransformation and elimination are not saturated (e.g., benzodiazepines, tricyclic antidepressants, lithium carbonate).

First-pass metabolism (first-pass effect) The passage of the drug from the portal circulation into hepatocytes and conversion there into metabolites. These metabolites may have a pharmacological profile different from that of the parent drug. They are typically then excreted by the hepatocytes into the biliary system and pass back into the small bowel where enterohepatic recirculation may occur (e.g., benzodiazepines, bupropion, nefazodone, neuroleptics, tricyclic antidepressants).

Percent protein binding Percentage of the drug present in plasma that is bound to plasma protein under physiological conditions. Many drugs, especially acidic agents such as phenytoin, are bound to albumin. Basic drugs, such as tricyclic antidepressants, may bind extensively to $\alpha 1$-acid glycoprotein. Levels of this protein can rise during acute inflammatory reactions (e.g., infections) and cause a temporary increase in plasma drug levels of no clinical consequence.

Pharmacodynamics What the drug does to the body. The mechanisms of action exerted by the drug such as cholinergic receptor blockade (e.g., benztropine).

Pharmacokinetics What the body does to the drug. The process of drug absorption from the site of administration, distribution to the target organ and other bodily compartments, metabolism or biotransformation (if necessary), and eventual elimination.

Plasma drug concentration-time curve A plot of the changes in plasma drug concentration as a function of time following single or multiple doses of a drug. This curve represents the series of events that follow the absorption of the drug into the systemic circulation: (a) the rate and the magnitude of the rise of plasma drug concentration; (b) the decline in plasma drug concentrations as a result of distribution to the target site (i.e., the brain for psychotropic drugs) and other tissue compartments where the drug may be active (e.g., the heart) or simply stored (e.g., the adipose tissue); and (c) the eventual decline due to biotransformation (if necessary) and elimination.

Steady-state concentration (C_{SS}) The condition under which drug concentration does not change as a result of continued drug administration at the same dosing rate. The amount administered per dosing interval equals the amount eliminated per dosing interval.

Therapeutic drug monitoring (TDM) Based on the ability to quantitate the concentration of drug and its clinically relevant metabolites in a biological sample such as plasma. Using this information, the physician can rationally adjust the dose to achieve a plasma drug concentration within the range in which optimal response occurs for most patients, in terms of both efficacy and safety. Such monitoring is used primarily for drugs that have a narrow therapeutic index and wide interindividual variability in clearance rates (e.g., bupropion, clozapine, lithium, some anticonvulsants, tricyclic antidepressants).

Therapeutic index The difference between the maximally efficacious dose or concentration and the toxic dose or concentration.

Therapeutic range The concentration of drug in plasma that usually provides a therapeutically desirable response in the majority of individuals without substantial risk of serious toxicity. The target concentration for an individual patient is usually chosen from within the therapeutic range.

Time maximum (T_{max}) The time needed to reach the maximal plasma concentration following a dose. T_{max} can vary depending on the route of administration and formulation of the product (e.g., immediate versus sustained-release forms).

Volume of distribution (V_d) The apparent volume into which the drug must have been distributed to reach a specific concentration. Many psychotropic drugs have much larger apparent volumes of distribution than would be expected based on physical size of the body, because the drugs dissolve disproportionately more in lipid and protein compartments (i.e., tissue) than in the body's water compartment.

Zero order kinetics Situation in which only a fixed amount of drug eliminated per unit of time regardless of plasma concentration because all mechanisms mediating elimination are saturated.

REFERENCES

1. Seeman P, Tallerico T. Antipsychotic drugs which elicit little or no parkinsonism bind more loosely than dopamine to brain D2 receptors, yet occupy high levels of these receptors. *Mol Psychiatry* 1998;3:123–134.
2. Seeman P. Therapeutic receptor-blocking concentrations of neuroleptics. *Int Clin Psychopharmacol* 1995;10(suppl 3):5–13.
3. Farde L, Nordstrom A-L, Wiesel F-A, et al. Positron emission tomographic analysis of central D1 and D2 dopamine receptor occupancy in patients treated with classical neuroleptics and clozapine. *Arch Gen Psychiatry* 1992;49:538–544.
4. Holford NHG, Sheiner LB. Understanding the dose-effect relationship: clinical application of pharmacokinetic-pharmacodynamic models. *Clin Pharmacokinet* 1981;6:429–453.
5. Kenakin TP. *Pharmacologic analysis of drug-receptor interaction.* New York: Raven Press, 1987.
6. Ross EM. Pharmacodynamics: mechanisms of drug action and the relationship between drug concentration and effect. In: Hardman JG, Limbird L, Molinoff P, et al., eds. *The pharmacological basis of therapeutics.* New York: McGraw-Hill, 1996:29–42.
7. Baker GB. Drug metabolism and psychiatry: introduction. *Cell Mol Neurobiol* 1999;19:301–308.
8. Klotz U. Effect of age on pharmacokinetics and pharmacodynamics in man. *Int J Clin Pharmacol Ther* 1998; 36:581–585.
9. Thurmann PA, Hompesch BC. Influence of gender on the pharmacokinetics and pharmacodynamics of drugs. *Int J Clin Pharmacol Ther* 1998;36:586–590.
10. Coutts RT, Urichuk LJ. Polymorphic cytochromes P450 and drugs used in psychiatry. *Cell Mol Neurobiol* 1999;19:325–354.
11. Preskorn SH. Clinically relevant pharmacology of selective serotonin reuptake inhibitors. An overview with emphasis on pharmacokinetics and effects on oxidative drug metabolism. *Clin Pharmacokinet* 1997;32(suppl 1):1–21.
12. Janicak PG, Davis JM. Pharmacokinetics and drug interactions. In: BJ Sadock, V Sadock, eds. *Kaplan & Sadock's comprehensive textbook of psychiatry, Vol. 2,* 7th ed. Philadelphia: Lippincott Williams & Wilkins, 2000:2250–2259.
13. Greenblatt DJ, Ehrenberg BL, Gunderman JS, et al. Pharmacokinetic and electroencephalographic study of intravenous diazepam, midazolam and placebo. *Clin Pharmacol Ther* 1989;45(4):356–365.
14. Hegarty JE, Dundee JW. Sequelae after the intravenous injection of three benzodiazepines—diazepam, lorazepam and flunitrazepam. *Br Med J* 1977;22:1384–1385.
15. Greenblatt DJ, von Moltke LL, Shader RI. The importance of presystemic extraction in clinical psychopharmacology. *J Clin Psychopharmacol* 1996;16:417–419.
16. Benet LZ, Kroetz DL, Sheiner LB. Pharmacokinetics: the dynamics of drug absorption, distribution, and elimination. In: Hardman JG, Limbird L, Molinoff P, et al., eds. *The pharmacological basis of therapeutics.* New York: McGraw-Hill, 1996:3–28.
17. Greenblatt DJ, Shader RI. Clinical pharmacokinetics of the benzodiazepines. In: Smith DE, Wesson DR, eds. *The benzodiazepines: current standards for medical practice.* Lancaster, U.K.: MTP Press, 1985:43–50.
18. Vgontzas AN, Kales A, Bixler EO. Benzodiazepine side effects: role of pharmacokinetics and pharmacodynamics. *Pharmacology* 1995;51:205–223.
19. Schwartz LL. The debate over substitution policy. Its evolution and scientific bases. *Am J Med* 1985;79:38–44.
20. DeVane CL, Pollock BG. Pharmacokinetic considerations of antidepressant use in the elderly. *J Clin Psychiatry* 1999;60(suppl 20):38–44.
21. Weller R, Preskorn SH. Psychotropic drugs and alcohol: pharmacokinetic and pharmacodynamic interactions. *Psychosomatics* 1984;25:301–309.
22. MacKichan JJ. Protein binding drug displacement interactions: fact or fiction? *Clin Pharmacokinet* 1989;16:65–73.
23. Vallner JJ. Binding of drugs by albumin and plasma protein. *J Pharm Sci* 1977;66:447–465.
24. Routledge PA. The plasma protein binding of basic drugs. *Br J Clin Pharmacol* 1986;22:499–506.

25. Campion EW, deLabry LO, Glynn RJ. The effect of age on serum albumin in healthy males: report from the normative aging study. *J Gerontol* 1988;43:M18–M20.
26. Cusack B, O'Malley K, Lavan J, et al. Protein binding and disposition of lidocaine in the elderly. *Eur J Clin Pharmacol* 1985;29:232–329.
27. Goulden KJ, Dooley JM, Camfield PR, et al. Clinical valproate toxicity induced by acetylsalicylic acid. *Neurology* 1987;37:1392–1394.
28. Paxton JW. Effects of aspirin on salivary and serum phenytoin kinetics in healthy subjects. *Clin Pharmacol Ther* 1980;27:170–178.
29. Abernethy DR, Kertzner L. Age effects on alpha-1-acid glycoprotein concentration and imipramine plasma protein binding. *J Am Geriatr Soc* 1984;32:705–708.
30. Edelman JS, Leibman J. Anatomy of body water and electrolytes. *Am J Med* 1959;27:256–277.
31. Parker BM, Cusack BJ, Vestal RE. Pharmacokinetic optimisation of drug therapy in elderly patients. *Drugs Aging* 1995;7:10–18.
32. Cohen LJ. Principles to optimize drug treatment in the depressed elderly: practical pharmacokinetics and drug interactions. *Geriatrics* 1995;50(suppl 1):S32–S40.
33. Glotzbach RK, Preskorn SH. Brain concentrations of tricyclic antidepressants: single-dose kinetics and relationship to plasma concentrations in chronically dosed rats. *Psychopharmacology* 1982;78:25–27.
34. Kornhuber J, Retz W, Riederer P. Slow accumulation of psychotropic substances in the human brain. Relationship to therapeutic latency of neuroleptic and antidepressant drugs? *J Neural Transm Suppl* 1995;46:315–323.
35. Preskorn SH. *Clinical pharmacology of selective serotonin reuptake inhibitors.* Caddo, OK: Professional Communications, 1996:1–255.
36. Richelson E. Pharmacokinetic interactions of antidepressants. *J Clin Psychiatry* 1998;59(suppl 10):22–26.
37. Preskorn SH, Alderman J, Chung M, et al. Pharmacokinetics of desipramine coadministered with sertraline or fluoxetine. *J Clin Psychopharmacol* 1994;14:90–98.
38. Jandhyala B, Steenberg M, Perel J, et al. Effects of several tricyclic antidepressants on the hemodynamics and myocardial contractility of the anesthetized dogs. *Eur J Pharmacol* 1977;42:403–410.
39. Pippenger CE. Clinically significant carbamazepine drug interactions: an overview. *Epilepsia* 1987;28:571–576.
40. Spina E, Pisani F, Perucca E. Clinically significant pharmacokinetic drug interactions with carbamazepine. An update. *Clin Pharmacokinet* 1996;31:198–214.
41. Tanaka E, Hisawa S. Clinically significant pharmacokinetic drug interactions with psychoactive drugs: antidepressants and antipsychotics and the cytochrome P450 system. *J Clin Pharm Ther* 1999;24:7–16.
42. Naranjo CA, Sproule BA, Knoke DM. Metabolic interactions of central nervous system medications and selective serotonin reuptake inhibitors. *Int Clin Psychopharmacol* 1999;14(suppl 2):S35–S47.
43. Fonne-Pfister R, Meyer UA. Xenobiotic and endobiotic inhibitors of cytochrome P-450dbl function, the target of the debrisoquine/sparteine type polymorphism. *Biochem Pharmacol* 1988;37:3829–3835.
44. Wright JM, Stokes EF, Sweeney VP. Isoniazid-induced carbamazepine toxicity and vice versa: a double drug interaction. *N Engl J Med* 1982;307:1325–1327.
45. Ragheb M, Ban TA, Buchanan D, et al. Interaction of indomethacin and ibuprofen with lithium in manic pa-

tients under a steady-state lithium level. *J Clin Psychiatry* 1980;41:397–398.
46. Mehta BR, Robinson BHB. Lithium toxicity induced by triamterene-hydrochlorothiazide. *Postgrad Med J* 1980;56:783–784.
47. Coupland NJ, Bell CJ, Potokar JP. Serotonin reuptake inhibitor withdrawal. *J Clin Psychopharmacol* 1996; 16:356–362.
48. Kitanaka I, Ross RJ, Cutler NR, et al. Altered hydroxy-desipramine concentration in elderly depressed patients. *Clin Pharmacol Ther* 1982;31:51–55.
49. Nelson JC, Jatlow P. Nonlinear desipramine kinetics: prevalence and importance. *Clin Pharmacol Ther* 1987;41:666–670.
50. Preskorn SH. *Outpatient management of depression: a guide for the primary-care practitioner.* Caddo, OK: Professional Communications, 1999.
51. Shad MU, Preskorn SH. Antidepressants. In: Levy RH, Thummel KE, Trager WF, et al., eds. *Metabolic drug interactions.* Philadelphia: Lippincott Williams & Wilkins, 2000:563–577.
52. Bertilsson L, Dahl ML, Tybring G. Pharmacogenetics of antidepressants: clinical aspects. *Acta Psychiatr Scand Suppl* 1997;391:14–21.
53. Greenblatt DJ, von Moltke LL, Harmatz JS, et al. Human cytochromes and some newer antidepressants: kinetics, metabolism, and drug interactions. *J Clin Psychopharmacol* 1999;19:23S–35S.
54. von Moltke LL, Greenblatt DJ, Schmider J, et al. *In vitro* approaches to predicting drug interactions *in vivo*. *Biochem Pharmacol* 1998;55:113–122.
55. Schmider J, von Moltke LL, Shader RI, et al. Extrapolating *in vitro* data on drug metabolism to *in vivo* pharmacokinetics: evaluation of the pharmacokinetic interaction between amitriptyline and fluoxetine. *Drug Metab Rev* 1999;31:545–560.
56. Wrighton SA, Ring BJ. Predicting drug interactions and pharmacokinetic variability with *in vitro* methods: the olanzapine experience. *Drug Metab Rev* 1999;31:15–28.
57. Bertz RJ, Granneman GR. Use of *in vitro* and *in vivo* data to estimate the likelihood of metabolic pharmacokinetic interactions. *Clin Pharmacokinet* 1997;32:210–258.
58. Loiseau P. Treatment of concomitant illnesses in patients receiving anticonvulsants: drug interactions of clinical significance. *Drug Safety* 1998;19:495–510.
59. Crowley JJ, Cusack BJ, Jue SG, et al. Aging and drug interactions: II. Effect of phenytoin and smoking on the oxidation of theophylline and cortisol in healthy men. *J Pharmacol Exp Ther* 1988;345:513–523.
60. Greenblatt DJ, von Moltke LL, Harmatz JS, et al. Drug interactions with newer antidepressants: role of human cytochromes P450. *J Clin Psychiatry* 1998;59(suppl 15): 19–27.
61. Preskorn SH, Beber JH, Faul JC, et al. Serious adverse effects of combining fluoxetine and tricyclic antidepressants. *Am J Psychiatry* 1990;147:532.
62. Preskorn SH, Baker B. Fatality associated with combined fluoxetine-amitriptyline therapy. *JAMA* 1997;277:682.
63. Yonkers KA, Kando JC, Hamilton J. Gender issues in psychopharmacologic treatment. *Essent Psychopharmacol* 1996;1:54–69.
64. Bhanthumnavin K, Schuster MM. Aging and gastrointestinal function. In: Finch CE, Hayflick L, eds. *Handbook of the biology of aging.* New York: Van Nostrand Reinhold, 1977:709–723.

65. Evans MA, Triggs EJ, Cheung M, et al. Gastric emptying rate in the elderly: implications for drug therapy. *J Am Geriatr Soc* 1981;29:201–205.
66. Wallace SM, Verbeek RK. Plasma protein binding of drugs in the elderly. *Clin Pharmacokinet* 1987;12:41–72.
67. Shock NW, Watkin DM, Yiengst BS, et al. Age differences in the water content of the body as related to basal oxygen consumption in males. *J Gerontol* 1963;18:1–8.
68. Vestal RE, Cusack BJ. Pharmacology and aging. In: Schneider EL, Rowe JW, eds. *Handbook of the biology of aging.* San Diego: Academic Press, 1990:349–383.
69. Bupp S, Preskorn SH. The effect of age on plasma levels of nortriptyline. *Ann Clin Psychiatry* 1991;3:61–65.
70. Schmucker DL. Aging and drug disposition: an update. *Pharmacol Rev* 1979;30:445–456.
71. Klotz U, Avant GR, Hoyumpa A, et al. The effects of age and liver disease on the disposition and elimination of diazepam in adult man. *J Clin Invest* 1975;55:347–359.
72. Berlinger WJ, Goldberg MJ, Spector R, et al. Diphenhydramine: kinetics and psychomotor effects in elderly women. *Clin Pharmacol Ther* 1982;32:387–391.
73. Cusack B, Kelly J, O'Malley K, et al. Digozin in the elderly: pharmacokinetic consequences of old age. *Clin Pharmacol Ther* 1979;25:772–776.
74. Castleden CM, George CF. The effect of aging on the hepatic clearance of propranolol. *Br J Clin Pharmacol* 1979;7:49–54.
75. Feely J, Crooks J, Stevenson IH. The influence of age, smoking and hyperthydroidism on plasma propranolol steady state concentration. *Br J Clin Pharmacol* 1981;12:73–78.
76. Greenblatt DJ, Divoll M, Abernethy DR, et al. Antipyrine kinetics in the elderly: prediction of age-related changes in benzodiazepine oxidizing capacity. *J Pharmacol Exp Ther* 1982;220:120–126.
77. Hayes MJ, Langman MJS, Short AH. Changes in drug metabolism with increasing age: 2. Phenytoin clearance and protein binding. *Br J Clin Pharmacol* 1975;2:73–79.
78. Mucklow JC, Fraser HS. The effects of age and smoking upon antipyrine metabolism. *Br J Clin Pharmacol* 1980;9:612–614.
79. Woodhouse KW, Mutch E, Williams FM, et al. The effect of age on pathways of drug metabolism in human liver. *Age Aging* 1984;13:328–334.
80. Woodhouse KW, Wynne HA. Age related changes in liver size and hepatic blood flow: the influence of drug metabolism in the elderly. *Clin Pharmacokinet* 1988;15:287–294.
81. Wynne HA, Cope LH, Mutch E, et al. The effect of age upon liver volume and apparent liver blood flow in healthy man. *Hepatology* 1989;9:297–301.
82. Beers MH, Ouslander JG. Risk factors in geriatric drug prescribing: a practical guide to avoiding problems. *Drugs* 1989;37:105–112.
83. Preskorn SH. Tricyclic antidepressants: the whys and hows of therapeutic drug monitoring. *J Clin Psychiatry* 1989;50(suppl 7):34–42.
84. Preskorn SH, Mac D. The implication of concentration-response studies of tricyclic antidepressants for psychiatric research and practice. *Psychiatr Dev* 1984;3:201–222.
85. Preskorn SH, Fast GA. Therapeutic drug monitoring for antidepressants: efficacy, safety and cost effectiveness. *J Clin Psychiatry* 1991;52(suppl 6):23–33.
86. Miller DD. The clinical use of clozapine plasma concentrations in the management of treatment-refractory schizophrenia. *Ann Clin Psychiatry* 1996;8:99–109.
87. Eilers R. Therapeutic drug monitoring for the treatment of psychiatric disorders. Clinical use and cost effectiveness. *Clin Pharmacokinet* 1995;29:442–450.
88. Olesen OV. Therapeutic drug monitoring of clozapine treatment. Therapeutic threshold value for serum clozapine concentrations. *Clin Pharmacokinet* 1998;34:497–502.
89. Freeman DJ, Oyewumi LK. Will routine therapeutic drug monitoring have a place in clozapine therapy? *Clin Pharmacokinet* 1997;32:93–100.
90. Preskorn SH, Jerkovich GS. Central nervous system toxicity of tricyclic antidepressants: phenomenology, course, risk factors and role of therapeutic drug monitoring. *J Clin Psychopharmacol* 1990;10:88–95.
91. Preskorn SH, Fast GA. Tricyclic antidepressant induced seizures and plasma drug concentration. *J Clin Psychiatry* 1992;53:160–162.
92. Alldredge BK. Seizure risk associated with psychotropic drugs: clinical and pharmacokinetic considerations. *Neurology* 1999;53:S68–S75.
93. Hollister LE, Motzenbecker FP, Degan RO. Withdrawal reactions from chlordiazepoxide ("librium"). *Psychopharmacology* 1961;2:63–68.
94. Harrison M, Gusto U, Naranjo CA, et al. Diazepam tapering in detoxification of high-dose benzodiazepine abuse. *Clin Pharmacol Ther* 1984;36:527–532.
95. Miller LG, Greenblatt DJ, Barnhill JG, et al. Chronic benzodiazepine administrations: I. tolerance is associated with benzodiazepine receptor downregulation and decreased aminobutyric acid receptor complex binding and function. *J Pharmacol Exp Ther* 1987;246:170–176.
96. Miller LG, Greenblatt DJ, Roy RB, et al. Chronic benzodiazepine administration: II. Discontinuation syndrome is associated with upregulation of aminobutyric acid receptor complex binding and function. *J Pharmacol Exp Ther* 1987;246:177–182.
97. Madakasira S, Preskorn SH, Weller R, et al. Single dose prediction of steady state plasma levels of amitriptyline. *J Clin Psychopharmacol* 1982;2:136–139.
98. Lemmer B. Clinical chronopharmacology: the importance of time in drug treatment. *Ciba Found Symp* 1995;183:235–253.

4

Indications for Antipsychotics

The primary indication for this group of drugs is the presence of psychosis in such disparate disorders as:

- *Schizophrenia*
- *Schizophreniform* disorder
- *Schizoaffective* disorder
- *Delusional* (paranoid) disorder
- *Brief psychotic* disorder
- *Mood* disorders with mood-congruent or incongruent psychotic symptoms
- *Psychoses secondary* to a nonpsychiatric medical condition

Because the most common condition studied is schizophrenia, this is the primary disorder discussed. We also consider "schizophrenic spectrum" (e.g., delusional, schizophreniform, schizoaffective); mood disorders with psychotic features; and various nonpsychotic conditions (e.g., in the developmentally disabled) for which antipsychotics have been used (see Appendices A, C, E, F, and G).

SCHIZOPHRENIA

History of the Concept

The identification of this illness in modern psychiatry began with Kahlbaum, who described catatonia; Hecker, who described hebephrenia; and Emil Kraepelin, who described dementia praecox (1–4).

The syndrome identified by Kraepelin is similar to the *Diagnostic and Statistical Manual of Mental Disorders,* 4th ed., revised (DSM-IV) (5) diagnosis of schizophrenia and to the Research Diagnostic Criteria (RDC) definition of chronic schizophrenia. It usually begins in adolescence or young adulthood, and frequently follows a progressively deteriorating course, with few patients ever achieving complete recovery.

In contrast to Kraepelin, who emphasized the progressive course and poor outcome, the Swiss psychiatrist Eugen Bleuler (6) used a much broader concept of schizophrenia. Focusing on the thought disorder and the inconsistent, inappropriate, and disorganized affect, he identified four fundamental symptoms:

- Autism
- Ambivalence
- Abnormal thoughts
- Abnormal affect

He also emphasized the incongruent relationships among thought, emotions, and behavior. Unlike his predecessors, he did not believe hallucinations and delusions were fundamental to the schizophrenic process, considering them accessory symptoms.

Historically, the diagnosis of schizophrenia in the United States has been based on bleulerian and psychoanalytic theory, partly due to the greater influence of the latter group in the 1950's and 1960's. In contrast, European psychiatry used a narrower set of diagnostic criteria, similar to Kraepelin's approach.

Psychoanalytic theory conceptualized schizophrenia as the use of primitive defenses (e.g., denial) against anxiety in the presence of a weakened ego. Because these patients are unable to use more mature defenses against id-derived impulses, they regress to a more primitive level of functioning, with the intrusion of primary process thinking into consciousness. Because this condition was seen as a severe regression, almost any significantly ill patient could be diagnosed as schizophrenic. If this hypothesis were true, anxiolytics should have an antipsychotic effect, but that is typically not the case. Further, antipsychotics have a different biochemical action (e.g., dopamine and serotonin receptor blockade) than the antianxiety agents (e.g., modulation of γ-aminobutyric acid (GABA) receptor–chloride ion channels), constituting both a mechanistic and a clinical difference between these two drug classes. More importantly, the relative lack of efficacy with anxiolytics undermines the theory that anxiety is critical to the pathogenesis of schizophrenia.

Another perspective comes from *family systems theory,* which characterizes the schizophrenic patient's family as having disordered communication, with various members playing unusual or aberrant roles. According to this theory, patients experience "double binds" when faced with contradictory expectations (7). Related controversial hypotheses held that the "schizophrenogenic" mother was the critical factor and then later that the schizophrenic's father also played a significant role (8–10). Intensive therapy, in the context of in-hospital separation from the family, was considered the treatment of choice. In contrast to classic psychodynamic therapy, which focuses on the individual patient, this approach attempts to resolve conflicts in the family system, as well as in the patient's psyche. Typically, this involves sessions that include all or as many members as possible. Thus, even though one member is identified as the patient, it is the disturbed communication and interactions among all members that is the focus of therapy. This and subsequent therapeutic approaches may be most effective when medication is used concurrently.

One of the more bizarre theories of schizophrenia is the *"labeling" theory.* Proponents feel that what is called "schizophrenia" is a label for individuals who are unable to function successfully in society.

Descriptive-Phenomenological Approach

At one time, schizophrenia was broadly defined, and almost all patients with moderate-to-severe psychotic symptoms were given this diagnosis. In contrast, bipolar disorder was defined very narrowly and only diagnosed in classic cases. Indeed, the prevalence of hospitalized patients diagnosed with schizophrenia in the United States was once almost double that in Great Britain. Conversely, mood disorders were diagnosed five times more frequently in Great Britain than in the United States. To explore these differences, the United States and the United Kingdom conducted a systematic, structured interview research study of patients in Brooklyn, New York, and London (11, 12). The Present State Examination (PSE) was used to standardize the diagnostic process. As a result, many schizophrenic patients in New York were rediagnosed as having mood disorders, usually psychotic depression or mania. This project also demonstrated that many patients in the United States diagnosed with schizophrenia would have received a diagnosis of mania or depression in the United Kingdom.

American psychiatry's approach to diagnosis began to change substantially with the development of specific diagnostic criteria (as well as the availability of effective treatments for bipolar disorder). These criteria were initially formulated by Feighner and Robins (the Feighner criteria), and later expanded by Spitzer, Endicott, and Robins into the RDC, which were the basis of the DSM-III, DSM-III-R, and DSM-IV (13–15). In addition to being more descriptive in orientation, this approach recognized the importance of empirical data to develop explicit inclusion and exclusion criteria, which can then be studied for reliability and validity.

Epidemiology

Throughout the world, the lifetime prevalence of schizophrenia is about 1%. Although the prevalence is slightly higher in the lower socioeconomic classes, data from a number of countries indicate that the social class distribution of the parents of schizophrenic probands is similar to that of the general population (16–18). This supports the *"social drift" hypothesis,* which postulates that the increased concentration of patients with schizophrenia in the lower socioeconomic stratum is the result of their impaired functioning.

Schizophrenic patients tend to be born during the late winter or early spring in the Western hemisphere, an observation that suggests the possibility of a viral infectious process in the mother and the fetus, most probably during the first trimester (19). A recent epidemiological report, however, indicates that viral exposure in utero may not be as critical. Rather, postpartum stressors in relationship to the number and age distribution of siblings may be more important (20). Although women have an onset of illness about 6 years later than men and the course of illness is somewhat milder, they have an increased incidence of illness onset at menopause, so the lifetime incidence is essentially identical.

Symptoms

Many conceptualize schizophrenia as a heterogeneous condition. Within this general categorization, patients may present with symptoms that can vary over the life cycle. Thus, some may manifest soft neurological signs early in life, develop florid positive symptoms in adolescence or young adulthood, and ultimately experience predominantly negative symptoms later in life. Others may develop positive symptoms only later in life that do not develop into the full deficit syndrome. Implicit in these observations is the possibility of varying genetic, developmental, and environmental influences, with the common underlying diathesis being psychosis (21).

Schizophrenia as presently conceptualized is characterized by symptom complexes such as *positive symptoms* (e.g., delusions and hallucinations) occurring in a clear sensorium and in the absence of a significant mood disturbance. It is also associated with *cognitive disturbances* such as illogical or tangential thinking. *Negative symptoms* (e.g., alogia, asociality, anergy, avolition, etc.) may be primary to the disorder (i.e., the deficit syndrome) or secondary to such concurrent issues as dysphoria or medication-induced neurological side effects. *Mood disturbances* are also common. For example, depression frequently occurs, may worsen with neuroleptics, and may improve with novel antipsychotics or the addition of an antidepressant. This information is important, given the increased suicidal behavior in these patients (22).

Delusions are false beliefs that the patient maintains in the face of incontrovertible, contradictory evidence. The schizophrenic patient usually has no insight that these beliefs are not real, but rather maintains a firm conviction in them. Schizophrenia is characterized by a variety of delusions, of which the persecutory type predominates. Other delusions often involve bizarre bodily changes. In contrast to delusional disorder, these delusions are not as well formed and occur in the context of other psychotic symptoms (e.g., hallucinations, negative symptoms).

Hallucinations are false perceptions in the absence of a real sensory stimulus. They are typically auditory, consisting of voices that arise from both within and outside the body. They may be threatening, can ridicule, or may urge patients to objectionable acts (i.e., command hallucinations). Visual hallucinations are also relatively frequent, but olfactory (e.g., unpleasant smells arising from the patient's own body) or tactile hallucinations (e.g., animals crawling inside one's body or insects crawling over the skin) are uncommon.

Catatonia (withdrawn type) is characterized by prolonged immobility, waxy flexibility, posturing, and grimacing. Because catatonic symptoms can also occur in other types of psychosis, they are not specific to schizophrenia.

Schneiderian, first-rank symptoms describe hallucinations and delusions thought to be typical of schizophrenics (23, 24). Examples include the following:

- *Audible thoughts* (i.e., voices speak the patient's thoughts out loud)
- *Voices arguing* (e.g., two or more voices argue or discuss issues, sometimes referring to the patient in the third person)
- *Voices commenting* on the patient's behavior
- *Somatic passivity* believed to be imposed by outside forces
- *Thought withdrawal* by outside forces, leaving the patient feeling as if his or her mind is empty
- *Thought insertions* by outside forces
- *Thought broadcasting* (i.e., thoughts escape from the patient's mind and are overheard by others)
- *Impulses, volitional acts, or feelings* that are not one's own but are imposed by outside forces
- *Delusional perceptions* (i.e., the patient attributes delusional meaning to normal perceptions)

Although positive symptoms are usually the focus of acute intervention and are at least partially responsive to neuroleptics, cognitive, mood, and negative symptoms are generally more debilitating, are less responsive to conventional agents, and may be more responsive to novel antipsychotics (e.g., clozapine, risperidone, olanzapine, quetiapine, ziprasidone).

Course of Illness

Several studies investigated the outcome in schizophrenic patients before antipsychotics were available (25–27) and generally found that an early onset of insidious symptoms, most characterized by negativity and a gradual deterioration into psychosis without clear precipitating events, was predictive of a poor outcome. These patients often demonstrated asocial and bizarre behavior during childhood and typically never married (28–31).

Longitudinal follow-up of carefully defined schizophrenia shows that approximately 95% have a lifetime illness and are rarely rediagnosed later as having a mood disorder (32, 33). They also often had the following characteristics:

- Poor performance in *school*
- Slightly *lower IQs*
- Abnormalities in *cognitive* and *motor* development
- *Visual-motor* incoordination
- *Proprioceptive* and *vestibular* difficulties

In contrast, patients with good premorbid personalities and more typical functioning during childhood who later developed schizophrenic symptoms, especially in the face of massive precipitating events, had better outcomes. They also tended to have family histories of mood disorders as well as affective features as part of their own illness, which led to the concept of process versus reactive schizophrenia (i.e., poor prognosis versus good prognosis) (34, 35).

Biological Correlates

In 1976, Johnstone, Crow, and coworkers (36) applied the then newly developed computed tomography (CT) imaging technology to study schizophrenic patients and reported *slightly larger ventricles* as compared with matched control subjects. Indeed, these abnormalities were first noted in 1927, when Jacoby and Winkley

(37) reported enlarged ventricles using pneumoencephalography, with a number of open studies subsequently confirming this result in the 1930s. Furthermore, patients with larger ventricles were usually more cognitively impaired and had fewer positive and more negative symptoms. Crow's suggestion of enlarged ventricles in association with negative symptoms spurred even more interest in this distinction. Subsequent studies with CT imaging and later with magnetic resonance imaging have verified that many people with schizophrenia have enlarged ventricles and associated cortical atrophy, especially in the temporal lobe and the hippocampal nuclei (38–41). Although schizophrenics do not show a specific abnormality like hydrocephalus, blind measurements over many studies have replicated these changes with several different radiographic techniques. It is important to note that the ventricular enlargement and the cortical atrophy are statistical phenomena. Thus, although the abnormality is present in 30–40% of schizophrenics, there is significant overlap with normal control subjects, as well as with a wide variety of other psychiatric conditions.

There is also evidence that the mothers of schizophrenics have a higher incidence of *obstetric complications*. Furthermore, schizophrenics have more *soft neurological signs* and *developmental anomalies* associated with fetal damage. All these complications occur more frequently in schizophrenics with *enlarged ventricles*.

In summary, enlarged ventricles and cortical atrophy are positively correlated with the following:

- *Negative* symptoms
- *Poor performance* on some neuropsychological tests
- The presence of *soft neurological signs*
- *Poor response* to treatment
- A *worse prognosis*

Finally, there is evidence that *blood flow* is reduced in schizophrenics, particularly to the frontal lobes, and that glucose metabolism, as measured by positron emission tomography, is reduced in the same area. This is particularly evident when a patient is stimulated with a mental task that induces frontal lobe activity, such as the Wisconsin Card Sort Test.

The implication of these findings for nomenclature is that these patients tend to present clinically as the kraepelinian, poor prognosis type.

Familial and Genetic Issues

There is an extensive literature showing that this disorder has a familial and hereditary pattern (42–45). Therefore, the genetic relatives of schizophrenic patients have an increased risk of developing this disorder. Several reviews of twin studies find that 30% to 65% of monozygotic twins are concordant for schizophrenia, in contrast to 0% to 28% of dizygotic twins (46–52).

There are also cross-fostering studies of children of schizophrenic parents, adopted away by nonschizophrenic foster parents, who were compared with adopted children of normal parents raised by schizophrenic foster parents (53, 54). Invariably, those children whose biological parents had schizophrenia developed this disorder more frequently than the offspring of nonschizophrenic parents, even when the latter were reared by schizophrenic foster families. In addition, the concordance rate for the illness in schizophrenic monozygotic twins reared apart was comparable with monozygotic twins reared together. **These findings leave little doubt of a hereditary factor in schizophrenia.**

The advent of molecular genetics has provided powerful techniques for chromosomal localization of these disorders, and there is intense ongoing investigation to localize the responsible gene (or genes) associated with schizophrenia. Presently, it is believed that several small susceptibility genes may be contributory. Because the search for gene location is essentially a statistical screening, some chance findings are expected to occur. Further, it is quite probable that the disorder is determined by more than one gene locus (55), which in turn may control sensitivity to various environmental influences (56).

A related issue is pharmacogenetics, which considers genetic factors (e.g., pharmacokinetics, pharmacodynamics) that determine an individual's clinical response and adverse effects to drugs such as the antipsychotics (57).

Cost of Schizophrenia

Schizophrenia is a devastating illness crippling virtually every aspect of an individual's identity. Thus, it interferes with the ability to correctly interpret perceptions, to relate appropriately to others on both a cognitive and an emotional basis, and to articulate one's thoughts clearly. Individuals with schizophrenia rarely achieve as much in life as their nonaffected age cohort. Before the discovery of antipsychotics, about 50% of hospital beds were occupied by these patients, and even now, they still occupy 25% of all beds. The disorder usually begins relatively early in life (i.e., late teens or early twenties) and rarely remits. It produces severe social deficits and at times chronic hospitalization for some. A substantial number of the homeless suffer from schizophrenia, as well as many who live isolated, unproductive lives in structured facilities. **In summary, schizophrenia represents a tragedy for both patients and their families and is a major burden to society.**

OTHER PSYCHOTIC DISORDERS

Schizophreniform Disorder

Patients with this condition manifest the symptoms of an acute exacerbation of schizophrenia, with symptoms lasting at least one month, but they make a complete recovery, with the prodromal, active, and residual phases remitting in less than 6 months.

Schizoaffective Disorder

Schizoaffective (SA) disorder is characterized by both psychotic and mood symptoms, with patients meeting the inclusion diagnostic criteria for acute schizophrenia and a major mood disorder. They should also have had a period during the episode of at least 2 weeks when psychotic symptoms predominate in the relative absence of mood symptoms. In addition, mood symptoms should be present for a substantial portion of an episode. This disorder can be further divided into SA-bipolar or SA-depressed subtypes. Although this disorder is not well understood, it has been considered as:

- A *variant of schizophrenia* (58)
- A *variant of a mood disorder*
- A combination of *both disorders* (59)
- A *separate entity* (60)
- A disorder representing the middle range on a *continuum between schizophrenia and mood disorders*

A number of studies on the heredity of SA disorder have found that these patients have more relatives with both mood and schizophrenic disorders, when compared with normal control subjects (61, 62). Although they also had some relatives with SA, the predominant familial illnesses are schizophrenia or an affective disorder. The course of illness and the prognosis appear to fall somewhere between that of mood and schizophrenic disorders. Thus, a greater percentage of SA disorder patients recover, with better functioning than schizophrenics, but they do not improve as much as those with pure mood disorders (63–65). The number of SA disorder patients who have a progressively deteriorating course also falls somewhere between that of schizophrenic and mood disorders. SA disorder-bipolar-type patients tend to have a family history, prognosis, and response to mood stabilizers consistent with classic bipolar disorder. In contrast, SA-depressed patients generally respond better to an antipsychotic and have a prognosis and family history more consistent with schizophrenia.

Delusional Disorder

This category is attributed to Kahlbaum and Kraepelin, who saw paranoia as a chronic, unremitting system of delusions distinguished by both the absence of hallucinations and the deterioration seen in schizophrenia. This disorder is characterized by one or more nonbizarre delusions of at least 1 month's duration.

Delusional disorder is relatively uncommon, with an incidence 25 times less than that of schizophrenia, although the true incidence may be greater, given the fact that such patients do not readily acknowledge their delusions. Both sexes are equally affected. The term *late paraphrenia* refers to the development of delusions (often with hallucinations) in elderly patients (i.e., patients over age 55 without preexisting major psychiatric illness). Interestingly, deafness is present in a substantial number of persons with this disorder.

Delusions can be held throughout life despite considerable contradictory evidence, which is usually reinterpreted to coincide with one's false beliefs. They are usually highly systematized, interrelated by a common theme, and often encapsulated (i.e., a person's thinking remains unimpaired except for the systematized delusions, which depart markedly from reality).

Subtypes of Delusional Disorder

Examples of delusional subtypes include the following:

- Erotomanic
- Grandiose
- Jealous
- Persecutory
- Somatic
- Mixed
- Unspecified

Erotomanic Type

The central core of this delusional variant is that one is loved in a highly idealized, romantic, or spiritual manner. Sometimes the delusion is kept secret, but frequently, efforts (e.g., telephone calls, letters, gifts, visits) are made to contact the person who is the object of the delusion, often a famous person or a superior at work. Although female patients are usually seen clinically, many men with this erotomanic-type delusional disorder become involved with the legal system when they stalk or try to inappropriately contact the individual who is the focus of their delusion.

Grandiose Type

These delusions often take the form of a false belief that the patient possesses some great, unrecognized talent; is the son or daughter of a famous person; or actually is the famous person, whereas the true celebrity is an impostor.

Jealous Type

Patients with this subtype are convinced, despite overwhelming evidence to the contrary, that a spouse or lover is unfaithful. As evidence of infidelity, these patients may use seemingly unrelated events to support their delusional system, often confronting their spouse or lover, taking steps to intervene, or initiating investigations into the perceived infidelity.

Persecutory Type

These patients take on beliefs such as that they are being conspired against, poisoned, or drugged by someone. They may even take action against their perceived persecutors, on occasion resorting to violence.

Somatic Type

This delusional theme involves bodily functions or sensations. Patients may feel that they emit a foul odor from some part of their body; that they have insects crawling on their skin or suffer from internal parasites; or that certain parts of the body are misshapen or ugly. They have no insight and will persistently seek treatment from the appropriate medical specialist.

Course of Illness

Lifetime prevalence of delusional disorder is about 0.05% to 0.1%. Although it can occur at any age, onset is generally after the age of 40 years. The course is highly variable, with some patients holding their false beliefs all their lives; others may have episodes that can remit within a few months, or follow a waxing and waning course. Although these patients are generally intellectually and occupationally intact, frequently their delusional system interferes with social and marital functioning.

Although large-scale studies have not been done, anecdotal case reports indicate that some of these patients may be helped by antipsychotics, with late paraphrenics usually more responsive. Unfortunately, because many of these patients are paranoid, they may not seek medical help or cooperate with treatment recommendations.

Brief Psychotic Disorder

This is an acute psychotic response to a severe stressor that generally subsides in 1 day to 1 month. This phenomenon is frequently seen in adolescence or young adulthood without prodromal symptoms or lasting impairment. Little information is available about such factors as prevalence and heredity, other than that which is inherent in the diagnosis. The role of antipsychotics for this disorder has not been studied in controlled investigations.

Shared Psychotic Disorder

In shared psychotic disorder (e.g., *folie à deux*), a close friend or relative passively accepts the delusional belief system of the more dominant member. Thus, the symptoms may not necessarily be truly delusional, and often remit when the individual is separated from the "inducer" or "primary case."

Psychotic Disorders Due to a Nonpsychiatric Medical Condition or Substance-Induced

Although antipsychotics are also widely used to treat behavioral disturbances in the *developmentally disabled* and a large body of anecdotal evidence exists to support their efficacy, there are few data from well-controlled clinical trials. These agents have also been effective in treating a wide variety of *secondary psychoses*, including those resulting from various diseases that can affect brain function (e.g., metabolic dysregulation, HIV infection, primary degenerative dementia, delirium).

There are few controlled studies of antipsychotics used in a wide variety of organic psychoses; instead, most of the literature consists of anecdotal case reports (single cases or series of cases).

Agitation in the Elderly

Agitation in the older patient is common and frequently associated with dementia with or without psychotic features. Agitated patients on geriatric units of state hospitals suffer from a wide variety of organic psychoses and probably constitute a different population from the chronically demented group, inasmuch as many were admitted because of an acute exacerbation of their psychosis (see the section "The Elderly Patient" in Chapter 14).

Psychotic Mood Disorders

It is well established that monotherapy with various antidepressants or mood stabilizers is relatively ineffective (i.e., they are necessary but not sufficient) for treating mood disorders with associated psychosis. Thus, psychotically depressed patients are best managed with a combination of antipsychotic-antidepressant or with electroconvulsive therapy. Although antipsychotics have a more rapid onset of action than lithium in an acute manic episode, we are unaware of clinical trials that examine the differential effect of antipsychotics or lithium for nonpsychotic versus psychotic mania. This topic is discussed further in Chapter 10.

NONPSYCHOTIC DISORDERS

Although antipsychotics are often used for nonpsychotic disorders, the limited evidence for benefit and relative risk usually militate against such strategies.

Anxiolytics are the treatment of choice for *anxiety disorders,* and antipsychotics should not be used for this purpose. Previously, psychotropics were classified as major (i.e., antipsychotics) and minor (i.e., anxiolytics) tranquilizers, a categorization we now know to be conceptually incorrect. There is evidence, however, that adding benzodiazepines (BZDs) to antipsychotics might improve the treatment of various acute psychotic episodes complicated by agitation, although this has not been well studied (see Chapters 5 and 10).

CONCLUSION

A wide range of disorders can benefit from antipsychotic therapy. For example, since the introduction of antipsychotics, 25% fewer hospital beds are occupied by patients with schizophrenia. In particular, the newer antipsychotics hold the promise of benefitting patients once refractory to conventional treatment. Thus, negative, cognitive, and mood symptoms may improve with use of newer agents such as clozapine, risperidone, olanzapine, quetiapine, and ziprasidone.

Certain disorders may require combined therapy. For example, SA-bipolar type may best respond to the addition of mood stabilizers, and BZDs may be useful adjuncts for agitated psychoses. Conversely, some mood disorders may require augmentation with antipsychotics (e.g., delusional depression). Unfortunately, except for schizophrenia, most other psychotic conditions have not been systematically studied to determine the optimal use of these agents.

REFERENCES

1. Kahlbaum K. *Die Gruppirung der Psychischen Krankheiten.* Danzig:Kafemann, 1863.
2. Kahlbaum K. *Die Katatonie oder das Spannungsirresein.* Berlin: Hirschwald, 1874.
3. Hecker E. Die Hebephrenie. *Arch Pathol Ant Physiol Klin Med* 1871;52:394–429.
4. Kraepelin E. *Dementia praecox and paraphrenia.* Barclay RM, trans. Huntington, NY: Robert Krieger, 1971 (facsimile of 1919 edition).
5. American Psychiatric Association. *Diagnostic and statistical manual of mental disorders,* 4th ed. Washington, DC: American Psychiatric Press, 1994.
6. Bleuler E. *Dementia praecox or the group of schizophrenias.* Zinkin J, trans. New York: International Universities Press, 1950.
7. Bateson G, Jackson DD, Haley J, et al. Toward a theory of schizophrenia. *Behav Sci* 1956;1:251–264.
8. Lidz R, Lidz T. The family environment of schizophrenic patients. *Am J Psychiatry* 1949;106:332–345.
9. Lidz T. Intrafamilial environment of the schizophrenic patient: VI. The transmission of irrationality. *Arch Neurol Psychiatry* 1958;79:305–316.
10. Wynne LC, Ryckoff IM, Day J, et al. Pseudomutuality in the family relations of schizophrenics. *Psychiatry* 1958;21:205–220.
11. Cooper B. Epidemiology. In: Wing JK, ed. *Schizophrenia: toward a new synthesis.* New York: Grune & Stratton, 1978;31–51.
12. Cooper JE, Kendell RE, Gurland BJ, et al. *Psychiatric diagnosis in New York and London: a comparative study of mental hospital admissions. Institute of Psychiatry, Maudsley Monographs, no. 20.* London: Oxford University Press, 1972.
13. Feighner JP, Robins E, Guze SB, et al. Diagnostic criteria for use in psychiatric research. *Arch Gen Psychiatry* 1972;26:57–63.
14. Spitzer RL, Endicott J, Robins E. Research diagnostic criteria: rationale and reliability. *Arch Gen Psychiatry* 1978;35:773–786.

15. American Psychiatric Association. *Diagnostic and statistical manual of mental disorders,* 4th ed. Washington, DC: American Psychiatric Association, 1994.
16. Dunham HW. *Community and schizophrenia.* Detroit: Wayne State University Press, 1965.
17. Faris REL, Dunham HW. *Mental disorders in urban areas.* Chicago: University of Chicago Press, 1939.
18. Goldberg EM, Morrison SL. Schizophrenia and social class. *Br J Psychiatry* 1963;109:785–802.
19. Watson CG, Kucala T, Tilleskjor C, et al. Schizophrenic birth seasonality in relation to the incidence of infectious diseases and temperature extremes. *Arch Gen Psychiatry* 1984;41:85–90.
20. Westergard T, Mortensen PB, Pedersen CB, et al. Exposure to prenatal and childhood infections and the risk of schizophrenia: suggestions from a study of sibship characteristics and influenza prevalence. *Arch Gen Psychiatry* 1999;56:993–998.
21. Tsuang MT, Stone WS, Faraone SV. Toward reformulating the diagnosis of schizophrenia. *Am J Psychiatry* 2000;157:1041–1050.
22. Radomsky ED, Haas GL, Mann JJ, et al. Suicidal behavior in patients with schizophrenia and other psychotic disorders. *Am J Psychiatry* 1999;156:1590–1595.
23. Mellor CS. First rank symptoms of schizophrenia. *Br J Psychiatry* 1970;117:15–23.
24. Taylor MA. Schneiderian first-rank symptoms and clinical prognostic features in schizophrenia. *Arch Gen Psychiatry* 1972;26:64–67.
25. Astrup C, Fossum A, Holmboe R. *Prognosis in functional psychoses.* Springfield, IL: Charles C Thomas, 1962.
26. Astrup C, Noreik K. *Functional psychoses: diagnostic and prognostic models.* Springfield, IL: Charles C Thomas, 1966.
27. Belmaker R, Pollin W, Wyatt RJ, et al. Follow-up of monozygotic twins discordant for schizophrenia. *Arch Gen Psychiatry* 1974;30:219–222.
28. Albee G, Lane E, Reuter JM. Childhood intelligence of future schizophrenics and neighborhood peers. *J Psychol* 1964;58:141–144.
29. Offord DR. School performance of adult schizophrenics, their siblings and age mates. *Br J Psychiatry* 1974;125:12–19.
30. Jones MB, Offord DR. Independent transmission of IQ and schizophrenia. *Br J Psychiatry* 1975;126:185–190.
31. Pfohl B, Winokur G. Schizophrenia: course and outcome. In: Henn FA, Nasrallah HA, eds. *Schizophrenia as a brain disease.* New York: Oxford University Press, 1982;26–39.
32. Guze SB, Cloninger R, Martin RL, et al. A follow-up and family study of schizophrenia. *Arch Gen Psychiatry* 1983;40:1273–1276.
33. Tsuang MT, Woolson RF, Winokur G, et al. Stability of psychiatric diagnosis: schizophrenia and affective disorders followed up over a 30- to 40-year period. *Arch Gen Psychiatry* 1981;38:535–539.
34. Stephens JH. Long-term course and prognosis of schizophrenia. *Semin Psychiatry* 1970;2:464–485.
35. Stephens JH, Astrup C. Prognosis in "process" and "non-process" schizophrenia. *Am J Psychiatry* 1963;119:945–953.
36. Johnstone EC, Crow TJ, Frith CD, et al. Cerebral ventricular size and cognitive impairment in chronic schizophrenia. *Lancet* 1976;2:924–926.
37. Weinberger DR, Wyatt RJ. Brain morphology in schizophrenia: *in vivo* studies. In: Henn FA, Nasrallah HA, eds. *Schizophrenia as a brain disease.* New York: Oxford University Press, 1982.
38. Weinberger DR, Bigelow LB, Kleinman JE, et al. Cerebral ventricular enlargement in chronic schizophrenia: an association with poor response to treatment. *Arch Gen Psychiatry* 1980;37:11–13.
39. Luchins DJ. Computed tomography in schizophrenia: disparities in the prevalence of abnormalities. *Arch Gen Psychiatry* 1982;39:859–860.
40. Nasrallah HA, McCalley-Whitters M, Jacoby CG. Cerebral ventricular enlargement in young manic males: a controlled CT study. *J Affect Disord* 1982;4:15–19.
41. Rieder RO, Mann LS, Weinberger DR, et al. Computed tomographic scans in patients with schizophrenia, schizoaffective, and bipolar affective disorder. *Arch Gen Psychiatry* 1983;40:735–739.
42. Tsuang MT, Winokur G, Crowe RR. Morbidity risks of schizophrenia and affective disorders among first degree relatives of patients with schizophrenia, mania, depression, and surgical conditions. *Br J Psychiatry* 1980;137:497–504.
43. Fowler RC, Tsuang MT, Cadoret RJ. Parental psychiatric illness associated with schizophrenia in the siblings of schizophrenics. *Compr Psychiatry* 1977;18:271–275.
44. Fowler RC, Tsuang MT, Cadoret RJ. Psychiatric illness in the offspring of schizophrenics. *Compr Psychiatry* 1977;18:127–134.
45. Wahlberg KE, Wynne LC, Oja H, et al. Gene-environment interaction in vulnerability to schizophrenia: findings from the Finnish Adoptive Study of Schizophrenia. *Am J Psychiatry* 1997;154:355–362.
46. Karlsson JL. Genealogic studies of schizophrenia. In: Rosenthal D, Kety SS, eds. *The transmission of schizophrenia.* Oxford: Pergamon Press, 1968:85–94.
47. Kendler KS. Overview. A current perspective on twin studies of schizophrenia. *Am J Psychiatry* 1983;140:1413–1425.
48. Fischer M. Psychoses in the offspring of schizophrenic twins and their normal co-twins. *Br J Psychiatry* 1971;118:43–52.
49. Fischer M, Harvald B, Hauge M. A Danish twin study of schizophrenia. *Br J Psychiatry* 1969;115:981–990.
50. Kallmann FJ. The genetic theory of schizophrenia. An analysis of 691 twin index families. *Am J Psychiatry* 1946;103:309–322.
51. Kringlen E. Twin studies in schizophrenia with special emphasis on concordance figures. *Am J Med Genet* 2000;97:4–11.
52. Cardno AG, Gottesman II. Twin studies of schizophrenia: from bow-and-arrow concordances to Star Wars MX and functional genomics. *Am J Med Genet* 2000;97:12–17.
53. Gottesman II, Shields J. Contributions of twin studies to perspectives in schizophrenia. In: Maher BA, ed. *Progress in experimental personality research. Vol. 3.* New York: Academic Press, 1966:1–84.
54. Kety SS, Rosenthal D, Wender PH, et al. The biologic and adoptive families of adopted individuals who became schizophrenic: prevalence of mental illness and other characteristics. In: Wynne LC, Cromwell RL, Matthysse S, eds. *The nature of schizophrenia: new approaches to research and treatment.* New York: John Wiley & Sons, 1978:25–37.
55. Kennedy JL, Pato MT, Bauer A, et al. Genetics of schizophrenia: current findings and issues. *CNS Spectrum* 1999;4:17–21.

56. Levinson DF, Mahtani MM, Nancarrow DJ, et al. Genome scan of schizophrenia. *Am J Psychiatry* 1998;155:741–750.

57. Cichon S, Nothen MM, Rietschel M, et al. Pharmacogenetics of schizophrenia. *Am J Med Genet* 2000;97:98–106.

58. Evans JD, Heaton RK, Paulsen JS, et al. Schizoaffective disorder: a form of schizophrenia or affective disorder: *J Clin Psychiatry* 1999;60:874–882.

59. Grossman LS, Harrow M, Goldberg JF, et al. Outcome of schizoaffective disorder at two long-term follow-ups: comparisons with outcome of schizophrenia and affective disorders. *Am J Psychiatry* 1991;148:1359–1365.

60. Maier W, Lichtermann D, Minges J, et al. Schizoaffective disorder and affective disorders with mood-incongruent psychotic features: keep separate or combine? Evidence from a family study. *Am J Psychiatry* 1992;149:1666–1673.

61. Tsuang MT, Woolson RF. Mortality in patients with schizophrenia, mania, depression, and surgical conditions. *Br J Psychiatry* 1977;130:162–166.

62. Coryell WH, Tsuang MT. DSM-III schizophreniform disorder: comparisons with schizophrenia and affective disorder. *Arch Gen Psychiatry* 1982;39:66–69.

63. Pope HG, Lipinski JF, Cohen BM, et al. "Schizoaffective disorder": an invalid diagnosis? A comparison of schizoaffective disorder, schizophrenia and affective disorder. *Am J Psychiatry* 1980;137:921–927.

64. Tsuang MT, Woolson RF, Fleming JA. Long-term outcome of major psychoses. I. Schizophrenia and affective disorders compared with psychiatrically symptom-free surgical conditions. *Arch Gen Psychiatry* 1979;36:1295–1301.

65. Bleuler M. *The schizophrenic disorders: long-term patient and family studies.* Clemens S. trans. New Haven, CT: Yale University Press, 1978.

5

Treatment With Antipsychotics

As in other areas of clinical science, serendipity, as well as careful investigation, have contributed to our knowledge about antipsychotics, including their:

- *Discovery*
- *Potential mechanisms of action*
- Range of *complications*

Chlorpromazine's (CPZ) efficacy was discovered primarily by chance in exploratory clinical trials after it had been initially synthesized as an antihistamine. Its discovery, however, was not entirely fortuitous, because it was chosen for human investigation since it was mildly sedating. The concept of an antipsychotic, however, was unknown. CPZ's sedative properties then led the French anesthesiologist and surgeon Henri Laborit to use it in a lytic cocktail to reduce autonomic response with surgical stress (1). He also persuaded many clinicians to try it for the treatment of a wide variety of other disorders. In this context, he encouraged John Delay and Pierre Deniker (1952), who then administered CPZ to schizophrenic patients. The rest is history (2, 3).

Even though CPZ did not produce a permanent cure for schizophrenia (or for any other psychotic disorder), it had a dramatic impact, benefitting many as no other treatment had before (4). News of its effectiveness spread rapidly, and within 2 years, CPZ was used worldwide, altering the lives of millions of psychotic patients in a positive manner.

The relocation of treatment from chronic hospital settings to outpatient community mental health centers is, in great part, due to the efficacy of antipsychotics. Naturalistic studies before the era of psychotropics revealed that two of three psychotic patients (primarily schizophrenic) spent most of their lives in state asylums. Before the mid-1950's, there had been a steady increase in state hospital populations, which paralleled the general population growth,

but after the introduction of antipsychotics, there was a marked reduction in those hospitalized for various psychoses. Presently, more than 95% of these patients live outside of the hospital, even though many continue to relapse or demonstrate residual symptoms. Thus, although the antipsychotics have not been a panacea, they make community-based care a reality for many who would otherwise have remained chronically institutionalized.

Reserpine, used as a folk medicine in India, was found to have antipsychotic properties at about the same time as CPZ. Both agents affected the dopaminergic system, albeit in different ways, but the functional results were similar (i.e., lowering dopamine activity). This phenomenon has continued to be an important factor in hypotheses about the mechanism of action of these drugs and for biological theories about the pathophysiology of psychotic disorders.

The revolutionary idea that drugs could exert a specific antipsychotic effect, coupled with a growing recognition of their significant drawbacks, led to the search for other substances with similar beneficial properties and fewer adverse effects. Thus, pharmacological animal screens, followed by systematic clinical investigations with chemically or structurally related compounds, has led to a variety of effective, better tolerated drugs for schizophrenia and other major psychotic disorders.

The therapeutic efficacy of clozapine, the first truly different antipsychotic, has spawned the development of a succession of novel agents (e.g., risperidone, olanzapine). In addition to the more recently approved quetiapine (Seroquel) and ziprasidone (Geodon), other new compounds (e.g., aripiprazole, iloperidone) may also receive Food and Drug Administration (FDA) marketing approval in the near future (5, 6).

Table 5-1 presents the classes, names, and typical doses for the most commonly used

TABLE 5-1. *Antipsychotic agents*

Class/trade name	Generic name	Dosage (average range, orally, per day)
Phenothiazines		
Aliphatics		
Thorazine	Chlorpromazine	100–1,000 mg
Sparine	Promazine	25–1,000 mg
Vesprin	Triflupromazine	20–150 mg
Piperidines		
Mellaril	Thioridazine	30–800 mg
Serentil	Mesoridazine	20–200 mg
Quide	Piperacetazine	20–160 mg
Piperazines		
Stelazine	Trifluoperazine	2–60 mg
Prolixin	Fluphenzine	5–40 mg
Trilafon	Perphenazine	2–60 mg
Tindal	Acetophenazine	40–80 mg
Compazine	Prochlorperazine	15–125 mg
Thioxanthenes		
Navane	Thiothixene	6–60 mg
Taractan	Chlorprothixene	10–600 mg
Dibenzoxiazepines		
Loxitane	Loxapine	20–250 mg
Butyrophenones		
Haldol	Haloperidol	3–50 mg
Inapsin	Droperidol	2.5–10 mg (i.m)
Dihydroindolones		
Moban	Molindone	15–225 mg
Dibenzodiazepines		
Clozaril	Clozapine	100–900 mg
Benzisoxazole		
Risperdal	Risperidone	2–10 mg
Zomaril[a]	Iloperidone	4–16 mg
Thienobenzodiazepines		
Zyprexa	Olanzapine	5–20 mg
Dibenzothiazepines		
Seroquel	Quetiapine	75–750 mg
Benzisothiazolyls		
Geodon	Ziprasidone	40–160 mg
Quinolinones		
Habilitat[a]	Aripiprazole	10–30 mg
Diphenytbutyrylpiperidines		
Semap[b]	Penfluridol	100 mg/week
Orap	Pimozide	1–10 mg

[a]Tentative, [b]Long-acting oral agent. Not approved in United States

antipsychotics, as well as for the newest agents recently (or anticipated to be) available in the United States (6). Figures 5-1 and 5-2 present the basic chemical structure of agents with antipsychotic effects.

MECHANISM OF ACTION

One common denominator of all antipsychotics is the blockade of central dopamine (DA) receptors. As a result, extrapyramidal

Radical
Chain
Base
2 }R1
A
S
B
10 N
(CH2)n
N
}R2
C

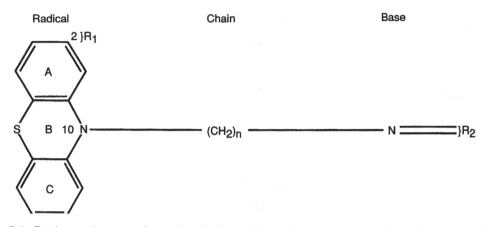

FIG. 5-1. Basic requirements for antipsychotic activity, with neuroleptics; distance between N_{10} of radical and the base N atom must equal at least three carbons *(n = 3)*, with a suitable substituent R_2 mainly determining the qualitative properties of the group; the A_2 substituent R_1 mainly determines the quantitative properties of the individual compounds.

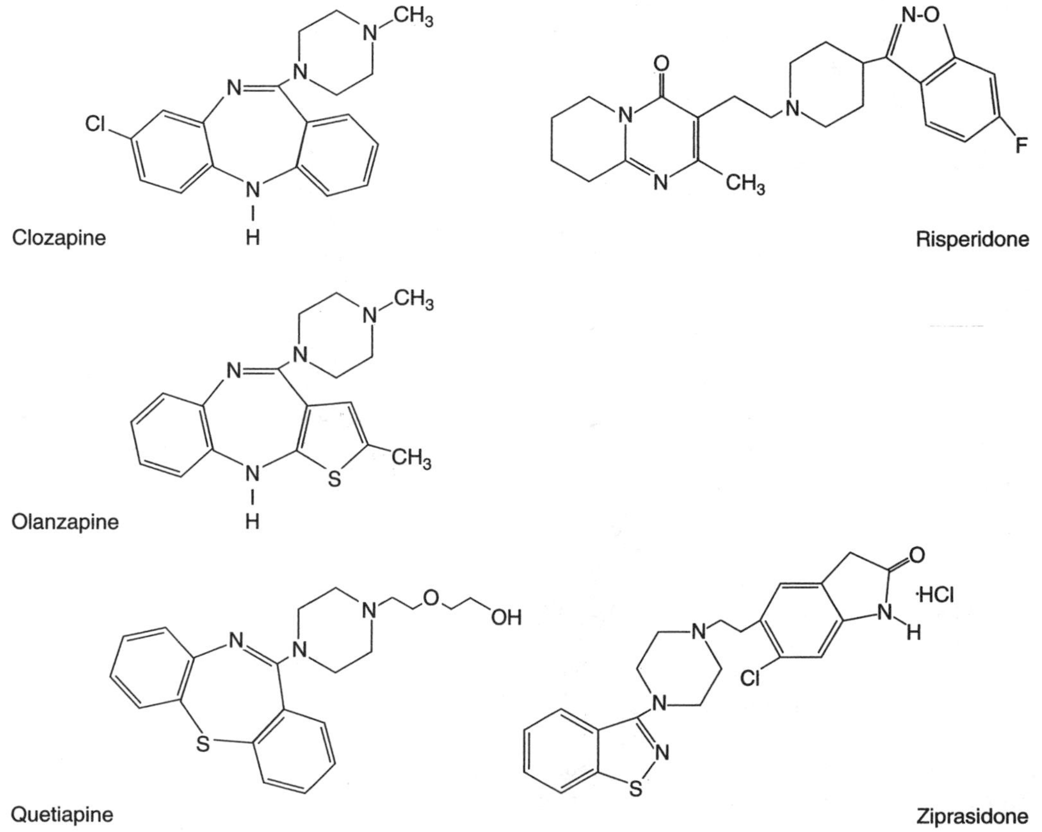

Clozapine
Risperidone
Olanzapine
Quetiapine
Ziprasidone
·HCl

FIG. 5-2. Chemical structures of novel antipsychotics.

reactions, particularly parkinsonian symptoms, are a major adverse effect of many of these drugs, as well as an important clue to their mechanism of action. True Parkinson's disease is caused by a DA deficiency in the nigrostriatal system. Further, crystallographic data have demonstrated that CPZ's molecular configuration is similar to that of DA, which could explain its ability to block this neurotransmitter's receptors. Drugs with similar structures that do not block DA receptors (e.g., promethazine, imipramine) do not have antipsychotic activity. Another example is the isomer of flupenthixol, which blocks DA receptors is an effective antipsychotic, but the isomer that does not is ineffective (7). The other family of dopamine receptors, D_1 and D_5, have not yet been implicated in psychosis.

Interestingly, some of the novel antipsychotics in their usual clinical dosing range do not produce extrapyramidal side effects. This is an important observation, because it offers the hope that these two effects can be dissociated. Generally, "neuroleptic" is applied to all drugs that produce both extrapyramidal and antipsychotic effects, but agents such as clozapine, risperidone, olanzapine, quetiapine, ziprasidone, and others may be antipsychotics without being neuroleptics, making the interchangeable use of the terms "neuroleptic" and "antipsychotic" no longer appropriate.

The evidence that antidopaminergic agents ameliorate psychosis and that DA agonists can produce psychosis or worsen preexisting disorders supports a central role for DA in any theory about pathophysiology. Further, there is a high correlation among directly measured D_2-*type receptor binding,* the clinical potency of these agents, animal behavioral models, and data about DA blockade.

Other drug effects that decrease DA activity also support this position. Thus, when DA synthesis is blocked by α-methyl-p-tyrosine (AMPT), the dose necessary for an antipsychotic effect is reduced (i.e., the dose-response curve is shifted to the left by the interaction between dopamine and AMPT). A drug such as reserpine that can deplete DA stores also has relatively mild antipsychotic properties. Also, aripiprazole, which has D_2 presynaptic agonist properties, de-

creases the production of DA, as well as blocking D_2 postsynaptic receptors.

Dopaminergic Pathways of the Central Nervous System

Because the existing evidence strongly implicates the DA system in psychosis, it is pertinent to discuss this neurotransmitter's central pathways. There are five tracts:

- The *striatal* system (A-9)
- The *mesolimbic* system (A-10)
- The *mesocortical* system (A-10)
- The *retinal* system
- The *neurohypophyseal* system

The last system is of interest in regard to the elevation in prolactin, an effect most closely associated with neuroleptics.

Postmortem studies of patients with idiopathic Parkinson's disease demonstrate cell loss in the striatal system (A-9), directly implicating this tract vis-à-vis the neuroleptic-induced pseudoparkinsonian side effects. The assumption that psychosis is related to the A-10 system is made by exclusion. Evidence also indicates that clozapine may differentially block DA pathways. Specifically, it seems to act on the mesolimbic dopaminergic system (A-10), while being relatively inactive in the striatal system (A-9); however, this remains controversial. Chronic administration of clozapine decreases the firing rate of A-10 mesocortical tract dopamine neurons while sparing A-9 neurons of the nigrostriatal pathway. By contrast, neuroleptics reduce the firing rate of both A-9 and A-10 neurons (8).

Because clozapine may block specific DA receptors, its antipsychotic activity could be consistent with an antidopaminergic mechanism of action. Conversely, clozapine does not typically induce extrapyramidal symptoms, which are presumably subserved by the A-9 system. Thus, while clozapine is known to block striatal DA receptors, in positron emission tomography (PET) studies, resolution is not sufficient to clarify effects on other tracts. Furthermore, low doses of metoclopramide, which significantly decrease the number of DA neurons spontaneously active in A-9, do not have antipsychotic effects (except at high doses) but can induce tardive dyskinesia (TD), as well as acute extrapyramidal side effects (EPS).

Neurophysiological Studies

Another way to measure striatal (A-9) or mesolimbic (A-10) activity is through neurophysiological studies involving the firing rate of these neurons. The acute administration of antipsychotics will cause DA neurons to initiate a burst pattern of firing, with the opposite occurring when a DA agonist is administered. Eventually, some degree of tolerance develops and the enhanced DA synthesis decreases with time on drug, as demonstrated in both human cerebrospinal fluid (CSF) studies and rat brain slices. On a more chronic basis, repeated drug administration results in a dramatic decrease in the proportion of spontaneously active dopaminergic neurons (i.e., excitation-induced depolarization blockade of the DA neuron spike-generating region). Both the depolarization blockade and the antipsychotic effects of these drugs develop slowly. Neuroleptics induce nigrostriatal and mesolimbic DA neurons into depolarization blockade, whereas the clozapine only induces depolarization in the mesolimbic-mesocortical DA neurons.

The working assumption that the striatal system is only involved with extrapyramidal function (e.g., parkinsonian side effects, dystonias, and TD) and that the mesolimbic or mesocortical systems are only involved with psychosis may be an oversimplification. Many of the neuroanatomical studies on the identified dopaminergic tracts are done with rats. In the monkey, by contrast, there are many more DA tracts that are either absent in the rat or at least markedly different; human systems could be different from the rat's or monkey's. Understanding the neuropharmacology of the antipsychotics is further complicated, given that neither the mesolimbic-mesocortical nor the striatal systems are homogeneous but may also include various subsystems.

Dopamine Autoreceptors

There are also dopaminergic presynaptic receptors (or autoreceptors) that generally play a negative feedback role. These autoreceptors sense the level of neurotransmitter and produce a negative feedback influence on DA synthesis and release. Thus, high DA release results in high intrasynaptic concentrations, which stimulate the autoreceptors, ultimately inducing a slowing of DA synthesis and release. Conversely, blockade of the postsynaptic receptors may lead to positive feedback loops, which can:

- Activate *tyrosine hydroxylase* in the presynaptic dopaminergic neuron.
- Increase DA *synthesis.*
- Increase the *firing rate.*
- Increase the levels of DA metabolites, such as *homovanillic acid* (HVA).

Further complicating the picture is the induction of autoreceptor supersensitivity with chronic neuroleptic administration, as well as the fact that at least one tract–the mesocortical, which projects to the prefrontal cortex–may lack such autoreceptors. Some of the authors conducted preliminary, single-dose studies with apomorphine at a dose that stimulated presynaptic DA autoreceptors that reduced synthesis and NT release, producing a measurable acute antipsychotic effect (9, 10).

Decreasing Dopaminergic Activity

Given the typical time course of adaptation to the biochemical and electrophysiological effects induced by antipsychotics in most dopaminergic systems, it is important to consider the time course for their efficacy. While an apparent clinical benefit can be seen within a few hours after treatment is initiated, the rate of improvement is roughly linear for the first 14 days, at which point it gradually levels off.

Time-dependent changes in plasma HVA (a major metabolite of DA) during neuroleptic treatment are consistent with the hypothesis that these agents' mechanism involves a slowly developing decrease in presynaptic DA synthesis and release. Whereas decreases in plasma HVA appear to parallel the time course of antipsychotic efficacy, peripheral DA systems may also contribute to plasma or urine HVA levels. Further, because different brain areas may or may not develop tolerance, it is quite possible that CSF HVA levels reflect those areas producing most of the HVA, but are not relevant to the psychotic process. With these caveats in mind, human CSF and plasma data are generally consistent with the animal studies, both of which have contributed considerable evidence implicating DA blockade and its aftermath. The relevance of these findings to the biological mechanisms subserving psychosis, however, has yet to be determined.

Tolerance

It is important to examine whether tolerance develops to the antipsychotic effect of these agents. For example, Sharma et al. (11) found that "nontolerant" psychotic patients had a significantly inferior clinical response to antipsychotics, in contrast to their "tolerant" counterparts. Further, they found an earlier age of illness onset and a more refractory course in the "nontolerant" group. Although biochemical and electrophysiological tolerance (i.e., return of HVA to more normal levels and depolarization inactivation, respectively) develop in most DA systems, they do not occur in all. Prefrontal and cingulate cortices, for example, may be spared, perhaps because of the absence of autoreceptors in these tracts. Evidence also indicates that many areas in nonhuman, primate brains develop biochemical tolerance to the neuroleptic-induced HVA rise, but other areas do not. Thus, with chronic neuroleptic treatment, certain areas (cingulate, dorsal frontal, and orbital frontal cortex) maintain their HVA increases. Patients who were examined postmortem after chronic antipsychotic therapy were found to have increased HVA levels in certain areas, such as the cingulate and perifalciform cortex. It is also interesting that stress and benzodiazepine receptor agonists can selectively stimulate DA neurons in the meso-prefrontal area, but not in other dopaminergic tracts.

By using D_2-blocking isotopes in a PET scanner, it is possible to image the striatum in psychotic patients. Earlier evidence from one PET scan study indicated that some drug-free schizophrenics manifested an increase in D_2 dopamine receptors, but another study failed to find such an alteration (12, 13). These studies used different receptor ligands, different assumptions, and both had a small sample size, so definitive conclusions are not possible. Finally, when PET scans are done on patients receiving clinically effective doses of novel and neuroleptic antipsychotics, all of these agents (including haloperidol, clozapine, risperidone, and olanzapine) produced varying levels of D_2 receptor occupancy in the striatum (14–16). Furthermore, they do so at the typical doses used to treat schizophrenic patients. Further, Kapur and colleagues (17) found that only *transiently* high D_2 receptor occupancy occurred with quetiapine, suggesting that this was sufficient for efficacy, while minimizing the possibility of EPS or elevated prolactin levels.

Increasing Dopaminergic Activity

If decreasing dopaminergic activity benefits psychosis, what is the effect of increasing dopaminergic activity? **Potentiation of DA by a variety of mechanisms is a common denominator for inducing paranoia, hallucinations, and other manifestations of psychosis.** For example:

- L-*Dopa* (3,4-dihydroxyphenylalanine), which is converted to DA in the body, can produce psychosis as a side effect.
- *Amantadine,* another dopaminergic drug, can also induce psychotic symptoms.
- *Stimulants,* such as amphetamine and methylphenidate, are potent releasers of DA, while cocaine also interferes with its reuptake, increasing DA concentrations at synaptic sites. All can produce paranoid reactions in some abusers.
- Bromocriptine, apomorphine, lisoride, and *other direct-acting DA agonists* benefit Parkinson's disease and can also cause psychotic reactions at high doses.

As noted above, large doses of amphetamine, cocaine, and other sympathomimetics can cause acute paranoid reactions, either spontaneously in abusers or experimentally in normal volunteers. An injection of a large amphetamine dose, for example, often produces a paranoid psychosis within hours. Frequent smaller doses over several days can also produce a paranoid psychotic reaction. An episode's duration usually parallels the length of time the drug remains in the body.

Additional evidence comes from studies of increasing dopaminergic activity in patients with active psychosis. Small i.v. doses of methylphenidate (e.g., 0.5 mg/kg) can result in a marked exacerbation of an acute schizophrenic episode (18). By contrast, such doses usually do not produce psychotic symptoms in normal control subjects or in remitted patients. The phenomenon of worsening a preexisting psychosis may be different from that of producing a paranoid reaction in normal subjects. Thus, specific preexisting psychotic symptoms worsen (e.g., catatonic patients become more catatonic), but patients without paranoia do not demonstrate such "new" symptoms. Methylphenidate is more potent in this regard than dextroamphetamine, consistent with the hypothesis that it intensifies psychotic symptoms by releasing central intraneuronal stores of norepinephrine and DA from the reserpine-sensitive pool (19).

Finally, sensitivity to an amphetamine test dose in recovered patients may predict an impending relapse (20).

Other Pathways

Interestingly, when physostigmine, a drug that increases brain acetylcholine, is administered before methylphenidate, it prevents the exacerbation, indicating that the worsening may be mediated by a dopaminergic-cholinergic imbalance (21). Physostigmine itself, however, does not reduce psychosis, suggesting that the underlying process is not amenable simply to altering cholinergic tone. Subsequently, nicotinic cholinergic receptors have been reported to play an important role in the inhibition of extraneous environmental noise. This observation has implications for deficits in gating sensory stimuli reported in schizophrenic patients (22).

Other systems (e.g., neurotransmitter, neuropeptides, neurohormonal) may also play important central or modulating roles in the psychotic process (Tables 5-2 and 5-3). In addition to dopamine, the following have been implicated:

- Serotonin (5-HT)
- Norepinephrine (NE)
- γ-Aminobutyric acid (GABA)

TABLE 5-2. *New drug treatments for psychosis classified by biochemical activity[a]*

Dopamine system
Nonspecific D_2 antagonists
Neuroleptics
Clozapine
Specific D_2 antagonists
Benzamides
Pimozide
Sulpiride
Raclopride
D_1 antagonists
SCH 23390
SCH 39166
D_2 antagonists/presynaptic DA autoreceptor agonist
Aripiprazole
Partial D_2 agonists
SDZ HDC912
Terguride
Serotonin system
Nonspecific $5\text{-}HT_2$ antagonists
Neuroleptics
Clozapine
Specific $5\text{-}HT_2$ antagonists
Ritanserin
Serotonin/Dopamine system
Specific $5\text{-}HT_2/D_2$ antagonists
Risperidone

[a]Bold type indicates agents available for clinical use in the United States or elsewhere.

- Glutamate (GLU)
- Neuropeptides

Indeed, a leading hypothesis as to why newer agents produce fewer EPS and perhaps provide greater benefit for negative symptoms is a more potent effect on the serotonin $5\text{-}HT_2$ receptor subtype. Thus, the ratio of $5\text{-}HT_2/D_2$ blockade has become an important measure of an agent's potential "atypicality" (5, 6). In addition, these novel antipsychotics have a neuroreceptor profile that differs substantially from the neuroleptics. For example, clozapine (Clozaril) is a dibenzothiazepine derivative with affinity for a variety of neurotransmitter receptors, including several serotonin receptors ($5\text{-}HT_{1C}$, $5\text{-}HT_3$, $5\text{-}HT_6$, and $5\text{-}HT_7$) that may modulate dopamine activity and contribute to this agent's atypical action. In addition, it is likely that clinically effective doses of clozapine antagonize $5\text{-}HT_{2A}$ and $5\text{-}HT_{2C}$ receptors (23). The resulting increased

TABLE 5-3. *Atypical antipsychotic receptor binding profiles*[a]

Receptor	Clozapine	Risperidone	Olanzapine	Quetiapine	Ziprasidone	Aripiprazole	Iloperidone
D_1	High	Low	High	Low/Mod	Low	Low	Low
D_2	Low	High	High	Low/Mod	High	Very high	Mod/High
D_3		High	High		High	High	High
D_4	High	High	High	None	Mod	Low	
D_6		Mod					
D_7		High					
$5\text{-}HT_{1A}$				Low/Mod	High	High	Mod
$5\text{-}HT_{2A}$	High	High	High	Low/Mod	High	High	High
$5\text{-}HT_{2A}/D_2$ Ratio	High	High	High	High	Very high	Low	High
$5\text{-}HT_{2C}$	High				High	High	High
$5\text{-}HT_3$	High		High		Very low		
$5\text{-}HT_{1D}$					High		
$5\text{-}HT_6$	High		High		High		High
$5\text{-}HT_7$		High			High		High
Alpha$_1$	Mod/High	High	Mod/High	Mod/High	Mod	Mod	High
Alpha$_2$	Mod	High	Low	Mod/High	Very low		High
Histamine$_1$	High	High	High	High	Mod	High	
Muscarinic$_1$	High	Low	High	None	Very low	Very low	Low

[a]Based on K_i data.
Mod, moderate.

$5\text{-}HT_{2A}/D_2$ ratio may be one basis for clozapine's unique antipsychotic efficacy (24). At clinical doses, clozapine also has a somewhat lower affinity for D_2 receptors, which may account for its low propensity to evoke EPS, as well as its negligible neuroendocrine effects (25, 26).

Conclusion

All clinically effective antipsychotics block DA receptor activity. Further, stimulation of this neurotransmitter can induce psychotic symptoms de novo or exacerbate an existing psychotic disorder. Atypical agents have differential impacts on other systems (e.g., 5-HT) in comparison with the earlier neuroleptic agents. They also selectively target specific DA tracts that may mediate the pathological condition, while sparing those tracts that mediate the unwanted adverse effects (e.g., EPS, TD).

EFFECTS ON COGNITION AND BEHAVIOR

Investigators have attempted to assess the impact of antipsychotics on the cognitive and the behav-

ioral disturbances characteristic of schizophrenia. The antipsychotics decrease typical, but nonspecific, positive symptoms such as hallucinations and delusions (Table 5-4). Thus, labeling them as "antischizophrenic" agents is too restrictive inasmuch as they also benefit such disparate disorders as psychotic depression or mania, late-onset paraphrenia, and organic-induced psychosis. As the symptoms reduced by neuroleptics are typical of psychosis in general, these agents are best conceptualized as a type of antipsychotic.

Serious mental disorders fundamentally alter one's personality. Evidence from controlled studies demonstrates that antipsychotics can "normalize" thought processes. Some claim that the involuntary administration of these drugs violates a patient's freedom of speech. In fact, with the onset of a psychotic episode, patients' "normal" mental processes become loose, rambling, illogical, circumstantial, incoherent, and inappropriately concrete and are often characterized by bizarre thought and speech patterns. Delusional ideas may dominate, with or without visual or auditory hallucinations.

TABLE 5-4. *Effect of neuroleptics on symptoms of schizophrenia*[a]

Bleuler's classification of schizophrenic symptoms	VA study no. 1	VA study no. 3	Kurland, 1962	NIMH-PSC no. 1	Gorham and Pokorny, 1964, vs. group psychotherapy
Fundamental symptoms					
Thought disorder	++	++	++	++	++
Blunted affect–indifference				++	+
Withdrawal–retardation	++	++	0	++	++
Autistic behavior–mannerisms	++	++	0	++	+
Accessory symptoms					
Hallucinations	++	++	+	+	0
Paranoid ideation	0	++	0	+	+
Grandiosity	0	0	0	0	+
Hostility–belligerence	++	++	H/R	+	+
Resistiveness–uncooperativeness	++	++	H/R	++	++
Nonschizophrenic symptoms					
Anxiety–tension–agitation	0	0	H/R	+	0
Guilt–depression	++	0	0	0	0
Disorientation				0	
Somatization					0

[a]++, symptom areas showing marked drug control group differences; +, those showing significant but less striking differences; 0, areas not showing differential drug superiority; H/R, heterogeneity of regression found on analysis of covariance of the measures indicated. (This invalidates this particular statistical procedure but does not mean that there was *no* drug effect.)
Adapted from Klein D, Davis JM. *Diagnosis and drug treatment of psychiatric disorders.* Baltimore: Williams & Wilkins, 1969:90.

There are several studies measuring cognitive performance before (drug-free) and after treatment that find a marked improvement on medication. Whereas it is true that some drugs have sedative properties, this is more than counteracted by their ability to correct disturbances of thought. The net effect is that a patient's cognitive functions are much improved, at times approaching premorbid status.

Antipsychotics can activate retardation or diminish excitation; therefore, "tranquilizer" is a misnomer. These agents do not, in any real sense, produce a state of tranquility in normal or psychotic individuals; in fact, normal control subjects often find their effects unpleasant. An appropriate analogy may be aspirin, which reduces an elevated temperature but typically does not alter normal temperature. Another example is insulin, which replaces the absent endogenous supply and restores a diabetic to normal glucostasis. So, too, antipsychotics normalize cognition and behavior.

In 1977, Spohn and coworkers (27) studied the effect of these agents in 40 chronic patients, who underwent a 6-week, placebo washout phase and were then randomly assigned to CPZ or placebo. In contrast to placebo, CPZ was found to:

• Enhance *concentration.*
• Reduce *overestimation and fixation* time on a perceptual task.
• Increase the *accuracy of perceptual judgment.*

The common denominator was the patients' ability to attend appropriately to a given task. Further, attentional dysfunction, information-processing impairment, and autonomic dysfunction were improved more in the drug-treated group.

In another study, drug-induced improvement in schizophrenic symptoms was also measured using the Brief Psychiatric Rating Scale (BPRS) and the Holtzman-Johnstone Thought Disorder Index (which elicits responses to standardized stimuli, i.e., the Rorschach test and the Wechsler

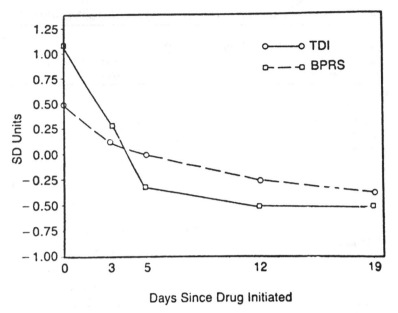

Days Since Drug Initiated

FIG. 5-3. Effects of neuroleptics on thought disorder and behavioral symptoms of schizophrenia. BPRS, Brief Psychiatric Rating Scale; TDI, Thought Disorder Index. (From Davis JM, Barter JT, Kane JM. Antipsychotic drugs. In: Kaplan HI, Sadock BJ, eds. *Comprehensive textbook of psychiatry,* 5th ed. Baltimore: Williams & Wilkins, 1989:1604, with permission.)

Adult Intelligence Scale) (28). Each response to the index was blindly categorized to quantify the level of thought disorder, which, although substantial before treatment, showed a marked improvement with adequate drug therapy. Further, thought disorder improved during the same period and to the same degree as the other symptoms (Fig. 5-3).

systems, which may underlie more classic or "positive" psychotic symptoms (Table 5-5) (29). Terminology should reflect available data, particularly because the cause of schizophrenia is not known, nor is it known how, in general, an antidopamine action benefits psychotic disorders. PET studies of obsessive-compulsive disorder

Conclusion

Assuming antipsychotics work (at least in part) by blocking DA receptors, it is not known why such blockade leads to a lessening of psychosis, but clearly, these agents do more than control agitation. Further, neuroleptics are most effective for positive symptoms. Novel agents may also inhibit mesocortical dopamine neurons, which, in turn, would enhance frontal lobe function, perhaps explaining why novel antipsychotics may reduce negative symptoms. This latter effect is also consistent with the hypothesis that the dorsal lateral prefrontal cortex may be particularly important when considering negative symptoms, as opposed to the anterior cingulate or limbic

TABLE 5-5. *Schizophrenia: symptom complexes*

Psychosis
  Hallucinations
  Delusions
Cognition
  Dissociative thinking
  Disorganization of thoughts
  Attentional impairments
Negative symptoms (e.g., deficit syndrome)
  Primary
  Secondary
    Dysphoria
    Neuroleptic-induced
Mood symptoms
  Dysphoria
  Depression

TABLE 5-6. *Efficacy of antipsychotics*

Degree of remission	Degree of change	Drug (%)	Placebo (%)
Remitted	Very much improved	16	1
Only borderline symptoms remain	Improved	29	11
Mild symptoms still present	Improved	16	10
Moderately ill	Slightly improved	31	31
Moderately ill	Not improved	6	15
Severely ill	Worse	2	33

From Cole JO, Davis JM. Antipsychotic drugs. In: Bellak L, Loeb L, eds. *The schizophrenic syndrome*. New York: Grune & Stratton, 1969:478–568, with permission.

find increased activity in the basal ganglia, which may prolong the "on-line" time of obsessive ideation. It is tempting to speculate that antipsychotics, also working through their effects on the basal ganglia, allow thought patterns to stay "on-line" for longer periods, thus approximating a more normal pattern. The practical consequence of drug treatment is that patients become less psychotic, as manifested by an improvement in all aspects of the syndrome, including thought disorder, cognition, mood, and behavior (30).

MANAGEMENT OF ACUTE PSYCHOSIS

Efficacy for Acute Treatment

Neuroleptics

Most double-blind studies evaluating the efficacy of antipsychotics find them superior to placebo for the treatment of acute and chronic psychotic disorders (primarily schizophrenia). For example, a classic double-blind, random-assignment investigation by Cole et al. (31) compared the response of schizophrenics treated with antipsychotics or placebo. In a reexamination of the data, we compared the fate of the 10% to 20% who had the best outcome (32). A small percentage recovered completely without residual symptoms in 6 weeks, representing about 16% of those on an active drug, but only about 1% on placebo. This is a remarkable difference, and although some did relatively well without medication, it is likely that they would have done even better with active drug therapy. Further, in the drug-treated group, only 2% deteriorated, in contrast to 33% in the placebo group. It is true that some patients showed little improvement with antipsychotics, but if they

had been given only placebo, these patients most likely would have deteriorated even more. Thus, at both ends of the prognostic spectrum, there appears to be a substantial benefit from drugs.

In some of the studies, the dosage was too low to produce an effect; but when adequate, these agents were consistently superior to placebo. The magnitude of improvement in the drug-treated group was considerable whether evaluated by the degree of change (e.g., worse, no change, slight improvement, marked improvement) or degree of remission (e.g., full remission, only minimal symptoms, still mildly ill, moderately ill, or severely ill). Results from a National Institute of Mental Health (NIMH) Collaborative Study, combining both types of evaluation, are presented in Table 5-6 (31, 32). These results can be summarized as follows:

- Sixteen percent of the drug-treated versus only 1% of the placebo-treated groups were *in complete remission* or *very much improved.*
- Twenty-nine percent of the drug-treated and 11% of the placebo group were evaluated as *improved, with only borderline symptoms.*
- Sixteen percent of the drug-treated and 10% of the placebo group were evaluated as *improved, with mild symptoms remaining.*
- Eight percent of patients *did poorly* on active drug (i.e., rated as not improved or still ill), compared with 48% on placebo.
- Only 2% of those on an antipsychotic versus 33% of the placebo patients *deteriorated* during 6 weeks of treatment.
- The *largest differences* between the drug- and the placebo-treated patients are *seen at both ends of the outcome spectrum.*

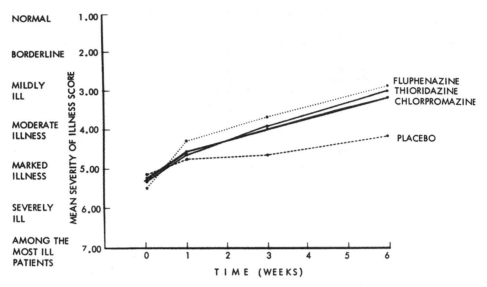

FIG. 5-4. Severity of illness over time in patients treated with phenothiazines. (From Cole JO, Davis JM. Antipsychotic drugs. In: Bellak L, Loeb L, eds. *The schizophrenic syndrome.* New York: Grune & Stratton, 1969:478–568, with permission.)

This study also found that new schizophrenic symptoms often emerged during the 6 weeks of placebo treatment, whereas worsening of symptoms was prevented by antipsychotics. **Heinz Lehmann (33) coined the term "psychostatic" to describe the ability of phenothiazine antipsychotics to prevent the reemergence of symptoms.**

The time course of improvement for most acutely psychotic patients on these agents (Fig. 5-4) demonstrates that most therapeutic gain occurs during the first 6 weeks, although further progress can be realized much later (e.g., clozapine). Thus, some patients improve rapidly, within a few days, whereas others show gradual changes over several months. There is no evidence for clinical tolerance, for if there were, one would have to increase the dose over time. Fixed-dose studies, however, show that the initial effective amount of drug does not lose efficacy. In addition, patients do not require higher doses after several weeks of treatment; instead, the reverse appears to be true. It is also clear that antipsychotics do not produce dependency of the barbiturate, stimulant, or narcotic type.

In the hope of developing either a more effective agent or one with fewer adverse effects, medicinal chemists have synthesized a number of new compounds. Preclinical animal model studies are used to select potentially useful drugs, using a profile of pharmacological properties reflecting differential blockade of dopamine, as well as other neurotransmitter systems (e.g., 5-HT). This research has led to the development of several new classes, as noted earlier in this chapter.

The question immediately arises as to whether any of the drugs in these various classes are superior to CPZ for the typical patient, for particular symptoms, or for subgroups of patients. With the exception of promazine and mepazine, all neuroleptics are clearly superior to placebo or nonspecific sedatives (e.g., phenobarbital; Tables 5-7 to 5-10). Comparisons with CPZ in controlled trials found mepazine and promazine inferior to CPZ, but all other agents were equal to CPZ in therapeutic efficacy (Table 5-10). Other controlled trials using thioridazine or trifluoperazine as standards also found all other neuroleptics to be comparable with these agents (Table 5-10). Whereas there were trends at times favoring one agent over another, they were usually not statistically significant, and an inspection of the data finds no agent to be consistently superior to any other. Furthermore, all these drugs produced consistent changes in the same

TABLE 5-7. Neuroleptic versus placebo in controlled studies of schizophrenia[a]

Drug	Number of studies in which drug was	
	More effective than placebo	Equal to placebo
Chlorpromazine	55	11
Reserpine	20	9
Triflupromazine	9	1
Perphenazine	5	0
Prochlorperazine	7	2
Trifluoperazine	16	2
Fluphenazine	15	0
Butaperazine	4	0
Thioridazine	7	0
Mesoridazine	3	0
Carphenazine	2	0
Chlorprothixene	4	0
Thiothixene	2	0
Haloperidol	14	0
Molindone	1	0
Loxapine	5	1
Phenobarbital	0	3

[a]Adapted from Klein D, Davis JM. *Diagnosis and drug treatment of psychiatric disorders.* Baltimore: Williams & Wilkins, 1969.

symptoms. These similarities are quite striking and support the theory that they work through a common mechanism of action (e.g., dopamine blockade). Furthermore, relevant differences are primarily related to their side effect profiles.

Pimozide is FDA-labeled for Tourette's disorder and is particularly interesting in that it is a highly specific DA antagonist that may produce fewer adverse effects than haloperidol. In open studies with adequate doses, this agent has demonstrated efficacy for acute schizophrenia. Several double-blind trials comparing pimozide with other neuroleptics also found it to be an equally effective maintenance therapy (34–38).

We consider this agent to be as effective as the other standard agents, with the same, but perhaps less severe, side effects.

Novel Antipsychotics

All the novel antipsychotics have an enhanced 5-HT$_2$ to D$_2$ receptor affinity ratio and a lower, though not negligible, affinity for the D$_2$ receptor.

Based on both preclinical and clinical data, the following apply to the novel antipsychotics:

- Each may have *antipsychotic efficacy below EPS thresholds* for many patients.
- Each has a *favorable efficacy/adverse effects ratio.*
- Therapeutic doses of each usually evoke *minimal or no extrapyramidal reactions.*
- Each is effective in alleviating *positive and negative symptoms,* particularly drug-induced secondary negative symptoms of schizophrenia.
- Most have *minimal or no endocrine effects.*

Clozapine

Receptor-Binding Studies. Clozapine (Clozaril) is the first clinically effective antipsychotic with an atypical profile (39, 40). Using PET scanning, Farde and coworkers (41, 42) demonstrated that patients receiving neuroleptics exhibit striatal D$_2$ receptor occupancy in the 70% to 89% range. Further, those agents with greater propensity to induce EPS had higher D$_2$ receptor occupancy rates ($82 \pm 4\%$ versus $74 \pm 4\%$), whereas no patients with occupancy rates below 75% had any EPS (41). Farde and colleagues then demonstrated that the D$_2$ occupancy rate of clozapine (125 to 600 mg/day) was between 20% and 67%. Thus, clozapine's low incidence of EPS may well be due to a subthreshold level of D$_2$ occupancy at clinical doses (25).

TABLE 5-8. Later generation neuroleptics versus placebo for schizophrenia: acute treatment

Number of studies	Number of subjects	Responders (%)		Difference (%)	χ^2	p value
		Drug (%)	Placebo (%)			
Loxapine versus placebo						
5	197	61	34	27	16.8	4×10^{-5}
Molindone versus placebo						
1	29	20	0	20	3.12	0.08

TABLE 5-9. *Neuroleptics versus phenobarbital for schizophrenia: acute treatment*

Number of studies	Number of subjects	Responders (%)		Difference (%)	χ^2	p value
		Antipsychotics (%)	Phenobarbital (%)			
2	153	50	14	36	17.4	3×10^{-5}

Because clozapine is an effective D_4 receptor blocker, there has been speculation that its superior efficacy may be a consequence of this property. Several D_4 antagonists or $D_4/5\text{-}HT_2$ antago- nists have been studied in early clinical investigations; however, they failed as effective treatments for schizophrenia in phase II trials. There is a striking correlation between clinical efficacy and

TABLE 5-10. *Effectiveness of other neuroleptics compared with chlorpromazine, thioridazine, and trifluoperazine*

Drug	Number of studies in which drug was		
	More effective than chlorpromazine	As effective	Less effective
Mepazine	0	0	4
Promazine	0	2	4
Triflupromazine	0	10	0
Perphenazine	0	6	0
Prochlorperazine	0	10	0
Trifluoperazine	0	11	0
Butaperazine	0	2	0
Thioridazine	0	12	0
Mesoridazine	0	7	0
Fluphenazine	0	9	0
Carphenazine	0	2	0
Acetophenazine	0	1	0
Thiopropazate	0	1	0
Chlorpromazine	0	6	0
Thiothixene	0	4	0
Haloperidol	0	4	0
Molindone	0	6	0
Loxapine	0	14	1
	More effective than thioridazine	As effective	Less effective
Mesoridazine	0	2	0
Carphenazine	0	1	0
Haloperidol	0	2	0
Piperacetazine	0	3	0
	More effective than trifluoperazine	As effective	Less effective
Mesoridazine	0	1	0
Carphenazine	0	3	0
Acetophenazine	0	1	0
Butaperazine	0	3	0
Chlorprothixene	0	1	0
Haloperidol	0	4	0

Adapted from Klein D, Davis JM. *Diagnosis and drug treatment of psychiatric disorders.* Baltimore: Williams & Wilkins, 1969.

D_2 blockade with most antipsychotics. Clozapine is a partial exception because it is a weaker D_2 antagonist than other agents at usual clinical doses. Although the pharmacological reason for clozapine's greater efficacy has not been elucidated, there is little evidence that its greater efficacy is explained by D_4 antagonism.

In summary, compared with neuroleptics, clozapine:

- Has a lower affinity for *D_2 receptors.*
- Binds proportionately more to *D_1 and D_4 receptors.*
- Appears to act selectively on *cortical* and *mesolimbic* DA neuronal systems (in preference to the nigrostriatal and tuberoinfundibular areas).
- Blocks *5-HT_2 receptors.*
- Has *few or no EPS effects* across the recommended dosing range.
- Has effects on several *other neurotransmitter systems* (e.g., NE, acetylcholine).
- Has a decreased rate of *sexual* and *reproductive dysfunction.*

More than 25 years' experience has established that clozapine is an effective treatment for:

- *Acute* and *maintenance* therapy of schizophrenia
- Neuroleptic *treatment-responsive* and *treatment-refractory* psychoses
- *Negative symptoms,* including EPS-related (43, 44)

Because of the difficulty in differentiating primary from secondary negative symptoms, however, continued assessment of clozapine's benefit is needed (45–48). Furthermore, clozapine's ability to improve cognitive function may be even more pronounced than its effects on negative symptoms (47–51).

The long-term effects of clozapine were documented after 18 months of treatment that led to substantial improvement in symptoms and social functioning in approximately 70% of previously treatment-refractory patients. This study used a mirror-image design that compared response to neuroleptics over a similar earlier period of time (52). Another study of 96 previously treatment-resistant patients treated with clozapine for at

least 2 years revealed marked improvement in the BPRS total scores, as well as positive and negative symptom subscale scores; Global Assessment Scale scores; Quality of Life scores; work functioning; capacity for independent living; and rehospitalization rates (53).

Clozapine also has been shown to benefit schizoaffective and bipolar patients with treatment-refractory mania (54); patients with Parkinson's disease; and those with other neurological disorders with psychoses, such as Huntington's disease. Although clozapine has been shown to be an effective agent in the elderly, its usefulness in this population is limited because of its anticholinergic, sedative, cardiovascular, and potentially toxic effects on the bone marrow (55). In a study of 12 elderly female psychotic patients on clozapine (maximal daily dose, 300 mg), for example, five were taken off clozapine because of postural hypotension, one had a nonfatal episode of agranulocytosis, and one had leukopenia (56).

Therapeutic Efficacy. Early evidence supporting clozapine's efficacy came from one double-blind, placebo-controlled study and six other neuroleptic-controlled, random-assignment studies (43, 57–60; Novartis, unpublished data). When compared with neuroleptics such as CPZ and haloperidol, clozapine was found to be more effective (i.e., three studies found clozapine significantly superior and two others found a trend favoring clozapine ($p = 0.10$)). When the results of these studies were combined, the probability that clozapine is superior to neuroleptic antipsychotics was highly statistically significant ($p = 1 \times 10^{-10}$) (Tables 5-11 and 5-12).

Remembering that when a large number of patients are studied, a relatively small effect can become statistically significant, this evidence seems to establish that clozapine is more effective than conventional agents. Because clozapine is marketed in over 20 countries, there has been wide clinical experience and several open trials supporting its efficacy as well.

Even though this agent has been found to be superior to neuroleptics, as well as to placebo, and beneficial in a substantial proportion of nonresponders, its side effect profile has been a major obstacle to its widespread use. Specifically,

TABLE 5-11. *Clozapine versus neuroleptics for schizophrenia: acute treatment*

Number of studies	Number of subjects	Responders (%) Clozapine (%)	Standard drug (%)	Difference (%)	χ^2	*p* value
1	25	85	75	10		
1	102	92	80	12		
1	216	70	57	13		
1	79	31	10	21		
1	267[a]	30	4	26		
1	50	92	60	32		
6	739	57%	36%	21%	41.7	1×10^{-10}

Meta-analysis of six random assignment double-blind studies (43, 57–60, Novartis, unpublished data) comparing clozapine to neuroleptics.

agranulocytosis (approximately 0.5 % to 1% incidence) and seizures (usually with higher doses) are the most serious side effects.

Given clozapine's significant adverse effects, Lieberman and colleagues (39) recommend its use only in psychotic patients who are clear nonresponders to other agents, in that they:

- *Failed three trials* of different agents from at least two chemical classes.
- Were treated for at least *6 weeks.*
- Received *doses in excess of 1,000 mg chlorpromazine equivalents.*
- Had *therapeutic drug monitoring (TDM)* or *parenteral administration* to control for rapid metabolism or a large first-pass effect.

More recently, some have advocated for adequate trials with at least one other novel agent and one neuroleptic before a trial with clozapine.

Clozapine For Comorbid Substance Abuse or Dependency. Comorbidity of alcohol/substance abuse or dependency with schizophrenia is substancial. In this context, Green and coworkers (61) made an interesting observation in two patients with schizophrenia and excessive alcohol abuse. These patients experience a dramatic decrease in alcohol use coincidental with beginning treatment with clozapine. Buckley and colleagues (62), as well as Marcus and Snyder (63), also observed a similar phenomenon in patients with comorbid schizophrenia and substance abuse treated with clozapine. Furthermore, Yovell and Opler (64) noted a decrease in craving for cocaine in clozapine-treated patients with schizophrenia. Several groups have also reported decreased smoking in schizophrenic patients treated with clozapine. It is likely that dopamine mediates the euphoria that is the common denominator of substance abuse. Through various mechanisms, an increase in dopamine release may be the common denominator for the pleasure of smoking, narcotic addiction, cocaine abuse, and alcoholism. Subsequently, Drake et al.

TABLE 5-12. *Clozapine versus neuroleptics for schizophrenia: acute treatment—summations*

Number of studies	Number of subjects	Responders (%) Clozapine (%)	Standard drug (%)	Difference (%)	χ^2	*p* value
Low difference groups						
4	422	31	45	15	10.4	0.001
High difference groups						
2	317	40	12	28	39.6	3×10^{-10}

(65) conducted several systematic observational studies. For example, 151 patients who were comorbid for alcohol use disorder were followed in a psychosocial treatment study. Of this group, 36 patients were treated with clozapine, which produced a significant reduction in the severity of alcohol use that was correlated with improvement of negative symptoms. The remission rate of alcohol abuse was 79% in patients comorbid for alcohol use disorder taking clozapine as compared with only 34% of those not on clozapine. These researchers also conducted a retrospective survey of 36 dual-diagnosis, schizophrenic patients with comorbid substance use disorder, and 85% demonstrated a decrease in symptoms. Although definitive, controlled, randomized studies have yet to be reported, this study is an interesting lead.

Starting doses should be in the range of 25 to 50 mg/day and titrated up slowly to minimize hypotension. The usual therapeutic range is 300 to 500 mg/day (the recommended maximal dose is 900 mg/day). The usual therapeutic dose is typically achieved in 2 to 5 weeks and should be maintained for several more before considering an increase. In this context, Perry and colleagues found a therapeutic threshold clozapine plasma level of 350 ng/mL (i.e., 64% with levels above this responded, versus only 22% with levels below this point), which required an average dose of 380 mg/day (66).

Risperidone

Receptor-Binding Studies. Risperidone (Risperdal) is a benzisoxazole derivative that has a relatively high $5\text{-}HT_{2A}/D_2$ ratio and relatively fewer and milder EPS than neuroleptics at its clinically effective doses. Receptor-binding studies of risperidone and its active metabolite, 9-OH-risperidone, in comparison with other novel antipsychotics revealed that:

In vitro:

- *Risperidone, 9-OH-risperidone,* and *ziprasidone* had the highest affinity for human D_2 receptors.
- *Olanzapine* was slightly less potent at D_2 receptor sites.
- *Clozapine* and *quetiapine* showed two orders of magnitude lower D_2 affinity (67).

In vivo:

- *Risperidone, 9-OH-risperidone, olanzapine, and clozapine* maintained a higher potency for occupying $5\text{-}HT_{2A}$ than D_2 receptors.
- *Risperidone* had a $5\text{-}HT_{2A}$ versus D_2 potency ratio of about 20.
- High potency for $5\text{-}HT_{2A}$ occupancy was observed for *risperidone* and *olanzapine*.

All the various compounds also displayed high to moderate occupancy of adrenergic a_1-receptors, with clozapine occupying even more a_1-receptors than D_2 receptors. Clozapine also showed predominant occupancy of H_1 receptors and occupied cholinergic receptors with equivalent potency to D_2 receptors.

A stronger predominance of $5\text{-}HT_{2A}$ versus D_2 receptor occupancy, combined with a more gradual occupancy of D_2 receptors, differentiated risperidone and 9-OH-risperidone from the other novel compounds. The predominant $5\text{-}HT_{2A}$ receptor occupancy probably plays a role in the beneficial action of risperidone on the negative symptoms of schizophrenia, whereas maintenance of a moderate occupancy of D_2 receptors seems adequate for treating the positive symptoms. Combined $5\text{-}HT_{2A}$ and D_2 occupancy and the avoidance of excessive D_2 receptor blockade are believed to reduce the risk for EPS (67–71). While risperidone also has a high affinity for the $5\text{-}HT_7$ but not for the $5\text{-}HT_6$ receptor, the importance of this differential activity is not clear.

Nyberg and colleagues (72) were the first to demonstrate that risperidone induces marked occupancy of central $5\text{-}HT_2$ and D_2 receptors *in vivo*. About 60% (range, 45% to 68%) of the $5\text{-}HT_2$ receptors in the frontal cortex and about 50% (range, 40% to 64%) of the D_2 receptors in the striatum were occupied 4 and 7 hours, respectively, after a single oral dose of 1 mg. These results indicate that $5\text{-}HT_2$ receptor occupancy should be very high at doses of 4 to 10 mg daily.

Because antipsychotic-induced EPS is related to the level of D_2 receptor occupancy, Kapur and his colleagues (73) used [11C]raclopride PET scans to determine *in vivo* D_2 receptor-binding characteristics in nine patients receiving 2 to 6 mg/day of risperidone. **These authors found that the mean level of receptor occupancy was 66% at 2 mg, 73% at 4 mg, and 79% at 6 mg.**

Further, the three patients who had the highest receptor occupancies experienced mild EPS that did not require antiparkinsonian medication. These results suggest that risperidone 4 to 6 mg daily achieves a D_2 receptor occupancy similar to that of neuroleptics and higher than that of clozapine. The occurrence of EPS at higher levels of D_2 receptor occupancy in this study and in previous clinical trials indicates that risperidone's high 5-HT_2 affinity provides some protection against EPS. Clinical and laboratory data suggest that when the D_2 receptor occupancy exceeds a certain threshold, any 5-HT_2-mediated protection against EPS may be lost. **Risperidone's low propensity to evoke EPS is progressively diminished as its dose increases and its occupancy of D_2 receptors rises. Thus, there is a dosage range between inducing and not inducing EPS.** Kapur (14) concluded that "5-HT_2 converts the erstwhile neuroleptic threshold for EPS into a 'neuroleptic foyer'" that provides "a larger window of treatment above the therapeutic threshold, but it does not guarantee freedom from EPS."

Therapeutic Efficacy. The therapeutic efficacy of risperidone for schizophrenia has been well established in several controlled trials conducted worldwide (74, 75). The clinical efficacy trials performed to support approval of risperidone by regulatory agencies have all been published. Therefore, it is appropriate to combine these data using meta-analytic techniques to explore the efficacy of risperidone compared with neuroleptics. For most drugs, the relationship of dose and response is defined by the classic sigmoidal curve. Thus, as the dose (or plasma level) increases beyond a threshold and reaches the linear portion of the curve, response increases. Once the dose is high enough to produce maximal clinical response, the dose-response curve then levels off.

Because a therapeutic window has been hypothesized to exist for neuroleptics, its existence for risperidone is a reasonable supposition. Indeed, evidence to support such a window was established in the North American Clinical Trial and the International Collaborative Study, both of which found doses of 4, 6, and 8 mg superior to higher or lower doses of risperidone.

In a study design with multiple groups, there will always be one group with a better outcome because of statistical variations. Therefore, a meta-analysis focusing on the 4–8-mg dose range of risperidone may only take advantage of such a statistical artifact (i.e., a best-case scenario). If we assume that doses of 4 mg or above are sufficient to produce an optimal response, then averaging all the doses above 4 mg may be the best estimate of the true efficacy of risperidone (i.e., a worst-case scenario). We calculated both scenarios using a meta-analysis on the published double-blind, random-assignment, controlled studies of risperidone versus neuroleptics to explore whether there is a difference in efficacy. Additionally, we performed a meta-analysis comparing doses of 10 mg or higher versus the dose range of 4 to 8 mg to see whether there is statistical evidence for a therapeutic window.

There are two basic types of meta-analysis: one is based on the number of patients who respond or do not respond to medication; the other is based on the mean improvement in the drug and the control groups. The former analysis can be considered a fourfold table of responders or nonresponders to the experimental treatment versus placebo or a standard treatment. The latter uses the method of Hedges and Oklin, which is based on the mean improvement score (and then the standard deviation) of patients receiving new drug versus conventional drug in each investigation. We performed both types of analysis (see also Chapter 2).

All these studies essentially use the same definition for responder (i.e., 20% improvement on a standard rating instrument, usually the Positive and Negative Symptoms Scale [PANSS]). Because this criterion is the standard and was decided beforehand, there is no statistical problem of a post hoc choice of optimal cutoff points for dichotomization.

It is important to first examine the possible superiority of a new versus conventional drug on the PANSS or the BPRS total scores before examining the effect on positive, negative, and general symptoms. If the overall effect is not significant, greater efficacy on one subscale may be balanced by a lesser outcome on another subscale. **Our**

TABLE 5-13. *Risperidone versus placebo for schizophrenia: acute treatment*

No. of studies	No. of subjects	Responders (%)		Difference (%)	χ^2	p value
		Risperidone	Placebo			
3	365	51	17	34	31	10^{-8}

Risperidone versus haloperidol for schizophrenia: acute treatment

No. of studies	No. of subjects	Responders (%)		Difference (%)	χ^2	p value
		Risperidone	Haloperidol			
12	2103	59	52	7	35.1	10^{-9}

Risperidone versus clozapine for schizophrenia: acute treatment[a]

No. of studies	No. of subjects	Responders (%)		Difference (%)	χ^2	p value
		Risperidone	Clozapine			
4	175	53%	58%	−5%	0.4	NS

[a] Meta-analysis of four random assignment double-blind studies (77, 78, 81, 82) comparing clozapine to risperidone.

meta-analysis clearly shows risperidone to be significantly superior overall to both placebo and haloperidol for general symptoms (76) (Table 5-13). This outcome is consistent with our reanalysis of the North American Clinical Trial data, which found risperidone superior to haloperidol for both positive and negative symptoms.

Risperidone Versus Clozapine. Several studies have also compared the efficacy and the safety of risperidone with clozapine in treatment-refractory schizophrenia (77–82). The results indicate that both agents may be comparably effective. Bondolfi et al. (82), for example, conducted an 8-week randomized, double-blind trial of risperidone versus clozapine in 86 treatment-resistant, physically healthy, chronic schizophrenics, each of whom had a total score of 60 to 120 on the PANSS. After a 1-week washout period, risperidone was increased to 6 mg/day or clozapine to 300 mg/day for the first segment of double-blind administration. At treatment endpoint, the mean daily doses were risperidone 6.4 mg (range, 3 to 10 mg/day) versus clozapine 291.2 mg (range, 150 to 400 mg/day). Patients were examined on days 7, 14, 21, 28, 42, and 56, and evaluated with the PANSS and the Clinical Global Impression (CGI) scales. Clinical improvement was defined as 20% or greater reduction in the total PANSS score. EPS was also

assessed by means of the Extrapyramidal Symptom Rating Scale (ESRS), while other adverse effects were rated by the UKU side effect rating scale. Both risperidone and clozapine were effective and safe. Although the overall incidence of treatment-emergent adverse effects was generally the same in both groups, significantly more patients on clozapine reported asthenia, lassitude, or increased fatigability, as well as weight gain. A meta-analysis of four randomized comparison trials found no difference in efficacy between these two agents. The doses of clozapine, however, were relatively low (Table 5-13).

Mood Disorders. Risperidone has also been reported to benefit major depressive disorder with psychosis, bipolar mania, and schizoaffective disorder (83–87).

In a few bipolar or schizoaffective patients, behavioral stimulation may be a prodrome to hypomania or mania. In this context, Dwight and colleagues (88) reported on eight consecutive patients with schizoaffective disorder by DSM-III-R criteria (six bipolar type, two depressive type). Of the six patients with bipolar schizoaffective disorder, four received risperidone alone, one had risperidone added to lithium (1,200 mg/day), and one had risperidone added to valproate (3,000 mg/day). The two patients with the depressive subtype of schizoaffective disorder received risperidone alone. The six patients in the bipolar group exhibited an increase in manic symptoms after 7 days of risperidone treatment, whereas all patients with substantial depressive symptoms displayed significant reductions in Hamilton Depression Rating Scale (HDRS) scores. The authors conclude that at least two possibilities may account for these observations: risperidone may have been ineffective in reducing manic symptoms in this small series of patients and symptomatic worsening may have been caused by progression of illness alone, or risperidone may have precipitated or exacerbated symptoms of mania. Several indications support the latter possibility. First, risperidone is a potent $5\text{-}HT_2$ receptor antagonist, which may imbue it with antidepressant activity (89, 90). Second, three patients who were depressed at the time of risperidone administration experienced an apparent switch into mania, reflected by an increase in their Young Mania Rating Scale scores and a decrease in their HDRS scores over the same interval. Third, in two patients, the addition of valproate reduced manic symptoms. Last, all patients with depressive symptoms had considerable improvement.

In contrast, other reports have indicated that risperidone may have precisely the opposite effect in bipolar and schizoaffective patients, with good-to-excellent mood-stabilizing and antipsychotic effects noted and no emergent cases of mania or hypomania. Tohen and coworkers (91), for example, effectively treated 20 bipolar I patients with a mean risperidone dosage of 5.1 ± 1.6 mg/day for more than 6 weeks with no induction of mania. Madhusoodanan and colleagues (92) also reported on two elderly schizoaffective, bipolar type, and two elderly bipolar patients who received a mean risperidone dosage of 1.9 ± 0.9 mg/day for about 3 weeks with a good response and no induction of mania or hypomania.

Janicak et al. (87) studied the relative efficacy and safety of risperidone versus haloperidol in the treatment of schizoaffective disorder. Sixty-two patients (29 depressed type, 33 bipolar type) entered a randomized, double-blind, 6-week trial of risperidone (up to 10 mg/day) or haloperidol (up to 20 mg/day). They found no difference between risperidone and haloperidol in the amelioration of psychotic and manic symptoms

nor any significant worsening of mania with either agent. For the total PANSS, risperidone produced a mean decrease of 16 points from baseline, compared with a 14-point decrease with haloperidol. For the total CARS-M scale, risperidone and haloperidol produced mean change scores of 5 and 8 points, respectively; and for the CARS-M mania factor, 3 and 7 points, respectively. Additionally, risperidone produced a mean decrease of 13 points from the baseline 24-item HAM-D compared with an 8-point decrease with haloperidol. In those patients who had more severe depressive symptoms (HAM-D baseline score >20), risperidone produced at least a 50% mean improvement in 12 of 16 (75%) patients, in comparison with 8 of 21 (38%) patients receiving haloperidol. Haloperidol produced significantly more EPS and resulted in more dropouts due to any side effect.

Although the data are relatively limited, we believe that risperidone may be a potential mood-stabilizing agent, and that lower doses and a slower escalation can substantially reduce any risk of a switch in mood phases (93).

Other Disorders. Risperidone therapy has been tried in several other conditions with mixed results, including:

- *Tic* disorders
- Mental retardation or pervasive *developmental disorders*
- *Psychiatric disorders caused by a medical condition* (e.g., acquired immune deficiency syndrome [AIDS]; organic delusional disorders)
- *Agitated or aggressive* states, including those associated with dementia
- *Anorexia nervosa*
- *Personality disorders* (e.g., borderline and schizotypal)
- *Obsessive-compulsive disorder*
- *Posttraumatic stress disorder*
- *Various other psychotic disorders,* such as brief psychotic disorder, delusional disorder, shared psychotic disorder, substance-induced psychotic disorder, and psychotic disorder not otherwise specified (94)

Developmentally disabled. The effect of risperidone in 63 adult, developmentally disabled men with disruptive, agitated, aggressive, or self-injurious behaviors was compared with their previous behavior on neuroleptics, usually haloperidol (95). Although not blinded, the clinical staff observed behavior without knowledge of medication. Targeted behaviors were measured for 6 months before treatment with risperidone began and then for each month after treatment. The mean dose of risperidone was 5.6 mg/day, and the mean duration was 643 days. Risperidone lowered ratings of self-injurious behavior from 55 to 18 and aggressive behavior from 23 to 9, while also producing a modest increase in appropriate social behaviors. The most striking finding of this mirror-image study was the reduction of aggression, which was not due to sedation because social interactions also increased.

In another study, 118 children with IQs ranging from 35 to 84 who demonstrated conduct disorder were randomized to risperidone (at a mean dose of 1.23 mg/day) versus placebo in a double-blind design (96). In comparison with placebo, risperidone produced a statistically significant reduction in insecure/anxious behavior, hyperactivity, self-injurious/stereotyped behavior, irritability, and aggressive/destructive behavior, as well as an increase in adaptive social behavior. The latter is important because it shows that the changes are not due to sedation, although more somnolence was apparent with risperidone.

Conduct disorder. The response of aggressive behavior in 20 patients with conduct disorder was evaluated in a double-blind, random-assignment, 10-week study comparing placebo with risperidone (dose range, 1.5-3 mg/day) (97). Children 5-15 years of age without mental retardation (i.e., IQ >80) and without attention deficit hyperactivity disorder (ADHD) were studied. The primary outcome variable was the Rating of Aggression against People and/or Property Scale. A 5 on this scale indicates that a person frequently attacks others and destroys property; 4, occasional attacks on people and destroys property; 3, a person either fights or is destructive; 2, someone is verbally abusive; 1, no aggression reported. At baseline, the children's mean score was about 3.7. At 10 weeks, those on placebo had scores of about 3.5, but those on risperidone had dropped to about 2.0.

Switching from Clozapine to Risperidone

Patients often switch from clozapine to risperidone because of:

- Clozapine's *side effects*
- The weekly *venipunctures* required for hematological monitoring
- The *cost* of clozapine and laboratory testing
- The hope that risperidone will be *safer* and *at least as effective*

Early after the introduction of risperidone, many patients who were doing reasonably well on clozapine risked deterioration by abruptly switching to risperidone. Indeed, a number of case reports have been published of patients who switched from clozapine to another atypical antipsychotic such as risperidone and then relapsed. Clinical evidence exists for a clozapine withdrawal syndrome manifested by worsening psychosis. Because it is possible that clozapine is uniquely effective for some patients, before switching a previously neuroleptic-refractory patient benefiting from clozapine, the clinician should *very carefully* weigh the risk of clozapine discontinuation with the possibility of a safer, as well as comparable, therapeutic response to an agent such as risperidone. This discontinuation is done best by cross-tapering or overlapping clozapine with the alternate agent (e.g., starting with a low risperidone dose [0.5 mg/day]) and gradually increasing it while reducing the clozapine over many weeks (98).

Switching from Risperidone to Clozapine

As noted earlier, this switch should always be done by cross-tapering, thus overlapping risperidone with clozapine. We suggest starting with a low clozapine dose (12.5 or 25 mg/day), with gradual increments, paralleled by a gradual reduction of the risperidone until it is totally discontinued.

Clozapine Plus Risperidone

In this context, there is anecdotal clinical data indicating that risperidone and clozapine can be overlapped or used concomitantly

with beneficial results and no serious adverse reactions (99–102). This strategy has been used successfully for residual positive symptoms during clozapine therapy and in patients who relapsed when a neuroleptic was withdrawn from combined therapy with clozapine. Indeed, up to 60% of clozapine-treated patients receive additional medication, including a second antipsychotic.

Among the reports on overlapping or combining clozapine and risperidone, some pharmacokinetic interactions have been reported (100, 103–105).

Case Example: Because of a patient's partial response to 5 months of clozapine therapy at 600 mg/day, risperidone was added for augmentation (started with 0.5 mg b.i.d. and increased to 1 mg b.i.d. after 1 week). Before this addition, the clozapine plasma level was 344 ng/mL, but after 2 weeks of risperidone augmentation, the level was elevated to 598 ng/mL with no adverse effects and substantial clinical benefit. In another report, there was an increase in the steady-state plasma levels of clozapine (675 mg/day) and its active metabolite norclozapine after the addition of risperidone 2 mg/day in a patient treated for 2 years. Before the addition of risperidone, her clozapine and norclozapine levels were 829 and 1,384 ng/mL, respectively. Two days after risperidone was added, these levels rose to 980 and 1,800 ng/mL. Clozapine dosage was reduced to 500 mg/day, and after 5 days of combined treatment with 4 mg/day of risperidone, the clozapine and norclozapine levels were 110 and 760 ng/mL, respectively. Aside from some mild oculogyric crises, she had no symptoms of clozapine toxicity or clinical changes during the period of cross-tapering. In another case, risperidone was added to clozapine because the patient had relapsed after discontinuation of fluphenazine and had not responded to clozapine. The addition of risperidone resulted in an acute remission of psychosis (100).

Because coadministered clozapine and risperidone may result in elevated plasma levels of clozapine and norclozapine, plasma levels should be monitored when these drugs are prescribed concurrently. Not all patients receiving risperidone as an adjunct to clozapine therapy, however, experience significant increases in blood levels. For example, in an open clinical trial, 12 patients were treated with clozapine (mean daily dose, 479.2 ± 121.5 mg; range 250 to 700 mg/day) and risperidone (mean daily dose, 3.8 ± 1.4 mg; range 2 to 6 mg) (66). In seven patients, clozapine serum concentrations assayed before and after 4 weeks of risperidone treatment increased nonsignificantly by 2.2% (i.e., from 374.6 ± 143.9 ng/mL to 382.9 ± 218.3 ng/mL). The addition of risperidone to clozapine was well tolerated and produced significant reduction of symptoms on the total BPRS and the psychotic, negative symptom, and depression subscales. No patients complained of dizziness or demonstrated changes in their blood pressure or pulse.

Combined risperidone and electroconvulsive therapy (ECT) produced a remarkable improvement in one patient's refractory depression, but it also caused a return of prior TD symptoms (106). When clozapine was added to the ECT-risperidone regimen and risperidone was tapered gradually, the patient's TD signs and symptoms remitted, and she responded well to combined ECT and clozapine.

Olanzapine

Receptor-Binding Studies. Olanzapine (Zyprexa) is a thienobenzodiazepine derivative with a receptor-binding profile similar to that of clozapine (Table 5-2) (107). The effects of olanzapine in several animal behavioral tests (e.g., conditioned avoidance response, apomorphine-induced climbing, 5-HTP-induced head twitch, punished responding, and drug discrimination studies), neuroendocrine assays, and electrophysiological studies suggest that it has a pharmacological profile similar to that of clozapine, and therefore may have similar antipsychotic effects in humans (108–110). Furthermore, as with clozapine, chronic olanzapine administration selectively decreases the number of spontaneously active A-10, but not the A-9, dopamine neurons (110).

In contrast to risperidone, which has a high affinity for the newly cloned 5-HT$_7$ receptor, olanzapine has a greater affinity for the 5-HT$_6$ receptor (68).

In 1996, Pilowsky and coworkers (111) found that olanzapine-treated patients showed significantly lower occupancy of striatal D$_2$ receptors compared with neuroleptic-treated patients. In support of the clinical trial data, PET studies have shown that 5-HT$_2$ and D$_2$ receptor occupancies with olanzapine and clozapine are comparable, and that olanzapine should have a low propensity to evoke acute EPS (112).

Therapeutic Efficacy. Data from a North American and European multicenter, fixed-dosing range, controlled study demonstrated that olanzapine significantly reduced symptoms in schizophrenic patients with a trend to be superior to that produced by haloperidol (15 ± 5 mg/day) (113, 114). These dose-finding studies found that a mean olanzapine dose of 10 mg/day produced a therapeutic benefit clearly superior to placebo (115). Although this dose does not necessarily guarantee full efficacy, all but one patient had a therapeutic response, as determined by a greater than 20% improvement in total BPRS scores. It also produced less acute EPS and reduced negative symptoms to a statistically superior extent than haloperidol (116).

An international, multicenter, double-blind trial addressed the acute efficacy and safety of a single-dose range of olanzapine (5 to 20 mg/day) compared with a single-dose range of haloperidol (5 to 20 mg/day) (116). A total of 1996 patients with a DSM-III-R diagnosis of schizophrenia (83.1%), schizophreniform disorder (1.9%), or schizoaffective disorder (15%) participated in this study. The primary overall efficacy analysis (i.e., the difference in baseline to endpoint [last observation carried forward [LOCF]] mean change on the BPRS) found olanzapine to be statistically superior to haloperidol (HPDL) (i.e., -10.98; -7.93; $p < 0.015$).

Our meta-analysis (best/worst case scenarios) of olanzapine studies shows that it is superior to haloperidol by a substantial degree, as well as superior for negative symptoms (Table 5-14). This is also consistent with the results of a path analysis suggesting that primary negative symptoms of schizophrenia were responsive to olanzapine (117). In interpreting these results, it is important to remember that none of the individual studies or the meta-analyses provides absolute improvement rates; rather, they provide information on the relative improvement with a new drug in comparison with placebo or a conventional agent. Therefore, it is not statistically valid to interpret effect-size changes as absolute measures.

In addition, in the international trial, the 300 patients with schizoaffective disorder (177 bipolar type and 123 depressive type) were the focus of a separate analysis (118). At the end of the maintenance phase, the bipolar subgroup had significantly greater improvement in mean change scores on the BPRS total score, the PANSS total score, the PANSS negative symptom subscale score, the CGI severity, and the Montgomery-Asberg Depression Rating Scale (MADRS). For the depressed subgroup, the magnitude of the improvement in BPRS total, PANSS total, and PANSS negative symptom scores was even greater than that observed in the bipolar subgroup. **Overall, these results indicate that olanzapine may be significantly superior to haloperidol in the treatment**

TABLE 5-14. *Olanzapine versus neuroleptics for schizophrenic: acute treatment*

Study	Effect size	Z statistic	p value
Best dose total score			
Positive symptoms	0.19	4.39	0.00001
Negative symptoms	0.12	2.74	0.01
Total symptoms	0.19	4.31	0.00002

of patients with schizoaffective disorder (113).

Olanzapine Versus Clozapine. Beasley et al. reported the results of a large, collaborative (41 centers), random-assignment, parallel-group, double-blind, placebo-controlled study of clozapine versus olanzapine in 180 patients who were nonresponsive to previous antipsychotics (119). A mean modal dose of 22 mg/day of olanzapine demonstrated a nonsignificant trend to produce more improvement than a mean modal dose of 354 mg/day of clozapine. For example, on the PANSS total score, olanzapine displayed an improvement of 26 points and clozapine showed an improvement of 22 points. Because patients were on neuroleptics before the study began, many had EPS at the start of the study and consequently were treated with anticholinergics. Those on olanzapine displayed a greater amelioration of EPS than clozapine, thereby decreasing the use of anticholinergics in this group. Ten percent of patients required anticholinergics while on clozapine, and 4.4% of patients needed anticholinergics on olanzapine. Additionally, olanzapine displayed a lower incidence of other side effects. There was, however, no significant difference in weight gain between the two drugs (i.e., olanzapine produced an average weight gain of 1.8 kg, whereas clozapine produced an average weight gain of 2.3 kg).

Olanzapine Versus Risperidone. Several naturalistic studies compared olanzapine with risperidone, usually finding these drugs produced the same overall efficacy. One study conducted at Riverview Hospital in British Columbia, however, found that 60% of risperidone patients were responders, compared with only 27% of olanzapine patients, and that the speed of response to risperidone was 14 days compared with 23 days with olanzapine. The mean dose of risperidone was 4.8 mg/day and for olanzapine 14.3 mg/day (120).

Conley et al. (121) reported a large, double-blind study comparing risperidone with olanzapine. This study included about 400 patients randomly assigned to a flexible dose of risperidone (2 to 6 mg) or olanzapine (5 to 20 mg) for 8 weeks. On many measures, clinical improvement was the same; however, risperidone did produce a slightly greater improvement than olanzapine on positive symptoms and on the anxiety/depression subscale. Most patients on risperidone received 4 to 6 mg/day, whereas half the patients on olanzapine received 10 mg and 10% received 5 mg. The mean dose of risperidone was 4.8 mg/day and for olanzapine 14.3 mg/day. Thus, it is possible that the dose of olanzapine was less than optimal and that the dose of risperidone was optimal.

Tran et al. (122) reported a double-blind, random-assignment study of olanzapine and risperidone in 331 inpatients and outpatients. At end point of this 28-week study, 37% responded to olanzapine and 27% to risperidone ($p = 0.05$), with the response criteria being a total PANSS score on the LOCF end point. If the 20% criteria were used, however, there was no difference between drugs. The PANSS (total score, positive, negative, and general symptoms scores) and the CGI scores showed no difference between drugs, but olanzapine produced slightly more improvement in the depression item on the PANSS and on the SANS summary score. Survival analysis also found that more olanzapine patients maintained their response in the last several weeks of the trial. Olanzapine patients had more weight gain and fewer EPS, as well as less blurred vision, early waking, and delayed ejaculation in comparison with risperidone. This latter side effect is interesting in view of the sustained plasma prolactin elevation seen with risperidone. There were other minor differences, but, in general, both drugs had similar efficacy and side effects.

The most interesting aspect of these two studies is that overall, both reported similar outcomes with either agent.

Quetiapine

Receptor-Binding Studies. Quetiapine (Seroquel) is also a dibenzothiazepine derivative produced by altering the structure of clozapine. This agent has an affinity for multiple brain receptors, a low propensity to evoke EPS in preclinical tests considered predictive of antipsychotic activity, and does not produce sustained plasma prolactin levels.

In vitro binding studies demonstrate that quetiapine has low-to-moderate affinity for D_1, D_2,

5-HT$_{1A}$, and 5-HT$_{2A}$ receptors, and moderate-to-high affinity for a$_1$- and a$_2$-adrenergic receptors. Like other novel agents, quetiapine also has greater relative affinity for 5-HT$_{2A}$ receptors than for D$_2$ receptors, only weakly induces catalepsy in rats, and causes few EPS in humans (123, 124). Quetiapine lacks appreciable affinity for muscarinic cholinergic and benzodiazepine binding sites and causes selective activation of the A-10 dopamine neurons when given acutely and depolarization inactivation of A-10 dopamine neurons when given chronically (125, 126). PET studies of quetiapine receptor occupancy suggest that once-daily dosing may be feasible (127).

In summary, findings from preclinical behavioral pharmacology and electrophysiological studies, as well as phase II and III data, indicate that quetiapine has an atypical profile, is effective, and is well-tolerated.

Therapeutic Efficacy. The efficacy and safety of quetiapine were tested in 109 schizophrenic patients in a multicenter, randomized, double-blind, placebo-controlled, parallel-group trial (128). Subjects randomized to quetiapine initially received 25 mg three times a day for 1 to 2 days. Thereafter, the dose was titrated upward, using a combination of 25, 50, 100, and 200-mg tablets, until an adequate therapeutic effect could be achieved. The maximal daily dose was 750 mg, but daily doses greater than 500 mg were limited to 14 days. Patients given placebo treatment received matching tablets administered in the same manner as quetiapine.

Psychiatric symptomatology was assessed by the BPRS, the CGI, and the SANS before trial entry, on the last day of the single-blind placebo phase, and weekly thereafter for 6 weeks. If treatment was discontinued before day 42, all efficacy assessments were completed at the time of dropout.

Analysis of BPRS factor scores showed that treatment with quetiapine resulted in selective improvement in the psychosis-related factors of thought disturbance and hostility/suspiciousness, as well as improvement in the mean BPRS positive-symptoms cluster score. By day 21, quetiapine was clinically and statistically superior to placebo in moderating negative symptoms.

Arvanitis and Miller (129) reported a multiple fixed-dose, placebo-controlled, double-blind study of quetiapine in comparison with haloperidol and placebo in acutely exacerbated patients with chronic schizophrenia. Quetiapine was administered in five doses: 75, 150, 300, 600, and 750 mg/day; haloperidol was given at 12 mg/day. The study design had slightly more than 50 patients in each group. The 75-mg dose of quetiapine was clearly less efficacious than the higher doses. Doses of 150 to 750 mg/day were superior to placebo and comparable with haloperidol in reducing positive symptoms and 300 mg/day was superior to placebo and comparable with haloperidol for negative symptoms.

Using meta-analytic techniques based on the means and the standard errors presented graphically in the poster, we estimated pooled data of the four effective dosages of quetiapine both for the BPRS and the CGI severity of illness change scores from baseline to endpoint. Quetiapine produced an improvement of 0.43 effect-size units in comparison with placebo, a difference that was highly statistically significant and about the same improvement as haloperidol. Thus, based on the BPRS or PANSS, quetiapine was similar to neuroleptics in efficacy (i.e., differences were nonsignificant). Based on our meta-analysis, quetiapine is clearly superior to placebo, but more data are needed to compare its efficacy with conventional agents (Table 5-15).

TABLE 5-15. *Quetiapine versus placebo or haloperidol for schizophrenia: acute treatment*

Quetiapine/placebo difference				Quetiapine/haloperidol difference			
No. of studies	n	Effect size units	p	No. of studies	n	Effect size units	p
3	547	0.43	10^{-5}	3	904	−0.07	NS

Ziprasidone

Receptor-Binding Studies. Among the newer atypical antipsychotics, ziprasidone (Geodon) has a distinctive pharmacological profile (Fig. 5-2). Binding studies indicate that ziprasidone has a high affinity for D_2 receptors, approximately equal to that of risperidone. *In vitro,* ziprasidone:

- Is a moderately potent D_2 *receptor antagonist* ($pK_i = 8.32$).
- Has a high affinity for the D_3 *receptor* ($pK_i = 8.14$).
- Shows a 100-fold lower affinity for the D_1 *receptor* (approximately equivalent to that of risperidone and haloperidol) than for the other dopamine receptor subtypes.

Ziprasidone also has a significant affinity for several 5-HT receptor sites, including very potent antagonistic activity at $5\text{-}HT_{2A}$ receptors ($pK_i = 9.38$) (130). *Ziprasidone has potent antagonistic action at the $5\text{-}HT_{2C}$ receptor, which may contribute to its capacity to alleviate the positive symptoms of schizophrenia. Its $5HT_{1A}$ agonism may improve negative and cognitive symptoms* (131).

Of the clinically tested new antipsychotics, ziprasidone has the highest $5\text{-}HT_{2A}/D_2$ receptor-affinity ratio. Ziprasidone is an antagonist at the a_1-adrenoreceptor, but its affinity is half that of its D_2 affinity. In addition, compared with its affinity for D_2 and $5\text{-}HT_{2A}$ receptors, ziprasidone has a relatively low affinity for histamine$_1$ receptors ($pK_i = 7.33$). *In vitro,* ziprasidone is a moderately potent inhibitor of neuronal reuptake of norepinephrine, serotonin, and, to a lesser extent, dopamine. This property is shared with some antidepressants, and contrasts with risperidone, which is inactive at all three monoamine uptake sites.

PET studies of ziprasidone's displacement of [^{11}C]raclopride at D_2 receptors have revealed decreased raclopride binding in a dose-dependent manner up to single doses of 60 mg. Ziprasidone receptor occupancy was >65% after single doses of 20 to 40 mg, with occupancy reaching a maximum of approximately 80% following a single dose of 60 mg (132). In addition, D_2 receptor occupancy remains high (>50%) 12 hours after a single dose of 40 mg.

The time course and proportion of CNS $5\text{-}HT_2$ receptor occupancy by single doses of ziprasidone (40 mg) was determined using the PET ligand [^{18}F]setoperone (133). Serum ziprasidone concentrations ranging from approximately 4 to 125 ng/mL at time points 4 to 18 hours postdose were associated with $5\text{-}HT_2$ occupancy rates from about 50% to nearly 100%. Receptor occupancy was related to plasma concentration, suggesting that twice daily administration of 20 mg or more to steady-state levels would be expected to provide greater than 80% occupancy of $5\text{-}HT_2$ receptors.

Ziprasidone's pharmacokinetics permit rapid and predictable dose adjustment, with metabolites that are considered to be clinically inactive (134). The results of PET pharmacokinetic and pharmacodynamic studies indicate that a twice daily dosage regimen is appropriate.

Therapeutic Efficacy. Ziprasidone (daily dose range, 40 to 160 mg given on a B.I.D. schedule with food) has been evaluated in patients with schizophrenia or schizoaffective disorder. A summary of the clinical literature on ziprasidone is published electronically by the FDA. Based on this data set, we combined 4 studies showing that ziprasidone in doses of 120 to 200 mg (Table 5-16) is both clinically and statistically superior to placebo and as effective as haloperidol, with beneficial effects

TABLE 5-16. *Ziprasidone versus placebo or haloperidol for schizophrenia: acute treatment*

Ziprasidone/placebo difference				Ziprasidone/haloperidol difference			
No of studies	n	Effect size units	p	No of studies	n	Effect size units	p
4	608	+0.46	0.00000002	1	165	−0.29	0.04

on both positive and negative symptoms. Data comparing ziprasidone to haloperidol is available from one study. When combining the two doses of ziprasidone utilized, improvement was similar to that seen with haloperidol. Further, a short-acting parenteral preparation has also been developed, and initial studies are promising; indicating 10 to 20 mg i.m. may be the optimal dose range (135, 135a, 135b).

In one double-blind, randomized, placebo-controlled study, patients were given a daily dose of 40 or 120 mg ziprasidone or placebo for 28 days in 132 patients (136). There was a statistically significant improvement in psychotic symptoms versus placebo in the 120 mg/day ziprasidone group as measured by the total BPRS and the CGI scores. Evaluations for parkinsonian symptoms, akathisia, abnormal movements, and sedation did not reveal any notable treatment effects. No significant differences existed between drug and placebo in the total number of adverse events, laboratory test abnormalities, or more serious adverse events. Thus, this study documented that 60 mg ziprasidone twice daily was an effective strategy with negligible risks.

A second report involved a 6-week, multicenter, double-blind, placebo-controlled study that compared the efficacy, safety, and tolerability of two fixed-dose regimens of ziprasidone in patients with an acute exacerbation of schizophrenia or schizoaffective disorder (137). Patients were randomized to receive ziprasidone, 104 patients, or placebo, 92 patients. Both the 80-mg and the 160-mg dose groups demonstrated statistically significant changes from the baseline BPRS, CGI severity, and PANSS total scores. Negative symptoms on the PANSS subscale also showed statistically significant differences favoring the ziprasidone groups over placebo. **This trial also demonstrated efficacy for affective symptoms, as measured by the MADRS.** In this context, a recent review of two placebo-controlled trials for schizoaffective disorder suggested that ziprasidone may be useful both for affective and psychotic symptoms (137a).

Aripiprazole

Another agent with apparently low EPS potential is aripiprazole (Habilitat). While it antagonizes $5HT_2$ receptors, it differs from other agents, in that it exhibits *selectivity for DA_2 receptors both postsynaptically as an antagonist and presynaptically as an agonist*. These differing actions at DA receptor subtypes in distinct cellular locations may produce different functional results in comparison with drugs that are DA_2 postsynaptic receptor antagonists only (138).

Iloperidone

Iloperidone (Zomaril) is a benzisoxazole derivative, similar in configuration to risperidone. Radiological studies find that this agent is a mixed $5HT_2/D_2$ antagonist with a preferential affinity for $5HT_{2A}$ receptors in humans. Like risperidone, it also has a very high affinity for alpha$_1$ adrenoreceptors. Preclinical, as well as phase II and III preclinical data, suggest that this agent may have antipsychotic effects improving both positive and negative symptoms associated with schizophrenia.

Dosing Strategies

The goal of drug therapy is to achieve maximal improvement by treating the underlying disease process rather than a given symptom. Retarded schizophrenic patients may respond dramatically, for example, even in the absence of more obvious target symptoms such as agitation and aggression. Although the goal is to treat the underlying process, the monitoring of more typical psychotic symptoms serves as a barometer for assessing a drug's effect.

In general, lower doses (e.g., risperidone 2 to 6 mg/day; olanzapine 5 to 20 mg/day) are preferable, usually sufficient, and help avoid toxicity. At these doses, results suggest that olanzapine has a substantially lower propensity than neuroleptics to evoke EPS, and perhaps TD. Indeed, early clinical trials were unable to distinguish olanzapine from placebo for EPS or akathisia. Further, there is some indication that doses of risperidone ≥10 mg may produce less improvement and more side effects than doses in the 4-8 mg dose range.

Because the onset of improvement is approximately 1 to 2 weeks with the antipsychotics, many clinicians prefer to start with a low to moderate dose and maintain the dose for that period. Whereas dosage can be adjusted more frequently to control adverse effects, it should not be adjusted daily on the basis of therapeutic effect because of the length of these agents' half-lives.

Some clinicians prescribe a loading dose to achieve a steady-state concentration more rapidly, and then taper off slowly to a lower maintenance regimen. Others prefer to start with a low dose and gradually increase it as needed. There is no strong evidence as to which approach produces a quicker or better long-term result. Under either regimen, the reduction of overt psychotic symptoms and a gradual cognitive reorganization are the goals. Initially, the clinician often administers a drug several times a day, but later phases of treatment usually require only once-a-day dosing because of the longer half-lives of most of these agents (20 to 24 hours). A single bedtime dose is convenient and practical inasmuch as the peak sedative effect occurs shortly thereafter.

Although studies have generally failed to find that "megadoses" (e.g., haloperidol, 100 to 150 mg/day) produced a better response than standard dosages, anecdotal information indicates that an occasional patient will benefit from this approach. Some recover more slowly, however, and improvement might be erroneously attributed to the later, high-dose strategy (i.e., in time, they might have responded equally well to a lower dose). Megadose trials of novel antipsychotics have not been conducted. Although nonresponders can be tried on moderately high doses, in view of the dose-response curve, there is no reason to treat most patients with heroically high doses. **Whenever higher doses are prescribed, therapeutic drug monitoring should also be used to avoid excessively high and potentially toxic blood levels.**

Toxicity

The toxicity dose-response curve is similar to the therapeutic dose-response curve. There are slightly more adverse effects at higher doses, but very high doses generally fail to produce appreciably greater toxicity. Thus, patients who received high-dose treatment for several months (e.g., 1,200 mg fluphenazine or 700 mg trifluoperazine) had the same incidence of adverse effects as those on standard doses and no significant increase in toxicity (139, 140). Even though serious complications may not occur with high doses, this does not mean they are a good idea. Although there is only a weak correlation between neuroleptic dose and TD, assuming it is at least partially dose and time-on-drug related, lifetime drug exposure is an important consideration. Whereas TD may also be associated with short-term, high doses, there is no definitive evidence to support this hypothesis. Although long-term, high-dose treatment might produce more TD, it is unlikely to occur during short-term higher dosing if clinically necessary. In fact, length of time on treatment is probably more important than dose.

Choice of Antipsychotic

The introduction of clozapine, risperidone, quetiapine, and ziprazidone has had a dramatic impact on the decision-making process in choosing an antipsychotic. Thus, these agents both minimize neurological adverse effects and may qualitatively improve some psychotic symptoms to a greater degree than neuroleptics.

Risperidone and olanzapine are more effective than neuroleptics and safer than neuroleptics and clozapine, so they represent first-line choices. Quetiapine and ziprasidone are safer but may only be equal in efficacy to neuroleptics. The timing for clozapine is less certain with arguments put forth for earlier versus later introduction based on efficacy and safety issues, respectively. Clozapine is an important drug for the patients who have not fully remitted with "first line" drugs.

All neuroleptics are equally effective and represent the next drug choices. Due to the clinical similarity of the neuroleptics, there is no reason to expect a given patient to respond differentially to a particular agent. So the critical consideration usually involves differences in adverse effects. Thioridazine and mesoridazine, for example, are more likely to produce cardiac complications making them a fourth-line choice, whereas haloperidol has fewer sedative and cardiovascular effects. In this context, the clinical myth exists that agitated patients respond best to a sedating agent (such as CPZ) and that withdrawn patients respond best to a less sedating agent (such as trifluoperazine, fluphenazine, or haloperidol). This has never been proven, and, indeed, evidence from early NIMH collaborative studies indicated that a second-order factor, labeled "apathetic and retarded," predicted a differentially good response to CPZ (141). This finding, however, was not replicated in another large clinical trial (142). Several schema have been developed to predict which patients would respond to which antipsychotics, but validation studies uniformly failed to support these initial findings.

Determining whether a particular subtype of patient responds differentially to a given drug is an empirical question. Despite the lack of clear differential indications, clinicians continue to encounter patients who respond to one antipsychotic but not another. It is also possible that patients maintained on the original agent may have done equally well. Some patients may preferentially improve on a particular drug due to differences in:

- *Absorption*
- *Distribution*
- Accumulation at *receptor sites*
- *Pharmacodynamic* actions
- *Metabolism* of its derivatives
- *Adverse cognitive effects,* such as sedation

It is also important to consider that improvement in some patients too quickly switched to another agent may be falsely attributed to the latter drug, rather than a delayed response to the first medication. Thus, it is unwise to change too rapidly or too frequently. The optimal dose of a single agent should be ascertained empirically and then allowed a reasonable time to exert its full effect. At some point (i.e., several days or weeks in a severely disturbed patient, or several weeks or months in a less dramatically impaired patient), however, a trial with a second drug (preferably from a different class) is warranted. The effectiveness of this strategy, however, has not been demonstrated in controlled clinical trials.

Cost of Treatment

The pharmaceutical industry generally markets a drug, so that a three-times-a-day dosage is much more expensive than once-a-day dosing (143). Thus, cost is primarily determined by the number of tablets rather than the milligram dose in each tablet. For example, 25 mg CPZ costs almost as much as a 100-mg tablet, and four 25-mg tablets cost nearly three times as much as one 100-mg tablet. Therefore, when the half-life is of sufficient duration, giving the largest available dose in a once-a-day regimen will save considerable expense while also substantially reducing nursing time and other related hospital costs. Further, for outpatients, a bedtime dose may be easier to remember and monitor, thus improving compliance. Usually, once-a-day dosing can be achieved with standard tablets. Delayed-release, oral forms are also available for some agents, but there is no evidence that these more expensive formulations have any advantage over standard preparations.

The clinician needs to know a patient's financial status when considering a dosing regimen. In a patient with limited financial means, the cost of medication may be a deterrent to compliance, and arrangements should be made to minimize any economic obstacles. From a societal point of view, the cost of medication is small in comparison with an outpatient visit, and both of these are negligible in comparison with the expense of hospitalization. Indeed, recent pharmacoeconomic studies indicate that although the initial costs of newer agents are substantially higher, the savings realized over months to years may exceed this initial cost differential (144–146).

Treatment of Psychotic Agitation

Rapid control of acutely disruptive behavior, often associated with an exacerbation of various types of psychotic disorders, is desirable to achieve the following:

- *Lessen* the propensity toward *violence*
- *Avoid* physical *restraints*
- Expedite diagnostic *assessment*
- Facilitate *more definitive treatment*

Violent behavior may have numerous causes, yet in many cases treatment must be initiated before an accurate diagnosis can be made. Nevertheless, a tentative diagnosis should be attempted. The most common causes of such behavior in emergency room settings include psychosis, personality disorder, and alcohol or drug intoxication or withdrawal. In medical or surgical wards, delirium is the more likely cause.

Psychosis. Schizophrenia or mania should be suspected when there is a history of psychiatric illness, onset of symptoms has been gradual, there is evidence of hallucinations, delusions, or disorganized thought, and orientation is intact.

Drug intoxication. Cocaine and amphetamine intoxication may cause an agitated paranoid psychotic episode. Physical signs include dilated pupils, slurred speech, ataxia, hyperreflexia, and nystagmus, as well as evidence of drug use (e.g., needle "tracks," nasal septum erosion). Vital signs, if obtainable, include elevated blood pressure, pulse rate, and temperature (see also the section "The Alcoholic Patient" in Chapter 14).

Delirium. Characteristics include the sudden onset of symptoms, disorientation, visual hallucinations, and transient, often paranoid, delusions. The intensity of symptoms often fluctuates, and the patient may have a known medical illness but no psychiatric history.

Antipsychotic Drug Therapy Strategies

Antipsychotics alone or in combination with BZDs are the treatment of choice for achieving rapid control of acute agitation. While aggressively administered high-dose antipsychotics can control extremely disruptive behavior, their adverse effects may be significant (147–151). At times, anxiolytics may be effective when used alone or in combination for prompt control, while lessening the chance for adverse events. If both are used, lower dosages of each may be adequate.

Route of administration depends on a variety of factors, including the degree of patient agitation and the availability of the various formulations of given drugs (Table 5-17). Although oral medication is preferable whenever possible, if a patient refuses or is unable to cooperate, parenteral administration may be required. Although i.v. administration produces the most rapid effect, it may not be feasible in extremely agitated, uncooperative patients.

Parenteral Administration

The primary indication for standard i.m. administration is when a patient is too disturbed to take oral medication. Because drugs are more rapidly absorbed when given parenterally and their effect occurs about 60 minutes faster than with oral administration (i.e., 30 vs. 90 minutes), violent or otherwise dangerously disturbed patients should initially receive i.m. injections. Further, because orally administered drugs are metabolized in the gut, as well as during their first pass through

TABLE 5-17. *Possible routes of administration of various psychotropics to manage psychotic agitation*

Liquid	Tablet	Intramuscular	Intravenous
Thiothixene	Lorazepam	Droperidol	Droperidol
Haloperidol	Diazepam	Haloperidol	Haloperidol
Loxapine	Chlordiazepoxide	Lorazepam	Diazepam
Risperidone	Risperidone	Olanzapine[a]	Lorazepam
		Ziprasidone[a]	

[a] In development.

the liver, less than 50% may reach the systemic circulation for ultimate availability at the intended brain sites.

Extremely psychotic, explosive patients usually respond (at least partially) to i.m. treatment in 15 to 30 min, often avoiding any serious incidents that might occur with oral administration's slower onset of action. Although orally administered drugs take longer to act, they may still be used for emergency titration after one (or several) i.m. injections have produced a rapid onset of action.

Intravenous administration of low-dose, high-potency agents is also an option in certain clinical situations. For example, i.v. haloperidol, alone or in combination with i.v. lorazepam, has been safe and effective in managing delirium in critically ill, medical patients (152, 153). At times, effective doses of haloperidol may be as low as 0.5 to 1 mg when given by this route. Alternatively, droperidol may offer some advantages over haloperidol, including overall efficacy, safety, and rapidity of onset (154).

Dosing Strategies

Some clinicians prefer a sedating agent, such as CPZ, whereas others prefer a high-potency agent, such as haloperidol, fluphenazine, or thiothixene, because their side effect profiles may allow for more aggressive dosing (e.g., low sedation, low anticholinergic, low hypotension). For example, Janicak et al. (155) conducted a controlled trial in acute, psychotically manic patients who required concomitant antipsychotics. In addition to lithium, they were randomly assigned to oral CPZ or thiothixene. The results between the two drug treatments over a 2-week period were very similar, with no clinically or statistically significant differences. The experimental design of this study dictated that the need for an additional dose of antipsychotic be reassessed every 2 hours during the day. While such highly excited, manic patients are often treated with augmenting agents, they are not usually monitored as frequently. By having their status reevaluated every 2 hours (according to the study design), most patients improved with relatively low doses of either agent, and as a result, none experienced intolerable ad-

verse effects. Had they not been monitored as frequently, higher than necessary doses may have been given (see also Chapter 10).

Although some clinicians rapidly escalate the dose of antipsychotic to higher levels (a strategy referred to as rapid tranquilization or a loading dose approach), we encourage flexibility in the:

- *Route* of administration
- *Dose* required to control the patient's clinical state, with lower doses combined with a BZD preferable to more aggressive antipsychotic doses
- *Frequency of reevaluations* assessing drug response and adverse effects

Repeated high i.m. doses over several days are inadvisable inasmuch as most patients do not require such aggressive intervention, and this strategy may increase the risk for severe EPS and the neuroleptic malignant syndrome (NMS). Finally, it is preferable to switch patients to oral treatment as quickly as possible to manage the remainder of an acute episode.

Benzodiazepines

Benzodiazepines (BZDs) may be given to patients with moderate agitation. These agents also are the treatment of choice in alcohol withdrawal states, characterized by agitation, tremors, or change in vital signs (see also the section "The Alcoholic Patient" in Chapter 14) (156).

Lorazepam. Lorazepam has been increasingly studied for control of psychotic aggressivity (157–167). One reason is that, of all the BZDs available in parenteral form, lorazepam has a pharmacokinetic profile (quick, reliable absorption) that makes it particularly suitable for this type of use. Open, retrospective, and controlled studies indicate that oral or parenteral lorazepam added to an antipsychotic controls disruptive behavior safely and effectively for most patients. The combination may also permit an overall reduction of the antipsychotic dose, although this assumption requires further study (162, 164, 166).

An open, comparative study of 14 acutely psychotic patients treated with lorazepam alone ($n = 8$, mean dose, 20.9 mg/day) or lorazepam plus haloperidol (mean dose, 15 mg/day; mean dose, 5.2 mg/day, respectively) demonstrated a significant decrease in psychotic symptoms over 48 hours (118). Although the improvement in both groups was equal, the doses of haloperidol were low, and there was no comparative placebo group.

Another *retrospective chart review* reported on patients treated in a 24-hour psychiatric emergency unit during two separate 6-month periods (162). During the first period (1982), patients usually received standard i.m. haloperidol for behavioral control; during the second period (1984), they received either i.m. haloperidol or a combination of i.m. haloperidol plus i.m. lorazepam. Further, the doses used during the second period (with or without lorazepam) were significantly lower, compared with the 1982 period. Although the authors concluded that the BZD allowed for lower doses of antipsychotics, it is difficult to determine its influence because all patients received lower doses of antipsychotics during the second period.

In another *open study*, agitated patients were randomly assigned to receive i.m. alprazolam (4 mg), i.m. haloperidol (5 mg), or a combination of the two (168). Agitation, assessed every 30 minutes, was better managed with the combination than either treatment alone.

Lorazepam (2 mg i.m.) was found to be equivalent to haloperidol (5 mg i.m.) either alone or when added to ongoing antipsychotic treatment, and significantly reduced the likelihood of akathisia and dystonia (167). In the treatment of acute mania, lorazepam has also been reported useful as an adjunct to lithium, as well as antipsychotics (157, 163, 165, 168, 169).

Clonazepam. Case reports and one small double-blind study indicate that oral clonazepam may be useful for psychotic agitation when combined with lithium or an antipsychotic (see also the section "Management of an Acute Manic Episode" in Chapter 10) (170, 175).

Midazolam. Intramuscular midazolam, another BZD with reliable parenteral absorption, has produced rapid sedation in acutely psychotic patients with marked agitation (176, 177).

Alprazolam. In a review of high-potency BZDs for psychotic disorders, Bodkin recommended avoidance of alprazolam for psychotic agitation because it may be activating and may induce belligerence or mania (178–186).

Complications of Benzodiazepines

Sedation, ataxia, and cognitive impairment may occur with higher BZD dosages. Other adverse effects reported in the treatment of schizophrenia include the following:

- Behavioral *disinhibition*
- *Increase in anxiety* and *depression* (163, 187–195)

Concomitant use of a BZD and clozapine may increase the risk of sedation, dizziness, collapse with loss of consciousness, respiratory distress, and fluctuating blood pressure (196).

Other Strategies

Before the discovery of the neuroleptics, episodes of psychotic excitement were usually managed with i.v. amobarbital in doses sufficient to heavily sedate or actually put patients to sleep. Upon awakening, they were often much less excited. The role that sleep deprivation plays in the onset of psychotic symptoms may be a partial explanation for this beneficial effect. Although sedatives have no specific effect on the underlying psychosis, they can calm psychotic excitement. Because the extreme excitement, rage, and explosivity often associated with a psychotic exacerbation are amenable to intervention with sedatives, this raises the possibility that these symptoms may have a different underlying mechanism than that subserving the psychosis itself.

Finally, *lithium, β-blockers, and anticonvulsants such as valproate, carbamazepine, and gabapentin* may be effective for the management of assaultiveness and agitation (197–204).

Conclusion

The authors have developed a treatment strategy to manage an acute psychotic exacerbation (outlined in Fig. 5-5) (5, 6). This approach is compatible with various published guidelines (205). When possible, the judicious, time-limited use of

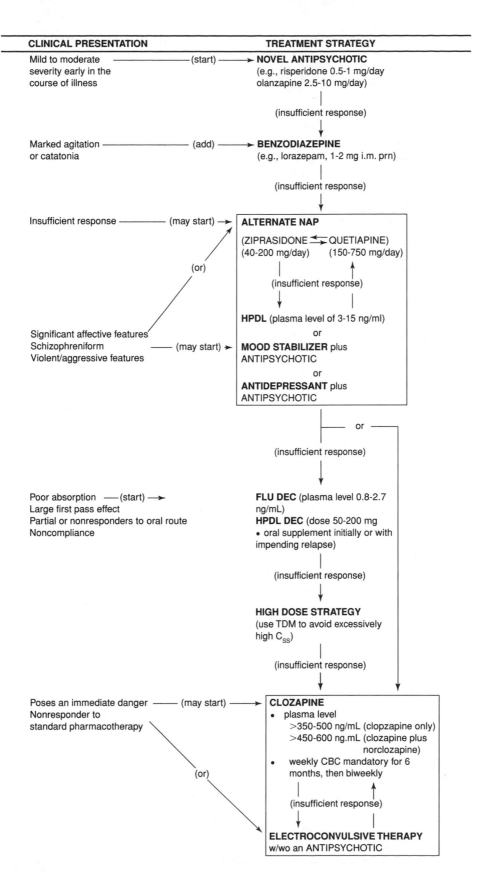

CLINICAL PRESENTATION   **TREATMENT STRATEGY**

Mild to moderate ——————(start)————→ **NOVEL ANTIPSYCHOTIC**
severity early in the   (e.g., risperidone 0.5-1 mg/day
course of illness   olanzapine 2.5-10 mg/day)

                                           (insufficient response)

Marked agitation ——————(add)————→ **BENZODIAZEPINE**
or catatonia   (e.g., lorazepam, 1-2 mg i.m. prn)

                                           (insufficient response)

Insufficient response ———— (may start) → **ALTERNATE NAP**

                                           (ZIPRASIDONE ⇌ QUETIAPINE)
                              (or)   (40-200 mg/day)   (150-750 mg/day)

                                           (insufficient response)

Significant affective features   HPDL (plasma level of 3-15 ng/ml)
Schizophreniform   —— (may start) ➤   or
Violent/aggressive features   **MOOD STABILIZER** plus
                                           ANTIPSYCHOTIC
                                                 or
                                           ANTIDEPRESSANT plus
                                           ANTIPSYCHOTIC

                                           ———— or ————

                                           (insufficient response)

Poor absorption ——(start)——→   **FLU DEC** (plasma level 0.8-2.7
Large first pass effect   ng/mL)
Partial or nonresponders to oral route   **HPDL DEC** (dose 50-200 mg
Noncompliance   • oral supplement initially or with
                                           impending relapse)

                                           (insufficient response)

                                           HIGH DOSE STRATEGY
                                           (use TDM to avoid excessively
                                           high C_{ss})

                                           (insufficient response)

Poses an immediate danger —— (may start) → **CLOZAPINE**
Nonresponder to   • plasma level
standard pharmacotherapy   >350-500 ng/mL (clopzapine only)
                                               >450-600 ng.mL (clozapine plus
                                                               norclozapine)
                                           • weekly CBC mandatory for 6
                              (or)   months, then biweekly

                                           (insufficient response)

                                           ELECTROCONVULSIVE THERAPY
                                           w/wo an ANTIPSYCHOTIC

FIG. 5-5. Strategy for the treatment of an acute psychotic episode.

sedatives in combination with an antipsychotic may bring about a more rapid and qualitatively better effect than aggressively increasing the dose of an antipsychotic. Parenteral administration is frequently required during the earliest phases of treatment and may avoid serious sequelae in the explosive, assaultive, or violence-prone patient. There is also a distinction between the use of augmenting sedatives for the acutely agitated or violent patient versus the chronically agitated or assaultive patient. In the former situation, sedatives might be added initially, and in the latter, after several weeks of antipsychotic therapy to improve the final result. Alternatively, β-blockers, anticonvulsants, or lithium may also be beneficial with or without a concurrent antipsychotic to manage the chronically aggressive patient.

MAINTENANCE/PROPHYLAXIS

Because the majority of psychotic patients have a chronic disorder, the issue of maintenance therapy becomes critical. Shortly after the introduction of antipsychotics, it became apparent that many patients quickly relapsed when their medications were withdrawn; conversely, maintenance pharmacotherapy could prevent such relapses.

There may be exceptions, however, to this general rule. For example, a brief reactive psychosis in response to a severe stressor may occur only once, making long-term maintenance treatment unnecessary. Before the era of antipsychotics, there were many naturalistic investigations that identified acute-onset, floridly psychotic episodes in patients who had a good premorbid history and subsequently made a full recovery. Because there are no systematic data on maintenance medication in such patients, it is hard to determine the optimal course of action after a first episode. Given the possibility that psychotic episodes in reaction to an overwhelmingly stressful event will not recur, delaying maintenance medication may be the most prudent course to avoid long-term adverse effects such as TD or weight gain. Thus, under certain circumstances, it may also be reasonable to use short-term treatment for 6 to 12 months to avoid a relapse and to ensure a solid recovery without

resorting to longer-term treatment to prevent a recurrence.

In this light, Robinson et al. (206) performed a study of 104 first-episode patients who were followed for a minimum of 2 months (mean, 207 weeks). The protocol was later limited to a maximal 5-year follow-up. Patients who wished to discontinue drug could do so. The rate of relapse was determined by the Cox Proportional Hazard Regression model. The cumulative life table relapse rate at 5 years was 82%. Most importantly, despite use of medication by many, there were only four unrelapsed patients after 5 years. Although medication was not controlled, the patients who discontinued had a fivefold increase in the relapse rate. This finding suggests that almost all first admission patients will relapse within the next 5 years, suggesting that most should be on maintenance medication.

Efficacy of Maintenance Antipsychotics

The efficacy of antipsychotics in preventing relapse is supported by at least 35 random-assignment, double-blind studies, which reported the number who relapsed on placebo versus maintenance medication (Table 5-18). A total of 3,720 patients were randomly assigned to either placebo or a neuroleptic (at least 6 weeks with oral therapy or 2 months with i.m. depot treatment), with 55% on placebo relapsing, compared with only 21% on maintenance medication. On the basis of the Mantel-Haenszel test, the combined studies indicated a highly significant difference ($\chi^2 = 483; df = 1; p < 10^{-107}$). **This finding represents overwhelming statistical evidence that in schizophrenia, antipsychotics prevent relapse.**

Some of these studies included remitted patients in outpatient trials, while others were still symptomatic inpatients or outpatients. In those fully remitted for several years, the antipsychotics could be characterized as having a clear prophylactic effect. In those partially remitted, this effect could be characterized as continued maintenance treatment. In the latter case, symptomatology worsened substantially with drug discontinuation. In each study, the placebo group is compared with the drug group, thus randomizing all of the earlier mentioned factors. Even

TABLE 5-18. *Efficacy of antipsychotics in preventing relapse*[a]

Study	Year of study	Number of subjects	Relapsed (%)		Difference (%) (placebo minus drug)
			Placebo (%)	Drug (%)	
Schauver et al.	1959	80	18	5	13
Diamond and Marks	1960	40	70	25	45
Blackburn and Allen	1961	53	54	24	30
Gross and Reeves	1961	109	58	14	44
Adelson and Epstein	1962	281	90	49	41
Freeman and Alson	1962	94	28	13	15
Troshinsky et al.	1962	43	63	4	59
Whitaker and Hoy	1963	39	65	8	57
Caffey et al.	1964	259	45	5	40
Kinross-Wright and Charalampous	1965	40	70	5	65
Garfield et al.	1966	27	31	11	20
Melnyk et al.	1966	40	50	0	50
Englehardt et al.	1967	294	30	15	15
Morton	1968	40	70	25	45
Prien and Cole	1968	762	42	16	26
Prien et al.	1969	325	56	20	36
Baro et al.	1970	26	100	0	100
Rassidakis et al.	1970	84	58	34	24
Clark et al.	1971	19	70	43	27
Leff and Wing	1971	30	83	33	50
Hershon et al.	1972	62	28	7	21
Hirsch et al.	1973	74	66	8	58
Hogarty et al.	1973	374	67	31	36
Gross	1974	61	65	34	31
Chien and Cole	1975	31	87	12	75
Clark et al.	1975	35	78	27	51
Schiele	1975	80	60	3	57
Andrews et al.	1976	31	35	7	28
Rifkin et al.	1977	62	68	7	61
Levine et al. (p.o.)	1980	33	59	33	26
Levine et al. (i.m.)	1980	34	30	18	12
Cheung	1981	28	62	13	49
Wistedt	1981	38	63	38	25
Nishikawa et al.	1982	55	100	85	15
Ruskin and Nyman	1991	18	50	13	37

[a] Summary statistics, $p < 10^{-107}$.
Adapted from Davis JM, Andriukaitis S. The natural course of schizophrenia and effective maintenance drug treatment. *J Clin Psychopharmacol* 1986;6:2s–10s.

though many populations from several countries were used, the drug-placebo difference was still evident.

To illustrate the effectiveness of long-term medication, we will summarize two critical studies. Hogarty and Goldberg (207) reported on 374 schizophrenic outpatients who, after discharge and a stabilization period on phenothiazines, were randomly assigned to CPZ or placebo. Half of each group also received psychotherapy from an individual caseworker plus vocational rehabilitation counseling. After 1 year, relapse had occurred in 73% of those receiving placebo without psychotherapy and in 63% of those given placebo plus psychotherapy. In contrast, only 33% of the CPZ-only and 26% of the CPZ-plus-psychotherapy group suffered a relapse. Overall, 31% of the drug-treated group relapsed, compared with 67% on placebo. Furthermore, the relapse rate with CPZ dropped to 16% when those who abruptly stopped their medication were excluded. Thus, almost half of the drug-treated relapses may have been secondary to medication noncompliance. While the psychotherapy groups had only slightly fewer relapses than patients not receiving psychotherapy, those who received drug plus psychotherapy functioned better than those on drug alone. Psychotherapy may take more time to work, because its effect was more apparent after 18 months of treatment. **It appears that these two treatments complement each other, with psychotherapy improving psychosocial functioning and drugs preventing relapses.**

The second study was a Veterans Administration (VA) collaborative project (208), which included 171 patients who received a placebo and 88 who received either CPZ or thioridazine (total subjects = 259). In this study, compliance was assured by including only inpatients, with nurses administering the medication. Relapse occurred in 45% of the placebo group, in contrast to only 5% of the drug-treated group.

Finally, the specific DA antagonist *pimozide* may have merit as a maintenance medication because of its long half-life and minimal side effect profile (209, 210).

Time Course of Relapse

An important issue in maintenance treatment is the rate of relapse upon discontinuation of therapy. This differs markedly from study to study, perhaps due to their varying durations. In addition, the definition of relapse varied, so that the rate was higher when defined as a modest reemergence of psychotic symptoms rather than an exacerbation sufficient to cause rehospitalization. Using the former criteria, the relapse rate may be as high as 5% to 20% per month, whereas the more conservative criteria might yield a 1% to 10% rate.

The number of patients not yet relapsed versus time was plotted in Figure 5-6 to address the question of whether recurrence occurred at a constant or varying rate. When the data for long-term placebo treatment were analyzed, relapses tended to occur along an exponential function analogous to that seen with the half-life of drugs in plasma (211). This indicates that relapse occurs at a constant rate.

Beginning with a fixed number of patients in a study group, the number relapsing at fixed time points will always be a constant percentage of the overall number remaining in the study. Thus, over time the actual number of patients relapsing will decrease because of a diminishing pool, but the rate does not change. If we begin, for example, with 100 patients and a constant relapse rate of 10% per month, 10 will relapse at the end of the first month, leaving 90 in the trial. In the second month, 10% of 90, or 9, will relapse, leaving 81 patients, and so on.

Data from several large collaborative studies were plotted, with results fitting the exponential model (for constant relapse rate) more accurately than a linear model. The relapse rates for these studies were as follows:

- A *constant relapse rate of 15.7%* per month in a VA hospital collaborative study (208) (Fig. 5-7).
- A *constant relapse rate of 10.7%* for those on placebo in the NIMH-Hogarty and Goldberg study (207) (Fig. 5-8).
- A *constant relapse rate of 8%* per month in the collaborative NIMH study (212) (Fig. 5-9).

The *least-squares analysis* of these data provided an excellent fit, with r^2 approaching 0.95.

In a long trial, it is expected that all at risk will have relapsed. Those not at risk will not, leaving a constant number of "5-year survivors." In an attempt to clarify this point, Hogarty et al. (213, 214) followed their placebo group for 2 or more years after the initial study and found that almost all had relapsed or were lost to follow-up. Indeed, after 18 months, the data hinted that the relapse rate was decreasing, but so few remained that the placebo group did not yield a sufficient number of unrelapsed patients for reasonable conclusions.

An important related question is if one prevents an exacerbation for 2 to 3 years, are patients less likely to relapse or will the rate remain about 10% per month (i.e., does maintenance of remission for a sustained interval fundamentally alter the course of illness)? In the drug-treated groups of Hogarty and Goldberg (207) and Hogarty and Ulrich (214), there were ample subjects for this type of assessment. **When antipsychotics were withdrawn after 2 to 3 years of successful treatment,**

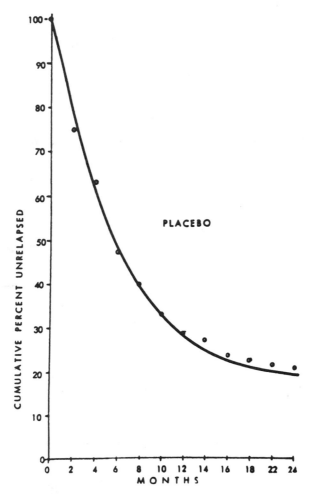

FIG. 5-6. Relapse rate of schizophrenic patients after 24 months on placebo. (From Prien RF, Cole JO, Belkin NF. Relapse in chronic schizophrenia following abrupt withdrawal of tranquilising medication. *Br J Psychiatry* 1969;115:679–686, with permission.)

the relapse rates were similar to those whose maintenance medications were stopped after only 2 months of therapy (213).

Evidence also indicates that patients with *inadequate plasma levels* are more likely to relapse, with the most frequent reason being inadequate compliance. A drop in a plasma level that was previously constant usually indicates poor compliance. Ironically, the act of drawing blood levels often encourages patient compliance.

A false conclusion frequently states that 50% of patients relapse without drugs, whereas 50% do not and, therefore, may not need medication; however, the follow-up period in most studies was only 4-6 months, at which time a rate of

10% per month yields about a 50% relapse rate per year. If the period had been extended to 1 year, the rate would have increased to 75% (211). **If the observation of a constant rate is true, the great majority of patients will relapse when active medication is discontinued, if followed long enough.**

Novel Antipsychotics

Clozapine, risperidone, olanzapine, quetiapine, and ziprasidone have all been approved for the treatment of schizophrenia. Data from long-term open evaluations of *clozapine* demonstrate that improvement is maintained over time, even when

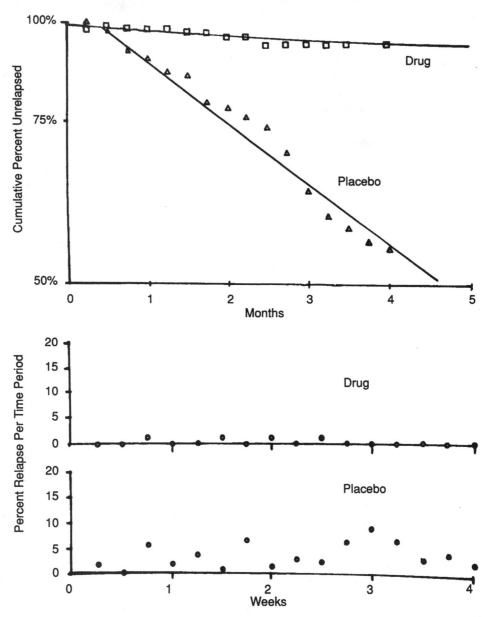

FIG. 5-7. Relapse rate of schizophrenic patients after 4 months on active drug or placebo. Bottom panels present hazard rate per week. (Adapted from Davis JM, Janicak PG, Chang S, Klerman K. Recent advances in the pharmacologic treatment of the schizophrenic disorders. In: Grinspoon L, ed. *Psychiatry 1982. The American Psychiatric Association annual review.* Washington, DC: APPI Press, 1982:192.)

the dose is reduced. Further, patients did not develop tolerance to its antipsychotic effect. Naturalistic reports indicate that an adequate trial for acute response in some patients may be at least 6 months. Further, a small number (8 of 14) of previously refractory patients were success-

fully maintained on clozapine for up to 2 years (215).

In an open-label study, 32 schizophrenic patients were treated with *risperidone* for 1 year and 19 were treated for 2 years (216). The mean dose was 9.4 mg/day in the 1-year follow-up

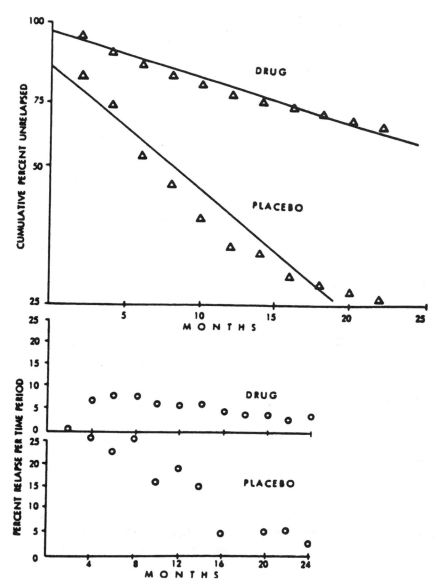

FIG. 5-8. Relapse rate of schizophrenic patients after 2 years on active drug or placebo. Bottom panels present hazard rate per 2-month period. (Adapted from Davis JM, Janicak PG, Chang S, Klerman K. Recent advances in the pharmacologic treatment of the schizophrenic disorders. In: Grinspoon L, ed. *Psychiatry 1982. The American Psychiatric Association annual review.* Washington, DC: APPI Press, 1982:193.)

and 8 mg/day in the 2-year follow-up. At the end of the first and second years, there was improvement on the total PANSS scores, on four PANSS factors (positive, negative, excited, and cognitive), and the CGI scale. Severity of EPS, based on ESRS scores, was also reduced. Clinical improvement (defined as a 20% or more reduction in the total PANSS score) was shown by

54% of the patients at end point. Social functioning (as assessed by the modified Strauss-Carpenter scale) also improved significantly after 2 years. Number of days spent in the hospital decreased significantly during the 2 years of treatment, while the number of days in group homes increased significantly. Although the results of this study indicate that up to 2 years of

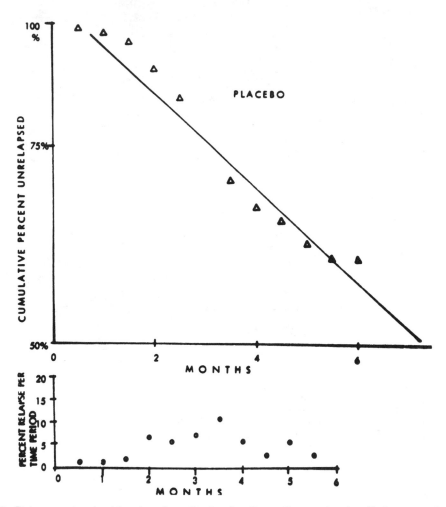

FIG. 5-9. Relapse rate of schizophrenic patients after 6 months on placebo. Bottom panel presents hazard rate per month. (Adapted from Davis JM, Janicak PG, Chang S, Klerman K. Recent advances in the pharmacologic treatment of the schizophrenic disorders. In: Grinspoon L, ed. *Psychiatry 1982. The American Psychiatric Association annual review.* Washington, DC: APPI Press 1982:194.)

risperidone therapy can be efficacious and safe, more maintenance studies are needed to clearly establish its long-term efficacy.

In another study by Csernansky et al. (217), risperidone was found to be superior to haloperidol in a long-term (>1 year), parallel-group, random-assignment design of 365 patients. Forty percent of these patients relapsed on haloperidol and 25% on risperidone ($p = 0.002$) (217). Risperidone produced a greater decrease in all five factors of schizophrenic symptomatology (i.e., positive and negative symptoms, disordered thought, impulsive-hostility, and anxiety-depression). These two results are somewhat conceptually different in that:

• Risperidone produced a better outcome because more patients *did not relapse.*
• Risperidone also produced a *greater decrease in the symptoms* of schizophrenia in all patients.

The latter would be an advantage even if there were no difference in the relapse rate. It is possible that the wider range of symptoms that benefit from atypical antipsychotics may have implications for long-term outpatient treatment. The

TABLE 5-19. *Percent clinically deteriorated or relapsed by current medication dose and length of hospitalization in schizophrenia[a]*

Chronicity	CPZ eq (mg)	Number of subjects	Relapsed (%)
Very chronic[a]	>300	45	22
Chronic[b]	>300	54	53
Very chronic[a]	<300	108	70
Chronic[b]	<300	64	73

[a]Very chronic = 15 years or over.
[b]Chronic = less than 15 years.
CPZ eq, chlorpromazine equivalents.
From Prien RF, Levine J, Switalski RW. Discontinuation of chemotherapy in chronic schizophrenia. *Hosp Community Psychiatry* 1971;22:4–7.

better social functioning observed in treatment with atypical agents and improvement in negative symptoms may be particularly important.

There is every reason to expect that this property would exist with *olanzapine*. Three fixed-dose ranges of olanzapine (5.0 ± 2.5 mg, 10.0 ± 2.5 mg, 15.0 ± 2.5 mg) and one fixed-dose range of haloperidol (15.0 ± 5 mg) were compared with placebo for up to 52 weeks of therapy (218). Survival analysis of time to rehospitalization for psychotic symptoms indicated that *olanzapine* was comparable to haloperidol and significantly better than placebo ($p = 0.007$). Kaplan-Meier estimation showed that 71.5% of olanzapine-treated patients *did not relapse,* compared with 32.8% for those on placebo. Further, another survival analysis demonstrated that significantly fewer patients in the olanzapine treatment group experienced relapse at any given time than those in the haloperidol group (i.e., $p = 0.048$; 80.9% for olanzapine compared with 72.2% for haloperidol).

Conclusion

After several recurrences, substantial evidence indicates that maintenance treatment is necessary. Patients who have had many episodes but make a good recovery from the acute exacerbation benefit most from maintenance medication. Those who have the least drug-psychotherapy versus no treatment difference tend to benefit least from maintenance pharmacotherapy (219). For example, Prien and his colleagues (212, 220, 221) found that chronically hospitalized patients

maintained on low-dose antipsychotics had fewer relapses than those who needed more medication (relapse percentages by categories of medication dose and chronicity; Table 5-19).

It is also possible that in some chronic patients their illness "burns out" and they no longer require medication. To test this possibility, Morgan and Cheadle (222) selected 74 of 475 patients who were clinically judged to be appropriately suitable for nondrug management, but only five remained stable after several years. Relapse occurred an average of 4.5 months after cessation of therapy, indicating that even better-functioning psychotic patients are at high risk if not maintained on active drug therapy. **In conclusion, although maintenance therapy may not always be appropriate, especially after a single acute reactive episode, its discontinuation poses a complicated clinical decision (223). Given the existing evidence, the majority of patients should receive indefinite maintenance medication.**

Effects on Natural Course of Illness

In addition to the prevention of relapse or recurrence is the related, critical question of whether relapses or untreated episodes affect the natural course of a psychotic disorder. Two studies by May and collaborators (224, 225), who investigated the outcome of 228 hospitalized schizophrenic patients randomly assigned to five treatment plans, provide data on the long-term effects of treating or not treating an acute episode. These patients were initially assigned to one of the following regimens: ECT; a phenothiazine alone; psychotherapy alone; a phenothiazine in combination with psychotherapy; or no specific treatment (control group).

Following stabilization, they were discharged into the community. Those with poor responses were generally in the groups not receiving drug or ECT. After 6 to 12 months, the remaining 48 nonresponding, hospitalized patients from all treatment groups then received pharmacotherapy and psychotherapy. Only two did not respond to the combination, and all were eventually discharged. **The principal difference among the groups at this point was that those initially assigned to the no drug or no ECT groups had their episode prolonged for 6 or more months until a drug was started.**

The patients were then followed for 3 to 5 years after the index admission. When the total number of days rehospitalized was compared, those who received only psychotherapy spent about twice as much time in the hospital as those who received pharmacotherapy plus psychotherapy. This was despite the fact that poststudy treatment was similar in both groups (i.e., current treatment was then an uncontrolled, clinically determined variable). Those who received no drug/no psychotherapy also did substantially worse than the drug/no psychotherapy group. It is of particular interest that the patients who initially received ECT and who were then maintained on antipsychotics as needed did as well as those who received drug treatment throughout. A critical aspect of May's study was the random assignment to an initial drug-free period (6 to 12 months), because it is presently impossible to have patients go unmedicated for such a long period due to ethical concerns.

This study provides significant evidence that antipsychotics and ECT positively alter the natural course of illness and that experiencing a psychotic episode without early definitive therapy is harmful. The precise mechanism involved in producing this harm is unknown, but we would assume that:

- A psychotic episode may induce some *lasting damage,* making future episodes more likely.
- The *disruptive psychotic behavior plus the long hospital stay* may have irreparable effects on social or family functioning.
- *Both scenarios may contribute* to the prognosis.

In another study, Greenblatt et al. (226) compared four variations of drug and social therapies in chronic schizophrenic patients continuously hospitalized and randomly divided them into drug and nondrug groups. The patients were also subdivided into those receiving intensive or minimal social therapy. Because they had been continuously hospitalized for many years, the outcome of the two nondrug groups is critical in evaluating the effect of a long drug-free period on ultimate status. At the 6-month point, the greatest improvement occurred in the two medication groups (drugs with or without social therapy). After 6 months, there was a trend toward greater symptomatic improvement in the drug plus intensive social therapy group (33%) when compared with the drug plus minimal social therapy group (23%). Those receiving intensive social therapy and no drugs fared poorly during this 6-month period, and then received 6 more months of psychosocial treatment plus drugs. In the final evaluation, intensive social therapy without drugs impeded improvement. When finally placed on medication, this group never gained the same benefit achieved by those initially treated with drugs plus intensive social therapy. In contrast, the therapy plus drug intervention combination was helpful, with intensive social therapy facilitating discharge into the community. As in the May studies, the 6-month drug-free period seemed to produce a carryover negative effect.

Early Intervention

An important implication of this observation is the suggestion that early intervention in schizophrenia could substantially alter the natural course of the illness. To investigate this idea, early-intervention projects have been developed. In one, primary physicians were trained to recognize the early symptoms of a mental disorder and to arrange consultation with an intervention team who assessed and treated the disorder. If early symptoms were present, the functional psychotic disorder was treated with low doses of the appropriate medication, often for a relatively short period of time (i.e., several weeks), and then tapered when symptoms abated while psychosocial intervention was continued. In some patients, symptoms returned and medication was reinstituted. The psychosocial program, social skills training, and social casework were continued for some time, and all patients were monitored for at least 2 years. Epidemiological data established that over the lifetime of this project, 7.5 new cases would be expected for 100,000 patients (227, 228).

The actual incidence of schizophrenia was reduced approximately 10-fold. The number of prodromal episodes in which a functional psychosis was expected was slightly higher than the expected number of schizophrenic cases, suggesting that the expected number of schizophrenic episodes did occur, but that these cases were identified and treated at an early prodromal phase and did not progress to a full episode. The fact that there would be a slightly higher incidence of prodromal events than expected full episodes was not surprising because not all patients with prodromal episodes would ultimately progress to schizophrenia. However, these findings suggest that prodromal events were actually the first presentation of schizophrenia, and further suggest that acute treatment without maintenance follow-up was able to prevent progression of the disease. One patient had a recurrence of the same symptoms on three different occasions and responded to medication and psychosocial interventions each time.

Benefits of early intervention with medication include the following:

• *Preventing social deterioration*
• *Keeping families intact*
• Allowing the *educational process to proceed*
• Helping "patients" to *develop the necessary social and vocational skills* for adequate functioning in the community

One interpretation of these results is that preventive, assertive case management may indeed be much easier than attempts to repair the social disfunction after deterioration has taken place. In this context, a 4-year study

comparing risperidone with haloperidol in first-episode patients is in progress (229). Preliminary results indicate that the time interval between the first prodromal symptoms and the first psychotic episode is 16 months, which is essentially equal to the interval between the first psychotic episode and diagnosis. Thus, it takes nearly 3 years from onset of prodromal symptoms to diagnosis. Particularly interesting is the finding that 70% of the patients have prior experience with antipsychotic medication, suggesting that clinicians were treating patients for psychosis before diagnosis. Several research efforts are now under way to bring early treatment to patients during their prodromal phase. At this time, we do not know whether such interventions will prevent progression. It is possible, however, that the pathophysiological process in schizophrenia is such that treatment in the prodromal phase might be effective and that some irreversible change takes place over the period of 3 to 4 years from prodromal symptoms to a definitive diagnosis.

Methods of Drug Administration

Targeted Treatment Strategy

Prophylaxis may act by treating episodes as they occur, thus attenuating a major exacerbation. In this light, an alternate drug maintenance approach may be to carefully follow patients longitudinally, and only medicate to abort an episode when there are early warnings of a relapse. Unfortunately, many relapses occur abruptly, and it is doubtful that an episode can be halted once the process has started. Yet, some episodes may be preceded by a week or two of prodromal signs.

In targeted treatment, pharmacotherapy is only used when prodromal symptoms become manifest, in the few days or weeks preceding a recurrence. Such nonspecific symptoms may include:

• Increased *anxiety, dysphoria,* lability of mood
• Loss of *interest,* reduced *energy, discouragement* about the future
• Reduced *attention,* increased *internal preoccupation,* increased *illusions, racing thoughts*
• Vague *digressive speech*, eccentric *behavior*
• *Nightmares*

A targeted treatment strategy uses these symptoms as cues to restart drug therapy, thus avoiding continual antipsychotic exposure. One important problem with this approach is that the organ needed to do the monitoring (i.e., the brain) is the organ that is dysfunctional.

There are four double-blind studies targeting treatment to an impending relapse as an alternative strategy to continuous maintenance medication. Jolley et al. (230, 231) reported that of 25 patients in a continuous-medication control group, only three relapsed, with two requiring hospitalization. In contrast, of 24 patients in a targeted treatment group, 12 relapsed, and eight required hospitalization. Herz et al. (232) compared over 100 patients on continuous or targeted therapy and observed more relapses in the targeted group. Using a survival analysis, they found a significant superiority for continuous medication. Herz and his coworkers (233) then studied another group of 101, finding 15 of 50 targeted patients relapsed, with 12 rehospitalized. In contrast, only eight of 51 maintenance-treatment patients relapsed, with three hospitalized.

Gaebel and his coworkers (234) reported a 2-year multicenter study in Germany using random assignment to early intervention, crisis intervention, or maintenance therapy. Of 364 patients, 159 completed the trial and 23% of the maintenance-medication group relapsed, contrasted to 63% of the crisis intervention and 45% of the early-intervention groups. It should be noted that the early-intervention group also received substantially more drug than the crisis intervention group. Their targeted treatment was a variant of low-dose therapy, with patients on antipsychotics much of the time when they were manifesting prodromal symptoms.

Based on the published abstract of their work, we multiplied the 23% who did not relapse with maintenance medication times the assumed 121 in each arm of the trial, averaged the 63% and 45% for the two nonmedication strategies, and then multiplied this mean (i.e., 53.5%) by the 242 in these two arms of the trial. The results indicated that 25% of continuously medicated patients relapsed, in contrast to 50% in the targeted treatment groups, a highly statistically significant difference.

Carpenter et al. (235) performed a similar unblinded comparison study. Of the 57 targeted patients, 53% relapsed, compared with only 36% of the 59 continuous-therapy patients. Survival analysis demonstrated again that a continuous regimen was clearly more effective than targeted therapy (i.e., relapse rate with continuous therapy was 1.6 versus 3.18 for the targeted therapy). Schooler et al. (236) found that 46% of the targeted group relapsed, in contrast to only 25% of the continuously treated group.

Analyzing only the four published studies with explicit data, 22% of the continuous group and 42% of the targeted group required hospitalization. The Mantel-Haenszel test also found this difference statistically significant ($\chi^2 = 21; df = 1; p = 0.00001$). **In summary, the five controlled studies of targeted versus continuous treatment found that outcome was poorer with the targeted strategy.**

Low-Dose Strategy

An alternate strategy would be to maintain patients on a continuous lower dose of antipsychotics (either long-acting parenteral or oral) that is then increased only when prodromal signs occur. Studies have shown that standard doses are more effective than lower doses, but again, many factors should be considered before embarking on a given approach.

There have been four dose-response studies of maintenance depot medication (see also "Long-Acting Antipsychotics" later in this chapter). Generally, most groups used a standard dose of 25 mg fluphenazine decanoate given i.m. every 2 weeks, although some compared standard with lower doses. The lowest doses were used by Kane and his coworkers (237), who chose 1.25 to 5 mg. In their study, three patients in the standard dose group relapsed and 61 patients remained well, while 26 patients in the low-dose group relapsed and 36 remained well. Marder et al. (238) used doses of 25 mg in comparison with 5 mg, but patients who showed very early signs of relapse could have their dose slightly increased. For purposes of our discussion, we consider the 5 or 25 mg their fixed starting dose. Of those on the standard dose of 25 mg, 10 relapsed and 21 remained well, whereas 22 relapsed and 13 remained well on the lower dose. When the patients had early signs of relapse, their dose was increased, and as a result, the dose-response relationship began to level out to no difference. Hogarty et al. (239) used doses of 25 mg versus an average of 3.8 mg, and found a nonsignificant difference between the two groups. Thus, in the standard dose group, 19 did not relapse and six did, whereas in the low-dose group 21 did not relapse and nine did. Johnson et al. (240) used flupenthixol decanoate, so there is the question of exact equivalence, but their low-dose group was roughly equivalent to the Hogarty and Marder groups. Of those on the standard, four of 31 relapsed in 18 months, and of those who received half of the standard dose, 12 of 28 relapsed in this time period. Davis et al. (241) reviewed the 6-month relapse rate in patients randomly assigned to 25, 50, 100, or 200 mg haloperidol decanoate on a monthly schedule. The relapse rate was lowest for those on 200 mg monthly. **If all studies are considered collectively, we see an increased relapse rate at the lower dose levels, with the threshold for a minimally effective dose probably slightly higher than the lowest used.**

When patients are randomly assigned to a lower than standard dose, the relapse rate rises slightly, but there are substantially fewer adverse effects. With a greater decrease in dose, however, there is a substantial increase in the relapse rate. The question is further complicated, in that different patients may require different doses. Given these tradeoffs, clinicians must often rely on trial and error. In studies demonstrating a slight increase in the relapse rate with slightly lower doses, an increase in dose almost always aborted a relapse, without the need for rehospitalization.

To supplement depot medication, oral preparations can be used when early warning signals of an impending relapse occur because the pharmacokinetics of depot preparations require months to reach steady-state (see also "Pharmacokinetics/ Plasma Levels" later in this chapter). By contrast, oral administration brings about an altered steady state in several days. **We recommend treating most patients with the minimally effective dose to avoid more serious adverse effects, even at the cost of a few more relapses, provided this strategy does not lead to rehospitalization or produce serious impairment in functioning.**

In conclusion, clinicians must balance several factors when choosing the proper therapy, including the following:

- Problem of *dysphoric adverse effects*
- Disruption of a *minor relapse*
- Likelihood of a *severe relapse*
- Long-term risk of *tardive dyskinesia*
- Likelihood of *suicide* during a relapse
- Likelihood of *compliance* with an oral versus parenteral depot formulation

Complications

Postpsychotic Depression

There is a significant difference between unremitted or partially remitted patients with pronounced negative symptoms and those in remission who experience a depressive episode. Siris et al. (242) selected candidates with a history of schizophrenia who recovered and then experienced a major depression that resolved with antidepressant therapy. Thirty-three patients receiving both maintenance antipsychotics and antidepressants were studied in a double-blind design that included an antipsychotic plus random administration of either an antidepressant or placebo. The group receiving both types of psychotropic had a statistically superior outcome ($p = 0.020$; two-tailed Fisher's test) on their global scores for each of the subscales in the depression ratings, but there was no difference in the measure of psychosis or adverse effects between the two groups. Siris et al. (243) also conducted a follow-up study on the previous antidepressant-treated group, maintaining them on fluphenazine decanoate and benztropine, as well as adjunctive imipramine. After 6 months, their imipramine was tapered to a placebo or they continued on the same medication regimen for 1 more year. All six who were tapered off active drug relapsed into a depressive state, in contrast to only two of the eight remaining on imipramine ($p = 0.009$). Of note is that those who relapsed again improved once adjunctive imipramine was reinstituted. Johnson (244) studied 50 schizophrenics in remission who were randomly assigned to receive nortriptyline or placebo for a 5-week trial. More subjects in the nortriptyline group (i.e., 28%) were free of depression at the end of the trial than in the placebo group (i.e., 8%). Prusoff et al. (245) studied 40 schizophrenic outpatients with depressive episodes treated with amitriptyline or placebo in addition to their maintenance perphenazine. In general, improvement in depression was modest, not statistically impressive, and there was a suggestion of worsening in psychosis.

In summary, episodes of superimposed depression benefit from intervention with concurrent antidepressant therapy, but these agents do not appear to help patients who suffer from a more chronic, negative symptom presentation.

Supersensitivity Psychosis

Supersensitivity psychosis (SSP) has been described as the rapid reemergence of psychotic symptoms upon discontinuation of long-term antipsychotic treatment. Chouinard and Steinberg's (246) criteria for the diagnosis are presented in an abbreviated form in Table 5-20, and descriptions of patients who meet these criteria can be found in Hunt et al. (247). This phenomenon is thought to be secondary to an upregulation of DA receptors in the neural circuits subserving psychosis. This concept is analogous to the hypothesis regarding TD, which postulates a DA receptor supersensitivity secondary to striatal drug blockade (i.e.,

dopaminergic receptor upregulation in the neural tract relevant to movement). Thus, withdrawal of these drugs may induce a rebound psychosis, just as it may cause TD.

Peet (248), in a chart review study of 55 outpatients, found seven who met the criteria for SSP. Singh et al. (249) compared five patients with a history of SSP and five without, predicting that those with SSP would relapse more rapidly upon discontinuation. In the study design, antipsychotic medication was abruptly replaced by placebo without any tapering, and the emergence of psychosis or TD was evaluated. The authors found no evidence of relapse into psychosis over a 2-week period. As the relapse rate of untreated schizophrenics is about 10% per month, we might expect some relapses during this time, but the sample size of this study was too small for definitive conclusions (i.e., 10 patients). To prove the existence of SSP one would have to show that there is an *increased relapse rate* or at least a worsening of symptoms greater than would otherwise be expected. Although the clinician must remain alert to this possibility, we would give this hypothesis the "Scotch verdict" of not proven, with the burden of proof resting on those who have proposed this syndrome.

Conclusion

Continuous, moderate-dose maintenance antipsychotics afford the best chance of preventing relapse in psychotic patients. Low doses of neuroleptics should theoretically diminish the possibility of TD, but, in fact, are only weakly correlated. Further, with too low a dose, patients are at risk of developing more frequent exacerbations, which usually require increased doses and may contribute to higher levels of psychopathology not amenable to future drug intervention. The availability of atypical agents with a lower propensity for EPS (and perhaps TD) may make these the drugs of choice in patients compliant with oral regimens.

The use of maintenance strategies must always be considered in the context of the long-term consequences to minimize more serious adverse effects (e.g., TD, weight gain). There is a trade-off between the risk of TD using adequate dose

---

TABLE 5-20. *Criteria for supersensitivity psychosis*

Inclusion criteria
    History of receiving neuroleptics or
        antipsychotics for at least 6 months
    Patient has had a decrease or
        discontinuation of medication with
        appearance of psychosis or
    Patient has had no decrease or
        discontinuation of medication during
        treatment but has more relapses or
        increased tolerance to antipsychotic effects
Exclusion criteria
    Patients in the acute phase of the illness
    Patients with continued psychotic illness who
        did not respond to neuroleptic treatment

long-term medication and the higher risk of relapse with lower dose strategies. The ongoing development of long-acting novel antipsychotics (e.g., risperidone, 9-OH-risperidone; olanzapine) should diminish the risk of TD substantially (40a). Because a recurrence of psychotic behavior may interfere with vocational and social functioning and, at the extreme, result in violence or suicide, the cost of an episode to patients, their families, and society must be carefully considered. Finally, psychosocial therapies can enhance the beneficial effects of medication, improving the overall quality of life.

Figure 5-10 outlines a recommended strategy for managing the chronic, relapsing psychotic patient (5, 6, 250).

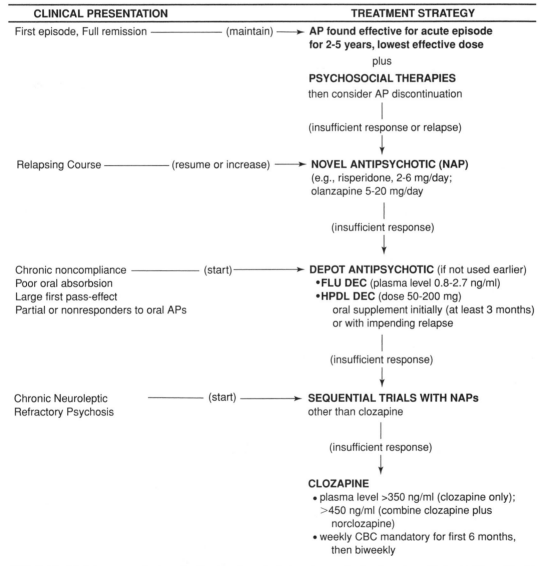

CLINICAL PRESENTATION	TREATMENT STRATEGY

First episode, Full remission —————— (maintain) ——▸ **AP found effective for acute episode for 2-5 years, lowest effective dose**

plus

PSYCHOSOCIAL THERAPIES

then consider AP discontinuation

(insufficient response or relapse)

Relapsing Course ————— (resume or increase) ——▸ **NOVEL ANTIPSYCHOTIC (NAP)** (e.g., risperidone, 2-6 mg/day; olanzapine 5-20 mg/day

(insufficient response)

Chronic noncompliance ————— (start)————▸ **DEPOT ANTIPSYCHOTIC** (if not used earlier)
Poor oral absorbsion   •**FLU DEC** (plasma level 0.8-2.7 ng/ml)
Large first pass-effect   •**HPDL DEC** (dose 50-200 mg)
Partial or nonresponders to oral APs   oral supplement initially (at least 3 months) or with impending relapse

(insufficient response)

Chronic Neuroleptic ————— (start) ————▸ **SEQUENTIAL TRIALS WITH NAPs**
Refractory Psychosis   other than clozapine

(insufficient response)

CLOZAPINE
• plasma level >350 ng/ml (clozapine only); >450 ng/ml (combine clozapine plus norclozapine)
• weekly CBC mandatory for first 6 months, then biweekly

FIG. 5-10. Maintenance strategy for the treatment of chronic psychotic disorders. (Adapted from Davis JM, Janicak PG, Preskorn S, Ayd FJ Jr. Advances in the pharmacotherapy of psychotic disorders. In Janicak PG, ed. *Principles and practice of psychopharmacotherapy update. Vol 1.* Baltimore, Williams & Wilkins, 1994:1.)

LONG-ACTING ANTIPSYCHOTICS

A parenteral, depot antipsychotic is one that can be administered in such a way that, after a single dose, a therapeutically efficient tissue concentration of at least 1 week's duration is achieved (251, 252). Slow release of the active drug is produced by combining the base antipsychotic with a fatty acid (decanoic acid). The alcohol group of the antipsychotic is esterified by the acid, producing a lipophilic compound whose solubility in oil is increased. An oil, usually sesame, is then used as a vehicle for intramuscular injection, where the ester, which is not pharmacologically active, is hydrolyzed by tissue esterases, slowly releasing the active compound. An alternative technique is the use of microspheres (e.g., risperidone).

Depot preparations should be considered for patients who have experienced several relapses, either due to inadequate oral regimen caused by pharmacokinetic factors (e.g., poor absorption) or ongoing problems with noncompliance. Because many patients stop their oral drugs, often precipitating a relapse, long-acting, depot preparations represent a major tactical advantage in chemoprophylaxis (253). In open trials, many who fared poorly on oral management were greatly benefitted by i.m. depot medication. This improvement was presumably because of previous noncompliance with their oral regimens, but it is also possible that some patients rapidly metabolize oral preparations (e.g., a large first-pass effect), never achieving adequate plasma levels by this route of administration.

Although these preparations are an important addition to the therapeutic armamentarium, particularly for outpatients, they may also occasionally benefit inpatients. It is important to appreciate the different pharmacokinetic properties of long-acting injectable drugs, especially the longer time period (i.e., 3 to 4 months) required to achieve steady-state concentrations, which must be taken into account when titrating dose.

Therapeutic Efficacy

Table 5-21 shows the difference in the percentage of patients who relapsed while on oral or depot antipsychotics from six random-assignment, double-blind studies (34, 253–257). Although the outcome is mixed, three of the studies found an appreciable difference between the two regimens. For example, one study found a 3% relapse rate per month on oral versus a 1% rate on depot fluphenazine. The three other studies, however, found little difference, but they also may have had more compliant patients. Combining these data with the Mantel-Haenszel test reveals a significantly lower relapse percentage on depot versus oral medication ($\chi^2 = 13.5$; $p < 0.0002$). The usefulness of depot medication is also supported by Johnson et al. (258–260), who used matched control subjects, as well as by Marriott and Hiep (261), Tegeler and Lehmann (262), and Freeman (263), all of whom used mirror-image control subjects (i.e., relapse rates in patients on oral medication versus relapse rates later when on depot medication).

Several longitudinal studies have also found that patients stabilized on depot fluphenazine relapsed when switched to an oral antipsychotic preparation (264). Mirror-image studies also found depot fluphenazine (decanoate or enanthate) reduced the incidence of relapse, as well as the number of days hospitalized, when compared with oral therapy. These open, crossover studies switched patients from oral to depot forms, and the outcome with each approach was evaluated.

Complicated research protocols make significant demands on patients; therefore, only those who can give informed consent, and are thus *more likely to be compliant*, enter such trials. Further, the *Hawthorne effect* may be operative, in that the interest of the investigator may effectively communicate to patients the importance of taking their medication. For example, tuberculosis is a major health problem in many parts of the world; a half million people die of this disease in India alone every year. Health workers who directly observe patients taking an antituberculosis drug have proven to be quite successful in improving the rate of recovery. When direct observed treatment is not used, patients are seven times more likely to die of this disease. Therefore, it seems reasonable that increased compliance by directly observing or some equivalent clinical management technique might improve outcome in schizophrenia on a long-term basis. The *increased quality of clinical care,* which is often a byproduct of research, may inspire some to become better educated about their disorder and its treatment and more highly motivated to take medication. Thus, such factors could cloud any differences in efficacy between oral and depot formulations.

Standard Depot Preparations

Fluphenazine

Whereas the fluphenazine depot preparations are superior to placebo in preventing relapse in groups of remitted schizophrenic patients, their advantage over oral fluphenazine is less clear. Rifkin et al. (255), for example, followed remitted schizophrenics for 1 year and found that 63% treated with placebo relapsed, whereas only 5% on depot and 4% on oral fluphenazine relapsed during that period. Schooler et al. (265) treated schizophrenic patients with either fluphenazine decanoate or oral fluphenazine for 1 year and again found no significant difference in relapse rates between these two groups (i.e., 24% versus 33%, respectively) during that time. By contrast, at least two other controlled studies conducted in a typical clinical setting found a clear difference favoring depot over oral preparations (Table 5-21).

Kane et al. (266) point out that some studies may not have effectively evaluated the potential benefit of depot fluphenazine. Thus, patients volunteering for such studies are those who might be compliant whether they took oral or depot medications; therefore, these studies may underrepresent the noncompliant population. In addition, inasmuch as relapse may not occur for 3 to 7 months after medications have been completely discontinued, a 1-year study period may not be long enough to evaluate the relative effectiveness of a depot versus oral antipsychotic.

In this context, Hogarty et al. (256) followed patients who were treated with either i.m. fluphenazine hydrochloride or i.m. fluphenazine decanoate for 2 years. After the first year, the relapse rate did not differ between the two groups (i.e., 40% for hydrochloride and 35% for decanoate). During the second year, however, 42% of those remaining in the hydrochloride group relapsed, as compared with only 8% of those remaining in the decanoate group. Although the difference was not statistically significant, the figures suggest an advantage favoring the depot preparation in minimizing relapse during the second year of treatment.

Fluphenazine enanthate and decanoate are similar in potency, efficacy, and adverse effects. They differ only in that the decanoate preparation is slightly more potent and slightly longer acting, requiring lower doses and less frequent administrations. Because the decanoate form manifests marginally fewer adverse effects, it is probably preferable.

Dose

When initiating depot fluphenazine, a conservative dose should be chosen, realizing that it may take several months to establish steady-state levels. It may also be necessary to supplement treatment with oral fluphenazine during this early phase until the required maintenance level

TABLE 5-21. *Percent difference in relapse between depot and oral preparations*

Study	Number of subjects	Study duration	Relapsed (%) Oral (%)	Relapsed (%) Depot (%)	Difference (Oral minus depot) (%)
Crawford and Forest (1974)	29	40 weeks	27	0	27
del Guidice et al. (1975)	82	1 year	91	43	48
Rifkin et al. (1977)	51	1 year	11	9	2
Falloon et al. (1978)	41	1 year	24	40	−16
Hogarty et al. (1979)	105	2 years	65	40	25
Schooler et al. (1979)	214	1 year	33	24	9

Mantel-Haenszel: $p < 0.0002$.

Adapted from Davis JM, Andriukaitis S. The natural course of schizophrenia and effective maintenance drug treatment. *J Clin Psychopharmacol* 1986 (suppl 1);6:2s–10s.

is ascertained. If psychotic symptoms should reemerge, oral or acute parenteral fluphenazine can also be used to establish control and the depot dosage increased accordingly at the next scheduled injection. If the depot dose is too high, as evidenced by the appearance of persistent adverse effects, then appropriate symptomatic treatment should be initiated and the dose reduced or injection intervals extended until adverse effects are controlled. The goal is to establish the lowest effective maintenance dose, mindful that too low a dose may increase the risk of relapse and rehospitalization (267). Conversely, too high a dose may expose the patient to unnecessary adverse effects and non-compliance.

Haloperidol

Haloperidol decanoate is an effective depot agent comparable with standard oral preparations (268–271). It can be given monthly, and has a marginally lower incidence of EPS compared with the fluphenazine formulations.

Clinically, haloperidol decanoate has been administered to hundreds of chronic schizophrenic patients in several open studies to determine its efficacy, pharmacokinetics, safety, and adverse effects. The trials ranged from 4 months to 2 years, with dosages ranging from 25 to 500 mg given once every 4 weeks. The results of these studies have consistently shown that depot haloperidol:

- Is as *effective in controlling psychotic symptoms* in chronic schizophrenic patients as oral haloperidol, other oral antipsychotics, or depot fluphenazine.
- Has not produced any clinically significant changes in *hematological* or *biochemical* values.
- Produces a *steady plasma* level that declines slowly by one-half during the interinjection interval.
- Does not increase and may even decrease the incidence of *extrapyramidal* and *other adverse effects* when compared with those produced by oral preparations (271–277).

Dose

The calculation of an appropriate dosage for the depot form requires converting from a given oral dose of haloperidol. Earlier observations found the bioavailability of oral haloperidol to be 60% to 70%, indicating that this would correspond to a monthly dose of haloperidol decanoate of about 20 times the daily oral dose (272). For example, if a patient is stabilized on a daily oral dose of 10 mg, then a corresponding monthly dose of the decanoate formulation would be 200 mg. Kane and others (278), however, suggest a lower starting ratio of 10–15:1. Doses will usually need to be adjusted individually, however, based on a given patient's response and the emergence of adverse effects.

Fluphenazine Depot Versus Haloperidol Depot

In general, double-blind comparisons have found the two depot formulations to be equieffective in the maintenance treatment of schizophrenic patients. Kissling et al. (279) evaluated both fluphenazine and haloperidol decanoate in a 6-month double-blind study involving 31 schizophrenic patients. These authors found both were equally effective in preventing relapse, with a slight advantage for haloperidol decanoate as reflected by fewer adverse effect-related dropouts and a decreased need for antiparkinsonian medications with this latter agent. Wistedt (280) compared fluphenazine decanoate with haloperidol decanoate in a double-blind study involving 51 schizophrenic patients over a 20-week treatment period. He found no difference between the drug groups on ratings of global clinical changes, with both showing a significant improvement over the course of the study. The haloperidol-treated group, however, did show a greater degree of improvement in ratings on a clinical psychopathology scale, and less depressive symptomatology compared with the fluphenazine group. Although there was no difference in EPS between groups, the patients on fluphenazine required higher doses of antiparkinsonian medication during the study, perhaps indicating a greater severity of EPS. Chouinard et al. (281) randomly assigned 12 schizophrenic outpatients to receive either haloperidol decanoate or fluphenazine decanoate in a dose ratio of 3:1. This was a double-blind study over an 8-month period, and it found no significant differences between the drug groups on any of the psychopathology ratings, parkinsonian symptoms, or the need for antiparkinsonian medication.

Fluphenazine decanoate may cause more acute EPS than haloperidol decanoate due to a phenomenon known as "dose dumping." Here, a small amount of depot formulation is released into the systemic circulation shortly after an injection. There may be a tendency for haloperidol to be more effective for a subset of schizophrenic symptoms, less depressogenic, and slightly less likely to exacerbate extrapyramidal symptoms. These effects, however, are not large, may not be clinically significant, and are not consistently evident in all studies.

Conclusion

Long-acting, parenteral, antipsychotic administration remains an important option in various clinical situations. Presently, only neuroleptics are available in this formulation, but it is anticipated that depot formulations of novel antipsychotics (e.g., risperidone, olanzapine) may soon be approved. The advent of such agents should significantly improve the efficacy and safety of this strategy.

PHARMACOKINETICS/PLASMA LEVELS

Clinically relevant pharmacokinetic factors involving antipsychotics include the following:

- Good *absorption* from the gastrointestinal tract
- An extensive *"first-pass"* hepatic effect
- *Subsequent high systemic clearance* due to a large hepatic extraction ratio each time the plasma recirculates through the liver
- *Extensive distribution* (V_D) due to highly lipophilic character
- *Plasma half-life* ($t_{1/2}$) of typically about 20 hours
- Primary *route of elimination* is hepatic metabolism

- The presence of *metabolites* with varying pharmacological profiles (e.g., some may be more effective than their parent compound [e.g., mesoridazine]: some may not reach the brain [e.g., sulfoxides], and some may have greater toxicity than the parent compound)

Antipsychotics are a chemically diverse group of drugs having in common the ability to ameliorate psychotic symptoms. Unfortunately, a significant percentage of patients fail to respond adequately or may develop adverse effects such as acute EPS, various tardive syndromes (e.g., TD, dystonia, etc.), and, less commonly, even more serious adverse events such as NMS and agranulocytosis.

The use of drug plasma levels to effect optimal clinical response and to minimize adverse or toxic effects is standard practice in general medicine (e.g., phenytoin, digoxin), as well as in psychiatry (e.g., lithium, tricyclic antidepressants, valproate; see Chapter 3). The theoretical basis for plasma level monitoring rests on several factors, including:

- The existence of a *long interval* between drug administration and clinical response
- *Large interindividual differences* in response to the same dose for the same diagnosis, in part reflecting differences in plasma levels achieved on a given dose
- Possible usefulness in helping to establish the *minimally effective dose*
- Possible usefulness in helping to *estimate the average dose* required to achieve a certain concentration when a positive correlation exists between a given steady-state concentration (C_{SS}) and the dose required.

Unfortunately, for a number of methodological and clinical reasons, the success achieved with this strategy for other classes of drugs (e.g., certain mood stabilizers) has not been achieved with the monitoring of antipsychotic steady state plasma concentrations. Difficulties in study design have contributed to this uncertainty, including:

- *Insufficient sample sizes*, especially at the low and the high ranges

- Inclusion of *refractory, nonhomogeneous, noncompliant* patients
- *Nonrandom adjustment* of the dose based on response, side effects, or initial presentation
- *Concurrent treatments*
- Too brief an *observation period* for clinical effects to occur
- Variable time of *blood sampling*
- *Inadequate evaluation* of clinical response, as well as the indefinite nature of response
- Presence of numerous *active metabolites*
- Inadequate *assay methods,* such as radioreceptor assays

Interpolation from Plasma to Brain Levels

It would be desirable to measure CNS antipsychotic levels in human beings. Although this will become possible with emerging imaging techniques, at present the only direct measurements that can be made are on postmortem tissue of patients who had recently discontinued drug or were on antipsychotics at the time of death (282). Haloperidol is concentrated in the brain at levels about 10 to 30 times higher than the expected plasma level. Animal studies find a brain:plasma ratio of about 20. Limited information from animal studies after drug withdrawal also shows a rapid disappearance from plasma. Although the half-life of haloperidol is about 24 hours in plasma, even several days after cessation of oral dosing significant CNS D_2 receptor activity is still evident. Indeed, PET studies indicate that after withdrawal of haloperidol or fluphenazine decanoate, D_2 blockade can persist for several months. Thus, it is likely that these agents stay in the human brain longer than in plasma and that brain levels are approximately 10 to 20 times higher than plasma levels.

Plasma Level Study Designs

While large interindividual variability in the steady-state plasma concentrations among patients treated with similar doses of a given antipsychotic is well established, the existence of a critical range of plasma concentration for therapeutic response or significant adverse effects remains controversial. A body of data from a number of fixed-dose studies, however, indicates a possible threshold for response or a linear or curvilinear relationship between plasma levels and clinical response for agents such as:

- Chlorpromazine (283)
- Fluphenazine (284, 285)
- Trifluoperazine (286)
- Thiothixene (287)
- Haloperidol (288–296)
- Clozapine (66, 291)
- Risperidone (297)
- Olanzapine (298)

In addition, prospective studies targeting large numbers of acutely ill patients to certain plasma levels to test a putative therapeutic threshold or range have been conducted with haloperidol (299).

Chlorpromazine

Curry et al. (300, 301) found a wide range of effective plasma drug levels in schizophrenics treated with comparable doses of CPZ, establishing that an upward or downward shift of 50% in dose usually produced adverse effects or a psychotic exacerbation, respectively. May et al. (302) found no relationship between plasma levels and response in 48 patients on fixed doses of CPZ (6.6 mg/kg/day). This agent is particularly problematic, however, because of its many, potentially confounding, metabolites, which are typically not measured.

Fluphenazine

Several groups have investigated fluphenazine plasma levels with either the oral or the parenteral, depot form. In one study, clinical response as a function of the mean C_{SS} of oral fluphenazine suggested an upper therapeutic end based on three nonresponding patients who had a mean C_{SS} above 2.8 ng/mL (285). Further, a lower end was suggested by two nonresponders and one partial responder whose levels were below 0.2 ng/mL. Van Putten et al. (303) found that higher fluphenazine plasma levels (up to 4.23 ng/mL) were significantly associated with a higher rate of improvement; however, 90% (65 of 72 patients) experienced disabling adverse effects with levels greater than 2.7 ng/mL.

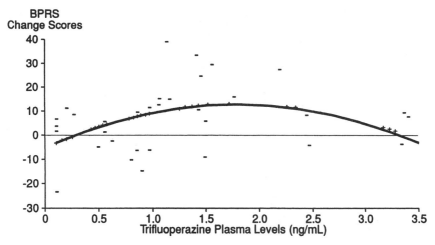

FIG. 5-11. Brief Psychiatric Rating Scale (BPRS) change scores in relationship to trifluoperazine plasma levels. (From Janicak PG, Javaid JI, Sharma RP, et al. Trifluoperazine plasma levels and clinical response. *J Clin Psychopharmacol* 1989;9:340–346, with permission.)

In a 2-year, double-blind comparison of 5 or 25 mg fluphenazine decanoate, Marder et al. (304) found a significant relationship between fluphenazine plasma levels and psychotic exacerbations after 6-9 months of maintenance therapy. Thus, those with levels less than 0.5 ng/mL did much worse than those with levels above 1.0 ng/mL. These data suggest that levels between 1.0 and 2.8 ng/mL may be the ideal range for many patients.

Serum levels ranged from 3 to 45 ng/mL, with a linear relation between clinical response during the first week of treatment and serum ($r = 0.5$), as well as RBC levels ($r = 0.64$). By contrast, Mavroidis et al. (287) found a curvilinear relationship between thiothixene plasma levels and clinical response. Thus, levels ranging between 2.0 and 15 ng/mL, measured 10–12 hours after the last dose, were associated with clinical improvement.

Trifluoperazine

Some of the authors reported on a potential therapeutic window with the commonly used phenothiazine, trifluoperazine (286). Specifically, there was evidence for a lower therapeutic threshold, around 1 ng/mL, and a suggestion of an upper end around 2.3 ng/mL (Fig. 5-11). Based on a review of dose-response studies, we concluded that 9 to 15 mg of trifluoperazine would be comparable to 300 mg of CPZ and should fall near the lower part of the linear portion of the dose-response curve.

Thiothixene

Yesavage et al. (305) treated 48 acute schizophrenics with thiothixene (80 mg/day), measuring serum and red blood cell (RBC) concentrations 2 hours after the morning dose.

Haloperidol

Haloperidol, the most commonly prescribed conventional neuroleptic, has only one pharmacologically active metabolite (i.e., reduced haloperidol). We reviewed the literature on HPDL plasma levels and summarized the outcome (306). While there are several studies examining the relationship between HPDL steady-state plasma levels and clinical response, they have used varying methodologies in terms of patient selection, symptom profile, diagnostic criteria, assay techniques, and the use of variable or fixed-dose schedules. Hence, the results of these studies are difficult to interpret collectively. As with other agents, the results with the fixed doses of HPDL have also been conflicting, although at least six early studies demonstrated a curvilinear relationship (i.e., therapeutic window)

TABLE 5-22. *Early fixed-dose studies finding a curvilinear relationship between haloperidol plasma levels and clinical response*

Study	Assay method	Therapeutic range	Rating scale	Study duration
Garver (1984)/ Mavroidis (1983)	GLC	4–11 ng/mL	NHSI	14 days
Smith (1984)	GLC (RRA)	7–17 ng/mL	BPRS Psychosis factor	24 days
Potkin (1985)	RIA	4–26 ng/mL	CGI	6 weeks
Van Putten (1985)	RIA	5–16 ng/mL	BPRS	7 days
Van Putten (1988)	RIA	2–12 ng/mL	BPRS Psychosis factor	4 weeks
Santos (1989)	RIA	12–35.5 ng/mL (7.4–24.9 in subchronic group)	BPRS Total score	21 days

Adapted from Janicak PG, Javaid JI, Davis JM. Neuroleptic plasma levels: methodological issues, study design, and clinical applicability. In: Marder SR, Davis JM, Janicak PG, eds. *Clinical use of neuroleptic plasma levels.* Washington DC: APPI Press, 1993:17–44.

between HPDL plasma levels and clinical response. Whereas optimal levels differed slightly among these studies, the mean low end was 4.2 ng/mL, and the mean high end was 16.8 ng/mL (Table 5-22) (288–294, 296). By contrast, some studies have not found a correlation between plasma HPDL levels and clinical response (314, 315).

Bleeker et al. (307) and Shostak et al. (308) also attempted to study the low end of a putative HPDL plasma level therapeutic window and found that none of three and two of five patients with low plasma levels, respectively, were responders. This contrasted with the outcome in their middle ranges, where five of 23 and five of six, respectively, responded. Conversely, five other studies deliberately probed the upper end of the therapeutic window. Doddi et al. (309), Kirch et al. (310), and Bigelow et al. (311), using medium or high HPDL doses, failed to find any evidence for an upper end of the therapeutic window in newly admitted patients. Rimon et al. (312) used extremely high HPDL doses (120 mg/day) in very chronic patients, but also failed to find an upper end of the therapeutic window. Coryell's group (313) prospectively assigned patients to fixed HPDL doses for at least the first 2 weeks of treatment to yield a distribution of plasma levels above and below a hypothesized therapeutic window of 18 ng/mL. They found a significant negative linear relationship (i.e., as dose increased, response decreased) between HPDL plasma levels and outcome at week 1, which did not persist into weeks 2, 3, and 4.

Targeted Plasma Level Designs

One can pool data from several fixed-dose studies to achieve an adequate sample size that would define the optimal cutoff point for a lower end and possibly for an upper end as well. These data can then be used to design a targeted plasma level study.

Using such a design, Volavka et al. (314) failed to find evidence for a therapeutic window after randomly assigning 111 schizophrenic or schizoaffective patients to one of three HPDL plasma levels (i.e., 2 to 13, 13.1 to 24, or 24.1 to 35 ng/mL). Interpretation of their results, however, may be complicated by too high a level for the low and perhaps middle ranges and a prolonged period of time to titrate to the middle and high HPDL plasma levels.

In a subsequent report, Volavka et al. (315) targeted acutely psychotic patients to a low (mean = 2.2 ng/mL) or a middle (mean = 10.5 ng/mL) HPDL plasma level group. Twenty-five patients with levels <3 ng/mL showed minimal response over 3 weeks.

Janicak et al. (316) attempted to address these issues by prospectively reassigning initial HPDL nonresponders to the putative therapeutic range (Fig. 5-12). During phase A, 25-30% of patients in the low, middle, and high HPDL plasma levels responded. Further, in the second phase of this study, initial partial or nonresponders to low or high plasma levels benefited from a dose adjustment (i.e., average = 25 mg/day) to achieve plasma levels of about 12 ng/mL (Fig. 5-13).

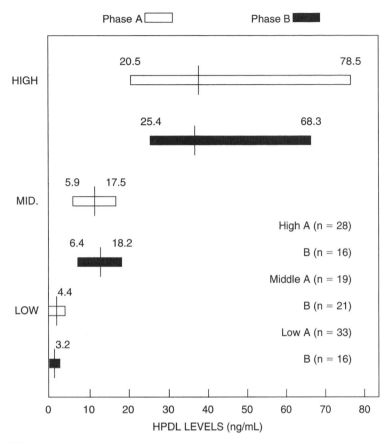

FIG. 5-12. Haloperidol (HPDL) plasma level ranges by targeted groups.

When they analyzed only the phase A nonresponders in phase B, the sample size was smaller; but those in the middle range demonstrated significantly more improvement on both the total BPRS and the positive symptom subscale scores, in contrast to those who remained in the low or the high groups. Further, no benefit was achieved by raising plasma levels beyond the defined middle range.

Case Examples: A 29-year-old woman was admitted to our research unit due to an exacerbation of her schizoaffective disorder. After giving informed consent, the patient participated in the targeted HPDL plasma level study. She was randomly assigned to the high plasma level and began treatment with 60 mg/day HPDL for 3 weeks. She scored a 40 on the BPRS at baseline (after an 11-day medication-free period). Her mean HPDL plasma level was 38.4 ng/mL for the first

3 weeks, and her BPRS score was 39 at the end of that period. She was then randomly reassigned to a middle plasma level, with a reduction of HPDL to 16 mg/day. At the end of this phase (24 days later), the patient's BPRS score was 22, with an average plasma level of 14.2 ng/mL. After no improvement in the first phase, the patient experienced a 45% decrease from her total baseline BPRS score during the second phase. Keeping in mind the lowest score on the BPRS is 18, this was an 82% drop in ratable symptoms.

A 29-year-old male schizophrenic patient was admitted to our research unit due to a worsening in his paranoid delusions and auditory hallucinations. After giving informed consent and undergoing a 12-day medication washout, he scored a 48 on the BPRS. He was randomly assigned initially to a low plasma level and received 2 mg/day

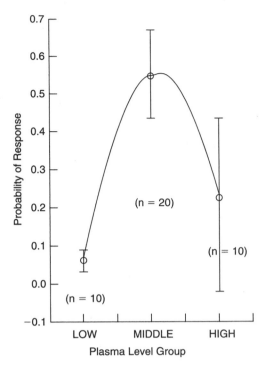

FIG. 5-13. Clinical response based on plasma level assignment in Phase B. (From Janicak et al. *Acta Psychiatr Scand* 1997;95:343–350, with permission.)

haloperidol, with an average plasma level of 1.29 ng/mL over 3 weeks. He demonstrated a slight improvement, scoring a 37 on the BPRS at that point (i.e., a 23% change). He was then randomly reassigned to a middle plasma level, and the dose of haloperidol was increased to 18 mg/day. After 27 days, he had an average plasma level of 12.0 ng/mL, and rated a 21 on the BPRS, or a 55% improvement from his baseline symptoms. Again, considering 18 is the lowest total BPRS score possible, this was an 84% drop in ratable symptoms.

Both patients demonstrated clinically relevant and statistically significant decreases in psychotic symptoms after their plasma HPDL concentrations were targeted within the 10 to 15 ng/mL range. Although it is possible they improved during the second phase solely due to time on treatment, their scores on the BPRS dropped rapidly once switched into the middle range. In addition, they demonstrated minimal improvement during the first 3 weeks.

Scores on the Simpson-Angus side effect scale were in the mild range for both patients, and did not change during either phase. Thus, this would not support decrease in toxicity as the reason for improvement, especially when the dose and blood levels were reduced in the first patient.

As part of this study a dose-prediction formula was developed to more rapidly achieve the desired HPDL C_{SS}. For this purpose, the first 28 patients, before receiving the initial assigned dose for achieving their targeted level, received a 15-mg "test"dose (p.o.) of HPDL, and blood samples were drawn 24 and 48 hours afterwards. Data analysis indicated a strong linear relationship between the targeted log C_{SS} achieved and the dose required when the 24-hour log transformed plasma level was included in a linear regression model ($r = 0.933$) (317). This formula was then prospectively tested and found to be valid in determining the dose required to achieve the desired HPDL C_{SS} (318).

The neuroleptic threshold data generated by McEvoy and colleagues (319) support the phase A findings of this study. This group determined the neuroleptic threshold (NT) dose (i.e., 3.7 ± 2.3 mg/day) for 106 schizophrenic and schizoaffective patients by starting with a low dose and increasing it until mild rigidity developed. The phase A results of the previous study were quite consistent with these data in that plasma levels as low as 2 ng/mL (mean dose = 3.3 mg/day) did not clearly fall below a therapeutic threshold for response. After a 2-week open trial at this dose, McEvoy then randomly assigned the 95 remaining patients under double-blind conditions to remain at the NT dose or to be switched to a higher dose of HPDL (mean = 11.6 ± 4.7 mg/day) for an additional 2 weeks. While there were similar rates of improvement on the total BPRS in phase A, and with McEvoy et al. at comparable time points, the Janicak study found a greater improvement in phase B (8.1 BPRS points) than in McEvoy et al.'s second phase (2.9 BPRS change score points). In McEvoy's study, while higher doses of HPDL did not produce greater improvement in measures of psychosis, they did lead to slightly better improvement in hostility.

These results also complement a series of PET studies by Nordstrom et al. (320)

and Nyberg et al. (72), which support a potential optimal striatal D_2 occupancy level. Thus, below 60% D_2 occupancy, response may be suboptimal, and greater than 80% D_2 occupancy may lead to increased EPS. In addition, Wolkin et al. (321) found that HPDL plasma levels of 5 to 15 ng/mL led to rapid increase in striatal D_2 blockade up to 80%. In a sample of seven acutely psychotic patients, Kapur et al. (322) in a prospective controlled trial found that 2 mg haloperidol for 2 weeks produced a 66% ± 7% D_2 receptor occupancy level. These first-episode psychotic patients achieved HPDL plasma concentrations ranging from 0.6 to 1.5 ng/mL ($\chi^2 = 1.1 \pm 0.4$). At these levels, five patients showed "much improvement" per the CGI, including a 45% improvement in positive symptoms and a 55% improvement in negative symptoms.

Whereas some studies using higher plasma levels find a modest decrement in clinical effect and others find a response plateau, none find evidence that higher plasma levels lead to enhanced efficacy. In addition, while not a marked phenomenon, with unnecessarily high neuroleptic plasma levels (or doses) there is an increased risk of adverse events. For example, there is evidence that rapid dose escalation may predispose to neuroleptic malignant syndrome (323, 324). **In this context, we emphasize the consistent agreement among studies that there is no additional benefit to using higher neuroleptic doses or plasma levels.**

For newer agents, defining the plasma level or dose-response relationship should be a priority to avoid using excessive doses for prolonged periods of time. This information may also be relevant for designing clinical trials using appropriate doses of neuroleptics for comparison trials against novel antipsychotics (i.e., parallel dose-response studies).

Clozapine

Clozapine Plasma Level-Drug Interactions

Clozapine is principally metabolized to *N*-desmethylclozapine (norclozapine). It is also metabolized to and n-oxide, other hydroxyl metabolites, and a protein-reactive metabolite. The n-oxide can be converted back to clozapine. The enzyme responsible for the metabolism of clozapine to norclozapine is the cytochrome P450 1A2 enzyme (325). This is consistent with a study showing that caffeine, a marker for 1A2, is cleared in relationship to the conversion of clozapine to norclozapine (326). Discontinuation of coffee intake can decrease the clozapine plasma levels by more than 50%, and increasing caffeine intake can produce a reemergence of the side effects (e.g., drowsiness, excess salivation). Additionally, smoking, which induces 1A2, lowers clozapine plasma levels. Fluvoxamine, an inhibitor of 1A2, dramatically increases plasma levels, and on occasion, adverse effects are seen (327). This phenomenon can lead to clozapine intoxication in patients on high doses of fluvoxamine.

Case Example: One patient ingested clozapine on two different occasions. On the first occasion she took clozapine and recovered in 6 hours from a comatose state. Two months later, while on therapeutic doses of fluvoxamine, she exhibited a state of fluctuating consciousness; on most occasions she was unable to gesture a simple request, but on some occasions she was able to react adequately. She was bothered by vivid and frightening visual hallucinations of tigers under her bed and serpents on her pillow. Her speech was disturbed, and she could not sit up because of truncal ataxia. Twenty-four hours after the intoxication, the overdose symptomatology declined significantly. The patient was able to walk a few steps and her speech was normal. Peak plasma levels were >9,000 ng/ml, falling to 4,000 by day 1 and under 1,000 by day 3. This excretion rate is slower than normally observed in overdoses, presumably because of the pharmacokinetic interaction with fluvoxamine through cytochrome P450 1A2 (328).

Phenytoin, an enzyme inducer, can reduce clozapine plasma levels. There have been two reported cases of risperidone causing an increase in clozapine plasma levels; however, because this agent is not an inhibitor of 1A2, the mechanisms for this increase are unclear. Nefazodone administered with clozapine has had minimal effects on clozapine's metabolism (329).

Clozapine Dose-Response Relationship

As with most of the older psychotropic drug, dose-response curves for clozapine have not been developed until recently. In a blinded, controlled study, Simpson and coworkers (330) randomized patients into three doses of clozapine 100, 300, and 600 mg. These researchers found that 600 mg was more effective than 300 mg and that doses up to 400 mg/day usually produce inadequate plasma levels. Thus, the results of this dose-response study are consistent with the plasma level studies. This provides some evidence that therapeutic drug monitoring may help ensure that patients receive a clozapine dose high enough to develop an adequate plasma level.

Clozapine Plasma Level-Response Relationship

Dose-response and plasma level-response information is conceptually very similar. In dose-response terms, it is important to know the average therapeutic threshold dose, the minimal dose to produce a full response. When plasma levels correlate with clinical response and there is a wide range of plasma levels for a given dose, then it is important to know the minimal therapeutic plasma levels to produce the optimal response for most patients. Several reports have indicated that plasma concentrations of clozapine above 350 to 450 ng/mL may be required to maximize response in treatment refractory schizophrenic patients (66, 291, 331, 332). Clozapine plasma levels, however, vary substantially from patient to patient. For example, Potkin et al. (291) found a 45-fold (40 to 911 mg/mL) range in plasma levels after a fixed dose of 400 mg/day. Initially, Perry et al. (66) did a plasma level study assigning patients to a dose of 400 mg/day for 4 weeks and identified 350 ng/mL as a threshold for response. At or above this plasma level, 64% of patients responded, as compared with only 23% of patients below that level. This group followed up these original results with a larger sample and in a follow-up of the existing samples, five of seven patients had an unsatisfactory response to a dose of 400 mg/day. When the dose was increased to achieve a plasma level above the threshold 350 ng/mL, however, most then responded (333).

Potkin et al. (291) also used a fixed dose of 400 mg/day in a study of 58 schizophrenic patients and found that very few (8%) patients with low clozapine plasma levels (<420 ng/mL) responded, in comparison with 60% of those with plasma levels >420 ng/mL. This group used a targeted plasma level design so that patients with originally low plasma levels had these levels increased above 420 ng/mL in a double-blind, random-assignment procedure. Response rate increased to 73%, compared with 29% of those whose plasma levels remained low. This result is particularly impressive because it was a randomized prospective change in dose, which provides important confirmation of the relationship between clozapine plasma levels and clinical efficacy. Kronig et al. (332) also found a therapeutic level of 350 ng/mL. Although the chosen level varies from study to study, there is general agreement that a threshold therapeutic plasma level exists somewhere between 350 and 450 ng/mL.

It is important to consider whether parent compound levels only or the sum of clozapine plus norclozapine plasma levels are measured, because in the latter case, the threshold would be higher. Note that a quality control study has been done comparing different laboratories on the assay reliability of clozapine plasma levels with split samples finding good agreement. Clinically, it is important to start with a small dose and gradually increase to avoid side effects. Even so, it is desirable to move rapidly to the correct level in patients who may need a slightly higher than average dose. Perry (334) has provided a prediction formula: the clozapine plasma level equals 111 × smoking (0 for smoker, 1 for nonsmoker) plus $0.464 x + 145$ for males, and $111 \times$ smoking status plus $1.59x - 149$ for females.

Risperidone and Olanzapine

Plasma-Level Response Relationship

Methods have also been developed to measure plasma levels of risperidone and olanzapine (297, 335). Preliminary data indicate that olanzapine levels ≥ 9.3 ng/mL at 24 hours and ≥ 23.2 ng/mL at 12 hours may be associated with improved response in schizophrenic patients (298, 298a). One small study found that dose reduction of risperidone from 6 to 3.6 ($\pm$0.9) mg/day lessened side effects and improved response rates but did not substantially alter risperidone (plus 9-OH-risperidone) plasma concentrations (i.e., 40.4 $\pm$ 31 versus 49.7 $\pm$ 13.4) (336).

Conclusion

In summary, the value of routine plasma level monitoring with antipsychotics remains uncertain; however, TDM can be useful in the following situations:

- To determine *patient compliance*
- To establish *adequacy* of the pharmacotherapy in nonresponders
- To *avoid toxicity* due to unnecessarily high plasma levels
- To monitor patients with other *medical disorders* or on *concurrent psychotropics* or *other medical drugs*
- To *maximize the clinical response* where the drug plasma level-response relationship has been elucidated
- To help define the *dose-response relationship*
- To safeguard clinicians in potential *medico-legal situations*

ALTERNATIVE TREATMENT STRATEGIES

In partially responsive or nonresponsive patients, the first issue is to determine whether an individual is truly treatment-resistant, because many receive nontherapeutic doses and the potential for improvement may not be adequately tested. Thus, in some situations, more aggressive treatment (dose increase, augmentation) may be appropriate, if not precluded by adverse effects. In selected cases, it may also be helpful to monitor plasma levels to ensure that they are in a reasonable range (see "Pharmacokinetics/Plasma Levels" earlier in this chapter). If a patient continues to demonstrate significant symptoms after a sufficient trial (2 to 3 weeks), alternatives to switching to another antipsychotic may include the addition of lithium, an anticonvulsant, or a second

antipsychotic agent. An antidepressant or anxiolytic may also be helpful, especially if affective or anxiety symptoms are prominent.

While there is no evidence that combining two neuroleptics is superior to comparable amounts of a single agent, the combined use of a neuroleptic plus a novel antipsychotic or, alternatively, the combination of two different novel agents (e.g., clozapine plus risperidone) may be beneficial in certain circumstances. Preliminary reports indicate that the pharmacology of novel antipsychotics may be sufficiently different that, when combined with each other or with neuroleptics, a better overall effect can be achieved in selected patients (100). Thus, potential scenarios include:

- Overlapping of two antipsychotics when *transitioning* from one agent to another
- *Supplementing of neuroleptic depot* therapy when symptoms worsen temporarily
- *Enhancing efficacy and/or decreasing adverse effects* when combining two different antipsychotics (101)

Dosing Strategy

Whereas lower doses are desirable and often sufficient, some patients may require short-term moderate to higher doses. Many clinicians are reluctant to use this approach, concerned about the potential for more significant adverse effects, and as a result may prematurely seek alternative strategies. These concerns may not be entirely warranted, however. Dubin et al. (337), for example, reviewed 10 papers addressing the prevalence of adverse effects during rapid tranquilization in 676 cases. Overall, their prevalence was extremely low (8%) and consisted mostly of EPS or hypotension (with low-potency agents). Again, when available, TDM of blood levels may be a more useful guide to adequacy of treatment than the dose used.

Tardive dyskinesia is also frequently mentioned as a reason to minimize exposure, but this condition usually develops after more chronic exposure. The relationship between TD and prior neuroleptic dosing is uncertain at this time, and the authors are not aware of any studies indicating that an acute, time-limited use of higher neuroleptic doses increases the prevalence of this disorder (338). Fortunately, the occurrence of NMS is an infrequent event (less than 1.5%), with no occurrences noted in the 676 cases reviewed by Dubin. In the discussion on adverse effects (later in this chapter), however, we note a higher incidence has been found by others during rapid dose increases.

Antipsychotics Plus Other Psychotropics

A second major question is the relative benefit of other concurrent psychotropic agents. Issues that are often raised include:

- Do adjunctive *benzodiazepines* (BZDs) help aggressivity in psychotic patients?
- Do adjunctive *mood stabilizers* help depressed, excited, or apathetic schizophrenic patients?
- Do adjunctive *anticonvulsants* help with seizure-related complications, associated aggression, or affective symptoms?

Benzodiazepines Plus Antipsychotics

Despite the advent of the atypical antipsychotic agents, efforts continue to identify other adjunctive medications that may improve response to standard treatments. In this context, we note that there is no consistent evidence that BZD monotherapy benefits schizophrenia. Another strategy, however, is the *addition of BZDs* to an antipsychotic regimen. This pharmacological approach is partially based on the evidence that GABA, which is facilitated by BZDs, inhibits

certain dopamine tracts and that these medications may attenuate the dopamine system via a different route (339–342).

Efficacy

It is important to distinguish between acute (e.g., 1 day) and longer term treatment with a BZD. Most of the literature addressing this issue consists of anecdotal reports, retrospective chart reviews, and uncontrolled studies in small patient samples, plus a small number of controlled trials for short-term acute BZD therapy. To our knowledge, at least 12 studies (including more than 450 patients) have evaluated the efficacy of *adjunctive* BZDs in nonresponsive schizophrenics (Table 5-23). Two of three open studies showed positive results, as did two controlled, single-blind studies (343-347). In seven double-blind, crossover studies (six with placebo controls), the results are more contradictory, in that five showed no advantage to an adjunctive BZD, and one of the two positive studies had a small sample size (188, 189, 348–351).

A *chart review* of 380 patients discharged from the Boston Veterans Administration Hospital found one group who were prescribed either an antipsychotic alone ($n = 22$; mean dose = 560 mg/day CPZ eq.) or combined with lorazepam ($n = 8$; mean dose = 265 mg/day CPZ eq.; 2.75 mg/day lorazepam) (163). Although it was concluded that the addition of lorazepam necessitated less antipsychotic, the patient distribution was quite unequal (only eight patients were on antipsychotic-BZD treatment), and this trend may have disappeared with a larger, more equalized sample size. A second group

TABLE 5-23. *Benzodiazepines (type/dose range) used in controlled treatment trials of schizophrenia*

As sole agent	In conjunction with antipsychotics
Chlordiazepoxide (20–700 mg/day) Diazepam (15–400 mg/day)	Alprazolam (0.5 mg/day to highest dose tolerated) Camazepam (40 mg/day) Chlordiazepoxide (30–300 mg/day) Clonazepam (1 mg/day to optimum dose) Diazepam (15–200 mg/day) Estazolam (6 mg/day) Lorazepam (0.75 mg/day to highest dose tolerated)

of 32 patients, discharged during the same time period, were prescribed an antipsychotic (mean dose = 771 mg/day CPZ eq.) and benztropine, or an antipsychotic (933 mg/day CPZ eq.), benztropine, and lorazepam. Those treated with the antipsychotic-BZD combination plus benztropine were actually on higher doses of an antipsychotic in comparison with the antipsychotic-alone group, contradicting the earlier results.

The Spring Grove State Hospital group compared a phenothiazine plus a benzodiazepine with a phenothiazine alone *in a double-blind, random-assignment trial* and found the combination inferior to the single agent (188, 189). Clinicians could increase the dose of the blinded medication until the patient became sedated. As a result, a much lower dose of phenothiazine was used when combined with the BZD than when given alone, probably because of the excessive sedation. Thus, the lower doses of phenothiazine in the combination group could have contributed to their poorer response.

Catatonia. Catatonia is a syndrome that can present as a symptom of several disorders. A large number of case reports have found that BZDs are effective in the treatment of catatonia. Specifically, lorazepam, clonazepam, and diazepam have been reported to induce temporary remission of catatonic symptoms (352–359). BZD treatment of catatonia is usually considered diagnostic, however, because symptoms return as the drug's therapeutic effect wanes. Continuing BZD treatment may produce longer symptom remission, but treatment should be directed to the underlying cause of the catatonia (177). In a review of 30 cases (with various psychiatric diagnoses), only two organic patients failed to demonstrate a significant clinical response (354, 360). **Based on these reports, lorazepam appears to be effective in "functional" catatonia.** Further, i.v. diazepam (10–20 mg) has also been reported to be effective (358). All these cases are consistent, in that patients tended to demonstrate a marked response to i.m. or i.v. administration of a BZD, and this response persisted when the medication was given on a maintenance basis (usually p.o.). In contrast, patients tended to relapse within 24 hours if the BZD was discontinued before initiating treatment for the underlying psy-

chopathology. The motivation to use lorazepam is its safe and rapid onset of action. BZDs may also benefit catatonia for longer periods of time if adequate results are not seen quickly (i.e., after 4 to 8 hours of 2 mg i.m. q 2 hours). ECT should also be considered if the patient is rapidly deteriorating or in a life-threatening crisis. Catatonia is an infrequent event, and for obvious ethical reasons, controlled studies would be impossible. Thus, although many of these case reports are impressive and indicate the effectiveness of parenteral BZDs, confirmatory controlled trials are unlikely.

Adverse Effects

Although generally less toxic than antipsychotics, benzodiazepines can also produce significant adverse effects (168, 190, 361–363). Ataxia, sedation, dysarthria, nausea, vomiting, confusion, excitation, disinhibition, and/or assaultiveness have all been reported. In one study, 32% experienced sedation and drowsiness, and 34% demonstrated arousal, excitation, or assaultiveness resembling a manic state, although this was higher than reported in most other studies (163). Thus, although BZDs may benefit some patients, they may be counterproductive in others (see also the section "Adverse Effects of Anxiolytics" in Chapter 12).

Conclusion

In summarizing the results, there appears to be no clear advantage to an antipsychotic-BZD combination in most patients. There was a consistent, although small, group of individuals, however, who demonstrated a rapid, dramatic, and sustained response (e.g., those who were catatonic) when treated with this combination. Some attribute this to a placebo effect, but the quick onset, lasting effect, and degree of improvement speak against this. Another possibility is that improvement may actually be secondary to relief from EPS such as akathisia; however, it is unlikely that the dramatic improvement in some patients could be explained by this alone. Finally, there may be a small subpopulation that experiences a true drug effect. Thus, schizophrenia, viewed by many as a heterogeneous disease, may encompass subgroups that benefit from the BZDs (193). Definitive controlled studies using adequate doses of antipsychotics in both groups (i.e., antipsychotics alone versus an antipsychotic plus BZD) have yet to be done. In part, this is due to the excessive sedation seen in the combined drug group, which may be avoided by using less-sedating low-dose, high-potency agents such as HPDL or risperidone.

In clearly nonresponding, nonaffective, psychotic patients, BZDs may be of benefit, but presently, there is no way to predict which patients will be helped. Although there is no evidence that any particular BZD is more effective than another, we would recommend the use of higher potency agents such as lorazepam or clonazepam.

Antidepressants Plus Antipsychotics

A collaborative VA study (364) found that the addition of imipramine or a monoamine oxidase inhibitor to CPZ did not benefit chronic psychotic patients any more than CPZ alone. Further, the addition of an amphetamine was slightly harmful. This finding has since been replicated in several studies on apathetic schizophrenic patients (365). A study of chronic ambulatory schizophrenics compared amitriptyline plus perphenazine with perphenazine alone (366). While they found the combination slightly better in ameliorating depressive symptoms, it was at the cost of a slight increase in patients' thought disorder.

Because it can be difficult to distinguish a severe, apathetic depression from a patient with catatonic features, an augmenting antidepressant should be considered. These agents may also help a post-psychotic depression, suggesting the importance of identifying subgroups that might benefit from this approach. This combination is also much more effective than antidepressant monotherapy in depression with psychotic features (see also Chapters 6 and 7).

Preliminary findings indicate that the addition of fluoxetine may increase response or benefit treatment-resistant schizophrenic patients (367–369). Further, deficit symptoms seemed to improve in some patients, supporting a possible

role for $5\text{-}HT_2$ hypersensitivity as the underlying mechanism (370). Care must be taken to monitor plasma levels of antipsychotics, which may rise when combined with this selective serotonin reuptake inhibitor (SSRI) or other related antidepressants due to their ability to inhibit various CYP 450 isoenzymes.

Mood Stabilizers/Anticonvulsants Plus Antipsychotics

Lithium

Because there is some evidence that lithium may help patients with schizoaffective or schizophreniform disorders, the question of whether lithium added to an antipsychotic would produce a better overall response has been studied. For example, Biederman et al. (371) compared HPDL alone with HPDL plus lithium in a group of 36 schizoaffective patients and found four of 18 improved with HPDL alone, versus 11 of 18 on the combination.

While the role of lithium in treating schizophrenia has not been well delineated, it may be useful in certain patients with aggression, agitation, or psychomotor excitement. Most, however, do not believe it has inherent antipsychotic properties. Clinical evidence from a small number of controlled trials finds lithium alone is not beneficial for process schizophrenia. For example, an earlier double-blind, controlled trial of lithium versus CPZ for chronic schizophrenics found lithium completely ineffective and possibly harmful in the more chronic patients, while the antipsychotic had its expected beneficial effect (372).

For many years, schizophrenia was divided into process (core) and reactive types. More recent investigations indicate that the reactive psychotic group has many affective, as well as schizophrenic features (e.g., family histories). This distinction is recognized in the DSM-IV (373) by such disorders as schizophreniform, schizoaffective, and brief reactive psychosis.

It is possible that there are three major functional disorders:

- Core *schizophrenia*
- Reactive *schizophreniform* disorder

- *Mood* disorders

But the present nosological system only recognizes two categories:

- *Schizophrenia*
- *Mood* disorders

Although schizophreniform disorder is usually classified in the schizophrenic spectrum, some would categorize it as a mood disorder. For many years, patients in the United States were diagnosed manic if they met narrowly defined criteria, and schizophrenia was a broader, more inclusive category. Recently, however, the DSM-IV criteria for schizophrenia have become more restrictive, and the pendulum has swung, with some defining this diagnosis narrowly and mood disorders more broadly. The picture is further complicated by patients with mixed schizophrenic and mood symptoms, some of whom are then diagnosed as schizoaffective disorder.

A limited body of evidence indicates that lithium helps atypical mania, schizoaffective disorder, or schizophreniform disorder, both as an acute treatment and for prevention of recurrence. There are younger patients who demonstrate both schizophrenic and manic features early in the course of their illness. When in doubt about the diagnosis, lithium may be preferable for an acute episode because, if successful, it will most likely be an effective prophylaxis as well. Clearly, some patients are so disturbed that the clinician cannot wait until lithium becomes fully effective, and an antipsychotic must be added, but often it can be discontinued after a brief period to determine whether lithium alone is sufficient.

Little work has been done on the drug treatment of schizophreniform or brief reactive psychosis. Hirschowitz et al. (374) further explored the range of lithium's efficacy by systematically treating patients with schizophrenic or schizophreniform disorders. They found that "poor-prognosis" schizophrenia rarely responded to lithium, whereas some with "good-prognosis" schizophrenia did benefit. Because there was no control group, it is possible that some were placebo responders.

This group investigated patients presenting with acute schizophrenic symptoms who underwent a drug-free washout period, received lithium only initially, and then antipsychotics later (374). Lithium was ineffective for classic schizophrenia, but some patients who met criteria for schizophreniform disorder did respond to lithium. Whether schizophreniform illness is a variant of mood disorders (a reasonable hypothesis in view of their lithium response) or a separate entity that is lithium-sensitive is still unclear. It is known that these patients have family histories that include mood-disordered as well as schizophrenic relatives. In a small pilot study, physostigmine (a drug with possible antimanic but no antipsychotic properties) benefited schizophreniform patients who responded to lithium, but had no effect in those who did not (Garver DL, personal communication).

Antipsychotics have a broad-spectrum effect, improving psychosis in schizophrenia, schizophreniform disease, mania, and organic psychosis; but response to lithium suggests an affective core. **Whereas almost all schizophreniform patients are presently treated with antipsychotics, it is possible that lithium may be more specific and safer in the management of at least some of these patients.**

Carbamazepine

Limited evidence indicates that carbamazepine plus an antipsychotic may also benefit some schizophrenic patients. This is an interesting possibility in view of the similar antimanic properties of lithium and carbamazepine (375). This area requires further research, especially to clarify the indications for combining anticonvulsants with an antipsychotic. For example, mania complicated by psychotic features may benefit from lithium, valproate, or carbamazepine augmented by antipsychotics. Because carbamazepine induces the metabolism of at least some antipsychotics (e.g., haloperidol, thiothixene), dose adjustment based on TDM may be necessary to achieve the optimal effect.

Valproate

Valproate seems to benefit behavior disorders associated with epilepsy and other neurological disorders, including episodic aggression associated with psychomotor epilepsy. There are case reports of patients suffering from mental retardation or stroke with aggressive outbursts who have been helped by treatment with valproate. It is unclear, however, whether valproate benefits schizophrenia where aggression is a prominent symptom. In this context, New York State has a computerized record-keeping system and a recent survey of medications used for schizophrenia showed that adjunctive valproate has been increasingly used. Its role as an augmentation for treating schizophrenia has shown promise (375a).

Valproate Monotherapy. One group studied valproate in newly admitted, acute schizophrenia patients (376). All had a history of prior episodes and were drug-free for a period of approximately 1 week before valproate monotherapy was started. Psychiatric condition changed very little during the drug-free period, but six of the eight patients substantially deteriorated, with an exacerbation of the psychotic symptoms while on valproate monotherapy. Exacerbation of psychotic symptoms occurred at a threshold doses of 1.5–2 grams and were dose related after that. Mean baseline BPRS scores were approximately 38 and rose to 50 while on valproate. This is the only study reported on valproate monotherapy in antipsychotic drug-free patients.

Valproate Augmentation. There are very few studies of valproate when given in combination with neuroleptics. A double-blind, placebo-controlled, crossover study looked at 32 chronically psychotic patients with TD (377). The patients had been on stable doses of neuroleptics, often for many years, and these neuroleptics were continued through the trial. Valproate (900 mg/day) was added, and some improvement was observed. Valproate relieved dystonic spasms more than placebo but did not seem to have a consistent effect on TD. In contrast, a small group of patients treated at the NIMH, using an AB design, found essentially no change with valproate (378). There have been case histories of patients improving with valproate augmentation but other anecdotal reports show no change. As noted earlier, a double-blind study comparing valproate with placebo augmentation of olanzapine or risperidone is now under way.

Non-antipsychotic Alternatives

Benzodiazepines

Although numerous controlled trials have examined the role of selected BZDs, their effects range from deterioration, to no change in most patients, to striking improvement in a rare patient when using BZDs either as the sole agent or as an adjunct to antipsychotics (172, 187–195, 346, 48–352, 379–394). Reported effects include:

- *Amelioration of anxiety and tension* superimposed over chronic schizophrenia in three of six patients, a finding not replicated by others (195, 351, 352)
- The benzodiazepine sedative-hypnotic estazolam added to an antipsychotic *reduced auditory hallucinations* in selected chronic schizophrenics (191)
- Beneficial effects in a few studies, but *no significant benefit or even deterioration* with BZD treatment in most studies.

When it occurs, onset of therapeutic activity may be rapid (within hours, days, or 1 to 2 weeks). Even in those few patients with good initial response, however, therapeutic effects attributable to BZDs may be temporary. Several controlled studies have found that tolerance developed by the fourth week of treatment (172, 188, 189, 349, 350, 387). High doses appear to be associated with more favorable response, but data are limited, contradictory, and inconclusive (177, 190, 347, 362).

There is little evidence available indicating that one BZD is more effective than another. Because the duration of most controlled studies has been 8 weeks or less, data on more prolonged treatment are anecdotal.

Sedation, ataxia, and cognitive impairment occur more frequently with high BZD dosages. Other adverse effects reported when BZDs were used to treat schizophrenia include behavioral disinhibition, exacerbation of psychosis, and increase in anxiety and depression (163, 188–195, 351). Concomitant use of a BZD and the atypical antipsychotic clozapine may increase the risk of sedation, dizziness and collapse with loss of consciousness (196). Respiratory compromise has also been reported with this combination (395, 396).

Propranolol

Propranolol may have specific antiaggressive effects for mentally retarded, organic, and certain schizophrenic patients with episodic violence. High-dose propranolol in patients with episodic aggression has been recommended, but this is based primarily on case reports. These indications should be distinguished from its use with or without an antipsychotic as a specific treatment for schizophrenia. For example, some open studies using high doses of propranolol (i.e., 500 mg to 2 g) reported success in an occasional schizophrenic patient, but not all studies confirmed this outcome (397–404).

In a review of the literature, we found three controlled trials, one demonstrating propranolol to be slightly superior to an antipsychotic, but two others finding it no better than placebo for schizophrenia (405).

When given concurrently, limited evidence indicates that this agent may increase an antipsychotic's plasma level, which could explain the enhanced effect. Thus, three controlled studies found propranolol plus an antipsychotic superior to propranolol alone; two studies, however, found the combination no more effective than an antipsychotic alone. In view of these negative studies, propranolol's efficacy remains doubtful, but there is sufficient positive evidence to consider it potentially helpful for some patients.

Electroconvulsive Therapy

Antipsychotics have long since replaced ECT for the treatment of schizophrenia. Several studies, however, have found ECT equal in efficacy to these agents, while one large-sample, controlled trial found it less effective than drugs, but more effective than psychotherapy (406). Some clinicians believe that selected patients may benefit when ECT is given concurrently with an antipsychotic. One controlled study, for example, found that ECT in combination with a phenothiazine led to a more rapid remission than the phenothiazine alone (407). Clinical experience has clearly documented an important role for ECT in catatonic

excitement or withdrawal, as well as for other severe, life-endangering psychotic states. More recently, ECT combined with novel antipsychotics has been reported to benefit previously poorly responsive psychotic patients and was well tolerated (106, 408, 409).

Conclusion

Figure 5-5 demonstrates a strategy to manage an acute psychotic exacerbation, with alternate interventions if response is insufficient or complications, such as aggression, catatonia, or mood disturbances, occur.

ROLE OF PSYCHOSOCIAL THERAPIES

There is virtually unanimous agreement among experienced mental health workers regarding the unique benefit of antipsychotics. Some with limited patient experience, however, are critical of these agents. Unfortunately, this attitude is based on inaccurate information that schizophrenia is a psychological condition and, as a logical deduction, that drugs are at best an ancillary therapy and at worst harmful. Another reason for increasing one's knowledge about this issue is that some members of the legal profession, at times supported by misguided mental health activists, have attempted to make drug therapy illegal, claiming that the definitive treatment is psychotherapy because it addresses the basic cause. This argument is less than compelling, because although the exact cause of schizophrenia and other psychotic conditions are unknown, they are almost certainly biological disorders.

Having established the primary role of antipsychotics, evidence indicates that psychosocial therapies, when administered with these agents, improve long-term prognosis. Because chronically psychotic patients have difficulties with social adjustment, reason dictates that they and their families could benefit from such interventions. Regardless of theoretical orientation, it is clear that practitioners should provide psychosocial therapy as part of a comprehensive treatment strategy.

In this context, the type of psychosocial interventions used in schizophrenia has changed

TABLE 5-24. *Assessment of outcome in patients with schizophrenia treated with and without antipsychotic drugs and psychotherapy*

	No drugs		Drugs	
	No psychotherapy	Psychotherapy	No psychotherapy	Psychotherapy
Percent released	59%	64%	95%	96%
Nurses' rating MACC total	38	38	48	48
Menninger nurses' health-sickness rating	26	23	29	30
Nurses' idiosyncratic symptoms (×125)[a]	37	29	66	74
Therapists' rating on symptoms rating sheet (×50)[a]	22	21	27	27
Analysis rating of insight	3.4	3.3	3.7	4.1

MACc, Massachusetts Mental Health Center.
Adapted from Davis JM, Janicak PG, Chang S, Klerman K. Recent advances in the pharmacologic treatment of the schizophrenic disorders. In: Grinspoon L, ed. *Psychiatry 1982. American Psychiatric Association annual review*. Washington DC: APPI Press, 1982:221.
[a]A higher number reflects greater improvement. To have the two scales fit with this convention, scores were subtracted from an arbitrary constant.

radically in the last 15 years. In the 1950's and 1960's, the emphasis was on psychodynamic psychotherapy, and in particular long-term psychoanalysis was practiced in institutions such as Chestnut Lodge or the Menninger Clinic. Schizophrenia was conceptualized as a behavior taught to a child by a "schizophrenogenic" parent. Patients were then isolated from their families for long-term hospital care. In recent years, the approach has been to effect social rehabilitation with active involvement of the family. We will first review evidence pertinent to earlier approaches and then discuss the more recent assertive case management model.

Efficacy of Psychosocial Therapies

Psychotherapy Only Versus Drug Therapy

There is no empirical evidence that long-term, in-hospital psychotherapy without drugs is beneficial. Indeed, in any study that compared psychotherapy only to drug therapy, the psychotherapy group always did more poorly. For example, the classic study by May found that patients receiving psychotherapy alone did poorly, both initially as well as during follow-up (224, 225). The study found that psychotherapy did not increase improvement scores over that observed in the control group, and indeed, there was a nonsignificant trend in the other direction. Because patients received only 24 hours of psychotherapy

by relatively inexperienced counselors; however, this did not constitute a definitive test of this intervention's potential efficacy (Table 5-24).

R. D. Laing and colleagues (410) used *family-oriented therapy* with schizophrenic patients, reporting that 25% received no "tranquilizers" at all (implying that 75% did receive medication!). Further, he and his coworkers used a broad definition of schizophrenia, much less restrictive than that which was common in Great Britain at the time, so it is possible that all core schizophrenic patients received medication (in a personal communication to J. M. Davis, Laing acknowledged that he did refer his patients to a competent psychiatrist for drug treatment).

Drug Therapy Only Versus Drug Plus Psychotherapy

At the Massachusetts Mental Health Center (MMHC), a small group of chronically ill schizophrenic patients who were treated by senior psychoanalysts deteriorated when a placebo was substituted for thioridazine. Further, there was no evidence that the drugs made patients less responsive to psychoanalytically oriented psychotherapy and, in fact, many were more responsive to the psychotherapeutic process when on thioridazine (411–413).

In another MMHC study, chronic state hospital patients were randomly assigned to four variations of drug and social therapies: *high-intensity social therapy with drugs; high-intensity social therapy* without drugs; *low-intensity social therapy with drugs*; or *low-intensity social therapy without drugs*. High-intensity social therapy consisted of a variety of psychotherapies, social work intervention, occupational therapy, psychodrama, and "total push" therapies. The low-intensity social therapy consisted of milieu interventions administered in a state hospital. Improvement rates in the drug-treated patients were significantly higher than the rates observed in the nondrug groups, either in the state hospital milieu or at the MMHC. Further, there was no significant symptomatic improvement in the *drug-plus-high-intensity* social therapy group (33%), when compared with the drug-plus-low-intensity social therapy group (23%) (Table 5-25). If anything, the high-intensity social therapy without drugs impeded improvement, because this group, even after being placed back on drugs after a 6-month hiatus, never caught up with the continuously drug-treated groups.

The VA performed a double-blind study comparing group therapy alone, group therapy plus an antipsychotic, and antipsychotic therapy alone (414). In most cases, drug treatment with or without group therapy, produced substantially better improvement than group therapy only. Again, as in the earlier studies of social therapy, the antipsychotics proved crucial. The VA also performed a comparable study in chronic, elderly schizophrenic patients with similar results (415). Three other studies have compared psychotherapy or group therapy plus drug therapy with drug therapy alone in hospital settings and found that

those receiving psychotherapy plus medication did marginally better (416–418).

John Rosen (419–420) claimed that *direct analysis* (a psychoanalytic-like technique) produced improvement in 37 cases of deteriorated schizophrenia. He defined improvement as the ability to live comfortably outside of an institution, with the achievement of psychological integrity, emotional stability, and character structure such that a patient could withstand as much environmental stress as one who never experienced a psychotic episode. The credibility of this claim, however, was shattered by an independent evaluation of these patients' outcome. Five years later, a follow-up of Rosen's group found that 37% had not been initially diagnosed as schizophrenic, but rather as psychoneurotic, manic-depressive, or possibly hyperthyroid (e.g., one patient recovered after her thyroid was removed). The remainder met criteria for schizophrenia, and during the next 10 years, 75% had between two and five subsequent readmissions. Thus, Rosen's initial claims were not substantiated because many did not have schizophrenia, and most of those who did were not able to sustain their improvement.

Drug Therapy Plus Various Psychotherapies

In a 2-year, collaborative study of psychotherapy in hospitalized, acute schizophrenic patients, investigators compared *exploratory* and *insight-oriented psychotherapy* (E-IO) with a control treatment of *reality-adaptive-supportive* (RAS) psychotherapy (i.e., essentially a placebo psychotherapy). All study patients were also placed

TABLE 5-25. *Results of four treatments in chronic schizophrenia*

	High social therapy[a]	Low social therapy[b]
Percentage showing high improvement at 6 months' evaluation		
Drug therapy	33%	23%
No drug therapy	0%	10%
Percentage showing high improvement after 36 months		
Drug therapy	35%	19%
No drug therapy for 6 months, then drug therapy	26%	6%

Adapted from Klein D, Davis JM. Diagnosis and drug treatment of psychiatric disorders. In: *Review of antipsychotic drug literature*. Baltimore: Williams & Wilkins, 1969:92.
[a]Patients transferred to Massachusetts Mental Health Center.
[b]Patients remaining in state hospitals.

on antipsychotics. A total of 164 patients entered the study, but 42% dropped out before the required minimal participation of 6 months, and only one third of the initial sample remained at the end of 2 years. Seventy-two patients (35 E-IO and 37 RAS) at 12 months and 47 (22 E-IO and 25 RAS) at 24 months were available for analyses. Although the differences between the E-IO and RAS groups were very small, the RAS patients, over a 2-year follow-up period, spent more time functioning independently and spent less time in the hospital, but the E-IO patients showed better self-understanding. The results indicated only a minimal outcome difference between the two types of psychotherapy, regardless of the outcome measure examined. These results are consistent with several other small studies of psychotherapy plus drug therapy versus drug therapy alone.

In another study, psychotherapy with and without drug therapy was compared with a *"no formal psychotherapy"* control group (421–423). No valid conclusions can be drawn from this study, however, because there was no adequate control group with respect to medication. Further, the majority of the psychotherapy group received medication and the control group was treated in an entirely different milieu, with many apparently transferred to a chronic facility.

Another study evaluating two types of *behaviorally oriented therapy* is open to the same criticism because it did not include adequate information about the drug treatment of those remaining in the state hospital (424, 425). It is known that at the beginning of the trial most patients were not on adequate doses of appropriate drugs, and some were not even receiving an antipsychotic. At various times during the study, a variable percentage (at times as great as 50%) of the psychological treatment groups also received medication. Thus, no valid conclusions can be drawn because the psychological treatment groups received drug therapy and many in the control group may not have received adequate drug therapy. Although this study is important in supporting the usefulness of specific behavioral interventions in comparison with milieu treatment, any conclusion concerning the role of drugs is not possible.

Maintenance Drug Therapy Plus Psychotherapy

Table 5-26 shows the effect of psychosocial treatment on relapse rates in seven studies (256, 426–431). All patients received maintenance antipsychotics, and the experimental variable was the presence or absence of some form of psychosocial therapy. Thus, these studies assessed

TABLE 5-26. *Outcome of patients treated with antipsychotic drugs with and without psychosocial treatment*[a]

Study	Evaluation interval	Drugs alone (number of subjects)		Drugs and psychosocial therapy (number of subjects)	
		Well	Relapsed	Well	Relapsed
Hogarty et al. (1974)	2 years	73	22	80	15
Goldstein et al. (1978)	6 weeks	42	8	44	2
Hogarty et al. (1979)	2 years	25	27	30	23
Falloon et al. (1982)	9 months	9	9	16	2
Tarrier et al. (1988)	9 months	8	8	29	3
Leff et al. (1990)	2 years	3	9	6	6
Hogarty et al. (1991)	2 years	11	10	39	15
Total		171	93	244	66
% Well/Relapsed		65%	35%	79%	21%

[a]MH $\chi^2 = 16.5$; $df = 1$; $p = 0.00005$.
Adapted from Davis JM; Andriukaitis S. The natural course of schizophrenia and effective maintenance drug treatment. *J Clin Psychopharmacol* 1986;6:2s–10s.

whether psychoeducation and family intervention have any additional benefit beyond that produced by medication. The number who relapsed in each treatment group was reported, so we combined the data from all seven studies and found a consistently better outcome for those with psychoeducation and family therapy intervention as compared with those on maintenance drug therapy only $(\chi^2 = 16.5; df = 1; p = 0.00005)$. Whereas the psychosocial treatments used in these seven studies employed similar techniques, not all were focused exclusively on lowering the family's expressed emotion toward the patient. Nevertheless, the consistently better outcome for those receiving some type of social therapy, in addition to antipsychotics, is a promising finding. Because they cannot be truly "blind," we would emphasize that these trials have been conducted by proponents of psychotherapy. Therefore, until they are replicated by others, we need to interpret the results cautiously. **These results underscore the importance of a careful transition from an inpatient to outpatient environment in preventing relapse.**

Other Approaches

Brief Hospitalization

Four controlled, random-assignment studies comparing brief hospital treatment with relatively longer periods of hospital-based psychological intervention found that the brief hospital stays produced comparable results to the longer stay regimen (432–437).

Family Therapy

It appears that patients from families with high expressed emotion (e.g., demanding, critical, high expectations) have a higher relapse rate than those from families with low expressed emotion (438–441). These findings suggested that certain patients may be vulnerable to emotional confrontations and led to the use of family therapy to reduce high expressed emotion. Families are taught techniques for coping with the patient and, perhaps more importantly, are educated about the disorder and the need for medication compliance.

Assertive Case Management

A trained case manager works to achieve social rehabilitation using the support of a multidimensional team that provides liaisons with medical and social agencies at all stages of the patient's illness. This includes intensive crisis management in the community setting as an alternative to inpatient care, as well as working with the inpatient team when necessary (228, 236). The emphasis is on assertive case management (ACM) to provide active support to work for effective solutions. A prominent part of the case manager's duty is to ensure that patients take their medications and receive adequate psychiatric care. Much of the success of this model is based on achieving adequate maintenance medication in patients and then building on this with social rehabilitation. A case manager can intervene at any stage of the illness using various practical efforts to achieve stable health, nutrition, and housing. The key concept is the "assertiveness" of the case manager in doing what is necessary to make sure that the patient receives appropriate care. Various add-ons such as stress reduction, cognitive-behavior therapy, and social skills training, are all important in an effective rehabilitation program. Another important aspect of ACM is the qualitative nature of the outcome. Patients in such programs have a much higher quality of life than those in regular hospital-based programs.

Hospitalization is extraordinarily expensive, and although ACM costs less than hospitalization, the overall difference is not as great as was once hoped. Although ACM has not proven to be significantly less expensive than hospital care in the short term, it is possible that once the patient is rehabilitated, subsequent costs will be substantially decreased. Furthermore, it may require several years for true rehabilitation to occur; hence, short-term studies may underestimate the total cost saving.

Part of ACM is educating patients and their families about the nature of their illness. Studies, however, have shown that education alone has no specific benefit in reducing clinical morbidity. Thus, ACM must include crisis intervention to realize a better quality of life and to avoid hospitalizations.

Specific studies suggest *psychosocial stress management* added to medication and ACM produces a beneficial effect for patients with schizophrenia. This includes training in communication skills and practical problem-solving strategies to enhance coping capacities and natural support networks. In addition, training in *living skills* has also proven helpful, particularly if integrated into real-life practice sessions. *Cognitive-behavior therapy* attempts to counteract some of the cognitive deficits seen in patients with schizophrenia, building on the base of medication and ACM.

Representative Payee Programs. One of the most aggressive aspects of this treatment is the representative payee program. This is usually a family member, case worker, or other responsible individual who is assigned control of the patient's disability income checks. Very frequently, patients with chronic schizophrenia will not use these funds appropriately. In many programs, a bank is appointed and will automatically take out money for rent. Some of the patient's money may be managed by the representative, so the patient does not become homeless or cannot afford to buy food. Instituting such a program can dramatically reduce readmission to a hospital or jail. For example, in a 1-year, randomized study of involuntary outpatient commitment, readmission was reduced by almost 75% and patients who were hospitalized required fewer inpatient days (442).

A Methodological Caution

The great majority of psychosocial studies are not adequately controlled. For example, some randomized studies with control groups are not blind. Patients and evaluators know who is in the experimental group and who is in the control group because each knows what psychosocial interventions are made on the patient's behalf. In some cases, blinded "graders" are used, but it is hard to blind psychosocial treatments. Considerable progress in experimental methodologies, however, has been made, and it is possible to provide incrementally/equally powerful control groups and disguise evaluations.

Conclusion

There is a very large psychotherapy community in the United States composed of professionals trained in various disciplines (e.g., psychologists, social workers, psychoanalysts). Some believe that psychotherapy is the treatment of choice for severe mental illness, although drugs may be necessary in extreme cases. We have reviewed in some detail the evidence on efficacy of psychotherapy with and without medication. Psychotherapy on its own has proven ineffective, but assertive case mangement plus medication is more effective than medication alone. Thus, the psychological approach for managing schizophrenia has undergone a paradigm shift and present tactics are in many ways the direct opposite of what was taught 50 years ago.

In the hospital setting, several groups failed to find psychotherapy without drugs effective, and the addition of psychotherapy to drug treatment produced marginal and inconsistent gains. In general, psychotherapeutic interventions are more appropriate in the outpatient setting. The role of these therapies can be analogized to the treatment of a broken leg, with medication comparable to casting the fracture and psychosocial therapies to the physical therapy that then facilitates the healing process.

Clinicians must be thoughtful in choosing the appropriate psychosocial treatment for specific patients. Any such intervention should be proven helpful, rather than chosen solely on the basis of a theoretical model. Finally, more complicated psychological strategies, often costlier in terms of time and expense, appear to offer no advantage over many more economical sociotherapeutic models.

ADVERSE EFFECTS

A long list of adverse effects may imply that most patients experience many of them to a significant degree. In fact, although almost all patients will experience some mild side effects with these drugs, such as dry mouth or tremor, they are usually transitory and disappear with time, medication reduction, or discontinuation. Fortunately, these effects are rarely serious or irreversible, and on average, the typical complications with antipsychotics are no worse than with medications prescribed for other medical disorders.

Central Nervous System

Acute Extrapyramidal Side Effects

Acute EPS can be classified into three categories:

* Parkinsonian syndrome
* Acute dystonias
* Akathisia

Lower potency neuroleptics, such as thioridazine and chlorpromazine, have a decreased incidence of EPS when compared with higher potency agents, such as haloperidol or fluphenazine. Novel agents, such as clozapine and quetiapine, are virtually devoid of EPS effects when given at their recommended dosing range.

The *parkinsonian syndrome* is characterized by a mask-like facies, resting tremor, cogwheel rigidity, shuffling gait, and psychomotor retardation. A more subtle form may present as emotional blunting (e.g., an apathetic appearance lacking in spontaneity) and a relative inability to engage in social activities, which can be confused with the emotional withdrawal, apathy, and retardation that are part of the deficit syndrome associated with a schizophrenic disorder or a post-psychotic depression. The syndrome is symptomatically identical to idiopathic parkinsonism and responds to antiparkinsonian medications (e.g., benztropine). Parkinsonian rigidity and akinesia may also respond to amantadine. Rarely, neuroleptics have been reported to produce a catatonic-like state, similar to akinetic mutism, which may also be responsive to amantadine.

The *dystonias* are involuntary contractions of major muscle groups and are characterized by symptoms such as torticollis, retrocollis, oculogyric crisis, and opisthotonos. *Akathisia* is a motor restlessness manifested by the urge to move about and/or an inability to sit still. This can be confused with psychotic agitation because patients are driven by a restlessness which is primarily motor and cannot be controlled by their own volition. Unlike psychotic agitation, however, akathisia is accompanied by subjective distress, worsened by increasing the antipsychotic dose, and often benefited by a decrease or the addition of a β-blocker or a BZD.

The parkinsonian syndrome and akathisia often occur early in therapy and tend to persist if not treated. They can also appear years later after prolonged treatment, frequently coexisting with TD. EPS, in general, occur equally in both sexes and all ages, however, there are age- and sex-related differences in the incidence of various types of EPS.

Although these adverse effects have fairly characteristic presentations, their diagnosis can occasionally be missed. For example:

* *Dystonia* can be confused with bizarre mannerisms.
* *Akathisia* can be confused with agitation.
* Parkinsonian *akinesia* can be confused with negative symptoms such as schizophrenic apathy or a retarded depression.

Treatment: Acute

An accurate diagnosis is important because these symptoms may be mistaken for an exacerbation of the psychosis, prompting an escalation in dose when a decrease or an antiparkinsonian drug should be considered. At times, a therapeutic trial with an agent such as procyclidine, benztropine, or diphenhydramine can be diagnostic, because acute dystonic reactions usually respond in minutes to parenteral administration of these agents.

EPS often present a clinical quandary because options can include blocking them with an antiparkinsonian drug, reducing the dose, changing to another agent, or some combination of these three. The decision should be based partly on clinical improvement, so if a patient's psychosis is stabilized, a decrease in the dose would be reasonable. If the patient is still quite psychotic, however, adding an antiparkinsonian drug or switching to another antipsychotic may be more appropriate. If adverse effects limit a clinically appropriate dose increase, switching to another agent is recommended (e.g., from a neuroleptic to a novel agent).

Acute dystonias are typically seen in the first few days to weeks of treatment and can occur with even limited exposure (e.g., children treated with a single dose of prochlorperazine for nausea). Although dystonias may disappear spontaneously, they should be treated aggressively, as they are often painful and upsetting to the patient. Rarely, laryngeal dystonias may seriously compromise respiration. Occasionally, an acute dystonic reaction is resistant to standard treatment but may respond to parenteral diazepam, caffeine sodium benzoate, or barbiturate-induced sleep.

Akathisia may respond to β-blockers (e.g., propranolol, atenolol), BZDs, amantadine, anticholinergics, or by lowering the dose or switching to a different antipsychotic. The fact that á-blockers benefit akathisia is an important observation, suggesting that it is mediated by noradrenergic mechanisms. The observation that propranolol is beneficial is supported by several double-blind studies, suggesting that this class of agents may be the treatment of choice (443-446). Although akathisia is generally thought of as an extrapyramidal reaction, the beneficial effects of propranolol may suggest a more complex etiology.

Although β-blockers are considered the treatment of choice for akathisia, low doses of clonazepam, diazepam, or lorazepam may also reduce its severity (172, 389, 445, 447–450). These BZDs may be a useful alternative when á-blockers are contraindicated (e.g., in patients with asthma, insulin-dependent diabetes mellitus, cardiac conduction abnormalities) or as an adjunct when akathisia persists despite stepwise escalation of these agents (177).

Treatment: Prophylaxis

Prophylactic antiparkinsonian medication for all patients on antipsychotics is controversial. Arguments against this approach include:

- Many patients *never manifest EPS*.
- There are *side effects associated with these medications,* such as dry mouth, blurred vision,

confusion, urinary retention, and, very rarely, paralytic ileus.
- *Dental caries* and diverticula may occur with chronic use.
- Patients can develop *behavioral toxicity,* which in its severe form may be characterized by disorientation, loss of immediate memory, and florid hallucinations.
- The *expense* of treatment is increased.
- Anticholinergics can produce a feeling of euphoria and *can be abused.*

Arguments in favor of their prophylactic use include the following:

- *EPS are often distressing,* particularly when they occur outside the hospital, and on rare occasions can be life-threatening (e.g., oculogyric crisis or opisthotonos when alone or while driving, laryngeal dystonia).
- Diagnosis can be difficult because *EPS may be subtle and easily confused with psychotic symptoms.*
- More *serious complications are uncommon* with the addition of antiparkinsonian drugs.

Studies in which antiparkinsonian medications were discontinued have significant methodological problems. One specific issue is that patients placed on prophylactic therapy, who then fail to develop symptoms when their antiparkinsonian medication is withdrawn, may never have developed EPS at all. Still, up to 70% of patients have been noted to exhibit EPS after discontinuation of their antiparkinsonian drug, indicating that these agents indeed provide long-term efficacy.

The appropriate study design to address their prophylactic efficacy is the random assignment of patients to active drug or placebo. The Spring Grove study, using this design, found that 27% of patients on perphenazine without an antiparkinsonian drug developed an EPS event, in contrast to only 10% of those on an antiparkinsonian drug (451). Further, those on the perphenazine-benztropine combination had therapeutic improvement comparable with those on perphenazine-placebo.

Comaty et al. (452) conducted a prospective double-blind, placebo-controlled trial of low-dose benztropine (i.e., 2 mg/day) maintenance therapy. After an acute EPS had been stabilized with 2 days of active antiparkinsonian medication, the recurrence of EPS did not differ significantly between those maintained on active drug or those switched to placebo over the next 8 days. While there was a trend favoring the active drug group, low-dose maintenance benztropine (i.e., 2 mg/day) afforded little benefit in comparison with placebo.

A classic study by Chien et al. (453) randomly assigned chronic schizophrenics to three groups: fluphenazine enanthate plus daily antiparkinsonian drugs; antiparkinsonian drugs for 5 days after each fluphenazine injection; or no prophylactic antiparkinsonian drug. In all groups, EPS were treated when they occurred. Neither the daily-antiparkinsonian-drug group nor the 5-days-after-fluphenazine-injection group showed complete abolition of EPS, with 8% to 20% experiencing symptoms. Nevertheless, the rates were substantially less than the 54% EPS incidence in those on no prophylactic drugs.

There is also evidence of the prophylactic effect of antiparkinsonian drugs from a chart review study showing that they substantially prevented EPS (454).

Patients who have been on antiparkinsonian drugs for longer than 3 months and have no signs of EPS should have them slowly tapered and, if possible, stopped. Those who redevelop symptoms should have their antiparkinsonian drug therapy resumed, with periodic attempts to reduce the dosage. Again, an alternate strategy is to switch to an antipsychotic with lesser EPS potential. Clozapine, quetiapine, ziprasidone, olanzapine, and lower doses of risperidone produce the fewest EPS; haloperidol, thiothixene, perphenazine, trifluoperazine, and fluphenazine produce the most; with thioridazine, chlorpromazine, chlorprothixene, and acetophenazine occupying an intermediate position.

Finally, there has been considerable interest in the use of vitamin E to combat EPS, including TD, based on the oxidative-stress hypothesis. A randomized trial of 12 patients receiving supplementary vitamin E and haloperidol versus 12 receiving haloperidol alone revealed that vitamin E had no prophylactic effect on acute drug-induced

EPS, nor did it interfere with the antipsychotic's therapeutic efficacy (455).

Late-Onset (Tardive) Extrapyramidal Side Effects

TD presents with abnormal involuntary movements, usually associated with chronic (i.e., longer than 2 years) antipsychotic therapy (456). Although there is some debate whether the antipsychotics are either necessary or sufficient to produce this syndrome in psychiatric patients, the consensus is that they at least play an important role. TD is characterized by the following:

- Buccolinguomasticatory movements
  - Sucking, smacking of *lips*
  - Choreoathetoid movements of the *tongue*
  - Lateral *jaw* movements
- Choreiform or athetoid movements of the *extremities* and/or *truncal areas*
- Any *combination* of these symptoms

TD varies in presentation, and should always be considered in the differential diagnosis of any abnormal involuntary movements in patients exposed to antipsychotics or DA-receptor blocking agents used for other medical conditions (e.g., prochlorperazine or metoclopramide).

Whereas TD usually occurs after several years of drug therapy, some patients can develop symptoms within less than 1 year of cumulative drug exposure. In Kane's (457) study of younger adult patients (mean age 29 years), the incidence of TD was about 4% per year of cumulative drug exposure for at least the first 5 years. The incidence is higher in older persons treated for similar lengths of time and lower in younger age groups. Longitudinal studies find that the incidence of TD may decrease and the prevalence remain constant at steady-state drug levels. Thus, the number of new cases is balanced by those who spontaneously remit. Frequently, TD first becomes evident with dose reduction or withdrawal, but also can appear on stable doses. Symptoms disappear during sleep, while varying in intensity during the waking hours. Movements may be more pronounced in stressful or emotional situations, but can also be apparent in relaxed states.

Although many cases are relatively mild and nonprogressive, a small percentage are so severe that they result in significant disability. Because reliable predictors to identify patients who will develop the more severe forms have not been established, antipsychotic therapy should always be cautiously used in every patient. Recent data suggest that TD may improve in some patients despite continued drug treatment, particularly if the doses are lowered; and that atypical agents (e.g., clozapine, risperidone) may have antidyskinetic effects in some patients. Clearly, a comprehensive assessment of the relative, long-term risks and benefits must be an integral part of the treatment plan for any patient on maintenance therapy.

Other Tardive Syndromes

Late-onset or tardive dystonia, akathisia, and possibly other types of EPS have also been described as separate disorders from classic TD. Tardive dystonia is characterized by the late appearance of dystonias that persist even though neuroleptics are discontinued. It is rare, with a prevalence of about 1.5%. It is probably a separate diagnostic entity inasmuch as anticholinergics benefit tardive dystonia, whereas these drugs can worsen TD. The onset of tardive dystonia occurs after a shorter total drug exposure time than generally seen with TD.

Associated Risk Factors

Several variables appear to increase the chance of developing TD, with advancing age being the single most important risk factor in terms of incidence, severity, and persistence. Older females appear to be at greater risk, as do older patients with mood disorders. This last category (i.e., mood disorders) emphasizes the importance of an accurate diagnosis and consideration of alternate treatments when the diagnosis is unclear (e.g., mood stabilizer rather than an antipsychotic). The incidence and type of acute EPS may also predict the future development of TD (458, 459).

Treatment Issues

For vulnerable patients, dose and duration of drug treatment are important variables, underscoring the preventative benefit of using the minimal effective dose for long-term treatment. Antiparkinsonian medications may aggravate TD, while reserpine-like drugs and those that raise brain acetylcholine levels (e.g., physostigmine, choline, lecithin) may help. Caution is required in interpreting the results of such treatments, however, because many patients recover spontaneously when the offending drug is discontinued. TD is infrequent in those not exposed to long-term, high-dose therapy. Further, spontaneous development of TD has been reported and can be as high as 50% in some patient populations (460). Dyskinesias in schizophrenic patients, for example, were also described by Kraepelin almost a century before the discovery of neuroleptics.

In summary, treatments for tardive dyskinesia include cessation of the neuroleptic; switching to a novel agent; cholinergic agents; and dopamine depleting drugs, such as reserpine or tetrabenazine.

Acute Extrapyramidal Side Effects, Tardive Dyskinesia, and the Atypical Antipsychotics

Clozapine

It is thought that neuroleptic-induced DA-receptor blockade produces a denervation supersensitivity, ultimately increasing the number of receptor sites. As noted earlier, clozapine does not typically induce EPS. For example, we are not aware of any documented, unequivocal reports of clozapine-induced dystonia or parkinsonian rigidity or tremor. In blind studies, a small number of patients are rated as having a mild degree of parkinsonian symptoms (i.e., hypokinesis, rigidity, tremor, akathisia), but this incidence is comparable with that seen with placebo and should be considered "background noise." Because it is difficult to distinguish akathisia from psychotic agitation, or social withdrawal and apathy from hypokinesis, these symptoms may actually have been misidentified as EPS. If clozapine produces EPS, then unequivocal reactions such as dystonia should occur. It is remotely possible, however, that clozapine produces very mild EPS, at a much lower rate than observed with neuroleptics. A placebo-clozapine comparison with blind ratings would be required to clarify this question, but to date, there have been no such large-scale studies with sufficient statistical power.

A number of patients have been exposed to clozapine for several years and TD has not developed. Studies have also investigated patients with TD who were switched to clozapine for periods of 3 weeks to 6 months (461–464). Some appeared to improve, but these findings are difficult to interpret because control groups would be needed to demonstrate conclusively that clozapine does not cause TD. **Theoretically, if clozapine does not cause acute EPS, then it should not cause TD.** Other novel agents such as risperidone, olanzapine, quetiapine, and ziprasidone await longer term exposure to assess their propensity to induce TD. Thus, we agree with Casey, who wrote: "it is possible that compounds associated with a low rate of EPS may also produce less TD, but prospective studies are needed to confirm this premise" (465).

In this light, an important indication for clozapine may be for patients who develop severe EPS or TD on another antipsychotic. Not only is clozapine unlikely to produce TD, as noted earlier, a body of clinical evidence indicates that it may benefit TD.

Although clozapine has been reported to ameliorate TD and dystonia (including coexisting tardive dystonia), as well as other movement disorders, all antipsychotics that have purported antidyskinetic properties have also been associated with the occurrence of TD (461, 466–468). Hence, clinicians should monitor all patients treated with a novel antipsychotic for the emergence of signs and symptoms of TD. Although this adverse effect (and other neuroleptic-evoked EPS) can be suppressed with higher doses of clozapine given over extended periods of time, the antipsychotic effect with this drug can be achieved in many patients below the TD-suppressing threshold. Although there is no established causative relationship between clozapine and TD, in theory it may occur (469).

Neuroleptics may also cause blepharospasm, which is a forcible closure of the eyelids and when severe can interfere with activities such as driving; this condition can also be socially disabling and disfiguring. In addition, there are a few cases indistinguishable from idiopathic Meighs syndrome, which presents with blepharospasm and oromandibular dystonia (470). Of interest, clozapine has been reported to be beneficial for these symptoms.

Risperidone

Fixed-dose studies initially established that 6–8 mg/day of risperidone produced fewer EPS, that lower doses may not be as effective, and that higher doses (>10 mg/day) may cause more EPS, approaching that seen with neuroleptics (74, 471). One review, however, found that doses below 10 mg/day did not produce more EPS than placebo (472). Furthermore, doses in excess of 16 mg/day offer no more therapeutic gains, but are associated with a significantly greater incidence of acute EPS (75). Hence, some argue that risperidone should be considered an atypical antipsychotic only at lower doses. These clinical findings prompted Casey to observe: "Although the clinical data with risperidone indicate a relatively narrow range for exploiting the antipsychotic-EPS ratio, this drug offers an advantage with respect to many of the conventional antipsychotics that have an even more narrow therapeutic:side effect index" (465). In this context, subsequent clinical experience has found that mean doses of 1–4.5 mg/day of risperidone are often effective and further decrease the potential for EPS.

Further data supporting the long-term safety of risperidone (mean doses of 7.6 to 9.4 mg/day) were reported by Brecher (471). He assessed seven 1-year studies, which included more than 1,100 patients, and compared outcomes with the short-term safety established in 8-week trials. Adverse events were similar to those listed in the package insert, reflecting the findings from the short-term double-blind studies. The emergence of EPS was also similar to that reported in the double-blind, short-term studies, with only two (<0.2%) cases of TD reported. No significant changes were observed with respect to ECG, routine chemistry and hematological tests, and vital signs. Long-term treatment was associated with mild weight gain (1.8 to 3.3 kg).

Olanzapine

Preclinical and clinical data indicate that olanzapine may have antipsychotic effects at doses below its EPS threshold. Although early clinical results substantiated a lesser propensity to cause EPS at the low end of the dose-response curve, with dose escalation there was a concomitant increase in the use of antiparkinsonian medication (473). In this context, it should be noted that studies that used higher olanzapine doses found them to be more effective than low to intermediate doses (117). Thus, olanzapine may be similar to risperidone in that both drugs have a therapeutic dose range in which the antipsychotic effect can be achieved without inducing significant EPS.

In the international, multicenter, double-blind trial of olanzapine, the Simpson-Angus Scale and the Barnes Akathisia Scale were used to monitor treatment-emergent EPS. The acute phase was followed by a 52-week, double-blind, maintenance phase, during which there were significantly lower rates of treatment-emergent Parkinsonism and akathisia ($p > 0.001$), as well as TD ($p < 0.003$) in comparison with haloperidol (117). These results suggest that olanzapine has a substantially lower propensity than neuroleptics to evoke EPS, and perhaps TD.

The integration of data from the multicenter trial cited above revealed that 894 olanzapine-treated patients had received up to 20 mg/day for a median of 237 days and 261 haloperidol-treated patients received up to 20 mg/day for a *median* of 203 days (474). Both groups were chronically-ill (mean >10 years) and there were no between-group differences for age on admission, age of first episode, or previous therapy. The Schooler and Kane criteria for TD and the Abnormal Involuntary Movement Scale (AIMS) were used to define long-term, treatment-emergent dyskinetic symptoms (LTTEDS) (475). Among olanzapine-treated patients, the incidence of LTTEDS at any postbaseline visit, at endpoint, or at the final two AIMS assessments was significantly less compared with the haloperidol-treated patients at all three time points ($p < 0.001$, $p < 0.001$, $p = 0.003$, respectively). The incidence of LTTEDS in a subset of patients (olanzapine = 707; haloperidol = 197) without a history of dyski-

nesia or TD at baseline and treated with olanzapine was also significantly lower at all three time points compared with the haloperidol-treated patients ($p < 0.001$, $p = 0.001$, $p = 0.003$, respectively). These findings support the unique EPS profile of olanzapine and its contribution to a decreased incidence of LTTEDS. Although they also support olanzapine's antidyskinetic properties, we note that it is difficult to prove that any new agent does not cause TD because it may take years of well-documented exposure to establish a causative linkage.

In this context, Lilly (474) reported a meta-analysis of three controlled studies of patients with TD who were treated with olanzapine. These authors found an 11-fold decrease in TD on olanzapine versus haloperidol based on the AIMS scale. There were a few patients who developed TD in the first 6 weeks of olanzapine, but this could have been from previous drug exposure, now not suppressed by the neuroleptic. Interestingly, there were no new cases (0/375) of TD developing in patients on long-term olanzapine treatment, whereas there were three of 83 cases on haloperidol. It is very difficult to arrive at definitive evidence about TD because most patients have received previous neuroleptic therapy and because TD-like symptoms occur spontaneously, providing an alternative explanation. It is clear that it is difficult to prove that olanzapine causes TD but equally difficult to prove that it does not. The 11-fold decreased incidence, however, is strong evidence that at least it produces much less TD.

Quetiapine

Clinical trials indicate that quetiapine has a low propensity to evoke EPS (128, 476). Treatment with quetiapine did not induce EPS in the dose range studied, as determined by the following:

- Analysis of *Simpson-Angus Scale* total scores
- Lack of treatment-emergent *acute dystonic reactions*
- Limited use of *anticholinergic medications*
- Limited incidence of *motor system adverse events*

Because very few patients had abnormal involuntary movements at baseline, the ability of

ACUTE EPS WITH ANTIPSYCHOTICS

Maximum			Minimum
◄ ··· ►			
HALOPERIDOL	RISPERIDONE	OLANZAPINE	CLOZAPINE
	(DOSE RELATED)		ZIPRASIDONE
			QUETIAPINE

FIG. 5-14. Relative risk of extrapyramidal side effects (EPS) among the available novel agents and haloperidol.

quetiapine to ameliorate such movements was inconclusive.

Ziprasidone

Preclinical studies of ziprasidone indicate that it also has a low propensity to induce EPS, which was confirmed in subsequent phase II and III studies. Furthermore, the motor symptoms evoked by ziprasidone were seldom sufficiently troublesome to warrant anticholinergic medication. In one phase III trial, not more than 25% of patients receiving 160 mg/day were prescribed an anticholinergic at any time during the 6-week treatment period. **These results indicate that therapeutic doses of ziprasidone not only induce a low incidence of acute EPS, but when they occur, they are often mild and do not require antiparkinsonian medication** (137).

Summary

Figure 5-14 depicts the relative risk of extrapyramidal side effects (EPS) among the available novel agents and haloperidol.

Other Central Nervous System Side Effects

Seizures

Most antipsychotics lower the seizure threshold in animals, but this complication rarely occurs in humans, even on high doses of these compounds. They are usually not contraindicated in those with seizure disorders, but should be used cautiously. In the absence of controlled data, it is our clinical opinion that epileptic patients who also require these agents generally show improvement in both their psychosis and seizure disorder. When seizures do occur, it is generally on higher doses and they consist of a single, isolated episode. A slightly lower dose or the addi-

tion of an anticonvulsant can bring about control of both disorders. An investigation into other possible medical conditions as the cause of a seizure episode should also be conducted.

Clozapine. Clozapine produces seizures at a greater rate than other antipsychotics, especially in the dose range of 600 to 900 mg/day. Fortunately, these levels are substantially above the usual therapeutic range of 300 to 400 mg/day, but seizures can occur on lower doses, as well. A more rapid escalation of the clozapine dose may also predispose to the development of seizures. According to the drug's manufacturer, the reported incidence of seizures, based on daily dosage, is as follows:

- 1% to 2% on less than 300 mg
- 3% to 4% on 300 to 599 mg
- 5% on 600 to 900 mg

Withdrawal Syndrome

The antipsychotics do not produce a classic withdrawal syndrome of the type seen with barbiturates or opioids; nor do they produce psychological dependency, as seen with psychostimulants (e.g., cocaine, amphetamine). Addicts and patients both dislike these drugs and do not spontaneously increase their dose. Indeed, they are more likely to discontinue them without medical advice.

Abrupt discontinuation, however, may be associated with certain symptoms, usually within 2 to 7 days, including:

- *Nausea* and *vomiting*
- Increased *sweating*
- Sensations of *heat* or *cold*
- *Insomnia*
- *Irritability*
- *Headache*

Patients abruptly withdrawn from an antipsychotic-antiparkinsonian drug combination generally experience one or two of these symptoms, usually to a mild degree, and rarely develop all of them. One study that randomly assigned patients to abrupt discontinuation of both drugs, or to abrupt discontinuation of the antipsychotic only, found that symptoms occurred almost entirely in the group withdrawn from both drugs. When the antipsychotic alone was discontinued, no withdrawal symptoms were experienced, presumably due to the continuation of the antiparkinsonian drugs. Patients who had their antiparkinsonian drugs abruptly discontinued 4 weeks later also experienced withdrawal symptoms, again suggesting that this syndrome results from the antiparkinsonian drug withdrawal. Because withdrawal phenomena have also been reported in patients on antipsychotics alone, we cannot exclude the possibility that their discontinuation (possibly because of their anticholinergic properties) can also produce these symptoms. We note that parkinsonian patients who discontinue their anticholinergic, antiparkinsonian drugs, experience a marked rebound in their symptoms. Although this syndrome is mild, we recommend tapering both drugs gradually, perhaps at a slightly slower rate for the antiparkinsonian agent.

Clozapine. Withdrawal symptoms after the abrupt discontinuation of clozapine differ from those noted with other antipsychotics (98, 477). Thus, rapid discontinuation may result in the following:

- A marked *exacerbation of the psychosis*
- A worsening of preexisting *TD* (primarily lingual movements)
- A number of *somatic symptoms*
- A more *rapid onset* than with neuroleptic discontinuation

For example, withdrawal of haloperidol in one patient revealed little change in either mental status or involuntary movements 3 weeks after discontinuation (478). In contrast, there was a marked deterioration in mental status and involuntary movements in this same patient 1 week after clozapine withdrawal. This "rebound psychosis" was attributed to increased dopamine re-

lease, a mechanism suggested by earlier observations made after withdrawal studies in humans and animals. For example, a study of the effects of abrupt withdrawal in rats showed increased and decreased striatal basal dopamine release with discontinuation of clozapine and haloperidol, respectively (479). The exacerbation of dyskinesia after clozapine withdrawal suggests that human nigrostriatal dopamine receptors (putatively involved in the emergence of dyskinetic movements) may be altered pharmacologically by this drug.

Clozapine withdrawal symptoms occur after stopping therapeutic doses (range 200 to 900 mg/day) administered from 4 months to several years. In a study, one-third of patients who were switched directly from clozapine to risperidone remained stable, one-third had to be switched back to clozapine, and one-third were treated with combined risperidone-clozapine or risperidone-neuroleptic (480).

Reports of cholinergic rebound with clozapine discontinuation also exist (481). For example, a single-blind crossover study compared the side effect profiles of clozapine and risperidone in 20 patients who were initially stabilized on clozapine (dose not stated) (482). Ten patients received risperidone first, and 10 continued clozapine for 6 weeks. Even though clozapine was tapered over a week before risperidone was started, 13 patients still complained of one or more of the following symptoms: malaise, nausea, vomiting, diarrhea, anorexia, depressed mood, agitation, and insomnia. These symptoms were not consistently ameliorated by the addition of risperidone alone, but usually remitted gradually over time. **Because there is strong evidence that abrupt cessation of more than 300 mg clozapine daily can cause intense withdrawal symptoms (in part caused by a "cholinergic rebound"), the use of anticholinergic medications should be considered.**

Another study considered the effects of discontinuing clozapine abruptly; during slow taper over 3 weeks; with cross-tapering; or without the addition of a neuroleptic (483). In eight of nine neuroleptic-responsive patients who had received clozapine for 2 years, relapse occurred despite dosage tapering. Relapse also occurred in six of eight patients despite cross-tapering with perphenazine, as well as in one of two patients who stopped clozapine abruptly and were immediately started on risperidone. Other major findings included the following:

- Some relapsed patients' *response to retreatment with neuroleptics* was decreased.
- *Antiserotonergic drugs* (e.g., risperidone and cyproheptadine) were of some value in treating the withdrawal psychosis and other somatic withdrawal symptoms.
- *Rapidity* and *severity of relapse* were significantly greater than that due to the withdrawal of neuroleptics in the same subjects 2 years previously.
- Relapse was significantly *more common in neuroleptic-responsive patients* than in neuroleptic-resistant patients.
- In all cases, response to *restarting clozapine* was rapid and robust.
- *Vulnerability to relapse* after clozapine discontinuation increased with the length of clozapine treatment.

Patients who relapsed after clozapine discontinuation exhibited a full range of psychotic symptoms, including paranoid delusions, auditory hallucinations, and disorganized thinking. A brief prodromal period of nonpsychotic symptoms (feeling strange, insomnia, difficulty concentrating, and agitation) preceded the emergence of positive symptoms in most patients. In addition, EPS occurred in seven of 19 patients, five of whom developed symptoms when perphenazine was added to clozapine, indicating that the latter agent was unable to block these neuroleptic-induced effects. EPS was also more severe than that experienced during prior treatment with neuroleptics. Withdrawal dyskinesia did not occur in any of these cases.

The accumulating data from reports on clozapine withdrawal support these important facts:

- Clozapine should be discontinued by *slow taper.*
- If *abrupt clozapine withdrawal* is necessary, clinicians should be prepared to treat a rapid and possibly severe psychotic relapse.
- Withdrawal *"rebound psychosis"* should not be attributed to an antipsychotic prescribed during or immediately after clozapine withdrawal.
- Patients stabilized on clozapine may be *switched safely* and *effectively* to another antipsychotic by gradually tapering clozapine for several weeks and/or adding another antipsychotic during tapering.

Thus, ample support exists for the recommendation of an NIMH panel that schizophrenic patients who have responded well to clozapine should not be taken off without a valid reason (102). **Based on the existing data, the best method for stopping clozapine is by a slow taper with prior addition of an alternate antipsychotic.**

Risperidone. Based on their review of the available data on the efficacy and safety of risperidone, Umbricht and Kane (472) concluded that the adverse effects most commonly associated with risperidone treatment discontinuation in the United States and Canadian studies were dizziness (1.5%), nausea (1.2%), and agitation (1.0%).

A hypertensive crisis in a 29-year-old man after abrupt discontinuation of risperidone is the only report to date of any serious withdrawal reaction that we are aware of (484). Although the episode was attributed to risperidone's a_1-blocking effect, this is debatable because the hypertension was first detected within hours of discontinuation, the patient had been given multiple drugs, and he used cannabis in the hospital.

Sedation

Sedation is a common adverse behavioral change that usually occurs during the first few days after starting an antipsychotic, with some patients rapidly developing tolerance. While patients should be warned about driving or operating machinery, the drowsiness is generally not troublesome. In general, sedative side effects are inversely proportional to the milligram potency of these drugs. Thus, clozapine, chlorpromazine, and thioridazine usually produce more sedation than risperidone, fluphenazine, haloperidol, thiothixene, or trifluoperazine. When necessary, it can be controlled by reducing the dose, switching to a less-sedating agent, or giving the entire dose at bedtime. These agents typically produce sedation in normal subjects, but paradoxically enhance the mental functioning of patients due to the reduction in their psychosis.

Cognitive Effects

It is difficult to evaluate cognitive changes in psychotic patients because deficits caused by the disorder must be separated from drug-induced impairment. Symptoms such as insomnia, bizarre dreams, impaired psychomotor activity, aggravation of psychosis, confusional states, and somnambulism can be seen on or off drug treatment. An apparent worsening of psychosis, which is thought to be an ideational analogue or variant of akathisia, may also occur. Some confusional states, particularly in the elderly, are due to the anticholinergic properties of these drugs, which are often compounded when anticholinergics are given to manage EPS, at times resulting in a central anticholinergic syndrome.

Temperature Dysregulation

The *neuroleptic malignant syndrome* (NMS) is an acute disorder of thermoregulation and neuromotor control carrying a mortality rate of about 21% when untreated. **The term neuroleptic malignant syndrome is probably a misnomer, and a better name might be the "hypodopaminergic, hyperpyrexia syndrome."**

The most frequent symptoms of NMS include:

- *Fever,* often greater than 40°C or 104°F
- Severe *muscle rigidity,* typically "lead pipe" or "plastic"
- *Altered consciousness*, usually with clouding of the sensorium, at times progressing to stupor or coma
- *Autonomic changes* characterized by symptoms such as fluctuating blood pressure, tachypnea, diaphoresis

NMS can occur with a wide variety of agents, including atypical antipsychotics such as tiapride, sulpiride, and clozapine. Although a few reports of NMS have been associated with risperidone therapy, there is also a report of one patient with a history of NMS while on neuroleptics who tolerated and responded well to risperidone (86, 485, 486). In addition, NMS occurs with DA-blocking agents used for other purposes, such as phenothiazine antiemetics (e.g., prochlorperazine), antipsychotics as adjuncts to anesthesia (e.g., droperidol), or amoxapine, an antidepressant with a neuroleptic-like metabolite. DA-depleting agents (e.g., reserpine) and combined antagonist-depleting agents (e.g., tetrabenazine) also may cause NMS. It can also occur when antiparkinsonian agents (e.g., amantadine) are decreased or discontinued. This suggests that NMS is caused by a decrease in dopaminergic tone, and supports the therapeutic benefit of dopaminergic agonists. Paradoxically, NMS has also been reported with amphetamine or cocaine use.

Keck et al. (487) reported an incidence of NMS ranging from 0.02% to 2.4% in a large number of neuroleptic-treated patients and found there was a 0.67% pooled mean estimate. Such studies probably overestimate the incidence, because cohorts without NMS are usually not reported. Large-scale epidemiological studies are required to obtain a more precise figure. Further, a significant proportion (i.e., 40%) of these patients were diagnosed as having mood disorders. The ratio of male to female patients who developed NMS was 3:2, and the mean reported age was about 40 years old.

Other possible risk factors include the following:

- Presence of an *organic mental disorder*
- *Agitation*
- *Dehydration*
- The rate, route, and dose of neuroleptic *administration*
- The use of *concurrent psychotropics* (e.g., lithium)

Although 80% of NMS cases occur within the first 2 weeks of initiation or an increase in the dose, it must be emphasized that NMS can occur at any time. Typically, the syndrome progresses rapidly, fully developing in 24 to 48 hours, and lasts for an average of 7 to 14 days, but up to 30 days is not unusual. The duration is usually twice as long when depot agents are involved.

Patients with NMS almost always have elevated creatine phosphokinase (CPK) levels.

Increases are usually in the 2,000 to 15,000 v/L range and rarely above 100,000 v/L. The absence of an elevation in CPK speaks against the diagnosis of NMS; however, it is nonspecific and can also be markedly increased with agitation, many forms of strenuous physical exercise, dystonic reactions, or intramuscular injections (i.e., CPK is a high-sensitivity, low-specificity test). Often agitated psychotic patients are given intramuscular injections, further increasing CPK levels. Serum glutamic-oxaloacetic transaminase (SGOT), serum glutamic-pyruvic transaminase (SGPT), and lactate dehydrogenase (LDH) are usually elevated, indicating liver involvement. White cell elevations range from 15,000 to 30,000/L, with a shift to the left occurring in about 40% of cases. The EEG is usually normal but may show diffuse slowing or other nonspecific abnormalities.

Neuroleptic Malignant Syndrome with Atypical Antipsychotics

As noted earlier, evidence indicates that atypical antipsychotics may also produce NMS (488). Several patients have developed NMS after treatment with clozapine, risperidone, or olanzapine. A few of these cases are classic NMS, with symptoms such as markedly elevated temperature and CPK levels. For each drug, approximately a dozen reported cases fulfill a reasonably stringent criteria for NMS, whereas the rest can be considered borderline. The number of NMS cases, however, appears low relative to use. In addition, some of the patients on clozapine who developed NMS were also receiving neuroleptics. There are cases of patients who had NMS on clozapine alone, however, and when rechallenged with clozapine experienced another NMS episode. Similarly, rechallenge with olanzapine- or risperidone-induced NMS has resulted in either questionable or definite reemergence of NMS.

Differential Diagnosis

In *malignant hyperthermia* (MH), muscle rigidity and fever develop rapidly, following exposure to inhalation anesthetic agents or succinylcholine. The gene for this disorder was recently described. Other differential diagnostic considerations include:

- Lethal *catatonia*
- *Heat stroke*
- Viral *encephalitis*
- *Tetanus*
- Other *infections*

Treatment

The most important step to effective treatment of NMS is early recognition and prompt withdrawal of the offending agent. In addition, supportive measures should be instituted as quickly as possible. If the patient is receiving an antiparkinsonian agent, it probably should be continued; however, data are lacking to support their usefulness, and care must be taken to avoid an anticholinergically induced worsening of mental status and perhaps further temperature increase. If there is reasonable certainty that the syndrome is NMS, the patient should be transferred to a medical setting in which intensive observation and treatment can be provided.

A variety of supportive measures can be used, including cooling blankets, ice packs, or an ice-water enema. The goal should be to return the temperature as close to normal as possible. One should also be ready to treat complications and give supplemental oxygen with or without mechanical ventilation (the amount of oxygen and the method of delivery will depend on the patient's needs).

Drug Treatment. Because of the nature of the disorder, there are no controlled studies; however, most investigators suggest a trial with one or more of these agents:

- Dantrolene
- Bromocriptine
- Amantadine
- Benzodiazepines
- Some combination of these agents

The initial dose of *dantrolene* should be 2 to 3 mg/kg over 10 to 15 minutes. The total dosage should not exceed 10 mg/kg/day because of the increased risk of hepatotoxicity. The dosage range reported as effective is 0.8 to 10 mg/kg/day. The typical oral dosage of *bromocriptine* is 2.5

to 10 mg three times daily; with increases up to 60 mg/day. Some have used bromocriptine in conjunction with dantrolene, with similar dosage patterns. The oral dose of *amantadine* is 200 to 400 mg/day in divided doses. *Levodopa plus carbidopa* is infrequently used, and efficacy is not well documented. Dosage of carbidopa is 25 mg plus levodopa 100 mg (three to eight times daily). The *calcium channel blocker* nifedipine has also been used to treat NMS, and further data on this drug are important, given its beneficial effect in a single case report (489). Benzodiazepines have not been well studied, but some clinical evidence indicates that when given in adequate doses (often parenterally) they may also benefit NMS.

We found that the specific drug treatment with dantrolene and/or dopaminergic agonists significantly reduced the mortality rate from NMS (i.e., 10% versus 21%), and did so uniformly in mild, moderate, and severe cases (490). To test the significance of this finding, we performed case-controlled analyses using as a control the mortality rate of NMS patients who had not received any specific treatment. Thus, by definition, the control group consisted of patients who had not received bromocriptine, amantadine, other DA agonists, dantrolene, any form of dopa or ECT.

Electroconvulsive Therapy. ECT is an effective treatment for more severe mania, depression, catatonia, schizophrenic excitement, and schizoaffective disorder. However, its use for the treatment of NMS is controversial because some patients have died or developed cardiac arrest during ECT, whereas others benefited when it was given during or shortly after an episode had resolved (491). Davis et al. (492) reviewed the world literature and found a mortality rate of 11% when ECT was used during an episode of NMS. This compares with a 10% rate in patients treated with specific drug therapy (e.g., dantrolene, DA agonists) and a 21% rate in patients who received only nonspecific treatment for their episode. Further, in the three deaths with ECT, high potency antipsychotics were continued before, during, and after ECT. Thus, the failure of the NMS to improve may have been due to the continued administration of the offending drug. There were also other cases when antipsychotics were continued with ECT throughout the episode

of NMS and the outcomes were not favorable, though the patients survived. **Again, these drugs should be discontinued whenever the possibility of NMS is suspected.** Although there are insufficient case report data to prove ECT helps NMS, this therapy clearly does not worsen the condition. Because some acutely psychotic patients require immediate intervention, ECT may be lifesaving, whereas premature reintroduction of an antipsychotic may worsen an NMS episode.

Retreatment After an Episode of Neuroleptic Malignant Syndrome. Retreatment strategies after an episode of NMS include the following:

- *ECT* for psychotic depression or other emergencies (493).
- *Lithium* or *alternate treatments,* such as valproate or carbamazepine, for bipolar, manic; schizoaffective; and schizophreniform disorders (alternate nonneuroleptic interventions may be better in light of reports that affectively disordered patients with psychotic features may be more susceptible to TD and NMS).
- In psychotic manic episodes, *lower doses of antipsychotic* in combination with lithium may be as effective as higher doses and perhaps diminish the possibility of an NMS recurrence (155).

If an antipsychotic is necessary, treatment should be instituted as long as possible after an episode (i.e., at least 2 weeks). Because as many as 50% of patients reexposed to an antipsychotic again develop the syndrome, an antipsychotic from a different family, and preferably a lower potency agent should be administered. Alternatively, the patient could be switched to a novel agent (e.g., clozapine, risperidone, olanzapine, quetiapine, ziprasidone) that may be less likely to induce NMS.

Further, it is best to *start with a very low dose and titrate up slowly* in a hospital setting to carefully monitor clinical response, temperature, and neurological and mental status. Using low doses will not necessarily jeopardize chances for an adequate clinical response. We found, for example, evidence for a therapeutic effect with low-dose trifluoperazine (285). This finding is consistent with the growing recognition that "less may indeed be more" when it comes to the dose of an antipsychotic.

Although *clozapine* has been considered an alternate agent, as mentioned earlier there is also a risk with this agent (494–496). An unusual adverse effect of clozapine, apparently unrelated to NMS, is *hyperthermia* in 10% to 15% of patients (usually 0.5°C to 1°C, but virtually never above 40°C [104°F]). This symptom usually occurs between the fifth and the fifteenth days of treatment, after which, temperature returns to normal. *Benzodiazepines* (e.g., lorazepam) have also been recommended to either avoid or at least minimize the dose of antipsychotic.

We would also suggest *prophylactic concomitant bromocriptine* for several weeks, with gradual tapering after that time period. Such prophylactic approaches during the retreatment phase have been attempted in a few patients, but there are no controlled studies. Nevertheless, it seems like a sensible strategy and poses little additional risk.

Autonomic Adverse Effects

Anticholinergic Effects

Certain antipsychotics and antidepressants block central and peripheral muscarinic cholinergic receptors, producing many anticholinergic adverse effects, such as:

- Blurred vision
- Dry mouth
- Constipation
- Urinary retention (497)

Patients may develop some tolerance to these effects, which tend to be most troublesome during the early stages of treatment. Dry mouth is one of the most frequent complaints, and patients should be advised to *rinse* their mouths frequently and to use *sugarless* gum or candy. The latter is because sugar products provide a good cultural medium for fungal infections, such as moniliasis, and may also increase the incidence of dental cavities. Further, dry mouth, in general, can predispose to infections, because saliva is bacteriostatic. *Urecholine* can alleviate urinary retention.

Hypersalivation

Approximately one third of patients on clozapine experience *hypersalivation,* both during the day and particularly at night (e.g., patients often complain of waking up with a wet pillow). Its mechanism is not well understood. This is believed to be mediated by M_4 agonist properties (498). While generally mild-to-moderate in intensity, it can be more severe, even warranting discontinuation of the drug. The increased salivation *may disappear with time* or with a reduction in dose, but can also persist. *Pirenzepine,* an $M_{1,4}$ antagonist, is used in Europe and *intranasal ipratropium bromide* is an anticholinergic available in the United States. *Anticholinergics* (e.g., trihexylphenidine) or *amitriptyline* have also been used, but their effectiveness is unclear (499).

Cardiovascular Effects

Orthostatic Hypotension

Agents with a-adrenergic blocking effects (e.g., clozapine, CPZ, risperidone) produce a dose-related postural hypotension and related tachycardia, most pronounced with rapid escalation and moderate to higher doses (500). This can occur after the first dose, worsen on the second or third day, but then subside due to tolerance. It also tends to be more problematic in the elderly and those on higher doses of parenteral medication. It is prudent to monitor blood pressure (lying and standing) after the first dose and during the first few days of treatment. Management of this effect begins with a gradual increase in a drug like clozapine (e.g., 12.5 mg b.i.d. or t.i.d. for 2 days, then 25 mg t.i.d. for several days), with a slower escalation over the next week to 10 days until the minimal therapeutic level (e.g., 300 mg/day in divided doses) is achieved. Such a schedule produces significant hypotension in only 3% to 5% of patients on clozapine, although many will experience milder degrees of hypotension.

Risperidone may also cause hypotension via its a-adrenergic blocking actions (501). In the elderly, hypotensive side effects can occur, especially if there is any of the following:

- A history of *hypotension*
- Preexisting *cardiac disease*

- *ECG* abnormalities
- The current use of either a *calcium channel blocker* or an *angiotensin-converting enzyme* (ACE) inhibitor

In a report of 122 elderly patients on risperidone, hypotension was noted in 28.7% and symptomatic orthostatic hypotension was noted in 9.8%. Significant decreases in blood pressure occurred with risperidone treatment ($p = 0.0001$) and were common in patients with cardiovascular disease and those taking an SSRI or valproate ($p = 0.03$) (502). Hence, like other antipsychotics, risperidone should be prescribed cautiously for elderly patients and those with preexisting cardiac disease. Its hypotensive versus its orthostatic hypotensive effects may be an age-related pharmacodynamic response. Blood pressure, including orthostatic blood pressure, should be monitored routinely until the risperidone dosage is stabilized. Furthermore, when risperidone therapy is initiated in the elderly, dosage should be titrated from 0.25 to 0.5 mg two times a day with increments of 0.25 to 0.5 mg weekly (92).

The chief danger with this adverse effect is fainting or falling, although such occurrences are rare. This is an important complication because injuries related to such falls can produce significant morbidity.

Treatment

Patients should be instructed to:

- *Rise* from bed *gradually*
- *Sit* with *legs dangling* for a brief period
- *Wait* at least *1 minute* before standing
- Sit or lie down if feeling *faint*
- Use *support hose* if hypotension persists

Rarely is it necessary to keep a patient in bed for prolonged periods. Those with serious cardiovascular disease, should have their doses increased even more slowly, with blood pressure frequently monitored. Acute orthostasis can usually be managed by having the patient lie down with feet elevated. On rare occasions, volume expanders or vasopressors may be required.

Cardiac Rhythm Disturbances

Patients with known or suspected cardiac disease should have a pretreatment ECG. An abnormality consisting of broadened, flattened, or clove T waves, with increased Q-R intervals has been described with thioridazine at doses as low as 300 mg/day, but does not seem to be associated with any significant clinical consequences. The point prevalence of drug-induced changes was obtained from the ECGs of 101 normal reference subjects plus 495 psychiatric patients. Thioridazine had by far the highest prevalence of prolonged *QTc intervals,* which were prolonged by tricyclic antidepressants as well. No other psychotropic was found to produce prolonged QTc in this study (503). Recently, the FDA (504) has added a box warning to the PDR and the package insert stating that thioridazine (Mellaril) has been shown to prolong QTc interval in a dose-related manner and is now only indicated for treatment-resistant or treatment-intolerant patients. A similar FDA letter (505) and box warning have been issued for mesoridazine (Serentil), an active metabolite of thioridazine.

"Torsades des pointes" has also been described with thioridazine and is characterized by a peculiar type of ventricular tachycardia in which the amplitude of successive beats fluctuates in a sine wave pattern (502). Thioridazine is now contraindicated when combined with fluvoxamine, propranolol, pindolol, or drugs that inhibit cytochrome P450 (e.g., fluoxetine and paroxetine), as well as other drugs known to prolong the QTc interval. Thioridazine is contraindicated in patients with reduced P450 2D6 levels, who have congenitally long QT syndrome, or who have a history of cardiac arrhythmias. Before starting thioridazine, patients should have an ECG that demonstrates a QTc interval shorter than 450 ms. Once started, thioridazine should be discontinued if the QTc interval increases to 500 ms. A prolonged QT_c interval has also been reported with novel agents such as ziprasidone. The clinical relevance of this, however, has yet to be clarified. We recommend a baseline ECG with more careful monitoring, particularly in patients with preexisting cardiac conditions.

Clozapine also produces nonspecific inverted T waves, but again, this is not considered clinically relevant. As far as is known, abrupt discontinuation of antipsychotics, including clozapine, does not produce serious adverse cardiac effects, although common sense dictates a gradual reduction over several days (39).

Sudden death is a rare phenomenon with the antipsychotics. An accurate assessment as to whether these drugs are causally or coincidentally involved cannot be made, because sudden death can occur in young, apparently healthy persons on no medication. For example, every year in the United States, some 600,000 people die suddenly. Although the most commonly postulated cause of sudden death is ventricular fibrillation, it can also result from:

* *Asphyxia* caused by regurgitated food
* An endobronchial *mucous plug in asthmatics*
* *Shock* in patients with *acquired megacolon*
* As a complication of *seizures*
* Slowed *intracardiac conduction* (similar to that induced by Type II antiarrhythmics and tricyclic antidepressants)

In the past, sudden death was thought to be the result of myocardial infarction, but with more patients surviving such episodes, it appears that many had ventricular arrhythmias without evidence of cardiac muscle damage.

Statistically, the incidence of sudden death in mental patients has not increased since the introduction of antipsychotics, and no one type is more implicated, with deaths occurring on high- and low-potency agents. Medical examiners should refrain from attributing sudden death to these drugs, or to any other cause for that matter, until research clearly establishes a causal rather than coincidental link.

Dermatological and Ocular Effects

A variety of *dermatological effects*–including urticarial, maculopapular, petechial, and edematous eruptions–occurs infrequently and usually early (in the first few weeks) in treatment. A contact dermatitis can even occur in person-

nel who handle CPZ. Because sunlight plays a role, difference in incidence may relate to variations in sun exposure. Photosensitivity of the phototoxic type resembles severe sunburn (most often occuring with CPZ); therefore, patients on antipsychotics should be encouraged to avoid excessive sunlight and to use sunscreens (499).

Chlorpromazine: Specific Skin and Eye Effects

Both the dermatological and ocular changes are a reaction to high levels of sunlight and chronic CPZ use. Dermatological effects specific to CPZ include a blue-gray, metallic discoloration in areas exposed to sunlight (face, neck, and the dorsum of hands), beginning with a tan or golden brown color and progressing to slate gray, metallic blue, or purple. Histological studies of skin biopsies reveal pigmentary granules similar, but not identical, to melanin.

Eye changes have been noticed after chronic, high-dose CPZ and are described as whitish brown granular deposits concentrated in the anterior lens and posterior cornea, visible only by slit lamp examination (these are quite different from, and in no way related to, senile cataracts). Statistically, opacities occur more frequently with skin discoloration, but retinal damage does not occur and vision is virtually never impaired. The occurrence and severity of both effects are related to the duration and total lifetime dose of CPZ (e.g., usually greater than a total dose of 1 to 3 kg). In the past two decades, with the increased use of high-potency agents, these adverse effects have virtually disappeared, but it is not clear that they are totally absent, because this complication is only apparent under a slit lamp. Treatments consist of minimizing exposure to the sun and switching to a different class of antipsychotic.

Thioridazine: Specific Eye Effects

Thioridazine poses a potentially greater danger to the eyes than CPZ. At doses greater than 800 mg/day, a *retinitis pigmentosa* may appear,

WEIGHT GAIN WITH ANTIPSYCHOTICS

Maximum				Minimum
◄ ··· ►				
CLOZAPINE	OLANZAPINE	QUETIAPINE	RISPERIDONE	HALOPERIDOL
				ZIPRASIDONE

FIG. 5-15. Relative risk of weight gain with various novel agents and haloperidol.

leading to substantial visual impairment or even blindness. In some cases, the condition does not fully remit when the drug is stopped; therefore, thioridazine doses of more than 800 mg/day are never recommended to allow for a reasonable margin of safety (499).

Endocrine Effects

A large body of preclinical research exists on the neuroendocrine effects of antipsychotics in a variety of species. Clinical studies find that they induce small, inconsistent effects on sex, adrenocortical, thyroid, and pituitary hormone-related activity. Although much of this literature is not directly relevant to humans, two important effects are *increased lactation* and *possible sexual dysfunction*. These agents presumably induce their effects by blocking DA receptors in the pituitary, producing a marked increase in prolactin (particularly in females, but also in males). This increase causes breast engorgement and lactation in female patients. If every patient were checked for lactation by manual pressure on the breast, the incidence could be as high as 20% to 40%, but complaints of overt lactation are relatively rare (i.e., less than 5%). *Gynecomastia* in male patients is also described. There is no clear evidence that sustained elevated prolactin levels produce serious consequences, and treatment usually involves dose reduction or switching to another antipsychotic.

Delayed ejaculation has been reported with agents such as thioridazine, perhaps due to its greater autonomic effects. Clinicians must be sensitive to these issues because many patients are embarrassed to talk about them.

Cases of drug-induced *diabetes* have also been reported (e.g., clozapine, olanzapine).

Glucose-tolerance curves may also be shifted by at least some novel antipsychotics in a fashion consistent with diabetes, and recently, cases of *ketoacidosis* have been reported (507, 508).

Weight Gain

The marked weight gain sometimes associated with drug therapy has not been explained on any endocrine basis. Theories promulgated include:

- *Increased calorie* consumption
- *Decreased calorie* use
- *Receptor* dysregulation (e.g., 5-HT$_{2c}$, H$_1$)
- *Glucose* and *insulin* dysregulation

On average, *clozapine* causes the largest weight gain in both men and women. One study found rates of 6 kg for women and 10 kg for men, with a similar degree of increase in the body mass index (BMI). A recent meta-analysis reviewing random-assignment blind studies of antipsychotics shows that the weight gain with antipsychotics is quite substantial over placebo and varies among novel agents (506). Due to the health consequences of obesity, weight gain is a significant side effect. In addition, with our culture's emphasis on slimness, weight gain may be socially disabling. Figure 5-15 depicts the relative risk of weight gain with various novel agents and haloperidol.

When particularly problematic, one may consider switching to molindone or ziprasidone, both of which may not cause weight gain.

Gastrointestinal Effects

Hepatic

Shortly after the introduction of CPZ, *jaundice* was noted to occur in about one of every 200 patients. Subsequently, its incidence inexplicably decreased to one in 1,000, although accurate data are often lacking. Jaundice is most often seen about 1 to 5 weeks after the initiation of therapy and is usually preceded by a flu-like syndrome (malaise, abdominal pain, fever, nausea, vomiting, and diarrhea), resembling mild gastroenteritis or infectious hepatitis. Important clinical factors include the following:

- *Temporal association* between jaundice and the recent initiation of drug therapy
- Lack of an enlarged or tender *liver*
- Chemical evidence of *choleostasis,* such as an increase in direct, relative to indirect, bilirubin
- Increased *alkaline phosphatase*
- A reduction of *esterified cholesterol*
- Moderately increased *aminotransferases*
- Peripheral blood smears demonstrating *eosinophilia*
- Liver biopsies showing *bile plugs in the canaliculi,* with eosinophilic infiltration in the periportal space

This disorder usually disappears after several weeks, with a complete return to normal liver function expected. Rarely, a longer-lasting exanthematous biliary cirrhosis occurs, characterized by a more chronic course of 6 months to 1 year, but also eventually clears. This may be an allergic phenomenon, as evidenced by:

- *Onset* in the first few weeks of treatment
- Frequent association with *other allergic reactions*
- Association with peripheral *eosinophilia* and eosinophilic infiltrations in the liver
- *Prolonged retention of sensitivity* on the challenge test
- Development of a *second episode* as long as 10 years after the first

The majority of cases reported in the literature have occurred with CPZ and rarely with other agents such as promazine, thioridazine, mepazine, prochlorperazine, fluphenazine, and triflupromazine. There is no convincing evidence that haloperidol or other nonphenothiazine agents produce this type of jaundice. It is occasionally useful to obtain baseline liver function tests on patients with increased susceptibility (e.g., prior history of hepatitis) in the unlikely event that jaundice may develop. Routine serial liver function tests have never proven useful or necessary. The offending drug should be discontinued if a patient develops jaundice, but the value of this practice is also unproven, because many patients have been maintained on CPZ throughout an episode of jaundice without adverse consequences (509).

Hematological Effects

Leukopenia is a reduction in the white blood cell count (WBC) to less than 3,500/mm^3 and a granulocyte count of at least 1,500/mm^3. Granulocytopenia is a reduction in the granulocyte count below 1,500/mm^3, whereas *agranulocytosis* is defined as a reduction below 500/mm^3. Antipsychotics induce leukopenia or granulocytopenia in up to 15% of patients, but this phenomenon has no clinical significance. In comparative studies, the incidence of clozapine-induced leukopenia and granulocytopenia was less than that with CPZ or haloperidol. Patients on any of these drugs may experience a WBC drop below 5,000 that shortly returns to a normal range, or a drop below 5,000 that then remains between 3,500 and 5,000, with some fluctuation. This drop in WBC does not typically progress to agranulocytosis.

Agranulocytosis occurs rarely but can be assumed to arise with any phenothiazine. It is usually seen in older females with other complicating systemic diseases and is considerably rarer in young, healthy adults. It generally occurs in the first 6 to 8 weeks of treatment, with an abrupt onset consisting of a sore throat, ulcerations, and fever. **Without rapid, aggresive intervention, the mortality rate is high, often exceeding 30%.**

The offending drug should be discontinued immediately, the patient transferred to a setting with reverse isolation facilities, and aggressive treatment of any infection immediately instituted. Cross-sensitivity to other phenothiazines is assumed to be possible, but supporting data are lacking. The value of routine complete blood counts is highly questionable because agranulocytosis develops so rapidly. On occasion, phenothiazines may temporarily reduce the total WBC count by as much as 30% to 60%, but this is a different and more benign hematological phenomenon, requiring neither special treatment nor discontinuation of drug therapy. Rarely, thrombocytopenic or nonthrombocytopenic purpura, hemolytic anemias, and pancytopenia are precipitated by phenothiazines, necessitating a switch to another antipsychotic in a different chemical class.

Clozapine-Related Agranulocytosis

Agranulocytosis has been reported worldwide with clozapine. While many other drugs also cause agranulocytosis, and in some cases patients were receiving such agents in addition to clozapine, a number of patients were not on any other potential offending drug, implicating clozapine as the primary cause (39, 43).

The WBC count of patients on clozapine must be followed closely (i.e., with weekly or even twice weekly complete blood counts), especially during the period of greatest risk (i.e., weeks 5 to 25). After the first 6 months, the FDA requires only biweekly CBC monitoring. If a patient's WBC count drops below:

- **3,500 (or has dropped by a substantial amount from baseline): counts should be repeated**
- **3,500 and/or the granulocyte count falls below 1,500**: monitor twice weekly with differentials
- **3,000 and/or granulocyte count <1,500**: interrupt treatment and obtain CBC and differentials daily. May resume if no symptoms of infection and WBC return to >3,000 plus >1,500 granulocyte count. Continue twice weekly monitoring until WBC >3,500
- **2,000 or granulocytes below 1,000**: stop clozapine and place the patient in reverse isolation with daily CBC and differential until levels return to normal. Do not rechallenge with clozapine

Risk Factors

Two of three patients suffering from agranulocytosis are female, but any relationship to age or dose of clozapine is unclear. Agranulocytosis is rare in the first 4 weeks of treatment, peaking in incidence during the period between the 5th and 25th weeks of treatment.

Initially, the mortality rate from clozapine-induced agranulocytosis was about 40%, but it has decreased by more than half. Now, while the mortality rate of agranulocytosis complicated by infection is still 40%, without infection, it is approximately 15%. In U.S. clinical trials, the incidence is about one per 100, but because this outcome is based on only 1,000 patients, it may not be an accurate estimate. It is notable that some who developed clozapine-induced agranulocytosis were later able to tolerate other antipsychotics without a recurrence, again implying a different underlying mechanism.

In a review of clozapine after its release in the United States, Alvir et al. (510) found that the cumulative incidence of clozapine-related agranulocytosis was 0.80% (95% confidence interval, 0.61 to 0.99) at 1 year and 0.91% (95% confidence interval, 0.62 to 1.20) at 1.5 years. Furthermore, of 73 patients (11,555 total patients were studied) who developed this dyscrasia, two died from infectious complications. In 61 of these patients, episodes of agranulocytosis began within 3 months of initiating drug therapy, and the risk was greater with increasing age and among women. Although the prodromal period leading to this condition was typically long in most patients, 16 developed it within 8 days of demonstrating WBC counts greater than 3,500 mm^3. Only three patients developed agranulocytosis after 6 months and one after 18 months. When clozapine is discontinued, the WBC count gradually returns to normal levels over 2 to 4 weeks. As mentioned earlier, treatment usually requires reverse isolation and management of intercurrent infections with appropriate antibiotics.

In addition, two recombinant hematopoietic factors–granulocyte colony-stimulating factor (G-CSF) and granulocyte-macrophage colony-stimulating factor (GM-CSF)–have been used to manage this condition. Chengappa et al. sought to determine whether the administration of G-CSF to patients who developed clozapine-associated agranulocytosis could shorten the course of this life-threatening complication (511). They examined the medical records of 11 patients over a 5-year period with clozapine-associated agranulocytosis. The patients had been diagnosed with chronic undifferentiated schizophrenia ($n = 4$), chronic paranoid schizophrenia ($n = 4$), and schizoaffective disorder ($n = 3$). The average dose of clozapine was 416 ± 219 mg/day. Seven (64%) of the 11 cases of agranulocytosis occurred during the high-risk period (i.e., during the first 12 to 18 weeks of clozapine treatment), two cases occurred approximately 6 months after the start of treatment, and two cases occurred after 1 year of treatment. There were no fatalities, and seven patients developed no clinical symptoms associated with agranulocytosis; thus, weekly blood cell counts provided the only clue. Six patients received G-CSF, and five did not. The overall clinical outcomes were similar between the two groups, although the G-CSF-treated patients had a significantly shorter duration of hospitalization. The authors observed that a history of leukopenia, agranulocytosis, or thrombocytopenia caused by the ingestion of neuroleptics, carbamazepine, or clozapine may increase the risk of clozapine-induced agranulocytosis. The concomitant use of clozapine and other drugs toxic to bone marrow may also increase this risk. Others have reported that the treatment of clozapine agranulocytosis with G-CSF decreases the duration of agranulocytosis by up to 50% (512, 513). Once the clozapine has been discontinued, it is important to start the G-CSF as soon as possible. They believe that clozapine should be stopped and a consultation obtained if a patient's absolute neutrophil count (ANC) falls below 1,500/μL. These authors recommend that G-CSF or GM-CSF be initiated within 48 h of the development of agranulocytosis and discontinued when the ANC exceeds 500/μL.

Clozapine-Related Thrombosis

Another example of a serious adverse effect that can surface through close systematic monitoring is the association of clozapine treatment with venous thromboembolytic complications (514, 515). Six cases of pulmonary embolism and six cases of venous thrombosis were reported to the Swedish Adverse-Reaction Committee. Most cases of venous thrombosis occurred in the first several months, and five resulted in death.

TABLE 5-27. *Pharmacokinetics of risperidone, olanzapine, quetiapine, and ziprasidone*

Risperidone
Absorption: rapid and complete
Time to peak concentration: 1–3 hours
Serum elimination half-life: about 20 hours
Time to steady-state concentration (C_{SS}):
  5–7 days
Protein binding: 89%/77% for metabolite
Metabolism: CYP 2D6
Active metabolite: 9-OH-risperidone

Olanzapine[a]
Absorption: well absorbed
Time to peak concentration: 5 hours
Serum elimination half-life: 20–70 hours
Time to steady-state concentration (C_{SS}):
  7 days
Protein binding: 93%
Metabolism: CYP 1A2 and 2D6
No active metabolites

Quetiapine
Absorption: rapid
Time to peak concentration: about 1.5 hours
Serum elimination half-life: 3–7 hours
Time to steady-state concentration (C_{SS}):
  2–3 days
Protein binding: 80%
Metabolism: primarily by CYP 3A4
No active metabolite

Ziprasidone[b]
Absorption: rapid with food
Time to peak concentration: 3.8–5.2 hours
Serum elimination half-life: 5–10 hours
Time to steady-state concentration (C_{SS}):
  1–3 days
Protein Binding: >99%
Metabolism: CYP 3A4
No active metabolites

---

[a] From Jibson M, Tandon R. *J Psychiatr Res* 1998; 32:215–228, and Stephenson et al. *Br J Psychiatry* 1999;174:52–58, with permission.
[b] From Tandon R, Harrigan E, Zorn S. Ziprasidone: a novel AP with unique pharmacology and therapeutic potential. *J Serotonin Res* 1997;4:159–177, and Davis R, Markham A. Ziprasidone. *CNS Drugs* 1997;8:153–159, with permission.

Drug Interactions with Antipsychotics

Drug interactions can be based on pharmacokinetics, pharmacodynamics, or both (326). To fully appreciate the risk:benefit ratio, any combination therapy requires extensive clinical experience. This is because most of the initial information is derived from well-controlled studies on carefully chosen patients, who clearly differ from chronically ill patients, whose response to a given treatment is influenced by multiple potential moderating problems such as:

- Comorbid *medical conditions* requiring other drug therapies
- Concurrent use of *other psychotropic medications*
- *Altered physiology* as during pregnancy
- Comorbid *substance* and *alcohol abuse*

Thus, information about clinically significant interactions may be limited at first; as a result, special vigilance is required to recognize, manage, and report potentially serious adverse (or therapeutic additive) interactions.

When antipsychotics are used in conjunction with a variety of anticonvulsants, their plasma levels may be significantly altered due to *pharmacokinetic interactions*. For example, when CBZ and haloperidol are coadministered, their interaction may cause a significant decrease in the neuroleptic's serum levels, sometimes resulting in clinical decompensation (516). Conversely, the cessation of CBZ may lead to increased antipsychotic plasma levels.

SSRIs such as fluoxetine and paroxetine may inhibit the metabolism of antipsychotics, increasing their plasma levels and the chance for toxicity (517, 518). While antipsychotics may inhibit the metabolism of tricyclic antidepressants, or,

in turn, have their metabolism inhibited by tricyclic antidepressants, the clinical relevance is uncertain.

Common *pharmacodynamic interactions* involve the additive anticholinergic or antidopaminergic effects of antipsychotics. Thus, concomitantly administered antiparkinsonian agents (e.g., benztropine) may increase the chances of toxicity (e.g., delirium); while dopamimetic agents (e.g., levodopa) may counteract the antipsychotic or neurotoxic effects of these agents.

The ideal strategy to avoid potential adverse drug interactions is to use monotherapy whenever feasible. Unfortunately, this is often not possible and combination drug therapies are required to achieve optimal outcome. Thus, it is paramount that the prescribing physician *consider the possibility* of deleterious pharmacokinetic and/or pharmacodynamic interactions. When feasible, *lowering the doses* of either or both drugs used in combination may help. When available, choosing an *alternate agent* (i.e., amantadine vs. benztropine to reduce anticholinergic effects) is also a viable strategy. Finally, *therapeutic drug monitoring* may be useful to avoid subtherapeutic levels or toxicity with certain drug combinations (e.g., SSRI plus antipsychotic).

Clozapine

This agent has a "broad spectrum" of activity encompassing several neurotransmitter systems. In this light, clozapine is similar to such phenothiazines as CPZ and thioridazine (519). It is

(*Text continues on page 177.*)

TABLE 5-28. *Novel antipsychotics: pharmacodynamics*

	Ris	9-OH-Ris	CLZP	OLZP	QUET	ZPSD
5-HT$_{2A}$	0.16	0.25	3.3	1.9	120	0.31
D$_2$	3.3	4.0	150	17	310	9.7
D$_1$	620	670	540	250	4,240	330
α_1	2.3	4.0	23	60	58	12
α_2	7.5	17	160	230	87	210
H$_1$	2.6	10	2.1	3.5	19	5.3

Adapted from Schotte et al. *In vitro* receptor binding profile in animal brains (K_i values in nM). *Psychopharmacology* 1996;124:57–73.

TABLE 5-29. Adverse effects of antipsychotics

Adverse effects	Clinical alerts	Treatment approaches	Most common offenders
1. Central nervous system			
A. Acute EPS			
• Pseudoparkinsonism	• Rigidity, bradykinesia, tremor, masked facies	• Decrease dose • Add antiparkinsonian agent • Switch to another agent • Parenteral antiparkinsonian agent	All neuroleptics, especially Haloperidol Fluphenazine
• Dystonias	• Retrocollis, oculogyric crisis, opistothonus, torticollis • Rarely, laryngeal spasm		
• Acute dyskinesias	• Rapid, involuntary, coordinated stereotypical movements, usually of mouth, tongue, face		
• Akathisia	• Restlessness, inability to sit still, pacing	• β-blockers; diazepam	
B. Late-onset (tardive) syndromes	• Dyskinesias (usually of tongue, mouth, lips) • Dystonic symptoms	• Stop drugs, if possible • Switch to NAP	All antipsychotics, especially neuroleptics
C. Decrease in seizure threshold	• Convulsion(s)	• Minimize dose • Slowly increase, if necessary • Add anticonvulsants (CBZ, VPA)	Chlorpromazine Promazine Clozapine
D. Withdrawal syndrome	• GI symptoms, irritability, headaches, psychosis	• Slowly taper AP drug	Clozapine
E. Drowsiness, oversedation		• Give as bedtime dose • Increase caffeine intake • Decrease dose • Change to less-sedating agent	Chlorpromazine Thioridazine Clozapine
F. Cognitive effects • Central anticholinergic syndrome	• Toxic psychosis • Delirium	• Stop or decrease anticholinergic agents • Physostigmine (?)	Thioridazine Chlorpromazine Clozapine (?) Olanzapine (?)
G. Temperature dysregulation • Neuroleptic malignant syndrome	• Hypothermia • Hyperthermia, rigidity, autonomic instability	• Stop drug • Cooling techniques, antipyrctics, other supportive treatment • Dantrolene, bromocriptine, other DA agonists, ECT	All antipsychotics

(continued)

TABLE 5-29. Continued.

Adverse effects	Clinical alerts	Treatment approaches	Most common offenders
2. Autonomic **A. Anticholinergic** • Difficulty in accommodation; increased intraocular pressure	• Pupillary changes, blurred vision	• Eyeglasses needed (rare) • Decrease dose • Decrease or stop concomitant anticholinergic agent(s)	Thioridazine Mesoridazine Chlorpromazine Clozapine Olanzapine
• Dry mouth	• May develop oral fungal infection	• Frequent, small sips of water • Sugarless candy or gum	
• Constipation	• Absent bowel sounds, can progress to paralytic ileus	• Bulk laxatives • Increase fluids • Switch to agent with less anticholinergic effect	
• Hesitancy, urinary retention • Nasal congestion	• Delayed or inhibited ejaculation		
B. Secondary to α-receptor blockade • Hypotension • Tachycardia • Pallor	• Dizziness, syncope • Postural hypotension	• Decrease dose • Change to higher potency agent • Support hose N.B. epinephrine should be avoided	Chlorpromazine Thioridazine Risperidone Quetiapine
3. Cardiovascular A. ECG changes B. Torsade des pointes C. QT prolongation D. Sudden death (?)	• Flattening of T wave • Ventricular tachycardia • Possible lethal arrhythmia	• No clinical significance • Stop drug • Avoid lower potency agents, if possible	Thioridazine Mesoridazine Ziprasidone Risperidone Haloperidol
4. Dermatologic-Ocular A. Dermatoses • Contact • Systemic • Photosensitivity	• Urticarial, maculopapular, petechial, edematous eruptions • Severe sunburn	• Stop drug • Prevent by using sunscreens	Phenothiazines (especially chlorpromazine)
B. Discoloration of skin and corneal or lens opacities	• Blue-gray metallic discoloration of skin • Whitish deposits on ocular exam (do not interfere with vision)	• Decrease dose • Switch drug • Avoid sunlight	Chlorpromazine Thiothixene
C. Pigmentary retinopathy	• Brownish discoloration of vision • Decrease in visual acuity • Pigmentation of fundi	• Do not exceed 800 mg/day of thioridazine • Stop drug if symptoms appear	Thioridazine

5. Endocrine system A. Galactorrhea, gynecomastia	• Lactation • Breast enlargement	• Decrease or change agent	Especially phenothiazines
B. Amenorrhea	• Menstrual irregularities	• Check for pregnancy • Decrease or change agent • Decrease or change agent	Risperidone
C. Disturbances in sex drive D. Disturbances in glucose metabolism	• Unexplained elevated blood sugar or abnormal G.T.T.		
E. Weight gain F. Ketoacidosis		• Restrict caloric intake • Increase exercise • Consider molindone or ziprasidone if gain is excessive	Clozapine Olanzapine
6. Gastrointestinal	• Decreased bowel motility and associated constipation		Chlorpromazine
Hepatic	• Jaundice, followed in 1-7 days by fever, nausea, RUQ pain, malaise	• Stop drug, switch to a nonphenothiazine	
7. Hematological A. Agranulocytosis B. Leukopenia	• Unexplained sore throat, fever, petechiae, malaise	• Weekly CBC with clozapine • Stop drug • Reverse isolation • Antibiotics, supportive care	Clozapine Chlorpromazine (rare with other phenothiazines)
8. Drug/drug interactions • Antacids • Barbiturates • Lithium	• Unexplained decrease in efficacy or increase in toxicity	• Avoid concomitant use of agents known to have synergistic or antagonistic effects	All antipsychotics
9. Overdose	• Signs and symptoms: effects maximum within 4–6 hours • CNS: agitation, confusion, delirium, twitching, dystonic movements, EPS, convulsions, hyperthermia • C-V: increased HR, decreased BP, arrhythmias, C-V collapse	• Supportive, gastric lavage (H_2O soluble) • Antiparkinsonian drugs (diphenhydramine) • Forced diuretics and hemodialysis not helpful • Lipoid dialysis may be beneficial	All antipsychotics

AP, antipsychotic; CBC, complete blood cell count; DA, dopamine; ECT, electroconvulsive therapy; EPS, extrapyramidal side effects; NAP, novel antipsychotic. Adapted from Davis JM, Janicak PG, Lindon R, et al. Neuroleptics and psychotic disorders. In: Coyle JT, Enna SJ, eds. *Neuroleptics: neurochemical, behavioral and clinical perspectives.* New York: Raven Press, 1983:15–64.

TABLE 5-30. Common antipsychotic–drug interactions

Class of drug	Possible mechanisms	Comment
Antacids Aluminum hydroxide Magnesium hydroxide	Decreased absorption	Better to give APs a few hours after their use
Anticholinergics	Antagonism of muscarinic cholinergic receptors	(a) Additive effects with low potency agents such as: • Chlorpromazine • Thioridazine • Clozapine (b) Amantadine may be an alternative
Anticonvulsants Carbamazepine and others (e.g., phenytoin)	Induce microenzymes (e.g., P450 2D6)	(a) Increase metabolism leading to clinically significant decrease in antipsychotic levels (e.g., haloperidol) (b) Possible increased incidence bone marrow toxicity with clozapine (c) May increase AP plasma levels
Valproate	Inhibits microenzymes Displaces drug from protein binding sites	
Antidepressants Tricyclics (TCAs)	Competitive inhibition of microsomal oxidation	(a) AP may increase TCA levels to toxic concentrations (b) TCA may increase AP levels (c) May increase AP levels
SSRIs	Competitive inhibition of microsomal oxidation	
Benzodiazepines	Possible interaction between GABA and DA systems	Possible respiratory arrest with clozapine
Histamine₂ receptor antagonists	Inhibits oxidative system of P450 cytochrome system	(a) Cimetidine more likely to cause this effect (b) Ranitidine (150 mg BID) may be preferable
Lithium	?	Possible neurotoxicity similar to NMS
Nicotine	(a) Pharmacodynamic actions on central cholinergic and dopaminergic systems (b) ?	Decrease AP-induced EPS Increase clearance of HPDL and lluphenzine

AP, antipsychotic; DA, dopamine; EPS, extrapyramidal side effects; GABA, γ-aminobutyric acid; HPDL, haloperidol; NMS, neuroleptic malignant syndrome; SSRI, selective serotonin reuptake inhibitor.

also subject to a hepatic first-pass effect, which produces metabolites with low or unknown pharmacological activity. It has an elimination half-life ranging from 6 to 33 hours and a volume of distribution (V_d 5 L/kg) lower than most other antipsychotics. This last quality indicates less drug is sequestered in tissue sites. Plasma levels of the parent compound at or above 350 ng/mL may be associated with a better clinical response (66, 520). Plasma levels are lower in men than women, especially male smokers (329).

In general, concomitant drugs with potent anticholinergic (e.g., benztropine) or bone marrow effects (e.g., carbamazepine) should be avoided. Toxicity with BZDs has been reported, including symptoms such as excessive sedation, sialorrhea, ataxia, and, in some instances fainting, loss of consciousness, and respiratory arrest (521–523). Other potentially significant interactions reported in the literature include:

- *Anticonvulsants* such as phenytoin and carbamazepine may lower clozapine levels (524–526).
- *Erythromycin* may increase clozapine levels, predisposing to seizures (527).
- *Cimetidine* may increase clozapine levels (528).
- Clozapine may increase *nortriptyline* levels (529).

Other Novel Antipsychotics

Tables 5-27 and 5-28 summarize the clinically relevant pharmacokinetic and pharmacodynamic properties of other novel antipsychotics (326). Drug interactions with these agents were not systematically evaluated because controlled clinical trials usually prohibit concurrent medications. There are also many special circumstances (e.g., patients with comorbid medical diseases, substance abuse, epilepsy, or atypical indications such as agitation associated with mental retardation or dementia) that are not usually addressed in clinical research trials. Thus, much remains to be learned about significant drug interactions in these patient groups. To our knowledge, however, no consistent, serious, clinically relevant interactions have been reported.

For the present, given their primary CNS effects, caution should be used when these agents are taken in combination with other centrally acting drugs or alcohol. For example, because of the potential for inducing hypotension, via a_1-antagonism, risperidone may enhance the effects of certain antihypertensive agents. Theoretically, it could also antagonize the effects of levodopa and dopamine agonists, used for such conditions as Parkinson's disease. Finally, because these agents are metabolized by the P450 cytochrome microenzyme system, any drugs that stimulate (e.g., carbamazepine) or inhibit (e.g., valproate) this system may affect their clearance (6).

In conclusion, although it is difficult to quantify discomfort, the adverse effects of antipsychotics most often experienced are less severe than symptoms associated with the common cold. Serious adverse events are much less common. There is a risk to every treatment, but it is erroneous to suggest that because a serious event may occur, it is likely to occur. One of the most dangerous activities we engage in, for example, is driving or riding in an automobile, yet that does not mean that every time we drive to work there is a high probability that we will experience a serious injury or death.

Table 5-29 summarizes the important adverse events seen with antipsychotics and Table 5-30 summarizes common, potentially clinically relevant, drug interactions with antipsychotics.

CONCLUSION

We have updated our treatment strategies for both acute and maintenance drug treatment of a psychotic disorder (Figs. 5-5 and 5-10). Each may have antipsychotic efficacy below EPS threshold for most patients and some may have little to no EPS at all. Some atypical antipsychotics (clozapine, risperidone, olanzapine, and amisulpride) are more effective than typical neuroleptics on positive symptoms, but particularly on negative symptoms, thought disorder (cognitive symptoms), impulsive hostility, and anxiety depression. Thus, we would attempt trials with risperidone and olanzapine first and later possibly quetiapine and ziprasidone before using clozapine, due to their more benign side effect profile. Thus, we would attempt trials with risperidone, olanzapine, quetiapine, and ziprasidone before using clozapine, due to their more benign side effect profile. Others, however, would argue that after one or two unsuccessful trials with other novel agents and/or a neuroleptic, a clozapine trial should be instituted to minimize long-term deterioration. We would emphasize that one should move to clozapine with reasonable dispatch before too much deterioration has taken place, if initial treatment does not lead to a full remission.

REFERENCES

1. Laborit H, Huguenard P, Alluaume R. Un nouveau stabilisateur végétatif, le 4560 RP. *Presse Med* 1952;60:206–208.
2. Delay J, Deniker P. Le traitement des psychoses par une methode neurolytique derivee de l'hibermotherapie. Congres des médecins alienistes et neurologistes de France, Luxembourg, July 1952:497–502.
3. Delay J, Deniker P. Trente-huit cas de psychoses traitees par la cure-prolongee et continue de 4560 RP. Le Congres de AL et Neurologie de Langue Francaise, in Compte Rendue Congress. Paris: Marson et Cie, 1952.
4. Lehmann HE, Ban TA. The history of the psychopharmacology of schizophrenia. *Can J Psychiatry* 1997;42:152–163.
5. Davis JM, Janicak PG, Preskorm S, Ayd FJ Jr. Advances in the pharmacotherapy of psychotic disorders. In: Janicak PG, ed. *Principles and practice of psychopharmacotherapy. Update 1.* Baltimore: Williams & Wilkins, 1994, 1–14.
6. Ayd FJ Jr, Janicak PG, Davis JM. Advances in the pharmacotherapy of psychotic disorders II: the novel antipsychotics. In: Janicak PG, ed. *Principles and practice of psychopharmacotherapy. Update 5.* Baltimore: Williams & Wilkins, 1997, 1–22.
7. Johnstone EC, Crowe TJ, Frith CD, et al. Mechanism of the antipsychotic effect in the treatment of acute schizophrenia. *Lancet* 1978;1:848.
8. Meltzer HY. Role of serotonin in the action of atypical antipsychotic drugs. *Clin Neurosci* 1995;3:64–75.
9. Smith RC, Tamminga C, Davis JM. Effect of apomorphine on schizophrenic symptoms. *J Neural Transm* 1977;40:171–176.
10. Schaffer MG, Davis JM, Tamminga CA. Apomorphine's antipsychotic activity. *Arch Gen Psychiatry* 1985;42:927.
11. Sharma RP, Javaid JI, Janicak PG, et al. Homovanillic acid in the cerebrospinal fluid: patterns of response after four weeks of neuroleptic treatment. *Biol Psychiatry* 1993;34:128–134.
12. Sedvall GC, Farde L, Persson A, et al. Imaging of neurotransmitter receptors in the living brain. *Arch Gen Psychiatry* 1986;43:995–1005.
13. Wong DF, Wagner HN, Tune LE, et al. Positron emission tomography reveals elevated D-2 dopamine receptors in drug naive schizophrenia. *Science* 1986;234:1558–1563.
14. Farde L, Wiesel FA, Holldin C, et al. Central D2-dopamine receptor occupancy in schizophrenic patients treated with antipsychotic drugs. *Arch Gen Psychiatry* 1988;45:71–76.
15. Kapur S, Zipursky R, Jones C, et al. Relationship between dopamine D_2 occupancy, clinical response, and side effects: a double-blind PET study of first-episode schizophrenia. *Am J Psychiatry* 2000;157:514–520.
16. Kapur S, Zipursky RB, Remington G. Clinical and theoretical implications of 5-HT_2 and D_2 receptor occupancy of clozapine, risperidone, and olanzapine in schizophrenia. *Am J Psychiatry* 1999;156:286–293.
17. Kapur S, Zipursky R, Jones C, et al. A positron emission tomography study of quetiapine in schizophrenia: a preliminary finding of an antipsychotic effect with only transiently high dopamine D_2 receptor occupancy. *Arch Gen Psychiatry* 2000;57:553–559.
18. Sharma RP, Javaid JL, Pandey GN, et al. Behavioral and biochemical effects of methylphenidate in schizophrenic and non-schizophrenic patients. *Biol Psychiatry* 1991;30:459–466.
19. Lieberman JA, Kane JM, Gadaleta D, et al. Methylphenidate challenge as a predictor of relapse in schizophrenia. *Am J Psychiatry* 1984;141:633–638.
20. Angrist B, Preselow E, Rubinstein M, et al. Amphetamine response and relapse risk after depot neuroleptic discontinuation. *Psychopharmacology* 1985;85:277–283.
21. Janowsky DS, El-Yousef MK, Davis JM. Antagonistic effects of physostigmine and methylphenidate in man. *Am J Psychiatry* 1973:130:1370–1376.
22. Leonard S, Adams C, Breese CR, et al. Nicotinic receptor function in schizophrenia. *Schizophr Bull* 1996;22:431–445.
23. Meltzer HY. Pre-clinical pharmacology of atypical antipsychotic drugs: a selective review. *Br J Psychiatry* 1996;168(suppl 29):23–31.
24. Meltzer HY, Matsubara S, Lee LC. Classification of typical and atypical antipsychotic drugs on the basis of dopamine D_1, D_2 and serotonin$_2$ pKi values. *J Pharmacol Exp Ther* 1989:25:238–246.
25. Kapur S. 5-HT_2 antagonism and EPS benefits: is there a causal connection? *Psychopharmacology* 1996;124:35–39.
26. Meltzer HY, Goode D, Schyve P, et al. Effect of clozapine on human serum prolactin levels. *Am J Psychiatry* 1979;136:1550–1555.
27. Spohn HE, Lacousiere R, Thompson K, et al. Phenothiazine effects on psychological and psychophysiological dysfunction in chronic schizophrenics. *Arch Gen Psychiatry* 1977;34:633.
28. Hurt SW, Holzman PS, Davis JM. Thought disorder. *Arch Gen Psychiatry* 1983;40:1281–1285.
29. Andreasen NC, Arndt S, Alliger R, et al. Symptoms of schizophrenia: methods, meanings, and mechanisms. *Arch Gen Psychiatry* 1995;52:341–351.
30. Marder SR, Davis JM, Chouinard G. The effects of risperidone on the five dimensions of schizophrenia derived by factor analysis: combined results of the North American trials. *J Clin Psychiatry* 1997;58:538–546.
31. Cole JO, Goldberg SC, Klerman GL. Phenothiazine treatment in acute schizophrenia. *Arch Gen Psychiatry* 1964;10:246–261.

32. Cole JO, Goldberg SC, Davis JM. Drugs in the treatment of psychosis: controlled studies. In: Solomon P, ed. *Psychiatric drugs*. New York: Grune and Stratton, 1966:153–180.
33. Lehmann HE. Drug treatment of schizophrenia. *Int Psychiatr Clin* 1965;2:717–751.
34. Falloon I, Watt DC, Sheperd M. A comparative controlled trial of pimozide and fluphenazine decanoate in the continuation therapy of schizophrenia. *Psychol Med* 1978;8:59–70.
35. Janssen P, Brugmans J, Dony J, et al. An international double-blind clinical evaluation of pimozide. *J Clin Pharmacol* 1972;12:26–34.
36. Gross H. A double-blind comparison of once-a-day pimozide, trifluoperazine, and placebo in the maintenance care of chronic schizophrenic outpatients. *Curr Ther Res* 1974;16:696–705.
37. Clark ML, Huber W, Hill D, et al. Pimozide (and thioridazine) in chronic schizophrenic outpatients. *Dis Nerv Syst* 1975;36:137–141.
38. Clark ML, Huber W, Serafetinides EA, et al. Pimozide (Orap): a tolerance study. *Clin Trials J* 1971;8(suppl 2):25–32.
39. Lieberman JA, Kane JM, Johns CA. Clozapine: guidelines for clinical management. *J Clin Psychiatry* 1989;50:329–338.
40. Baldessarini R, Frankenburg FR. Clozapine: a novel antipsychotic agent. *N Engl J Med* 1991;324:746–754.
41. Farde L, Nordstrom A-L, Wiesel FA, et al. PET analysis of central D_1 and D_2 dopamine receptor occupancy in patients treated with classical neuroleptics and clozapine: relation to extrapyramidal side effects. *Arch Gen Psychiatry* 1992;49:536–544.
42. Farde L, Nordstrom A-L, Nyberg S, et al. D1-, D2-, and 5-HT2-receptor occupancy in clozapine-treated patients. *J Clin Psychiatry* 1994;55:1–3.
43. Kane J, Honigfeld G, Singer J, et al. Clozaril collaborative study group: clozapine for the treatment-resistant schizophrenic: a double-blind comparison with chlorpromazine. *Arch Gen Psychiatry* 1988;45:789–796.
44. Meltzer HY, Zureick JL. Negative symptoms in schizophrenia: a target for new drug development. *Psychopharmacol Ser* 1989;7:68–77.
45. Brier A, Buchanan RW, Kirkpatrick B, et al. Effects of clozapine on positive and negative symptoms in outpatients with schizophrenia. *Am J Psychiatry* 1994;151:20–26.
46. Carpenter WT Jr. Serotonin-dopamine antagonists and treatment of negative symptoms. *J Clin Psychopharmacol* 1995;15(suppl 1):30S–35S.
47. Carpenter WT Jr. The treatment of negative symptoms: pharmacological and methodological issues. *Br J Psychiatry* 1996;168(suppl 29):17–22.
48. Rosenheck R, Dunn L, Peszke M, et al. Impact of clozapine on negative symptoms and on the deficit syndrome in refractory schizophrenia. Department of Veterans Affairs Cooperative Study Group on Clozapine in Refractory Schizophrenia. *Am J Psychiatry* 1999;156:88–93.
49. Lee MA, Thompson PA, Meltzer HY, et al. Effects of clozapine on cognitive function in schizophrenia. *J Clin Psychiatry* 1994;55(suppl B):82–87.
50. Weinberger DR, Gallhofer B. Cognitive function in schizophrenia. *Int Clin Psychopharmacol* 1997;12(suppl 4):S29–S36.
51. Meltzer HY. Dimensions of outcome with clozapine. *Br J Psychiatry* 1992;160(suppl 17):46–53.
52. Jonsson D, Walinder J. Cost-effectiveness of clozapine treatment in therapy-refractory schizophrenia. *Acta Psychiatr Scand* 1995;92:199–201.
53. Meltzer HY, Cola PH, Way L, et al. Cost effectiveness of clozapine in neuroleptic-resistant schizophrenia. *Am J Psychiatry* 1993;150:1630–1638.
54. Calabrese JR, Kimmel SE, Woyshville MJ, et al. Clozapine for treatment-refractory mania. *Am J Psychiatry* 1996;153:759–764.
55. Frankenberg FR, Kalunian D. Clozapine in the elderly. *J Geriatr Psychiatry Neurol* 1994;7:131–134.
56. Chengappa KN, Baker RW, Kreinbrook SB, et al. Clozapine use in female geriatric patients with psychoses. *J Geriatr Psychiatry Neurol* 1995;8:12–15.
57. Fischer-Cornelssen KA, Ferner UJ. An example of European multi-center trials: multispectral analysis of clozapine. *Psychopharmacol Bull* 1976;12:34–39.
58. Honigfeld G, Patin J, Singer J. Clozapine: antipsychotic activity in treatment-resistant schizophrenics. *Adv Ther* 1984;1:77–97.
59. Shopsin B, Klein H, Aaronson M, et al. Clozapine, chlorpromazine, and placebo in newly hospitalized, acutely schizophrenic patients: a controlled, double-blind comparison. *Arch Gen Psychiatry* 1979;36:657–664.
60. Claghorn J, Honigfeld G, Abuzzahab FS, et al. The risks and benefits of clozapine versus chlorpromazine. *J Clin Psychopharmacol* 1987;7:377–384.
61. Green AI, Zimmet SV, Strous RD, et al. Clozapine for comorbid substance use disorder and schizophrenia: do patients with schizophrenia have a reward deficiency syndrome that can be ameliorated by clozapine? *Harvard Rev Psychiatry* 1999;6:287–296.
62. Buckley P, Thompson P, Way L, et al. Substance abuse among patients with treatment-resistant schizophrenia: characteristics and implications for clozapine theory. *Am J Psychiatry* 1994;151:385–389.
63. Marcus P, Snyder R. Reduction of comorbid substance abuse with clozapine [Letter]. *Am J Psychiatry* 1995;152:959.
64. Yovell Y, Opler LA. Clozapine reverses cocaine craving in a treatment-resistant mentally ill chemical abuser: a case report and a hypothesis. *J Nerv Ment Dis* 1994;182:591–592.
65. Drake RE, Xie H, McHugo GJ, et al. The effects of clozapine on alcohol and drug use disorders among patients with schizophrenia. *Schizophr Bull* 2000;26:441–449.
66. Perry P, Miller D, Arndt SV, et al. Clozapine and norclozapine concentrations and clinical response in treatment refractory schizophrenic patients. *Am J Psychiatry* 1991;148:231–235.
67. Schotte A, Janssen PFM, Gommeren W, et al. Risperidone compared with new and reference antipsychotic drugs: *in vitro* and *in vivo* receptor binding. *Psychopharmacology* 1996;124:57–73.
68. Roth B, Craigo S, Choudhary S, et al. Binding of typical and atypical antipsychotic drugs to 5-hydroxytryptamine-6 and 5-hydroxytryptamine-7 receptors. *J Pharmacol Exp Ther* 1994;268:1403–1410.
69. Leysen JE, Janssen PM, Gommeren W, et al. *In vitro* and *in vivo* receptor binding and effects on monoamine

turnover in rat brain regions of the novel antipsychotics risperidone and ocaperidone. *Mol Pharmacol* 1992;41:494–508.

70. Seeman P, Van Tol H. Dopamine receptor pharmacology. *Trends Pharmacol Sci* 1994;15:264–270.

71. Sleight AJ, Kock W, Bigg DC. Binding of antipsychotic drugs at alpha$_{1A}$-and alpha$_{1B}$-adrenoceptors: risperidone is selective for the alpha 1B-adrenoceptors. *Eur J Pharmacol* 1993;238:407–410.

72. Nyberg S, Farde L, Eriksson L, et al. 5-HT$_2$ and D$_2$ dopamine receptor occupancy in the living human brain. A PET study with risperidone. *Psychopharmacology* 1993;110:265–272.

73. Kapur S, Remington G, Zipursky RB, et al. The D$_2$ dopamine receptor occupancy of risperidone and its relationship to extrapyramidal symptoms: a PET study. *Life Sci* 1995;57:103–107.

74. Chouinard G, Jones B, Remington G, et al. A Canadian multicenter placebo-controlled study of fixed doses of risperidone and haloperidol in the treatment of chronic schizophrenic patients. *J Clin Psychopharmacol* 1993;13:25–40.

75. Marder SR, Meibach RC. Risperidone in the treatment of schizophrenia. *Am J Psychiatry* 1994;151:825–835.

76. Davis JM, Janicak PG. Risperidone: a new, novel (and better?) antipsychotic. *Psychiatr Ann* 1996;26:78–87.

77. Small JG, Miller MJ, Klapper MH, et al. Risperidone versus clozapine in resistant schizophrenia. Poster presentation at the 146th Annual Meeting of the American Psychiatric Association, San Francisco, May 27, 1993.

78. Heinrich K, Klieser E, Lehmann E, et al. Risperidone versus clozapine in the treatment of schizophrenic patients with acute symptoms: a double-blind, randomized trial. *Prog Neuro-Psychopharmacol Biol Psychiatry* 1994;18:129–137.

79. Chouinard G, Vainer JL, Belanger M-G, et al. Risperidone and clozapine in the treatment of drug-resistant schizophrenia and neuroleptic-induced supersensitivity psychosis. *Prog Neuro-Psychopharmacol Biol Psychiatry* 1994;18:1129–1141.

80. Daniel DG, Weinberger DR, Kleinman JE, et al. Risperidone versus clozapine in psychosis. Presented at the 147th Annual Meeting of the American Psychiatric Association, Philadelphia, May 1994.

81. Klieser E, Lehmann E, Kinzler E, et al. Randomized double-blind, controlled trial of risperidone versus clozapine in patients with chronic schizophrenia. *J Clin Psychopharmacol* 1995;15(suppl 1):45S–51S.

82. Bondolfi G, Baumann P, Patris M, et al. A randomized double-blind trial of risperidone versus clozapine for treatment-resistant chronic schizophrenia. Presented at the 148th Annual Meeting of the American Psychiatric Association, Miami, May 1995.

83. Lee H, Cooney JM, Lawlor BA. The use of risperidone, an atypical neuroleptic, in Lewy body disease. *Int J Geriatr Psychiatry* 1994;9:415–417.

84. Raheja RK, Bharwani I, Penetrante AE. Efficacy of risperidone for behavioral disorders in the elderly: a clinical observation. *J Geriatr Psychiatry Neurol* 1995;8:159–161.

85. Goldberg R, Goldberg J. Antipsychotics for dementia-related behavioral disturbances in elderly institutionalized patients. *Clin Geriatr* 1996;4:58–68.

86. Joshi UP, Joshi PM. Risperidone in geriatric patients with chronic psychoses and concurrent medical illnesses. New research 387. Presented at the 149th Annual Meeting of the American Psychiatric Association. New York, May 1996.

87. Janicak PG, Keck PE Jr, Davis J, et al. A double-blind, randomized, prospective evaluation of the efficacy and safety of risperidone versus haloperidol in the treatment of schizoaffective disorder. *J Clin Psychopharmacol* (in press).

88. Dwight MM, Keck PE, Stanton SP, et al. Antidepressant activity and mania associated with risperidone treatment of schizoaffective disorder. *Lancet* 1994;344:554–555.

89. Livingston MG. Risperidone. *Lancet* 1994;343:457–460.

90. Keck PE, McElroy SL, Strakowski SM, et al. Pharmacologic treatment of schizoaffective disorder. *Psychopharmacology* 1994;114:529–538.

91. Tohen M, Zarate CA, Centorrino F, et al. Risperidone in the treatment of mania. *J Clin Psychiatry* 1996;57:249–253.

92. Madhusoodanan S, Brenner R, Araujo L, et al. Efficacy of risperidone treatment for psychoses associated with schizophrenia, schizoaffective disorder, bipolar disorder, or senile dementia in 11 geriatric patients: a case series. *J Clin Psychiatry* 1995;56:514–518.

93. Stoll AL. Risperidone induction of mania: fact or fallacy? *Int Drug Ther Newsl* 1996;31:5-6.

94. Findling RL, Roth BL, Schulz SC. Risperidone: broadening clinical indications. In: Ayd FJ Jr, ed. *The art of rational risperidone therapy.* Baltimore: Ayd Medical Communications, 1996, 21–39.

95. Sandman C, Haney Copley K, Marion S, et al. Risperidone in patients with developmental disabilities reduces maladaptive and increases prosocial behavior amon adults. Presented at the 38th Annual Meeting of the American College of Neuropsychopharmacology, Acapulco, December 12–16, 1999.

96. Aman M, Findling R, Derivan A, et al. Risperidone versus placebo for severe conduct disorder in children with mental retardation [Abstract]. Presented at the 38th Annual Meeting of the American College of Neuropsychopharmacology, Acapulco, December 12–16, 1999.

97. Findling RL, McNamara NK, Branicky LA, et al. Risperidone in children with conduct disorder. Presented at the 37th Annual Meeting of the American College of Neuropsychopharmacology, Las Croabas, Puerto Rico, December 14–18, 1998.

98. Baldessarini RJ, Gardner DM, Garver DL. Conversion from clozapine to other antipsychotic drugs [Letter]. *Arch Gen Psychiatry* 1995;52:1071–1072.

99. Risch SC, Jackson C, Ware M, et al. Case reports of combined clozapine and risperidone pharmacotherapy: pharmacokinetic and pharmacodynamic interactions. Poster presentation at the 33rd Annual Meeting of the American College of Neuropsychopharmacology, San Juan, Puerto Rico, December 1994.

100. McCarthy RH, Terkelson KG. Risperidone augmentation of clozapine. *Pharmacopsychiatry* 1995;28:61–63.

101. Janicak PG, Tandon R. The use of combination antipsychotic therapies: PRO and CON. *J Psychotic Disord* 1998;2(1):15–17.

102. Shore D, Matthew S, Cotte J, et al. Clinical implications of clozapine discontinuation: report of an NIMH workshop. *Schizophr Bull* 1995;21:333–338.

103. Tyson SC, Devane CL, Risch SC. Pharmacokinetic interaction between risperidone and clozapine [Letter]. *Am J Psychiatry* 1995;152:1401–1402.

104. Koreen AR, Lieberman JA, Kronig M, et al. Cross-tapering clozapine and risperidone [Letter]. *Am J Psychiatry* 1995;152:1690.

105. Henderson DC, Goff DC. Risperidone adjunct to clozapine therapy in chronic schizophrenics. *Psychopharmacology Bull* 1995;31:578.

106. Farah A, Beale MD, Kellner CH. Risperidone and ECT combination therapy - a case series. *Convuls Ther* 1995;11:280–282.

107. Bymaster FP, Calligaro DO, Falcone JF, et al. Radioreceptor binding profile of the atypical antipsychotic olanzapine. *Neuropsychopharmacology* 1996;14:87–96.

108. Moore NA, Tye NC, Axton MS, et al. The behavioral pharmacology of olanzapine, a novel "atypical" antipsychotic agent. *J Pharmacol Exp Ther* 1992;262:545–551.

109. Fuller RW, Snoddy HD. Neuroendocrine evidence for antagonism of serotonin and dopamine receptors by olanzapine (LY170053), an antipsychotic drug candidate. *Res Commun Chem Pathol Pharm* 1992;77:87–93.

110. Stockton ME, Rasmussen K. Electrophysiological effects of olanzapine, a novel atypical antipsychotic, on A9 and A10 dopamine neurons. *Neuropsychopharmacology* 1996;14:97–104.

111. Pilowsky LS, Busatto GF, Taylor M, et al. Dopamine D_2 receptor occupancy *in vivo* by the novel atypical antipsychotic olanzapine–a 123IBZM single photon emission tomography (SPET) study. *Psychopharmacology* 1996;124:148–153.

112. Nyberg S, Farde L, Halldin C. A PET study of 5-HT_2 and D_2 receptor occupancy induced by olanzapine in healthy subjects. *Neuropsychopharmacology* 1997;16:1–7.

113. Beasley CM, Tollefson GD, Sanger T, et al. Olanzapine versus placebo and haloperidol: acute phase results of the North American double-blind olanzapine trial. *Neuropsychopharmacology* 1996;14:105–118.

114. Beasley CM Jr, Hamilton SH, Crawford AM, et al. Olanzapine versus haloperidol: acute phase results of the international double-blind olanzapine trial. *Eur Neuropsychopharmacol* 1997;7:125–137.

115. Beasley CM Jr, Sanger T, Satterlee W, et al. Olanzapine versus placebo: results of a double-blind, fixed-dose olanzapine trial. *Psychopharmacology* 1996;124:159–167.

116. Tollefson GD, Beasley CM, Tran PV, et al. Olanzapine versus haloperidol in the treatment of schizophrenia, and schizoaffective and schizophreniform disorders: results of an international collaborative trial. *Am J Psychiatry* 1997;154:457–465.

117. Sanger TM. Negative symptoms: a path analytic approach to a double-blind, placebo- and haloperidol-controlled clinical trial with olanzapine. *Am J Psychiatry* 1997;154:466–474.

118. Tran P, Lu Y, Sanger T, et al. Olanzapine in the treatment of schizoaffective disorder. Presented at the 36th Annual NCDEU Meeting. Boca Raton, FL, May 1996.

119. Beasley CM Jr, Beuzen JN, Birkett MA, et al. Olanzapine versus clozapine: an international double-blind study of the treatment of resistant schizophrenia. New Research, Annual Meeting of the American Psychiatric Association, Washington, DC, May 15–20, 1999;NR260:136.

120. Procyshyn RM, Zerjav S. Drug utilization pattern and outcomes associated with in-hospital treatment with risperidone and olanzapine. *Clin Ther* 1998;20:1203–1217.

121. Conley RR, Brecher M, the Risperidone/Olanzapine Study Group. Risperidone versus olanzapine in patients with schizophrenia or schizoaffective disorder [Abstract]. 37th Annual Meeting of the American College of Neuropsychopharmacology, San Juan, Puerto Rico, 1998.

122. Tran PV, Hamilton MS, Kuntz AJ, et al. Double-blind comparison of olanzapine versus risperidone in the treatment of schizophrenia and other psychotic disorders. *J Clin Psychopharmacol* 1997;17:407–418.

123. Saller CF, Salama AI. Seroquel: biochemical profile of a potential atypical antipsychotic. *Psychopharmacology* 1993;112:285–292.

124. Migler BM, Warawa EJ, Malik JB. Seroquel: behavioral effects in conventional and novel tests for atypical antipsychotic drug. *Psychopharmacology* 1993;112:299–307.

125. Hirsch SR, Link CGG, Goldstein JM, et al. ICI 204,636: a new atypical antipsychotic drug. *Br J Psychiatry* 1996;168(suppl 29):45–56.

126. Goldstein JM, Litwin LC, Sutton EB, et al. Seroquel: electrophysiological profile of a potential atypical antipsychotic. *Psychopharmacology* 1993;112:293–298.

127. Fleischhaker WW, Linkz CGG, Hurst BC. ICI 204,636 ("Seroquel") a putative new atypical antipsychotic: results from Phase III trials [Abstract V.D.1]. *Schizophr Res* 1996;18:132.

128. Borison RL, Arvanitis LA, Miller BG, et al. ICI 204.636, an atypical antipsychotic: efficacy and safety in a multicenter, placebo-controlled trial in patients with schizophrenia. *J Clin Psychopharmacol* 1996;16:158–169.

129. Arvanitis LA, Miller BG, and the Seroquel Trial 13 Study Group. Multiple fixed doses of "Seroquel" (quetiapine) in patients with acute exacerbation of schizophrenia: a comparison with haloperidol and placebo. *Biol Psychiatry* 1997;42:233–246.

130. Bench CJ, Lammertsma AA, Dolan RJ, et al. Dose dependent occupancy of central dopamine D_2 receptors by the novel neuroleptic CP-88,059-01: a study using positron emission tomography and ^{11}C-raclopride. *Psychopharmacology* 1993;112:308–314.

131. Sharma RP, Shapiro LE. The $5HT_{1A}$ receptor system: possible implications for schizophrenic negative symptomatology. *Psychiatric Annals* 1996;26:88–92.

132. Bench CJ, Lammertsma AA, Grasby PM, et al. The time course of binding to striatal dopamine D_2 receptors by the neuroleptic ziprasidone (CP-88,059-01) determined by positron emission tomography. *Psychopharmacology* 1996;124:141–147.

133. Fischman AJ, Bonab AA, Babich JW, et al. Positron emission tomographic analysis of receptor occupancy

in healthy volunteers treated with the novel antipsychotic agent, ziprasidone. *J Pharmacol Exp Ther* 1996;279:939–947.

134. Zorn SH, Seegar TF, Seymour PA, et al. Ziprasidone (CP-88,059). Preclinical pharmacology review. *Jpn Neuropsychopharmacol* 1995;17:701–708.

135. Bagnall A, Lewis RA, Leitner ML, et al. Ziprasidone for schizophrenia and severe mental illness. *Cochrane Database Syst Rev* 2000;(2):CD001945.

135a. Brook S, Lucey JV, Gunn KP. Intramuscular ziprasidone compared with intramuscular haloperidol in the treatment of acute psychosis. *J Clin Psychiatry* 2000;61:933–941.

135b. Lesem MD, Zajecka JM, Swift RH, et al. Intramuscular ziprasidone, 2 mg versus 10 mg, in the short-term management of agitated psychotic patients. *J Clin Psychiatry* 2001;62:12–18.

136. Harrigan E, Morrissey M, and the Ziprasidone Working Group. The efficacy and safety of 28-day treatment with ziprasidone in schizophrenia/schizoaffective disorder. Presented at the XXth Collegium Internationale Neuropsychopharmacologicum, Melbourne, Australia, June 1996.

137. Daniel DG, Zimbroff DL, Potkin SG, et al. Ziprasidone 80 mg/day and 160 mg/day in the acute exacerbation of schizophrenia and schizoaffective disorder: a 6-week placebo-controlled trial. Ziprasidone Study Group. *Neuropsychopharmacology* 1999;20:491–505.

137a. Keck PE, Jr., Reeves KR, Harrigan EP. Ziprasidone in the short-term treatment of patients with schizoaffective disorder: results from two double-blind, placebo-controlled, multicenter studies. *J Clin Psychopharmacol* 2001;21:27–35.

138. Lawler CP, Prioleau C, Lewis MM, et al. Interactions of the novel antipsychotic aripiprazole (OPC-14597) with dopamine and serotonin receptor subtypes. *Neuropsychopharmacology* 1999;20:612–627.

139. Quitkin F, Rifkin A, Klein DF. Very high dosage vs. standard dosage fluphenazine in schizophrenia: a double-blind study of nonchronic treatment-refractory patients. *Arch Gen Psychiatry* 1975;32:1276–1281.

140. Wijsenbeek H, Steiner M, Goldberg SC. Trifluoperazine: a comparison between regular and high doses. *Psychopharmacology (Berl)* 1974;36:147–150.

141. Goldberg SC, Mattison N, Cole JO, et al. Prediction of improvement in schizophrenia under four phenothiazines. *Arch Gen Psychiatry* 1967;16:107–117.

142. Goldberg SC, Frosch WA, Drossman AK, et al. Prediction of response to phenothiazines in schizophrenia: a cross-validation study. *Arch Gen Psychiatry* 1972;26:367–373.

143. Jurman RJ, Davis JM. Comparison of the costs of psychotropic medications: an update. *Psychiatr Med* 1991;2:349–359.

144. Meltzer HY, Cola PA. The pharmacoeconomics of clozapine: a review. *J Clin Psychiatry* 1994;55(9, suppl B):161–165.

145. Revicki DA. Pharmacoeconomic evaluation of treatments for refractory schizophrenia: clozapine-related studies. *J Clin Psychiatry* 1999;60(suppl 1):7–11; discussion 28–30.

146. Foster RH, Goa KL. Risperidone. A pharmacoeconomic review of its use in schizophrenia. *Pharmacoeconomics* 1998;14:97–133.

147. Reschke RW. Parenteral haloperidol for rapid control of severe, disruptive symptoms of acute schizophrenia. *Dis Nerv Syst* 1974;35:112–115.

148. Anderson WH, Kuehnle JC, Catanzano RM. Rapid treatment of acute psychosis. *Am J Psychiatry* 1976;133:1076–1078.

149. Salzman C, Hoffman SA. Rapid tranquilization. *Hosp Community Psychiatry* 1982;33:346.

150. Huyse F, Van Schijndel RS. Haloperidol and cardiac arrest. *Lancet* 1988;2:568–69.

151. Modestin J, Krapf R, Boker W. A fatality during haloperidol treatment: mechanism of sudden death. *Am J Psychiatry* 1981;138:1616–1617.

152. Tesar GE, Murray GB, Cassem NH. Use of high-dose intravenous haloperidol in the treatment of agitated cardiac patients. *J Clin Psychopharmacol* 1985;5:344–347.

153. Adams F. Emergency intravenous sedation of the delirious, medically ill patient. *J Clin Psychiatry* 1988;49(suppl 12):22–27.

154. Chambers RA, Druss BG. Droperidol: efficacy and side effects in psychiatric emergencies. *J Clin Psychiatry* 1999;60:664–667.

155. Janicak PG, Bresnahan DB, Sharma R, et al. A comparison of thiothixene with chlorpromazine in the treatment of mania. *J Clin Psychopharmacol* 1988;8:33–37.

156. Dubin WR, Weiss KJ. *Handbook of psychiatric emergencies.* Springhouse, PA: Springhouse Corporation, 1991.

157. Modell JG, Lenox RH, Weiner S. Inpatient clinical trial of lorazepam for the management of manic agitation. *J Clin Psychopharmacol* 1985;5:109–113.

158. Bick PA, Hannah AL. Intramuscular lorazepam to restrain violent patients. *Lancet* 1986;1:206.

159. Ward ME, Saklad SR, Ereshefsky L. Lorazepam for the treatment of psychotic agitation. *Am J Psychiatry* 1986;143:1195–1196.

160. Dever A, Schweizer E. Rapid remission of organic mania after treatment with lorazepam. *J Clin Psychopharmacol* 1988;8:227–228.

161. Modell JG. Further experience and observations with lorazepam in the management of behavioral agitation. *J Clin Psychopharmacol* 1986;6:385–387.

162. Salzman C, Green AI, Rodriguez-Villa F, et al. Benzodiazepines combined with neuroleptics for management of severe disruptive behavior. *Psychosomatics* 1986;27(suppl):17–23.

163. Arana GW, Ornsteen ML, Kanter F, et al. The use of benzodiazepines for psychotic disorders: a literature review and preliminary clinical findings. *Psychopharmacol Bull* 1986;22:77–87.

164. Campbell R, Simpson GM. Alternative approaches in the treatment of psychotic agitation. *Psychosomatics* 1986;27(suppl):23–26.

165. Lennox RH, Newhouse PA, Creelman WL, et al. Adjunctive treatment of manic agitation with lorazepam versus haloperidol: a double-blind study. *J Clin Psychiatry* 1992;52:47–52.

166. Garza-Trevino ES, Hollister LE, Overall JE, et al. Efficacy of combinations of intramuscular antipsychotics and sedative-hypnotics for control of psychotic agitation. *Am J Psychiatry* 1989;146:1598–1601.

167. Salzman C, Solomon D, Miyawaki E, et al. Parenteral lorazepam versus parenteral haloperidol for the control

of psychotic disruptive behavior. *J Clin Psychiatry* 1991;52:177–180.

168. Cohen S, Khan A, Johnson S. Pharmacological management of manic psychosis in an unlocked setting. *J Clin Psychopharmacol* 1987;7:261–264.

169. Busch FN, Miller FT, Weiden PJ. A comparison of two adjunctive strategies in acute mania. *J Clin Psychiatry* 1989;50:453–455.

170. Freinhar JP. Clonazepam in the treatment of mentally retarded persons. *Am J Psychiatry* 1986;143:1324.

171. Freinhar JP, Alvarez WH. Clonazepam: a novel therapeutic adjunct. *Int Psychiatry Med* 1985–86;15:321–328.

172. Altamura AC, Mauri MC, Mantero M, et al. Clonazepam/haloperidol combination therapy in schizophrenia: a double-blind study. *Acta Psychiatr Scand* 1987;76:702–706.

173. Freinhar JP, Alvarez WH. Use of clonazepam in two cases of acute mania. *J Clin Psychiatry* 1985;46:29-30.

174. Chouinard G, Young SN, Annable L. Antimanic effect of clonazepam. *Biol Psychiatry* 1983;18:451–466.

175. Chouinard G. The use of benzodiazepines in the treatment of manic depressive illness. *J Clin Psychiatry* 1988;49(suppl):15–19.

176. Mendoza AR, Djenderedjian AH, Adams J, et al. Midazolam in acute psychotic patients with hyperarousal. *J Clin Psychiatry* 1987;48:291–292.

177. Bodkin JA. Emerging uses for high-potency benzodiazepines in psychotic disorder. *J Clin Psychiatry* 1990;5(suppl):41–46.

178. Feighner JP, Aden GC, Fabre LF, et al. Comparison of alprazolam, imipramine and placebo in the treatment of depression. *JAMA* 1984;249:3057–3064.

179. Fawcett J, Edwards JH, Kravitz HM. Alprazolam: an antidepressant? *J Clin Psychopharmacol* 1987;7:295–310.

180. Gardner DL, Cowdry RW. Alprazolam-induced dyscontrol in borderline personality disorder. *Am J Psychiatry* 1985;142:98–100.

181. Rosenbaum JF, Woods SW, Groves JE, et al. Emergence of hostility during alprazolam treatment. *Am J Psychiatry* 1984;141:792–793.

182. Arana GW, Pearlman C, Shader RI. Alprazolam-induced dyscontrol in borderline personality disorder. *Am J Psychiatry* 1985;142:369.

183. Goodman WK, Charney DS. A case of alprazolam, but not lorazepam, inducing manic symptoms. *J Clin Psychiatry* 1987;48:117–118.

184. France RD, Krishnan KRR. Alprazolam-induced manic reaction. *Am J Psychiatry* 1984;141:1127–1128.

185. Pecknold JC, Fleury D. Alprazolam-induced manic episodes in two patients with panic disorder. *Am J Psychiatry* 1986;143:652–653.

186. Strahan A, Rosenthal J, Kaswan M, et al. Three cases of acute paroxysmal excitement associated with alprazolam treatment. *Am J Psychiatry* 1985;142:859–861.

187. Michaux MH, Kurland AA, Agallianos DD. Chlorpromazine-chlordiazepoxide and chlorpromazine-imipramine treatment of newly hospitalized, acutely ill psychiatric patients. *Curr Ther Res* 1966;8(suppl):117–152.

188. Hanlon TE, Ota KY, Agallianos DD, et al. Combined drug treatment of newly hospitalized, acutely ill psychiatric patients. *Dis Nerv Syst* 1969;30:104–116.

189. Hanlon TE, Ota KY, Kurland AA. Comparative effects of fluphenazine, fluphenazine-chlordiazepoxide and fluphenazine-imipramine. *Dis Nerv Syst* 1970;31:171–177.

190. Jimerson DC, van Kammen DP, Post RM, et al. Diazepam in schizophrenia: a preliminary double-blind trial. *Am J Psychiatry* 1982;139:489–491.

191. Lingjaerde O. Effect of the benzodiazepine derivative estazolam in patients with auditory hallucinations: a multi-centre double-blind, crossover study. *Acta Psychiatr Scand* 1982;65:339–354.

192. Karson CN, Weinberger DR, Bigelow L, et al. Clonazepam treatment of chronic schizophrenia: negative results in a double-blind, placebo-controlled trial. *Am J Psychiatry* 1982;139:1627–1628.

193. Pato CN, Wolkowitz OM, Rapaport M, et al. Benzodiazepine augmentation of neuroleptic treatment in patients with schizophrenia. *Psychopharmacol Bull* 1989;25:263–266.

194. Bacher NM, Lewis HA, Field PB. Combined alprazolam and neuroleptic drug in treating schizophrenia. *Am J Psychiatry* 1986;143:1311–1312.

195. Dixon L, Weiden PJ, Frances AJ, et al. Alprazolam intolerance in stable schizophrenic outpatients. *Psychopharmacol Bull* 1989;25:213–214.

196. Sassim N, Grohmann R. Adverse drug reactions with clozapine and simultaneous application of benzodiazepines. *Pharmacopsychiatry* 1988;21:306–307.

197. Shader RI, Jackson AH, Dodes LM. The antiaggressive effects of lithium in man. *Psychopharmacologia* 1974;40:17–24.

198. Sheard MH, Marini JL, Bridges CI, et al. The effect of lithium on impulsive aggressive behavior in man. *Am J Psychiatry* 1976;133:1409–1413.

199. Williams DT, Mehl R, Yudofsky S, et al. The effect of propranolol on uncontrolled rage outbursts in children and adolescents with organic brain dysfunction. *J Am Acad Child Psychiatry* 1982;21:129–135.

200. Ratey JJ, Morrill R, Oxenkrug G. Use of propranolol for provoked and unprovoked episodes of rage. *Am J Psychiatry* 1983;140:1356–1357.

201. Yudofsky SC, Stevens L, Silver J, et al. Propranolol in the treatment of rage and violent behavior associated with Korsakoff's psychosis. *Am J Psychiatry* 1984;141:114–115.

202. Greendyke RM, Kanter DR, Schuster DB, et al. Propranolol treatment of assaultive patients with organic brain disease. *J Nerv Ment Dis* 1986;174:290–294.

203. Sorgi PJ, Ratey JJ, Polakoff S. Beta-adrenergic blockers for the control of aggressive behaviors in patients with chronic schizophrenia. *Am J Psychiatry* 1986;143:775–776.

204. Hyman SE, Arana GW. *Handbook of psychiatric drug therapy.* Boston: Little, Brown, 1988.

205. American Psychiatric Association Practice Guidelines for the treatment of patients with schizophrenia. *Am J Psychiatry* 1997;154(suppl):1–63.

206. Robinson D, Woerner M, Alir J, et al. Predictors of relapse following response from a first episode of schizophrenia or schizoaffective disorder. *Arch Gen Psychiatry* 1999;56:241–246.

207. Hogarty GE, Goldberg SC. Collaborative study group. Drug and sociotherapy in the aftercare of schizophrenic patients. One-year relapse rates. *Arch Gen Psychiatry* 1973;28:54–64.

208. Caffey EM, Diamond LS, Frank TV, et al. Discontinuation or reduction of chemotherapy in chronic schizophrenics. *J Chronic Dis* 1964;17:347–358.

209. Clark ML, Huber W, Serafetinides EA, et al. Pimozide (Orap). A tolerance study. *Clin Trial J* 1971;2(suppl):25–32.

210. Clark ML, Huber W, Hill D, et al. Pimozide in chronic outpatients. *Dis Nerv Syst* 1975;36:137–141.

211. Davis JM, Dysken MW, Haberman SJ, et al. Use of survivial curves in analysis of antipsychotic relapse studies. In: Cattabeni F, Racogni G, Spano P, eds. *Longterm effects of neuroleptics*. New York: Raven Press, 1980:471–481.

212. Prien RF, Cole JO, Belkin NF. Relapse in chronic schizophrenics following abrupt withdrawal of tranquilizing medication. *Br J Psychiatry* 1969;115:679–686.

213. Hogarty GE, Ulrich RF, Mussare F, et al. Drug discontinuation among long-term successfully maintained schizophrenic outpatients. *Dis Nerv Syst* 1976;37:494–500.

214. Hogarty GE, Ulrich RF. Temporal effects of drug and placebo in delaying relapse in schizophrenic outpatients. *Arch Gen Psychiatry* 1977;34:297–301.

215. Mattes JA. Clozapine for refractory schizophrenia: an open study of 14 patients treated up to 2 years. *J Clin Psychiatry* 1989;50:389–391.

216. Inanaga K, Miura C, Kuniyoshi M, et al. The effect of continuation therapy of risperidone in the treatment of schizophrenia. The relationship between the clinical efficacy and the plasma level of monoamine metabolites. *Jpn J Neuropsychopharmacol* 1993;15:617–631.

217. Csernansky J, Okamoto A. Risperidone vs haloperidol for prevention of relapse in schizophrenia and schizoaffective disorder. Presented at the Annual Meeting of the American College of Neuropsychopharmacology, Acapulco, December 12–16, 1999.

218. Tollefson GD. Clinical experience with long-term continuation treatment with olanzapine. Presented at the World Psychiatric Association meeting, Madrid, September 23–28, 1996.

219. Goldberg SC, Schooler NR, Hogarty GE, et al. Prediction of relapse in schizophrenic outpatients treated by drug and sociotherapy. *Arch Gen Psychiatry* 1977;34:171–184.

220. Prien RF, Cole JO. High dose chlorpromazine therapy in chronic schizophrenia. Report of National Institute of Mental Health Psychopharmacology Research Branch Collaborative Study Group. *Arch Gen Psychiatry* 1968;18:482–495.

221. Prien RF, Levine J, Switalski RW. Discontinuation of chemotherapy for chronic schizophrenics. *Hosp Community Psychiatry* 1971;22:4–7.

222. Morgan R, Cheadle J. Maintenance treatment of chronic schizophrenia with neuroleptic drugs. *Acta Psychiatr Scand* 1974;50:78–85.

223. Davis JM, Marder S, Kane JM. Antipsychotic drugs. In: Kaplan HI, Sadock BJ, eds. *Comprehensive textbook of psychiatry. Vol. 2*, 5th ed. Baltimore: Williams & Wilkins, 1989:1591–1626.

224. May PRA, Tuma AH, Dixon WJ. Schizophrenia. A follow-up study of results of treatment. I. Design and other problems. *Arch Gen Psychiatry* 1976;33:474–478.

225. May PRA, Tuma AH, Yale C, et al. Schizophrenia–a follow-up study of results of treatment. II. Hospital stay over two to five years. *Arch Gen Psychiatry* 1976;33:481–486.

226. Greenblatt M, Solomon MH, Evans AS, et al., eds. *Drug and social therapy in chronic schizophrenia*. Springfield, IL: Charles C Thomas, 1965.

227. Falloon IRH, Coverdale JH, Laidlaw TM, et al. Early intervention for schizophrenic disorders. Implementing optimal treatment strategies in routine clinical services. *Br Med J* 1998;172(suppl 33):33–38.

228. Kuipers E, Fowler D, Garety D, et al. London-East Anglia randomised controlled trial of cognitive-behavioural therapy for psychosis. *Br J Psychiatry* 1998;173:61–68.

229. Murray RR. Living with schizophrenia. In Murray RR, Schooler NR (chairs). Novel antipsychotic use in schizophrenia [Academic Highlights]. *J Clin Psychiatry* 2000;61:223–232.

230. Jolley AG, Hirsch SR, McRink A, et al. Trial of brief intermittent neuroleptic prophylaxis for selected schizophrenic outpatients: clinical outcome at one year. *Br Med J* 1989;298:985–990.

231. Jolley AG, Hirsch SR, Morrison E, et al. Trial of brief intermittent neuroleptic prophylaxis for selected schizophrenic outpatients: clinical and social outcome at two years. *Br Med J* 1990;301:837–842.

232. Herz MI, Glazer WM, Mostert MA, et al. Intermittent vs. maintenance medication in schizophrenia. Two year results. *Clin Neuropharmacol* 1990;13(suppl 2):426–427.

233. Herz MI, Glazer WM, Mostert MA, et al. Intermittent vs. maintenance medication in schizophrenia. *Arch Gen Psychiatry* 1991;48:333–339.

234. Gaebel W, Kopcke W, Linden M, et al. 2-Year outcome of intermittent vs. maintenance neuroleptic treatment in schizophrenia. *Schizophr Res* 1991;4:288.

235. Carpenter WT, Hanlon TE, Heinrichs DW, et al. Continuous versus targeted medication in schizophrenic outpatients: outcome results. *Am J Psychiatry* 1990;147:1138–1148.

236. Schooler NR, Keith SJ, Severe JB, et al. Relapse and rehospitalization during maintenance treatment of schizophrenia: the effects of dose reduction and family treatment. *Arch Gen Psychiatry* 1997;54:453–463.

237. Kane JM, Rifkin A, Woerner M, et al. Low dose neuroleptic treatment of outpatient schizophrenics. I. Preliminary results for relapse rates. *Arch Gen Psychiatry* 1983;40:893–896.

238. Marder SR, Van Putten T, Mintz J, et al. Low- and conventional-dose maintenance therapy with fluphenazine decanoate. Two-year outcome. *Arch Gen Psychiatry* 1987;44:518–521.

239. Hogarty GE, McEvoy JP, Munetz M, et al. Dose of fluphenazine, familial expressed emotion, and outcome in schizophrenia. Results of a two-year controlled study. *Arch Gen Psychiatry* 1988;45:797–805.

240. Johnson DAW, Ludlow JM, Street K, et al. Double-blind comparison of half-dose and standard-dose flupenthixol decanoate in the maintenance treatment of stabilised outpatients with schizophrenia. *Br J Psychiatry* 1987;151:634–638.

241. Davis JM, Kane JM, Marder SR, et al. Dose response of prophylactic antipsychotics. *J Clin Psychiatry* 1993;54(suppl):24–30.

242. Siris SG, Morgan V, Fagerstrom R, et al. Adjunctive imipramine in the treatment of postpsychotic depression: a controlled trial. *Arch Gen Psychiatry* 1987;42:533–539.

243. Siris SG, Mason SE, Beranzohn PC, et al. Adjunctive imipramine maintenance in post-psychotic depression/negative symptoms. *Psychopharmacol Bull* 1990;26:91–94.

244. Johnson DAW. Studies of depressive symptoms in schizophrenia. *J Psychiatry* 1981;139:89–101.

245. Prusoff BA, Williams DH, Weissman MM, et al. Treatment of secondary depression in schizophrenia. A double-blind, placebo-controlled trial of amitriptyline added to perphenazine. *Arch Gen Psychiatry* 1979;36:569–575.

246. Chouinard G, Steinberg S. New clinical concept on neuroleptic-induced supersensitivity disorders. In: Stancer HC, Garfinkel PE, Rakoff VM, eds. *Guidelines for use of psychotropic drugs*. New York: Spectrum Publications, 1984:205–227.

247. Hunt JI, Singh H, Simpson GM. Neuroleptic-induced supersensitivity psychosis: retrospective study of schizophrenic inpatients. *J Clin Psychiatry* 1988;49:258–261.

248. Peet M. Supersensitivity psychosis [Letter]. J Clin Psychiatry 1991;52:90.

249. Singh H, Hunt JL, Vitiello B, et al. Neuroleptic withdrawal in patients meeting criteria for supersensitivity psychosis. *J Clin Psychiatry* 1990;51:319–321.

250. Green B. Focus on risperidone. *Curr Med Res Opin* 2000;16(2):57–65.

251. Comaty JE, Janicak PG. Depot neuroleptics. *Psychiatr Ann* 1987;17:491–496.

252. Knudsen P. Chemotherapy with neuroleptics. Clinical and pharmacokinetic aspects with a particular view to depot preparations. *Acta Psychiatr Scand* Suppl 1985;322(2):51–75.

253. del Guidice J, Clark WG, Gocka EF. Prevention of recidivism of schizophrenics treated with fluphenazine enanthate. *Psychosomatics* 1975;16:32–36.

254. Crawford R, Forrest A. Controlled trial of depot fluphenazine in out-patient schizophrenics. *Br J Psychiatry* 1974;124:385–391.

255. Rifkin A, Quitkin F, Rabiner CJ, et al. Fluphenazine decanoate, fluphenazine hydrochloride given orally, and placebo in remitted schizophrenics. I. Relapse rates after one year. *Arch Gen Psychiatry* 1977;34:43–47.

256. Hogarty GE, Schooler NR, Ulrich R, et al. Fluphenazine and social therapy in the aftercare of schizophrenic patients. Relapse analyses of a two-year controlled study of fluphenazine decanoate and fluphenazine hydrochloride. *Arch Gen Psychiatry* 1979;36:1283–1294.

257. Schooler NR, Levine J, Severe JB. NIMH-PRB collaborative fluphenazine study group. Depot fluphenazine in the prevention of relapse in schizophrenia: evaluation of a treatment regimen. *Psychopharmacol Bull* 1979;15:44–47.

258. Johnson DAW. Further observations on the duration of depot neuroleptic maintenance therapy in schizophrenia. *Br J Psychiatry* 1979;135:524–530.

259. Johnson DAW, Pasterski JM, Ludlow JM, et al. The discontinuance of maintenance neuroleptic therapy in chronic schizophrenic patients: drug and social consequences. *Acta Psychiatr Scand* 1983;67:339–352.

260. Johnson DAW, Wright NF. Drug prescribing for schizophrenic outpatients on depot injections: repeat surveys over 18 years. *Br J Psychiatry* 1990;156:827–834.

261. Marriott P, Hiep A. A mirror image outpatient study at a depot phenothiazine clinic. *Aust NZ J Psychiatry* 1976;10:163.

262. Tegeler J, Lehmann E. A follow-up study of schizophrenic outpatients treated with depot neuroleptics. *Prog Neuropsychopharmacol* 1981;5:79–90.

263. Freeman H. Twelve years' experience with the total use of depot neuroleptics in a defined population. In: Cattabeni F, et al., eds. *Long-term effects of neuroleptics (Advances in Biochemical Psychopharmacology)*. New York: Raven Press, 1980:559–564.

264. Davis JM, Andriukaitis S. The natural course of schizophrenia and effective maintenance drug treatment. *J Clin Psychopharmacol* 1986;6(suppl 1):2S–10S.

265. Schooler NR, Levine J, Severe JB, et al. Prevention of relapse in schizophrenia. An evaluation of fluphenazine decanoate. *Arch Gen Psychiatry* 1980;37:16–24.

266. Kane JM, Woerner M, Sarantakos S. Depot neuroleptics: a comparative review of standard, intermediate, and low-dose regimens. *J Clin Psychiatry* 1986;47(suppl):30–33.

267. Kane JM. The use of depot neuroleptics: clinical experience in the United States. *J Clin Psychiatry* 1984;45:5–12.

268. Zissis NP, Psaras M, Lyketsos G. Haloperidol decanoate, a new long-acting antipsychotic, in chronic schizophrenics: double-blind comparison with placebo. *Curr Ther Res* 1982;31:650–655.

269. Viukari J, Salo H, Lamminsivu U, et al. Tolerance and serum levels of haloperidol during parenteral and oral haloperidol treatment in geriatric patients. *Acta Psychiatr Scand* 1982;65:301–308.

270. Zuardi AW, Giampietro AC, Grassi ER, et al. Double-blind comparison between two forms of haloperidol. An oral preparation and a new depot decanoate in the maintenance of schizophrenic patients. *Curr Ther Res* 1983;34:253–261.

271. Nair NPV, Suranyi-Cadotte B, Schwartz G, et al. A clinical trial comparing intramuscular haloperidol decanoate and oral haloperidol in chronic schizophrenic patients: efficacy, safety, and dosage equivalence. *J Clin Psychopharmacol* 1986;6(suppl 1):30S–37S.

272. Deberdt R, Elens P, Berghmans W, et al. Intramuscular haloperidol decanoate for neuroleptic maintenance therapy. Efficacy, dosage schedule and plasma levels. An open multicenter study. *Acta Psychiatr Scand* 1980:62:356–363.

273. Reyntjens AJM, Heykants JJP, Woestenborghs RJH, et al. Pharmacokinetics of haloperidol decanoate. A 2-year follow-up. *Int Pharmacopsychiatry* 1982;17:238–246.

274. Gelders YG, Reyntjens AJM, Ash CW, et al. 12-month study of haloperidol decanoate in chronic schizophrenic patients. *Int Pharmacopsychiatry* 1982;17:247–254.

275. Suy E, Woestenborghs R, Heykants J. Bioavailability and clinical effect of two different concentrations of haloperidol decanoate. *Curr Ther Res* 1982;31:982–991.

276. Youssef HA. A one-year study of haloperidol decanoate in schizophrenic patients. *Curr Ther Res* 1982;31:976-981.
277. Bucci L, Marini S. Haloperidol decanoate in chronic schizophrenic patients. *Curr Ther Res* 1985;37:1091-1097.
278. Kane JM. Dosage strategies with long-acting injectable neuroleptics, including haloperidol decanoate. *J Clin Psychopharmacol* 1986;6(suppl):20S-23S.
279. Kissling W, Moller HJ, Walter K, et al. Double-blind comparison of haloperidol decanoate and fluphenazine decanoate effectiveness, adverse effects, dosage and serum levels during a six months' treatment for relapse prevention. *Pharmacopsychiatry* 1985;18:240-245.
280. Wistedt B, Persson T, Hellbom E. A clinical double-blind comparison between haloperidol decanoate and fluphenazine decanoate. *Curr Ther Res* 1984;35:804-814.
281. Chouinard G, Annable L, Campbell W, et al. A double-blind, controlled clinical trial of haloperidol decanoate and fluphenazine decanoate in the maintenance treatment of schizophrenia. *Psychopharmacol Bull* 1984;20:108-109.
282. Kornhuber J, Schultz A, Wiltfang J, et al. Persistence of haloperidol in human brain tissue. *Am J Psychiatry* 1999;156:885-890.
283. Wode-Helgodt B, Borg S, Fyro B, et al. Clinical effects and drug concentrations in plasma and cerebrospinal fluid in psychotic patients treated with fixed doses of chlorpromazine. *Acta Psychiatr Scand* 1978;58:149-173.
284. Chang SS, Javaid JI, Dysken MW, et al. Plasma levels of fluphenazine during fluphenazine decanoate treatment in schizophrenia. *Psychopharmacology* 1985;87:55-58.
285. Dysken MW, Javaid JI, Chang SS, et al. Fluphenazine pharmacokinetics and therapeutic response. *Psychopharmacology* 1981;73:205-210.
286. Janicak PG, Javaid JI, Sharma RP, et al. Trifluoperazine plasma levels and clinical response. *J Clin Psychopharmacol* 1989;9:340-346.
287. Mavroidis ML, Kanter DR, Hirschowitz J, et al. Clinical relevance of thiothixene plasma levels. *J Clin Psychopharmacol* 1984;4:155-157.
288. Smith RC, Baumgartner R, Misra CH, et al. Haloperidol. Plasma levels and prolactin response as predictors of clinical improvement in schizophrenia. Chemical versus radioreceptor plasma level assays. *Arch Gen Psychiatry* 1984;41:1044-1049.
289. Garver DL, Hirschowitz J, Glicksteen GA, et al. Haloperidol plasma and red blood cell levels and clinical antipsychotic response. *J Clin Psychopharmacol* 1984;4:133-137.
290. Mavroidis ML, Garver L. Plasma haloperidol levels and clinical response: confounding variables. *Psychopharmacol Bull* 1985;21:62-65.
291. Potkin SG, Bera R, Gulasekaram B, et al. Plasma clozapine concentrations predict clinical response in treatment resistant schizophrenia. *J Clin Psychiatry* 1994;55(9, suppl B):117-121.
292. Potkin SG, Shen Y, Zhou D, et al. Does a therapeutic window for plasma haloperidol exist? Preliminary Chinese data. *Psychopharmacol Bull* 1985;21:59-61.
293. Van Putten T, Marder SR, May PRA, et al. Plasma levels of haloperidol and clinical response. *Psychopharmacol Bull* 1985;21:69-72.
294. Van Putten T, Marder SR, Mintz J, et al. Haloperidol plasma levels and clinical response: a therapeutic window relationship. *Psychopharmacol Bull* 1988;24:172-175.
295. Davis JM, Ericksen SE, Hurt S, et al. Haloperidol plasma levels and clinical response: basic concepts and clinical data. *Psychopharmacol Bull* 1985;21:48-51.
296. Santos JL, Cabranes JA, Vasquez FF, et al. Clinical response and plasma haloperidol levels in chronic and subchronic schizophrenia. *Biol Psychiatry* 1989;26:381-388.
297. Aravagiri M, Marder SR, Van Putten T, et al. Determination of risperidone in plasma by high-performance liquid chromatography with electrochemical detection: application to therapeutic drug monitoring in schizophrenic patients. *J Pharm Sci* 1993;82:447-449.
298. Perry PJ, Sanger T, Beasley C. Olanzapine plasma concentrations and clinical response in acutely ill schizophrenic patients. *J Clin Psychopharmacol* 1997;17:472-477.
298a. Perry PJ, Lund BC, Sanger T, et al. Olanzapine plasma concentrations and clinical response: acute phase results of the North American olanzapine trial. *J Clin Psychopharmacol* 2001;21:14-20.
299. Marder S, Davis JM, Janicak PG, eds. *Clinical Use of Neuroleptic Plasma Levels.* Washington, DC: American Psychiatric Press, 1993:137-142.
300. Curry SH. Determination of nanogram quantities of chlorpromazine or its metabolites in plasma using gas liquid chromatography with an electron capture detector. *Anal Chem* 1968;40:1251-1255.
301. Curry SH, Marshall JHL, Davis JM, et al. Chlorpromazine plasma levels and effects. *Arch Gen Psychiatry* 1970;22:289-296.
302. May PRA, Van Putten T, Jenden DJ, et al. Chlorpromazine levels and the outcome of treatment in schizophrenic patients. *Arch Gen Psychiatry* 1981;38:202-207.
303. Van Putten T, Aravagiri M, Marder SR, et al. Plasma fluphenazine levels and clinical response in newly admitted schizophrenic patients. *Psychopharmacol Bull* 1991;27:91-96.
304. Marder SR, Van Putten T, Aravagiri M, et al. Fluphenazine plasma levels and clinical response. *Psychopharmacol Bull* 1990;26:256-259.
305. Yesavage JA, Holman CA, Cohn R, et al. Correlation of initial serum levels and clinical response. *Arch Gen Psychiatry* 1983;40:301-304.
306. Janicak PG, Javaid JI, Davis JM. Neuroleptic plasma levels: methodological issues, study design, and clinical applicability. In: Marder SR, Davis JM, Janicak PG, eds. *Clinical use of neuroleptic plasma levels.* Washington, DC: American Psychiatric Press, 1993:17-44.
307. Bleeker JAC, Dingemans PM, Frohne-de Winter ML, et al. Plasma level and effect of low dose haloperidol in acute psychosis. *Psychopharmacol Bull* 1984;20:317-319.
308. Shostak M, Perel JM, Steller RL, et al. Plasma haloperidol and clinical response: a role for reduced haloperidol in antipsychotic activity. *J Clin Psychopharmacol* 1987;7:394-400.

309. Doddi S, Rifkin A, Karajgi B, et al. Blood levels of haloperidol and clinical outcome in schizophrenia. *J Clin Psychopharmacol* 1994;14:187–195.

310. Kirch GG, Bigelow LB, Korpi ER, et al. Serum haloperidol concentration and clinical response in schizophrenia. *Schizophr Bull* 1988;14:283–289.

311. Bigelow L, Kirch DG, Braun T, et al. Absence of relationship of serum haloperidol concentration and clinical response in chronic schizophrenics: a fixed-dose study. *Psychopharmacol Bull* 1985;21:66–68.

312. Rimon R, Averbuch I, Rozick P, et al. Serum and CSF levels of haloperidol by radioimmunoassay and radioreceptor assay during high-dose therapy of resistant schizophrenic patients. *Psychopharmacology* 1981;73:197–199.

313. Coryell W, Kelly M, Perry P, et al. Haloperidol plasma levels and acute clinical change in schizophrenia. *J Clin Psychopharmacol* 1990;10:397–402.

314. Volavka J, Cooper T, Czobor P, et al. Haloperidol blood levels and clinical effects. *Arch Gen Psychiatry* 1992;49:354–361.

315. Volavka J, Cooper TB, Czobor P, et al. Plasma haloperidol levels and clinical effects in schizoprenia and schizoaffective disorder. *Arch Gen Psychiatry* 1995;52:837–845.

316. Janicak PG, Javaid JI, Sharma RP, et al. A two-phase, double-blind randomized study of three haloperidol blood levels for acute psychosis with reassignment of initial non-responders. *Acta Psychiatr Scand* 1997;95:343–350.

317. Javaid JI, Janicak PG, Hedeker D, et al. Steady-state plasma level prediction for haloperidol from a single test dose. *Psychopharmacol Bull* 1991;27:83–88.

318. Javaid JI, Janicak PG, Sharma RP, et al. Prediction of haloperidol steady-state levels in plasma after a single test dose. *J Clin Psychopharmacol* 1996;16:45–50.

319. McEvoy JP, Hogarty GE, Steingard S. Optimal dose of neuroleptic in acute schizophrenia. A controlled study of the neuroleptic threshold and higher haloperidol dose. *Arch Gen Psychiatry* 1991;48:739–745.

320. Nordstrom A-L, Farde L, Halldin C. High 5-HT2 receptor occupancy in clozapine treated patients demonstrated by PET. *Psychopharmacology* 1993;110:365–367.

321. Wolkin A, Brodie JD, Barouche F, et al. Dopamine receptor occupancy and haloperidol plasma levels [Letter]. *Arch Gen Psychiatry* 1989;46:482–483.

322. Kapur S, Remington G, Jones C, et al. What is the lowest effective dose of haloperidol? Evidence from PET studies. *Biol Psychiatry* 1996;39:513.

323. Ericksen SE, Hunt SW, Davis JM. Dosage of antipsychotic drugs [Letter]. *N Engl J Med* 1979;294:1296–1297.

324. Keck PE, Harrison GP, Cohen BM, et al. Risk factors for neuroleptic malignant syndrome. A case study. *Arch Gen Psychiatry* 1989;46:914–918.

325. Janicak PG, Davis JM. Pharmacokinetics and drug interactions. In: Sadock BJ, Sadock VA (eds), *Kaplan & Sadock's comprehensive textbook of psychiatry. Vol. 2,* 7th ed. Philadelphia: Lippincott Williams & Wilkins, 2000:2250–2259.

326. Bertilsson L, Carrillo JA, Dahl M-L, et al. Clozapine disposition covaries with CYP1A2 activity determined by a caffeine test. *Br J Clin Pharmacol* 1994;38:471–473.

327. Koponen HJ, Leinonen E, Lepola U. Fluvoxamine increases the clozapine serum level significantly. *Eur Neuropsychopharmacol* 1996;6:69–71.

328. Haring C, Barnas C, Saria A, et al. Dose-related plasma levels of clozapine [Letter]. *J Clin Psychopharmacol* 1989;9:71–72.

329. Taylor D, Bodani M, Hubbeling A, et al. The effect of nefazodone on clozapine plasma concentrations. *Int Clin Psychopharmacol* 1999;14:185–187.

330. Simpson GM, Josiassen RC, Stanilla JK, et al. Double-blind study of clozapine dose response in chronic schizophrenia. *Am J Psychiatry* 1999;156:1744–1750.

331. Miller DD, Fleming F, Holman TL, et al. Plasma clozapine concentrations as a predictor of clinical response: a follow-up study. *J Clin Psychiatry* 1994;55(9, suppl B):117–121.

332. Kronig MH, Munne RA, Szymanski S, et al. Plasma clozapine levels and clinical response for treatment refractory schizophrenic patients. *Am J Psychiatry* 1995;152:179–182.

333. Perry PJ, Miller DD, Fleming F, et al. Plasma clozapine concentrations as a predictor of clinical response: a follow-up study. *J Clin Psychopharmacol* 1994;55(suppl B):117–121.

334. Perry PJ, Bever KA, Arndt S, et al. Relationship between patient variable and plasma clozapine concentrations: a dosing nomogram. *Biol Psychiatry* 1998;44:733–738.

335. Aravagiri M, Ames D, Wirshing WC, et al. Plasma level monitoring of olanzapine in patients with schizophrenia: determination by high-performance liquid chromatography with electrochemical detection. *Ther Drug Monit* 1997;19:307–313.

336. Lane HY, Chiu WC, Chou JC, et al. Risperidone in acutely exacerbated schizophrenia: dosing strategies and plasma levels. *J Clin Psychiatry* 2000;61:209–214.

337. Dubin WR. Rapid tranquilization: antipsychotic or benzodiazepine. *J Clin Psychiatry* 1988;49:5–11.

338. Casey DE. Tardive dyskinesia. In: Meltzer HY, ed. *Psychopharmacology: the third generation of progress.* New York: Raven Press, 1987:1411–1419.

339. Fornum F. Biochemistry, anatomy, and pharmacology of GABA neurons. In: Meltzer HY, ed. *Psychopharmacology: the third generation of progress.* New York: Raven Press, 1987:173–182.

340. Garbutt J, VanKammen DPO. The interactions between GABA and dopamine: implications for schizophrenia. *Schizophr Bull* 1983;9:336–353.

341. Lloyd KG, Murselli PL. Psychopharmacology of GABAergic drugs. In: Meltzer HY, ed. *Psychopharmacology: the third generation of progress.* New York: Raven Press, 1987:183–195.

342. Meldrum B. Pharmacology of GABA. *Clin Neuropharmacol* 1982;5:293–316.

343. Mohler IJ, Evans SJ. γ-Aminobutyric acid (GABA), receptors and their association with benzodiazepine recognition sites. In: Meltzer HY, ed. *Psychopharmacology: the third generation of progress.* New York: Raven Press, 1987:265–272.

344. Csernansky JG, Lombrozo L, Gulevich GD, et al. Treatment of negative schizophrenic symptoms with alprazolam: a preliminary open-label study. *J Clin Psychopharmacol* 1984;4:349–352.

345. Douyon R, Angrist B, Peselow E, et al. Neuroleptic augmentation with alprazolam: clinical effects and pharmacokinetic correlates. *Am J Psychiatry* 1989;146:231–234.

346. Nestoros JN, Nair NPV, Pulman JR, et al. High doses of diazepam improve neuroleptic-resistant chronic schizophrenic patients. *Psychopharmacology* 1983;81:42–47.

347. Weizman A, Tyano S, Wijsenbeek H, et al. High dose diazepam treatment and its effect on prolactin secretion in adolescent schizophrenic patients. *Psychopharmacology* 1984;82:382–385.

348. Wolkowitz OM, Breier A, Doran A, et al. Alprazolam augmentation of the antipsychotic effects of fluphenazine in schizophrenic patients. *Arch Gen Psychiatry* 1988;45:664–671.

349. Csernansky JG, Riney SJ, Lombrozo L, et al. Double-blind comparison of alprazolam, diazepam, and placebo for the treatment of negative schizophrenic symptoms. *Arch Gen Psychiatry* 1988;45:655–659.

350. Holden JMC, Itil TM, Keskiner A, et al. Thioridazine and chlordiazepoxide, alone and combined, in the treatment of chronic schizophrenia. *Compr Psychiatry* 1968;9:633–643.

351. Kellner R, Wilson RM, Muldawer MD, et al. Anxiety in schizophrenia: the responses to chlordiazepoxide in an intensive design study. *Arch Gen Psychiatry* 1975;32:1246–1254.

352. Ruskin P, Averburch I, Buchman RW, et al. Benzodiazepines in chronic schizophrenia. *Biol Psychiatry* 1979;14:557–558.

353. Salam SA, Pillai A, Beresford TP. Lorazepam for psychogenic catatonia. *Am J Psychiatry* 1987;144:1082–1083.

354. Salam SA, Kilzich N. Lorazepam in psychogenic catatonia: an update. *J Clin Psychiatry* 1988;49(suppl):16–21.

355. Greenfeld D, Conrad C, Kincare P, et al. Treatment of catatonia with low-dose lorazepam. *Am J Psychiatry* 1987;144:1224–1225.

356. Walter-Ryan WG. Treatment for catatonic symptoms with intramuscular lorazepam. *J Clin Psychopharmacol* 1985;5:123–124.

357. Wetzel H, Heuser I, Benker O. Stupor and affective state: alleviation of psychomotor disturbances by lorazepam and recurrence of symptoms with RO 15-1788. *J Nerv Ment Dis* 1987;175:240–242.

358. Martenyi F, Harangozo J, Laszlo M. Clonazepam for the treatment of catatonic schizophrenia. *Am J Psychiatry* 1989;146:1230.

359. McEvoy JP, Lohr JB. Diazepam for catatonia. *Am J Psychiatry* 1984;141:284–285.

360. Menza MA, Harris D. Benzodiazepines and catatonia: an overview. *Biol Psychiatry* 1989;26:842–846.

361. Saltana AS, Kilzieh N. Lorazepam treatment of psychogenic catatonia: an update. *J Clin Psychiatry* 1988;49:16–21.

362. Hass S, Emrich HM, Beckmann H. Analgesic and euphoric effects of high dose diazepam in schizophrenia. *Neuropsychobiology* 1982;8:123–128.

363. Mondell JG. Further experience and observations with lorazepam in the management of behavioral agitation [Letter]. *J Clin Psychopharmacol* 1986;6:385–387.

364. Salzman C. Use of benzodiazepines to control disruptive behavior in inpatients. *J Clin Psychiatry* 1988;49(suppl 12):13–15.

365. Casey JF, Hollister LE, Klett CJ, et al. Combined drug therapy of chronic schizophrenics. Controlled evaluation of placebo, dextro-amphetamine, imipramine, isocarboxazid, and trifluoperazine added to maintenance doses of chlorpromazine. *Am J Psychiatry* 1961;117:997–1003.

366. Davis JM. The treatment of schizophrenia. *Curr Opin Psychiatry* 1990;3:29–34.

367. Weissman M. The psychological treatment of depression. Evidence for the efficacy of psychotherapy alone, in comparison with, and in combination with pharmacotherapy. *Arch Gen Psychiatry* 1979;36:1261–1269.

368. Goff DC, Brotman AW, Waites M, et al. Trial of fluoxetine added to neuroleptics for treatment-resistant schizophrenic patients. *Am J Psychiatry* 1990;147:492–494.

369. Goldman MB, Janecek HM. Adjunctive fluoxetine improves global function in schizophrenia. *J Neuropsychiatry Clin Neurosci* 1990;2:429–431.

370. Arango C, Kirkpatrick B, Buchanan RW. Fluoxetine as an adjunct to conventional antipsychotic treatment of schizophrenic patients with residual symptoms. *J Nerv Ment Dis* 2000;188:50–53.

371. Biederman J, Lerner Y, Belmaker RH. Combination of lithium carbonate and haloperidol in schizo-affective disorder. A controlled study. *Arch Gen Psychiatry* 1979;36:327–333.

372. Shopsin B, Kim SS, Gershon S. A controlled study of lithium vs. chlorpromazine in acute schizophrenics. *Br J Psychiatry* 1971;119:435–440.

373. American Psychiatric Association. *Diagnostic and statistical manual of mental disorders,* 4th ed., revised. Washington, DC: American Psychiatric Press, 1994.

374. Hirschowitz J, Casper R, Garver DL, et al. Lithium response in good prognosis schizophrenia. *Am J Psychiatry* 1980;137:916–920.

375. Okuma T, Yamashita I, Takahashi R, et al. A double-blind study of adjunctive carbamazepine versus placebo on excited states of schizophrenic and schizoaffective disorders. *Acta Psychiatr Scand* 1989;80:250–259.

375a. Wassef AA, Hafiz NG, Hampton D, et al. Divalproex sodium augmentation of haloperidol in hospitalized patients with schizophrenia: clinical and economic implications. *J Clin Psychopharmacol* 2001;21:21–26.

376. Lautin A, Angrist B, Stanley M, et al. Sodium valproate in schizophrenia: some biochemical correlates. *Br J Psychiatry* 1980;137:240–244.

377. Linnoila M, Viukari M, Hietala O. Effect of sodium valproate on tardive dyskinesia. *Br J Psychiatry* 1976;129:114–119.

378. Ko GN, Korpi ER, Freed WJ, et al. Effect of valproic acid on behavior and plasma amino acid concentrations in chronic schizophrenia patients. *Biol Psychiatry* 1985;20:199–228.

379. Smith ME. A clinical study of chlorpromazine and chlordiazepoxide. *Conn Med* 1961;25:153–157.

380. Hankoff LD, Rudorfer L, Paley HM. A reference study of ataraxics: a two-week double blind outpatient evaluation. *J New Drugs* 1962;2:173–178.

381. Azima H, Arthurs D, Silver A. The effects of chlordiazepoxide (Librium) in anxiety states. *Can Psychiatr Assoc J* 1962;7:44–50.

382. Merlis S, Turner WJ, Krumholz W. A double-blind comparison of diazepam, chlordiazepoxide and chlorpromazine in psychotic patients. *J Neuropsychiatry* 1962;3(suppl):S133–S138.

383. Rao AV. A controlled trial with "Valium" in some psychiatric disorders. *Indian J Psychiatry* 1964;4:188–192.

384. Maculans GA. Comparison of diazepam, chlorprothixene and chlorpromazine in chronic schizophrenic patients. *Dis Nerv Syst* 1964;25:164–168.

385. Stonehill E, Lee H, Ban TA. A comparative study with benzodiazepines in chronic psychotic patients. *Dis Nerv Syst* 1966;27:411–413.

386. Gundlach R, Engelhardt DM, Hankoff L, et al. A double-blind outpatient study of diazepam (Valium) and placebo. *Psychopharmacologia* 1966;9:81–92.

387. Hekimian LJ, Friedhoff AJ. A controlled study of placebo, chlordiazepoxide and chlorpromazine with thirty male schizophrenic patients. *Dis Nerv Syst* 1967;28:675–678.

388. Guz L, Moraea R, Sartoretto JN. The therapeutic effects of lorazepam in psychotic patients treated with haloperidol: a double-blind study. *Curr Ther Res* 1972;14:767–774.

389. Marneros A. Anxiolytische Zusatzbehandlung bei den affektbetonten Schizphrenien. *Therapiewoche* 1979;29:7533–7538.

390. Lingjaerde O, Engstrand E, Ellingsen P, et al. Antipsychotic effect of diazepam when given in addition to neuroleptics in chronic psychotic patients: a double blind clinical trial. *Curr Ther Res* 1979;26:505–514.

391. Lerner Y, Lwow E, Levitin A, et al. Acute high-dose parenteral haloperidol treatment of psychosis. *Am J Psychiatry* 1979;136:1061–1064.

392. Nishikawa T, Tsuda A, Tanaka M, et al. Prophylactic effect of neuroleptics in symptom-free schizophrenics. *Psychopharmacology* 1982;77:301–304.

393. Nestoros JN, Suranyi-Cadotte BE, Spees RC, et al. Diasepam in high doses is effective in schizophrenia. *Prog Neuropsychopharmacol Biol Psychiatry* 1982;6:513–516.

394. Wolkowitz OM, Pickar D. Benzodiazepines in the treatment of schizophrenia: a review and reappraisal. *Am J Psychiatry* 1991;148:714–726.

395. Frankenburg FR, Kalunian D. Cardiorespiratory problems with clozapine. *J Clin Psychiatry* 1996;57:548–549

396. Klimke A, Kleiser E. Sudden death after intravenous application of lorazepam in a patient treated with clozapine. *Am J Psychiatry* 1994;151:780.

397. Atsmon A, Blum I. Treatment of acute porphyria variegata with propranolol. *Lancet* 1970;24:196–197.

398. Atsmon A, Blum I. The discovery. In: Roberts E, Amacher P, eds. *Propranolol and schizophrenia.* New York: Alan R. Liss, 1978;5–38.

399. Atsmon A, Blum I, Steiner M, et al. Further studies with propranolol in psychotic patients. *Psychopharmacologia* 1972;27:249–254.

400. Atsmon A, Blum I, Wijsenbeek H, et al. The short-term effects of adrenergic-blocking agents in a small group of psychotic patients. *Psychiatr Neurol Neurochir* 1971;74:251–258.

401. Yorkston NJ, Zaki SA, Havard CWH. Propranolol in the treatment of schizophrenia: an uncontrolled study with 55 adults. In: Roberts E, Amacher P, eds. *Propranolol and schizophrenia.* New York: Alan R. Liss, 1978;39–68.

402. Yorkston NJ, Zaki SA, Malik MKU, et al. Propranolol in the control of schizophrenic symptoms. *Br Med J* 1974;4:633–635.

403. Yorkston NJ, Zaki SA, Themen J, et al. Propranolol to control schizophrenic symptoms. *Adv Clin Pharmacol* 1976;12:91–104.

404. Yorkston NJ, Zaki SA, Themen J, et al. Safeguards in the treatment of schizophrenia with propranolol. *Postgrad Med J* 1976;52(suppl 4):175–180.

405. Davis JM, Janicak PG, Chang S, et al. Recent advances in the pharmacologic treatment of the schizophrenic disorders. In: Grinspoon L, ed. *Psychiatry 1982. The American psychiatric association annual review.* Washington, DC: APPI, 1982, 178–228.

406. Langsley DG, Enterline JD, Hickerson GX. A comparison of chlorpromazine and EST in treatment of acute schizophrenic and manic reactions. *Arch Neurol Psychiatry* 1959;81:384–391.

407. Smith K, Surphlis WRP, Gynther MD, et al. ECT and chlorpromazine compared in the treatment of schizophrenia. *J Nerv Ment Dis* 1967;144:284–290.

408. Benaton R, Sirota P, Megged S. Neuroleptic-resistant schizophrenia treated with clozapine and ECT. *Convuls Ther* 1996;12:117–121.

409. Kupchik M, Spivak B, Mester R, et al. Combined electroconvulsive-clozapine therapy. *Clin Neuropharmacol* 2000;23:14–16.

410. Esterson A, Cooper DG, Laing RD. Results of family-oriented therapy with hospitalized schizophrenics. *Br Med J* 1965;2:1462–1465.

411. Grinspoon L, Ewalt JR, Shader RI. *Schizophrenia: pharmacotherapy and psychotherapy.* Baltimore: Williams & Wilkins, 1968:67–74.

412. Grinspoon L, Ewalt JR, Shader RI. *Schizophrenia: pharmacotherapy and psychotherapy.* Baltimore: Williams & Wilkins, 1972.

413. Messier J, Finnerty R, Botvin C, et al. A follow-up study of intensively treated chronic schizophrenic patients. *Am J Psychiatry* 1969;125:1123–1127.

414. Gorham DR, Pokorny AD. Effects of a phenothiazine and/or group psychotherapy with schizophrenics. *Dis Nerv Syst* 1964;25:77–86.

415. Honigfeld G, Rosenbaum MP, Blumenthal IJ, et al. Behavioral improvement in the older schizophrenic patient: drug and social therapies. *J Am Geriatr Soc* 1965;8:57–72.

416. Dvangelakis MG. De-institutionalization of patients. *Dis Nerv Syst* 1961;22:26–32.

417. Rogers CR, Gendlin EG, Kiesler DJ, et al., eds. *The therapeutic relationship and its impact: a study of psychotherapy with schizophrenics.* Madison: University of Wisconsin Press, 1967.

418. Gunderson JG, Frank AF, Katz HM, et al. Effects of psychotherapy in schizophrenia: II. Comparative outcome of two forms of treatment. *Schizophr Bull* 1984;10:564–598.

419. Rosen JN. The treatment of schizophrenic psychoses by direct analytic therapy. *Psychiatr Q* 1947;21:117–119.

420. Rosen JN. *Direct analysis: selected papers.* New York: Grune & Stratton, 1953.
421. Karon B, O'Grady P. Intellectual test changes in schizophrenic patients in the first six months of treatment. *Psychother Theory Res Pract* 1969;6:88–96.
422. Karon BP, Vandenbos GR. Experience, medication and the effectiveness of psychotherapy with schizophrenics. *Br J Psychiatry* 1970;116:427–428.
423. Karon BP, Vandenbos GR. The consequences of psychotherapy to schizophrenic patients. *Psychother Theory Res Pract* 1972;9;111–119.
424. Paul GL, Lentz RJ. *Psychosocial treatment of chronic mental patients: milieu vs. social learning programs.* Cambridge: Harvard University Press, 1977.
425. Paul GL, Tobias LL, Holly, BL. Maintenance psychotropic drugs in the presence of active treatment programs: a "triple-blind" withdrawal study with long-term mental patients. *Arch Gen Psychiatry* 1972;27:106–115.
426. Falloon IRH, Boyd JL, McGill CW, et al. Family management in the prevention of exacerbations of schizophrenia. A controlled study. *N Engl J Med* 1982;306:1437–1440.
427. Goldstein MJ, Rodnick EH, Evans JR, et al. Drug and family therapy in the aftercare of acute schizophrenics. *Arch Gen Psychiatry* 1978;35:1169–1177.
428. Hogarty GE, Goldberg SC, Schooler NR, et al. Collaborative Study Group. Drug and sociotherapy in the aftercare of schizophrenic patients. II. Two-year relapse rates. *Arch Gen Psychiatry* 1974;31:603–608.
429. Hogarty GE, Anderson CM, Reiss DJ, et al. Family psychoeducation, social skills training, and maintenance chemotherapy in the aftercare treatment of schizophrenia. II. Two-year effects of a controlled study on relapse and adjustment. *Arch Gen Psychiatry* 1991;48:340–347.
430. Leff J, Berkowitz R, Shavit N, et al. A trial of family therapy versus a relatives' group for schizophrenia. Two-year follow-up. *Br J Psychiatry* 1990;157:571–577.
431. Tarrier N, Barrowclough C, Vaughn C, et al. The community management of schizophrenia. A controlled trial of a behavioural intervention with families to reduce relapse. *Br J Psychiatry* 1988;153:532–542.
432. Knight A, Hirsch S, Platt SD. Clinical change as a function of brief admission to a hospital in a controlled study using the present state examination. *Br J Psychiatry* 1980;137:170–180.
433. Herz MI, Endicott J, Spitzer RL, et al. Day vs. inpatient hospitalization: a controlled study. *Am J Psychiatry* 1971;127:1371–1382.
434. Herz MI, Endicott J, Spitzer RL. Brief hospitalization: a two year follow-up. *Am J Psychiatry* 1977;134:502–507.
435. Glick ID, Hargreaves WA, Drues J, et al. Short vs. long hospitalization: a prospective controlled study. IV. One-year follow-up results for schizophrenic patients. *Am J Psychiatry* 1976;133:509–514.
436. Glick ID, Hargreaves WA, Raskin M, et al. Short vs. long hospitalization: a prospective controlled study. I. The preliminary results of a one year follow-up of schizophrenics. *Arch Gen Psychiatry* 1974;30:363–369.
437. Caffey EM, Jones RB, Diamond LS, et al. Brief hospital treatment of schizophrenia: early results of a multiple hospital study. *Hosp Community Psychiatry* 1968;19:282–287.
438. Brown GW, Birley JLT, Wing JK. Influence of family life on the course of schizophrenic disorders: a replication. *Br J Psychiatry* 1972;121:241–258.
439. Leff JP, Wing JK. Trial of maintenance therapy in schizophrenics. *Br Med J* 1971;2:599–604.
440. Vaughn CE, Leff JP. The influence of family and social factors on the course of psychiatric illness. A comparison of schizophrenic and depressed neurotic patients. *Br J Psychiatry* 1976;129:125–137.
441. Vaughn CE, Snyder KS, Jones S, et al. Family factors in schizophrenic relapse. Replication in California of British research on expressed emotion. *Arch Gen Psychiatry* 1984;41:1169–1177.
442. Conrad KJ, Matters MD, Hanrahan P, et al. Characteristics of persons with mental illness in a representative payee program. *Psychiatr Serv* 1998;49:1223–1225.
443. Adler LA, Rieter S, Corwin J, et al. Differential effects of propranolol and benzotropine in patients with neuroleptic-induced akathisia. *Psychopharmacol Bull* 1987;23:519–521.
444. Kramer MS, Gorkin RA, Johnson C, et al. Propranolol in the treatment of neuroleptic-induced akathisia(nia) in schizophrenics: a double-blind, placebo-controlled study. *Biopsychiatry* 1988;24:823–827.
445. Lipinski JF, Zubenko GS, Cohen BM, et al. Propranolol in the treatment of neuroleptic-induced akathisia. *Am J Psychiatry* 1984;141:412–415.
446. Adler L, Angrist B, Peselow E, et al. A controlled assessment of propranolol in the treatment of neuroleptic-induced akathisia. *Br J Psychiatry* 1986;149:42–45.
447. Adler L, Angrist B, Peselow E, et al. Efficacy of propranolol in neuroleptic-induced akathesia. *J Clin Psychopharmacol* 1985;5:164–166.
448. Donlan PT. The therapeutic use of diazepam for akathisia. *Psychosomatics* 1973;14:222–225.
449. Kutcher S, Williamson P, MacKenzie S, et al. Successful clonazepam treatment of neuroleptic-induced akathisia in older adolescents and young adults: a double-blind, placebo-controlled study. *J Clin Psychopharmacol* 1989;9:403–406.
450. Gagrat D, Hamilton J, Belmaker RH. Intravenous diazepam in the treatment of neuroleptic-induced acute dystonia and akathisia. *Am J Psychiatry* 1978;135:1232–1233.
451. Hanlon TE, Schoenrich C, Frenck W, et al. Perphenazine benzotropine mesylate treatment of newly admitted psychiatric patients. *Psychopharmacologia* 1966;9:328–339.
452. Comaty JE, Janicak PG, Rajaratnam J, et al. Is maintenance antiparkinsonian treatment necessary? *Psychopharmacol Bull* 1980;26:267–271.
453. Chien CP, DiMascio A, Cole JO. Antiparkinsonian agents and depot phenothiazine. *Am J Psychiatry* 1974;131:86–90.
454. Lapolla A, Nash LR. Treatment of phenothiazine-induced parkinsonism with biperiden. *Curr Ther Res* 1965;7:536–541.
455. Adler LA, Rostrosen J, Edson R, et al. Vitamin E treatment for tardive dyskinesia. *Arch Gen Psychiatry* 1999;56:836–841.
456. Crane GE. Dyskinesia and neuroleptics. *Arch Gen Psychiatry* 1968;19:700–703.

457. Tardive Dyskinesia. A Task Force Report of the American Psychiatric Association. Washington, DC: American Psychiatric Press, 1992.
458. Muscettola G, Barbato G, Pampallona S, et al. Extrapyramidal syndromes in neuroleptic-treated patients: prevalence, risk factors, and association with tardive dyskinesia. *J Clin Psychopharmacol* 1999;19:203–208.
459. van Harten PN, Hoek HW, Matroos GE, et al. The inter-relationships of tardive dyskinesia, parkinsonism, akathisia and tardive dystonia: the Curacao Extrapyramidal Syndromes Study II. *Schizophr Res* 1997;26:235–242.
460. Owens DG, Johnstone EC, Frith CD. Spontaneous involuntary disorders of movement. *Arch Gen Psychiatry* 1982;39:452–461.
461. Caine ED, Polinsky RJ, Kartzinel R, et al. The trial use of clozapine for abnormal involuntary movement disorders. *Am J Psychiatry* 1979;136:317–320.
462. Cole JO, Gardos G, Tarsay D, et al. Drug trials in persistent dyskinesia. In: Fann WE, Davis JM, Domino E, Smith RC, eds. *Tardive dyskinesia: research and treatment.* New York: Spectrum Medical, 1980;419–428.
463. Gerbino L, Shopsin B, Collora M. Clozapine in the treatment of tardive dyskinesia: an interim report. In: Fann WE, Davis JM, Domino E, Smith RG, eds. Tardive dyskinesia: research and treatment. New York: Spectrum Medical, 1980;475–490.
464. Lieberman JA, Saltz BL, Johns CA, et al. Clozapine effects on tardive dyskinesia. *Psychopharmacol Bull* 1989;25;57–62.
465. Casey DE. Extrapyramidal syndromes and new antipsychotic drugs: findings in patients and non-human primates models. *Br J Psychiatry* 1996;168(suppl 29):32–39.
466. Levin H, Reddy R. Clozapine in the treatment of neuroleptic-induced blepharospasm: a report of 4 cases. *J Clin Psychiatry* 2000;61:140–143.
467. Friedman J. Clozapine treatment of psychosis in patients with tardive dystonia. *Movement Disord* 1994;9:321–324.
468. Lieberman J, Saltz B, John C, et al. The effects of clozapine in tardive dyskinesia. *Br J Psychiatry* 1991;154:503–510.
469. Adityanjee AM, Estrera AB. Successful treatment of tardive dystonia with clozapine. *Biol Psychiatry* 1996;39:1064–1066.
470. Casey DE. Clozapine: neuroleptic-induced EPS and tardive dyskinesia. *Psychopharmacology* 1989;99:S47–S53.
471. Brecher M. Long-term safety of risperidone: results of seven 1-year trials. Presented at the 149th Annual Meeting of the American Psychiatric Association, New York, May 1996.
472. Umbricht D, Kane JM. Risperidone: efficacy and safety. *Schizophr Bull* 1995;21:593–606.r
473. Beasley CM, Tollefson G, Tye NC, et al. Olanzapine: a potential "atypical" antipsychotic agent. *Proc Am Coll Neuropsychopharmacol* 1993;32:23.
474. Beasley CM Jr, Deliva MA, Tamura RN, et al. Randomised double-blind comparison of the incidence of tardive dyskinesia in patients with schizophrenia during long-term treatment with olanzapine or haloperidol. *Br J Psychiatry* 1999;174:23–30.
475. Schooler NR, Kane JM. Research diagnosis for tardive dyskinesia. *Arch Gen Psychiatry* 1982;39:486–487.
476. Small JG, Hirsch SR, Arvanitis LA, et al. Quetiapine in patients with schizophrenia: a high- and low-dose double-blind comparison with placebo. *Arch Gen Psychiatry* 1997;54:549–557.
477. Simpson GM, Lee LH, Shrivastava RK. Clozapine in tardive dyskinesia. *Psychopharmacology* 1978;56:78–80.
478. Alphs LD, Lee HS. Comparison of withdrawal of typical and atypical antipsychotic drugs: a case study. *J Clin Psychiatry* 1991;52:346–348.
479. Ichikawa J, Meltzer HY. Differential effects of repeated treatment with haloperidol and clozapine and dopamine release and metabolism in the striatum and the nucleus accumbens. *J Pharmacol Exp Ther* 1991;256:348–357.
480. Abuzzahab FS, Gillund JM. Clozapine and risperidone in schizophrenia. Poster presentation at the 33rd Annual Meeting of the American College of Neuropsychopharmacology, San Juan, Puerto Rico, December 1994.
481. DeLeon J, Stanilla JK, White AO, et al. Anticholinergics to treat clozapine withdrawal [Letter]. *J Clin Psychiatry* 1994;55:119–120.
482. Daniel DG, Goldberg TE, Weinberger DR, et al. Different side effect profiles of risperidone and clozapine in 20 outpatients with schizophrenia or schizoaffective disorder: a pilot study. *Am J Psychiatry* 1996;153:417–419.
483. Meltzer HY, Lee MA, Ranjan R, et al. Relapse following clozapine withdrawal: effect of neuroleptic drugs and cyproheptadine. *Psychopharmacology* 1996;124:176–187.
484. Krasucki CG, Mackeith JAC. Severe hypertension associated with risperidone withdrawal [Letter]. *Psychiatr Bull* 1995;19:452–453.
485. Meterissian GB. Risperidone-induced neuroleptic malignant syndrome: a case report and review. *Can J Psychiatry* 1996; 41:52–54.
486. Tarsy D. Risperidone and neuroleptic malignant syndrome. *JAMA* 1996;275:446.
487. Keck PE, McElroy SL, Pope HG. Epidemiology of NMS. *J Clin Psychiatry* 1991;21:148–151.
488. Caroff SN, Mann SC, Campbell EC. Atypical antipsychotics and neuroleptic malignant syndrome. *Psychiatr Ann* 2000;30:314–321.
489. Mesh H, Molcho A, Aizenberg D, et al. The calcium antagonist nifedipine in recurrent neuroleptic malignant syndrome. *Clin Neuropharmacol* 1988;II:552–555.
490. Sakkas P, Davis JM, Hau J, et al. Pharmacotherapy of NMS. *Psychiatr Ann* 1991;21:157–164.
491. Addonizio G, Susman VL. ECT as a treatment alternative for patients with symptoms of neuroleptic malignant syndrome. *J Clin Psychiatry* 1987;48:102–105.
492. Davis JM, Janicak PG, Sakkas P, et al. Electroconvulsive therapy in the treatment of the neuroleptic malignant syndrome. *Convuls Ther* 1991;7:111–120.
493. Janicak PG, Easton MS, Comaty JE, et al. Efficacy of ECT in psychotic and nonpsychotic depression. *Convuls Ther* 1989;5:314–320.
494. Miller DD, Sharafuddin MJA, Kathol RG. A case of clozapine-induced NMS. *J Clin Psychiatry* 1991;52:99–101.

495. Anderson ES, Powers PS. NMS associated with clozapine use. *J Clin Psychiatry* 1991;52:102-104.

496. DasGupta K, Young A. Clozapine-induced NMS. *J Clin Psychiatry* 1991;52:105–107.

497. Cole JO, Davis JM. Antipsychotic drugs. In: Bellak L, ed. *The schizophrenic syndrome.* New York: Grune & Stratton, 1969:478–568.

498. Calderon J, Rubin E, Sobota WL. Potential use of ipatropium bromide for the treatment of clozapine-induced hypersalivation: a preliminary report. *Int Clin Psychopharmacol* 2000;15:49–52.

499. Fritze J, Elliger T. Pirenzepine for clozapine-induced hypersalivation. *Lancet* 1995;346–1034.

500. Boshes RA, Davis JM. Medical side effects of psychoactive drugs. In: Berger PA, Brodie HK, eds. *American handbook of psychiatry. Vol. 8.* New York: Basic Books, 1986.

501. Land W, Salzman C. Risperidone: a novel antipsychotic medication. *Hosp Community Psychiatry* 1994;45:131–134.

502. Zarate CA, Baldessarini RJ, Siegel AJ, et al. Risperidone in the elderly: a pharmacoepidemiologic study. *J Clin Psychiatry* 1997;58(7):311–317.

503. Reilly JG, Ayis SA, Ferrier IN, et al. QTc-interval abnormalities and psychotropic drug therapy in psychiatric patients. *Lancet* 2000;35:1048–1052.

504. "FDA Dear Doctor Letter." Washington, DC: Food and Drug Administration, July 7, 2000.

505. Bess A, Cunningham S. "FDA Dear Doctor Letter." Washington, DC: Food and Drug Administration, September 22, 2000.

506. Allison DB, Mentore JL, Heo M, et al. Antipsychotic-induced weight gain: a comprehensive research synthesis. *Am J Psychiatry* 1999;156:1686–1696.

507. Colli A, Cocciolo M, Francobandiera R, et al. Diabetic ketoacidosis associated with clozapine treatment. *Diabetes Care* 1999;22:176–177.

508. Lindenmayer JP, Patel R, et al. Olanzapine-induced ketoacidosis with diabetes mellitus. *Am J Psychiatry* 1999;156:836–837.

509. Davis JM, Janicak PG, Linden R, et al. Neuroleptics and psychotic disorders. In: Coyle JT, Enna SJ, eds. *Neuroleptics: neurochemical, behavioral, and clinical perspectives.* New York: Raven Press, 1983, 15–64.

510. Alvir JMJ, Lieberman JA, Safferman AZ, et al. Clozapine-induced agranulocytosis: incidence and risk factors in the United States. *N Engl J Med* 1993;329:162–167.

511. Chengappa KNR, Gopalani A, Haught MK, et al. The treatment of clozapine-associated agranulocytosis with granulocyte colony-stimulating factor (G-CSF). *Psychopharmacol Bull* 1996;32:111–121.

512. Pollmacher T, Fenzel T, Mullington J, et al. The influence of clozapine treatment on plasma granulocyte colony-stimulating (G-CSF) levels. *Pharmacopsychiatry* 1997;31:118–121.

513. Gerson SL, Gullion G, Yeh H-S, et al. Granulocyte colony-stimulating factor for clozapine-induced agranulocytosis. *Lancet* 1992;340:1097.

514. Hagg S, Spigset O, Soderstrom TG. Association of venous thromboembolism and clozapine. *Lancet* 2000;355:1155–1156.

515. Coodin S, Ballegeer T. Clozapine therapy and pulmonary embolism. *Can J Psychiatry* 2000;45:395.

516. Kidron R, Averbuch I, Klein E, et al. Carbamazepine-induced reduction of blood levels of haloperidol in chronic schizophrenia. *Biol Psychiatry* 1985;20:219–222.

517. Jann MW, Fidone GS, Hernandez JM, et al. Clinical implications of increased antipsychotic plasma concentrations upon anticonvulsant cessation. *Psychiatr Res* 1989;28:153–159.

518. Goff DC, Midha KK, Brotman AW, et al. Elevation of plasma concentrations of haloperidol after the addition of fluoxetine. *Am J Psychiatry* 1991;148:790–792.

519. Goff DC, Baldessarini RJ. Drug interactions with antipsychotic agents. *J Clin Psychopharmacol* 1993;13:57–67.

520. Spina E, Avenoso A, Facciola G, et al. Relationship between plasma concentrations of clozapine and norclozapine and therapeutic response in patients with schizophrenia resistant to conventional neuroleptics. *Psychopharmacology (Berl)* 2000;148:83–89.

521. Cobb CD, Anderson CB, Seidel DR. Possible interaction between clozapine and lorazepam [Letter]. *Am J Psychiatry* 1991;148:1606–1607.

522. Grohmann R, Ruther E, Sassim N, et al. Adverse effects of clozapine. *Psychopharmacology* 1989;99(suppl):S101–S104.

523. Friedman LJ, Tabb SE, Sanchez CJ. Clozapine–a novel antipsychotic agent [Letter]. *N Engl J Med* 1991;325:518.

524. Miller DD. Effect of phenytoin on plasma clozapine concentrations in two patients. *J Clin Psychiatry* 1991;52:23–25.

525. Finley P, Warner D. Potential impact of valproic acid therapy on clozapine disposition. *Biol Psychiatry* 1994;36:487–488.

526. Wilson WH. Do anticonvulsants hinder clozapine treatment? *Biol Psychiatry* 1995;37:132–133.

527. Funderburg LG, Vertrees JE, True JE, et al. Seizure following addition of erythromycin to clozapine treatment. *Am J Psychiatry* 1994;151:1840–1841.

528. Szymanski S, Lieberman JA, Picou D, et al. A case report of cimetidine-induced clozapine toxicity. *J Clin Psychiatry* 1991;52:21–22.

529. Smith T, Riskin J. Effect of clozapine on plasma nortriptyline concentration. *Pharmacopsychiatry* 1994;27:41–42.

6

Indications for Antidepressants

DEPRESSIVE DISORDERS

Major depression is one of the most debilitating and common illnesses in medicine, having a major impact on social, emotional, and occupational functioning. The incidence of major depression dramatically increases from adolescence to early adulthood. The average age at onset is the late 20s, but the disorder may begin at virtually any age. It has long been recognized to run in families, suggesting the potential for a biological predisposition.

The symptoms of major depression typically evolve over a period of days to weeks. Prodromal depressive and nondepressive symptoms (e.g., generalized anxiety, panic attacks, phobias), however, may be present for months to years before the onset of a full depressive syndrome. An episode may also develop in association with severe psychosocial stress (e.g., bereavement). Although some individuals have only a single episode with full return to premorbid functioning, 50% to 85% have recurrences (1).

In summary, major depression is a heterogeneous group of disorders bound together by the presence of low mood plus disturbances in vegetative symptoms, such as:

- Sleep
- Appetite
- Sex drive
- Energy level
- Interest
- Concentration/attention (2)

This chapter provides an overview of these various conditions.

Diagnostic Criteria

A major depressive episode consists of mood changes accompanied by neurovegetative symptoms on a daily basis for at least 2 weeks. Our nosology also lists inclusion and exclusion criteria for major depressive disorder (MDD) (Table 6-1; Appendices G and H), but there are problems with these.

First, this classification takes a "Chinese menu" approach, in that a patient needs to meet only five of nine criteria in category A, and should have none in categories D or E. Thus, substantially different symptom clusters may still meet criteria for the same diagnosis. This approach increases diagnostic heterogeneity and impedes research by including patients in clinical trials with similar syndromic diagnoses but with different symptom constellations, and possibly with different pathophysiologies. The more immediate impact is to impair prediction about the natural outcome and to complicate the choice of appropriate treatment strategies. Improved diagnostic criteria would require the presence of the complete neurovegetative syndrome to meet the diagnosis of MDD. Otherwise, one could code conditions as a partial MDD, or use a completely different designation. Nonetheless, the *Diagnostic and Statistical Manual of Mental Disorders,* 4th edition (DSM-IV) (3), is an advance over the earlier diagnostic systems, which essentially based the diagnosis on the presence of a depressed mood alone.

The *reliance on a syndromic diagnosis* of MDD rather than a symptomatic diagnosis is important for prognostic and treatment planning purposes. The use of syndromes comes from factor analysis of characteristics that distinguished drug versus placebo responders in clinical trials conducted in the early 1960's, when depressed mood was the singular criterion for entry. From these studies, a mood change alone was highly predictive of a placebo response, whereas the presence of neurovegetative signs and symptoms predicted a poor response to placebo.

TABLE 6-1. _DSM-IV diagnostic criteria for a major depressive episode_

- Presence of at least five of the following symptoms during the same 2-week period (nearly every day), representing a change from previous functioning; at least one symptom is either (a) depressed mood, or (b) loss of interest or pleasure. Exclude symptoms due to a general medical condition, or mood-incongruent delusions or hallucinations
  - Depressed mood (irritable mood in children and adolescents)
  - Markedly diminished interest or pleasure in almost all activities
  - Significant weight loss or gain (failure to attain expected weight gain in children)
  - Insomnia or hypersomnia
  - Observable psychomotor agitation or retardation
  - Fatigue or loss of energy
  - Feelings of worthlessness, or of excessive or inappropriate guilt (which may be delusional)
  - Diminished ability to think or concentrate, or indecisiveness
  - Recurrent thoughts of death; recurrent suicidal ideation, plans, or attempts
- Symptoms are not due to physiologic effects of a substance or a general medical condition
- Symptoms are not better accounted for by bereavement
- Symptoms do not meet criteria for mixed episode
- Symptoms cause clinically significant distress or impairment in social, occupational, or other important areas
- Not superimposed on schizophrenia; schizophreniform disorder, delusional disorder, or psychotic disorder not specified

Melancholic Type
- The presence of at least five of the following:
  - Loss of interest or pleasure
  - Lack of reactivity to usually pleasurable stimuli
  - Depression worse in the morning
  - Frequent early awakening
  - Observable pyschomotor retardation or agitation
  - Significant weight loss or gain
  - No significant personality disturbance before first major depressive episode
  - One or more previous major episodes; previous good response to psychotropics or somatic therapy resulting in complete or nearly complete recovery

Seasonal Pattern (SAD)
- Regular temporal relationship between the onset of an episode (bipolar or major depression) and a particular 60-day period of the year
- Full remissions (or switch from depression to mania or hypomania) also occur within a particular 60-day period of the year
- Occurrence of at least three episodes of mood disturbance in three separate years (at least two consecutive) that demonstrated temporal seasonal relationship
- Seasonal episodes of mood disturbance outnumber nonseasonal episodes

Adapted from _American Psychiatric Association. Diagnostic and Statistical Manual of Mental Disorders_, 4th ed. Washington, DC: American Psychiatric Association, 1994.

An additional problem with the DSM-IV criteria is the _short duration_. In earlier nosologies (e.g., Washington University criteria), a minimum of 4 weeks was required. In double-blind, placebo-controlled trials, a duration of less than 3 months is often associated with a higher placebo response rate. **Thus, the longer an episode, the greater the clinician's confidence that a patient will need and will respond to medical intervention.**

Epidemiology

The Epidemiologic Catchment Area study found that MDD has a 1-month prevalence of 2.2% and a lifetime prevalence of 5.8% in Americans 18 years of age and older (4). However, the most recent estimate from the National Comorbidity Survey is that the 1-year prevalence rate for unipolar major depression and dysthymia is 10.3% among community residents 15 to

54 years of age (5), which translates into approximately 27 million Americans suffering from either condition in a given year. In addition, another estimated 11% of the community who do not meet full criteria for either condition have substantial depressive symptoms.

Major depression is up to three times more common in first-degree relatives of a proband with major depression when compared with the general population. It frequently occurs in individuals with co-morbid psychiatric syndromes and/or medical illness. A survey of psychiatrists found that

- 84% of their patients with major depression had *at least one co-morbid condition.*
- 61% had a *concomitant Axis I disorder.*
- 30% had an *Axis II diagnosis.*
- 58% had a *co-morbid Axis III illness* (6).

Klerman and Weissman (7) reported an increase in the rates of MDD for all ages in the years between 1960 and 1975, and an even greater increase in cohorts born after World War II. This latter observation was associated with several factors, including the following:

- A *lowering of the age of onset*, with an increase in the late teenage and early adult years
- A *persistent gender effect,* with the risk of depression consistently two to three times higher among women than men across all adult ages
- The *suggestion of a narrowing in the differential risk to men and women* because of a greater increase in the risk of depression among young men
- A *persistent family effect*, with the risk about two to three times higher in first-degree relatives as compared with control subjects, suggesting a genetic predisposition for at least some forms of depression.

Differential Diagnosis

A depressive episode may result from a diverse group of psychiatric and nonpsychiatric conditions (Table 6-2) that differ in their natural course as well as in their response to treatment. Hence, a differential diagnosis is critical to the workup of an episode.

TABLE 6-2. *Diagnostic indications for antidepressants (DSM-IV categories)*

- Mood disorders
  - Major depressive disorder
    - Single or recurrent
    - With or without melancholia
    - Seasonal pattern
  - Bipolar disorder
    - Depressed
    - Mixed
  - Cyclothymic disorder
  - Dysthymic disorder
- Psychotic disorders (e.g., schizoaffective disorder, depressive type)
- Mood disorder due to a general medical condition (e.g., dementia with depression)
- Substance-induced mood disorder (e.g., amphetamine or similarly acting sympathomimetic intoxication or withdrawal)

This workup should include all the elements outlined in Chapter 1. In the case of a patient with a major depressive episode, heightened attention should be paid to the following:

- Current or past *symptoms of mania*
- Current and past *treatment history*
- History of *substance abuse disorders*
- General *medical history*
- Thorough *review of symptoms* (particularly in elderly patients with a first-time episode)
- *Personal history* (e.g., psychologic development, response to life transitions, major life events)

Masked Depression

The first step is the recognition that a depressed mood is not synonymous with a depressive episode. Conversely, an episode of depression may not present with a mood complaint, but rather with associated symptoms such as insomnia or other somatic complaints. This is particularly true for the elderly and for those seen in primary care settings. Even when a mood complaint is prominent, it may not be described as "depressed," but instead as "irritable" or "anxious." Thus, patients with MDD may have a variety of complaints other than depressed mood, including the following:

TABLE 6-3. *Presenting complaints of depression beyond the typical symptoms*

- Prepubertal children
  - Somatic complaints
  - Agitation
  - Anxiety
  - Phobias
- Adolescents
  - Substance abuse
  - Antisocial behavior
  - Restlessness
  - Truancy and other school difficulties
  - Promiscuity
  - Rejection hypersensitivity
  - Poor hygiene
- Adults
  - Somatic complaints, particularly cerebrovascular, gastrointestinal, genitourinary
  - Low back pain or other orthopaedic symptoms
- Elderly
  - Cognitive deficits
  - Pseudodementia
  - Somatic complaints as described above for adults

- Insomnia
- Fatigue
- Various somatic complaints, such as headache or gastrointestinal distress

Failure to recognize that MDD underlies such complaints can lead to unnecessary and costly tests, as well as a delay in effective treatment. Complaints may also vary by age group. Common symptomatic issues are listed in Table 6-3.

Subsyndromal Mood Disorders

Some patients are first seen with a condition other than MDD (e.g., alcohol abuse), but the history often suggests the possibility of an underlying affective condition. Thus, a positive family history in first-degree relatives or reports consistent with an earlier, but apparently resolved, depressive episode may be critical to making the proper diagnosis. These patients may also have positive results on biological markers associated with MDD (e.g., the dexamethasone suppression test, the thyrotropin-releasing hormone test, or shortened rapid eye movement latency on the electrooculogram). In addition, a substantial percentage respond to antidepressant therapy.

Treatment-Resistant Depression

We define treatment nonresponse as the persistence of a significant depression for at least 6 weeks despite appropriate treatment (8). Appropriate treatment is defined by four D's:

- Diagnosis
- Drug
- Dose
- Duration

Incorrect diagnosis is the most common cause for nonresponse to antidepressants. Two common examples are dual depression, in which a superimposed MDD improves with antidepressant therapy but dysthymic symptoms persist and are mistaken for unimprovement, and affective disturbances associated with alcohol or drug abuse, which may persist even though symptoms of the MDD improve with drug therapy.

Noncompliance with the medication regimen is the next most common factor. Therapeutic drug monitoring can be useful to confirm suspected noncompliance. The physician can then address the reasons for noncompliance with the patient.

Subtherapeutic doses are often prescribed, especially by nonpsychiatrists. One study (9) found that 60% of depressed elderly patients were not given antidepressants, either while in the hospital or on outpatient follow-up (median interval of 45 weeks). Furthermore, most of those who were given antidepressants received doses that were generally suboptimal.

Time on treatment is another issue. Even though patients can show improvement at 2 to 3 weeks, many require at least 6 weeks before an adequate response occurs. If, however, there has not been at least partial benefit by 4 weeks, we recommend pursuing an alternative strategy.

Treatment approaches for nonresponders are discussed in more detail in Chapter 7, "Alternative Treatment Strategies."

Types of Depressive Disorders

There are several ways to subtype mood disorders (Table 6-4). *One system distinguishes functional psychiatric disorders from other medical conditions.* In DSM-III, depressive disorders occurring presumably as a consequence of

TABLE 6-4. *Subtypes of depressive disorder*

- Bipolar depression vs. unipolar depression
- Psychotic vs. nonpsychotic
- Primary psychiatric vs. secondary to other medical conditions
- Uncomplicated vs. complicated by other comorbid disorders.

medical conditions were referred to as *organic mood disorders*, which was misleading because it implied that primary mood disorders were neither "organic" nor "medical conditions." Neither conclusion was accurate because, like other medical "organic" disorders, these conditions have associated morbidity and mortality risks. As clinical neuroscience provides a better understanding of their pathophysiology, the "organic" basis will become more apparent. Thus, the DSM-IV dropped the distinction between "functional" and "organic" forms of mood disorders; instead, it distinguishes depressions that are primarily psychiatric from those that are primarily related to nonpsychiatric, medical conditions.

A second model is the primary versus secondary dichotomy (see "Secondary Type" later in this chapter).

Both the primary/psychiatric versus nonpsychiatric/medical disorder dichotomy and the uncomplicated versus complicated dichotomy are considered.

Primary Type: Major Depressive Disorder

Bipolar Versus Unipolar

The crucial element of both a bipolar and a unipolar disorder is the occurrence of an affective episode. The critical distinction is that *bipolar disorder* includes hypomanic/manic, depressive, and mixed episodes, whereas a *unipolar disorder* includes only depressive episodes. The diagnosis proceeds in a stepwise fashion:

- A patient has a *complaint* (e.g., insomnia).
- The physician determines through *questioning* that the patient has a full depressive syndrome.
- Next, the physician *rules out medical causes* for the depressive syndrome through further history taking, a physical examination, and laboratory tests.

- Finally, the physician must assess whether the patient has a *unipolar or bipolar disorder,* because patients with the latter disorder are often first seen with a depressive episode.

Although this differentiation can be difficult and sometimes not possible until a manic episode occurs, there are some clues that should help, including the following:

- The patient's age—the *younger the patient,* the greater the chance that the course will be that of a bipolar disorder on longitudinal follow-up
- A *positive family history* for bipolar disorder, particularly in first-degree relatives
- A *hypomanic phase before* the onset of the depressive episode

Hypomania consists of disturbances in the same neurovegetative functions found in depression; they are, however, qualitatively different. Moreover, they generally are not viewed as a problem by the patient. This means that patients are unlikely to complain spontaneously about such an episode, and the clinician must be alert and screen for its occurrence.

Although hypomanic and manic episodes are discussed comprehensively in Chapter 9, it is important to note that the disturbance in mania (and hypomania), as well as in depression, includes the same core symptoms, differing only in the direction of change. Complicating the diagnosis, unipolar patients may also present with classic melancholia or atypical (nonclassic) symptoms. The latter, in particular, can overlap considerably with hypomania. Similarly, bipolar patients in a depressive phase may demonstrate classic or nonclassic symptoms (Table 6-5).

Subtypes of Major Depressive Disorder

There are three subtypes of MDD: *melancholia,* or classic depression; *atypical,* or nonclassic depression; and *psychotic* depression. These three subtypes have construct validity based on differences in the following:

- *Phenomenology* (Table 6-5)
- *Family history* of the illness, especially in first-degree relatives
- *Age of onset* distributions

TABLE 6-5. *Signs and symptoms of different types of affective episodes*

Sign/Symptom	Melancholia	"Atypical" or nonclassic depression[a]	Hypomania
Mood	Depressed Anxious Irritable	Irritable Anxious Depressed	Irritable Euphoric
Affect	↓ Reactivity	↑ Reactivity	↑ Reactivity
Energy (subjective)	↓	↓	↑
Activity (objective)	↓	↑	↑
Sleep	↓	↑	↓
Appetite	↓	↑	↓
Sex drive	↓	↓	↑
Concentration/attention	↓	↓	↓
Interest	↓	↓	↑

[a] Additional signs/symptoms of "atypical" depression include leaden paralysis and rejection hypersensitivity. From Preskorn SH, Burke M. Somatic therapy for major depressive disorder: selection of an antidepressant. *J Clin Psychiatry* 1992;53 [9, Suppl.] 5–18, with permission.

- *Response rates* to specific types of drug or somatic therapies
- Incidence of positive *biological markers*

There are several reasons to acknowledge these different subtypes:

- Melancholia is considered the classic depressive disorder; thus, *nonclassic types can be misdiagnosed* (e.g., as a personality disorder), particularly because frequent and prominent symptoms include irritability, demanding demeanor, and hostility.
- *Psychotic episodes* may be misdiagnosed as schizophrenia in younger patients or dementia with paranoia in the elderly.
- *Failure to identify the specific subtype may delay the most effective treatment,* particularly with psychotic depression.
- Failure to consider *differing natural courses* of each subtype handicaps the clinician in anticipating sequelae or responding quickly when they occur.

Patients with these different subtypes also differ in terms of the likelihood that they will demonstrate abnormalities on various biological tests for MDD. Thus, these markers are most likely to be positive in psychotic depressions and least likely to be positive in "atypical" MDD, with melancholia falling between these two groups. A meta-analysis of reports on dexamethasone suppression tests found that nonsuppression was found in substantially more patients with psychotic versus nonpsychotic depression (64% versus 41%) and in only 12% of outpatients with nonmelancholic major depression (10). The fact that these tests are most often positive in psychotic MDD is also consistent with the observation that they predict a low placebo response.

Melancholia (Classic Depression). The features that distinguish melancholia from the other subtypes of MDD include the following:

- *A profoundly depressed* mood and appearance
- *Anhedonia*
- Accompanying feelings of *helplessness, hopelessness, worthlessness,* and *guilt* over imagined "sins"
- Problems with initial, middle, and terminal (or early morning awakening) *insomnia*
- Significant *anorexia,* often with appreciable *weight loss* (usually 20 or more pounds)
- Obvious *psychomotor retardation* or *agitation*
- An *absence of mood reactivity*
- A *diurnal variation* in the severity of symptoms
- Age of onset in the *mid-40s*
- *Female-to-male* ratio of 2:1

This disorder tends to occur most often in patients with a positive family history of depression, although it can occur in the absence of such a history.

Atypical (Nonclassic Depression). Another subtype has been termed "atypical" MDD to denote that the clinical presentation is different from that of the classic form, as follows:

- *Hypersomnia* rather than insomnia
- *Hyperphagia* rather than anorexia
- *Psychomotor agitation* rather than psychomotor retardation
- *Anxious* or *irritable mood* rather than dysphoria
- A *younger age of onset* than for melancholia, with a mean in the mid-20s
- *Female-to-male ratio* of about 3-4 : 1

In addition, these patients often exhibit *rejection hypersensitivity,* and a *"leaden paralysis."* They may be misdiagnosed as having a personality disorder because of the associated irritability and demanding demeanor. The presence of long-standing irritability and hostility may reflect a chronic depressive disorder and not necessarily "character" pathology. With this type of MDD, the patient tends to have a family pattern that has been designated "depressive-spectrum." Here, first-degree female relatives experience depression, whereas male relatives exhibit alcohol abuse or other unstable character traits reminiscent of antisocial personality disorder.

In 1997, a large epidemiological study found that 11.3% of individuals with lifetime major depression had only episodes meeting "atypical" criteria (11). These patients (especially male patients) may also be at greater risk for sedative-hypnotic abuse. If the clinician is cognizant of these probabilities, preventive steps can be taken (e.g., education about sedative-hypnotics). **The identification of the nonclassic forms, as well as their differences in clinical presentation, has substantial implications for their differential treatment** (see Chapter 7).

Psychotic or Delusional Depression. Psychotic depression is often characterized by the presence of mood-congruent (the symptom is consistent with the mood state) delusions or hallucinations. Age of onset tends to follow a bimodal distribution, occurring either in the young or the old. Younger patients often have a family history of bipolar disorder. The female-to-male ratio tends to approximate 1 : 1. This disorder usually has fewer psychotic symptoms than ma-

nia or schizophrenia, most often a single, mood-congruent hallucination or delusion. Delusions are more common than hallucinations, which is why the term "delusional depression" has also been used. Whether the patient presents with delusions or hallucinations has no apparent prognostic significance. Examples include the false belief that

- One has *cancer* as a punishment from God for some earlier perceived sin.
- One is *bankrupt* because of fiscal irresponsibility.
- Others have malicious intent toward one because one is *perceived as evil.*
- One is of such little value that one has *ceased to exist.*

The last two examples are often referred to as nihilistic delusions, frequently seen in older patients, who may even be convinced that their bodies have started to decay.

The presence of delusions may lead to an erroneous diagnosis of schizophrenia in younger patients or of dementia with paranoia in the elderly. Nihilistic delusions may be more subtle, particularly in the elderly, appearing as a profound sense of worthlessness and despair. When probed further, the delusional quality of their thinking becomes more apparent, facilitating the appropriate therapeutic intervention. When a patient has not benefited from antidepressant monotherapy and demonstrates significant feelings of worthlessness and hopelessness, the possibility of a psychotic MDD should be entertained.

A retrospective study of 52 delusionally depressed patients suggested that there may be various subgroups: bipolar, early onset; unipolar; and possibly unipolar, late onset (12). As with previous reports, there was a remarkably high rate of psychotic relapse in those patients who manifested psychotic symptoms at the index admission (i.e., depression or mania with psychotic features). Moreover, psychotic features were more common in bipolar than in unipolar depression.

Treatment Implications. A review of response rates found that only 35% of patients with psychotic depression responded to treatment

TABLE 6-6. *Literature review of psychotic and nonpsychotic depressed patient response to tricyclic antidepressants*

| Study | Psychotic | | | Nonpsychotic | | | Difference % recovery |
	Responders N	%	Nonresponders N	Responders N	%	Nonresponders N	
Friedman, 1961	0	0	8	11	65	6	65
Hordern, 1963	4	15	23	89	81	21	66
Simpson, 1976	8	53	7	31	86	5	33
Glassman, 1977							
adequate plasma levels	3	33	6	19	95	1	62
inadequate plasma levels	3	38	5	6	27	16	−11
Avery, Winokur, 1977	2	9	20	18	25	53	16
Davidson, 1977	0	0	3	3	100	0	100
Avery, Lubrano, 1979	72	40	109	174	68	82	28
Charney, Nelson, 1981	2	22	7	32	80	8	58
Brown, 1982	3	17	15	17	74	6	57
Nelson, 1984	2	15	11	7	58	5	43
Howarth, Grace, 1985	21	62	13	9	41	13	−21
Chan, 1987	7	44	9	48	81	11	37
Summary Results	127	35%	236	464	67%	227	32%

N, number. Adapted from Chan CH, Janicak PG, Davis JM, et al. Response of psychotic and nonpsychotic depressed patients to tricyclic antidepressants. *J. Clin Psychiatry* 1987;48:197–200.

with a tricyclic antidepressant alone versus 67% of patients with nonpsychotic depression (Table 6-6) (13). Yet these patients have a better response to electroconvulsive therapy (ECT) (14). These patients have also been found to respond to combined treatment with an antidepressant and an antipsychotic in comparison with either an antidepressant or antipsychotic alone (15). Despite these data, one study found that less than 50% of patients with psychotic depression referred to an ECT service had been treated with an antipsychotic and only 15% had received a daily dose equivalent to 200 mg or more or chlorpromazine (16).

For these reasons, we recommend that such patients receive either combination treatment with an antidepressant and an antipsychotic or ECT. Even when treated appropriately, however, patients with psychotic major depression may have a substantially higher frequency of relapse or recurrence and a shorter time to these events

when compared with nonpsychotic patients (17).

Primary Type: Other Depressive Disorders

Dysthymia (Depressive Neurosis)

Dysthymia represents a chronic but less severe form of depression. Depressed mood and partial neurovegetative symptoms are typically present for sustained periods (e.g., years). The major differences between this condition and MDD are the duration of the mood disorder, the absence of feelings of low self-esteem, worthlessness, and hopelessness, and the absence of a full neurovegetative syndrome.

There are still many questions about this condition, including the following:

• Is it a fundamentally *different condition* than MDD?

- Does it share a common *pathophysiology* or *etiology* with MMD?
- Is it the *precursor* of an MDD?
- Is it the *residue* of an incompletely remitted MDD episode?
- Is it the *sequelae* of an MDD episode that did not receive prompt and aggressive treatment?

If the answer to the last question is positive, dysthymia could represent a phenomenon consistent with the concept of "learned helplessness," which would underscore the importance of early detection and aggressive therapy of MDD.

Clinical trials have found that patients with dysthymia without a concurrent major depressive episode had a higher response rate to treatment with either a selective serotonin reuptake inhibitor (SSRI) or a tricyclic antidepressant than to placebo. These patients also experienced improvement in psychosocial functioning (18).

Dual Depression

Patients who meet criteria for both MDD and dysthymia are referred to as having a "double" or "dual" depression. This term, however, should not be used for a first episode until an adequate trial of at least three different classes of antidepressants or two classes of drug and ECT has been tried. Retrospective distortion is common in these patients, who may report having always been depressed, but remit completely with adequate therapy. Assuming a valid designation of dual depression, most clinicians manage the neurovegetative syndrome with medication while simultaneously using psychotherapeutic approaches specifically developed for mood disorders (e.g., cognitive or interpersonal psychotherapy).

Co-morbid Anxiety Disorder

The anxiety symptoms or disorders most often co-morbid with major depression include the following:

- *Panic disorder*
- *Panic attacks*
- *Obsessive-compulsive disorder*
- *Generalized anxiety* (19)

Frequently, distinguishing between depressive and anxiety disorders is difficult because patients have an admixture of symptoms. This issue has gained considerable attention because the DSM-IV diagnosis must be compatible with the International Classification of Diseases, Clinical Modification (ICD-CM) system, which includes a category termed "mixed anxiety and depression." There are, however, many unanswered questions about this category, including its incidence, etiology, natural course, and treatment response, especially as distinguished from MDD alone or various anxiety disorders alone (20).

Clarifying this matter is complicated by several issues. One has to do with the structure of assessments (e.g., Hamilton Anxiety and Depression Rating Scales), which were developed to quantitate severity and treatment-related changes, but not to determine diagnosis. Nevertheless, these scales are often used for the latter purpose in clinical trials requiring preset scores to determine enrollment. Because the scales were not designed for diagnostic purposes, they have substantial overlap, giving the impression that depressive and anxiety disorders frequently present with a mixture of symptoms.

Another issue is that many primary care physicians have difficulty distinguishing between depressive and anxiety disorders. This has led to the impression that patients in a general medical setting are more likely to have an admixture of symptoms, rather than a clearly defined condition. That depressed patients have anxiety symptoms and anxiety-disordered patients have depressive symptoms, as assessed by the Hamilton scales, are used to support this clinical impression, which ignores the fact that these scales were developed to quantitate symptoms *only after a definitive syndromic diagnosis had been made.*

Rather than postulating a new category, there may be other explanations for the phenomenon of mixed symptoms. Patients are frequently not forthright about psychiatric-related complaints because of the associated stigma. Furthermore, in the primary care setting, the amount of time a physician can spend with a patient is limited. Thus, given a reluctant historian, the ability to make the proper diagnosis is often limited.

Making an appropriate diagnosis is also complicated by the minimal psychiatric training many primary care physicians receive, compounded by the fact that many practicing physicians received their only formal exposure to psychiatry at a time when diagnosis was not emphasized, a point that deserves some elaboration. Psychiatry has undergone fundamental philosophical changes in the past 20 years. At the beginning of the 20th century, most specialties had adopted the medical model as their guiding principle for diagnosis. In this model, empirically based diagnoses are the cornerstone upon which the understanding and treatment of medical illnesses are based. In contrast, the psychoanalytic approach, which dominated psychiatry until the early 1970's, espoused principles of ego psychology, believed to be common to all psychiatric conditions. With this philosophy, the cause for all conditions was known and the treatment was the same (i.e., psychoanalytically oriented psychotherapy), making diagnosis less important.

Given this context, it is not surprising that general physicians find psychiatric differential diagnosis difficult. Whether there is a unique condition consisting of mixed anxiety and depression is not known, but before it is added to our nomenclature, there should be evidence supporting its construct validity. The following are the standard tests of such validity:

- Demonstration of a *unique clustering* of signs and symptoms
- *Reproducibility* over time (i.e., temporal stability)
- *Unique course of illness*
- *Predictability of treatment response*
- Evidence of a *common pathophysiology or etiology* (e.g., does it breed true within a given family?)

Whereas such data exist for MDD and the various anxiety-related disorders, such data do not exist for the proposed mixed anxiety and depression category.

There are also possible adverse consequences to establishing such a category (21). First, it may contribute to an even more casual practice of making a differential diagnosis by providing an ill-defined syndrome in which patients with complaints of depression and/or anxiety can be read-

ily placed. Thus, such a categorization could contribute to a decreased recognition of MDD, place patients at greater risk for sequelae such as suicide, and delay the implementation of effective treatment.

Although there is considerable overlap in drug therapies for depressive and anxiety-related disorders, there are also important differences. For example, there is no convincing evidence that benzodiazepines are effective for MDD. Even so, benzodiazepines are often the first-line treatment in the primary care setting for patients with anxiety symptoms, regardless of their psychiatric diagnosis. Finally, such a category could impede research by blurring the distinctions between MDD and anxiety-related disorders, creating a heterogenous, rather than homogeneous, grouping of patients for clinical studies. In terms of treatment, monotherapy with an antidepressant (e.g., SSRI) is often sufficient to control symptoms while also clarifying the diagnosis (see also Chapter 7).

Panic Associated with Major Depression

Approximately 25% of patients with major depression have associated past or current panic attacks. The adverse consequences of severe anxiety have been relatively unrecognized, but the possible association between panic symptoms and suicidality dramatically underscores this problem. Panic episodes have four major components:

- *Physical complaints*, such as tachycardia, dyspnea, dizziness, flushing, tremor, and sweating
- *Cognitive complaints* usually characterized as a sense of catastrophic fear of dying, losing control, or going "crazy"
- *Affective symptoms* including terror, heightened arousal, marked anticipatory anxiety, and feelings of despair and failure
- *Behavioral symptoms*, such as social withdrawal, excessive dependency, and phobic avoidance

Agoraphobia may also develop in depressed patients with panic symptoms.

Standard doses of antidepressants, especially in the earliest phases of therapy, can heighten anxiety, irritability, and restlessness. As a result, it is best to start with low doses (e.g., 5 to 10 mg per day of fluoxetine), using a gradual upward dose adjustment, as tolerated. Thus, a slower adjustment schedule in the earliest phases of treatment or the judicious addition of an anxiolytic may be helpful.

Avoiding drugs that lower the threshold for panic symptoms, such as caffeine or over-the-counter stimulants, may also help. Some phobic symptoms are managed by *in vivo exposure* or *cognitive therapy*. In general, the best approach is a combination of pharmacotherapy and psychotherapy, in particular, cognitive behavioral techniques.

Finally, because patients with panic disorder and major depression are frequently sensitive to any adverse effects of antidepressants, it is generally advisable to start at a reduced dose and gradually adjust the dose to the usually effective level to achieve the intended benefit.

Seasonal Affective Disorder

Seasonal affective disorder (SAD) is a recurrent depressive illness that regularly coincides with particular seasons (22–25). Such a phenomenon is consistent with the influence of seasonal and other environmental factors on mood changes, which have been described for more than two millennia. The two predominant presentations have bimodal peaks of depression onset, either in the spring or in the fall. The spring-onset type (SOSAD) is usually more severe, albeit less frequent, and is associated with a greater risk of suicide, hospitalization, and the need for somatic therapies (i.e., electron convulsive therapy [ECT]). The fall-onset type (FOSAD) is more common, results in less severe depressive episodes, is typically managed on an outpatient basis, and poses less danger of suicide. Full remission in the summer months is a diagnostic criteria for FOSAD, with patients noting significant increases in energy and productivity during this period. As many as 25% of patients actually meet clinical criteria for hypomania, perhaps precipitated by a sudden resolution of the depressive episode in the late winter–early spring period (see Table 6-1 for DSM-IV criteria).

Wehr and Rosenthal (26) have reported both differences and similarities between SOSAD and FOSAD. Specifically, vegetative signs differ between these two seasonal conditions, with atypical symptoms predominating in FOSAD and more typical and more severe symptoms in SOSAD. Furthermore, studies indicate that FOSAD may be precipitated by light deficiency and responds to treatment with bright light. Contributing factors to SOSAD are less well established, but some preliminary data indicate that warmer ambient temperature may be one possible triggering mechanism. At higher latitudes, FOSAD tends to be longer and more severe. In contrast, SOSAD is more severe at lower latitudes (27). More recently, Schwartz and colleagues (28) followed up a group of 59 patients with SAD for an average interval of 8.8 years and noted that the pattern of winter depression and summer remission remained fairly persistent.

Epidemiology. SAD appears to have a prevalence rate of about 4% to 6%, with a female-to-male ratio of about 4:1. Another 20% of the population describe symptoms consistent with SAD that do not meet diagnostic criteria for severity. There appears to be a correlation with age, such that the mean age of onset is in the mid-20s.

Although there appears to be a familial pattern, there are no definitive data demonstrating a hereditary component. Studies from four different centers have found a greater incidence of mood disorders in the first-degree relatives of SAD patients. For example, in 294 subjects studied, Rosenthal and Wehr (29) found a family history of mood disorders in 55% and of alcoholism in 36%. The majority of patients (i.e., about 80%) tend to be female, young, white, and in the middle to upper middle class socioeconomically. Many fall in the mild-to-moderate level of severity in terms of their depression, and few have previous histories of antidepressant therapy or hospitalization for their mood disturbance. Severity of episodes may relate to their length, which varies from an average of 5 months in Maryland to 6 months in the Chicago area, perhaps reflecting differences in latitude and the relative length of winter.

Clinical Presentation. Rosenthal and Wehr (29, 30) have described SAD as an MDD but noted that many who suffer from this condition have atypical symptoms, including the following:

- *Increased* rather than decreased *sleep*
- *Increased* rather than decreased *appetite,* with increased food intake
- *Carbohydrate craving*
- Marked *increases in weight*, as well as more typical symptoms, such as *decreased energy* or fatigue and *social withdrawal*

Reports vary as to the predominant picture, which ranges from one quite similar to melancholia to one more consistent with an atypical depressive disorder or a bipolar II disorder (Table 6-5). Complaints usually involve a diminution in energy, followed by an increased need for sleep, increased appetite and weight, and a lack of involvement or interest in one's activities. Only toward the end of the episode onset does the patient become aware of the depressed mood and such classic symptoms as poor concentration, feelings of self-worthlessness, and multiple somatic complaints. Insomnia often develops over the next 1 to 2 months. Whereas this atypical picture is more characteristic of the early phases of the illness, reminiscent of certain bipolar subtypes, the affective episode appears to evolve toward a more classic depressive syndrome as it progresses over multiple seasons.

Conclusion. Evidence for the syndromal validity of SAD is strong, and perhaps even stronger than for other established diagnoses such as dysthymia. *Phototherapy* has been shown to be effective for SAD but does not produce as much improvement as occurs with the season change to summer, suggesting that some factor other than light may be operable (31). *Circadian hypotheses* have been most frequently used to explain the mechanism of action of bright light therapy, as well as the pathophysiology of SAD; results, however, are inconclusive (see Chapter 8).

Patients with SAD have been found to be resistant to exacerbation of depressive symptoms following acute tryptophan depletion (32), suggesting that dysfunction of central serotonin mechanisms may be less relevant to the pathophysiology of SAD than other forms of major depression.

Secondary Type: Complicating Disorders

Another model of mood disorder subtyping is the primary versus secondary dichotomy. This model distinguishes a primary depressive disorder from a syndrome chronologically secondary to another psychiatric or medical condition. "Secondary" simply designates the timing of the mood disorder in reference to another psychiatric or medical problem. The concept of "secondary" is not meant to suggest causality, although such an inference is often assumed. This dichotomy found its major use in identifying mood disorders alone versus those associated with another "co-morbid" psychiatric condition such as alcohol dependence. The distinction is valuable because mood disorders complicated by another illness have a poorer natural prognosis and a poorer response to therapy.

Before making a definitive diagnosis of a primary depression or concluding the existence of treatment resistance, one must consider the possibility of another concurrent, confounding medical or psychiatric disorder, in addition to depression.

Medical Disorders

Physical problems that may complicate or underlie a depressive condition include the following:

- Subclinical *hypothyroidism*
- *Malabsorption* resulting from various gastrointestinal conditions (e.g., Crohn's disease)
- Unrecognized *malignancies*
- Chronic *renal failure*
- Coexisting *dementia*
- *Autoimmune disorder* (e.g., systemic lupus erythematosus).

Most of these conditions are chronic and debilitating, and their underlying mechanisms are not well understood. Postulated relationships include demoralization and depression resulting from the anorexia and malaise caused by profound systemic effects. These disorders may also affect the amine systems that are thought to mediate the depressive syndrome.

Malignancies, particularly of neural crest origin, are known to affect brain function adversely through remote (presumably hormonal) effects on neural tissue. For example, ovarian adenocarcinoma can selectively induce a profound cerebellar syndrome caused by the selective death of Purkinje cells (presumably from a neurotoxic hormonal factor). Such phenomena simply illustrate the complicated nature of CNS functioning and the need to be cautious about explanations in the absence of systematic data.

Brain lesions that produce depression can be divided into structural and biochemical types. Any disease that produces a mass lesion or deficit in the frontal lobes can cause a depressive syndrome. Typically, occurrence and severity are correlated with proximity to the tip of the frontal lobe rather than to the extent of motor function loss. The most extensively studied lesions are *strokes*, but *tumors* and *plaques* related to multiple sclerosis can both produce similar results.

Lesions on the left side, closer to the tip of the frontal lobe, are the most likely to produce depression. Such lesions result in bilateral cortical depletion of CNS amines, again implicating these neurotransmitters in the pathogenesis. Furthermore, treatments that potentiate norepinephrine transmission have been effective in reversing such syndromes.

Biochemical lesions that induce depressive syndromes include such classic examples as *Parkinson's* and *Huntington's* diseases, especially early in their courses. These disorders involve derangements of central amine systems (i.e., in Parkinson's, there is a disturbance in both dopamine and norepinephrine; in Huntington's, dopamine is affected, as well as other nonbiogenic amine neural circuits). Furthermore, antidepressants and ECT, which potentiate central neurotransmission, have effectively relieved depression associated with Parkinson's disease.

Treatment of these disorders has received less systematic study, in part because these patients are more diverse in terms of their health status, leading to potentially complicating alterations in the pharmacokinetics and pharmacodynamics of antidepressants.

As with any decision to initiate an antidepressant trial, it should be based on the potential risks and benefits. The limited evidence that exists indicates that both drugs and ECT can be used safely and effectively in such patients when appropriate allowances are made for health status. Empirical trials are wanting but clearly warranted.

Concurrent Psychiatric Disorders

Concurrent psychiatric disorders frequently occur in the context of depression. For example, as noted earlier, there is a high incidence of *anxiety disorders* co-morbid with depression.

Personality disorders can complicate management (e.g., borderline disorder with a superimposed MDD). *Dual depression* occurs in patients who have chronic dysthymic disorder and then experience a superimposed MDD. *Substance abuse and dependence* are frequently comorbid with mood disorders and substantially increase depression-related morbidity and mortality rates (see "Drug-Induced Syndromes").

Concurrent Psychosocial Issues

Significant *psychosocial stressors* that are not addressed and ameliorated are frequently assumed to contribute to persistent depressive symptomatology despite adequate pharmacologic intervention. In such situations, supportive, interpersonal, and cognitive therapy may be necessary adjuncts to medication.

Drug-Induced Syndromes

Conditions mimicking MDD can occur secondary to a wide variety of prescribed and illicit agents. With some drugs, the syndrome occurs as a direct and immediate effect. For example, some *antihypertensive agents* (e.g., reserpine, α-methyldopa) acutely antagonize central biogenic amine neurotransmitter systems.

This phenomenon is one of the pillars of the biogenic amine hypothesis of depression (see "Suicide" later in this chapter). An intriguing finding with reserpine is that those susceptible to a depressive syndrome while on this agent also have an increased likelihood of a personal or family history of MDD, in comparison with those who are not susceptible. This finding suggests an interaction between a constitutional predisposition and the biochemical effects of this drug. Because depression is a common disorder, we would expect some cases to occur by chance alone with every medical drug (e.g., depression has been reported in patients on clonidine, propranolol, and calcium antagonists). Thus, the development of a depressive episode on a drug (e.g., propranolol) could be coincidence, or there could be a causal relationship. To establish a causal relationship would require adequately controlled and powered studies, but such work is rarely done.

Other agents may also produce a depressive syndrome after lengthy or repeated use. This is generally true with certain drugs of potential abuse such as *psychostimulants and sedative-hypnotics*. Again, antagonistic effects on biogenic amines appear to be critical in the pathophysiology of the resultant depression.

Acutely, *psychostimulants* (e.g., cocaine, amphetamines) act as indirect agonists of biogenic amines, causing their release and inhibiting their neuronal reuptake. Repeated exposure, however, causes a depletion of central amines, similar to the action of reserpine. The syndrome produced by cocaine is initially reversible with the addition of higher doses, but over time, profound neurotransmitter depletion occurs that cannot be ameliorated by further drug increases. This phenomenon has been termed "burnout" and creates a vicious cycle critical to the addiction potential of this agent, as well as other psychostimulants. The first step in treatment is to discourage drug abuse through education. When the condition is more advanced, treatment often involves detoxification with an antidepressant (e.g., desipramine) that potentiates the effects of any remaining central biogenic amines. Antidepressants have also been used to reduce cocaine craving, thereby decreasing the likelihood of relapse. This is important because higher levels of depressive symptoms during substance abuse treatment are associated with a greater urge to use cocaine and other drugs, as well as a higher likelihood of relapse (33).

Alcohol abuse and dependence are the most common causes of drug-induced depressive syndromes. As with psychostimulants, alcohol's effect requires chronic, sustained exposure, but unlike with psychostimulants, symptoms generally occur as a result of withdrawal and are reversed by its reinstitution. Gradual depletion of central amines, particularly serotonin, appears to be an important pathogenic factor. With chronic exposure, alcohol produces a decrease in cerebrospinal fluid (CSF) 5-hydroxyindoleacetic acid (5-HIAA) and an increased density of serotonin-2 (5- HT_2) receptors in the neocortex, similar to the findings observed in at least a subset of naturally occurring depressive disorders. Thus, chronic alcohol exposure may produce a phenocopy of MDD because it causes a derangement in central neurotransmitter systems similar to that underlying primary mood disorders.

Nevertheless, depressive episodes among alcohol-dependent men and women are heterogeneous in terms of both causation and clinical course. Studies have shown differences between patients with the onset of major depression before alcohol dependence or during a long abstinence period (i.e., independent major depression) versus those who experience depressive symptoms only in association with alcohol use (34). Specifically, the former are more likely to:

- Be married
- Be white
- Be female
- Have attempted suicide
- Have a close relative with a major mood disorder

For such patients, aggressive treatment of their mood disorder may be particularly important in achieving and maintaining sobriety.

Other *sedative-hypnotics* (e.g., benzodiazepines) are also capable of producing a phenomenologically similar syndrome during the withdrawal phase of addiction, but the mechanisms responsible are not well understood. The possibility that common mechanisms are involved is supported by the fact that a depression induced by one class of sedative-hypnotics can be reversed by another class. For example, benzodiazepines can reverse the syndrome induced by alcohol withdrawal.

TABLE 6-7. *Indications for antidepressants: other mood disorders*

- Alzheimer's dementia with depression
- Vascular dementia with depression
- Premenstrual dysphoric disorder
- Postpartum depression
- Adjustment disorder with depressed mood
- Bereavement

Other Disorders

Antidepressants may also be useful for other mood and nonmood disorders (Tables 6-7 and 6-8).

SUICIDE

Major depression is a significant risk factor for suicide. The presence of suicidal ideation should be assessed initially and repeatedly over the course of treatment. **In this respect, depressive disorders are a major health care problem, contributing to 70% of suicide-related deaths** (with a 15% mortality risk associated with suicide in untreated recurrent major episodes).

Epidemiology

Suicide is the ninth leading cause of death in the United States for all ages. Among teenagers and young adults, it is the third most frequent cause of death. Approximately 40,000 to 50,000 Americans die every year by their own hand. Thus, suicide claims more lives annually in the United States than leukemia or kidney disease. Suicide also seriously affects relatives, friends, and co-workers who were close to the victim. Suicide potential is the highest among middle-aged men and women, is more prevalent among whites, and is frequently preceded by work or legal problems, which themselves could be the result (as opposed to the cause) of antecedent and often untreated psychiatric disorders.

There has been an alarming increase in the rate of suicide over the past 30 years, especially for young men, both white and black. Suicide deaths in this cohort (i.e., the ages of 18 to 30 years) increased nearly 150% between 1960 and 1980, paralleled by increased substance abuse and depressive disorders. A possible new factor is the report of social contagion, as evidenced by clusters or miniepidemics of suicide that mimic the original method.

Assessment of Suicide Potential

Clinicians may be reluctant to ask about suicidal ideation because of their own discomfort with the topic, or for fear of offending the patient. The latter virtually never occurs when the topic is approached in a stepwise, empathic manner. Instead, such an approach typically generates relief

TABLE 6-8. *Indications for antidepressants: other psychiatric and medical conditions*

- Sleep disorders (see Chapters 11 and 12)
  - Insomnia
  - Somnambulism
  - Night terrors
  - Sleep apnea
  - Narcolepsy (including cataplexy)
  - Functional enuresis
- Anxiety disorders (see Chapters 11–13)
  - Phobic disorders
  - Panic disorder
  - Obsessive-compulsive disorder
  - Generalized anxiety disorder
  - Posttraumatic stress disorder
- Eating disorders (see Chapter 14, "The Eating Disordered Patient")
  - Bulimia
  - Anorexia
- Attention deficit and disruptive behavior disorder (see Chapter 14, "The Child and Adolescent Patient")
- Substance-related disorder
  - Cocaine craving
  - Certain paraphilias
  - Pain syndromes
    - Headaches (e.g., intractable migraine)
    - Bone pain secondary to metastases (see Chapter 14, "The Dying Patient")
    - Pain disorder (see Chapter 13, "Somatoform Disorder"),
    - Chronic pain
- Gastrointestinal
  - Irritable bowel syndrome
- Genitourinary
  - Enuresis
- Cardiovascular
  - Arrhythmias
- Miscellaneous
  - Mild immune dysfunction
  - Some dermatologic disorders

and appreciation that the clinician has recognized the seriousness of a patient's complaints. The first step is to elicit the depressive symptoms and acknowledge the patient's distress. Next, the examiner empathically inquires whether these symptoms have ever led to feelings that life is not worth living. At this point, patients often spontaneously discuss suicide. If not, they may acknowledge that life seems hopeless and bleak, allowing the clinician to inquire about any death wishes or thoughts about taking one's life. The importance of a clinician's sensitivity to the potential for suicide is borne out by studies showing that many victims (more than 70%) visit a physician within 2 months preceding their death (35). Because suicide is usually the result of a treatable illness, its identification and appropriate management can avert an unnecessary tragedy.

Risk Factors

Although direct inquiry about suicide is the single most critical part of an evaluation, one should also ask about other risk factors associated with completed suicide. Although there is no fail-safe method for identifying all patients at serious risk, knowledge of these factors can help estimate its likelihood.

Psychiatric-Related Risk Factors

By far, the most important contributor to suicide is a serious psychiatric disorder, with MDD, bipolar disorder, schizophrenia, and substance abuse being most closely associated with suicide. The male-to-female ratio is less pronounced among psychiatric patients than in the general population, with a higher rate in unmarried psychiatric patients living alone. The lifetime probability of death by suicide in various psychiatric disorders is estimated to be between 10% and 15%, contrasting with less than a 1% lifetime probability in those without a psychiatric disorder.

Older persons account for one-third of all suicides in the United States even though this group represents only 12% of the population (36). Suicide is even more often related to major depression in the elderly than in younger individuals in whom other causes such as substance abuse,

bipolar disorder, schizophrenia, and personality disorders often play a major role. In fact, suicide rates are highest in older white men relative to any other segment of the population. For example, white men older than 85 years age commit suicide 30 times as frequently as black women.

Black and colleagues (37) studied suicide in subtypes of major mood disorders and compared them with the general population in Iowa. They found an increased risk in all psychiatric groups except for female patients with bipolar mood disorder, which was associated with a lower risk in comparison with unipolar disorders. Seventy-three percent of all suicides occurred during the first few years of follow-up. This trend was particularly pronounced in primary unipolar female patients and bipolar male patients.

Beck et al. (38) reported that hopelessness in the context of major depression was the MDD symptom most often associated with suicide. This finding was replicated by Fawcett et al. (39), who found that hopelessness with anhedonia, mood cycling within an episode, loss of mood reactivity, and psychotic delusions were high-risk factors for a subsequent suicide. Soloff and associates (40) also found that hopelessness and impulse aggression independently increased the risk of suicidal behavior in patients with borderline personality disorder and in patients with major depression. Negative life events (e.g., the death of a loved one or humiliating events such as financial ruin) often precede suicide.

Johnson and co-workers (41) found that the lifetime rate of suicide attempts with uncomplicated panic disorder was about 7%, which is consistently higher than that of the general population without a psychiatric disorder (i.e., about 1%). The researchers concluded that panic disorder, either uncomplicated or as a "co-morbid" illness, led to a risk of suicide attempts comparable with those of major depression ("co-morbid" or uncomplicated). Their data were derived from the Epidemiologic Catchment Area Study, with a probability sample of more than 18,000 adults living in five United States communities.

In a second review of these data, Weissman et al. (42) found that 20% of patients with panic disorder and 12% of those with panic attacks had made suicide attempts. These results could not be explained by the coexistence of major depression, nor the presence of alcohol or drug abuse. They concluded that panic disorder or attacks were associated with an increased risk of suicidal ideation and attempts.

One-fourth to one-half of all completed suicides were by psychiatric patients who had a history of a prior attempt. Thus, the majority of those who attempted suicide did not ultimately go on to complete the act, with estimates placing the ratio of attempters to completers at approximately 8:1. The absence of past suicide attempts does not guarantee or substantially reduce the risk of suicide if other risk factors are present. This risk factor is counterintuitive and, therefore, deserves special mention. Most individuals who die of suicide do so on their first or second attempt. Thus, the absence of a prior attempt should not minimize concern about its risk. In fact, the absence of previous attempts in a first-time, profoundly depressed middle- or late-life patient who has other risk factors (as discussed) should increase rather than diminish concern. Because suicide completions usually occur on the first or second attempt, multiple attempters (i.e., greater than five) are at greater risk for future attempts rather than completion.

In summary, the *risk factors for suicide in psychiatric patients* include the following:

- *Male* sex
- *Middle age,* in contrast to the general population, where the elderly are at greatest risk
- *Race*–whites are at a much higher risk than blacks
- *Depression* and *schizophrenia*–the primary psychiatric diagnoses associated with completed suicides
- *History of a suicide attempt* (but not multiple attempts)
- *Adverse life events*
- *Hospitalization*
- The *6- to 12-month period after discharge* (this interval risk is particularly true among women in the first 6 months after hospitalization)

Treatment-Related Risk Factors

One noteworthy naturalistic study (43) compared the incidence of suicidal behavior with the prescribed dose of heterocyclic antidepressant (HCA) and found the rate was 22% for low doses (i.e., less than 75 mg per day) but decreased progressively as the HCA dose was increased (i.e., 11% at 75 to 149 mg per day; 1% at 150 to 249 mg per day; and 0.5% at 250+ mg per day). This finding is even more remarkable considering that the more severely ill patients would be receiving the higher doses.

Epidemiologic Risk Factors

Middle-aged or older individuals who complete suicide tend to suffer from a depressive disorder. Younger individuals who complete suicide usually suffer from schizophrenia or a bipolar disorder. The risk factors for suicide attempts versus completions are the following:

- **For suicide attempts**
  - Female sex
  - Recent stressful life event
  - Impulsivity
  - Previous attempts
- **For suicide completions**
  - Male sex
  - A psychiatric disorder
  - A family history of suicide
- **For suicide completions in patients younger than age 30 years**
  - Male sex
  - American Indian or white
  - Depression and other mood disorders
  - Current substance abuse
  - Eating disorders
  - A history of prior attempts (but not more than five)
  - Social contagion (perhaps most critical in American Indians)
  - A family history

Generally, the clinical and the psychosocial factors that combine to increase the risk of suicide have a high sensitivity but a low specificity. Because only a small minority who meet these criteria successfully complete suicide, the clinician's task of accurately assessing risks is exceedingly difficult.

History-Related Risk Factors

Some data indicate that those who make multiple attempts (i.e., greater than five) are different from those who will die from suicide. Multiple suicide attempters tend to be younger and to have a diagnosis other than a depressive disorder (e.g., antisocial, histrionic, or borderline personality). Although they are likely to make future attempts, they do not constitute a substantial proportion of those who die of suicide.

Medical Risk Factors

Most patients with medical disorders who commit suicide, even those with terminal disorders, have concurrent treatable major depression. In addition, the type of medical condition may increase risk. Thus, patients with respiratory diseases are three times more likely to commit suicide than patients with other medical conditions. Those on hemodialysis or who suffer from cancer also constitute high-risk groups, in comparison with the general population.

Substance Abuse-Related Risk Factors

The relationship between alcohol abuse and suicide has been recognized for many years, with at least one in five suicide victims being intoxicated at the time of their death. Alcohol may lower inhibitions, serving as a precipitant to the act, or the disease of alcoholism itself could be a risk factor. Alcohol also induces biochemical changes (e.g., lowers CSF 5-HIAA and decreases 5-HT_2 receptors in the neocortex), similar to changes observed in at least a subset of depressive disorders. Thus, alcohol may aggravate or contribute to the pathophysiology that mediates the depressive syndrome and leads to suicide completions.

Roy and colleagues (44) studied approximately 300 alcoholics, of whom 20% attempted suicide. In comparing the attempters with nonattempters, there were a number of predictors:

* Sex and age: *younger women*
* Lower *socioeconomic status*
* Consumption of greater *alcohol amounts*

* Onset of alcohol-related problems at an *earlier age*
* An apparent increase in *additional lifetime psychiatric diagnoses,* including
  * Major depression
  * Panic disorder
  * Phobic disorder
  * Generalized anxiety disorder
  * Antisocial personality disorder
  * Substance abuse
* Significantly more first- or second-degree alcoholic relatives

Murphy and Wetzel (45) concluded that the current estimate of 11% to 15% lifetime risk of suicide in alcoholics was not tenable based on a more careful examination of the data, and was probably more in the range of 2% to 3.4%. This percentage is still in contrast with the approximate 1% annual incidence of suicide in the United States. Much of the increase, however, could be related to another Axis I diagnosis (e.g., bipolar disorder).

The characteristics of alcoholic patients who committed suicide include the following:

* *Male* sex
* 20 to 40 years of *age*
* *Concurrent abusers of alcohol plus other drugs of abuse* (e.g., opiates, sedatives, psychostimulants, amphetamines, cocaine)

The relationship between suicide and other drugs of abuse typically involves a pattern of chronic use, an earlier age of onset, and a prior history of drug overdose. Often there is a childhood history of hyperactivity or parental abuse or a family history of depression, suicide, or alcoholism. As with alcohol, other substances can decrease inhibition or markedly impair judgment, turning a gesture into a completed suicide. **Clinicians should assume that patients with a history of substance abuse are at a higher risk for impulsive behavior that may place them or others in jeopardy.** In obtaining a history, specific questions in addition to suicidal ideation or behavior should include the following:

* Prior *drug overdoses*
* *Accidents*

TABLE 6-9. *Hidden cost of not treating major depressive disorder*

Mortality	Morbidity	Societal cost
• 30,000–35,000 MDD suicides per year • Accidents due to impaired concentration and attention • Death due to illnesses that can be sequelae (e.g., alcohol abuse)	• Suicide attempts • Accidents • Associated illnesses • Lost jobs • Failure to advance • Substance abuse	• Dysfunctional families • Absenteeism • Decreased productivity • Job-related injuries • Adverse effect on quality control

MDD, major depressive disorder.

- Serious *risk-taking behavior*
- *Legal difficulties*
- Recent increasing *pattern of abuse*
- Recent *interpersonal losses*

Because maintaining a drug habit often involves criminal activities, one should also inquire about access to guns or other lethal weapons. Every effort should be made to remove weapons from the home, if possible, especially if there is a serious risk of suicide in the near future.

Biological Risk Factors

There are a number of biochemical findings associated with suicide. One example is the 5-HT system, with such findings as the following:

- *Lower CSF 5-HIAA* concentrations in those who attempt violent and impulsive suicide
- *Lower brain serotonin or 5-HIAA* concentrations in suicide victims
- A greater frequency of *tryptophan hydroxylase U allele* in patients who had attempted suicide (46)
- Increased *density of serotonin receptors* (particularly 5-HT$_2$ receptors in the neocortex and in platelets), consistent with decreased activity of presynaptic serotonin
- Increased *platelet 5-HT$_{2A}$ receptors* in suicidal patients independent of diagnosis (47, 48)

The clinical implications of such data point to a relationship between abnormalities in the central serotonin system and self-injurious behavior. These findings have led to an interest in developing specific drugs that alter 5-HT activity to treat suicidality, impulsivity, and aggressivity independent of any specific psychiatric disorder.

Central serotonin function can be enhanced by agents such as lithium and various serotonin reuptake inhibitors. Recent studies have found that the use of such agents is associated with reductions in the likelihood of suicide attempts and completions in both patients with major depression and those with cluster B personality disorders (49, 50).

In summary, the issue of suicide should always be considered in depressed patients and gently but thoroughly explored during the initial evaluation. Subsequent reinquiry is also critical, given the possibility of an increased incidence of suicide during the early phases of treatment and recovery, as well as during the period just after hospitalization.

Other Causes of Death

Depressive disorders can lead to death in other ways (Table 6-9). For example, depressed individuals are more prone to accidents that result from their impaired concentration and attention. They also often attempt to self-medicate, particularly with alcohol or other sedative agents, which may lead to death as a result of organ toxicity, as well as accidents. Psychotic depressive patients may act irrationally, putting themselves at greater physical risk. Although rare today, patients have died of severe malnutrition secondary to catatonic symptoms that precluded the ability to care for their basic needs. Depression can also contribute to a higher morbidity and mortality rate in patients with co-morbid medical disorders. For example, a large database indicates that depression may predispose to the development of ischemic heart disease and increase the risk of cardiac-related death (51).

OTHER COSTS OF MAJOR DEPRESSION

Depressive disorders can also cause substantial morbidity. Injury or illness occurs secondary to suicide attempts, accidents, substance abuse, malnutrition, or irrational behavior resulting from psychosis. Failure to seek medical attention for intercurrent medical disorders may occur because of apathy, feelings of guilt, or low self-esteem. Finally, impaired concentration and attention, a lack of energy, or anhedonia can all substantially impair psychosocial functioning (e.g., failure to advance in one's career or in school; job loss; social isolation; dysfunctional home life, including divorce).

Attempts have been made to calculate the societal cost of MDD in terms of health care utilization, absenteeism from work, decreased productivity, job-related injuries, and adverse effects on quality control because of impaired concentration and attention. In a prospective study of 3,000 patients, depression was related to poorer physical health and increased health care utilization (52). In the same study, employed individuals had a five times greater risk of using disability days. In another study, disability because of major depression was similar to or worse than chronic medical illnesses such as hypertension, diabetes mellitus, and arthritis (53).

Conservative estimates of direct and indirect costs of major depression in the United States resulting from the associated morbidity and mortality exceed $30 billion. Most of this cost is due to indirect expenses to society, such as decreased productivity and increased need for social services because of disability. In addition, there is the cost to family caregivers, the failure to advance in one's career or education, lost leisure time, and the pain and suffering endured by depressed patients and their families (54, 55). The societal cost of depressive disorders is estimated to be approximately $45 billion annually (56).

Recognition of these costs has led to the concept of the "medical offset effect"; that is, the savings in medical care may be sufficient to outweigh the cost of mental health treatment. For example, depressed elderly medical inpatients have been found to use more hospital and outpatient medical services than nondepressed patients but are not more likely to receive more mental health services (57). This fact is remarkable when compared with other studies that have shown that depression treatment consumes only 8 cents of every health care dollar spent on patients with depression (58). Moreover, patients who stay on their antidepressant regimens for at least 6 months are more likely to experience significant reductions in the cost of medical care services (59). Given these findings, it is not surprising that a net mean annual economic savings of $877 was found when depression treatment was delivered in the mental health sector compared with the general medical sector (55). Thus, medical offset may make it counterproductive for health insurance companies to limit mental health care and to encourage primary care physicians to provide what care is permitted. In this context, a 15-year follow-up study found that 80% of depressed individuals had a poor outcome (i.e., committed suicide, remained ill, or experienced a recurrence) without effective treatment (60).

CONCLUSION

Depression is common, is frequently unrecognized or underestimated, and may be deadly. For example, 50% of completed suicides are associated with a major depressive episode. Furthermore, depression can adversely affect life activities in a variety of ways. Medical disorders such as cardiovascular disease are also affected by depression, often predicting future cardiac events and hastening death, which is unfortunate, given that there is a very specific set of diagnostic criteria and that there is a variety of effective pharmacologic and somatic therapies (see Chapter 7) (8).

REFERENCES

1. Mueller TI, Leon AC, Keller MB, et al. Recurrence after recovery from major depressive disorder during 15 years of observational follow-up. *Am J Psychiatry* 1999;156:1001–1006.
2. Kendler KS, Gardner CO Jr. Boundaries of major depression: an evaluation of DSM-IV criteria. *Am J Psychiatry* 1998;155:172-177.
3. American Psychiatric Association. *Diagnostic and Statistical Manual of Mental Disorders,* 4th ed. Washington, DC: American Psychiatric Press, 1994.

4. Regier D, Farmer M, Rae D, et al. One-month prevalence of mental disorders in the United States and sociodemographic characteristics: the Epidemiologic Catchment Area study. *Acta Psychiatr Scand* 1993;88:35–47.
5. Kessler RC, McGonagle KA, Zhao S, et al. Lifetime and 12-month prevalence of DSM- III-R psychiatric disorders in the United States: results from the National Comorbidity Survey. *Arch Gen Psychiatry* 1994;51:8–19.
6. Pincus HA, Zarin DZ, Tanielian TL, et al. Psychiatric patients and treatments in 1997: findings from the American Psychiatric Practice Research Network. *Arch Gen Psychiatry* 1999;56:442–449.
7. Klerman GL, Weissman MM. Increasing rates of depression. *JAMA* 1989;261:2229–2235.
8. Janicak PG, Martis B. Strategies for treatment-resistant depression. *Clin Cornerstone* 1999;1(4):58–71.
9. Koenig HG, George LK, Meador KG. Use of antidepressants by nonpsychiatrists in the treatment of medically ill hospitalized depressed elderly patients. *Am J Psychiatry* 1997;154:1369–1375.
10. Nelson JC, Davis JM. DST studies in psychotic depression: a meta-analysis. *Am J Psychiatry* 1997;154:1497–1503.
11. Levitan RD, Lesage A, Parikh SV, et al. Reversed neurovegetative symptoms of depression: a community study of Ontario. *Am J Psychiatry* 1997;154:934–940.
12. Aronson TA, Shukla S, Hoff A, et al. Proposed delusional depression subtypes: preliminary evidence from a retrospective study of phenomenology and treatment course. *J Affect Disord* 1988;14:69–74.
13. Chan CH, Janicak PG, Davis JM, et al. Response of psychotic and nonpsychotic depressed patients to tricyclic antidepressants. *J Clin Psychiatry* 1987;48:197–200.
14. Janicak PG, Easton M, Comaty JE, et al. Efficacy of ECT in psychotic and nonpsychotic depression. *Convuls Ther* 1989;5:314–320.
15. Spiker DG, Weiss JC, Dealy RS, et al. The pharmacological treatment of delusional depression. *Am J Psychiatry* 1985;142:430–436.
16. Mulsant BH, Haskett RF, Prudic J, et al. Low use of neuroleptic drugs in the treatment of psychotic major depression. *Am J Psychiatry* 1997;154:559–561.
17. Flint AJ, Rifat SL. Two-year outcome of psychotic depression in late life. *Am J Psychiatry* 1998;155:178–183.
18. Kocsis JH, Zisook S, Davidson J, et al. Double-blind comparison of sertraline, imipramine, and placebo in the treatment of dysthymia: psychosocial outcomes. *Am J Psychiatry* 1997;154:390–395.
19. Fogelson DL, Bystritsky A, Sussman N. Interrelationships between major depression and the anxiety disorders: clinical relevance. *Psychiatr Ann* 1988;18:158–167.
20. Boulenger JP, Lavallée YJ. Mixed anxiety and depression. Diagnostic issues. *J Clin Psychiatry* 1993;54[Suppl 1]:3–8.
21. Preskorn SH, Fast G. Beyond signs and symptoms: the case against a mixed anxiety and depression category. *J Clin Psychiatry* 1993;54:24–32.
22. Lahmeyer HW. Seasonal affective disorders. *Psychiatr Med* 1991;9:105–114.
23. Blehar MC, Rosenthal NE. Seasonal affective disorders and phototherapy: report of a National Institute of Mental Health-Sponsored Workshop. *Arch Gen Psychiatry* 1989;46:469–474.
24. Eagles JM, Wileman SM, Cameron IM, et al. Seasonal affective disorder among primary care attenders and a community sample in Aberdeen. *Br J Psychiatry* 1999;175:472–475.
25. Magnusson A. An overview of epidemiological studies on seasonal affective disorder. *Acta Psychiatr Scand* 2000;101:176–184.
26. Wehr TA, Rosenthal NE. Seasonality and affective illness. *Am J Psychiatry* 1989;146:829–839.
27. Rosen LN, Moghadam LZ. Patterns of seasonal change in mood and behavior: an example from a study of military wives. *Milit Med* 1991;156:228–230.
28. Schwartz PJ, Brown C, Wehr TA, et al. Winter seasonal affective disorder: a follow-up study of the first 59 patients of the National Institute of Mental Health Seasonal Studies Program. *Am J Psychiatry* 1996;153:1028–1036.
29. Rosenthal NE, Wehr TA. Seasonal affective disorders. *Psychiatr Ann* 1987;17:670–674.
30. Rosenthal NE, Sack DA, Gillin JC, et al. Seasonal affective disorder: a description of the syndrome and preliminary findings with light therapy. *Arch Gen Psychiatry* 1984;41:72–80.
31. Postolache TT, Hardin TA, Myers FS, et al. Greater improvement in summer than with light treatment in winter in patients with seasonal affective disorder. *Am J Psychiatry* 1998;155:1614–1616.
32. Neumeister A, Praschak-Rieder N, Hebelmann B, et al. Rapid tryptophan depletion in drug-free depressed patients with seasonal affective disorder. *Am J Psychiatry* 1997;154:1153–1155.
33. Brown RA, Monti PM, Myers MG, et al. Depression among cocaine abusers in treatment: relation to cocaine and alcohol use and treatment outcome. *Am J Psychiatry* 1998;155:220–225.
34. Schuckit MA, Tipp JE, Bergman M, et al. Comparison of induced and independent major depressive disorders in 2,945 alcoholics. *Am J Psychiatry* 1997;154:948–957.
35. Robins E. *The final months.* New York: Oxford University Press, 1981.
36. Anonymous. *Suicide and depression in late life: critical issues in treatment, research, and public policy.* New York: Wiley, 1996:176–186.
37. Black DW, Winokur G, Nasrallah A. Suicide in subtypes of major affective disorder: a comparison with general population suicide mortality. *Arch Gen Psychiatry* 1987;44:878–880.
38. Beck AT, Brown G, Berchick RJ, et al. Relationship between hopelessness and ultimate suicide: a replication with psychiatric outpatients. *Am J Psychiatry* 1990;147:190–195.
39. Fawcett J, Scheftner W, Clark D, et al. Clinical predictors of suicide in patients with major affective disorders: a controlled prospective study. *Am J Psychiatry* 1987;144:35–40.
40. Soloff PH, Lynch KG, Kelly TM, et al. Characteristics of suicide attempts of patients with major depressive episode and borderline personality disorder: a comparative study. *Am J Psychiatry* 2000;157:601–608.
41. Johnson J, Weissman MM, Klerman GL. Panic disorder, comorbidity, and suicide attempts. *Arch Gen Psychiatry* 1990;47:805–808.
42. Weissman MM, Klerman GL, Markowitz JS, et al. Suicidal ideation and suicide attempts in panic disorder and attacks. *N Engl J Med* 1989;321:1209–1214.
43. Keller MB, Klerman GL, Lavori PW, et al. Treatment received by depressed patients. *JAMA* 1982;248:1848–1855.

44. Roy A, Lamparski D, DeJong J, et al. Characteristics of alcoholics who attempt suicide. *Am J Psychiatry* 1990;147:761–765.

45. Murphy GE, Wetzel RD. The lifetime risk of suicide in alcoholism. *Arch Gen Psychiatry* 1990;47:383–392.

46. Mann JJ, Malone KM, Nielsen DA, et al. Possible association of a polymorphism of the tryptophan hydroxylase gene with suicidal behavior in depressed patients. *Am J Psychiatry* 1997;154:1451–1453.

47. Pandey GN, Pandey SC, Dwivedi Y, et al. Platelet serotonin-2A receptors: a potential biological marker for suicidal behavior. *Am J Psychiatry* 1995;156:850–855.

48. Pandey GN. Altered serotonin function in suicide: evidence from platelet and neuroendocrine studies. *Ann N Y Acad Sci* 1997;836:182–200.

49. Leon AC, Keller MB, Warshaw MG, et al. Prospective study of fluoxetine treatment and suicidal behavior in affectively ill subjects. *Am J Psychiatry* 1999;156:195–201.

50. Verkes RJ, Van der Mast RC, Hengeveld MW, et al. Reduction by paroxetine of suicidal behavior in patients with repeated suicide attempts but not major depression. *Am J Psychiatry* 1998;155:543–547.

51. Roose SP, Spatz E. Treatment of depression in patients with heart disease. *J Clin Psychiatry* 1999;60[Suppl 20]:34–37.

52. Broadhead WE, Blazer DG, George LK, et al. Depression, disability days, and days lost from work in a prospective epidemiologic survey. *JAMA* 1990;264:2524–2528.

53. Wells KB, Stewart A, Hays RD, et al. The functioning and well-being of depressed patients. *JAMA* 1989;262:914–919.

54. Kessler RC, Walter SEE, Forthofer MS. The social consequences of psychiatric disorders, III: probability of marital stability. *Am J Psychiatry* 1998;155:1092–1096.

55. Zhang M, Rost KM, Fortney JC. Earnings changes for depressed individuals treated by mental health specialists. *Am J Psychiatry* 1999;15:108–114.

56. Hirschfield RMA, Keller MD, Panico S, et al. The National Depressive and Manic Depressive Association consensus statement on the undertreatment of depression. *JAMA* 1997;277:333–340.

57. Koenig HG, Kuchibhatla M. Use of health services by hospitalized medically ill depressed elderly patients. *Am J Psychiatry* 1998;155:871–877.

58. Rost K, Zhang M, Fortney J, et al. Expenditures for the treatment of major depression. *Am J Psychiatry* 1998;155:883–888.

59. Thompson D, Hylan TR, McMullen W, et al. Predictors of a medical-offset effect among patients receiving antidepressant therapy. *Am J Psychiatry* 1998;155:824–827.

60. Kiloh LG, Andrews G, Neilson M. The long-term outcome of depressive illness. *Br J Psychiatry* 1988;153:752–757.

7

Treatment with Antidepressants

The 1990's could be termed the decade of antidepressants (1). A new antidepressant was marketed virtually every year for these 10 years. The groundwork for this explosion in antidepressant options began with the introduction of the monoamine oxidase inhibitors (MAOIs) and the tricyclic antidepressants (TCAs) in the 1950's.

The antidepressant properties of these earlier antidepressants were chance discoveries. Imipramine was first developed as a potential antipsychotic, but when Kuhn (2) tested the clinical efficacy of this agent, he found that it only benefited depressed schizophrenic patients. This observation prompted him to test it in patients who were suffering from melancholia. Iproniazid was developed as an antitubercular drug, but the observation that euphoria was a side effect led George Crane (3) to conduct clinical trials, which found it useful in purely depressed patients. A year later, Nathan Kline (4), following up on this observation, reported positive results when he administered iproniazid to another depressed group.

Paralleling these clinical developments were basic pharmacological studies, which noted that reserpine (5–8) and α-methyldopa produced depression in patients treated for hypertension (9–11). The fact that the MAOIs and TCAs functionally increased norepinephrine (NE) activity while reserpine lowered its activity led Schildkraut (12) and Bunney and Davis (13) to independently formulate the NE hypothesis of depression. This same line of reasoning was also applied to serotonin (5-HT) (14, 15).

Given two effective classes of antidepressants, pharmacologists developed animal models to screen new compounds in an attempt to predict efficacy. Thus, Everett (16) developed the *dopa test*, and others found that antidepressants reversed reserpine- or tetrabenazine-induced sedation in rodents (17, 18). The *learned helplessness test* is another paradigm in which an animal is put in an impossible situation and eventually gives up (19–21). For example, a dog repeatedly shocked and unable to escape gives up trying, even though an exit is subsequently made available to him. A similar model is a test in which animals are dropped into a tank of water (22, 23). At first, they actively try to escape by swimming for a given amount of time, but then give up and just float. Antidepressants cause the animals in both paradigms to struggle longer before capitulating. NE and 5-HT were hypothesized to be the mediating neurotransmitters in these behavioral models.

Because many have suggested that the beneficial effect of antidepressants is based on their ability to block the uptake of NE and 5-HT, pharmaceutical companies screen potential antidepressants for their ability to block neurotransmitter uptake. Partially as a result of this paradigm (i.e., reuptake blockade), the industry has developed agents that can specifically block NE uptake, 5-HT uptake, or both. More recently, drugs that also affect specific receptors or receptor subtypes have been developed (e.g, mirtazapine) (24).

MECHANISM OF ACTION

The expanded range of antidepressants that has appeared over the last decade constitutes both a benefit and a challenge for the prescriber. The primary advantage is that a better selection can be made to achieve specific effects for a specific patient. The challenge is that there is now much more information for the prescriber to consider. These issues are summarized in Table 7-1.

Mastering this information can be facilitated by understanding antidepressants from the perspective of their clinical pharmacology (i.e., their mechanisms of action). This is made easier by understanding how newer antidepressants were

TABLE 7-1. *STEPS when considering the selection of an antidepressant*

Safety	Tolerability	Efficacy	Payment	Simplicity
Acute therapeutic index	Acute tolerability index	Overall efficacy	Cost effectiveness	Ease of optimal dosing
Long-term safety	Late-emergent tolerability	Unique spectrum of efficacy		Need for dose adjustment
Pharmacokinetic interactions		Rate of onset of efficacy		Need for divided daily dosing
Pharmacodynamic interactions		Maintenance efficacy		Need for any specific monitoring
		Prophylactic efficacy		

From Preskorn S. Antidepressant drug selection: criteria and options. *J Clin Psychiatry* 1994; 55(suppl 9A):6–22, with permission.

developed using the older antidepressants as a blueprint about what mechanisms could mediate an antidepressant response and what mechanisms only mediated adverse effects. Thus, it is important to understand the concept of rational drug development in psychiatry.

Over the past decade, drug discovery and development in psychiatry have advanced well beyond serendipity as the first step. The process has become proactive in that molecular targets of interest in the CNS are chosen first, and then new candidate drugs are designed to stereospecifically interact only with these targets (25). In rational drug development, a target of interest is selected based on some knowledge or theory about how that mechanism might affect the pathophysiology underlying a specific disorder. Examples of specific mechanisms include:

- The *neuronal uptake pump* for a neurotransmitter
- A specific *neurotransmitter receptor subtype*
- A subunit of an *ion channel*

A new molecular entity is then developed to stereospecifically interact with one of these targets. At the same time, the molecule is modified structurally so that it does not affect other sites that mediate undesired effects, such as peripheral cholinergic receptors. Through this systematic approach, a new candidate drug is selected for clinical testing to support registration for marketing. This type of rational drug development has become possible in psychiatry because of the improved understanding of central

and peripheral mechanisms of action that are responsible for both the desired and the undesired effects of currently available psychotropics.

To put this issue in perspective, Table 7-2 illustrates the "cocktail" of drugs needed to reproduce the effects that occur in a patient receiving a single tertiary amine TCA, such as amitriptyline. The problem with tertiary amine TCAs is that the patient has to experience a large number of undesirable effects to receive the benefit from the mechanism that mediates antidepressant response.

At times, a drug that affects more than one target simultaneously may be preferable for specific

TABLE 7-2. *Polypharmacy with a single drug: "cocktail" of effects of the tricyclic antidepressant amitriptyline*

Drug	Action
Chlorpheniramine	H_1 receptor blockade
Benztropine	Acetylcholine receptor blockade
Desipramine	NE uptake inhibition
SSRI	5-HT uptake inhibition
Nefazodone	$5-HT_2$ receptor blockade
Cimetidine	H_2 receptor blockade
Prazosin	α_1 NE receptor blockade
Yohimbine	α_2 NE receptor blockade
Quinidine	Direct membrane stabilization

NE, norepinephrine; SSRI, selective serotonin reuptake inhibitor.

From Preskorn S. *Outpatient Management of Depression: a guide for the practitioner, 2nd ed.* Caddo, OK: Professional Communications, Inc., 1999, with permission.

indications because of desired consequences, such as enhanced potency, wider therapeutic efficacy (e.g., greater spectrum of activity in a heterogeneous condition such as major depression), faster onset of desired activity, or better tolerability. There are four goals of new drug development:

- Widen the *therapeutic index* of the drugs
- Improve their *tolerability profiles*
- Maintain or improve their *efficacy*
- Reduce the possible number of *pharmacodynamically* or *pharmacokinetically mediated drug-drug interactions*

Neurobiology of Depression

Considerable advances have been made over the past decade in this area at several levels including anatomy, chemistry, endocrinology, immunology, and genetics. There has been a synergy with regard to the advances in these areas and advances in antidepressant pharmacology. Advances in neurobiology have focused drug development on new potential mechanisms of action while advances in antidepressants have provided tools to further refine current knowledge of the neurochemistry and neurophysiology responsible for their clinical effect.

Indeed, hypotheses regarding the biological mechanisms subserving mood disorders have developed from observations on the clinical effects of drug and somatic therapies in humans, as well as drug-induced behavioral changes in animals (26). For the purpose of discussion, current theories can be divided into several categories:

- Neurotransmitter-receptor
- Membrane and cation
- Neurophysiological
- Biological rhythms
- Neuroendocrine
- Immunological
- Genetic

We emphasize that these theories are not mutually exclusive. Thus, a genetically determined membrane defect could produce a dysregulation in the neurotransmitter-receptor interaction. This, in turn, may impact second messenger systems within specific neural circuits, resulting in a disturbance of biological rhythms such as neuroendocrine function.

Neuroanatomy of Depression

Advances in this area have perhaps been the most profound over the past 5 to 10 years, occurring as a result of imaging studies followed by focused postmortem studies of the brains of patients with both bipolar and unipolar depression. Neuroimaging studies of patients with familial pure major depression have identified neurophysiological abnormalities in multiple areas of the orbital and medial prefrontal cortex (PFC), the amygdala, and related parts of the striatum and thalamus. Some of these abnormalities appear to be state dependent (i.e., present only when the patient is clinically depressed), whereas other abnormalities appear to be trait dependent (i.e., present whether the patient is depressed or not) (27).

The state-dependent areas are thus implicated in mediating the emotional, cognitive, and behavioral manifestations of a major depressive episode, whereas the latter are more likely to play a more fundamental role in the pathogenesis of the illness. Based on this work, a neural circuit has been proposed. The areas in the PFC include the ventrolateral, orbital and dorsomedial/dorsal anterolateral PFC, the anterior (agranular) insula, and the anterior cingulate gyrus. The areas in the striatum include the ventromedial caudate and the accumbens projecting to the ventral pallidum. Other areas include the ventral tegmentum, the bed nucleus of the stria terminalis, the nucleus tractus solitarius, the periaqueductal gray, and the locus ceruleus (28, 29).

The identification of these areas has focused other studies looking for microanatomical abnormalities in these areas, as well as changes in receptor physiology. For example, examination of the subgenual part of Brodmann's area has revealed marked reductions in the number of astroglial cells in patients with familial major depression and in those with bipolar disorder (30). Of interest, there was no change in either the number or the size of neurons in these areas.

These findings may indicate a primary dysfunction in glial cells as a causative factor in the pathogenesis of major depression. Astroglia are responsible for a number of important neural processes including regulation of extracellular potassium, glucose storage and metabolism, and glutamate uptake. All of these processes are, in turn, crucial for normal neuronal function. Thus, these findings may dramatically shift the focus of antidepressant therapy from mechanisms focused solely on neurons to those involving astroglial cells.

Nevertheless, receptor studies in these areas are consistent with a role for biogenic amine function in the pathophysiology of major depression. Two of the most replicated findings are increased 5-HT$_{2A}$ receptor binding in the PFC and reduced 5-HT$_{1A}$ receptor number and function in the brains of depressed suicide victims. These findings have led to positron emission tomography studies to quantitate the number of 5-HT$_2$ and 5-HT$_{1A}$ receptors in the brain of patients with clinical depression (31, 32). This work has documented a 42% and a 27% reduction in 5-HT$_{1A}$ receptors in the raphe and mesiotemporal cortex, respectively, in unmedicated patients with primary, recurrent, familial major depression.

This work holds the potential to develop an anatomical understanding of major depression. Such an understanding can provide a structure upon which to integrate somewhat disparate neurochemical and neurophysiological findings. At the same time, it can point to new areas such as the role of glial dysfunction in at least some forms of major depression.

Neurotransmitter and Related Hypotheses

Monoamine Theories of Depression

Catecholamine Hypothesis

This theory, first promulgated in the mid-1960's, postulated a diminished activity of catecholamines in the CNS (e.g., NE) (12, 13). Conversely, mania was explained as a relative increase in their activity.

The ascending NE pathway in the CNS begins with projections from the locus ceruleus, an anatomical site encompassing neurons (containing 85% to 90% of central NE stores) that project to the

- Hippocampus
- Cerebral cortex
- Amygdala
- Lower brainstem center (which controls sympathetic output)

The effect of antidepressants on this system was believed to subserve their efficacy. Whereas various agents may enhance, inhibit, or modulate NE activity, the heterocyclics (HCAs) and MAOIs increase the activity of this transmitter by two different mechanisms. HCAs generally block the uptake pump that recovers NE from the synaptic cleft shortly after its release from the presynaptic neuron. Thus, uptake inhibition is occurring during both the acute and the chronic phases of therapy. Interestingly, antidepressant response usually occurs during the chronic phase. MAOIs, by contrast, interfere with enzymatic deamination. In either case, the outcome is increased NE concentrations.

The earliest investigations of this hypothesis measured the major metabolites of NE [e.g., 3-methoxy-4-hydroxyphenylacetic acid (MHPG)] in cerebrospinal fluid (CSF), plasma, and urine. The purpose was to elucidate the biological mechanisms subserving mood disorders, to develop potential markers to facilitate diagnosis, and to aid in the prediction of treatment response. Although initially promising, this line of inquiry has been impeded by various methodological obstacles (e.g., the relative contribution of peripheral versus central sources) and conflicting results. Most studies, for example, find that CSF MHPG in depressed patients is identical to that in normal control subjects. Because it is in equilibrium with plasma MHPG, however, the failure to find low CSF or plasma MHPG does not negate the NE hypothesis. This is, in part, because CSF MHPG may not be an accurate reflection of NE activity in the CNS.

The Depression-Type (D-type) Score, developed as a predictive tool by Mooney et al. (33), exemplifies the most comprehensive attempt to pursue this line of investigation. Janicak et al. (34) summarized this issue while reporting negative results on the predictive value of urinary

MHPG in unipolar depressed patients treated with standard antidepressants. Because the value of MHPG has not been clearly established as a predictor of response, its routine commercial use is not warranted (35).

In animals, *subchronic treatment* (i.e., for several days or weeks) with HCAs, MAOIs, and electroconvulsive therapy (ECT) coincides more closely with the time to maximal clinical response (36–38). This time frame coincides with the most consistent adaptive change, which is a reduced sensitivity of postsynaptic receptors, leading to diminished adenylate-cyclase activity. In the original hypothesis, depression was postulated to be secondary to decreased NE levels, release, or subsensitive receptors. A downregulation (or reverse catecholamine) hypothesis has been subsequently proposed to explain the decreased numbers of postsynaptic β_2-adrenergic receptors in peripheral tissues (e.g., leukocytes) after chronic antidepressant treatment. Thus, depression may be the result of a hypoadrenergic state rather than a hyperadrenergic state (i.e., increased levels or release, or supersensitive receptors are the critical events). This hypothesis was further supported by the neuropharmacological effects of chronic antidepressant treatment, which decreased the following:

• Brain tyrosine hydroxylase and NE
• Postsynaptic β-adrenergic receptor sensitivity and density
• The basal firing rate of NE neurons in the locus ceruleus

Within this context, the original theory may still be valid, because a defect in presynaptic neurotransmission should result in a compensatory up-regulation of postsynaptic receptors. Thus, normalization of presynaptic activity should downregulate (or "normalize") postsynaptic receptor function.

In addition, β-adrenergic receptors are increased in the brains of suicide victims, as are the number of α_2-adrenergic receptor binding sites in the brain of suicide completers and in the platelets of depressed patients (39). The implication is that the pathological increased activity of these autoreceptors may reduce NE output secondary to a short loop, negative feedback

mechanism. Furthermore, Crews and Smith (40) found the α_2-adrenergic receptors adapted (i.e., downregulated) after 3 weeks of treatment with desipramine, ultimately enhancing NE transmission.

On balance, these actions could support a decrease rather than an increase in the functional state of CNS NE transmission, because depression can be conceptualized as a state of supersensitive catecholamine receptors secondary to decreased NE availability. This reasoning is consistent with the original hypothesis of diminished NE functioning, with antidepressants returning receptors to a more normal state of sensitivity. Siever and Davis (41) further elaborated on this concept by suggesting the possibility of dysregulation in the homeostatic mechanisms of one or more neurotransmitter systems, culminating in an unstable or erratic output.

Indolamine Hypothesis

The second neurotransmitter implicated in the monoamine theory was 5-HT (13). Indeed, more than 30 years ago, Bunney and Davis (13) noted that 5-HT may also be a candidate neurotransmitter involved in depression.

This neurotransmitter is contained in a few pathways, of which the midbrain raphe nuclei to the limbic-septal area (e.g., hippocampus and amygdala) is probably the most important. Serotonin abnormalities are widely reported in patients with depression, especially those with suicidal behavior, including the following:

• Decreased levels of *5-HT or its metabolite, 5-hydroxyindoleacetic acid (5-HIAA),* as well as decreased imipramine binding and increased 5-HT$_2$ binding sites are found in postmortem suicide brains (42).
• *Increased 5-HT$_2$ receptor binding sites* are found in the platelets of depressed and suicidal patients (43).
• *Decreased 5-HIAA CSF levels* are found in living, depressed patients who attempt suicide by violent means (44).
• *Decreased 5-HT uptake in the platelets* (V_{max}) of depressed patients is linked to a decrease in the number of platelet imipramine binding sites (45).

- *Blunting of the maximal prolactin response to i.v. tryptophan* (the precursor of 5-HT) is found in depressed patients. Similar results have also been observed with fenfluramine and m-chlorophenylpiperazine (mCPP) (46).
- *p-Chlorophenylalanine,* which decreases 5-HT synthesis, reverses the clinical efficacy of antidepressants (47, 48).
- *Depletion of plasma tryptophan precursors* may reverse antidepressant-induced remissions (49).
- *Tryptophan and 5-hydroxytryptophan,* the precursors of 5-HT, may have antidepressant effects, alone or in combination with other drugs (50).
- Analogous to β-adrenergic receptor downregulation, *antidepressants reduce 5-HT receptor number but not their affinity* (51).
- *ECT potentiates prolactin response to thyrotropin-releasing hormone* (TRH), which is mediated by serotonin (52).
- *Electroconvulsive shock (ECS) enhances 5-HT_2 receptor functional activity and binding* characteristics in postmortem studies on animals (53).

Partial Agonists

In the context of the receptor-ligand model, the role of partial agonists has been clarified. In essence, these ligands are partially stimulatory to a receptor in the absence of the natural, fully stimulating ligand. In the presence of the natural ligand, however, partial agonists reduce the degree of stimulation, in that they compete with full agonists (e.g., 5-HT) for binding sites, and in essence function as antagonists.

In this context, Eison (54) argues for a common underlying pathology for anxiety and depression. In support of this position, he cites the azapirones (e.g., buspirone, gepirone, tandospirone, ipsapirone), which appear to exert their beneficial effects by modulating the activity of 5-HT through partial agonism of 5-HT_{1A} receptors. In support of their antidepressant effects, he notes that members of this class can downregulate 5-HT_2 receptors, as well as de-

sensitize presynaptic, 5-HT_{1A} autoreceptors. He notes that 5-HT_{1A} receptors are also found postsynaptically, and azapirones may affect postsynaptic receptors differently than their presynaptic counterparts (i.e., buspirone is only a partial agonist of postsynaptic receptors). He concludes that in a given context of 5-HT activity (i.e., up or down), these drugs may be able to normalize neurotransmission, which is excessive in anxiety disorders and deficient in depressive disorders.

Other Neurotransmitters

Other neurotransmitter systems have also been implicated in depression, including γ-aminobutyric acid (GABA), the opioids, and, in particular, dopamine.

Dopamine

Randrup et al. (55) first postulated a role for dopamine in depressive disorders. More recently, a reanalysis of the data from several groups has found evidence for a bimodal distribution of CSF homovanillic acid (HVA) levels in depressed patients, with one group comparable with normal control subjects and the other with decreased levels (56). Roy and colleagues (57) also reported on the potential predictive value of lower urinary HVA output in depressed patients who attempted suicide versus those who did not. Both reports indicate a decreased turnover in dopamine.

Consistent with earlier studies, Muscat et al. (58) reported on chronic exposure to mild unpredictable stress in rats as a model to study the antidepressant-reversible decreases in the consumption of palatable sweets. Using this model, they found that certain dopamine agonists (i.e., quinpirole, bromocriptine) administered intermittently had the same positive effects as TCAs. They further postulated that the infrequent, intermittent administration of dopamine agonists (e.g., psychostimulants) may avoid problems with tolerance and abuse while providing a clinically relevant antidepressant strategy. A report by Kapur and Mann (59) comprehensively reviews the role of dopamine in depressive disorders. They discuss several lines of evidence, including the following:

- The *lower CSF HVA levels* in some depressed patients
- An increased incidence of *depression in Parkinson's disease*, as well as in patients receiving dopamine-depleting or antagonistic agents
- The *antidepressant effect* of agents that enhance dopamine transmission
- The *ability of various classes of antidepressants and ECS to enhance dopamine effects* in animal models

Interactional Theories of Depression

Permissive Hypothesis

Clearly, a single neurotransmitter theory does not suffice to explain all known evidence. As a result, models that include two or more systems have been developed to encompass their modulatory interactions. One of the most cogent is the "permissive" hypothesis, which proposes that a decreased function in central serotonin transmission sets the stage for either a depressive or manic phase (60). This circumstance itself is not sufficient to produce the mood disturbance, however, with superimposed aberrations in NE function required to determine the phase of an affective episode (i.e., decreased 5-HT and decreased NE subserves depression; decreased 5-HT and increased NE subserves mania). Data from animal studies to support this theory include the following:

- 5,6-Dihydroxytryptamine lesions of the serotonin nuclei are known to attenuate the reduction in β-noradrenergic receptor binding induced by chronic tricyclic treatment (61).
- 6-Hydroxydopamine lesions, which destroy NE neurons in the dorsal and ventral bundles as well as in the locus ceruleus, block the enhanced locomotor responses to quipazine after repeated ECS.

Adrenergic-Cholinergic Balance Hypothesis

A second interactional theory postulates an imbalance between the cholinergic and the noradrenergic systems (62). The central cholinergic system consists of projections primarily from the nucleus basalis. A relative increase in this system's activity in comparison to central NE activity is thought to play a role in producing depression. Conversely, a decrease relative to central NE activity is thought to play a role in producing mania. Clinically, agents with cholinomimetic effects (e.g., precursors, cholinergic agonists, cholinesterase inhibitors) have shown some benefit in mania (see Chapter 10, "Alternative Treatment Strategies"). Cholinergic abnormalities are also thought to underlie some of the abnormal sleep patterns [e.g., decreased rapid eye movement (REM) latency; increased REM density] found in depression. Also consistent with this theory is evidence that ECT

- Decreases brain acetylcholine (ACh) levels.
- Increases choline acetyltransferase activity, the enzyme most prominently involved in ACh breakdown.
- Causes release of CSF ACh.
- Produces cholinergically mediated electroencephalographic (EEG) slowing following a series of treatments.

Bidimensional Model

Proponents of this hypothesis identify three types of abnormal neurochemistry:

- Causative
- Phenomenological ("expressive")
- Epiphenomenological (possible useful state markers)

As others before them, Emrich and colleagues (63) propose that a single neurochemical imbalance is not sufficient to explain many of the inconsistencies and contradictions in studies with various mood stabilizers. Instead, they speculate that several neurotransmitter imbalances relating to different brain areas should be anticipated.

The possible differing mechanisms of action of three mood stabilizers (i.e., lithium, valproate, carbamazepine) are incorporated into a bidimensional model of mood regulation that postulates two "gating zones" (one for depression and one for mania). These zones are thought to be subserved by different neurochemical abnormalities, leading to a situation in which both could be impacted by certain agents (i.e., mood stabilizers) or, alternatively, could individually be affected by unidirectional compounds (e.g., HCAs).

Second Messenger Dysbalance Hypothesis

Receptors are glycoproteins imbedded in the lipid bilayer of neuronal membranes and can detect minute amounts of specific ligands (e.g., neurotransmitters, hormones). The ligand–receptor interaction sets in motion a transduction system (e.g., an enzyme, ion channel) that orchestrates various intracellular biochemical events.

More recently, investigators have looked beyond the receptor–ligand binding relationship to study intraneuronal events stimulated by this interaction. Two primary areas are the adenylate cyclase (AC) and the phosphoinositol second messenger systems. **Such investigations have led to the postulation that functional disturbances in intraneuronal signal transmission distal to the receptors of classic neurotransmitters (i.e., the first messengers) are pathogenetically important in mood disorders** (64). Furthermore, it suggests that these disorders are caused by a dysfunction in the "crosstalk" between major intraneuronal signal amplification systems (e.g., AC and the phospholipase C systems). Thus, depression may result from a diminished functioning in cyclic adenosine monophosphate (cAMP)-mediated effector cell responses, together with an absolute or relative dominance of the inositol triphosphate diacylglycerol-mediated responses. Mania is conceptualized as resulting from the reverse circumstances.

Work in this area has yielded results that link the changes in receptor physiology to changes in second messenger systems. For example, blunted β-adrenergic receptor responsivity of noradrenergic receptor-coupled AC occurs after repeated doses of most, but not all, antidepressants (36). Yet, an increase in AC activity has been demonstrated in the hippocampus and cortex following chronic antidepressant treatment and ECS (65, 66), which suggests that, even though there is a relative decrease in β-adrenergic receptors after chronic as compared with acute antidepressant administration, levels of cAMP remain elevated compared with the no treatment condition. Thus, despite downregulation of β-adrenergic receptor, there is an overall increase in the activity of the cAMP system because of an increase in biogenic amine levels in the synapse as a result of antidepressant action on amine uptake mechanisms. Thus, current antidepressants, including NE and serotonin reuptake inhibitors, may exert their effects through activation of the cAMP pathway, which in turn leads to regulation of cAMP-dependent protein kinase and subsequently to activation of the cAMP response element binding protein (CREB). This protein could, in turn, mediate its effect by inducing increased expression of neuroprotective neurotrophies such as brain-derived neurotropic factor (66). Along with CREB, this factor has been shown to be elevated following chronic antidepressant and ECS treatment (67, 68).

The effect of increased neurotrophins could mitigate hippocampal changes associated with exposure to stress. Although theoretical, this model of antidepressant action is supported by empirical studies of the pathophysiology of depression in patients (69, 70) as well as animal models (71, 72). These theories also link back to the neuroanatomical findings that began this section.

Membrane and Cation Hypothesis

The resting membrane potential, monoamine transport and reuptake, and other functions of the cellular membrane are partially related to cation transport mechanisms. This has led to a hypothesis proposing that there is a deficiency in one or more of these transport functions; that such a deficit is genetically determined; and that the resulting membrane dysfunction predisposes to a mood disorder.

The steady-state distribution of lithium has provided some evidence to support this hypothesis. Thus, patients with bipolar illness have higher mean intracellular and extracellular red blood cell to lithium ratios, as do their first-degree relatives (73). These findings have led to speculation about genetic control of the lithium ratio and its role in the pathogenesis, as well as pharmacotherapy, of mood disorders.

Biological Rhythm Hypothesis

Halberg (74) postulated a desynchronization of circadian rhythms in depression, whereas Goodwin and colleagues (75) found a phase advance in the rhythms of depressed patients, and Schulz and Lund (76) found a diminished amplitude. Perhaps most interesting is the ability of antidepressants to alter these rhythms, possibly by binding to receptor sites in the suprachiasmatic nucleus (77).

A clear example is the disturbance in the sleep–wake cycle that constitutes one of the hallmarks of depression. Thus, several non-REM components are disrupted, including the following:

• A decrease in *total sleep time*
• An increase in *sleep onset latency*
• A decrease in the *arousal threshold*
• An increase in *wakefulness*
• *Terminal insomnia* (early morning awakening)

as well as REM–related phenomena such as the following:

• A *decrease in REM onset latency*
• An *increase in REM density*
• A *redistribution of REM sleep* to earlier in the sleep phase

These last three items culminate in a state of "REM pressure," which can be viewed as a state of hyperarousal.

Theories explaining the mechanism of action of phototherapy and the biological basis of seasonal affective disorder (SAD) are also related to this area of investigation (i.e., infraradian rhythm disturbances) (78) (see also Chapter 8, "Bright Light Phototherapy"). For example, Skewerer

and colleagues (79) reported that plasma NE levels in SAD were inversely related to the level of depression, and these levels increased proportionally to the degree of therapeutic improvement. Depue et al. (80), in reporting their work on the possible role of dopamine in SAD, noted that basal serum prolactin values did not change as a function of season or after successful phototherapy. Furthermore, these values remained significantly lower in comparison to control subjects, suggesting they could serve as a trait marker for this disorder.

These findings do not exclude the possibility that the central serotonin system is also involved, given its influence on prolactin levels. In this regard, some data show an antidepressant response to dietary l-tryptophan and d-fenfluramine, an indirect serotonin agonist (81). In an open trial, Jacobsen reported a euphoric, energized reaction in 10 SAD patients given infusions of the serotonin agonist mCPP (82). Finally, Lacoste and Wirz-Justice (83) found evidence for seasonal rhythms in serotonin levels in their healthy control subjects, with the winter values being significantly lower than in their summer counterparts.

Neuroendocrine Hypotheses

Cortisol hypersecretion, blunted growth hormone and prolactin responses, blunted thyrotropin-stimulating hormone (TSH) response to TRH, reduced luteinizing hormone secretion, and disturbances in β-endorphin, vasopressin, and calcitonin have all been associated with depression.

As summarized by Gold and colleagues (84), acute behavioral and physiological changes that occur in the general adaptational syndrome are almost identical to those seen in the depressive syndrome. They suggest that melancholia may be conceptualized as an acute generalized stress response that has escaped the normal regulatory restraints. Furthermore, they implicate a dysregulation in glucocorticoid activity, which typically antagonizes corticotropin-releasing hormone neurons, as well as the locus ceruleus–NE system, in addition to mediating immunosuppression. This activity would normally restrain or counterregulate the effectors of the stress response, precluding excessive or extended activation.

Dysregulation of the hypothalamic-pituitary-adrenal axis is thought to cause a disturbance of the circadian rhythm of cortisol. Depression is associated with failure of feedback mechanisms to regulate cortisol secretion, resulting in high cortisol levels. The relationship between cortisol secretion and depression can be investigated through the use of the dexamethasone suppression test (DST) (85), because approximately 50% of patients with symptoms of major depressive disorder show nonsuppression of cortisol. Furthermore, patients who are improved but continue to have an abnormal DST result may be at a higher risk for relapse or suicidal behavior (49).

Dysregulation of the hypothalamic-pituitary-thyroid axis causes a reduction in thyroid function. There may be a relationship between an abnormal TSH response to TRH and depressive symptoms. Thus, unipolar patients undergoing the TRH-TSH test (which measures the difference between baseline TSH and peak postinfusion TSH after they are given synthetic TRH) reportedly have a blunted response, whereas bipolar, depressed patients have an elevated response (see also Chapter 1, "Role of the Laboratory").

Immunological Hypothesis

Two hypotheses about the relationship between mood and the immune system have been the suggestions that (a) depression may alter immunological function or (b) that an unidentified infectious process (e.g., viral) may induce affective disturbances. In support of the former postulate, Bartrop et al. (86) and Schleifer et al. (87) both reported suppression of the immune system following a period of bereavement.

Subsequently, Schleifer et al. (88) found significant age-related immunological differences between their group of 91 unipolar depressed patients and a group of matched control subjects. Specifically, mitogen responses and the number of T4 lymphocytes did not increase in the depressed group with advancing age, as was the

case with the normal control subjects. The impact of elevated cortisol levels on this phenomenon also needs further clarification.

More recently, Kronfol and Remick (89) reviewed the role of cytokines in various CNS activities and concluded that a better understanding of these immunological chemical messengers may help further understand pathological conditions such as depression, as well as provide for possible novel treatments.

Although the results of several lines of investigation have generally been inconclusive, there may be subtypes of depressive disorders that affect immune function. Furthermore, the question of a possible causative infectious process has yet to be adequately addressed.

Genetic Hypothesis

The evidence available from family, twin, and adoption studies supports the existence of genetic factors in the development of primary mood disorders.

There is clearly a higher incidence of both bipolar and apparent unipolar disorders in first-degree relatives of bipolar patients. We say "apparent" because "unipolar" patients from bipolar families may simply have not yet experienced a manic phase. Families of unipolar patients, however, show a higher incidence of unipolar, but not bipolar disease. Given that unipolar and bipolar disorders are inherited separately suggests that there are at least two variations of mood disorders. We do not know where the gene (or genes) for the disorders are located, however, or how such aberrant genes translate into a mood disorder. Linkage studies using recombinant DNA techniques have examined possible loci for association with mood disorders (e.g., the tenth or eleventh chromosomes) (90). Further confirmation is required, however, and it is possible that other loci may also be implicated (91). A more precise statement about the mode of genetic transmission, its contribution to pathogenesis, and environmental interactions is currently not possible.

In an effort to find a biological process that may identify a specific genotype, differences in various enzymes (e.g., monoamine oxidase, dopamine β-hydroxylase, and catechol-O-methyltransferase) have also been investigated.

Both unipolar and bipolar disorders tend to be recurrent and progressive. Post (92) postulates that early episode stress-related alterations in gene expression may subserve long-lasting changes in stress responsivity, episode sensitization, and differences in pharmacosensitivity as a function of the longitudinal course of an illness. He further proposes that adequate drug prophylaxis may interrupt the phenomenon of "episodes begetting episodes," but that subsequent exacerbations may overwhelm or circumvent previously effective treatments.

Conclusion

Since the original catecholamine hypothesis, which attempted to elucidate the biological mechanisms subserving mood disorders, there has been a gradual evolution from consideration of a single neurotransmitter system to the modulating interactions of various neurotransmitters. Next, the effects these "first messenger" systems have upon receptor subtypes and the intraneuronal "second messenger" or signal amplification system in postsynaptic cells have been explored. Most recently, the subsequent cascade of intraneuronal events culminating in altered gene expression are increasingly the focus of investigations of pathophysiology and as potential targets for drug therapy.

Furthermore, many of these neurotransmitters subserve or intimately interact with a number of neuroendocrine, circadian rhythm, and neurophysiological activities, which may be dysregulated in mood disorders. Genetic defects are quite likely the basis for such pathology.

MANAGEMENT OF AN ACUTE DEPRESSIVE EPISODE

The treatment of major depression in psychiatry is analogous to the treatment of many conditions in general medicine. Thus, patients with these various disorders can benefit from several classes of medications with different mechanisms of action and adverse effects. The development of newer agents with unique spectra of activity re-

quires the parallel development of specific strategies for their optimal use. Later, after a review of the efficacy literature, we suggest such a model to manage the depressed patient.

Throughout the rest of this chapter, response and remission rates are used. Therefore, these concepts are briefly discussed here. *Response* is most often defined as a 50% or greater reduction in symptom severity as measured by a standardized rating assessment such as the Hamilton Depression Rating Scale (HDRS). The drawback to this approach is that response does not differentiate between partial and complete response, particularly when the initial symptom severity is high. Thus, a patient could be classified as a responder and still be quite symptomatic. **In some instances, a patient could be classified as responder and still meet entry requirements for an antidepressant clinical trial based on their persistent symptom severity.**

Remission means that the symptom severity is below a predetermined cutoff on a standardized rating assessment (93). The cutoff score is generally such that nondepressed or never depressed individuals could reach that level. There is no universally agreed upon cutoff to define remission (94). For example, a cutoff of 5 is sufficiently low that the percentage of patients achieving this score is quite low, whereas a cutoff of 15 is so high that the difference between response and remission rates is virtually nonexistent. For these reasons, most studies use a cutoff between 7 and 10. Using a 50% reduction to define response and a cutoff of 7 to define remission, most positive, placebo-controlled antidepressant clinical trials will find response and remission rates of 50% to 65% and 35% to 45%, respectively, for the active antidepressant treatment and 30% to 45% and 20% to 30%, respectively, for placebo (Table 7-3) (95).

The 17-item HDRS is the most commonly used scale in antidepressant clinical trials. This version of the HDRS is heavily weighted toward melancholic symptoms. There are also 21-item, 24-item, and 28-item versions with the additional items assessing nonmelancholic symptoms. The Montgomery-Asberg Depression Scale (MADRS) is another instrument that is frequently used in antidepressant clinical trials.

TABLE 7-3. *Combined antidepressants versus placebo: acute treatment*

Number of studies	Number of subjects	Responders (%)		Difference (%)	Chi square	*p* value
		Drug (%)	Placebo (%)			
Combined Heterocyclic Antidepressants						
79	5,159	63	36	27	365	$<10^{-40}$
Combined Monoamine Oxidase Inhibitors						
16	1,697	66	32	35	49.9	2×10^{-12}

Severe depression is another term that is frequently seen in the literature discussing clinical depression and antidepressant trials. There is no uniform definition of this term. One or more of the following criteria may be used to differentiate patients with nonsevere versus severe depression:

- *Hospitalization*
- *Functional impairment* as assessed by a scale such as the Global Assessment Scale
- *Absolute symptom severity* as assessed by a standardized rating assessment
- *Depressive subtype, particularly psychotic* or *melancholic* as defined in *Diagnostic and Statistical Manual of Mental Disorders,* 4th ed (DSM-IV)

None of these definitions is ideal. Patients may be hospitalized for a suicide gesture or a comorbid condition such as a severe personality disorder or substance abuse rather than solely on the basis of their depression severity. A score of 25 or higher on the 17-item HDRS is the most commonly used cutoff to distinguish nonsevere from severe depression. This approach, however, is subject to the possibility of inflation of scores to qualify patients for the trial.

These issues must be kept in mind when interpreting claims made on the basis of clinical trial results. The variability in scales and definition of terms used in antidepressant trials also confounds attempts to make comparisons across studies and to do meta-analyses. With these caveats in mind, the next several sections review the acute and maintenance efficacy of the available antidepressant options, as well as some currently investigational antidepressants.

There are more than 400 well-controlled studies and many more partially controlled or open trials supporting the efficacy of standard antidepressants for major depression. In severely ill patients, these agents produce a striking improvement in behavior and a marked lessening of depression, generally beginning 3 to 10 days after their initiation. The rate of response is linear over time, with a "half-life to improvement" of about 10 to 20 days. Consequently, patients who do not demonstrate a satisfactory response after an adequate trial for a 4- to 6-week period, probably will not. The degree of response in the first 2 weeks of treatment may predict the ultimate outcome, with 60% to 80% of depressed patients substantially benefited by marketed antidepressants during this period, in contrast to 20% to 50% of those on placebo (96).

We have provided a summary of the results from double-blind, random-assignment studies (usually class I or II designs) comparing HCAs, selective serotonin reuptake inhibitors (SSRIs), other new antidepressants, and MAOIs with placebo or with each other for the acute treatment of depression. Each study was reviewed, and a global judgment made, based on all the evidence presented, as to whether a given drug was more effective than placebo or another control therapy.

Heterocylic Antidepressants

HCA is the term is used to refer to both TCAs and analogues of these agents, such as maprotiline and amoxapine. TCAs are by far the most commonly used HCAs and include tertiary amines such as amitriptyline, doxepin, and imipramine and secondary amines such as desipramine and nortriptyline. Most secondary amines could also be viewed as NE-selective antidepressants, while the hallmark of tertiary amine TCAs is their

TABLE 7-4. *Specific heterocyclic antidepressants versus placebo: acute treatment*

Drug	Number of studies	Number of subjects	Responders (%) Drug (%)	Placebo (%)	Difference (%)	Chi square	*p* value
First Generation							
Amitriptyline	8	292	60	26	34	30.9	3×10^{-8}
Imipramine	50	2,649	68	40	28	184.0	$<10^{-40}$
Second Generation							
Amoxapine	10	386	67	49	18	12.4	4×10^{-4}
Bupropion	4	425	55	29	26	26.6	2×10^{-7}
Lofepramine	3	135	79	48	31	4.6	0.02
Mianserin	5	336	60	28	31	31.0	2×10^{-8}
Trazodone	13	824	59	28	32	93.3	1×10^{-22}

effects on multiple neurotransmitters over their clinically relevant dosing range.

Efficacy for Acute Treatment

Imipramine

Studies comparing imipramine with placebo (including 2,649 depressed patients) found that 68% on active drug were substantially improved (i.e., responders), compared with 40% on placebo (i.e., an average drug–placebo difference of 28%) (Table 7-4). Imipramine was more effective than, or at least equal to, placebo in all studies, but placebo was never found to be better than imipramine. Generally, those studies that failed to show a definite active drug effect suffered from methodological inadequacies such as insufficient dose, inappropriate rating scales, and small, nonhomogeneous patient pop-

ulations (e.g., significant numbers of psychotic, schizoaffective, or neurotic patients). The probability of these results occurring by chance alone was nonexistent when calculated by the Mantel-Haenszel test.

Despite a clear advantage for drug over placebo, approximately 30% of patients on imipramine remained unimproved, indicating the need for alternative treatment methods in many of these patients.

Amitriptyline

Most studies comparing amitriptyline with placebo found the drug to be superior. Those comparing it with imipramine found these two agents to be equally effective (Tables 7-4 and 7-5). No studies found amitriptyline to be less effective than imipramine and two double-blind studies showed amitriptyline (200 mg) to be

TABLE 7-5. *Summary of controlled double-blind studies of heterocyclic antidepressants*

Drug	Number of Studies in Which the Effect Was More than placebo	Equal to placebo	More than imipramine	Equal to imipramine	Less than imipramine
Amitriptyline	9	2	2	5	0
Desipramine	3	2	0	6	1
Doxepin	2	0	0	3	0
Imipramine	30	14	—	—	—
Maprotiline	2	2	0	10	0
Nortriptyline	4	0	0	0	0
Protriptyline	2	0	0	2	0
Trimipramine	1	0	2	0	0

Adapted from Klein DF, Davis JM. *Diagnosis and drug treatment of psychiatric disorders.* Baltimore: Williams & Wilkins, 1969:193–194.

TABLE 7-6. *First versus second generation standard antidepressants: acute treatment*

| Drug | Number of studies | Number of subjects | Responders (%) | | Difference (%) |
			New antidepressant (%)	Standard antidepressant (%)	
Amoxapine	19	784	79	73	6
Bupropion	4	293	71	72	−1
Clomipramine	6	350	61	62	−1
Lofepramine	4	160	55	60	−5
Maprotiline	20	1,638	73	72	1
Mianserin	15	1,155	58	64	−6
Trazodone	18	913	62	58	4

superior to imipramine (200 mg) (97, 98). This finding, however, may be an artifact, in that the imipramine group included more delusional patients, who generally respond poorly to monotherapy with any antidepressant. When imipramine and amitriptyline were administered in different dose ratios—maximal dose of imipramine 240 mg per day and amitriptyline 150 mg per day—they were again found to be equally effective, raising the possibility that amitriptyline is slightly more potent than imipramine on a milligram per milligram basis.

Clomipramine

The Food and Drug Administration (FDA) has approved clomipramine for the treatment of obsessive-compulsive disorder. Clomipramine is also used in the United States, Europe, Canada, England, and, indeed, most of the world as an antidepressant. In six random-assignment, double-blind studies, this agent was equal in efficacy to standard tricyclics, with a side-effect profile comparable with other TCAs (Table 7-6).

Among HCAs, clomipramine is one of the more selective reuptake inhibitors of serotonin. Because plasma levels of its demethylated metabolite (which primarily works through the NE system) can in some patients exceed those of the parent compound, its therapeutic action cannot be solely attributed to serotonin uptake inhibition.

Doxepin

Doxepin was found to be superior to placebo and equal to other tricyclics (Table 7-5). Virtually all subjects were outpatients with mixed anxiety and depression, rather than inpatients with major depressive disorder. Despite this methodological limitation, a reasonable conclusion is that doxepin has significant antidepressant properties. Three studies comparing doxepin with imipramine, amitriptyline, and clomipramine found it to be equal to the other drugs, but there was a trend favoring imipramine (99–101). Doxepin is less potent than imipramine, and slightly higher doses are necessary to achieve optimal benefit, partly because doxepin has the highest first-pass effect of all the TCAs.

Trimipramine

Several small, double-blind studies show trimipramine to be superior to placebo and at least comparable with other standard TCAs (Table 7-5). There was a trend in one large, carefully controlled study favoring amitriptyline, but it did not supply data on percent improvement, so it was not included in our analysis (102). Considering all the data, we would conclude that trimipramine is equal in effect to other TCAs.

Desipramine and Nortriptyline

Based on comparisons with imipramine and amitriptyline, desipramine and nortriptyline (secondary amine compounds) are comparable in efficacy with their tertiary amine parent compounds and clearly superior to placebo (Table 7-5). **Clinically, they are often preferred to the tertiary amine compounds because of their less bothersome side-effect profiles.** The introduction of newer compounds (e.g., SSRIs) with a wider therapeutic index, however, has made this distinction less clinically relevant.

Protriptyline

This tricyclic drug is superior to placebo and equivalent to standard HCAs in outpatient populations. It is a more potent agent on a per milligram basis (i.e., average daily dose is 20 to 60 mg), partly because of its low first-pass effect and long half-life (Table 7-5). Hence, patients develop substantially higher plasma levels per milligram dose of protriptyline versus other TCAs.

Amoxapine

Amoxapine has been found to be effective in several double-blind studies (Tables 7-4 and 7-6). It is a dibenzoxazepine derivative that has both NE and serotonin uptake inhibiting properties. Amoxapine is converted into 8-hydroxyamoxapine, which has considerable dopamine receptor binding properties (i.e., radioreceptor bioassays on patients given amoxapine have found activity levels similar to those of patients on typical antipsychotics), a chemical structure similar to loxapine, and effects similar to antipsychotics (103). As a result of this metabolite, amoxapine theoretically may have unique beneficial effects in psychotically depressed patients. However, this possibility has never been adequately tested. Nevertheless, this metabolite is likely responsible for some of the antidopamine effects reported in patients taking amoxapine, including acute and chronic extrapyramidal side effects and elevated prolactin levels (104). Like TCAs, amoxapine can be lethal in overdoses.

Maprotiline

Two studies found maprotiline to be clearly superior to placebo and two other studies found trends in the same direction ($p < 0.001$, combined data) (Table 7-5) (105–108). More than 1,600 patients were randomly assigned to either maprotiline or a standard HCA: 660 on maprotiline did well, and 247 showed minimal improvement, no change, or worsened. For the HCAs (usually imipramine or amitriptyline), 640 patients did well, and 255 showed minimal improvement, no change, or worsened. In summary, 73% did well with maprotiline, and 72% did well with a standard antidepressant. Combining these data with the Mantel-Haenszel test indicated no difference in efficacy (Table 7-6). Maprotiline has a dose-dependent risk of seizures. As with TCAs and amoxapine, overdoses of maprotiline can be lethal.

Lofepramine

Well-controlled studies have found lofepramine to be superior to placebo and comparable with amitriptyline, imipramine, and maprotiline (109). It may be better tolerated than earlier HCAs, especially by elderly patients. Desipramine is its major metabolite (Tables 7-4 and 7-6).

Selective Serotonin Reuptake Inhibitors

During the past two decades, there has been increasing evidence that serotonin neurotransmission is diminished during an episode of depression. Drugs that modify 5-HT activity by inhibiting its uptake carrier have been the most clinically productive line of inquiry thus far.

Zimelidine was the first serotonin reuptake inhibitor available for clinical use, but in 1982 was withdrawn worldwide because of its toxicity (110). Despite this initial setback, five members of this class have been marketed in the United States and various countries around the world: *citalopram* (Celexa), *fluoxetine* (Prozac), *fluvoxamine* (Luvox), *paroxetine* (Paxil), and *sertraline* (Zoloft). All except fluvoxamine have marketed indications in the United States for the treatment of major depression. Fluvoxamine is marketed in the United States for the treatment of obsessive-compulsive disorder rather than major

TABLE 7-7. *SSRIs versus placebo: acute treatment*

Drug	Number of studies	Number of subjects	Responders (%)		Difference (%)	p value
			SSRI (%)	Placebo (%)		
Fluoxetine	9	1,365	65	41	24	10^{-22}
Fluvoxamine	3	125	67	42	25	0.008
Paroxetine	9	649	65	36	29	10^{-14}
Sertraline	3	575	78	48	30	10^{-12}

SSRI, selective serotonin reuptake inhibitor.

depression, although it is marketed in a number of other countries for major depression.

Efficacy for Acute Treatment

The overall efficacy among the SSRIs for major depressive disorder is remarkably similar, consistent with the hypothesis that they have the same mechanism of action (i.e., serotonin uptake inhibition).

Our meta-analysis (Tables 7-7 and 7-8), demonstrates that all SSRIs are superior to placebo beyond any reasonable doubt. Comparative studies also show that the SSRIs are equal in effectiveness to standard antidepressants. Even though the large number of patients studied and the failure to find a significant difference strongly suggest that these drugs are equal to all other comparative antidepressants, one important limitation is that the studies were generally based on depressed outpatients. Furthermore, even though the magnitude of the antidepressant effect seen with paroxetine across its dosing range is somewhat less, the results are consistent with those of sertraline and fluoxetine.

All of the SSRIs also show a flat dose–response curve, meaning that there is usually no advantage to increasing the dose above that which is the usually effective minimum dose. Of interest, the four SSRIs marketed as antidepressants in the United States at their usual effective therapeutic dose (i.e., 40 mg per day for citalopram, 20 mg per day for paroxetine and fluoxetine, and 50 mg per day for sertraline) produce comparable effects on either plasma serotonin levels or the serotonin uptake pump in platelets (25). These results are consistent with the conclusion that serotonin uptake inhibition is the mechanism responsible for the antidepressant efficacy of these agents.

Rate of Onset of Efficacy

There are several randomized, double-blind studies suggesting that fluoxetine has a slower onset of antidepressant activity than other antidepressants, including citalopram (111), moclobemide (112), paroxetine (113), and venlafaxine (114). This may be because it takes several weeks to reach steady-state of fluoxetine and norfluoxetine because of their long half-lives. Thus, effective

TABLE 7-8. *SSRIs versus standard antidepressants: acute treatment*

Drug	Number of studies	Number of subjects	Responders (%)		Difference (%)
			SSRI (%)	Standard AD (%)	
Citalopram	6	347	73	74	−1
Fluoxetine	16	1,549	63	64	−1
Fluvoxamine	4	137	70	66	+4
Paroxetine	16	1,322	62	60	+2
Sertraline	3	682	68	65	+3

AD, antidepressant; SSRI, selective serotonin reuptake inhibitor.

levels may not be achieved in a comparable interval of time as other SSRIs when the patient is started on the lowest, usually effective dose (i.e., 20 mg per day). Nevertheless, although the magnitude of the difference in early response was statistically greater for the comparative drug in these studies, the absolute magnitude of the effective dose was modest (113, 115).

Unique Spectrum of Efficacy

There is considerable debate as to how effective SSRIs are in patients with more severe clinical depression, particularly those who have been hospitalized. Part of this debate may be because the vast majority of studies done with SSRIs involved outpatients. As mentioned earlier, hospitalization is not simply determined by severity of an episode but may be driven by other variables such as concomitant substance abuse or a medical illness.

With this caveat in mind, each side of the debate has evidence to support its position. The evidence is first summarized supporting the position that SSRIs are less effective than are some other antidepressants (particularly those with dual effects on both serotonin and NE CNS systems) in patients with more severe depression or who are hospitalized. Danish investigators in two double-blind, active-controlled studies found that clomipramine produced a superior response with either paroxetine or citalopram in the treatment of patients hospitalized for major depression (116, 117). Two double-blind studies also have shown that venlafaxine and mirtazapine were more effective than fluoxetine in patients hospitalized with depression (114, 118). Finally, there are studies showing that the addition of desipramine (one of the most selective NE reuptake inhibitors) to an SSRI can convert nonresponders or partial responders to full response (119, 119a, 120).

Studies supporting the position that SSRIs are effective in severe depression were performed in patients hospitalized for major depression, those with severe depression (i.e., having a 17-item HDRS score of 25 or more), and those with melancholia. The following caveat should be kept in mind when interpreting some of these data. Some of these studies were active-controlled only and found no difference in efficacy between an SSRI and a TCA. This does not prove that the SSRI is as efficacious as the TCA, but instead only means the study was not able to disprove the null hypothesis of no difference. This can occur simply because not enough patients were entered in the study to adequately separate the two treatments. Thus, the finding of no difference is not as meaningful as finding a difference. That is true whether the comparison is an active control or a placebo. This issue is particularly important when interpreting the results of antidepressants clinical trials because of their considerable signal-to-noise problems (121).

There have been five double-blind studies comparing the antidepressant efficacy of different SSRIs versus different TCAs in patients with HDRS scores of 25 or more (122–126). Three of these studies permitted inclusion of both inpatients and outpatients (122–124), whereas the other two were solely done in outpatients (125, 126). Three were placebo-controlled (123, 125, 126). In these three studies, the SSRI (i.e., fluvoxamine, paroxetine, or sertraline) was either superior to both the TCA and placebo or was comparable with the TCA and superior to placebo. In the other two studies, the SSRI was not different from the TCA and there was no placebo control. There have also been four studies and one meta-analysis of European clinical trials which found no difference in antidepressant efficacy between several different SSRIs and several different tertiary amine TCAs in patients hospitalized for major depression (127–131). Finally, there have been two relatively small studies showing that fluoxetine and fluvoxamine both had antidepressant efficacy superior to placebo in patients with melancholia (132, 133). Another larger study failed to find a difference between paroxetine and amitriptyline in treating such patients (134).

There is also controversy over what to do if a patient does not respond to the first trial of an SSRI. If the reason for nonresponse is poor tolerability, then many clinicians try a second SSRI. Based on a recent survey, the course of action preferred by most psychiatrists is to switch to a drug with a different mechanism of action or a dual mechanism of action when a patient

TABLE 7-9. *Antidepressant effect (Δ change in Hamilton Depression Rating Scale [HDRS][a])* *as a function of dose in fixed-dose, placebo-controlled studies*

	Daily dose (mg/day)					
Fluoxetine	5	20	40	60		
Study I[b]						
Δ change	—	4.1[c]	3.9[c]	1.5		
Study II[d]						
Δ change	4.2[c]	3.0[c]	4.2[c]	—		
Sertraline[e]	—	50	100	200		
Δ change	—	2.7[c]	2.8[c]	3.9[f]		
Paroxetine[g]	10	20	30	40		
Δ change	−1.2	2.4[c]	1.5[c]	1.5[c]		
Venlafaxine[h]	62.5	75	175	182	225	375
Δ change	1.0	4.5[c]	2.0	4.0[c]	6[c]	5[c]
Nefazodone[i]	200–250	300	400	500	600	—
Δ change	1.7	2.0	2.7[c]	5.1[j]	0.6[j]	—

[a]Antidepressant effect = (baseline HDRS-final HDRS) on drug minus (baseline HDRS-final HDRS) on placebo.
[b]From Wernicke J, et al. Fixed dose fluoxetine therapy for depression. *Psychopharmacol Bull* 1987;23:164–168.
[c]$p < 0.05$ vs. placebo.
[d]From Wernicke J, et al. Low dose fluoxetine therapy for depression. *Psychopharmacol Bull* 1988;24:183–188.
[e]From Preskorn S, Lane R. 50 mg/day as the optimum dose for sertraline. *Int Clin Psychopharmacol* 1995; 10(3):129–141.
[f]$p < 0.001$ vs. placebo.
[g]From Dunner DL, Dunbar GC. Optimal dose regimen for paroxetine. *J Clin Psychiatry* 1992;53(suppl):21–26.
[h]From Preskorn S. Antidepressant drug selection: criteria and options. *J Clin Psychiatry* 1994;55(suppl 9A):6–22.
[i]From Nefazodone presentation to the Food and Drug Administration Psychopharmacology Advisory Committee. Washington DC, July 1993.
[j]$p < 0.01$ vs. placebo.

experiences inadequate efficacy from an adequate trial of an SSRI (135).

Few data are available to guide this decision beyond clinical experience. There is a modest amount of evidence that nonresponders to TCAs, principally desipramine or imipramine, alone may respond to a SSRI alone and vice versa (136). No compelling evidence exists showing that nonresponders to one SSRI as a result of a lack of efficacy will respond to a second trial with another SSRI. There is limited confidence in the results of studies that have been done switching nonresponders from one SSRI to another for two reasons. First, virtually all have been open label and, second, most were conducted by the manufacturer of the second SSRI. Until there is more substantive evidence that switching from one SSRI to another is worthwhile, it may be more prudent to switch to a class of antidepressants with a different putative mechanism of action.

Venlafaxine

Venlafaxine, a phenylethylamine, sequentially inhibits first the neuronal uptake pump for serotonin and then NE (137). In contrast to tertiary amine TCAs, which can also inhibit serotonin and NE uptake pumps, venlafaxine has low binding for most other neuroreceptors and does not inhibit Na^+ ion fast channels, making it relatively safe in overdoses compared with TCAs.

Venlafaxine is dependent on CYP 2D6 and 3A3/4 enzymes for its biotransformation and eventual clearance (138–140). CYP 2D6 converts venlafaxine into O-desmethylvenlafaxine (ODV), which is believed to have pharmacological activity comparable with the parent drug based on *in vitro* studies (141). Thus, this metabolite is to venlafaxine as norfluoxetine is to fluoxetine in that the half-life of ODV is longer than that of the parent drug, although it is only 12 hours versus 14 days for norfluoxetine.

Efficacy for Acute Treatment

In contrast to the SSRIs, venlafaxine has an ascending dose–response curve consistent with its sequential, concentration (and hence dose) dependent effects on serotonin and NE uptake pumps (Table 7-9). At 225 mg per day, the magnitude of the antidepressant effect is 50% higher than that seen with the SSRIs. Also consistent with its dual mechanism of action at higher concentrations, venlafaxine at a dose of 225 mg per day produced an antidepressant response in hospitalized patients with melancholia superior to both placebo and fluoxetine (114–142). In contrast to the flat dose–response curve seen with the SSRIs, the ascending dose–response curve seen with venlafaxine provides a stronger rationale to use higher doses in patients who have not responded or only partially responded to an initial lower starting dose (e.g., 75 mg per day).

A close examination of the efficacy data from the fixed dose study with venlafaxine affords an opportunity to comment on how study design can affect the results. In this study, the magnitude of the antidepressant effect of venlafaxine was smaller at 375 mg per day than at 225 mg per day (see Table 7-9). Although possibly a chance result, this is readily understood based on the design and data analysis used for this study. In fixed dose studies, patients are randomly assigned to predetermined doses, regardless of need, and dosage is adjusted rapidly to that predetermined dose. This approach is in contrast to clinical practice wherein patients are typically started on the lowest, usually effective dose and only adjusted upward as needed and tolerated. Such adjustment is frequently done much more gradually than in a fixed dose study and thus the patient may adjust to dose-dependent adverse effects. Most patients, for example, will adapt to the nausea produced by drugs that potentiate 5-HT, such as the SSRIs and venlafaxine.

This study, like most studies, are analyzed using a last-carried-forward approach. In this approach, the last observed data for a patient are carried forward if they dropped out before the final assessment is made. The reason is to avoid missing data and to avoid biasing the results by only looking at patients who completed the study and thus benefited from and tolerated the treatment whether placebo, investigational drug, or standard comparator drug. Based on this, a fixed dose design will often produce a curvilinear dose–response curve, with a better outcome in the middle than at either end. The reason for the decreased response at the lowest dose is that the dose is insufficient to produce therapeutic concentrations of the drug at the necessary site of action in most patients. The blunted response at the upper end reflects the early dropouts who could not tolerate the therapy. Thus, the results in such studies may well underestimate the efficacy of the drug at the highest doses, in contrast to a design in which only patients who needed the higher dose are advanced. This issue is a common problem in the interpretation of all fixed-dose studies.

Rate of Onset of Efficacy

There is no accepted way to determine the rate of onset of antidepressant action (148a). Perhaps the most stringent and clinically meaningful test is an examination of responder or remitter status (i.e., 50% decrease in symptom severity or full resolution of the syndrome, respectively) as a function of time. These dichotomized data address many of the methodological problems inherent in the group average difference approach. The venlafaxine database demonstrates a response rate on 375 mg per day that is five times that of placebo after 1 week of treatment (143). After 2 weeks of treatment, almost one of three patients receiving this dose had responded versus less than one of ten patients on placebo. This difference was both statistically significant (i.e., $p < 0.05$) and clinically meaningful (i.e., fivefold increase in response rate). In addition, there is a statistically significant early separation between venlafaxine and placebo in terms of average reduction in depressive symptoms over several double-blind, random-assignment clinical trials (144–147).

These data are consistent with the observation from basic studies showing that combined administration of drugs that individually inhibit either 5-HT or NE uptake pumps, or the administration of high-dose venlafaxine produces a more rapid β-adrenergic receptor subsensitivity (148). In addition, data from clinical studies using combined administration of NE and 5-HT reuptake inhibitors demonstrate a more rapid antidepressant action (119, 119a). These onset-of-response data provide physicians with clinically meaningful information when faced with severely ill patients for whom shortening the time to onset of antidepressant action is particularly important. In this context, it would be ideal to have similar data on all available antidepressants so that more comparative statements about the relative onset of action can be made (148a).

Unique Spectrum of Efficacy

An almost universal question when a new drug is marketed is whether it helps patients who have not responded to other medications. However, because of the following, there is rarely a good answer:

- There is *technical difficulty* in doing such studies.
- There is *high risk* involved in this type of study (i.e., finding an answer that is not favorable to the sponsor).
- Trials during clinical development are *designed to meet registration requirements* rather than to answer such questions.

As with other drugs, a methodologically rigorous study addressing this issue has not been done with venlafaxine. Nevertheless, there are data from an open-label trial of venlafaxine that warrant comment (149). In this study, high-dose venlafaxine produced an acute response in more than 30% of patients who had historically not adequately benefited from adequate trials of at least three antidepressants from different classes or two antidepressants plus ECT. Until more definitive data are available, this study does support a trial of high-dose venlafaxine in such patients.

Venlafaxine shares similar advantages with the SSRIs over the TCAs and the MAOIs. In addition, potential advantages of venlafaxine over the SSRIs are as follows:

- An *ascending dose–antidepressant response curve,* with possible greater overall efficacy at the higher doses
- Evidence of a clinically meaningful *more rapid onset* of antidepressant action
- Evidence of *superior efficacy in hospitalized patients* with major depression in comparison with placebo or fluoxetine
- *Minimal effects on any of the major CYP enzymes* in contrast to antidepressants such as fluoxetine, fluvoxamine, or paroxetine

Disadvantages relative to the SSRIs include the potential for blood pressure elevation at higher doses. The marketing of a once-a-day sustained release form of venlafaxine has effectively dealt with the need for a twice-a-day dosing schedule with the original immediate release version. That the venlafaxine dose can be adjusted is a pharmacological advantage, but it may be a marketing disadvantage, because many physicians may prefer the simplicity of a "one dose fits all" concept, as seen with the SSRIs.

Nefazodone

Nefazodone has a chemical structure related to trazodone and incorporates both 5-HT uptake properties plus 5-HT$_{2A}$ receptor blockade (150–153). There is evidence from controlled trials that this agent is an effective antidepressant with a favorable side-effect profile.

Nefazodone has some unusual pharmacological properties, not only inhibiting serotonin uptake, but also blocking the 5-HT$_{2A}$ receptor. It may be that the antidepressant effect of serotonin agents is due to mediation of 5-HT$_{1A}$ transmission in the absence (or even the blockade) of 5-HT$_{2A}$ transmission. As a result of these actions, nefazodone is even more specific in terms of affecting a subtype of serotonin receptor than are the SSRIs or venlafaxine.

Efficacy for Acute Treatment

The clinical trials of nefazodone differed from that of the SSRIs and venlafaxine in that the only truly fixed-dose study was done early in its development (154). That study had major limitations, such as the doses used were low (50 to 300 mg per day) compared with those later found to be optimally effective. Also, the number of subjects was small. Subsequent studies did not use a fixed dose design but rather a targeted dose range design (i.e., low dose = 50 to 300 mg per day and high dose = 300 to 600 mg per day) (154). Even though patients were randomly assigned to either range, the physician could adjust dosing within these ranges to maximize the treatment outcome. Although the use of fixed dose ranges is reasonable and valid, this design does not permit as straightforward an assessment of the dose–response curve as do conventional fixed dose studies. This difference should be kept in mind, particularly when comparing the antidepressant effect size seen with nefazodone with that of other antidepressants that were studied using truly fixed dose designs.

Using this fixed dose range design, a series of double-blind, controlled trials with placebo and standard drug (mainly imipramine or fluoxetine) were done (154–159). Nefazodone was found to be superior to placebo and equivalent to imipramine and fluoxetine in efficacy. A meta-analysis, including all the efficacy studies with nefazodone, examined the magnitude of the antidepressant response as a function of the average daily dose and found an ascending dose–antidepressant response curve. The magnitude of the antidepressant effect at doses of 300 to 400 mg per day is comparable with that seen with the SSRIs and lower doses of venlafaxine (Table 7-9). This finding suggests that nefazodone at these doses is effective in the same percentage of patients as the other comparative antidepressants. At doses of 500 mg per day, however, the magnitude of the response exceeds that seen with the SSRIs but is less than that seen with high-dose venlafaxine (i.e., 225 to 375 mg per day). Interestingly, at 600 mg per day, the response to nefazodone was virtually the same as to placebo. This finding may be an artifact of the study design, however, because the clinician could adjust dosage within the dose range based on efficacy and tolerability. Hence, dosages for patients who failed to respond should have been adjusted to the highest tolerated dose. Such a design produces a curvilinear dose–response curve with a diminution in response at the highest level because dosages for nonresponders are adjusted upward to the highest tolerated dose. In addition, there is the problem of dropouts, which occurs because of the acute nuisance adverse effects at high doses, as discussed in the sections on SSRIs and venlafaxine. **Nonetheless, this result indicates that there is generally no advantage to exceeding 500 mg per day of nefazodone.**

Rate of Onset of Efficacy

Nefazodone produced a rapid (i.e., by 1 week) and statistically significant improvement in sleep and anxiety symptoms associated with major depression (160). The full antidepressant response, however, takes an interval of time comparable with that of the SSRIs. Unlike venlafaxine, there is no evidence that higher doses produce a more rapid onset of full remission.

Unique Spectrum of Efficacy

No studies demonstrate unique efficacy for nefazodone in any subgroup of patients with major depression. There is also no rigorous evidence to support the position that nefazodone is effective in patients who have not benefited from an adequate trial of another antidepressant. However, there is a double-blind, placebo-controlled study showing nefazodone to be superior to placebo in patients hospitalized for major depression.

Advantages of nefazodone relative to SSRIs or venlafaxine include the following:

- An ascending dose–antidepressant *response curve* in contrast to SSRIs
- Perhaps a more benign *adverse effect profile,* particularly with regard to activation and sexual dysfunction, in contrast to the SSRIs and venlafaxine

- A potentially more rapid onset of *anxiolytic effect*
- A *lack of blood pressure elevation,* in contrast to venlafaxine

Disadvantages of nefazodone include the need for a twice-a-day dosing schedule and dose adjustment. Work is under way to develop a once-a-day sustained release version of nefazodone. The fact that nefazodone must be started at a lower than usually effective dose and then adjusted to an effective dose is a distinct disadvantage. That is made even more problematic because arguably more variability exists among patients in terms of the optimal dose of nefazodone as far as efficacy and tolerability than for virtually any other antidepressant. Finally, nefazodone produces substantial inhibition of CYP 3A3/4, leading to the potential for adverse pharmacokinetic interactions as well as possible unknown long-term consequences.

Trazodone

A review of several random-assignment, well-controlled trials found trazodone to be 32% more effective than placebo and a nonsignificant 4% more effective than tertiary TCAs (Tables 7-4 and 7-6). The therapeutic dose is 200 to 600 mg per day, and although it has fewer anticholinergic adverse effects, excessive sedation may limit the total dose. The absolute milligram dosage is higher than for HCAs, with some patients needing 400 to 600 mg to achieve adequate response. There are advantages and disadvantagees to trazodone, which include the following:

Advantages

- *No anticholinergic* effects
- *Sedation*; useful for agitation and hostility in geriatric patients
- May be used as a *hypnotic* agent
- Relative *safety with overdose*
- *No quinidine*-like effect

Potential disadvantages

- *Not antiarrhythmic*
- May induce or exacerbate *ventricular arrhythmia* (not proven)

- *Priapism*
- Postural *hypotension*

Bupropion

Bupropion has been found to be an effective antidepressant in several double-blind studies (Tables 7-4 and 7-6) (161). It is a weak dual reuptake inhibitor of DA and NE. There are a number of observations in animals that bupropion can *in vivo* block the uptake of both DA and NE, including the downregulation of postsynaptic β-noradrenergic receptors and protection against the dopamine neurotoxictiy of 6-hydroxydopamine (162). Bupropion is also self-administered in animals when using the paradigm for amphetamine-like drugs.

However, its relative weak affinity for these uptake pumps has raised questions as to whether either of these mechanisms is relevant to its antidepressant activity. The combined plasma concentration of bupropion and its three active metabolites are consistent with the conclusion that the inhibition of both of these uptake pumps likely occurs under clinically relevant dosing conditions. For comparison purposes, the combined levels of bupropion and its metabolites are in microgram per milliliter range versus the nanogram per milliliter range for almost all other antidepressants (163). The only other antidepressant that achieves plasma concentration comparable with bupropion is nefazodone and its metabolites (164). That observation is also consistent with the relatively weak *in vitro* affinity of nefazodone and its metabolites for 5-HT$_{2A}$ receptors and the serotonin uptake pump.

The high levels of bupropion and its metabolites achieved on usual therapeutic doses may also account for its narrow therapeutic index in terms of causing seizures. In other words, the levels are sufficiently high that bupropion through another relative weak mechanism is also capable of affecting neuronal firing thresholds.

The weak *in vitro* activity of bupropion is also consistent with its marginal evidence of antidepressant activity, particularly, because its maximal recommended daily dose was capped at 450 mg. Bupropion was initially marketed as an immediate release preparation with the recommendation to be taken on a three-times-per-day basis. That approval was based on efficacy studies using daily doses as high as 900 mg. After that approval, concern about its potential for causing seizures led to a decision to cap the dose at 450 mg. The FDA permitted reanalysis of the efficacy data using only those patients whose daily dose had not exceeded 450 mg in the original studies. The efficacy data were not as robust but the FDA still permitted marketing of the product. Many of the earlier studies in the literature report on data in patients with doses higher than 450 mg per day because they were published before the heightened concern about dose-dependent seizures with this drug.

These facts must be kept in mind when evaluating the efficacy data with this antidepressant. The best evidence supporting this warning is the recent approval of the sustained release version of bupropion. Three double-blind studies were done to support the submission of this formulation for approval. The FDA concluded that all three of these studies failed to show that the sustained release version of bupropion in the doses used (i.e., less than 450 mg per day) was superior to placebo in the treatment of outpatients with major depression (bupropion summary basis of approval). As a result, this formulation was approved on the basis of bioequivalence with the immediate release formulation. The FDA in its approval documents did not specify why it chose to approve this formulation without efficacy data. One possibility is that there are reasons to believe that the sustained release formulation is less likely to cause seizures than is the immediate release version at comparable doses. In contrast to these failed studies, two relatively small studies published in 1983 reported that immediate release bupropion at doses up to 600 mg per day was superior to placebo in the treatment of inpatients hospitalized for major depression (165, 166).

Despite the rather modest evidence of efficacy of this drug as an antidepressant at doses of 450 mg per day or less, it can be a useful option for several reasons:

- Bupropion appears to be *pharmacologically unique* relative to other conventional antidepressants and most closely resembles the action of psychostimulants.
- Evidence from its initial clinical development program indicates that it *works in patients who historically had not responded to TCAs* (167).
- Bupropion appears to be *relatively free of adverse effects on sexual function,* in contrast to the SSRIS or venlafaxine (168).
- Data support its *usefulness in conditions not typically responsive to other antidepressants,* specifically adult attention deficit hyperactivity disorder (ADHD) (169) and smoking cessation (170).
- This agent is *not sedating,* has a *low incidence of anticholinergic adverse effects, does not cause weight gain,* has *no effects on intracardiac conduction,* and has no significant safety risk beyond seizures in overdoses.

Mirtazapine and Mianserin

Mianserin and its analogue, mirtazapine (i.e., 6-azo-mianserin), are tetracyclic compounds and differ from other antidepressants in terms of the putative mechanism responsible for their antidepressant efficacy (171). Mianserin is the older drug and is marketed in several countries around the world but not in the United States.

Three double-blind studies found mianserin to be superior to placebo, but 15 studies found it to be slightly less effective than tertiary amine TCAs (Tables 7-4 and 7-6).

Mirtazapine has been on the market in the United States since August 1996, and it is available in several other countries. The putative mechanism of action mediating antidepressant activity is the blockade of several serotonin receptors (i.e., $5-HT_{2A}$ and $5-HT_{2C}$) and α_2-adrenergic receptors (172). The latter effect increases NE release by a direct effect on the presynaptic α_2-adrenergic autoreceptor and indirectly increases serotonin release via the tonic effect on the adrenergic input to raphe neurons. In addition to these mechanisms of action, mirtazapine and mianserin also block histamine and specific 5-HT receptors (i.e., $5-HT_{2A}$, $5-HT_{2C}$, $5-HT_3$) but have minimal affinity for muscarinic

ACh receptors or α_1-adrenergic receptors, and do not inhibit either NE or serotonin uptake pumps in contrast to TCAs, SSRIs, venlafaxine, or nefazodone.

The approval of mirtazapine in the United States was based on six double-blind, placebo- and amitriptyline-controlled studies in which it was found to be superior to placebo and comparable with amitriptyline in terms of antidepressant efficacy (173, 174). In a double-blind, crossover study, 63% of patients who failed to respond to 6 weeks of double-blind treatment with amitriptyline responded to mirtazapine (175). In two studies, mirtazapine was found to be efficacious in the treatment of patients hospitalized for major depression. In the first study, the antidepressant efficacy of mirtazapine was comparable with that of amitriptyline and superior to placebo (176). In the other study, the antidepressant efficacy was superior to that of fluoxetine (118). There are advantages and disadvantages to mirtazapine, including the following:

Potential advantages

- *Minimal anticholinergic* effects
- *Sedation;* may be useful for agitation and hostility in geriatric patients
- *Safety in overdose*
- *No quinidine-like effect*
- *No blood pressure effects,* including orthostatic hypotension

Potential disadvantages

- *Daytime sedation*
- *Increased appetite*
- *Weight gain*
- *Transient neutropenia* (typically presents and resolves within first 6 weeks of treatment)
- *Transient mild elevations of liver function tests,* particularly serum glutamic-pyruvic transaminase (SGPT) (typically presents and resolves within first 6 weeks of treatment)
- *Rare* adverse event of *severe neutropenia* (3 of 2,796 patients); uncertain causal relationship to mirtazapine treatment

Reboxetine

Efficacy for Acute Treatment

Reboxetine is a norepinephrine selective reuptake inhibitor (NSRI). Based on *in vitro* studies, reboxetine does not block the reuptake of either dopamine or serotonin. It has low affinity for adrenergic, cholinergic, histaminic, dopaminergic, and serotoninergic receptors (176). At a dose of 4 mg twice daily, reboxetine has exerted substantial inhibition of NE uptake in humans as witnessed by abolishment of the tyramine pressor response (177).

Reboxetine is marketed in several countries around the world. However, the FDA has recently rejected its new drug application (NDA) because of insufficient evidence of efficacy. Nevertheless, resubmission is planned after the completion of ongoing studies.

Although its mechanism of action is similar to that of desipramine and maprotiline, reboxetine is not a TCA, and, in contrast, does not inhibit electrically excitable membranes. For this reason, overdose of reboxetine should not carry a significant risk of cardiotoxicity or seizures. Although a distinct advantage, the aforementioned is based on preclinical data because there is minimal clinical experience with overdoses of this drug.

Most efficacy trials with reboxetine have so far only been published in review articles (178). Most of these articles did not have peer review and do not contain the full details concerning methodology or results. This fact limits the ability to accurately determine its relative efficacy and tolerability. In short-term (4 to 8 weeks), placebo-controlled clinical trials, reboxetine produced a response (defined as at least a 50% reduction in severity scores) in 56% to 74% of patients. These results were statistically superior to placebo in most studies. Reboxetine was also found to be as effective as imipramine and desipramine in four double-blind, randomized, active-controlled (but not placebo-controlled) studies involving more than 800 outpatients or inpatients with major depression. Reboxetine produced equivalent antidepressant response rates compared with fluoxetine in two clinical trials, one of which was also placebo-controlled. However, reboxetine was reported to have improved social motivation and behavior more than fluoxetine as assessed by the newly developed Social Adaptation Self-Evaluation Scale. In all of the studies, reboxetine had a similar time (i.e., 2 to 3 weeks) to onset of the antidepressant efficacy as do other antidepressants.

Monoamine Oxidase Inhibitors

Interest in drugs that inhibit monoamine oxidase has been spurred, not only by controlled studies that document their antidepressant efficacy, but also by the demonstration of their benefit in the treatment of the following:

- *Atypical depression*
- *Mixed anxiety* and *depressive disorders*
- *Panic disorder,* with or without agoraphobia
- *Eating disorders,* particularly bulimia (because of required dietary restrictions; however, this may not be a feasible therapy in many of these patients)

Iproniazid was the first widely prescribed MAOI. Realization that this drug can produce rare but dangerous liver toxicity led to the synthesis of the other hydrazine MAOIs, such as isocarboxazid, nialamide, and phenelzine, as well as the nonhydrazine MAOIs, tranylcypromine, and pargyline.

There are two types of monoamine oxidase (i.e., A and B), which represent different proteins. MAO-A preferentially deaminates serotonin and NE, whereas MAO-B preferentially deaminates dopamine, benzylamine, and phenylethylamine. Certain substrates (e.g., tyramine and tryptamine) are comparably deaminated by both types.

Important intraspecies differences are found in the relative proportions of MAO-A or MAO-B in tissues [e.g., human brain has more MAO-B (about 70%) activity; rat brain has more MAO-A]. After administration of an MAOI, intracellular levels of endogenous amines (e.g., NE) increase, but levels of amines not usually found in humans (tryptamine and phenylethylamine) also increase, followed by a compensatory decrease in amine synthesis because of feedback mechanisms. Levels of other amines or their metabolites (i.e., false transmitters) increase in storage vesicles and may displace true transmitters, while presynaptic neuronal firing rates decrease. After 3 to 6 weeks, brain serotonin may return to normal levels and NE levels may decrease. There is a compensatory decrease in the number of d_2 and β receptors, including β-adrenergic receptor-related functions (e.g., NE-stimulated adenyl cyclase).

Most presently available MAOIs are irreversible inhibitors of the enzyme, forming a chemical bond with part of the enzyme or the flavin adenine dinucleotide cofactor. When treatment is stopped, inhibition continues for a time until MAO levels return to normal as the new enzyme is synthesized. Thus, phenelzine, isocarboxazid, and tranylcypromine are all irreversible, nonselective MAOIs. *Clorgyline,* however, is an irreversible, selective MAO-A inhibitor; moclobemide is a reversible, selective MAOI; *l-deprenyl* and *pargyline* are relatively selective, irreversible MAO-B inhibitors.

Although the half-life of an MAOI is short (hours), the half-life of MAO inhibition is about 2 weeks because it takes that long for the new enzyme to be synthesized. Some have speculated that phenelzine may be metabolized by acetylation and that there are two hereditary types (i.e., slow and fast acetylators), with slow acetylators presumably having a greater degree of MAO inhibition. There is limited support for the theory that slow acetylators have a better response, whereas other investigators find no difference (179). More importantly, there is no evidence that phenelzine is indeed acetylated.

New Approaches to MAOIs

Given the unique efficacy of MAOIs, there have been several attempts to develop kinder and gentler versions. *A transdermal form of selegiline is one promising approach.* Another approach is the development of *selective and reversible MAOIs* (180).

Selegiline is an irreversible but relatively selective inhibitor of MAO-B. An oral preparation is

TABLE 7-10. *Characteristics of MAOIs*

Maoi	Selectivity	Substrate	Reversibility
Brofaromine (NA)	MAO-A	Serotonin and norepinephrine	Yes
Cimoxatone (NA)			Yes
Clorgyline (NA)			No
Moclobemide (NA)			Yes
Toloxatone (NA)			Yes
Pargyline (NA)	MAO-B	Phenylethylamine and benzylamine	No
Selegiline			No
Isocarboxazid	MAO A,B	Tyramine, dopamine, and tryptamine	No
Phenelzine			No
Tranylcypromine			No

MAOI, monoamine oxidase inhibitor; NA, not available in the United States.

currently marketed as a treatment for Parkinson's disease. An oral dose produces meaningful inhibition of MAO-B but not MAO-A. **The concept behind the transdermal patch is to preferentially deliver more selegiline to the brain than to the liver such that meaningful inhibition of both MAO-A and MAO-B is achieved in the brain but only MAO-B inhibition is achieved in the liver.** The goal is to have antidepressant efficacy *without the risk of tyramine-induced hypertensive crisis.* Recent studies have suggested that the selegiline transdermal system (STS) may have achieved this goal. Normal volunteers given STS 20 cm^3/20 mg for 13 days were able to consume more than 300 mg of tyramine without experiencing any clinically relevant increases in systolic or diastolic blood pressure (181). Yet, a double-blind study found that the same STS regimen was statistically superior to placebo in the treatment of outpatients with major depression (182). The response rate was 37% for STS versus a 24% response rate for placebo with response defined as at least a 50% reduction in HDRS scores. If further studies are positive, then physicians may be able to treat cases with an MAOI with an appreciable lower risk of causing hypertensive crises.

Another approach is to develop *selective and reversible MAOIs.* The goal again is to produce agents with a minimal risk of tyramine reactions and thus markedly diminish the need for the dietary restrictions that have plagued the use of nonselective and irreversible A, B inhibitors.

Collaborative clinical trials of the reversible inhibitors of monoamine oxidase A (RIMAs) in Europe have included more than 2,000 patients, many hospitalized for more severe, endogenous depressive episodes (183). In comparison trials with the TCAs, the onset of effect with RIMAs was also more rapid in some cases.

The best studied of this group is moclobemide, which has been equal in efficacy to tertiary amine TCAs and superior to placebo (Tables 7-10 and 7-11). Despite these promising results, the development of moclobemide in the United States was discontinued, presumably because of failure to separate from placebo in double-blind studies.

Other RIMAs under investigation include the following:

- Brofaromine
- Cimoxatone
- Toloxatone

If type A inhibitors eventually prove to be as efficacious as other MAOIs and non-MAOIs, there is no doubt that some clinicians will prescribe them with increasing frequency. In addition, if there is minimal risk of adverse interactions with tyramine and other substances (e.g., sympathomimetics), medical and legal concerns about their use will be appreciably reduced.

Table 7-10 summarizes the characteristics of several of RIMAs, which are either clinically available or under study. There are advantages and disadvantages to these agents, including the following:

TABLE 7-11. *MAOIs versus placebo: acute treatment*

Drug	Number of studies	Number of subjects	Responders (%) MAOI (%)	Placebo (%)	Difference (%)	Chi square	p value
Moclobemide	6	535	65	24	41	87.2	10^{-20}
Phenelzine	8	429	56	43	14	7.9	0.005

MAOI, monoamine oxidase inhibitor.

Potential advantages

- *No nonspecific biochemical or pharmacological actions*
- Antidepressant effect attributed to effect on *isoenzyme MAO-A* only; therefore, propensity to cause *tyramine potentiation* is substantially reduced
- Effective in *endogenous* and *atypical depression*
- The ability to *monitor the presumed mechanism of action* (i.e., monoamine oxidase inhibition) using platelets as a surrogate rather than monitoring the plasma drug level

Potential disadvantages

- Effective *dosage* is variable
- *Adverse effects*—loss of appetite, nausea, and other gastrointestinal disturbances; insomnia
- Shorter *duration* of action
- *Idiosyncratic responses* from time to time
- Substantially *different pharmacodynamic profiles* from earlier MAOIs

Efficacy for Acute Treatment

At one time, TCAs were thought to be more effective than the MAOIs, but recent investigation has found these two classes equally effective (184). The poorer showing in some of the earlier studies was the result of subtherapeutic doses of MAOIs administered to treatment-resistant populations (e.g., psychotic depressions, which are not usually responsive to any form of monotherapy).

The efficacy of phenelzine and tranylcypromine has now been well established by several large, double-blind studies, which found them equal to tertiary amine TCAs and clearly superior to placebo (Tables 7-11 and 7-12) (185). Other studies indicate that atypical depressions may respond better to MAOIs and typical depressions to TCAs; however, most find that their similarities are more obvious than their differences (186). One research group has suggested that anergic, bipolar patients respond particularly well to tranylcypromine and other MAOIs (187). Extensive clinical experience indicates the MAOIs are often effective when TCAs have failed.

TABLE 7-12. *Summary of controlled double-blind studies of MAOIs*

Drug	Number of studies in which the effect was More than placebo	Equal to placebo	More than imipramine	Equal to imipramine	Less than imipramine
Isocarboxazid	2	4	0	2	2
Pargyline	2	0	0	0	0
Phenelzine	11	4	0	4	3
Tranylcypromine	2	1	0	3	0

MAOI, monoamine oxidase inhibitor.
Adapted from Klein DF, Davis JM. Diagnosis and drug treatment of psychiatric disorders. Baltimore: Williams & Wilkins, 1969:207–208.

Other Drug Therapies

Psychomotor Stimulants

Cocaine, amphetamine, dextroamphetamine, methylphenidate, and pemoline are classified as psychomotor stimulants, producing an acute euphoria in control subjects, as well as a wide variety of responses in psychiatric patients. These stimulants are also effective in postponing the deterioration in psychomotor performance that often accompanies extreme fatigue, a property that may be useful in some carefully selected cases.

Although there is no doubt that amphetamines or other psychomotor stimulants induce an initial euphoria, there is considerable doubt that they can serve as long-lasting antidepressants. Cocaine, for example, produces a euphoria almost immediately after i.v. injection and within a few minutes after intranasal administration, but the euphoria, as well as the tachycardia, decrease at a slightly faster rate than the level of plasma cocaine. A second dose given 1 hour later fails to produce a similar level of euphoria or tachycardia, suggesting a rapid tachyphylaxis.

Amphetamines

One British study found amphetamine to be no different than placebo in the treatment of depressed outpatients (188); a second study found amphetamine *less effective* than phenelzine and no better than placebo (189); and a Veteran's Administration (VA) study found dextroamphetamine no more effective than placebo in hospitalized depressed patients (190). Uncontrolled clinical evidence indicates that amphetamine may occasionally be of value, but, except for a mild, early, transient benefit, there is no evidence that amphetamine can ameliorate moderate-to-severe depressive episodes.

Methylphenidate

The authors have encountered some patients refractory to all other therapies who had a dramatic, full, rapid, and sustained response to methylphenidate. One study found methylphenidate effective in treating mildly depressed outpatients, particularly those who drank three or more cups of coffee a day (191). A replication study did not find a drug–placebo difference on the physician's ratings, but did demonstrate one for the patients' subjective assessment of improvement (192). Another blind study of methylphenidate found improvement in an outpatient group (193). Finally, two of three trials of methylphenidate in apathetic, senile geriatric patients showed that this drug produced more improvement than placebo (194). To date, no evidence indicates that it is beneficial in cases of moderate-to-severe depression.

Complications

All psychostimulants can cause jitteriness, palpitations, and psychic dependence. Depression may arise after their discontinuance, and high doses can produce a florid psychosis. On occasion, even small doses of amphetamine can precipitate psychotic episodes in those with an underlying predisposition (e.g., schizophrenic disorder).

Summary

Five studies of amphetamine for depression were clearly negative, with none finding it more effective than placebo. Although there were occasional hints of efficacy, in one study amphetamine was even less effective than placebo.

The results with methylphenidate, however, are more impressive. Two of three studies found a significant effect and the third found improvement on the patients' subjective evaluation. Although amphetamine and methylphenidate are similar in their pharmacology, they differ in some respects. Amphetamine releases dopamine from newly synthesized pools (α-methyl-p-tyrosine-sensitive pool); whereas methylphenidate releases dopamine from storage sites (reserpine-sensitive sites). This pharmacological difference could be related to the apparent greater efficacy of methylphenidate.

In conclusion, there are also isolated reports of depressed patients who fail to respond to standard antidepressants but do well on low doses of stimulants. There are also some limited trial data supporting antidepressant efficacy for methylphenidate but not amphetamine.

TABLE 7-13. *Lithium versus placebo: acute treatment*

Disorder	Number of studies	Number of subjects	Responders (%) Lithium (%)	Placebo (%)	Difference (%)	Chi square	*p* value
Unipolar depression	4 (Uncontrolled)	79	39	27	12	0.5	NS
Unipolar depression	1 (Controlled)	27	57	38	19	0.9	NS
Bipolar depression	2 (Controlled)	38	76	35	41	5.5	0.02

Lithium

Lithium has been found to be superior to placebo, particularly as an acute treatment for the depressed phase of a bipolar disorder (Table 7-13). Mendels et al. (195) reviewed and Souza and Goodwin (196) statistically combined the data from many of the same trials. Their results also indicate that the marginal evidence for the acute antidepressant effect of lithium was in the bipolar depressed patient group.

In addition, the use of lithium as an augmentation to standard antidepressants has been the most effective strategy in partially responsive depressive episodes (see "Alternative Treatment Strategies" later in this chapter).

Antipsychotics

There are several early studies addressing the possible antidepressant effects of neuroleptics (e.g., chlorpromazine, thioridazine, chlorprothixene); however, interpretation of their results is complicated by the inclusion of patients with anergic schizophrenia, psychotic depression, or compensation neurosis (Table 7-14) (197). In general, antipsychotics seemed better for anxious or hostile, rather than retarded depressions. In contrast, a VA random-assignment, double-blind study found that imipramine was superior to placebo for retarded depression (198). It is not clear how to translate this finding into a clinically meaningful strategy for treating depression.

Benzodiazepines

Benzodiazepines (BZDs) have been used for the treatment of depression because their sedative effects can reduce insomnia, agitation, and anxiety symptoms that frequently accompany depressed states. Considerable evidence also indicates that major depression may accompany panic and agoraphobic disorders (199–201). *When depression precedes the onset of panic disorder, clinical experience suggests a better response to antidepressants than to BZDs, although no studies have directly addressed this issue* (202). Conversely, available evidence indicates that *when depression occurs after the onset of panic disorder,* treatment with either a BZD or a tricyclic may result in concomitant improvement of both the panic and depressive symptoms (198–203). Depression, however, has been reported to be an adverse effect of BZD treatment.

Compared with TCAs and MAOIs, BZDs have a rapid onset of action, have fewer unpleasant

TABLE 7-14. *Summary of controlled double-blind studies of neuroleptics for depression*

Drug	Number of studies in which the effect was More than placebo	Equal to placebo	More than imipramine	Equal to imipramine	Less than imipramine
Chlorpromazine	3	0	0	3	0
Chlorprothixene	0	0	0	1	0
Thioridazine	0	0	0	1	0

Adapted from Klein DF, Davis JM. *Diagnosis and drug treatment of psychiatric disorders.* Baltimore: Williams & Wilkins, 1969:208.

TABLE 7-15. *Benzodiazepines versus standard antidepressants: acute treatment*

| Number of studies | Number of subjects | Responders (%) | | Difference (%) | Chi square | *p* value |
		BZD (%)	Standard AD (%)			
19	1,275	51	72	21	65.3	6×10^{-16}

AD, antidepressants; BZD, benzodiazepine.

adverse effects, and are considerably less toxic. Despite these advantages, however, BZDs (with the possible exception of alprazolam, discussed later) generally appear devoid of true antidepressant effects. When the results of several well-controlled studies totalling 1,275 patients were summarized, the overall response to BZDs was 51% versus 73% for standard antidepressants. This generated a highly significant difference ($p < 10^{-16}$) on the Mantel-Haenzsel test in favor of the antidepressants (Table 7-15).

Schatzberg and Cole (204) reviewed 20 controlled studies of BZDs used in the treatment of a mixed profile of depressions and also concluded that, although anxiety and insomnia may be significantly relieved, core depressive symptoms (e.g., psychomotor retardation and diurnal variation) remain essentially unchanged. Some positive resolutions were seen in depressions associated with a high level of anxiety, but there was little evidence for efficacy in more severe depressions without prominent anxiety.

In addition, Cassano et al. (205) reviewed a series of studies comparing a TCA with a BZD for "neurotic" and "endogenous" depressions, as well as anxiety states. They concluded that BZDs were effective in reducing insomnia, agitation, and anxiety, and had some effect in elevating mood and improving social adjustment, but were not effective in improving core depressive symptoms. Furthermore, "endogenous" patients given BZDs often appeared to experience residual symptoms. Noting that these findings suggest that BZDs could be useful adjuncts to TCAs, Klerman, nevertheless, cautioned against this approach, because these agents have been reported to aggravate depression, possibly increase the risk of suicide, and may lead to a more chronic syndrome (204–210). By contrast,

Fawcett (211) suggests that treatment with anxiolytics may decrease suicidal behavior in anxious, depressed patients. Conceivably, the use of BZDs in anxious, agitated depression could lead to an association between suicide and BZD treatment on a statistical rather than a causative basis.

When BZDs, particularly those with short half-lives (e.g., alprazolam and lorazepam), are used with nonsedating antidepressants such as secondary amine TCAs (e.g., desipramine, nortriptyline), SSRIs, and venlafaxine to treat insomnia, patients may experience offset symptoms (dysphoric mood, agitation, increased insomnia) when they have trough blood levels the next day. They may then take a higher dose on following nights, possibly leading to increased physiological and psychological dependence, prolongation of depressive states, and social disability.

Alprazolam and Adinazolam

There were large development programs to test the efficacy of both of these triazolobenziapines (211–214). Neither drug was able to convincingly separate from placebo. Hence, their development was abandoned.

Complications

BZDs may exacerbate depression and possibly increase suicide risk. Case reports and clinical trials also indicate that BZD treatment of generalized anxiety and panic may result in emergence of depression (215–226). In some of these reports, depression is ill-defined, but in others, it met DSM-III criteria for a major depressive disorder, requiring treatment with an antidepressant (225, 226). Depression has been reported with a variety of BZDs (alprazolam, bromazepam, clonazepam, diazepam, lorazepam), but there is no evidence that one is more likely than another to cause or aggravate depressive illness.

Risk may be increased in patients with low trait anxiety or when higher than usual BZD doses are used (219, 222, 223, 225, 226). Depression may abate if dosage is decreased, although discontinuation and treatment with an antidepressant may be required (222, 225, 226).

Alprazolam has no significant anticholinergic or cardiovascular effects, but in almost all studies reporting adverse effects, alprazolam-induced sedation was comparable with or greater than that of the tertiary amine TCA. In one comparison with desipramine, drowsiness led to motor vehicle accidents in 2 of 16 outpatients taking alprazolam and required discontinuation in another 3 (212, 213).

The risk of dependency for any BZD and related compounds increases with longer use and higher dosages. The relative risk among members of this class for causing dependency and the severity of withdrawal appears to be related to two pharmacological characteristics: one pharmacodynamic and one pharmacokinetic. Pharmacodynamically, the risk is higher the greater the potency of the BZD for binding to the BZD binding site and thus potentiating the central effects of the neurotransmitter GABA. Pharmacokinetically, the risk appears to increase the shorter the half-life of the compound because it increases the likelihood that clearance can occur before compensatory readjustment. Both of these reasons appear to explain why the likelihood and the severity of withdrawal are greater with triazolobenzodiazepines such as alprazolam, than with the older, less potent and more long-lived BZDs such as diazepam.

Such withdrawal can be serious. For example, Goldberg and colleagues (227) reported the occurrence of a seizure in a patient who, against instructions, failed to taper alprazolam but instead abruptly discontinued it. Of note, the triazolobenzodiazepines probably have the highest withdrawal seizure rate of all BZDs, and possibly of all psychotropics.

Azapirones

Buspirone is the only member of this class marketed in the United States. Several compounds in this class, however, have been in active clinical trials in this country and include gepirone, ipsapirone, and tandospirone. The last is marketed in some countries as an anxiolytic. Members of this class are structurally, pharmacodynamically, and pharmacokinetically similar. They are all partial agonists at the 5-HT$_{1A}$ receptor, although there are some differences among them in terms of the degree to which they act as partial agonists. They also all have a relatively short half-life, generally in the range of 3 to 6 hours, and are metabolized by cleavage to compounds that do not have activity at the 5-HT$_{1A}$ receptor.

Each of these drugs unsuccessfully underwent extensive clinical trial testing for possible antidepressant activity. The inability to demonstrate such activity could have been due to the difficulty in achieving sufficiently stable plasma drug levels of these compounds over the dosing interval because of their short half-life. However, several sustained release formulations of these drugs also were unable to demonstrate superiority over placebo in double-blind trials. That fact calls into question whether partial agonism of the 5-HT$_{1A}$ receptor is a viable mechanism of antidepressant activity. Despite the current discouraging performance of this class of drugs as antidepressants, studies are currently under way with a sustained release version of gepirone.

Natural Remedies

An ironic consequence of the success of rational drug development in psychiatry has been the recent increased interest and use of natural compounds and herbs to treat clinical depression. All of the herbal remedies discussed herein contain pharmacologically active ingredients, which may produce beneficial or adverse effects. After all, opium, cocaine, and curare are herbal products. Being "natural" is not synonymous with being safe or ineffective. As a general rule, any chemical, which through its action on the human body can produce a beneficial effect, can also cause an adverse effect, often through the same mechanism of action. Many patients take these remedies without telling their physicians, setting the stage for potential untoward results caused by the natural remedy–drug interaction, either pharmacokinetic or pharmacodynamic.

The use of herbs has also been fueled by the increased awareness of clinical depression and its treatment as a result of the marketing efforts of major pharmaceutical companies. That effort has transformed prescription antidepressants into one of the largest dollar sales category in pharmaceuticals such that the sales for a "block buster" antidepressant can be more than 2 billion dollars per year. **Not surprisingly, then, herbal remedies or "phytomedicine" has also become a multibillion dollar industry in the United States with an estimated one in ten Americans having used herbal agents within the past year, with or without their physician's knowledge.**

Herbal remedies are used for a wide range of psychiatric and nonpsychiatric medical conditions, but a number are specifically touted as being useful in treating depression. These agents include the following:

- *Hypericum perforatum,* or St. John's Wort (also known as Klamath weed)
- *Ginkgo biloba*
- *Ginseng*
- *Lobelia inflata*
- *Mentat*
- *Morinda citrifolia* and *officinalis*
- *Rhazya stricta*
- *Valeria officinalis*

Herbal remedies currently are considered "dietary supplements" and, hence, are regulated under the same provisions as foods. Thus, to be marketed, these products do not have to meet the same stringent manufacturing or testing requirements as do patented drugs. The net result is twofold:

- There is the potential for *significant variability in the composition* of these remedies from producer to producer and even year to year variability for the same producer (just like good and bad years for wine from the same vineyard).
- There is limited information about the *clinically relevant pharmacology* of these products.

The variability in composition is because these are natural products and often are not pure extracts of a single chemical. Instead, they often contain multiple chemicals that may contribute to different beneficial or adverse effects. Composition may also vary as a function of what part of the plant is used to make the product (e.g., the root versus the stalk). In contrast to patented medications, there is no requirement to prove safety or efficacy to market it. There is also no requirement to define the basic pharmacology of the product. Hence, there is often little substantive knowledge about the pharmacodynamics or the pharmacokinetics of the compound or constituents.

Given the widespread use of herbal products, the current situation is gradually changing. Attempts are being made by some of the manufacturers of herbal remedies to establish good manufacturing standards and labeling that specifies the relative composition of the product. More research is also being done on their pharmacology. Nevertheless, these efforts pale in comparison with what is required for the approval of patented medications.

This situation is reminiscent of the early days of the approval of patented medications. In general, the history of the development of regulations governing drug approval has been the direct result of serious untoward events. Examples include the deaths of more than 100 children in 1938 as a result of the use of diethylene glycol in a solution of sulfanilamide or the thalidomide-induced birth defects in the early 1960's. Only time will tell whether self-regulation by the herbal industry will prevent such a disaster from rewriting the current rules that govern their marketing and promotion.

Hypericum perforatum (St. John's Wort)

This herbal product has the most data available to support its usefulness as an antidepressant. Nevertheless, only minimal information is available about its pharmacology and its relative risk–benefit ratio. At least seven different biologically active chemicals have been isolated from crude extracts of hypericum. Several are ubiquitous in the plant kingdom. The exceptions are hypericin and pseudohypericin, which have been assumed to be responsible for any antidepressant activity of this product. Nevertheless, there is the potential for one or more of these seven compounds and their metabolites to mediate desired or undesired effects, particularly when used in combination with other medications (i.e., herb–drug interactions).

Hypericum has several potential mechanisms of action, including affinity for multiple neuroreceptors, uptake pumps for all three biogenic amines, and monoamine oxidase (228, 229). Hypericum, based on *in vitro* studies, is equipotent at inhibiting the uptake pumps for serotonin, dopamine, and NE. No patented antidepressant can make that claim. However, hypericum has only weak affinity for these mechanisms in comparison with approved antidepressants such as the SSRIs and TCAs. Hence, the question remains as to whether hypericum under its usual dosing conditions achieves high enough concentrations to produce a magnitude of effect that is likely to be physiologically relevant or comparable with that seen with marketed antidepressants (230). Of interest, subchronic administration of hypericum produces downregulation of β-adrenergic receptors in rodent frontal cortex as do TCAs. However, it produces up-regulation of 5-HT$_2$ receptors, which is an effect opposite to that of SSRIs and TCAs (228, 231).

Although the actions of hypericum on biogenic amine mechanisms could mediate its potential antidepressant efficacy, these actions also raise the possibility that hypericum could interact with drugs that affect any one of the three principal biogenic amine systems (232). Thus, caution should be exercised when prescribing biogenic amine active drugs to individuals taking hypericum.

While little is known about the pharmacodynamics of hypericum, even less is known about its metabolism or its potential to affect the metabolism of other drugs. However, hypericum has recently been shown to produce substantial induction of CYP 3A3/4 such that a warning has been issued about its ability to decrease the levels of protease inhibitors to less than effective concentrations. Thus, physicians will likely need to prescribe higher doses of CYP 3A3/4 substrates when a patient is taking hypericum just as in patients on carbamazepine, a classic CYP 3A 3/4 inducer.

Several meta-analyses on the efficacy of St. John's Wort as an antidepressant have been published. The first involved 23 randomized trials (15 placebo-controlled and eight active-controlled) involving 1,757 outpatients. It concluded that there was preliminary evidence supporting hypericum extracts as being superior to placebo in patients with mild to moderate clinical depression (233). Two more recent reviews of subsequent, placebo-controlled studies also concluded that hypericum is more effective than placebo but possibly less effective than TCAs (234, 235). Recently, however, a U.S. multicentered, double-blind, placebo-controlled trial on 200 patients with major depression could not demonstrate significance for St. John's Wort over placebo (235a). A large-scale, multicenter, double-blind, placebo- and active-controlled study is still ongoing in the United States, testing the efficacy of hypericum versus an SSRI in patients with major depression.

The most common adverse effects of hypericum are similar to those of SSRIs and include the following:

- Gastrointestinal symptoms
- Dizziness
- Confusion
- Fatigue
- Sedation (236)

Its adverse effect profile suggests that hypericum may produce physiologically relevant serotonin uptake inhibition comparable with that seen with SSRIs. Photosensitivity has also been rarely reported (237).

Of interest, treatment with hypericum is more expensive than with TCAs. Although it is somewhat less expensive than fluoxetine and paroxetine, depending on the formulation of hypericum used, its cost is comparable with that of sertraline.

Ginkgo biloba

Standardized extracts of ginkgo have been studied in Europe for the treatment of vascular dementia (238), and the lay literature cites this agent as having antidepressant activity (239). The latter appears to be based on one double-blind trial in 40 elderly patients who had not responded to TCAs. The authors reported a statistically better response on ginkgo compared with placebo (240). Ginkgo has numerous actions, including effects on platelets (e.g., antagonism of platelet-activating factor, inhibition of platelet aggregation and degranulation, and inhibition of platelet adhesion) (238). In terms of CNS effects, ginkgo has been reported to inhibit MAO-A and -B, bind to 5-HT$_{1A}$, and normalize cholinergic transmission (238).

Consistent with these multiple actions, ginkgo is not innocuous, with adverse effects that include the following:

• Gastrointestinal disturbances
• Headache
• Restlessness
• Dermatitis (239)

Several case reports of spontaneous bilateral subdural hematomas associated with chronic ginkgo use have been reported (241, 242). Although these reports may simply reflect the underlying vascular problems for which ginkgo is most often taken, they may also be due to the effect of ginkgo on platelet function. There has also been one case of tonic-clonic seizures and loss of consciousness following a ginkgo overdose in an infant (243).

Ginseng

Ginseng is cited in the lay literature as effective for multiple symptoms including depression (239), yet, there are no controlled trials, and little is known about its pharmacodynamics or pharmacokinetics. There are reports that suggest it may decrease the effect of warfarin and increase levels of digoxin (244, 245). Two case reports have suggested that concomitant administration of ginseng and phenelzine can cause insomnia, headache, tremulousness, irritability, and visual hallucinations (246). It also has estrogenic and androgenic properties, including androgenization and unexplained vaginal bleeding in postmenopausal women.

Valeria officinalis

This herb has been part of folk medicine since pre-Christian times (247). It has been primarily used as a sedative and for the treatment of epilepsy. Consistent with this use, this herb reportedly can increase synaptic concentrations of GABA (248). GABA has also been isolated from valeria and extracts of valeria have been reported to bind to GABA receptors in rat brain. Although valeria has been reported to be active in rodent models of depression, there have been no efficacy trials in humans. The potential adverse effects of valeria include the sensation of strangeness (247) and several cases of liver damage (e.g., central lobular necrosis) (249). Mutagenicity in bacteria has been reported and attributed to unstable, water-insoluble valepotriates (238). As a result of these reports, many, but not all, commercial preparations of valeria use water-soluble extracts standardized for their content of valeric acid.

Other Herbal Remedies

Lobelia inflata, mentat, Morinda citrifolia and officinalis, and Rhazya stricta have all been suggested to have antidepressant properties. There are no controlled studies, however, with any of these herbal products to support these claims. Moreover, these products are not innocuous.

Lobelia is a nicotine-like herb that acts as an agonist at the nicotinic ganglion. Consistent with this action, it can be dangerous in an overdose, causing respiratory distress, rapid heart rate, sweating, decreased blood pressure, convulsions, and coma. As a result, the FDA has declared it to be an unsafe herb (238).

Mentat is used as a cognitive enhancer. Essentially no information on its pharmacology, efficacy, or safety in humans is available.

Morinda citroflia and *officinalis* is composed of multiple compounds including nystose, succinic acid, 1F-fructofurnaosylynytose, an inulin-type hexasaccharide, and hepatasaccharide

(250). This observation is useful when considering the complexity of trying to understand the pharmacology of herbal products. Essentially, no information on its pharmacology, efficacy, or safety in humans is available.

Rhazya stricta is a poisonous plant used as a traditional folk medicine in the United Arab Emirates. It has possible antineoplastic effects and may have considerable cytotoxicity. Although antidepressant activity has been suggested on the basis of animal studies (251), essentially no information on its pharmacology, efficacy, or safety in humans is available.

S-Adenosyl-l-Methionine

S-Adenosyl-l-methionine (SAMe) is a naturally occurring substance whose primary role appears to be that of a methyl donor in the CNS (252). It participates in the metabolism of various biogenic amines implicated in the pathogenesis of depressive disorders. Several investigations have indicated that it may be an effective antidepressant with minimal adverse effects.

We performed a Mantel-Haenszel test on three studies comparing SAMe with placebo and found that this agent was significantly better (i.e., chi square $= 26.0$; $p < 3 \times 10^{-7}$) (253). A second Mantel-Haenszel test on nine studies comparing SAMe with standard antidepressants revealed a chi square of 6.7 ($p < 0.01$). In sum, 109 of 142 SAMe-treated patients and 80 of 124 TCA-treated patients were classified as responders (i.e., a 12% difference favoring SAMe) (253).

Results of a literature review and metaanalyses were consistent with our preliminary findings, all of which show a greater efficacy for SAMe over placebo and comparable efficacy with TCAs. Furthermore, adverse effects with this agent were generally negligible in comparison with those associated with TCAs. Even though there was a trend in most studies favoring SAMe over the TCAs, the number of subjects was small. Furthermore, the significant difference with the metaanalysis was based principally on the results of two studies, suggesting caution in its interpretation. Unfortunately, difficulties in developing a stable oral preparation of this drug have impeded its development for routine clinical use.

Choice of Antidepressant

When selecting an antidepressant, the following should always be considered:

- Use of *monodrug therapy* whenever possible
- *Safety and tolerability,* keeping in mind that these are different concepts (i.e., a treatment may be safe but poorly tolerated, whereas another treatment is well tolerated but with a low margin of safety)
- *Class* and *spectrum of activity* of a given antidepressant
- *Likelihood of pharmacokinetic or pharmacodynamic interactions,* with the goal of minimizing adverse interactions with other drugs or medical conditions
- *Ease of administration* (to maximize the likelihood of treating with the optimal dose and to facilitate patient compliance)
- *Confidence in its use,* generally based on:
  - Years of patient exposure
  - Number and quality of controlled trials, including data on effectiveness for severe, as well as milder, episodes
  - Number and variety of patients treated in terms of age, health status, and concurrent medications
- *Cost* and *cost effectiveness*
- When *psychotic symptoms* are present, use of a combination of antidepressant plus antipsychotic or a trial with ECT

Certain clinical variables are also helpful in choosing a drug for an initial trial, including the following:

- If the patient (or a family member) has had a *previous positive response* to a particular drug, it should be considered as a first choice.
- If patients have predominant symptoms of *insomnia or psychomotor agitation*, a more sedating drug (e.g., trazodone or mirtazapine) may benefit initially but could be problematic later in therapy (i.e., cause excessive sedation once sleep normalizes).
- In psychomotorically *retarded* patients, many clinicians prefer to use a less sedating drug (e.g., an SSRI, venlafaxine, bupropion, or desipramine), but definitive evidence is lacking.

TABLE 7-16. *Classification of antidepressants by chemical structure and mechanisms of action*

Antidepressant	Chemical class	Mechanism of action
Tertiary amine (TCAs)	Heterocyclics	Norepinephrine (NE) and 5-HT uptake inhibition plus effects on numerous other receptors and on intracardiac conduction
Secondary amine TCAs	Heterocyclics	NE uptake inhibition
Mianserin		α_2 NE presynaptic
Mirtazapine		α_2 NE presynaptic 5-HT$_2$ presynaptic
Selective serotonin reuptake inhibitors		
Fluoxetine	Phenylpropylamine	5-HT > NE uptake inhibition
Sertraline	Naphthalenamine	5-HT $\gg$ NE uptake inhibition
Paroxetine	Phenylpiperidine	5-HT $\gg$ NE uptake inhibition
Venlafaxine	Phenylethylamine	5-HT and NE uptake inhibition
Triazolopyridines		
Nefazodone, trazodone	Phenylpiperazine	5-HT$_2$ receptor blockade > 5-HT update inhibition
Bupropion	Aminoketones	Dopamine and NE uptake inhibition
Monoamine oxidase inhibitors		
Phenelzine	Hydrazine	Nonselective irreversible monoamine oxidase inhibitors
Tranylcypromine	Nonhydrazine	

Adapted from Preskorn S. Antidepressant drug selection: criteria and options. *J Clin Psychiatry* 1994:55 (suppl 9A):6–22.

- Patients with *cardiovascular disorders* or those predisposed to *anticholinergic adverse effects* (e.g., elderly or diabetic patients) probably do best on drugs low in these effects (e.g., an SSRI, venlafaxine, or bupropion).
- Depressed patients with an *eating disorder* (i.e., anorexia or bulimia) or a *history of seizures* should not take bupropion or maprotiline because of an increased risk of *seizures*.
- *Highly suicidal* patients should be given agents posing less risk of lethality with overdose and less risk of interacting with other drugs taken in an overdose attempt (i.e., sertraline, citalopram, or venlafaxine).

For the same reason, sertraline, citalopram, and venlafaxine are the preferred antidepressants for elderly and medically ill patients.

Antidepressant Classes

With the preceding issues in mind, the clinician can begin to formulate a logical and systematic approach to antidepressant therapy. At present, several classes of antidepressants are available as defined by the presumed mechanism of action underlying their antidepressant efficacy (Table 7-16).

The benefit of having different classes to choose from includes the apparent difference in their mechanisms of action (which may lead to differences in their range of antidepressant activity), as well as differences in tolerability and safety. Knowledge about these differences can then be used to tailor drug treatment for a given patient, thus optimizing outcome.

The SSRIs and other newer antidepressants have replaced the TCAs as the antidepressants of first and even second choice for most physicians. The reason is that they have greater safety and better tolerability rather than efficacy. There is still no class of antidepressant, however, that is better than TCAs in terms of efficacy. Another advantage of all newer antidepressants, except the phenylpiperazines (i.e., nefazodone and trazodone) and bupropion over TCAs is the ability to start with a dose that is usually effective rather than having to start at a subtherapeutic dose and adjust upward later.

Selective Serotonin Reuptake Inhibitors

Members of this class have response and re-mission rates equal to the TCAs in outpatients with major depression. Fluoxetine, paroxetine, and sertraline can be started at their usually effective dose (Table 7-17). The recommendation for citalopram is to initiate treatment at 20 mg per day and then advance to 40 mg per day, which was the lowest dose to separate from placebo in the double-blind trials with this SSRI. As noted previously, fluvoxamine is not labeled as an antidepressant in the United States. Fluoxetine, paroxetine, and sertraline all have flat dose–antidepressant response curves based on double-blind, placebo-controlled, fixed-dose studies. This means that the magnitude of the antidepressant effect on average does not increase with higher doses; however, the dropout rate resulting from adverse effects does increase with higher initial starting doses. In fact, the average magnitude of the antidepressant effect in the fixed-dose studies with fluoxetine and paroxetine was somewhat lower at higher doses, because more patients dropped out before they had an opportunity to experience a full therapeutic effect.

Nevertheless, there is wide interindividual variability in the metabolism of SSRIs, comparable with that of TCAs. Therefore, some patients who rapidly or slowly clear these drugs may need a higher or lower dose, respectively, than the usually effective dose. This issue is further addressed in the section on therapeutic drug monitoring later in this chapter.

The need for dose adjustment presents a special problem for fluoxetine, because of the extended half-life of its active metabolite, norfluoxetine (i.e., 7 to 15 days). Because of autoinhibition of metabolism, these half-lives are even longer at higher doses. These half-lives are also longer in healthy individuals older than age 65 years. Because it takes as long as 1 to 2 months to achieve steady-state concentrations of norfluoxetine, it becomes difficult to determine the optimal dose for the patient who needs a dose other than 20 mg per day.

Virtually all patients can be treated using a once-a-day schedule with the SSRIs. The dose is typically given in the morning with or without meals, although taking the medication with meals may reduce the likelihood of nausea that can occur early in treatment. **Given the long half-life of norfluoxetine, fluoxetine could be given as infrequently as once a week and still achieve therapeutic steady-state plasma drug levels.** Thus, it could be used as a "depot" oral medication, allowing for a supervised once weekly dose administration for the noncompliant patient who is not in a setting that permits daily supervision of drug administration, similar to the use of depot neuroleptics for the noncompliant patient with psychosis.

Those who fail to respond to an SSRI may respond to a TCA, and vice versa. Thus, these two broad-spectrum classes can be used in a sequential strategy to adequately treat the majority of cases. However, many physicians try another newer antidepressant (e.g, venlafaxine, bupropion, nefazodone) in such patients because of the safety and tolerability problems associated with TCAs. Of note, the tolerability profile of secondary amine TCAs such as desipramine is as favorable as any of the newer antidepressants and probably better than nefazodone. Nevertheless, the secondary amine TCAs have a therapeutic index as narrow as tertiary amine TCAs (e.g., amitriptyline, imipramine) in terms of lethality in overdoses resulting from cardiotoxicity.

Venlafaxine

Optimal dosing with venlafaxine differs from that of both TCAs and SSRIs. Venlafaxine is like the SSRIs and different from the TCAs in that a therapeutic dose (i.e., 75 mg per day) can be started from the beginning. Unlike the SSRIs, however, dose escalation with venlafaxine does increase the magnitude of the antidepressant effect, which supports increasing the dose in the event of an inadequate response to the initial trial

TABLE 7-17. *Selective serotonin reuptake inhibitors: dose regimens*

Drug	Usual starting dose (MG)	Usual daily dose (MG)
Clomipramine	25	100–250
Fluoxetine	10–20	20–60
Fluvoxamine	50	150–300
Paroxetine	20	20–40
Sertraline	50	50–150

(Table 7-9). Venlafaxine in its sustained release formulation can be given once a day, just like the SSRIs and TCAs.

Because of its sequential, concentration-dependent effects on 5-HT and NE uptake pumps, venlafaxine may offer a wider spectrum of efficacy than SSRIs. Because of its absence of effects on other neuroreceptors and fast Na$^+$ channels, venlafaxine has a better safety and tolerability profile than do TCAs.

Nefazodone

Unlike venlafaxine and the SSRIs, nefazodone in adults is started at 200 mg per day and then requires at least a one time increase to 300 mg per day to achieve an effective dose. Similar to the immediate release formulation of venlafaxine, nefazodone requires twice-a-day administration and may induce a greater response rate with higher doses if the patient fails to respond initially. Thus, like venlafaxine, nefazodone appears to have a dual mechanism of action, although the specific mechanisms involved are different for these two agents. At lower doses, the most potent action of nefazodone is 5-HT$_{2A}$ blockade, whereas higher concentrations produce greater inhibition of the 5-HT uptake pump (254–256).

This drug has perhaps the most complicated dosing schedule of any antidepressant. The current dosing guidelines for the immediate release formulation is for twice daily dosing. For that reason, an extended release version is in development. The hope is that it will simplify dosing guidelines.

Of note, one of the authors (SHP) conducted a study showing that 85% of patients who responded to acute treatment with the immediate release formulation of nefazodone using a twice daily dosing schedule could be converted to once daily dosing. First, patients underwent treatment for 3 months using an equally divided twice daily schedule. Next, the dose was adjusted to 25% in the morning and 75% at night for 1 week. Then 100% of the dose was given at night. These patients were maintained on this schedule for 3 months with no evidence of loss of efficacy and evidence of improved tolerability.

Bupropion

The typical therapeutic dose range for bupropion is 225 to 450 mg per day. The latter is the maximally recommended daily dose because seizure risk above this level increases exponentially. The dosing recommendation with the immediate release formulation is to initiate treatment at 50 mg given on a thrice daily schedule and then to gradually adjust the dose upward with a minimal weekly interval between dose increases. To reduce the likelihood of seizures, the lowest effective daily dose of bupropion should be used; the daily dose should not exceed 450 mg per day; no individual dose should exceed 150 mg; and doses of the immediate release form should not be given closer than 4 hours apart. Bupropion sustained release tablets are now available. The recommended dosing strategy is 150 mg by mouth QAM (every morning), which is increased to 150 mg by mouth twice daily as early as day 4 of dosing. The maximal daily dose is 200 mg by mouth twice a day. Dose increments should be done slowly while observing for clinical efficacy and adverse effects (257–259).

Reboxetine

In countries where reboxetine is marketed, the dosing recommendation is to start with an oral dose of 4 mg twice daily in adults and 2 mg twice daily in elderly patients for at least 3 to 4 weeks (260). After that, the dose can be increased to 10 mg per day in adults and 6 mg per day in elderly patients as needed based on assessment of efficacy and tolerability. Lower doses are recommended for patients with severe renal or hepatic impairment

Tricyclic Antidepressants

As mentioned earlier, for certain patients there may be no class of antidepressants with better efficacy than the TCAs. For this reason alone, these medications remain a valuable part of the antidepressant armamentarium. When the dose of a TCA is adjusted based on clinic assessment of response, a TCA will produce at least a partial response in 60% to 70% of depressed patients and a full remission in 20% to 40%. When the dose is adjusted using therapeutic drug monitoring (TDM), the full remission rate may be higher.

Starting with a standard TCA such as imipramine, a typical dose is 25 mg three times daily. Dose may be increased by 25 mg every 2 or 3 days, as tolerated, and can usually be increased to 150 mg per day by the end of the first week in healthy adults. The elderly, medically compromised, those hypersensitive to side effects, or those with associated panic disorder may require lower doses and more gradual increases (see discussion in Chapter 6).

As discussed later in this chapter, optimal dosing of these medications requires TDM at least once early in treatment to adjust for the substantial, primarily genetically determined differences in the elimination rate of these drugs, even in physically healthy individuals. Generally, repeat monitoring is only done for cause, such as the following:

- *Suspected noncompliance*
- Addition of a drug that can induce or inhibit the *CYP enzymes* responsible for the metabolism of these drugs
- Development of significant *cardiac, hepatic,* or *renal dysfunction*

The physician may want to do repeat monitoring, however, if the patient requires doses above the generally recommended limit. Once the proper dose is established, most or all of the medication can generally be given once daily, usually 1 hour before bedtime. Exceptions to single daily dosing would be not to exceed 150 to 200 mg of a TCA at one time and to use divided, lower total daily doses in the elderly, in the very young, or in medically ill individuals, particularly those with cardiac disease.

Monoamine Oxidase Inhibitors

MAOIs may be the treatment of choice for atypical depressive disorders. As noted in Chapter 6, features of this subgroup usually include the following:

- *Reversed diurnal variation in mood* (i.e., worse in the afternoon or evening)
- *Mood reactivity* and *lability in the same depres-*

sive episode, ranging from irritability to mild dysphoria to severe depression
- *Hypersomnia, hyperphagia*
- *Somatization*
- *Rejection hypersensitivity*
- *Anxiety,* including panic episodes

Starting doses of various MAOIs are as follows:

- *Phenelzine*—15 mg twice daily; daily dose range = 45 to 90 mg
- *Tranylcypromine*—10 mg twice daily; daily dose range = 20 to 40 mg
- *Isocarboxazid*—10 mg twice daily; daily dose range = 020 to 60 mg
- *Moclobemide*—100 to 200 mg daily, three times per day (450 mg upper dose for outpatients)

In *major depression* (unipolar or bipolar), MAOIs, particularly nonselective and irreversible agents, are a fallback choice for major depressive disorder, improving response in nonpsychotic depressed patients whose symptoms fail to respond to the other classes of antidepressants and for whom ECT is not yet warranted.

These agents may also be used in *geriatric patients;* however, lower initial amounts are indicated (see Chapter 14, "The Elderly Patient"). In general, geriatric patients should initially receive one-half the adult dose. Phenelzine, for example, may be started at 15 mg two or three times daily in the healthy younger adult but should be started at 15 mg once daily in the elderly patient. Dose adjustments in the geriatric patient should be made less frequently than in the younger adult, and weekly changes should be sufficient to minimize untoward effects. MAOIs should not be used above 60 mg per day in this age group.

Contraindications for Monoamine Oxidase Inhibitors. Physical conditions that may preclude the use of MAOIs include the following:

- Advanced *renal disease*
- *Pheochromocytoma*
- Significant *hypertension*

Cautious use is required in patients with impairment in the following organ systems:

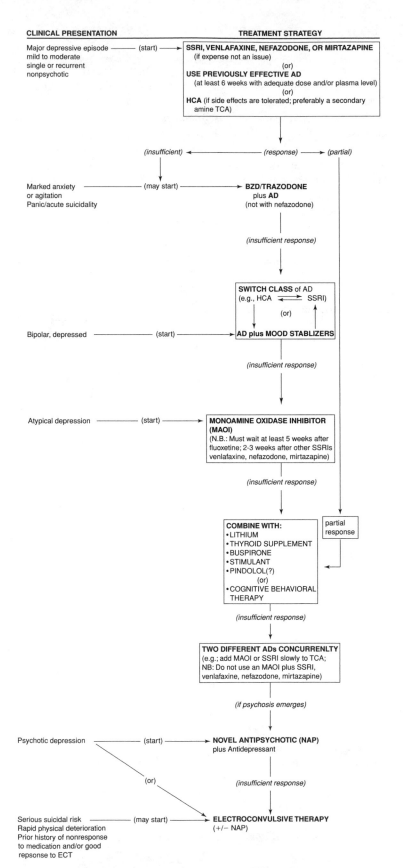

CLINICAL PRESENTATION

TREATMENT STRATEGY

Major depressive episode — (start) → | **SSRI, VENLAFAXINE, NEFAZODONE, OR MIRTAZAPINE**
mild to moderate
single or recurrent
nonpsychotic

SSRI, VENLAFAXINE, NEFAZODONE, OR MIRTAZAPINE
(if expense not an issue)
(or)
USE PREVIOUSLY EFFECTIVE AD
(at least 6 weeks with adequate dose and/or plasma level)
(or)
HCA (if side effects are tolerated; preferably a secondary
amine TCA)

(insufficient) ← *(response)* → *(partial)*

Marked anxiety — (may start) → **BZD/TRAZODONE**
or agitation
Panic/acute suicidality

BZD/TRAZODONE
plus **AD**
(not with nefazodone)

(insufficient response)

SWITCH CLASS of AD
(e.g., HCA ⇌ SSRI)
(or)

Bipolar, depressed — (start) → **AD plus MOOD STABLIZERS**

(insufficient response)

Atypical depression — (start) → **MONOAMINE OXIDASE INHIBITOR
(MAOI)**
(N.B.: Must wait at least 5 weeks after
fluoxetine; 2-3 weeks after other SSRIs
venlafaxine, nefazodone, mirtazapine)

(insufficient response)

COMBINE WITH:
• LITHIUM
• THYROID SUPPLEMENT
• BUSPIRONE
• STIMULANT
• PINDOLOL(?)
(or)
• COGNITIVE BEHAVIORAL
THERAPY

partial
response

(insufficient response)

TWO DIFFERENT ADs CONCURRENLTY
(e.g.; add MAOI or SSRI slowly to TCA;
NB: Do not use an MAOI plus SSRI,
venlafaxine, nefazodone, mirtazapine)

(if psychosis emerges)

Psychotic depression — (start) → **NOVEL ANTIPSYCHOTIC (NAP)**
plus Antidepressant

(or)

(insufficient response)

Serious suicidal risk — (may start) → **ELECTROCONVULSIVE THERAPY**
Rapid physical deterioration
Prior history of nonresponse
to medication and/or good
repsonse to ECT

ELECTROCONVULSIVE THERAPY
(+/− NAP)

FIG. 7-1. Treatment of an acute major depressive episode.

- *Hepatic*
- *Cardiovascular*
- *Respiratory* (e.g., asthma, chronic bronchitis)
- *Ocular* (e.g., narrow-angle glaucoma)

If a patient does not respond to one MAOI, or if there appears to be a loss of efficacy over time, it may be reasonable to try a second. When switching from a hydrazine-based MAOI (e.g., phenelzine or isocarboxazid) to a nonhydrazine MAOI (e.g., tranylcypromine), one should wait at least 2 weeks. **This is because the nonhydrazine MAOI, tranylcypromine, produces NE uptake inhibitory and sympathomimetic effects similar to dextroamphetamine and may cause a toxic reaction if initiated within 2 weeks following MAO inhibition by another agent (261).**

If a patient is to be switched to a TCA (e.g., amitriptyline), an MAOI should be discontinued for 2 weeks before beginning the new treatment. Because recovery of the MAO enzyme following irreversible inhibition takes up to 2 weeks, sympathomimetic agents given during that time may increase the risk of a hypertensive crisis. Special caution should be taken when switching from any potent inhibitor of serotonin uptake to an MAOI or vice versa. Potent inhibitors of serotonin uptake include all the SSRIs, venlafaxine, and clomipramine. Although nefazodone is not a potent serotonin uptake inhibitor, a similar warning appears with this drug in its U.S. package insert.

If MAOIs and drugs that block serotonin uptake are used in close proximity, there is a potential for the development of the serotonin syndrome (see "Adverse Effects" later in this chapter). Therefore, the physician should allow 2 weeks between stopping an irreversible and nonselective MAOI and starting a potent serotonin reuptake inhibitor. This interval is not to permit clearance of the drug, which occurs within hours, but rather to allow sufficient time for regeneration of the MAO enzyme. In contrast, the required interval between stopping the serotonin reuptake inhibitor and starting the MAOI is to permit clearance of the drug and thus is a function of the half-life of the specific SSRI. A 2-week interval is adequate for all of these drugs with the exception of fluoxetine. Because of the extended half-life of norfluoxetine, a minimum of 5 weeks should lapse between stopping fluoxetine (20 mg per day) and starting an MAOI. With higher daily doses, the interval should be longer. For example, a serotonin syndrome was reported following a 6-week washout in a patient who had been given fluoxetine (80 mg per day) (262). TDM revealed that she had a norfluoxetine level of 84 ng/mL, the average level at steady-state on 20 mg per day. This patient recovered without residual sequelae, although full recovery took 2 months. The seriousness of this interaction is underscored by the fact that three fatalities have occurred when tranylcypromine was started shortly after fluoxetine had been stopped (263).

Conclusion

Regardless of the specific agent, it is important to watch for improvement in target symptoms. Psychomotor agitation or retardation often improve first, followed by concentration and increased capacity for interpersonal contact. The patient's family (or nursing staff) may recognize an improvement before the patient does. However, the patient's subjective sense of depression, anhedonia, and hopelessness may not improve until the fourth to sixth week of treatment, often prompting them to pressure the physician to prematurely abandon a potentially successful antidepressant trial.

Figure 7-1 summarizes the strategy we would follow for patients who fail to adequately respond initially (see also "Alternative Treatment Strategies" later in this chapter).

Table 7-18 summarizes the various factors to consider when choosing a specific class of antidepressant.

MAINTENANCE/PROPHYLAXIS

After inducing remission from an acute depressive episode, the next phase of treatment is preventing a relapse back into that episode. The period of highest vulnerability for a relapse is the first 6 to 9 months after the induction of a

TABLE 7-18. Considerations when selecting an antidepressant: comparison of classes

Consideration	Tricyclic Antidepressants (e.g., Nortripyline)	Selective serotonin Reuptake inhibitors (e.g., Sertraline)	Phenylpiperazines (e.g., Nefazodone)	Aminoketones (e.g., Bupropion)	Monoamine oxidase Inhibitors (e.g., Tranylcypromine)	Venlafaxine
Likelihood of response	High	Equivalent to tricyclic antidepressants (TCA) in outpatients	Less than TCAs	Less than TCAs	Less than TCAs	Equivalent to TCAs: superior to placebo in inpatients and outpatients
Unique spectrum of activity	Can work in selective serotonin reuptake inhibitor (SSRI) failures	Can work in TCA failures	None demonstrated	Can work in TCA failures	Can work in TCA failures	Possible efficacy in cases not responsive to TCAs or SSRIs (open label studies)
Maintenance of response	Evidence from controlled studies	Evidence from controlled studies	Evidence from controlled studies	None demonstrated	None demonstrated	Evidence from controlled studies
Safety	Serious systemic toxicity can result from overdose, either acute ingestion or from gradual accumulation due to slow clearance	No serious systemic toxicity demonstrated	Minimal serious systemic toxicity due to acute overdose	Seizures as primary acute systemic toxicity due to acute overdose, easily managed in medical setting	Serious systemic toxicity can result from acute overdose acute ingestion	No serious systemic toxicity demonstrated; 3% incidence of dose-dependent hypertension
Tolerability	Good with secondary amine TCAs; fair to poor with tertiary amine TCAs	Good, especially if dose is kept to effective minimum dose Dose-dependent adverse effects include nausea, loose stools, sexual dysfunction.	Good Sedation and cognitive slowing are dose-dependent adverse effects	Generally good, especially if dose is kept to effective minimum dose	Generally good, except for the occurrence of hypotension and the dietary restrictions	Comparable to SSRIs at low dose; NE mediated adverse effects at higher doses
Pharmacokinetic interactions	Can be affected by other drugs (e.g., SSRIs) to a clinically significant extent but do not affect other drugs	Can inhibit oxidative metabolism of a variety of drugs. Substantial differences among SSRIs in terms of effects on CYP enzymes: Fluoxetine; fluvoxamine > paroxetine > citalopram, sertraline (Table 7-29). No known effect of other drugs on SSRIs that is clinically significant	Inhibits cytochrome P450 enzyme 3A3/4.	Can be affected by fluoxetine and probably others in a potentially clinically significant way. No known effect on the metabolism of other drugs	Neither is affected by other drugs nor affects other drugs in a clinically significant way	Has profile comparable to sertraline in terms of effects on CYP enzymes (i.e., limited to mild inhibition of CYP 2D6)

Pharmacodynamic interactions	Multiple, due to the large number of effects of TCAs. Can be agonistic (additive or potentiating) or antagonistic. Such interactions are more likely and more significant with tertiary as opposed to secondary amines	See MAOI interaction. May occur with other serotonin agonists. Can have agonistic interaction with dopamine agonists in terms of extrapyramidal effects.	Can have interaction with other agents with decreased arousal or impaired cognitive performance. Can interact with adrenergic agents affecting blood pressure regulation. Complex interactions with other serotonin-active agents	Can have interactions with dopamine agonists and antagonists	Clinically significant interactions with: Tyramine and sympathomimetic agents on blood pressure Serotonin-active agents, inducing the central serotonin syndrome	Comparable to SSRIs at low doses. NE mediated interactions possible at higher doses
Physician confidence	Excellent due to extensive database in terms of human exposure (e.g., patient-years of exposure, total number of patients exposed, variety of patients exposed)	Excellent due primarily to efficacy and safety profile. Less extensive database in terms of human exposure compared to TCAs but rapidly expanding	Satisfactory due to substantial database in terms of human exposure. Concerns are with spectrum of activity and tolerability	Reserved due to less extensive database concerning human exposure coupled with concerns about safety due to dose-dependent seizure risk	Caution due to safety concerns, primarily about patient compliance with dietary restrictions	Less extensive use than TCAs or SSRIs, but otherwise good
Ease of administration	Excellent, generally can be administered once a day	Excellent for sertraline and paroxetine due to once-a-day administration. Good for fluoxetine, typically administered once a day, but long half-life of parent compound and active metabolite can make dose titration difficult	Satisfactory but requires divided daily dosing for antidepressant effect	Satisfactory but requires divided daily dosing for antidepressant effect	Satisfactory, but clinical practice is to generally give in divided daily doses	Satisfactory with divided daily doses required for immediate release formulation; sustained release formulation in development

From Preskorn SH, Burke M. Somatic therapy for major depressive disorder: selection of an antidepressant. *J Clin Psychiatry* 1992; 53(suppl 9):5–18., with permission.

TABLE 7-19. *Tricyclic antidepressants versus placebo: maintenance therapy*

Number of studies	Number of subjects	Relapsed (%)		Difference (%)	Chi square	p value
		AD (%)	Placebo (%)			
18	2,225	23	50	27	150	10^{-34}

AD, antidepressant.

remission. For that reason, it is advisable to maintain the patient on the medication at full dose at least during this interval. This phase of treatment has been termed either *maintenance or continuation treatment.* Antidepressant treatment after this interval (i.e., *prophylactic therapy*) is generally reserved for patients who have a substantial risk of recurrent episodes.

Even through most countries, including the United States, do not require maintenance or prophylactic studies for marketing approval, the amount of such data is growing. Most of the maintenance studies use either a double-blind crossover or a double-blind continuation design.

In the *crossover design,* patients with an episode are given medication and brought into a remission, then maintained on medication for 2 to 3 months. Those who are successfully maintained in remission are then entered into a double-blind phase in which they are randomly assigned to either stay on the medication or switched to a placebo. Both groups are otherwise treated identically and followed up for a specified period of time, usually 1 year. The outcome measure is relapse into a depressive episode.

The *continuation design* differs in that patients with an acute depressive episode are randomly assigned to either drug or placebo treatment. Only those who respond, whether they received active medication or placebo, are then entered into the continuation phase. During this time, they receive the treatment to which they initially responded without breaking the blind. The outcome measure is relapse rate, but in drug responders versus placebo responders. Typically, the follow-up interval in these studies has also been for 1 year. The double-blind continuation design avoids the possibility of drug withdrawal affecting the likelihood of relapse, as well as interfering with the blinded nature of the study. The design of these two types of studies is then complementary. Imipramine is the antidepressant that has been most extensively studied using both types of designs and has typically been the active control in the continuation studies with newer antidepressants (Tables 7-19 through 7-21).

The decision to use prophylactic therapy should be based on the:

• *Severity* of the depressive episode
• *Frequency* of past depressions
• Risk of *suicide*
• Risk of potential *adverse effects*

TABLE 7-20. *Relapse prevention continuation studies: double-blind, random assignment to remain on SSRIs or crossover to placebo*

SSRI	Duration (WK)	Relapse rate (%) outcome			p Value
		Placebo	Drug	Difference	
Fluoxetine[a]	52	57	26	31	<0.01
Paroxetine[b]	52	43	16	27	<0.01
Sertraline[c]	44	46	13	33	<0.001

[a]From Montgomery S. Dufour H, Brion S, et al. The prophylatic efficacy of fluoxetine in unipolar depression. *Br J Psychiatry* 1988; 153(suppl 3):69–76.
[b]From Eric L. A prospective double-blind comparative multicentre study of paroxetine and placebo in preventing recurrent major depressive episodes. *Biol Psychiatry* 1991;29(suppl 11):245S–255S.
[c]From Doogan D, Caillard V. Sertraline in the prevention of depression. *Br J Psychology* 1992;160:217–222.
SSRI, selective serotonin reuptake inhibitor.

TABLE 7-21. *Relapse prevention continuation studies: double-blind continuation on treatment without crossover*

Treatment	Number	Relapse rate (%)
Venlafaxine Study[a]		
Imipramine	62	31
Trazodone	30	29
Venlafaxine	220	18
Placebo	119	32
Nefazodone Study[b]		
Imipramine	84	7
Nefazodone	63	10
Placebo	94	22

[a]From Entsuah R, Rudolph R, Dervian A, et al. A low relapse rate confirms the long-term efficacy of venlafaxine in the treatment of major depression [abstract]. Abstracts of Panels and Posters, Poster Session II. ACNP Meeting, Hawaii, Dec 1993;129.
[b]Nefazodone presentation to the Food and Drug Administration Psychopharmacology Advisory Committee. Washington, DC, July 1993.

Antidepressants do not prevent relapses into mania and may even precipitate a manic phase. For these reasons, a mood stabilizer (with or without concomitant antidepressants) is the prophylaxis of choice for bipolar depressions. If there is a reasonable hint of bipolarity (e.g., a family history of bipolar illness, a prior hypomanic episode, or drug-induced hypomania), a mood stabilizer should be considered (see Chapter 10 for more detailed discussion).

Preventing relapse is of critical importance in the life course of major depressive disorder, and every effort should be made to ensure patient compliance. Maintenance (i.e., continuation) therapy should be continued for 6 to 9 months after an acute episode, with recent data indicating that, for an acute episode, doses equivalent to 200 mg of imipramine may be optimal (264, 265).

After 6 to 9 months, the antidepressant can usually be tapered over a period of several weeks to avoid withdrawal symptoms, which may increase or even mimic relapse. If symptoms reemerge, medication should be reinstated and maintained for an additional 3 to 6 months before an attempt is made to taper them again. In patients with recurrent unipolar depressions, indefinite prophylactic treatment may be required.

Efficacy for Maintenance Treatment

Heterocyclics

Although considerable emphasis has recently been placed on maintenance therapy for major depression, there is a large body of evidence dating back more than 20 years that supports the usefulness of TCAs in preventing relapse after the induction of an acute remission (266). Imipramine has the most data of any antidepressant for being effective in terms of maintaining remission during the vulnerable 6 to 9 months after the induction of a remission. The next best studied is amitriptyline. There are marginal data with any of the other TCAs. Double-blind, fixed dose studies have shown that reducing the TCA dose during maintenance phase increases the likelihood of a relapse. For this reason, the dose that got the patient well is the dose that should be maintained during continuation treatment.

Selective Serotonin Reuptake Inhibitors

Evidence from six random-assignment, double-blind, placebo-controlled crossover studies with all of the SSRIs (except fluvoxamine) indicates that these agents can prevent relapse after a remission has been achieved (267, 268) (Table 7-20). These six studies involved 910 adults with major depression who had responded to acute treatment with an SSRI. Ten percent of the participants randomly assigned in a double-blind fashion to stay on their SSRI relapsed over 24 weeks versus 35% of those switched in a double-blind fashion to placebo. Three of these studies went beyond 24 weeks and lasted 44 and 52 weeks, respectively (267–269). In those studies, the advantage of being maintained on drug versus being switched to placebo was still apparent 44 and 52 weeks later. Over the course of 1 year, there is an approximately 30% greater relapse rate for those switched to placebo versus those maintained on an SSRI.

A relapse prevention study comparing the continuation efficacy of fluvoxamine with that of sertraline also found no difference (270).

Venlafaxine

The one study done to date with venlafaxine used a double-blind continuation design rather than a crossover design used with the SSRIs (Table 7-21). Responders in the double-blind, placebo- and active-controlled acute efficacy phase could elect to remain on double-blind treatment for a 1-year follow-up phase (271). The treatment arms in these studies included venlafaxine, tra- zodone, imipramine, and placebo. At the end of 1 year, 18% of patients on venlafaxine had re- lapsed versus 32% on placebo. The difference between the venlafaxine and the placebo groups was smaller than that seen between the SSRIs and their respective placebo groups (Table 7-20), consistent with the difference in the design of these studies.

A higher percentage of patients would be ex- pected to relapse in the crossover design for two reasons. First, a significant portion of the pa- tients in the crossover study had, in fact, re- sponded specifically to the drug treatment. Af- ter a period of stabilization, these patients were randomly reassigned to placebo and thus would be expected to relapse. Second, a basic prob- lem in the crossover design is that withdrawal symptoms can mimic the recurrence of depres- sive symptoms. That is true for the SSRIs, par- ticularly fluvoxamine and paroxetine, because of their relatively short half-lives.

In contrast, patients in the placebo arm of the double-blind continuation study done with venlafaxine had responded to placebo and then remained on placebo under double-blind con- ditions. Whereas a sizable percentage of the patients switched to placebo in the crossover studies likely required active drug treatment to experience a response, that is not necessarily true for placebo-treated patients in the double-blind continuation studies. Thus, the nature and the course of the illness in these two types of studies may not be the same, accounting for the differ- ence in relapse rates.

Another surprise finding from the double- blind continuation study with venlafaxine is that the relapse rates on imipramine and trazodone were comparable with placebo (Table 7-21). The number of patients on trazodone was relatively small and may have played a role in the results, because each person who relapsed in that arm added 3% to the total percentage versus only 0.5% and 1.0% in the venlafaxine and the placebo

arms, respectively. The higher incidence of ad- verse effects on these two drugs may have also contributed to poorer compliance during the con- tinuation phase, resulting in a higher relapse rate in the imipramine and the trazodone groups.

Nefazodone

As with venlafaxine, a double-blind continuation study has been done with nefazodone (see Ta- ble 7-21). Patients who responded to nefazodone, imipramine, or placebo in the acute phase were offered the option of remaining on double- blind treatment for 1 year (272). Those patients who chose to participate were then followed up monthly to assess whether efficacy persisted. The relapse rate was 22% on placebo versus 10% on nefazodone and 7% on imipramine. The absolute difference in relapse rates between nefazodone and placebo was similar to that of venlafaxine versus placebo (i.e., 12% to 14%). **Thus, main- tenance treatment with nefazodone, as with venlafaxine and the SSRIs, reduced the risk of relapse when compared with placebo even when the comparison group had initially re- sponded to placebo and remained on placebo for the maintenance period.**

Given their design differences, no direct com- parison can be made between the relative relapse efficacy of SSRIs, venlafaxine, and nefazodone. The bottom line, however, is that both designs demonstrated that maintenance therapy for up to 1 year is important in reducing the risk of a de- pressive relapse after an initial response.

Bupropion

Minimal data are available about whether main- tenance therapy with bupropion is efficacious; there has been only one recently completed open label study (273). No efficacy data, however, have been presented.

Mirtazapine

A double-blind continuation study has been con- ducted with mirtazapine. As with venlafaxine and nefazodone, patients in this acute, double- blind, placebo- and active-controlled study with mirtazapine could remain on the double-blind treatment at the end of the initial 6-week efficacy trial and were then followed up for up to 1 year. There was a statistically significant lower risk of relapse (defined as HDRS > 16) on both mirtazapine (18%) and amitriptyline (28%) in comparison with placebo (53%), indicating that mirtazapine has maintenance efficacy (274). More recently, a 40-week, double-blind, placebo-controlled crossover study was performed with mirtazapine (275). Patients maintained on this drug had less than half the likelihood of relapsing than those patients switched to placebo (i.e., 19.7% versus 43.8%, $p < 0.01$).

Reboxetine

In a 1-year, double-blind, placebo-controlled, long-term treatment study of 358 depressed patients, 22% of reboxetine-maintained patients relapsed versus 55% of those switched to placebo (276).

Monoamine Oxidase Inhibitors

Similar to patients on other antidepressants, patients on MAOIs should be maintained on MAOIs for a period of at least 6 months. If there is a history of recurrent depressive episodes following discontinuation, MAOI therapy should be extended for 2 years or more, as long as the patient is closely supervised and shows no significant adverse effects or toxicity. There is evidence that a few patients maintained on MAOIs for periods of 6 months or more may experience loss of therapeutic effect, which correlates with a decrease in adverse effects such as anorexia and insomnia (277). Of note, tolerance to the hypotensive effects does not seem to develop. Waning of therapeutic efficacy can be compensated for by increasing the dose, but this strategy may be limited by adverse effects, particularly hypotension.

Efficacy for Prophylaxis

Prophylaxis refers to continued antidepressant therapy for the prevention of new episodes, as opposed to maintenance therapy to prevent a relapse back into the current episode. As might be expected, there has been only a modest amount of research done on the prophylactic efficacy of antidepressants. Furthermore, the studies that do exist differ substantially in terms of their design and scientific rigor.

There is one major prospective, double-blind, random-assignment study comparing imipramine alone and interpersonal psychotherapy alone with placebo and with the combination (264, 265). This study provided compelling evidence for the prophylactic efficacy of continued imipramine therapy relative to either placebo or interpersonal psychotherapy in patients selected as being at high risk for relapse. While this study is highly commendable, there are significant limitations when attempting to translate the results to clinical practice. For example, even though the number of patients involved was adequate to distinguish between the efficacy of the different treatments, it was not sufficient to assess long-term safety. Fifty patients were assigned to imipramine alone or in combination with interpersonal psychotherapy and 75 were assigned to placebo alone or placebo in combination with interpersonal psychotherapy. Because the study was geared to answering the question of relapse prevention, the population selected had a highly recurrent form of the illness. Thus, the modest number of patients involved and the selection criteria raise significant questions about reliance on this study to support the "antidepressant forever" movement that exists within some psychiatric circles.

In a less rigorously designed, but nonetheless supportive British collaborative study, patients who had responded to either amitriptyline or imipramine were randomly assigned to either stay on the TCA (75 or 100 mg per day) or be switched to placebo. After 15 months, 22% of the TCA maintenance group had relapsed compared with 50% of those on placebo (278). Beyond this study, there is one small placebo-controlled study of phenelzine (276) and one small placebo-controlled study comparing phenelzine and nortriptyline in elderly patients (279, 280). The remaining data are limited to active-controlled studies comparing the prophylactic efficacy of continuation treatment with a TCA or related antidepressant with lithium carbonate

TABLE 7-22. *Lithium versus placebo: maintenance therapy (recurrent unipolar depression)*

Number of studies	Number of subjects	Relapsed (%)		Difference (%)	Chi square	*p* value
		Lithium (%)	Placebo (%)			
8	287	41	75	34	34.7	3×10^{-9}

(278, 281–289). In two of these studies, initial treatment was with ECT; in the others, treatment was with TCAs from the beginning. Maintenance treatment was then administered in a double-blind, random-assignment fashion.

No comparable long-term studies have been done with the SSRIs, bupropion, nefazodone, venlafaxine, or mirtazapine.

Lithium

In bipolar depressed patients, lithium (with or without concurrent antidepressants) is the maintenance treatment of choice, with divalproex (DVPX) or carbamazepine as potential alternatives (see also Chapter 10, "Maintenance/Prophylaxis"). Maintenance lithium has also been shown to prevent relapse in recurrent unipolar depression (Table 7-22).

Souza and Goodwin (196) studied the prophylactic value of lithium by combining data from both controlled and uncontrolled studies assessing the benefit of this agent over 3 months to 5 years. They found that lithium was significantly more effective than placebo in 263 unipolar depressed patients studied in eight controlled trials ($p < 0.0001$). In the uncontrolled studies, there was a similar effect size corresponding to an improvement rate of 70% for the lithium-treated group versus only 35% for the placebo-treated group. When lithium was compared with other antidepressants as a potential prophylactic therapy, there was a nonsignificant trend favoring lithium. Only two studies compared lithium alone to lithium plus imipramine, with the pooled results favoring the combination ($p < 0.02$).

An earlier study of 40 unipolar depressed patients by this same group found a cumulative probability of recurrence over 2 years to be 0.08 with lithium and 0.58 without lithium (290). These investigators concluded that the outcome strongly supported the value of lithium

prophylaxis in unipolar depression, contrasting this agent's lack of acute efficacy.

Psychotherapy

As mentioned earlier, concomitant interpersonal psychotherapy did not alter the likelihood of relapse in either the imipramine- or the placebo-treated group in the study by Frank and colleagues (264, 265). That finding replicated an earlier study, which found psychotherapy was ineffective for preventing depressive recurrence, although it was helpful in improving social adjustment (291). Taken together, these two studies indicated that both forms of treatment are important for some patients with major depression but that they accomplish different goals, analogous to the complementary roles of orthopedic surgery and physical therapy. This recognition is in direct opposition to the old approach of viewing pharmacotherapy and psychotherapy as an either/or situation or as being in competition with each other.

Conclusion

Two issues have emerged from the literature on maintenance treatment for depressive disorders. First, the condition is often recurrent and debilitating. Second, antidepressants (in doses comparable with acute treatment levels) with or without various psychotherapeutic approaches, can favorably alter the longitudinal course. Fig. 7-2 shows the strategy we recommend.

Our approach to both acute and maintenance therapy is consistent with the American Psychiatric Association guidelines for the treatment of major depressive disorder in adults (292).

PHARMACOKINETICS

As explained in Chapter 3, *pharmacodynamics* (i.e., a drug's affinity for various sites of action)

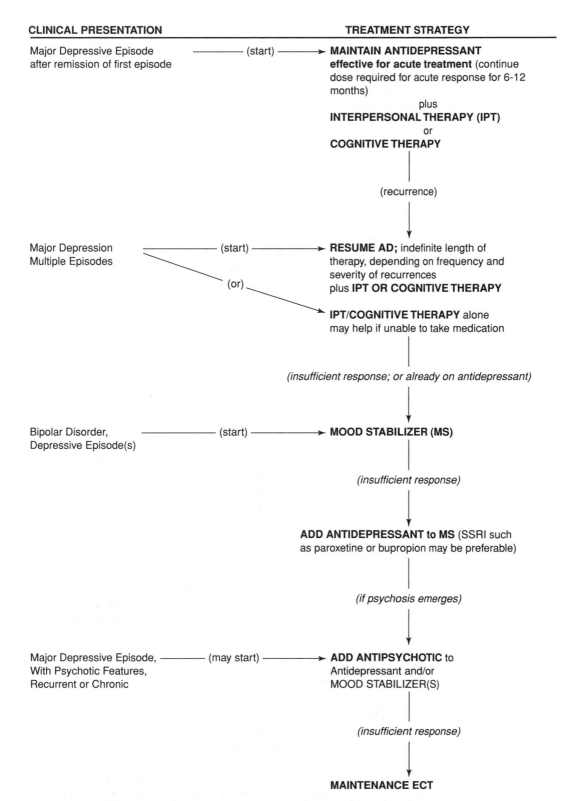

FIG. 7-2. Maintenance strategy for recurrent and/or chronic depression.

determines what the drug is capable of doing. *Pharmacokinetics* determines what the drug will do based on the concentration achieved under clinically relevant dosing conditions. Drug concentration determines what sites of action (i.e., what effect) will be engaged and to what degree (i.e., magnitude of the effect). The pharmacokinetics of a drug is also important because it determines whether a drug will be susceptible to specific types of drug–drug interactions and whether specific types of patients (e.g., those with hepatic or renal impairment) will be sensitive to the effects of the drug. This section briefly outlines the major points about the pharmacokinetics of specific antidepressants.

Tricyclic Antidepressants

TCAs are pharmacologically complex. They are slowly, but usually completely, absorbed from the small bowel, enter the portal blood, pass through the liver, where there is significant first-pass metabolism mediated by CYP 3A3/4 (40% to 70%). They then enter the systemic circulation for distribution. These agents are generally highly protein-bound (75% to 95%), as well as highly lipophilic, with a large volume of distribution. Their half-lives range from 16 to 126 hours, but are usually 24 to 30 hours.

The prolonged half-lives occur in individuals who are genetically different in CYP 2D6 or who have significant hepatic, renal, or left ventricular cardiac dysfunction.

TCAs are metabolized in the liver by three pathways:

- *N-Demethylation* (CYP 1A2, 2C19, and 3A3/4)
- *N-Oxidation* (CYP 2D6)
- *Aromatic hydroxylation* (CYP 2D6)

Aromatic hydroxylation is the most important of these three pathways because it is the principal pathway mediating the elimination of these drugs. This is true for all patients except those deficient in CYP 2D6, either because of genetics or because of inhibition by a coprescribed drug (e.g., fluoxetine).

The ratio of parent drug to desmethylated metabolite at steady-state has been reported to range from 0.47 to 0.70 for imipramine:

desipramine and from 0.83 to 1.16 for amitriptyline:nortriptyline. These typical ratios can be used to help distinguish between an acute overdose (increased ratios) versus a steady-state situation (normal ratios).

Selective Serotonin Reuptake Inhibitors

Whereas members of this class are quite similar in terms of their pharmacodynamics, they are quite different in terms of their pharmacokinetics (25). The clinically most important differences in the pharmacokinetics of the SSRIs are as follows:

- *CYP enzymes* responsible for their metabolism
- *Half-life*
- *Linear versus nonlinear* pharmacokinetics
- Changes in plasma drug levels as a function of *age* and *gender*

Given the significant structural differences, it should not be surprising that different CYP enzymes mediate the metabolism of different SSRIs. Desmethlyation of citalopram is principally dependent on CYP 2C19 and 3A3/4 (293), an important point when one considers that 20% of Asians are genetically deficient in CYP 2C19. Thus, higher levels of citalopram develop in such individuals on a given dose and they might benefit from starting on a lower dose that is adjusted more gradually.

Little has been established regarding which CYP enzymes mediate the metabolism of fluvoxamine and fluoxetine. These two SSRIs inhibit multiple CYP enzymes, which complicates studying their metabolism as well as being important when using these SSRIs in patients on other medications. Although some evidence suggests that CYP 1A2 may be important in the metabolism of fluvoxamine, more recent work is not consistent with that conclusion (294). There is some evidence suggesting that CYP 2D6 catalyses the metabolism of R- and S- fluoxetine and S-norfluoxetine but not R-norfluoxetine (295). Coupled with the substantial inhibition of CYP 2D6 produced by fluoxetine and norfluoxetine, this may account for the long half-lives of fluoxetine and its active metabolite. The potential role of other CYP enzymes in the metabolism of fluoxetine and norfluoxetine remains controversial.

Paroxetine at low concentration is dependent on CYP 2D6 for its clearance. However, this enzyme is almost completely saturated by paroxetine at low concentrations, which accounts for the nonlinear pharmacokinetics of paroxetine and why its half-life goes from 10 to 20 hours when the dose is advanced from 10 to 20 mg per day. At higher concentrations, paroxetine is most likely dependent on CYP 3A3/4 for its clearance. This dose-dependent change in the clearance of paroxetine probably accounts for the higher incidence of withdrawal reactions with this SSRI than might otherwise be expected for a drug with a half-life of 20 hours at steady-state on 20 mg per day (296, 297).

The N-demethylation of sertraline is catalyzed by multiple CYP isoforms, including CYP 3A3/4, 2C19, 2C9, 2D6, and 2B6 (298). In most patients, no one of these isoforms likely contributes to more than 40% of the overall metabolism of sertraline. This makes sertraline relatively immune to drug–drug interactions caused by the use of another drug that inhibits or induces the metabolism of CYP enzymes. Nevertheless, a dose adjustment of sertraline may be prudent when starting or stopping drugs that are substantial inducers or inhibitors of CYP 3A3/4 (299, 300).

All of the SSRIs (except fluoxetine) have half-lives of 15-30 hours. Fluoxetine and its equipotent metabolite, norfluoxetine, have half-lives of 2 to 4 and 7 to 15 days, respectively. These half-lives are such that it takes several weeks to achieve steady-state and a comparable interval to fully clear the drug once it has been discontinued. Hence, fluoxetine can take several weeks to reach maximal effect, which can persist for many weeks after its cessation, making it essentially an oral depot medication. This fact also complicates its use and must be taken into account when adjusting its dose or switching from fluoxetine to another medication. The latter is because the risk of an adverse drug-drug interaction can persist for weeks after this agent is discontinued (301, 302). For all of these reasons, fluoxetine should be reserved for cases in which the advantages of its long half-life outweigh its disadvantages. That is particularly true because there are other SSRIs available that do not pose these problems.

Fluvoxamine, fluoxetine, and paroxetine have nonlinear pharmacokinetics, which means that dose increases lead to disproportionately greater increases in plasma drug levels (25). In contrast, citalopram and sertraline have linear pharmacokinetics. For these reasons, dose increases with fluvoxamine, fluoxetine, and paroxetine can lead to greater than proportional increases in concentration-dependent effects such as serotonin-mediated adverse effects (e.g., nausea) and inhibition of specific CYP enzymes.

Citalopram and paroxetine have the largest age-related change in plasma drug levels in comparison with other SSRIs. Their levels can be up to 100% greater in physically healthy individuals older than 65 years of age versus younger individuals. For this reason, the recommendation is to start these two SSRIs at half the usual dose and adjust upward more slowly in elderly patients. Age-related changes in SSRI plasma levels are important because elderly patients are likely to be on concomitant medications and effects on specific CYP enzymes are concentration dependent.

The half-life of norfluoxetine is even longer in physically healthy elderly patients compared with younger patients (20 versus 15 days, respectively, on average) (303). However, the average plasma levels of fluoxetine and norfluoxetine are not appreciably higher in elderly patients versus younger patients because there is an apparent reduction in its bioavailability as a function of age. Nevertheless, the longer half-life in elderly patients further complicates the use of this SSRI, particularly in those who are on multiple medications. For this reason, fluoxetine should generally be avoided in elderly patients.

Although there is no age-related change in fluvoxamine plasma levels, fluvoxamine has nonlinear and sex-dependent pharmacokinetics (304). A doubling of the dose from 50 to 100 mg twice a day causes, on average, a 340% increase in fluvoxamine plasma levels, which is more pronounced in men (460%) than in women (240%).

Sertraline also has an age by gender interaction but it is considerably more modest (305). Young men (mean = 30.6, range = 21 to 43) develop levels that are 35% lower than those of young women (mean = 34.4, range = 20 to 45) or of older men (mean = 72.0, range = 67 to 82) or women (mean = 69.7, range = 65 to 82).

Venlafaxine

The biotransformation of venlafaxine to its active metabolite, ODV, is dependent on CYP 2D6 (138, 306). The further elimination of ODV is dependent on CYP 3A3/4. Venlafaxine and ODV have approximate half-lives of 5 and 11 hours, respectively. Because venlafaxine and ODV have virtually identical pharmacological profiles, both are believed to contribute equally to the patient's overall response in terms of both efficacy and adverse effects (141). The 11-hour half-life of ODV is consistent with the fact that the immediate release formulation of venlafaxine is efficacious when administered twice daily.

The sum of the concentration of venlafaxine and ODV is probably more important than their relative ratio. Thus, CYP 2D6 deficiency, which occurs in approximately 7% of caucasians, has fewer clinical implications for venlafaxine than for drugs that are biotransformed by this isoenzyme to either centrally inactive metabolites (e.g., paroxetine) or metabolites that have a different pharmacological profile than the parent drug (e.g., TCAs). The increase in venlafaxine plasma levels is offset by a parallel decline in ODV levels such that the sum is the same. Nevertheless, a substantial inhibition of CYP 3A3/4 could result in a meaningful increase in both venlafaxine and ODV plasma levels, particularly in patients who are CYP 2D6 deficient. Such an increase would be expected to result in an increase in the incidence or severity of the known dose-dependent effects of venlafaxine mediated by its inhibition of the neuronal uptake pumps for serotonin and NE.

Nefazodone and Trazodone

These drugs have complicated pharmacokinetics (307-309). More is known about the pharmacokinetics of nefazodone than trazodone, particularly regarding its metabolites and their activity. Both parent drugs have short half-lives of approximately 4 hours and are primarily metabolized by CYP 3A3/4 to form the active metabolite, mCPP, which has a pharmacological profile different from that of either nefazodone or trazodone. This metabolite is a 5-HT_{2C} agonist and is anxiogenic when administered alone, in contrast to the parent drugs (310, 311). Thus, a significant shift in the relative ratio of mCPP to the parent drug could paradoxically cause anxiety and stimulation instead of anxiety reduction and sedation. Whereas mCPP is formed by CYP 3A3/4, its elimination is dependent on CYP 2D6. Such a shift in the ratio of the parent drug to this metabolite could occur as a result of either genetically determined or drug-induced deficiency of CYP 2D6 activity. For example, drug-induced deficiency in CYP 2D6 activity and the resultant accumulation of mCPP may account for paradoxical reactions when switching from the long-lived fluoxetine to nefazodone.

Nefazodone is biotransformed into two other metabolites, hydroxynefazodone (OH-NEF) and triazolodione (312). These latter two metabolites cannot be formed from trazodone because of structural differences between it and nefazodone. *OH-NEF* is an active metabolite with a pharmacological profile similar to that of the parent drug and is believed to contribute comparably to the overall clinical response. Its half-life is also approximately 4 hours.

Triazolodione has only part of the pharmacological activity of nefazodone, being a relatively pure 5-HT_{2A} antagonist blocker. Thus, it would be expected to produce only part of the overall pharmacological effects of the parent drug. Nonetheless, this metabolite may be clinically important because it accumulates in concentrations 10 times that of nefazodone because of its considerably longer half-life (i.e., 18 to 33 hours).

Nefazodone has appreciable nonlinear pharmacokinetics because of its metabolism by and inhibition of CYP3A3/4 (313). At doses of 200 mg per day, nefazodone undergoes an extensive first-pass metabolism such that its bioavailability is only approximately 20%. At doses of 400 mg per day, its bioavailability is appreciably higher, as are its plasma drug levels. This phenomenon is most likely due to inhibition of its own first-pass metabolism by CYP 3A/4. For this reason, dose-dependent effects of nefazodone can increase nonlinearly with higher doses.

Bupropion

The dearth of information on the metabolism of bupropion may initially seem surprising; however, this drug is one of the oldest of the newer antidepressants, having entered clinical trials in the mid-1970's and having been approved before fluoxetine (308, 314, 315). Ironically, its marketing was delayed after its approval because of the risk of seizures, which, in turn, is almost undoubtedly a consequence of its complicated pharmacokinetics (163).

The parent drug has a half-life of 8 to 10 hours and is biotransformed by oxidative metabolism to three active metabolites:

- Hydroxybupropion
- Threohydrobupropion
- Erythrohydrobupropion

These metabolites all have half-lives of 24 hours or more, and thus accumulate to a greater extent than the parent drug. Although preclinical testing has demonstrated that these metabolites are pharmacologically active, their beneficial or adverse effects have not been tested beyond one clinical study, which showed that patients in whom higher levels of these metabolites developed had a poorer outcome than those with lower levels (316).

Substantial interindividual variability is seen in the plasma levels of bupropion, as well as in its three metabolites. There is a correlation between levels of threohydrobupropion and erythrohydrobupropion but not between the levels of these metabolites and those of either the parent drug or hydroxybupropion (315). **Thus, there can be substantial differences in plasma levels among patients on the same dose of bupropion.**

CYP 2B6 is responsible for the conversion of bupropion to hydroxybupropion (317, 318). The mechanisms responsible for the conversion of bupropion to its other two major metabolites are not known nor are the mechanisms that mediate the eventual elimination of hydroxybupropion from the body. Moreover, little is known about CYP 2B6, including any potential genetic polymorphisms, whether it is inhibited or induced by other drugs or substances, and whether genetic polymorphisms or pharmacokinetically mediated drug–drug interactions are risk factors for seizures during bupropion treatment. For the same reason, it is unknown whether coadministration of specific CYP enzyme inducers (e.g., carbamazepine) or inhibitors (e.g., fluoxetine) could alter the clearance of bupropion or its metabolites in a clinically meaningful way. Some case report data indicate that coadministration of fluoxetine can elevate levels of two bupropion metabolites (314).

Mirtazapine

Mirtazapine has a half-life of 20 to 40 hours (319). Its elimination is principally dependent on CYP enzyme-mediated biotransformation as a necessary step. Three CYP enzymes—CYP 1A2, CYP 2D6, and CYP 3A3/4—mediate mirtazapine biotransformation to approximately an equal extent (320). Mirtazapine is also about 25% dependent on elimination by way of a phase II conjugation reaction with glucuronic acid.

Mirtazapine exhibits linear pharmacokinetics over its clinically relevant dosing range. That finding suggests that mirtazapine does not inhibit the three CYP enzymes that mediate its biotransformation. That conclusion is further supported by *in vitro* studies, which demonstrate that mirtazapine is a weak inhibitor of these CYP enzymes (321). Together these two observations suggest that coadministration of mirtazapine will not alter the elimination of coadministered drugs that are dependent on these specific CYP enzymes for their elimination. Nonetheless, a definitive statement on this matter awaits appropriately designed *in vivo* pharmacokinetic studies testing the potential effect of mirtazapine on model substrates for these CYP enzymes.

Reboxetine

Maximal plasma concentrations occur 2 to 3 hours after oral administration of reboxetine (178). Reboxetine has linear pharmacokinetics over its clinically relevant dosing range and a half-life of approximately 12 hours. For this latter reason, a twice a day, equally divided dosing schedule was used during clinical trial development. Its clearance is reduced and half-life becomes longer as a function of advanced age (mean = 81 years of age) and renal and hepatic impairment (178, 322, 323). Reboxetine is principally metabolized by CYP 3A3/4 such that its dose should be reduced when used in combination with drugs that are substantial inhibitors of CYP (e.g., certain azole antifungals, certain macrolide antibiotics). Reboxetine itself, however, does not cause detectable inhibition of CYP 3A3/4 based on formal *in vivo* pharmacokinetic interaction studies as well as its own linear pharmacokinetics.

Monoamine Oxidase Inhibitors

Only minimal information is available about the pharmacokinetics of the traditional MAOIs (e.g., phenelzine, tranylcypromine) (308). Such data are probably less critical for these versus other antidepressants, because MAOIs are consumed by their mechanism of action (i.e., irreversible inhibition of MAO by covalently binding to the enzyme). This mechanism accounts for the fact that traditional MAOIs have half-lives of only 2 to 4 hours, but their effects persist for an extended period because of their irreversible inactivation of their target. These MAOIs undergo presystemic or "first pass" degradation, and, thus, genetic or acquired alterations in this metabolism could alter their bioavailability and hence their effects.

THERAPEUTIC DRUG MONITORING

In general, pharmaceutical companies see TDM as a marketing problem. They are concerned that physicians would avoid using a drug if they thought TDM was necessary. They are also concerned that their competitors would use such information to criticize their product by suggesting to physicians that it is too complicated to use. Thus, the subject of TDM is not a neutral, scientific issue, with companies often discouraging any suggestion that TDM could enhance the safe and optimal use of their product. The reader needs to keep that in mind when evaluating the literature in this area.

As discussed in Chapters 1 and 3, the basic concept underlying TDM is that a relationship must exist between drug concentration and the magnitude of its effect. Drug dose is simply the first approximation of what concentration is achieved in the average individual. TDM is a refinement of this approximation, establishing the concentration achieved in a specific individual on a given dose. Thus, TDM is principally a tool to determine how interindividual variability in pharmacokinetics could account for interindividual variability in drug response. TDM can also be used to determine whether the patient is compliant. Recall that drug concentration is determined by the following equation:

Drug concentration = dosing rate/clearance

Thus, TDM is a measure of an individual's ability to clear or eliminate a drug.

The physician can estimate the reciprocal of the patient's elimination rate for a drug by dividing the plasma drug level by the dosing rate (i.e., the daily dose that produced that particular plasma drug level). For example, with TCAs, patients fall into three groups:

- The majority (i.e., greater than 90%) are *normal or "extensive" metabolizers* in whom values of 0.5 to 1.5 ng/mL/mg/day develop.
- Members of a smaller group (i.e., 5% to 10%) are genetically deficient in CYP 2D6 and, hence, are *"poor" metabolizers* in whom plasma drug levels in the range of 4.0 to 6.0 ng/mL/mg/day develop.
- An even smaller group of patients (i.e., 0.5%) are *ultrarapid metabolizers* of TCAs in whom levels less than 0.5 ng/mL/mg/day develop (324).

There is a linear relationship between dose and plasma drug levels (i.e., linear or first-order pharmacokinetics) in normal and ultrarapid metabolizers. In these individuals, the earlier equation can be used to predict the daily dose needed to produce a specific plasma drug level once TDM has been done to estimate the patient's elimination rate. In poor metabolizers, TCAs follow nonlinear pharmacokinetics (i.e., disproportionate increases in plasma drug levels with dose increases) because they lack the CYP 2D6 and must use lower affinity enzymes to metabolize these drugs.

TDM enhances the clinician's ability to adjust the dose of medications rationally to compensate for interindividual differences in elimination rate. It represents a refinement of the dose–response relationship, taking into account interindividual differences in elimination. It is a step beyond the traditional but often inefficient and error-prone approach of dose adjustment based on assessment of clinical response.

The role of TDM for different antidepressants varies from being a standard of care issue with TCAs to a discretionary laboratory test with most of the newer drugs. The reason for this difference relates to the pharmacology of the various classes of antidepressants, particularly in terms of toxicity. TDM is essential for the safe use of TCAs because of their narrow therapeutic index and the substantial interindividual differences in elimination rates. These two factors result in the risk that serious toxicity can develop in poor metabolizers on standard doses. In contrast to TCAs, most new antidepressants have such a wide therapeutic index that serious toxicity is not a concern.

With newer antidepressants, the primary reason to use TDM is to improve efficacy. Methodological problems, however, make it virtually impossible to demonstrate a relationship between the plasma level of an antidepressant and response. This issue has been discussed in detail elsewhere (25, 324) and is briefly summarized here.

The methodological problem is that only one-third of patients in most clinical trials of an antidepressant respond specifically to the drug. Another one-third responds to the placebo condition and the last one-third are nonresponders. Thus, the signal-to-noise ratio is 1:2. Even if there was a perfectly linear relationship between antidepressant level and response, it would be virtually impossible to establish it by doing a clinical trial and plotting response as a function of drug level. Studies that find no relationship are thus

expected. The authors of such reports, however, erroneously conclude that the failure to find a relationship means that one does not exist. The way to determine the optimal plasma level range of a newer antidepressant with a large therapeutic index (i.e., the ratio of the toxic dose to the therapeutic dose) is to determine the mean plus one standard deviation of the plasma concentration range achieved on the usually effective, lowest dose. If a patient does not benefit from the usually effective, lowest dose and achieves a concentration below that range, then he or she may have not responded for that reason. In that case, a trial of a higher dose would be appropriate.

With the aforementioned caveats in mind, the relationship between plasma antidepressant levels and both beneficial and adverse clinical effects for older and newer antidepressants are reviewed in the following paragraphs.

TCA Plasma Levels and Antidepressant Response

These older antidepressants have a therapeutic range that is bound on the lower end by lack of efficacy and on the upper end by risk of serious toxicity. These drugs also have substantial interindividual variability in drug metabolism so that ineffective concentrations can develop in some patients on the usual dose and toxic concentrations can develop in others. For that reason, TDM is a standard of care issue when using TCAs to treat clinical depression (325).

Studies have attempted to demonstrate a relationship between concentration and antidepressant response for the following:

- Nortriptyline
- Desipramine
- Amitriptyline
- Imipramine (326)

Nortriptyline

Most studies found a curvilinear plasma concentration–antidepressant response relationship with an optimal range of 50 to 150 or 170 ng/mL depending on the study. Within this range,

70% of patients with primary major depressive disorder experience complete remission (e.g., a final HDRS score equal to or less than 6) versus only 29% of patients who had plasma concentrations outside this range (i.e., below or above 50 to 170 ng/mL). Of note, the response rate is generally higher in the lower end of this range than at the upper limit. For that reason, a modest reduction (rather than increase) might be the best course of action if the patient has not optimally benefited and their plasma level is near the upper limit.

Desipramine

The optimal therapeutic range for antidepressant response with this secondary amine TCA is 110 to 160 ng/mL. The studies have found a remission rate of 59% within versus 20% outside this range.

Amitriptyline

The results for this tertiary amine tricyclic are less convincing in terms of efficacy but quite robust with regard to toxicity. The optimal range for this medication in terms of antidepressant efficacy is approximately 80 to 150 ng/mL (amitriptyline plus nortriptyline). Studies generally found a nonsignificant trend with a remission rate of 48% within versus 29% outside this range.

Imipramine

This agent did not show a curvilinear relationship between concentration and antidepressant response in adult patients, with a threshold relationship best fitting the data. Based on the Perry et. al. analysis of the adult studies (326), the upper end for optimal antidepressant response to imipramine was close to the threshold for CNS and cardiac toxicity.

Thus, the upper limit to the therapeutic range is a function of toxicity rather than reduced efficacy in contrast to the other TCAs. Perry et al. (326) proposed a minimal threshold for this tertiary amine TCA of 265 ng/mL (imipramine plus desimipramine) with a remission rate of 42% above this threshold versus 15% below it. Of note, this threshold for optimal antidepressant response is closer to the threshold for CNS and cardiac toxicity than for any other TCA. Preskorn and colleagues (327) found a lower optimal threshold for imipramine plus desimipramine (125 ng/mL) when it was used to treat clinical depression in children and adolescents than when used in adults.

A summary of the plasma concentration–efficacy data with these four TCAs supports the use of TDM, at least once, as a routine aspect of therapy for major depressive disorder. The data are consistent across three of these agents that optimal plasma levels are associated with a greater likelihood of full remission after 4 weeks. Translated into clinical terms, **Perry et al. (326) find a 1.7- to 3-fold increase in clinical response to TCAs if the depressed patient obtains an optimal TCA plasma level**.

TCA Plasma Levels and Toxicity

Studies have also focused on issues of TDM and enhanced safety to avoid CNS or cardiac toxicity, as well as catastrophic outcomes.

Central Nervous System Toxicity

The relationship between TCA plasma concentration and CNS toxicity has been well established. The incidence of TCA-induced delirium varies from 1.5% to 13.3% (mean of 6%) when hospitalized patients take doses of 300 to 450 mg per day without the benefit of TDM-based dose adjustment (328). Furthermore, these symptoms often evolve insidiously, such that they can mimic the depressive episodes that these medications are being used to treat (329). *An increase in affective symptoms* (e.g., deterioration in mood, poor concentration, social withdrawal, and lethargy) may be the earliest warning signs of impending CNS toxicity. *Motor symptoms* (e.g., tremor and ataxia) frequently develop next, followed by *psychosis* (e.g., thought disorder, delusions, and hallucinations). All of these may lead the clinician to erroneously conclude that the depressive episode is worsening, prompting an increase in the TCA dose or the addition of an antipsychotic. The latter strategy, in turn, can increase the TCA plasma levels by inhibiting metabolism, further exacerbating toxicity. The last stage in the evolution of TCA-induced CNS toxicity is *delirium* (e.g., memory impairment, agitation, disorientation, and confusion) and/or *seizures*. TDM can detect the slow metabolizer who is at greater risk for developing this scenario.

In patients who are not neurologically compromised, TCA plasma concentrations less than 250 ng/mL rarely produce CNS manifestations. As this threshold concentration is exceeded, asymptomatic, nonspecific EEG abnormalities develop (330). With concentrations beyond 450 ng/mL, there is a significant increased risk of seizures and delirium (331). The relative risk of delirium increases 13- and 37-fold when TCA plasma levels exceed 300 and 450 ng/mL, respectively (328). Of note, peripheral anticholinergic effects (e.g., blurry vision, dry mouth, and constipation) cannot be used as a foolproof clinical means of detecting potentially toxic plasma levels of TCAs.

TCA-induced seizures typically have no prodrome and are a single generalized motor seizure that lasts several minutes. The incidence of seizures during treatment with standard doses is estimated at 0.5% in nonepileptic patients (332). Patients who experience TCA-induced seizures during routine chemotherapy and with no other risk factors for seizures generally have plasma TCAs levels well in excess of 450 ng/mL (331, 333).

Finally, the minimal threshold for development of coma is approximately 1,000 ng/mL (334). This occurs almost exclusively in acute overdoses, but nevertheless is consistent with the conclusion that TCA-induced CNS toxicity is concentration dependent.

Cardiovascular Toxicity

The cardiovascular effects of TCAs have also been well documented, and the mechanisms underlying these effects elucidated by *in vitro* and *in vivo* animal studies (335). Because the effects of TCAs on intracardiac conduction are concentration dependent and occur at levels above the upper therapeutic threshold, TDM can help avoid iatrogenic cardiotoxicity.

Although conduction disturbances are more likely to occur in persons predisposed to cardiac disease, data demonstrate that these effects also occur in healthy individuals if the appropriate threshold is exceeded. In healthy middle-aged subjects, TCA plasma concentrations of less than 200 ng/mL rarely induce intracardiac conduction defects. At 200 ng/mL, however, asymptomatic clinically nonsignificant slowing of the His bundle–ventricular system routinely occurs (336). At concentrations of more than 350 ng/mL, first-degree atrioventricular (A-V) block was found in 70% of physically healthy patients on desipramine or imipramine (337, 338). A number of case reports have demonstrated that TCA plasma levels near 1,000 ng/mL achieved as a result of slow clearance during routine treatment rather than from overdose can cause fatal arrhythmias (339–341). In some of these cases, malpractice suits have been filed alleging failure to diagnose TCA toxicity and specifically cited failure to use TDM to adjust the dose. As a result, there have been court awards in favor of the plaintiffs totaling millions of dollars.

Clinicians should be aware that significant postmortem changes in TCA plasma levels may occur, and interpretation must be done cautiously. Sudden death may only be coincidentally associated with a drug the patient was taking. Nevertheless, if a patient is found to have a toxic level postmortem and no anatomical cause of death at autopsy, the clinician may have a legal problem if TDM was not used at least once early in treatment to rationally adjust the dose.

Techniques for TDM with TCAs

Generally, the physician starts with a standard TCA dose (e.g., 50 to 75 mg per day of nortriptyline) in a physically healthy adult. After 1 week, most patients are at steady-state. A blood sample is then drawn 10 to 12 hours after the last dose to ensure that absorption and distribution of the drug are complete and because virtually all the data on optimal concentration ranges are based on this postdose time interval. If the sample cannot be drawn at 10 to 12 hours, obtaining it later is better than earlier, because these drugs have half-lives of approximately 24 hours. If the level is drawn at 16 hours rather than 10 to 12 hours, the drug is only 4 hours into its first postabsorption half-life, and even though this sample will underestimate the 10- to 12-hour level, the magnitude of the error is small. In contrast, too early a sample can overestimate the 10- to 12-hour level to a greater extent and in a less predictable way.

Single-dose prediction strategies can be used to more rapidly predict the dose required to achieve a therapeutic plasma concentration. Nomograms have been developed in which a 25-mg test dose of nortriptyline is given, and then blood is drawn 24, 36, or 48 hours later to obtain plasma concentrations. These data are then plotted on the nomogram to estimate the dose that would achieve a therapeutic plasma concentration. The utility of this approach is limited, however, because errors in technique (e.g., imprecise timing of blood draw) can be magnified, leading to miscalculations of the required dose.

Selective Serotonin Reuptake Inhibitor Plasma Levels and Antidepressant Response

Given the wide therapeutic index of the SSRIs, the safety issues that make TDM a standard of care with the TCAs are not applicable to this class. Although the risk and severity of their typical adverse effects (e.g., nausea) increase with dose escalation, there is almost no chance of life-threatening toxicity. Hence, physicians can adjust the dose of these drugs upward without this concern. The issue of TDM with the SSRIs, therefore, involves increasing the percentage of patients who will experience an optimal antidepressant response.

Although studies have been done with virtually all of the SSRIs attempting to correlate antidepressant efficacy with plasma drug levels, they have consistently failed to find a relationship (121, 342–348). However, a relationship has been found between the plasma levels of each SSRI achieved on the lowest, usually effective dose and the ability to inhibit approximately 70% to 80% of serotonin uptake (25). Thus, patients who have SSRI plasma levels below this threshold have probably not had an optimal trial of the SSRI as a result of rapid clearance, inadequate dose, or noncompliance.

A unique role for TDM with SSRIs is to determine the risk and magnitude of a CYP enzyme mediated drug–drug interaction. Like most drugs, the effect of SSRIs on CYP enzyme is concentration dependent. Thus, TDM could be used to determine the risk and likely magnitude of the effect of an SSRI on the metabolism of another drug. This would primarily involve fluoxetine, fluvoxamine, and paroxetine because of their substantial inhibitory effect on one or more CYP enzymes at their lowest, usually effective dose. This is particularly true for fluoxetine and its active metabolites, which because of their long half-lives can persist for several weeks after discontinuation. During this interval, there remains the risk of a drug–drug interaction. If the physician wishes to start another medication that could interact pharmacodynamically or pharmacokinetically with fluoxetine/norfluoxetine, then TDM could determine when the plasma levels decrease sufficiently so the patient is not at substantial risk (302). The same approach can be used to avoid pharmacodynamically mediated drug interactions after fluoxetine discontinuation (e.g., when is it safe to start an MAOI after stopping fluoxetine?)

In conclusion, TDM is not a standard of care issue with other SSRIs but can be used if a patient has not benefited from the lowest, usually effective dose and can be used to rule out persistent effects after stopping fluoxetine (300).

Other Antidepressants

Venlafaxine

As with SSRIs, TDM is not a standard of care issue with this agent. A recent study demonstrated that the sequential effects of venlafaxine on serotonin and then NE uptake pumps is dose and hence concentration dependent (137). Thus, TDM can be used with venlafaxine in the same manner as with the SSRIs.

Nefazodone and Trazodone

The pharmacokinetics of these two phenylpiperazines makes TDM technically difficult. The half-lives of the parent drugs (i.e., nefazodone and trazodone) are approximately 4 hours, which means that modest differences in sample timing (i.e., time after last dose) could cause significant differences in observed plasma levels of the parent compounds (156). These drugs also have nonlinear pharmacokinetics, such that modest differences in compliance could substantially affect plasma drug levels. Furthermore, they also undergo extensive biotransformation to form several active metabolites (312, 313, 349). In the case of nefazodone, one of these metabolites (hydroxynefazodone) has a pharmacological profile similar to the parent drug, another (triazolodione) reproduces only part of the pharmacology of the parent drug, and another (mCPP) has a pharmacological profile substantially different from the parent drug (350). Trazodone also undergoes extensive biotransformation, including the production of mCPP (310). This further complicates any attempt to relate drug plasma levels to clinical efficacy, because each metabolite is likely to contribute to the clinical outcome. Their contributions, however, may be different from and even opposite to that of the parent drug. For these reasons, TDM research would be exceedingly difficult and unlikely to generate clinically useful therapeutic ranges.

Bupropion

This antidepressant comes the closest to the TCAs in terms of the potential usefulness of TDM. As discussed previously, it has a narrow therapeutic index (i.e., the difference between the antidepressant dose and a dose that carries the risk of a significantly increased seizure risk). Considerable interindividual variability in plasma levels of bupropion and its active metabolites among patients on the same dose has been observed.

In addition, studies indicate a relationship between trough, steady-state plasma concentrations of 50 to 100 ng/mL and optimal response. Moreover, higher levels of the parent compound and its metabolites are associated with a poorer outcome (351, 352).

The following indicate that pharmacokinetics are a significant contributor to the occurrence of seizure in patients taking bupropion:

- The incidence of seizures is *dose related* (and, hence, must be concentration related).
- Seizures typically *occur within days of a dose change and a few hours after the last dose,* suggesting that peak plasma concentrations play a role.
- Individuals with *lean body mass* (i.e., smaller volume of distribution), such as anorexic-bulimic patients have an increased risk.

Thus, the clinician might use TDM with bupropion to guard against the development of unusually high plasma levels of the parent drug or its metabolites. That would be particularly true for the medically compromised or the patient on other drugs that could interfere with the clearance of bupropion. In such a case, the laboratory should assay the parent drug and its three major metabolites—hydroxybupropion, threohydrobupropion, and erythrohydrobupropion.

Monoamine Oxidase Inhibitors

Phenelzine has been studied for the treatment of anxiety, phobic and obsessive-compulsive disorders, as well as typical and atypical depressions. Its antidepressant efficacy has been correlated with an 80% to 85% inhibition of the MAO enzyme. Studies by Ravaris, replicated by this text's authors, indicate that 60 mg per day are usually needed to inhibit MAO by at least 80% (353, 354). Although monitoring of platelet MAO inhibition during treatment may permit more optimal dosing, the assay is not readily available commercially. This, coupled with the infrequent use of MAOIs, has hampered the widespread application of this specialized form of TDM.

Conclusion

There are three possible relationships between plasma concentration and efficacy:

- *None or a poor* relationship between plasma level and therapeutic response
- A *threshold for therapeutic response,* such that below this level there is less likelihood of response and above it there is a good chance for response
- A *threshold for toxicity* such that above this level the potential for increased adverse effects outweighs the likelihood of further therapeutic gain

TDM with antidepressants can be used for the following reasons:

- *Plasma levels are in the usual optimal range, but there is insufficient clinical response*: try another agent, an augmentation strategy, or ECT (see also "Alternative Treatment Strategies" later in this chapter).
- *Plasma levels are low* and there is insufficient response: increase the dose.
- *Plasma levels are high* and there is insufficient clinical response or severe adverse effects: reduce the dose or try another agent.
- Patient with *obsessive-compulsive symptoms* (or disorder) is *nonresponsive on adequate blood levels*: consider clomipramine or an SSRI (e.g., fluoxetine, sertraline, paroxetine).

ALTERNATIVE TREATMENT STRATEGIES

Treatment-Resistant Depression

Two major problems complicating the question of treatment-resistant depression are inappropriate diagnosis and inadequate treatment (355). Studies have found only a small proportion (<15%) of newly diagnosed depressed patients receive adequate antidepressant treatment as defined by dose and duration criteria (356, 357). Hence, a substantial number of "treatment-resistant" cases are actually the result of inadequate therapy (i.e., relative resistance). For example, in the MacEwan and Remick (358) study, 70% of those defined as treatment-unresponsive achieved complete remission with an adequate trial of an HCA, MAOI, or ECT. Patients who do not receive sufficient benefit from a trial of one antidepressant now have the option of newer agents whose activity does not necessarily overlap with earlier generation compounds (e.g., SSRIs, venlafaxine, nefazodone).

Guscott and Grof (359) list a series of variables, presented here with minor modifications, critical to the understanding and management of refractory depression:

- Is the *diagnosis correct* (e.g., both incorrect diagnosis or subtype, such as atypical depression)?
- Does the patient have a *psychotic* depression?
- Has the patient received *adequate treatment* (dose and duration)?
- Do *adverse effects* preclude adequate dosing?
- Is the patient *compliant?*
- Was a rational, *stepwise approach* used?
- How was *outcome measured?*
- Is there a *coexisting medical* or *psychiatric disorder* (e.g., substance abuse) that interferes with response to treatment?
- Are there *other factors* in the clinical setting that interfere with treatment?

Also of concern are the effects that nonresponse may have on the clinician, including the following:

- *Avoidance* of the patient (e.g., countertransference)
- *Affective disturbances,* resulting in feelings of dysphoria, anger, and decreased tolerance for patients' complaints
- An increased tendency to add or to *switch diagnosis to an Axis II disorder*

Guscott and Grof (359) consider the vast majority of these patients only *relatively refractory* and analogize this situation to other medical disorders, such as asthma, which is often underdiagnosed and undertreated. Thus, like asthma, morbidity and mortality associated with depression are increasing worldwide. Ironically, these complications occur at a time when the understanding of the pathophysiology of major depression has greatly advanced over the past 2 decades, and when appropriate diagnosis and aggressive drug therapy can improve outcome. Guscott and Grof recommend giving careful attention to an adequate treatment trial, using a rational, stepwise model, like those often used in other medical specialties to treat asthma, essential hypertension, and rheumatoid arthritis.

White and Simpson (360) caution that patients intolerant to TCAs should not be considered "treatment resistant" because another antidepressant with a different profile (e.g., an SSRI) can often bring about remission. Other strategies include a second trial using an HCA with a different biochemical profile (i.e., switching from a tertiary to a secondary TCA).

Evidence for this approach, however, is least from the perspective of improving tolerability and weak in terms of improving efficacy. Finally, Paykel and Van Waerkom (361) emphasize that, in addition to pharmacotherapy, other therapeutic modalities—including social support, environmental manipulation, and family, cognitive, or dynamic psychotherapy—are often helpful in managing these patients.

Patients tend to improve with time and the level of depression fluctuates from day to day. Sometimes when a second drug is added, improvement may have occurred simply because of the passage of time but is falsely attributed to the additional drug. It is difficult to do controlled studies in treatment nonresponders, because so many improve with the first treatment. Because there are many drugs and combinations used to achieve an adequate homogeneous sample of nonresponders to any given treatment, a large collaborative study mechanism would be necessary. Such a study, entitled Sequence Treatment Algorithm for Resistant Depression (STAR*D) is just beginning under National Institute of Mental Health sponsorship. This study is patterned after clinical treatment. It begins with open label treatment with an SSRI to prospectively determine cases of treatment-resistant depression. The nonresponders will then enter the randomized portion of the trial. This study should provide clinically useful information about what treatment is the best next option for the depressed patient who has not benefitted from a previous trial of a different antidepressant.

Specific Strategies to Manage Treatment Resistance

There are three major options available with true treatment nonresponse (362):

- *Switch* to another antidepressant.
- *Augment* with another medication.
- Use a *combination* of antidepressants.

Switch to Another Antidepressant

Perhaps the greatest research need in antidepressant pharmacotherapy is what to do when the first antidepressant trial fails to produce response. Indeed, in clinical trials, 35% to 40% of patients do not achieve a 50% reduction in their symptoms on any single antidepressant and the majority do not have a full remission. Thus, this discussion is relevant to the majority of patients with major depression.

Even so, the research in this area has been disappointingly sparse. The existing studies have serious limitations such as small numbers of subjects and design problems, including lack of blinding, random assignment, and an appropriate control group.

Although some physicians may try multiple members of the same class (e.g., multiple sequential trials of different SSRIs), a recent survey found that most psychiatrists prefer to switch to a different class of antidepressant for patients who have not experienced adequate benefit (135). We concur that this approach is more rational and more likely to be a productive strategy than switching among antidepressants with the same apparent mechanism of action. Although there have been a number of studies purporting that switching among SSRIs is a useful strategy, most of these studies, which were sponsored by the manufacturer of the second SSRI, are often methodologically flawed and are therefore of limited value (363).

The switching strategy with the most rigorous data to support its usefulness is between an SSRI and either desipramine or imipramine (either direction). Numerous double-blind crossover studies support this practice (136, 364). Although these studies are considerably more rigorous and less susceptible to bias than the open label SSRI switch studies, they still do not involve rerandomization of patients. Thus, the response rate could be confounded and inflated by the passage of time.

As a results of these studies, clinicians have proposed that switching to reboxetine or bupropion might a useful strategy given that these antidepressants share the ability with desipramine and imipramine to block NE uptake. Nevertheless, only one small open label study has been done to test this possibility (365). If bupropion is to be used in patients switched from an ineffective trial of fluoxetine, the dose should be kept low for several weeks to allow for the clearance of fluoxetine and norfluoxetine. Case reports indicate that fluoxetine can elevate levels of the active metabolites of bupropion, which, in turn, could mediate an increase risk of adverse effects (366).

The switch from an SSRI to high-dose venlafaxine is another theoretically appealing strategy, because high-dose venlafaxine blocks the uptake pumps for both serotonin and NE (137). To test this concept, a double-blind study has recently been completed testing the usefulness of switching SSRI nonresponders to either citalopram or venlafaxine. The results of that study are being analyzed.

Two open label studies have been done with nefazodone (367, 368). As discussed earlier, the value of such open label studies is dubious. Moreover, this strategy is limited by the divided dose schedule recommended for the immediate release formulation of nefazodone, the need for dose adjustment, and the potential for complicated drug–drug interactions, particularly when switching from fluoxetine to nefazodone.

In a single-site, open label study, Wheatley and colleagues (369) conducted a crossover study from fluoxetine to mirtazapine, principally to test for a pharmacokinetic interaction. These investigators noted that mirtazapine did produce a clinically meaningful antidepressant response in a sizable percentage of patients who had not benefited from fluoxetine. A subsequent multicenter, open label study made the same observation (370). These results are encouraging but must again be interpreted cautiously given the open label designs.

Augmentation Strategy

This approach is generally used when there has been at least some antidepressant response (355). It generally refers to the addition of a medication that is not formally labeled as an antidepressant, which is in contrast to the combined use of two antidepressants, as discussed later in this section.

Lithium. Lithium augmentation of standard antidepressants has been reported to significantly benefit previously treatment-resistant and psychotic depressions, particularly in bipolar patients (371, 372). There is substantial case report literature reporting that many patients have benefited when lithium was added to ongoing TCA therapy. Often these results occurred rapidly, sometimes with low doses of lithium. Although the results of controlled trials have not been as dramatic, they still support this approach, which should be seriously considered for treatment-resistant major depression.

Although initial reports concluded that low-dose lithium could augment the effect in patients partially responsive to an SSRI (373), subsequent reports have been less encouraging (374, 375). Furthermore, there is an increase in bothersome adverse effects when lithium is added to SSRI therapy (376). Both of these factors plus the need for TDM when using lithium has caused this approach to fall from favor in recent years.

Thyroid Hormone. Data from a limited number of controlled studies indicate that, particularly in women, adding triiodothyronine may produce remission in a nonresponder (377). However, most of these studies have been done with TCAs rather than the newer antidepressants.

Pindolol. The original intent for using pindolol in combination with an SSRI or similar antidepressant was to speed the onset of antidepressant activity. The value of that approach remains controversial as does the value of augmentation with pindolol. Most of the studies are not methodologically rigorous and the results are conflicting (378–380). A recent double-blind, placebo-controlled trial found no benefit with pindolol in accelerating response to fluoxetine in 86 predominantly recurrent, chronically depressed patients (381). When pindolol is used in combination with an SSRI, the dose is generally 2.5 mg given three times per day.

Buspirone. This has been an agent in search of a use. As with pindolol, most initial reports were open label. The only double-blind, placebo-controlled study did not support the usefulness of buspirone augmentation; however, the placebo response in patients with alleged treatment refractory depression was 47% (382). Generally, the dose of buspirone as an augmentation strategy has been 5 to 15 mg twice a day.

Even though buspirone is generally safe and well tolerated when used alone, it is susceptible to clinically meaningful drug–drug interactions. Buspirone is converted via CYP 3A3/4 to an active metabolite, l-phenylpiperzine (1-PP), which is, in turn, dependent on CYP 2D6 for its elimination. Thus, buspirone can interact with antidepressants and other drugs that cause substantial inhibition of CYP 3A3/4 (e.g., fluvoxamine and nefazodone) and CYP 2D6 (e.g., fluoxetine and paroxetine). However, the outcomes are different. Substantial inhibition of CYP 3A3/4 can increase both the bioavailability and prolong the clearance of the parent drug, buspirone. In contrast, substantial inhibition of CYP 2D6 can delay the clearance of its active metabolite, 1-PP, which has a substantially different pharmacology than the parent drug. Both types of interactions have been reported to cause significant behavioral toxicity (383).

Combined Use of Two Antidepressants

Faced with nonresponse to one or more trials of different antidepressants, many psychiatrists try combining antidepressants. As with most of the treatments in this section, rigorous data supporting the safety and efficacy of this approach is generally in short supply. In such an instance, the clinician faces the dilemma of doing nothing or trying a combination that is often based only on theoretical arguments or anecdotal case reports.

As one might expect, virtually every antidepressant has been tried in combination with every other antidepressant with the possible exception of MAOIs (384). The combined use of desipramine and an SSRI has the best data to support its usefulness (119, 120). However, other groups have not found as robust an effect as was initially reported.

Because reboxetine and bupropion share with desipramine the ability to block the NE uptake pump, some clinician may want to combine them with an SSRI. Bupropion, however, should be used cautiously with fluvoxamine, fluoxetine, and paroxetine because these three antidepressants inhibit one or more CYP enzymes to a substantial degree at their lowest, usually effective antidepressant dose. Therefore, the dose of bupropion should be kept low and TDM could be used to ensure that unusually high levels of bupropion or its active metabolites do not develop.

Although most physicians avoid the combination of an MAOI with most other antidepressants, a number of reports indicate that MAOIs combined with a TCA can be effective and safe in treatment-resistant patients. This combination should be used only by a physician skilled in their use and familiar with their potential adverse effects and drug interactions. Generally, tertiary amine TCAs have been used in combination with MAOIs. Once the dose of the TCA is established, the MAOI should be slowly added. Never attempt the reverse order without a 2-week delay. It may also be prudent to lower the TCA dose slightly before starting the MAOI. An example might be the addition of phenelzine to amitriptyline, starting with an initial dose of 15 mg and subsequent dose increments weekly as needed. The total dose of an MAOI, used in combination with TCA, is usually lower than when used alone (e.g., 30 to 60 mg per day). When the combination is discontinued, the MAOI should be stopped first.

Desipramine and maprotiline, which are selective NE reuptake inhibitors, should not be combined with an MAOI because of the risk of hypertensive crisis. The combination of an MAOI plus reboxetine and bupropion also blocks the NE uptake pump and thus theoretically should carry the same risk of a hypertensive crisis when combined with an MAOI. Thus, these combinations should also be avoided.

The combination of an MAOI plus an SSRI, venlafaxine, or nefazodone should not be attempted because of the risk of a serotonin syndrome.

No data are available on the safety or efficacy of combining mirtazapine or nefazodone with MAOIs. Until studies are available, it is prudent to avoid such combinations.

Combination Strategies in Special Patient Populations

Patients suffering from a psychotic depression usually do not benefit from antidepressant monotherapy and usually require the combination of an antidepressant and antipsychotic or

ECT. There is limited evidence that amoxapine, whose primary active metabolite (8-hydroxy-amoxapine) has antipsychotic-like properties, can be used as monodrug therapy (385).

Depression associated with panic attacks may benefit from the combination of an antidepressant-anxiolytic or the use of an SSRI (e.g., fluoxetine or paroxetine), which may have antipanic properties separate from their antidepressant effects.

Post and Kramlinger (386) have also suggested that lithium added to carbamazepine may be useful in treatment-resistant mood-disordered patients. One possible basis for this approach is that carbamazepine, which has a tricyclic ring structure similar to imipramine, may sensitize postsynaptic serotonin receptors in a similar way to standard drugs such as imipramine. A mood stabilizer (e.g., lithium, valproate, carbamazepine) plus antidepressant may benefit some rapid cycling or mixed bipolar patients, attenuating the propensity to switch from mania to depression.

Other Alternative Treatment Strategies

Alternative primary monotherapies include the following:

- ECT and other somatic therapies
- Lithium monotherapy
- Possibly lamotrigine
- Psychostimulants

ECT should be considered for more severe forms of depression (e.g., those associated with melancholic and psychotic features, particularly when the patient exhibits an increased risk for self-injurious behavior) or when there is a past, well-documented history of nonresponse or intolerance to pharmacological intervention. Limited data indicate that bipolar depressed patients may be at risk for a switch to mania when given a standard TCA. A mood stabilizer alone (i.e., lithium, valproate, carbamazepine, lamotrigine), or in combination with an antidepressant, may be the strategy of choice in these patients. Some elderly patients and those with acquired immunodeficiency syndrome may also benefit from low doses of a psychostimulant only (e.g., methylphenidate) (see also Chapter 14,

"The HIV-Infected Patient"). Fig. 7-1 summarizes the strategy for a patient whose depressive episode is insufficiently responsive to standard therapies.

Other promising, investigational, nondrug forms of somatic therapy for affective disorders include transcranial stimulation and vagus nerve stimulation. These treatments are also discussed in Chapter 8.

Drug-Induced Depressive Syndromes

Treatment of these disorders is first directed at the causative agent (e.g., reserpine, α-methyldopa). Withdrawing the offending compound and providing supportive care may be all that is required, with the symptoms dissipating in days to weeks. When such conservative measures are unsuccessful, most clinicians initiate an antidepressant.

With drugs that produce a depression after chronic exposure (e.g., alcohol), detoxification is instituted, in addition to supportive care and therapy for substance dependency. Even though most alcoholics will experience depression immediately after the cessation of heavy and prolonged consumption, the majority will remit within several weeks following detoxification and supportive care (see Chapter 14, "The Alcoholic Patient"). For those who do not, it is likely there had been a preexisting depressive disorder, which itself can lead to substance dependency, because patients frequently self-medicate before seeking professional intervention. This possibility should be evaluated through a review of the patient's personal medical and psychiatric history, as well as family history.

The recovering patient who remains depressed after appropriate treatment of the abstinence syndrome should be given an antidepressant trial. Treatment planning should take into account the patient's physical status, especially because it may affect the pharmacokinetics and pharmacodynamics of the agent selected (see Chapter 3).

ROLE OF PSYCHOSOCIAL THERAPIES

Because this book focuses on psychopharmacotherapy, it is not intended to exhaustively review the role of psychotherapy. Nonetheless, some form of counseling is usually necessary during the treatment of major depressive disorder. Broadly defined, psychotherapy covers a wide range of modalities, from simple education and supportive counseling to cognitive-behavioral to insight-oriented psychodynamically based therapy.

No illness occurs in a vacuum. There is a fluid interaction between an individual and his or her illness (e.g., life situations may aggravate the illness and vice versa). These disorders affect the way people think about themselves, as well as how other people view them. For these reasons, medications are not optimally prescribed in a vacuum as if they alone will resolve the problem. Although the good practitioner in any branch of medicine is mindful of these facts, this recognition is especially important in psychiatric disorders because of the difficulty patients have in separating themselves from the illness and its associated social stigma. Thus, patients may be able to view an illness such as cancer as something that has happened to them and therefore as something distinct from themselves. This distancing is much more difficult with a psychiatric disorder because it affects the fundamental processes (e.g., mood and cognition) that define one's self. This statement is particularly germane to major depressive disorder because it often involves feelings of guilt, worthlessness, low self-esteem, helplessness, and hopelessness. These symptoms, coupled with the delayed onset of drug action, make education and supportive counseling imperative.

Good clinical management requires that patient education about their illness and its treatment be given in a supportive manner, while simultaneously exploring whether life situations are aggravating the condition or vice versa. If medication is indicated, the patient should know why and what can be reasonably expected from this course of action. This education should include the following explanations:

- *How medications are believed to work* for their condition
- *How to take the medications*
- *What life activities,* if any, *need to be altered* while on the medication
- The *potential adverse effects,* as well as what to do if they occur

Education does not stop at this point, but is an ongoing process throughout treatment. Because major depressive disorder impairs concentration and attention, it is useful to repeat this information several times during the initial and follow-up visits. It is often helpful to query the patient about what has been explained and then clarify or expound on issues as indicated. **It is critically important to avoid patient discouragement by balancing optimism with the acknowledgment that antidepressants generally have a delayed onset of action.**

It is also prudent to explain other options, especially if the first medication trial is unsuccessful. Thus, it is crucial to reassure the patient before the first antidepressant trial that if unsuccessful, there is a good chance of responding to an alternative therapy. Patients understand and accept the concept of empirical trials. Educating and involving them in the decision-making process is not only "politically correct," but also therapeutic because this approach

- Addresses feelings of *loss of control and inadequacy.*
- Makes a patient an *active participant* of the treatment.
- Enhances *compliance.*

Education should continue even after the depressive episode has remitted. An explanation of the value of maintenance and prophylactic therapy, as well as when it is appropriate to discontinue treatment, is important. The early signs of relapse should be explained to both the patient and close family members or friends, if appropriate. The goal is to increase the likelihood of early detection in case of recurrence. This is based on the hope that early intervention may prevent or at least shorten the duration or intensity of an episode and lessen its consequences (387).

In addition, a number of studies have compared the efficacy of specific forms of psychotherapy, particularly cognitive-behavioral therapy (CBT), and antidepressants in the treatment of patients with an acute episode of major depression (388–395). Most studies have reported these forms of psychotherapy and antidepressants to be equally effective. As a result of disparate findings, spirited debate has arisen with regard to this issue. Issues raised in this debate have included relative efficacy in patients with mild versus more severe episodes of major depression and the adequacy of antidepressant treatment in these studies. A summary of these issues is presented in the following paragraphs.

The study by Elkin et al. (391) from the National Institute of Mental Health Treatment of Depression Collaborative Research Program suggested that antidepressants had superior efficacy in the treatment of moderate to more severe episodes of major depression (i.e., 17-item HDRS score of 20 or more). In response to that claim, DeRubeis et al. (396) performed a meta-analysis of four studies and found that CBT was as effective as several different antidepressants in such cases. More recently, Keller et al. (397) found that a variant of CBT called cognitive-behavioral analyses (CBAS) therapy was as effective as nefazodone (mean dose = 460 mg per day) in producing both response and remission in outpatients with moderate to more severe chronic depression.

Returning to the debate, Meterissian and Bradwejn (398) argued that pharmacotherapy was not adequate in the earlier studies comparing it with CBT. Klein (399) further argued that these studies were flawed because ineffective antidepressants were continued for 12 to 16 weeks (i.e., the length of time used to administer the CBT). According to Klein, two courses of antidepressants could have been conducted in this time period and hence a clinically meaningful comparison would be to permit the switching of patients who had not responded after 6 to 8 weeks to a different antidepressant. Recently, Thase et al. (395) have conducted such a study comparing 16 weeks of CBT (n = 52) with either fluoxetine (n = 10) or bupropion (n = 13). Their study permitted patients who had not responded to one of these antidepressants to be switched to the other after 8 weeks while CBT continued. Despite the limited statistical power resulting from the small numbers of patients on the antidepressants, these investigators found pharmacotherapy was superior to CBT on four of six measures and had a lower rate of nonresponse (i.e., 13% versus 46% for CBT and drug, respectively). The difference favoring pharmacotherapy over CBT emerged late in treatment and was principally due to the switching of nonresponders to the alternate antidepressant.

In summary, the debate continues over the relative efficacy of pharmacotherapy versus psychotherapy, particularly CBT. Although this argument may be of interest from a guild perspective, it does not advance current knowledge of the basic nature of the condition. Virtually all of the studies can be faulted on the grounds that they have been open label and hence susceptible to bias on the part of the investigators. There is also the problem of standardizing CBT, ensuring equivalent dosing of CBT versus pharmacotherapy, inadequate numbers, and generalizability.

Rather than pitting these two forms of treatment against each other in an "either/or" paradigm, another question is whether outcome is better when both treatments are used together. This issue was addressed in the study by Keller et al. (397), which found that a greater percentage responded to combined treatment with nefazodone and CBAS than to either treatment alone. That result is consistent with earlier studies comparing psychotherapy, TCA plus psychotherapy, and a control group of patients who called for emergency appointments only (demand-only psychotherapy) and served thus as a "low-contact" or a placebo group (400–403). In these studies, the combined treatment with a TCA plus psychotherapy also demonstrated greater efficacy on specific outcome measures than either treatment alone. Nevertheless, these results may not generalize to all forms of psychotherapy. For example, one study found that patients given medication experienced more benefit than those undergoing group psychotherapy (404).

Another issue is whether psychotherapy can prevent relapse. The classic study by Frank et al. (405) found that interpersonal psychotherapy (IPT) plus imipramine was not superior to imipramine alone and that IPT alone was not significantly better than placebo treatment in preventing relapse. Recently, however, Fava et al. (406) found that 40 randomly assigned patients with recurrent major depression (three or more episodes) did better on CBT than with routine clinical management after responding to antidepressant treatment. Thus, this question has also not been resolved.

In the absence of definitive evidence clearly supporting either side in these debates, many clinicians use the following general guidelines. If there are more complicated problems or persistent personal issues, then formal psychotherapy may be indicated. That decision needs to be made within the context of an individual's specific situation. When possible, a recommendation for more intense psychotherapy should be reserved until there has been a reasonable opportunity to assess response to drug therapy plus education and supportive counseling. Many life situations that seem insurmountable become more manageable when a depressive episode has remitted. This caveat is particularly important during the first episode in a patient with a good premorbid history and an illness duration of less than 1 year. It is also applicable to patients with recurrent major depressive disorder who have a good return to psychosocial functioning between episodes.

ADVERSE EFFECTS

An important aspect of antidepressant pharmacotherapy is selection based on the adverse effect profile of a specific medication, because most antidepressants are comparable in terms of efficacy. One of the major accomplishments of modern antidepressant development has been to improve the adverse effect profile of newer agents in comparison with TCAs and MAOIs without compromising efficacy (1). That has been accomplished by developing chemicals that retain the ability to affect sites of action that appear to be capable of mediating antidepressant efficacy (e.g., the serotonin uptake pump), but avoid effects on unnecessary sites of action (e.g., ACh receptor, fast sodium channels). This approach has led to both better tolerated and safer medications. Table 7-23 lists the common potential adverse affects of a number of antidepressants, as well as their relative severity.

Accurate identification of drug-induced adverse effects is complicated by the fact that many of these complaints (e.g., headaches, fatigue, dry mouth, dizziness) are associated with depression and, hence, can occur while on placebo (1). Some of these symptoms may have been present before the initiation of medications, whereas others emerge spontaneously but are still unrelated to the drug. Therefore, placebo-controlled studies are essential to determine whether the frequency of a given adverse effect occurs more on active medication than on placebo.

Whereas formal clinical trial data are the most rigorous information available about the adverse effects of a drug, it is often incomplete as a result of the limited range of patients included in such studies. **Formal clinical trials generally exclude patients who are very young or very old, medically ill, on multiple medications, drinking to excess, or using illicit drugs.** For that reason, most physicians prefer medications that have been on the market for a few years, unless the new medication has compelling advantages over existing agents. The more extensively a drug has been used in clinical practice, the more confident one can be in their safety and tolerability for a variety of patients with different illnesses and on multiple combinations of medications. Extensive clinical experience does exist for most of the newer antidepressants as well as TCAs.

Tricyclic Antidepressants

Secondary amine TCAs (e.g., nortriptyline, desipramine) are better tolerated and somewhat safer than their tertiary amine parent compounds (e.g., amitriptyline, imipramine) (407, 408). This is due to differences in the relative potencies of several pharmacological actions, which include their binding affinity for the following:

- *Muscarinic ACh receptors,* which mediate their atropine-like effects
- *Histamine receptors,* which may mediate their sedative and possibly the weight gain effects
- α-*Adrenergic receptors,* which mediate their orthostatic hypotensive effects (409)

In addition, their ability to stabilize electrically excitable membranes (i.e., quinidine-like properties) through inhibition of fast sodium channels is the action most likely responsible for their most important adverse effects: cardiotoxicity and neurotoxicity (410).

Whereas tertiary amine TCAs are more potent than secondary amine TCAs in terms of sites of action mediating adverse effects, they are less potent than secondary amine TCAs in terms of

TABLE 7-23. *Adverse effects of antidepressants*

Drugs	Sedation	Anticholinergic	Orthostatic hypotension	Cardiac effects
Heterocyclics				
Amitriptyline	High	High	Moderate	High
Clomipramine	High	High	Low	Moderate
Desipramine	Low	Low	Low	Moderate
Doxepin	High	Moderate	Moderate	Moderate
Imipramine	Moderate	Moderate	High	High
Maprotiline	Moderate	Moderate	Low	Moderate
Nortriptyline	Moderate	Moderate	Low	Moderate
Protriptyline	Low	Moderate	Low	Moderate
Trimipramine	High	High	Moderate	High
Selective Serotonin Reuptake Inhibitors				
Fluoxetine	Low	None	None	None
Paroxetine	Low	Low	None	None
Sertraline	Low	None	None	None
Fluvoxamine	Low	None	None	None
Citalopram	Low	None	None	None
Selective Norepinephrine Reuptake Inhibitors				
Reboxetine	Low	Low	Low	Low
Dibenzoxazepines				
Amoxapine	Low	Moderate	Low	None
Phenylpiperazines				
Trazodone	High	Low	Moderate	Low
Nefazodone	Low	Low	Low	Low
Aminoketones				
Bupropion	High	Very low	Very low–none	Low
Serotonin and Norepinephrine Reuptake Inhibitors				
Venlafaxine	Low	Very low	Very low	Low
Serotonin and Norepinephrine Receptor Activity				
Mirtazapine	Moderate	Low	Low	Low
Monoamine Oxidase Inhibitors				
Isocarboxazid	Low	None	High	None
Phenelzine	Low	Low	High	None
Tranylcypromine	High	Very low	Very low	None

Adapted from Ward M. Appendix B. In: Flaherty J, Davis JM, Janicak PG, eds. *Psychiatry: Diagnosis and Therapy.* 2nd ed. Norwalk, CT: Appleton & Lange, 1995:493-494.

antidepressant efficacy based on the results of the plasma drug level studies reviewed earlier in this chapter. That fact further increases the safety and tolerability of secondary amine versus tertiary amine TCAs (411). Nevertheless, secondary amine TCAs are still toxic when taken in overdose, and this issue must always be considered when applying treatment in a patient who poses a substantial suicide risk.

The most troublesome problems with TCAs involve the following:

• The *cardiovascular* system

• The *central nervous system*
• The *peripheral nervous* system
• *Overdose-related* issues

Cardiovascular Effects

Soon after the TCAs were introduced, it was noted that fatal overdoses were usually secondary to heart block or ventricular arrhythmias (412). This observation led to the concern that, in vulnerable patients, these drugs might produce similar complications at therapeutic plasma concentrations. Over the past 25 years, however, prospective trials have led to a more accurate understanding of their cardiac effects. The best way to review the present state of knowledge is to categorize these effects as follows:

* *Orthostatic* hypotension (significant, even at therapeutic doses)
* *Conduction* delays, arrhythmias (significant in many overdose cases)
* *Contractility* impairment (not significant except in rare overdose cases)

Orthostatic Hypotension

One of the most frequent and potentially serious adverse effects of TCAs (as well as MAOIs) is orthostatic hypotension. This effect leads to discontinuation of antidepressant therapy in approximately 10% of healthy depressed patients. Furthermore, fractures, lacerations, possible myocardial infarction, and sudden death have all been reported, especially in elderly patients.

By far, the most studied drug is *imipramine*. Fewer complete data are available for other TCAs. Existing studies, however, strongly imply that hypotension also occurs with *amitriptyline* and *desmethylimipramine*. Little is known about the potential of doxepin to lower blood pressure, although it is widely used. *Nortriptyline* is the only TCA currently on the market for which a reduced risk of orthostasis has been reported. For example, one study reported that this effect was negligible in 40 healthy, middle-aged depressed patients, and another documented a reduced risk (413).

Both the rate and the magnitude of drug-induced hypotension increase dramatically in depressed patients suffering from cardiac disease. In 25 depressed patients with preexisting congestive heart failure, imipramine-induced orthostasis was approximately 50%. In contrast, of 21 patients without preexisting congestive failure who were given therapeutic plasma concentrations of nortriptyline, this problem developed in only one patient (414). Furthermore, 19 of these 21 patients had previous trials of imipramine, with eight experiencing falls on this agent.

Mechanism. The mechanisms underlying this effect are not clear, but various investigators have implicated the following:

* *Peripheral* α-adrenergic blockade
* Enhanced stimulation of *central* α-adrenergic receptors
* *Direct* adrenergic vasodilation

If a drug possesses a given property *in vitro* or *in vivo,* this may be presumptive evidence, but it does not necessarily mean that the therapeutic or adverse effects are mediated by that property. What is needed is direct evidence in humans that postural hypotension is caused by the α-adrenergic blocking properties of these drugs.

A significant risk factor for the development of orthostasis with imipramine may be depression itself. For example, one study, found that, of 22 nondepressed cardiac patients with some degree of congestive heart failure (i.e., mean ejection fraction 33% by radionuclide angiography) who were given imipramine for control of their arrhythmia, only one (4%) discontinued the medication because of orthostasis (415, 416). This rate contrasts with a 50% incidence of hypotension among melancholic patients with a similar degree of left-ventricular impairment treated with comparable plasma concentrations of imipramine. Muller et al. (417) also found that 24 of 37 depressed cardiac patients experienced significant hypotension in contrast to none of the heart patients without depression.

Treatment. Patients should always be warned of this possible adverse effect and be instructed to rise carefully from a lying or sitting position by dangling their feet before standing or sitting, or quickly lying down when feeling faint. Because falls resulting in broken bones or concussions can occur, such common sense precautions are important.

When hypotension remains problematic, support hose, salt, and fluids can also be used. Some recommend the use of the mineralocorticoid fluorohydrocortisone (Florinef, 0.025 to 0.05 mg twice a day).

Conduction Delays, Arrhythmias

Sudden death has occurred in patients with preexisting heart disease on antidepressant therapy. It may be difficult, however, to separate a causally related drug effect from a cardiovascular incident precipitated by other factors and only by chance coincident with drug therapy. Furthermore, Roose (418), who has summarized the literature, noted that major depressive disorder occurs frequently after a myocardial infarct and may adversely affect the recovery process.

Early reports on imipramine noted that some patients developed first-degree heart block, as well as other bundle branch patterns, but it took almost 15 years to clarify that these conduction delays were the only adverse effects at therapeutic plasma concentrations. It is now well documented that increased PR, QRS, or QT intervals occur with all standard TCAs, at or slightly above their therapeutic plasma levels.

Electrophysiological studies have confirmed that the TCAs exert their major effect on the His-ventricular (HV) interval. Although they frequently prolong PR and QRS intervals in depressed patients with a normal pretreatment electrocardiogram (ECG), such moderate increases are not, by themselves, clinically significant. This propensity to reduce conduction velocity, however, raises the question of whether patients with preexisting disorders would be at increased risk for development of symptomatic A-V block. This concern was supported by the frequency of A-V block after overdose and by case reports of patients with preexisting bundle branch block in whom two-to-one block developed when given imipramine.

Roose et al. (419) conducted a prospective study of 41 depressed patients with first-degree A-V or bundle branch block (or both) who were compared with 151 patients with normal pretreatment ECGs. Both groups were given therapeutic plasma concentrations of imipramine or nortriptyline. The rate of two-to-one A-V block was significantly higher (9%) in patients with preexisting bundle branch block, as compared with the rate (0.7%) in those with normal pretreatment ECGs ($p < 0.05$ by Fisher's Exact Test). In fact, the one patient with a normal pretreatment ECG in whom two-to-one A-V block developed had an abnormal His conduction, apparent only by catheterization.

Therapeutic plasma concentrations of TCAs have clinically significant antiarrhythmic activity (420). Imipramine and nortriptyline (and probably other TCAs) share electrophysi-

ological properties characteristic of type I (A, B) compounds (e.g., quinidine, procainamide, disopyramide) and can even be used in cardiac patients free from depression, exclusively for the control of arrhythmia (421).

Because overdoses can cause severe arrhythmias, it had been previously thought that these drugs were contraindicated in patients with preexisting problems. A drug, however, may not produce the same cardiovascular effect at a therapeutic versus a toxic plasma concentration. For example, in one study, 17 of 22 nondepressed cardiac patients with ventricular arrhythmias had more than 75% premature ventricular contraction (PVC) suppression after imipramine treatment (422). Particularly important from the cardiologist's perspective, imipramine also suppressed PVCs with complex features, a more serious type of rhythm disturbance. Significant reductions also occurred in the frequency of bigeminy (85% ± 45%) pairs (89% ± 30%), and ventricular tachycardia (99% ± 2%). However, combining similar agents (e.g., imipramine plus quinidine) may produce a *proarrhythmic effect*.

Contractility Problems

TCAs may adversely affect left ventricular function (LVF). This phenomenon was addressed using the systolic time interval (STI), a measurement partly dependent on the QRS duration. However, TCAs prolong QRS, and hence the STI method can overestimate the effect of TCAs on LVF because of their prolongation of the QRS interval.

The introduction of radionuclide angiography has provided a more reliable means of assessing drug effects on LVF. Using this methodology, relatively low doses of imipramine and doxepin did not impair LVF in 17 depressed patients; however, only a few had ejection fractions less than 40%. Subsequently, Glassman et al. (423) reported radionuclide data on 15 depressed patients with moderate-to-severe LVF impairment (mean ejection fraction = 33%) treated with therapeutic plasma concentrations of imipramine. Although imipramine had no deleterious effect on any measure of LVF, as previously discussed, it produced intolerable orthostatic hypotension in about 50%.

This finding was replicated in a second series of ten depressed patients with heart failure (mean pretreatment ejection fraction = 31%), who also had no change in any measure of LVF when treated with therapeutic plasma concentrations of imipramine. TCAs should therefore be used cautiously in patients with congestive heart failure (CHF), principally because of their potential for causing clinically significant orthostatic hypotension and for delaying intracardiac conduction.

In summarizing the relationship between TCA therapy and cardiovascular effects, Roose and Glassman (424) concluded that TCAs

- Are *antiarrhythmic* agents and are effective in patients with ventricular ectopic activity
- Rarely have an adverse effect on *cardiac output* at usually therapeutic concentrations, even in patients with CHF
- *Slow conduction,* which places patients with bundle branch block at risk for development of conduction complications

Anticholinergic Effects

Typical autonomic effects resulting from the anticholinergic properties of TCAs include the following:

- *Dry mouth*
- *Impaired visual accommodation,* aggravation of narrow-angle glaucoma (rarely)
- *Palpitations, tachycardia, dizziness*
- *Urinary hesitancy* or retention; constipation; rarely paralytic ileus, which can be fatal if not detected early
- *Memory impairment*

Dry mouth is the most common autonomic adverse effect, and patients should be alerted to its possible occurrence. *Profuse sweating,* especially at night, can also occur, but the precise mechanism is unknown. There is an increased risk of *dental caries* as a result of the loss of the bacteriostatic effects of saliva. This problem is further compounded when patients attempt to relieve dry mouth by ingesting hard candy or soft drinks; therefore, sugar-free substances should be recommended.

These autonomic adverse effects are usually mild and typically become less bothersome after the first few weeks of treatment. In any event, they can be controlled by adjusting the drug dosage. Bethanechol (urecholine) at doses of 25 to 50 mg given three to four times a day can reverse the urinary retention.

Based on *in vitro* assay techniques to measure the binding of agents to muscarinic receptors, amitriptyline has the strongest anticholinergic properties, doxepin is intermediate, and desipramine the weakest (425). *In vitro* and animal studies have shown that none of the newer antidepressants have meaningful anticholinergic effects at their usual therapeutic dose (Table 7-23). Consistent with their pharmacology, clinical studies find that they produce no more anticholinergic problems than placebo. Although it is not known to what degree *in vitro* preparations correlate with *in vivo* activity, one can assume a positive correlation.

Central Anticholinergic Syndrome

This toxic reaction is manifested by the following:

- Florid visual *hallucinations*
- Loss of immediate *memory*
- *Confusion*
- *Disorientation*

Diagnosis is based on the typical symptom picture and reversibility by physostigmine, an agent that increases brain ACh, thus overcoming the atropine blockade. Discontinuance of anticholinergics usually ends the problem within a day or so. Rarely, in selected cases, physostigmine can produce a dramatic reversal, but it should not be used hastily, because error in diagnosis or too much of this drug may produce a cholinomimetic toxic syndrome.

Withdrawal Syndrome

There is no withdrawal problem with the TCAs of the type seen with narcotics, alcohol, sedatives, or serotonin reuptake inhibitors (i.e., SSRIs, venlafaxine). Nonetheless, abrupt discontinuation of

150 to 300 mg per day or more of a TCA, especially after 3 or more months of treatment, can induce an autonomic rebound (i.e., gastrointestinal disturbances, autonomic symptoms, anxiety, agitation, and disrupted sleep). The incidence varies, depending on dosage and duration of consumption. The higher the daily dosage and the longer it has been ingested, the more likely the occurrence. Onset usually begins by 48 hours after abrupt discontinuation. These symptoms may be related to the anticholinergic potency of the TCA. Withdrawal of the drug produces a state of muscarinic receptor supersensitivity, resulting in "cholinergic overdrive." If abrupt withdrawal is necessitated by a switch to hypomania or mania, temporary benztropine therapy can minimize the risk of autonomic symptoms. When possible, antidepressants should always be discontinued by gradual taper.

Noradrenergic Effects

Jitteriness, tachycardia, and *tremor* can occur early in the course of treatment, particularly in patients with co-morbid panic attacks. TCAs may cause a persistent, fine, rapid tremor, particularly in the upper extremities. Desipramine and protriptyline may be the most common offenders. Propranolol (60 mg per day) may help and is unlikely to worsen depression. Alternatively, switching to a drug with less NE activity may also help.

Central Nervous System Effects

Insomnia has been reported, especially in elderly patients, but it is usually transitory and responds to morning dosing or switching to a more sedating antidepressant. Even though all these drugs produce sedation, there are quantitative differences. For example, amitriptyline and doxepin are more sedating than most other antidepressants (Table 7-23). Patients should be cautioned that the sedation produced by alcohol may add to or potentiate the sedative effects of the drug. The pharmacological mechanism for sedation is most likely H_1-receptor blockade.

Although more "stimulating" antidepressants (e.g., bupropion, SSRIs, venlafaxine, or certain MAOIs) do not potentiate alcohol, they can produce insomnia. To minimize this problem, the dose may be given earlier in the day. TCAs may cause episodes of *excitement* (rare), confusion, or mania, usually in patients with an underlying psychotic illness, suggesting that a preexisting disorder must be present for these drugs to exert any psychotomimetic effects.

In addition to large overdoses of these drugs, amounts used clinically may occasionally produce *seizures*. Because convulsions may be unrelated to drug treatment, however, their origin should always be carefully evaluated. In this context, Preskorn and Fast (331) found that the only risk factor associated with seizures in eight patients on routine TCA therapy was an elevated plasma level (mean $= 734 \pm 249$ ng/mL; range $= 438$ to 1200 ng/mL).

Maprotiline and *bupropion* cause more seizures than agents such as imipramine, amitriptyline, and nortriptyline. This issue, plus other safety concerns, has significantly limited the use of maprotiline. If maprotiline is used, many clinicians start with a low dose (75 mg per day or less in elderly patients), gradually increasing by 25-mg increments over 2 or more weeks (the drug has a half-life of about 48 hours). Average doses in outpatients are 150 mg, with a maximum of 225 mg.

Davidson (426) found that the risk of seizures with bupropion was higher at doses greater than the recommended maximum (i.e., 450 mg per day). The seizure risk may be as low as one per 1,000 patients with the sustained release formulation when the dose is kept less than 450 mg per day, and the patient has no preexisting seizure history and is not on any medication that also can lower seizure thresholds or interfere with the metabolism of bupropion.

Twitching, dysarthria, paresthesia, peroneal palsies, and *ataxia* may also occur in rare instances. Disturbances of motor function are uncommon and are most likely to occur in elderly patients.

Overdose

For more than 25 years, TCAs were one of the leading causes of drug-related deaths, exceeded only by alcohol–drug combinations and heroin (427). The risk of fatality resulting from a TCA overdose has severely limited their use now that newer, safer antidepressants are available. Nevertheless, overdoses of these medications still occur. There is still no simple antidote for a TCA overdose. A TCA overdose produces a characteristic clinical picture consisting of the following:

• Temporary agitation, confusion, convulsions
• Hypotension, tachycardia, conduction delays
• Manifestations of anticholinergic blockade
• Bowel and bladder paralysis
• Disturbance of temperature regulation
• Mydriasis
• Delirium

Patients may progress to coma (generally lasting less than 24 hours) often complicated by shock and respiratory depression. Typically, a TCA-induced coma is usually short in duration.

The most characteristic and serious sequelae of overdose involve disturbances in cardiac conduction and repolarization. These disturbances are manifested clinically by

• A-V *block*
• Intraventricular *conduction* defects
• Prolongation of the *QT* interval

As conduction times are prolonged, the chance of developing reentry arrhythmias grows. Malignant ventricular arrhythmias are uncommon in mild or moderate overdoses, but they are more likely in severe cases.

All of these signs and symptoms may be present to some degree or may be absent, depending on the quantity of drugs ingested. The lethal dose has been estimated to be about 1 g, although overdoses as low as 500 mg have been fatal. All of the TCAs can be fatal in overdose, and the same is true for some of the newer HCAs, such as maprotiline (by a different mechanism) and amoxapine. In a series of 32 fatal ingestions, 14 victims died on the way to the hospital, nine were alive on arrival but already had major symptoms, and the remaining nine arrived without major symptoms, but such symptoms developed within 2 hours of arriving (428). All deaths from the direct toxicity of the drug occurred within the first 24 hours.

Disturbances of cardiac rhythm (e.g., tachycardia, atrial fibrillation, ventricular flutter, and A-V or intraventricular block) are the most frequent causes of death. Thus, management of cardiac function is critical. If the patient survives the early phase, recovery without sequelae is probable, and vigorous resuscitative measures are important. A major clinical problem is determining when a patient is no longer in danger. Many patients with mild overdose have been hospitalized unnecessarily or for inordinately prolonged periods because of this concern. Late deaths (2 to 5 days after overdose) have been seen; however, most of these involved complications that had presented earlier and were expected (429, 430). If no major symptoms have developed after 6 hours (depressed level of consciousness, hypotension, depressed respiration, seizures, conduction block, or arrhythmia), it is unlikely that they will develop. Although clinicians need to know about the rare possibility of late death, common sense is required when a decision is necessary regarding the discontinuation of more intensive medical care.

Although the literature indicates that seizures and arrhythmias are associated with TCA plasma levels greater than 1,000 ng/mL, the QRS duration might be a better early predictor than plasma levels in overdose cases. For example, in a series of 49 TCA overdoses, seizures occurred only in cases with a QRS duration above 0.10 second, and ventricular arrhythmia was seen with a QRS greater than 0.16 second (430). Thus, for acute overdose, the ECG may provide a reliable and quick measure of risk with TCA drugs; however, how well a QRS of less than 0.10 second predicts ultimate safety or how long after ingestion the ECG must be followed, is uncertain (431).

The most frequent cardiovascular effects of an acute overdose are tachycardia and hypotension. The hypotension is partially related to a relative volume depletion, but correction does not bring complete resolution. Even though radionuclide and catheterization studies have shown that TCAs do not impair LVF, either at therapeutic plasma levels or with overdose, data are not available for victims who died. One study describes two cases of fatal overdose in which ventricular pacing produced regular ventricular depolarization but minimal cardiac output, suggesting that at very high concentrations, TCAs might directly impair the myocardium (as demonstrated in animal studies) (429).

CNS toxicity is a serious problem with *maprotiline* and is the probable mechanism of death rather than cardiac complications.

Treatment

The one principle about which there is no dispute regarding TCA overdoses is the need for aggressive interventions to rapidly remove the drug. The contents of the stomach should be emptied in any suspected TCA overdose, because once absorbed, dialysis is less efficient in removing these drugs. Treatment should include the following:

- Induced *vomiting* or gastric aspiration
- *Lavage* with activated charcoal
- *Anticonvulsants* (such as intravenous diazepam)
- *Coma care*
- Support of *respiration*
- Attention to *cardiac* effects

A slurry of activated charcoal given repeatedly through a nasogastric tube, following the initial emptying of the stomach, greatly accelerates TCA elimination, probably because of the large enterohepatic circulation that is interrupted by the repeated charcoal (432). While encouraging, this technique has been subjected to only limited study in actual cases of overdose.

Treatment with quinidine or similar drugs might be considered for ventricular arrhythmias, but if the physician realizes that the TCAs themselves are type I antiarrhythmic agents, *the potential dangers* of this approach become apparent. Although systematic studies are not yet available, it seems reasonable to treat these victims as one would treat quinidine overdoses (i.e., with hypertonic sodium bicarbonate and cardiac pacing). This therapeutic regimen should significantly increase the percentage of surviving patients or, at least, ensure that the treatment will not unintentionally exacerbate the problem. Tachycardia is generally not a problem, and the use of physostigmine to counteract it is controversial.

Miscellaneous Adverse Effects

Weight Gain

Tertiary amine TCAs and mirtazapine are antidepressants that cause weight gain. The blockade of both the 5-HT$_{2C}$ and the H$_1$ receptors have been suggested as the possible mechanisms behind this effect. For patients who experience this problem, SSRIs, venlafaxine, and bupropion may be better options. Although there is mild weight loss on SSRIs during initial treatment (i.e., the first 6 to 8 weeks), this effect is not sustained with longer treatment. That fact thwarted efforts to develop these drugs for this indication.

Sexual Dysfunction

Priapism is an abnormal, painful, and persistent erection, not related to sexual arousal, which can be caused by a variety of conditions (e.g., neurological, hematological, local trauma, and scorpion or black widow spider bites). Its occurrence also has been associated with various drugs, including the following:

- *Antipsychotics,* such as chlorpromazine and thioridazine
- *Drugs of abuse,* such as marijuana or cocaine
- *Antihypertensives,* such as guanethidine and hydralazine
- *Antidepressants,* such as trazodone

Its occurrence should be considered an acute medical emergency, and in the first few hours after an episode the patient should be closely monitored. Increased penile tumescence should lead to immediate discontinuation of the drug and consultation with an urologist. If the condition persists, retained blood can lead to edema and eventual fibrosis of the corpora and permanent impotence. Thus, sustained penile tumescence is an emergency and may require direct injection into the cavernous bulbosa or surgical detumescence (306). Because this adverse effect is rare, many specialists have not had extensive experience, and it may be useful to contact the medical staff of the drug's manufacturer to help find an experienced urologist.

Hypersensitivity Effects

Skin reactions occur early in therapy but can subside with continued treatment. *Jaundice,* which can also occur early, is of the cholestatic type, similar to that attributed to chlorpromazine. *Agranulocytosis* is a rare complication, as are cases of leukocytosis, leukopenia, and eosinophilia. There are no data on the incidence of antidepressant-induced agranulocytosis, except to note that it is rare with all of the agents discussed in this chapter.

Selective Serotonin Reuptake Inhibitors

In 1988, fluoxetine became the first SSRI marketed in the United States. Since then, sertraline (1992), paroxetine (1993), fluvoxamine (1994) and citalopram (1998) have been marketed. Their widespread acceptance has added substantially to the patient-years of experience with these medications. Thus, the confidence in our knowledge of the adverse effect profile of these drugs in the general population and in special populations (e.g., the elderly, the medically ill) has grown substantially over the past decade.

Although the early clinical trials comparing SSRIs with tertiary amine TCAs found the newer agents to have better tolerated side-effect profiles, these differences were less evident when they were compared with secondary amine TCAs (433–438). The most important advantage of the SSRIs is the absence of severe adverse effects (e.g., cardiac conduction delays, seizures, postural hypotension) and death from overdose.

The adverse-effect profiles of SSRIs and TCAs are generally different, with those related to the former most consistent with serotonin agonism (434–436, 439). The most frequent early complications include the following:

- Headache, dizziness
- Nausea, loose stools, constipation
- Somnolence, insomnia
- Sweating, tremor, dry mouth
- Anxiety, restlessness

Whereas less frequent adverse effects include the following:

- Weight gain
- Inhibition of ejaculation or orgasm
- Bruxism, myoclonus, paraesthesia

The management of the most common adverse effects includes the following:

- *Nausea:* Usually transient and dose-related. May improve with dose reduction or symptomatic measures (e.g., food, antacids, addition of drugs that block 5-HT$_3$ receptors, such as cisapride). There has been increasing concern about using cisapride in combination with antidepressants that can substantially inhibit CYP 3A3/4 (i.e., fluvoxamine, nefazodone). The reason is that high levels of cisapride can cause arrhythmias as a result of delayed intracardiac conduction.
- *Anorexia:* More pronounced in overweight patients and those with carbohydrate craving. May lead to abuse in patients with bulimia or anorexia nervosa.
- *Increased anxiety and nervousness:* Occurs early in treatment, especially in patients with prominent anxiety symptoms. May improve with support, dose reduction, or concomitant treatment with a BZD.
- *Tremor:* May improve with dose reduction, a β-blocker, or a BZD

These adverse effects rarely require discontinuation, and several are dose related (e.g., anxiety, tremor, nausea) (439, 440). As with all other classes of antidepressants, the SSRIs often have a delayed onset of action, but unlike TCAs the effective dose can be given from the beginning, rather than by gradual adjustment. They also have flat dose–antidepressant response curves, meaning that, on average, there is no increased likelihood of response with higher doses. Realizing these facts can help to minimize adverse effects by resisting the temptation to increase the dose within the first 2 to 4 weeks of treatment.

In addition to a different side-effect profile, SSRIs differ from TCAs by virtue of their wider safety margin, because they do not cause life-threatening toxic effects (e.g., patients having survived acute ingestion of amounts equal to 10 times the daily dose) (434). For this reason, many

TABLE 7-24. *Placebo-adjusted incidence (%) of various forms of sexual dysfunction on new antidepressants[a]*

Adverse Effect	Fluoxetine (N = 1,730, N = 799)[b]	Sertraline (N = 861, N = 853)[b]	Paroxetine (N = 421, N = 421)[b]	Venlafaxine (N = 1,033, N = 1,033)[b]	Nefazadone (N = 393, N = 394)[b]
Abnormal ejaculation/orgasm[c]		13.3	12.9	12.0	
Other male gender disorders[d]			10.0		
Impotence[e]				6.0	
Decreased libido[f]	1.6		3.3	2.0	1.7/0.5
Sexual dysfunction	1.9				
Sexual dysfunction (female)		1.5			
Female genital disorder[g]				1.8	1.1
Menstrual disorder[h]		0.5			2.5
Painful menstruation		0.5			

[a]Incidence is based on gender whenever appropriate. Placebo incidence on average for each of the above categories less than 0.5%.
[b]The first number is the number on the medication, and the second is the number on the parallel placebo group.
[c]Incidence based on number of male patients.
[d]Includes anorgasmia, delayed orgasm, erectile dysfunction, impotence, and "sexual dysfunction."
[e]Includes mostly anorgasmia and difficulty reaching climax or orgasm.
[f]Separate values for males and females available for nefazodone but not for the other antidepressants.
[g]Includes vaginitis.
[h]Includes dysmenorrhea and menstrual complaints.
From Preskorn S. Comparison of the tolerability of bupropion, nefazodone, imipramine, fluoxetine, sertraline, paroxetine, and venlafaxine. *J Clin Psychiatry* 1995;56:17–25, with permission.

clinicians prefer these drugs in patients who may be a significant suicide risk.

This rationale, however, was brought into question by concerns that fluoxetine (and by inference other SSRIs) might increase the likelihood of suicide in some patients (441, 442). An analysis of clinical trial experience with several SSRIs, however, did not reveal an increased incidence of suicide attempts or completions in comparison with patients who were randomly assigned to placebo or a TCA (439, 443, 444). An excellent review by Mann and Kapur (443) concludes that depressed patients are at greater risk by virtue of their disorder. They found that the overall incidence of suicide did not differ significantly among the various types of antidepressants. Nevertheless, there has been speculation but no definitive evidence that there may be a subgroup of patients more susceptible to certain adverse effects of SSRIs such as agitation and akathisia, perhaps predisposing them to a paradoxical increase in suicidal ideation or behavior (443). Mann and Kapur further postulated that the biochemical mechanism may be a temporary decrease in firing rates of presynaptic 5-HT neurons. Careful monitoring of such symptoms and requesting the patient to inform the clinician immediately upon their emergence may be the best way to prevent such potential sequelae if they occur. Whether they are due to the underlying illness or aggravated by the drug treatment, the clinician will want to know.

Sexual Dysfunction

SSRIs and venlafaxine can cause of variety of sexual dysfunctions including delayed ejaculation, anorgasmia, and decreased libido (Table 7-24). For two reasons, the adverse effect of these medications on sexual function was underestimated during the early clinical trials. First, such trials rely on spontaneous reporting by participants. Second, these adverse effects appear to take several weeks to develop. These adverse effects develop in approximately 30% to 40% of patients on adequate doses of SSRIs and venlafaxine. Although all manufacturers of these medications endeavor to suggest that their product is less likely to cause these effects, there is no compelling evidence to indicate that is true. Comparisons of rates across studies are not fair comparisons because they may differ based on how these problems were assessed.

Many patients do consider these problems to be a nuisance rather than a reason to terminate SSRI therapy. Others find these problems intolerable. A wide range of treatments have been tried including dopamine agonists including bupropion, yohimbine, cyproheptadine, and sildenafil. Most of these treatments had only anecdotal and open label studies to support their usefulness. However, sildenafil was found to be superior to placebo in a double-blind study (445).

Other Antidepressants

Venlafaxine

Venlafaxine is the only marketed antidepressant that inhibits both the uptake pumps for serotonin and NE without affecting numerous neuroreceptors in contrast to tertiary amine TCAs. However, several have been or are under development, including duloxetine and milnicipram (446).

Acute Safety Index

Venlafaxine, like the SSRIs and nefazodone, does not have substantial effects on Na^+ fast channels and thus has a wide therapeutic index (447). During clinical trial development, patients survived acute ingestion of over 6,750 mg of venlafaxine without serious sequelae (147). These acute overdoses have required no specific therapeutic interventions beyond general nursing care, with nausea and vomiting being the most common adverse effects. Indeed, these effects further reduce the severity of a significant overdose by having an emetic effect.

Acute Tolerability

Venlafaxine inhibits both the neuronal uptake pumps for serotonin and NE over its clinically relevant dosing range. It is approximately five times more potent *in vitro* as an inhibitor of the serotonin versus the NE uptake pump, and its adverse effect profile is consistent with this fact (448). At the lower end of its clinically relevant dosing range, venlafaxine has an adverse effect profile (e.g., nausea and somnolence) similar to that of the SSRIs (Table 7-25). At higher doses, venlafaxine also causes dose-dependent increases in several other adverse effects including high blood pressure, sweating, and tremors (Table 7-26). The effect on blood pressure is consistent with the fact that higher doses of venlafaxine produce physiologically meaningful potentiation of NE via the inhibition of its uptake pump. The incidence of elevated blood pressure has been a cause of some concern; however, it is a dose-dependent effect and is rarely observed at less than 225 mg per day (147, 449). Approximately 3% of patients in the clinical trial development program experienced this complication, with less than 1% needing to discontinue as a result. The magnitude of the increase was, on average:

- 1 mm Hg for those receiving 75 mg per day of venlafaxine
- 2 mm Hg for those receiving 225 mg per day
- 7.5 mm Hg for those receiving 375 mg per day (450)

Age, sex, renal or hepatic function, and baseline blood pressure were not clinically meaningful predictors of risk (143, 147, 449, 450). It is not known whether unstable, elevated blood pressure is a serious risk factor because such patients were excluded from the venlafaxine studies. This exclusion criterion is standard for all such clinical trials and not unique to the venlafaxine studies. With this caveat in mind, patients in the clinical trials were grouped into quartiles by blood pressure. Those in the highest quartile actually had a reduction in blood pressure during treatment with this agent (147).

Since venlafaxine has been marketed, patients in whom clinically meaningful blood pressure elevations have developed in routine clinical practice have been able to remain on the drug while their blood pressure was managed with an antihypertensive. These patients were kept on venlafaxine, because their depressive syndrome had responded well to this agent but not to other antidepressants. When feasible, other management strategies include a dose reduction or a switch to another class of antidepressant. Thus, the main issue is detection of this adverse effect, because it is easily managed. Elevated blood pressure developed within 2 months of being stabilized at a given dose in virtually all patients in whom

TABLE 7-25. *Comparison of the placebo-adjusted incidence rate (%) of frequent adverse effects for fluoxetine, sertraline, paroxetine, venlafaxine, and nefazodone*

Item	Fluoxetine (N = 1,730, N = 799)[a]	Sertraline (N = 861, N = 853)[a]	Paroxetine (N = 421, N = 421)[a]	Venlafaxine (N = 1,033, N = 609)[a]	Nefazadone (N = 393, N = 394)[a]
Headache	4.8	1.3	0.3	1	3
Nervousness[b]	10.3	4.4	4.9	12	—
Tremors	5.5	8.0	6.4	4	1
Insomnia	6.7	7.6	7.1	8	2
Drowsiness[c]	5.9	7.5	14.3	14	11
Fatigue[d]	5.6	2.5	10.3	6	7
Anorexia	7	1.2	4.5	9	—
Confusion[e]	1.5	0.8	1.0	1	9
Dizziness[f]	4.0	5.0	7.8	12	23
Paresthesia[g]	−0.3	1.3	2.1	1	2
Vision disturbances	1.0	2.1	2.2	4	12
Palpitations[h]	−0.1	1.9	1.5	2	—
Respiratory[i]	5.8	0.8	0.8	—	9
Nausea[j]	11.0	14.3	16.4	26	11
Dyspepsia	2.1	3.2	0.9	1	2
Diarrhea[k]	5.3	8.4	4.0	1	1
Flatulence	0.5	0.8	2.3	1	—
Dry mouth	3.5	7.0	6.0	11	12
Constipation	1.2	2.1	5.2	8	6
Frequent micturition	1.6	0.8	2.4	1	1
Urinary retention[l]	—	0.9	2.7	2	1
Sweating	4.6	5.5	8.8	9	—
Rash[m]	0.9	0.6	1.0	1	2

[a] The first number is the number on the medication, and the second is the number on the parallel placebo group.
[b] Nervousness includes anxiety, agitation, hostility, akathisia, central nervous system stimulation.
[c] Drowsiness includes somnolence, sedated, drugged feeling.
[d] Fatigue includes asthenia, myasthenia, psychomotor retardation.
[e] Confusion includes decreased concentration, memory impairment.
[f] Dizziness includes lightheadedness, postural hypotension, hypotension.
[g] Paresthesia includes sensation disturbances, hypesthesia.
[h] Palpitations includes tachycardia, arrhythmias.
[i] Respiratory includes respiratory disorder, upper respiratory infection, flu, dyspnea, pharyngitis, sinus congestion, oropharynx disorder, fever and chills, rhinitis, cough or infection.
[j] Nausea includes vomiting.
[k] Diarrhea includes gastroenteritis.
[l] Urinary retention includes micturition disorder, difficulty with micturition, urinary hesitancy.
[m] Rash includes pruritus.
From Preskorn S. Comparison of the tolerability of bupropion, nefazodone, imipramine, fluoxetine, sertraline, paroxetine, and venlafaxine. *J Clin Psychiatry* 1995;56:17–25, with permission.

elevated blood pressure developed, so that this interval is the period for closest monitoring (143, 147, 449, 450). We recommend that patients on doses of 225 mg per day or more should have their blood pressure monitored at every visit during this interval.

Long-Term Safety Index

As with the SSRIs, there are no known long-term safety issues. Nonetheless, the caveat remains that clinicians should be vigilant, because there has been insufficient long-term exposure to rule out this possibility.

Late-Emergent Tolerability

Consistent with its pharmacology, venlafaxine produces a similar type and incidence of sexual dysfunction as do the SSRIs. This effect can become apparent after several weeks of treatment at a stable dose.

TABLE 7-26. *Placebo-adjusted, dose-dependent adverse effects of paroxetine, venlafaxine, and nefazodone (mg/d)*

	Paroxetine (mg/day)			
Adverse effect	10 (N = 102)	20 (N = 104)	30 (N = 101)	40 (N = 102)
Nausea	1.0	13.2	21.0	22.6
Sweating	−1.0	4.7	6.9	9.8
Dizziness	3.0	2.8	5.0	8.8
Somnolence	4.9	10.5	13.0	13.8
Abnormal ejaculation	5.8	6.5	10.6	13.0
Constipation	−1.0	1.8	4.0	6.8
	Venlafaxine (mg/day)			
Adverse effect	75 (N = 89)		225 (N = 89)	375 (N = 88)
Nausea	18.5		24.1	43.9
Sweating	1.3		7.0	13.9
Dizziness	14.8		18.2	19.6
Somnolence	12.6		13.7	21.8
Tremor	1.1		2.2	10.2
Hypertension	0		1.1	3.4
Yawning	4.5		5.6	8.0
Chills	1.1		4.5	5.7
	Nefazodone (mg/day)			
Adverse effect	<300 (N = 211)			300–600 (N = 209)
Nausea	2			11
Dizziness	3			15
Somnolence	7			18
Constipation	1			7
Confusion	1			8
Blurred vision	1			7
Abnormal vision[a]	−2			8
Tinnitus	−1			2

[a]Includes scotoma, visual trails.
From Preskorn S. Comparison of the tolerability of bupropion, nefazodone, imipramine, fluoxetine, sertraline, paroxetine, and venlafaxine. *J Clin Psychiatry* 1995;56:17–25.

Nefazodone and Trazodone

Acute Safety Index

Nefazodone, like the SSRIs and venlafaxine, has negligible effect on Na^+ ion fast channels and therefore does not slow intracardiac conduction. As a result, during clinical trials development, patients survived drug overdoses exceeding 11,200 mg without the need for any intervention beyond observation and routine nursing care (146, 451). One nonstudy patient who took 2,000 to 3,000 mg of nefazodone with methocarbamol and alcohol experienced a seizure (type not documented) but otherwise recovered uneventfully.

Acute Tolerability

In the analysis of the comparative adverse effects of the newer generation of antidepressants, dizziness was most common with nefazodone. Indeed, it occurred more often on this drug than with any of the others (1). These results are compatible with its preclinical pharmacology, which differs substantially from the other new antidepressants (i.e., most potent action is blockade of the 5-HT$_{2A}$ receptor).

Trazodone can be quite sedating, leading to complaints of fatigue, a "drugged" feeling, and cognitive slowing, limiting the ability to

TABLE 7-27. *Dropout rates (%) as a function of dose in fixed-dose, placebo-controlled studies*

Fluoxetine						
Daily dose (mg/day)	5	20	40	60		
% Dropout rate[a]	—	−9	−6	8		
% Dropout rate[b]	3	−1	7	—		
Sertraline						
Daily dose (mg/day)	—	50	100	200		
% Dropout rate[c]	—	7	12	24		
Paroxetine						
Daily dose (mg/day)	10	20	30	40		
% Dropout rate[d]	3	6	16	13		
Venlafaxine						
Daily dose (mg/day)	62.5	75	175	182	225	375
% Dropout rate[e]	6	12	4	12	19	25
Nefazodone						
Daily dose (mg/day)	200–250	300	400	500	—	—
% Dropout rate[f]	−2	6	4	12	—	—

[a]From Wernicke J, et al. Fixed dose fluoxetine therapy for depression. *Psychopharmacol Bull* 1987; 23:164–168.

[b]From Wernicke J, et al. Low dose fluoxetine therapy for depression. *Psychopharmacol Bull* 1988; 24:183–188.

[c]From Preskorn S, Lane R. 50 mg/day as the optimum dose for sertraline. *Int Clin Psychopharmacol* 1995;10(3):129–141.

[d]From Dunner DL, Dunbar GC. Optimal dose regimen for paroxetine. *J Clin Psychiatry* 1992;53(suppl):21–26.

[e]From Preskorn S. Antidepressant drug selection: criteria and options. *J Clin Psychiatry* 1994;55(9 suppl A):6–22.

[f]From Nefazodone presentation to the Food and Drug Administration Psychopharmacology Advisory Committee. Washington, DC, July 1993.

adjust the dose to an effective antidepressant level (308). Despite some structural similarity between nefazodone and trazodone, these adverse effects were not a common finding with nefazodone but instead occurred at an incidence comparable with that of other new antidepressants, possibly because nefazodone is less potent at blocking histamine receptors than is trazodone (452). **On a more positive note, because of this sedative effect, trazodone is frequently used as a non–habit-forming sleep aid, particularly in patients who experience insomnia with an SSRI.**

In comparison with the other new antidepressants, the incidence rate of the following adverse effects was appreciably lower on nefazodone:

- Nervousness
- Tremors
- Insomnia
- Anorexia
- Sweating (Table 7-25)

The incidence rate of nervousness, anorexia, and palpitations was lower on nefazodone than on placebo, suggesting this agent may have direct anxiolytic effects in patients with major depression. As with all antidepressants, the dropout rate resulting from adverse effects was higher with increasing doses of nefazodone. The magnitude of this phenomenon, however, may be underestimated because of the difference in study design (i.e., fixed dose range versus true fixed dose) (Table 7-27).

Nefazodone, like bupropion, causes a lower incidence of sexual dysfunction (e.g., lower sexual drive, anorgasmia) than do the SSRIs and venlafaxine. Thus, these two antidepressants can be a welcome alternative for patients who are troubled by these adverse effects (453–455).

In contrast to decreased libido seen with SS-RIs and venlafaxine, concerns about priapism invariably arise when trazodone is discussed. This adverse effect is rare, occurring in only 1 of 6,000 treated male patients (456, 457). If the patient is informed of this possibility and discontinues the drug promptly, priapism usually resolves without further intervention. Although earlier persistent cases were treated surgically, this approach carries a 50% chance of permanent impotence; pharmacological intervention via direct injections into the cavernous bulbosa is preferable (458, 459). Using this approach, the chance of permanent impotence is low and depends on the duration of symptoms before treatment (460). This latter fact is another reason to fully inform the male patient on trazodone, so that early detection and intervention can be implemented.

Trazodone can cause sedation and postural hypotension but is generally benign in acute overdoses as documented by a substantial number of overdoses occurring without death.

Long-Term Safety Index and Tolerability

Like for the SSRIs and venlafaxine, there are no known long-term safety or late-emergent tolerability issues with nefazodone and trazodone. Nonetheless, the caveat remains that clinicians should be vigilant, because there has not been sufficient long-term systematically studied exposure to rule out the possibility of such problems.

Bupropion

Acute Safety Index

Bupropion, the only marketed aminoketone antidepressant, also has a side-effect profile different from the other classes of antidepressants. It is essentially devoid of anticholinergic, antihistaminic, and orthostatic hypotensive effects. Its principal adverse effects are consistent with its indirect agonism of dopamine and NE via uptake inhibition and include the following:

- Restlessness
- Activation
- Tremors

- Insomnia
- Nausea (461)

These adverse effects bear some similarity to those of the SSRIs. Although these adverse effects rarely require discontinuation, aggravation of psychosis and seizures caused by this agent do (427, 462–464). In contrast to the SSRIs and venlafaxine, bupropion usually does not cause sexual dysfunction. As such, bupropion may be an alternative for patients bothered by these adverse effects (465). Bupropion may also be a useful antidote for SSRI-induced sexual dysfunction (453, 455, 466, 467).

In a review of 37 reported cases, Davidson (426) found that the risk of seizures with bupropion was higher at doses above the recommended maximum (i.e., 450 mg per day). An increased risk of seizures was also noted in eating-disordered patients (i.e., bulimics) on bupropion, leading to its temporary withdrawal from the market. With the immediate release formulation, the seizure risk is four per 1,000 patients when the dose is kept at or below 450 mg per day in those without known risk factors (426, 468). The seizure risk may be as low as one per 1,000 patients with the sustained release formulation when the dose is kept below 450 mg per day and the patient has no preexisting seizure history and is not on any medication that also can lower seizure thresholds or interfere with the metabolism of bupropion.

The pathogenesis of bupropion-induced seizures is in part pharmacokinetically mediated (314). This conclusion is based on several observations:

- Incidence of seizures is *dose dependent.*
- Seizures generally *occur within days of a dose increase.*
- Seizures generally *occur within the first few hours after the dose.*
- Bulimic patients with increased *lean body mass* may be at higher risk for seizures.

Acute Tolerability

In humans, bupropion undergoes extensive biotransformation to three metabolites that have pharmacological activity (469). During treatment, these metabolites accumulate in concentrations several times higher than the parent compound (352). High plasma levels of these metabolites, particularly hydroxybupropion, may be associated with an increased incidence of serious adverse effects, as well as poorer antidepressant response (314). These observations form the basis of the possible utility of using TDM to guide dose adjustment with bupropion.

Bupropion falls between TCAs and SSRIs in terms of safety in overdose. Death is a rare possibility with an overdose of bupropion alone because there are no adverse effects on the cardiovascular or the respiratory systems (461). Seizures may occur but are readily treatable in a hospital setting.

Mirtazapine

Acute Safety Index

Mirtazapine like the other new antidepressants has a wide therapeutic index and is generally safe in overdose (470). Twelve overdoses occurred during the clinical development program with mirtazapine. The largest amount ingested in such an acute overdose was 975 mg per day, which is more than 20 times the maximal recommended dose. There was only one death in these 12 cases and that occurred in a patient who also took amitriptyline and a neuroleptic in addition to mirtazapine. This death was most likely due to the amitriptyline, given the estimated amount she ingested, the manner of the death (cardiac arrhythmia), and the fact that toxic levels of amitriptyline and its metabolites were found at the time of postmortem examination. The remainder of these overdose cases recovered without sequelae and did not require any intervention beyond observation (471).

As mentioned earlier, severe neutropenia developed in three of 2,796 patients in the worldwide clinical trials database with mirtazapine and two of these cases met criteria for agranulocytosis (i.e., a granulocyte count less than 500 with either signs of infection or fever) (470; mirtazapine package insert). The granulocyte count returned promptly after mirtazapine discontinuation. That fact is inconsistent with a toxic effect on bone marrow or stem cells in contrast to the

more serious forms of drug-induced agranulocytosis such as with clozapine. The fact that the granulocyte count in these cases returned to normal within days of mirtazapine discontinuation suggests that mirtazapine may have been causally implicated in this event. Nonetheless, the rate in the clinical trials was too low (approximately one in 1,000) to make a definitive statement on this matter. In addition, the confidence intervals surrounding the apparent rate are too large to know for certain what the true rate might be. Furthermore, there have been no reports of agranulocytosis in patients on mirtazapine in The Netherlands even though the drug has been marketed there for more than 2 years. The data on the first 9,000 patients were covered in a review by Montgomery (472).

For these reasons, the drug was approved in the United States without the recommendation to do white blood cell (WBC) counts as a condition of treatment in contrast to clozapine, which has an established risk of causing agranulocytosis (see Chapter 5). Nonetheless, physicians should obtain a WBC count if signs of infection or fever develop in a patient on mirtazapine. If the granulocyte count is suppressed, the drug should be discontinued and a report filed with the appropriate drug regulatory agency.

During the clinical trials, a mild (i.e., >1.5 but <3.0 times the upper limit of normal), transient elevation of liver enzymes, particularly SGPT (i.e., ALT) was noted in 2% of patients (470). This elevation typically occurred within the first 3 to 4 weeks of treatment in the patients in whom it occurred and typically had resolved despite continued treatment by the end of the 6-week study. This elevation was asymptomatic and was detected only as a result of scheduled monitoring during the study. The mirtazapine studies did not screen for hepatitis C as an exclusionary criterion for study enrollment, so these elevations may have been due to the periodic exacerbations of this chronic infection rather than being caused by the drug.

For these reasons, a mild elevation of this type during treatment with mirtazapine does not necessarily mean that the drug should be discontinued but rather that repeated monitoring should be done to determine whether it resolves. The drug should be discontinued if the elevation exceeds

3.0 times the upper limit of normal. A workup may be indicated to determine whether the elevation is symptomatic of an underlying liver disease (e.g., hepatitis C) rather than necessarily assuming it is due to mirtazapine.

Acute Tolerability

The most frequent adverse effects leading to drug discontinuation during the U.S. clinical trials were sedation and increased appetite with weight gain (470). The former is consistent with the blockade of the histamine receptor, which is one of the most potent mechanisms of action of this drug. The weight gain is likely due to its blockade of the 5-HT$_{2C}$ receptor. Although these effects can result in drug discontinuation, they may also be a reason to prescribe the drug in specific patients (i.e., those with prominent insomnia and nervousness and those with significant anorexia and weight loss). Even though not all patients experience these effects, those who do typically experience them with the first dose and typically within 2 to 3 hours of drug administration, consistent with the time required to achieve peak plasma drug levels. These effects rarely occur on a delayed basis and would not be expected to occur as a new event after 1 week on a stable dose. In the clinical trials with mirtazapine, the prevalence of both sedation and increased appetite and weight gain decreased somewhat over the 6 weeks of treatment. That finding might be due to development of some level of tolerance or that sensitive patients were discontinued from the studies. From clinical experience, these effects can be persistent for many weeks on mirtazapine so the clinician should not count on the development of tolerance.

Reboxetine

As with most data for reboxetine, this information primarily comes from summary papers rather than primary sources (473, 474). With this caveat, the adverse-effect profile of reboxetine is consistent with its pharmacology as an NSRI. Thus, it is similar to that of desipramine and maprotiline but without the risk of serious CNS (i.e., seizures, delirium) or cardiac (i.e., conduction disturbances) toxicity. The most common adverse effects of reboxetine are dry mouth, constipation, urinary hesitancy, increased sweating, insomnia, tachycardia, and vertigo. Whereas the first three adverse effects are commonly called "anticholinergic," they are well known to occur with sympathomimetic drugs as well. In other words, these effects can be either the result of decreased cholinergic tone or increased sympathetic tone, although they tend to be more severe with the former than the latter. In contrast to TCAs, reboxetine does not directly interfere with intracardiac conduction. The tachycardia produced by reboxetine, however, can be associated with occasional atrial or ventricular ectopic beats in elderly patients.

In terms of comparative adverse effects, imipramine produces more dry mouth than reboxetine probably because imipramine blocks muscarinic cholinergic receptors as well as inhibiting NE uptake (475). Imipramine also produces more tremulousness and hypotension than reboxetine. Consistent with their pharmacology, fluoxetine produces more serotonin-mediated adverse effects than does reboxetine (i.e., nausea, loose stools, and somnolence), whereas reboxetine causes more sympathomimetic adverse effects (476). To date, reboxetine has not been reported to cause an increased incidence of laboratory abnormalities.

Monoamine Oxidase Inhibitors

Despite impressions to the contrary, MAOIs are generally well tolerated if patients observe the restricted diet and avoid medications that contain sympathomimetic amines. Adverse effects are rarely a treatment-limiting problem with the exception of hypotension. MAOIs also fall between TCAs and SSRIs in terms of overdose risk. Major toxic reactions to MAOIs are uncommon but require immediate discontinuation and symptomatic treatment.

Hypotension

In the absence of a dietary indiscretion, hypotension is the principle and potentially treatment-limiting adverse effect caused by MAOIs. It must be carefully managed to avoid precipitating a hypertensive rebound (477–480). Although most often orthostatic in nature, a general reduction in blood pressure can be seen in some patients. This adverse effect may present as fatigue or decreased motivation. Hence, the unsuspecting clinician may erroneously interpret it as a worsening of the depressive episode. Monitoring the blood pressure (both lying and standing) at every visit and making arrangements for blood pressure checks between physician visits is advisable until the optimal dose has been established with regard to efficacy, safety, and tolerability.

One pharmacological theory of the mechanism underlying postural hypotension is the false-transmitter theory. Tyramine may be metabolized to an inactive metabolite (octopamine) that partially fills the NE storage vesicles with a false (inactive) transmitter, but definitive proof is lacking.

The dose of MAOI can sometimes be reduced, but this adverse effect often occurs at the minimal therapeutic dose. A good fluid intake plus increased salt intake, support stockings, and a mineralocorticoid (e.g., fluorohydrocortisone at doses of 0.3 to 0.8 mg) can alleviate the problem.

Hepatotoxicity

This is an uncommon reaction, most frequently associated with iproniazid, a hydrazine-based MAOI that has been removed from general use. The reaction seemed to be related to the liberation of free hydrazine and does not occur with nonhydrazine MAOIs. The risk of hepatotoxicity with currently available hydrazine MAOIs (phenelzine, isocarboxazid) is extremely low.

Miscellaneous Adverse Effects

Other reactions include a lupus-like syndrome (again, primarily associated with iproniazid), rash, and total suppression of REM sleep.

Like some other antidepressants and lithium, the MAOIs can also cause weight gain. Because they do not affect cholinergic receptors, they produce less constipation, dry mouth, and blurred vision, typically associated with the tricyclics. MAOIs do produce some similar adverse effects, particularly urinary hesitancy, possibly because of their adrenergic effects.

The most common MAOI behavioral toxicity is the precipitation of a hypomanic or manic episode, but restlessness, hyperactivity, agitation, irritability, and confusion can also occur. Rare cases of paranoid psychosis have been reported.

DRUG–DRUG INTERACTIONS

Antidepressants are commonly used in combination with other medications. From 30% to 80% of patients on an antidepressant are on two additional medications (481–484). The following factors increase the likelihood that the patient will be on additional medications:

- Age, elderly patients *on more medication* than younger patients
- Concomitant *medical illness*
- Presence of *co-morbid psychiatric syndromes*
- More *refractory* forms of major depression
- Treatment of *adverse effects* that are troublesome and persistent but not otherwise treatment limiting

The frequency with which antidepressants are coprescribed with other psychotropic and nonpsychotropic medications makes the potential for drug–drug interactions a clinically meaningful concern.

For convenience, drug–drug interactions are commonly divided into two types: pharmacodynamic and pharmacokinetic (25). Advances in pharmaceutical science have made it possible to classify, and even anticipate, both pharmacodynamic and pharmacokinetic drug–drug interactions on the basis of the mechanism underlying the interaction.

Pharmacodynamic drug–drug interactions occur when the effect of one drug on its site of action either enhances or diminishes the clinical effect of a concomitantly prescribed drug on its site of action. *Pharmacokinetic drug–drug interactions* are when one drug alters the absorption, distribution, metabolism, or elimination of a concomitantly prescribed drug, thus altering its concentration or the concentration of an active metabolite at its site of action. The most common clinically meaningful pharmacokinetic drug–drug interactions occur when one drug alters (either by induction or inhibition) the functional activity of the cytochrome P450 (CYP) enzymes mediating the phase I oxidative metabolism of a concomitantly prescribed drug.

Pharmacodynamic drug–drug interactions are classified based on the sites of action of the drugs involved. If combined effects on these sites of action produce an enhanced or diminished effect, then that likelihood can be reasonably extrapolated to all drugs that share effects on those same sites of action. For example, both β-blockers and α_1-adrenergic receptor blockers are known to individually decrease blood pressure and to produce a greater effect when used in combination. Tertiary amine TCAs block α_1-adrenergic receptors and hence predictably cause decreased blood pressure. They can also produce a heightened effect when used in combination with β-blockers.

Most pharmacokinetic drug–drug interactions involve a change in the rate of oxidative drug metabolism and can be classified on the basis of the CYP enzyme involved (485, 486). These enzymes are responsible for the bulk of phase I oxidative drug metabolism, which is a necessary step in the eventual elimination of most drugs. Concomitantly prescribed drugs can alter the functional activity of CYP enzymes either through induction or inhibition. A given drug has specific effects on certain CYP enzymes, which, in turn, are responsible for the metabolism of various drugs. If a drug is known to alter the functional activity of a specific CYP enzyme, then it will alter the elimination rate of any drug dependent on that enzyme for its biotransformation. Thus, this type of pharmacokinetic drug–drug interaction can be classified on the basis of the CYP enzyme involved.

CYP enzymes are grouped into families and subfamilies based on amino acid homology, because function follows structure (487). Families are designated by the first Arabic number and subfamilies by the alphabetic letter. To be in the same family and subfamily, the enzymes must have at least 40% and 60% sequence homology, respectively. The last Arabic number identifies a given enzyme, which is a specific gene product.

The CYP enzymes are divided into two main groups: the steroidogenic enzymes, which are located in the mitochondria, and the xenobiotic enzymes, which are located in the endoplasmic reticulum (488, 489). The latter are responsible for the majority of oxidative drug metabolism. Drugs can induce (i.e., increase the rate of enzyme synthesis) or inhibit these enzymes, thus altering the rate of biotransformation of other drugs dependent on these enzymes for their elimination. The principal enzymes (in order of importance) implicated in such pharmacokinetic drug–drug interactions are the following:

- CYP 3A3/4 responsible for 50% of known oxidative metabolism
- CYP 2D6 responsible for 30% of known oxidative metabolism
- CYP 1A2 responsible for 5% to 10% of known oxidative metabolism
- CYP 2C9/10 responsible for 5% to 10% of known oxidative metabolism
- CYP 2C19 responsible for 5% to 10% of known oxidative metabolism

As a general rule, a change in the rate of biotransformation produces a comparable change in clearance and is the inverse of a dose change (i.e., a reduction in clearance is similar to an increase in the dosing rate). More complicated interactions can occur when the effect on the CYP enzyme produces a shift in the relative ratio of the parent drug to that of an active metabolite. Thus, a qualitative change in the response can occur when a pharmacokinetic drug–drug interaction shifts the relative ratio of the parent drug to an active metabolite with a different pharmacological profile.

Pharmacodynamic Drug–Drug Interactions

The serotonin syndrome and hypertensive crisis are the two most common serious pharmacodynamically mediated drug–drug interactions are discussed in the following paragraphs.

Serotonin Syndrome

This syndrome most often occurs as a result of the interaction of two or more drugs acting via different mechanisms to potentiate the central effects of serotonin at 5-HT$_{1A}$ receptors in the brainstem and spinal cord (490). It consists of the following symptoms:

- Gastrointestinal
  - Abdominal cramping
  - Bloating
  - Diarrhea
- Neurological
  - Tremulousness
  - Myoclonus
  - Dysarthria
  - Incoordination
  - Headache
- Cardiovascular
  - Tachycardia
  - Hypotension
  - Hypertension
  - Cardiovascular collapse—death
- Psychiatric
  - Hypomanic symptoms
  - Racing thoughts
  - Pressure of speech
  - Elevated or dysphoric mood
  - Confusion
  - Disorientation
- Other
  - Diaphoresis
  - Elevated temperature
  - Hyperthermia
  - Hyperreflexia

Hyperpyrexia and death may be the outcome of this rare drug–drug interaction. The classic cause of this syndrome is the coadministration of an MAOI with a serotonin uptake inhibitor such as an SSRI or venlafaxine. For this reason, it is mandatory to wait at least 2 weeks before switching from an SSRI to an MAOI, and at least 5 weeks when switching from fluoxetine to an MAOI, particularly tranylcypromine. Longer intervals are required if the dose of fluoxetine has been greater than 20 mg per day, because this drug inhibits its own clearance and hence has an even longer half-life at higher doses. Longer intervals are also advisable in elderly patients or individuals with significant hepatic, renal, or left ventricular cardiac dysfunction. It is probably safe to use a drug-free period of only a few days

when switching from a tricyclic to an MAOI. If the syndrome develops, management consists of discontinuation of the offending agents and waiting for resolution. Although not adequately documented in humans, methysergide (5-HT antagonist) or propranolol (a 5-HT$_{1A}$ antagonist) may be helpful.

Hypertensive Crisis

Hypertensive crisis often occurs as a result of the interaction of two or more drugs acting via different mechanisms to potentiate the cardiovascular effects of NE. It can also occur as a result of a drug–food interaction involving MAOIs and tyramine-containing foods. Like the serotonin syndrome, hypertensive crisis can be fatal. Prodromal symptoms include the following:

- Sharply *elevated blood pressure*
- Severe occipital *headaches*
- *Stiff neck*
- *Sweating*
- *Nausea* and *vomiting*

Because of this risk, a patient's ability to comply with the dietary restrictions should be carefully evaluated before starting treatment. Hospitalized patients should be placed on a tyramine-free diet and outpatients should be questioned about their history of compliance, suicidal potential, and ability to comprehend the dietary restrictions, which should be given in writing. Patients who cannot follow directions accurately or who may be manipulative or suicidal should not be considered for treatment with MAOIs.

Table 7-28 lists foods and drugs to be avoided while the patient is taking MAOIs. There can also be unexpectedly high tyramine content in some tap (especially lager) beers (491). For a complete description of the tyramine content of foods and beverages, see Shulman et al. (492). Case reports indicate that alcohol-free beer may pose a significant risk as well (493). It may be helpful to recommend that the patient keep a diary and record any untoward events that follow ingestion of certain foods or drinks. In this way, a personalized diet can be constructed while making the patient more aware of those foods that pose a risk.

TABLE 7-28. *Dietary and drug restrictions for monoamine oxidase inhibitors*

Foods	Drugs
HIGH tyramine content per serving—MUST BE AVOIDED	
Aged cheese, (e.g., English Stilton, cheddar, Camembert, blue)	Stimulants
Yeast products	Decongestants
Pickled or salted herring, snails	Antihypertensives
Aged meats, processed meats, any nonfresh meats	Antidepressants
Chicken liver or beef liver (more than 2 days old)	HCAs
Broad bean pods (fava beans)	SSRIs
Sauerkraut	Bupropion
Banana peel	Phenylpiperazines
Licorice	Venlafaxine
Tap beer	Narcotics
	Meperidine
MODERATE tyramine content per serving—LIMITED AMOUNTS ALLOWABLE	
Soy sauce	Dextromethorphan
Sour cream	Pressor agents
Cyclamates, monosodium glutamate	General anesthetics
	Sedatives
	Hypoglycemics
LOW tyramine content per serving—PERMISSIBLE	
Pasteurized cheeses, cream cheese	Over-the-counter
Alcohol (e.g., wine, distilled spirits, non-tap beer, and alcohol-free beer) in moderation	preparations containing caffeine
Caffeine-containing beverages (e.g., coffee, tea, cola drinks)	or other
Fresh liver (less than one serving per day)	stimulants
Smoked fish (salmon, carp, whitefish)	(e.g., ephedrine)

HCA, heterocyclic antidepressant; SSRI, selective serotonin reuptake inhibitor.
Adapted from Janicak PG, et al. Pharmacological treatment of depression. In: Flaherty J, Davis JM, Janicak PG, eds. *Psychiatry: diagnosis and therapy.* 2nd ed. Norwalk, CT: Appleton & Lange, 1993:54–61. SSRI, selective serotonin reoptake inhibitor; HCA, heterocyclics antidepressant

Written instructions in case of an adverse reaction usually require that the patient be directed to an emergency room for evaluation, monitoring, and treatment. Nonspecific treatment of a hypertensive crisis is as follows:

- Discontinuance of the MAOI
- Acidification of the urine to hasten elimination
- Maintenance of glucose and temperature balance

To control hypertension, phentolamine 5 mg i.v. is recommended, with repeated doses of 0.25 to 0.5 mg i.m. every 4 to 6 hours. Alternatively, chlorpromazine 50 mg i.m. is given, followed by 25 mg i.m. every 1 to 2 hours. **Nifedipine is not recommended.** Blood pressure should be monitored closely to avoid overcompensation and hypotensive episodes.

We studied platelet MAO levels after phenelzine was discontinued and found that the half-life of MAO regeneration was about 5 days (354). Nevertheless, one reliable patient required hospitalization for a hypertensive crisis precipitated by cheese ingested 12 days after phenelzine discontinuation. Patients should be asked to follow dietary restrictions for at least 2 weeks after discontinuation to allow regeneration of enzymes.

The MAO-B inhibitor, l-deprenyl, has been approved by the FDA for use in Parkinson's disease. At the lower dose range, it does not interact with tyramine. As mentioned earlier, there is preliminary evidence of antidepressant efficacy for a transdermal delivery system for selegiline. This formulation does not interact with tyramine to produce a hypertensive crisis (181).

Adverse Effects Related to Pharmacokinetic Interactions

There is a great disparity of current knowledge regarding the effects of antidepressants on CYP enzymes. There have been almost no studies to test the potential effects of TCAs, MAOIs, and trazodone on CYP enzymes. There has only been one study with bupropion but it demonstrated that bupropion produces substantial inhibition of CYP 2D6 comparable with the effect of fluoxetine and paroxetine. In contrast to studies in these antidepressants, there have been extensive *in vitro* and *in vivo* studies of SSRIs, nefazodone, and venlafaxine.

The *in vitro* studies determine the potency of the drug for inhibiting a specific CYP enzyme. The likelihood that a drug may produce sufficient inhibition of a CYP enzyme under clinically relevant dosing conditions can be estimated by knowing the *in vitro* potency of the drug and estimating the concentration of the drug that will occur at the enzyme under such dosing conditions (494, 495). Mathematical modeling can be used to decide whether formal *in vivo* pharmacokinetic interactions should be done for confirmatory purposes.

Table 7-29 summarizes the results of the *in vivo* studies that have been done examining the effects of the various SSRIs, nefazodone, and venlafaxine on specific CYP enzymes at their usually effective minimal dose. The effects are rated according to the extent to which these drugs will increase the plasma levels of a concomitantly administered drug that is dependent on that specific CYP enzyme for its metabolism:

• *Mild* indicates a 20% to 50% increase.
• *Moderate* indicates a 50% to 150% increase.
• *Marked* indicates more than a 150% increase.

Clearly, there are substantial differences among these new drugs in terms of their ability to inhibit specific CYP enzymes and hence their propensity for altering the clearance of specific drugs that may be coprescribed with them. Because drug inhibition of these enzymes is a concentration-dependent phenomenon, the effect of each drug at higher doses will, on average, be greater. Because fluoxetine, nefazodone, and paroxetine have nonlinear pharmacokinet-

ics, the degree of inhibition produced by these drugs would be expected to be disproportionately greater at higher doses.

The major distinguishing characteristic among the SSRIs is CYP enzyme inhibition. Fluvoxamine, fluoxetine, and paroxetine produce substantial inhibition of one or more CYP enzymes, whereas citalopram and sertraline do not (Table 7-29). In fact, fluvoxamine, fluoxetine, and paroxetine have all caused fatal drug–drug interactions via such CYP enzyme inhibition (339, 496, 497).

Given current knowledge in this area, fluvoxamine, fluoxetine, and paroxetine would likely not be developed for the current market, nor would they likely receive FDA approval for marketing. Virtually all companies currently screen for effects on CYP enzymes during preclinical development and substantial inhibition of a CYP enzyme is one criterion used to screen out potential drugs from further development. This criterion is overridden only when the potential beneficial effects of the drug clearly outweigh this disadvantage and there is no safer drug available that has the same benefit. The FDA has taken the same position in the approval process of drugs that made it into human testing before such preclinical screening was routine. In the case of SSRIs, citalopram and sertraline are SSRIs that have all the advantages of this class without the liability of substantial CYP enzyme inhibition. Given these facts, it is surprising that fluoxetine and paroxetine are still used to any extent.

Table 7-30 shows a partial list of which drugs are dependent on which CYP enzymes for their oxidative metabolism. Tables 7-29 and 7-30 can be used to determine whether a dose adjustment is needed in a concomitantly administered drug and approximately how much of an adjustment is needed when adding an SSRI or other new antidepressant to an ongoing drug regimen or vice versa. Therapeutic drug monitoring of the concomitant drug can then be done to further fine tune the dose adjustment. The relatively modest effects of citalopram, sertraline, and venlafaxine on CYP enzymes reduce the likelihood that these three antidepressants, when prescribed at their usually effective doses, will alter the pharmacokinetics of other drugs that the patient may be taking. That is an advantage, because patients

TABLE 7-29. Effects of specific SSRIs on specific CYP enzymes at their respective, usually effective, antidepressant dose[a]

Enzyme	Citalopram	Fluoxetine	Fluvoxamine	Paroxetine	Sertraline	Nefazodone	Venlafaxine
CYP 1A2	NCS	NCS	Substantial[b,c]	NCS	Unlikely[b]	NCS	Unlikely
CYP 2C9/10	?	?[d]	?	NCS[c]	NCS[c]	NCS	NCS
CYP 2C19	NCS	Moderate[c]	Substantial[c]	?	NCS[c]	NCS	NCS
CYP 2D6	Mild[b]	Substantial[b,c]	NCS[b,c]	Substantial[b,c]	Mild[b,c]	NCS	Mild
CYP 3A3/4	?	Mild[b,c]	Moderate[b,c]	NCS	NCS	Substantial	NCS

? = absence of or contradictory *in vitro* or *in vivo* data available for this selective serotonin reuptake inhibitor; Unlikely, unlikely to have a clinically meaningful effect based on in vitro studies; NCS, not clinically significant in most situations <20% change*; Mild, 20% to 50% change*; Moderate,* 50% to 150% change; Substantial, >150% change*. Change in the area under the curve (AUC) of the plasma level-time curve of a substrate (i.e., concomitantly administered drug) dependent on that CYP enzyme for its clearance.   [a]Table is a summary of other tables and data reviewed in References 84–86. Hence, it is based on effects observed or predicted based on the concentration of these drugs that would be usually produced by their usually effective, antidepressant dose. Since the inhibition of these enzymes is concentration dependent, the magnitude of the effect will be higher on average at higher doses, particularly for drugs with nonlinear pharmacokinetics.

[b]Predicted based on *in vitro* inhibitory rate constants and on knowledge about clinically relevant plasma drug levels.

[c]Based on the following *in vivo* data: A large number of well-documented, case reports principally involving theophylline for fluvoxamine's effect on CYP 1A2 and formal in vivo studies for effects on CYP 2D6 and on CYP 2C9/10, 2C19, and 3A3/4. Relative to CYP 3A3/4 studies have recently been completed demonstrating that paroxetine and sertraline do not inhibit the clearance of the following CYP 3A3/4 substrates: carbamazepine and terfenadine. A third recently completed study also documented that sertraline did not alter the clearance of alprazolam, which is another CYP 3A3/4 substrate (Preskorn S, unpublished data).

[d]Studies with tolbutamide and warfarin suggest no effects; but 23 cases with adequate data with phenytoin suggest a substantial effect of fluoxetine on CYP 2C9/10. The reasons for the discrepancy in these results are not clear.

The designation NCS is further supported by the linear pharmacokinetics of sertraline over its full dosing range (i.e., 50–200 mg/day) since sertraline is demethylated by CYP 3A3/4. Adapted from Reference 84 at the end of this section.

TABLE 7-30. *Drugs metabolized by specific cytochrome P450 (CYP) enzymes[a]*

CYP 1A2
Antidepressants—amitriptyline, clomipramine, imipramine *Antipsychotics*—clozapine
β-Blocker—propranolol
Miscellaneous—caffeine, paracetamol, theophylline, R-warfarin
CYP 2C9/10
Phenytoin, *S*-warfarin, tolbutamide
CYP 2D19
Antidepressants—citalopram, clomipramine, imipramine
Barbiturates—hexobarbital, mephobarbital, S-mephenytoin
Benzodiazepines—diazepam
β-Blockers—propranolol
CYP 2D6
Antiarrhythmics—encainide, flecainide, mexiletine, propafenone
Antipsychotics—haloperidol, perphenazine, risperidone, thioridazine
β-Blockers—alprenolol, bufarolol, metaprolol, propranolol, timolol
Miscellaneous—debrisoquin, 4-hydroamphetamine, perhexiline, phenformin, sparteine
Opiates—codeine, dextromethorphan, ethylmorphine
Selective Serotonir reuptake inhibitors—fluoxetine, N-desmethylcitalopram, paroxetine
Tricyclic antidepressents—amitriptyline, clomipramine, desipramine, imipramine,
    N-desmethylclomipramine, clomipramine, nortriptyline, trimipramine
Other antidepressants—venlafaxine, the mCPP metabolite of nefazodone and trazodone
CYP 3A3/4
Analgesics—acetaminophen, alfentanil, codeine, dextromethorphan
Antiarrhythmics—amiodarone, disopyramide, lidocaine, propafenone, quinidine
Anticovulsants—carbamazepine, ethosuximide
Antidepressants—amitriptyline, clomipramine, imipramine, nefazodone, sertraline,
    O-desmethylvenlafaxine
Antiestrogens—docetaxel, loratadine, terfenadine
Antipsychotics—clozapine
Benzodiazepines—alprazolam, clonazepam, diazepam, midazolam, triazolam
Calcium channel blockers—diltiazem, feodipine, nicardipine, nifedipine, niludipine, minodipine,
    nisoldipine, nitrendipine, verapamil
Immunosuppressants—cyclosporine, tacrolimus (FK506-macrolide)
Local anesthetics—cocaine, lidocaine
Macrolide antibiotics—clarithromycin, erythromycin, triacetyloleandomycin
Steroids—androstendione, cortisol, dihydroepiandrosterone, 3-sulfate, dexamethasone, estradiol,
    ethinylestradiol, progesterone, testosterone
Miscellaneous—benzphetamine, cisapride, dapsone, lovastatin, omeprazole (sulfonation)

---

[a]Major pathway for elimination of tricyclic antidepressants is ring hydroxylation which is almost exclusively mediated by CYP 2D6; N-desmethylation, a minor pathway, is mediated by several CYP enzymes (i.e., CYP 1A2 > CYP 3A3/4 > CYP 2C19).

NOTE: Tables such as this are limited by current knowledge. The CYP enzyme(s) responsible for biotransformation has been determined for only approximately 20% of marketed drugs. Many drugs were developed before the necessary knowledge and technology existed. Hence, these lists are first attempts but will become more comprehensive as we backfill our knowledge base. Also note that some drugs are listed under more than one CYP enzyme since different enzymes mediate either the same or different metabolic pathways. That does not necessarily mean that each of these enzymes contributes equally to the elimination of the drug. One enzyme may be principally responsible, based on the substrate affinity and the capacity and abundance of the enzyme.

Adapted from Reference 25.

---

on antidepressants are frequently on other medications.

Because most antidepressants require oxidative metabolism as a necessary step in their elimination, they can be the target of a pharmacoki-

netic drug–drug interaction, as well as the cause. The CYP enzymes mediating the biotransformation of the various antidepressants are also shown in Table 7-30. CYP 1A2 and 3A3/4 are induced by anticonvulsants such as barbiturates and carbamazepine. As expected, coadministration of these anticonvulsants has been shown to lower plasma levels of TCAs and would be predicted to have the same effect on nefazodone, sertraline, and venlafaxine.

The nature of the target drug, as well as the magnitude of the change, determines the clinical relevance of both induction and inhibition. The clinical implications will be greater for drugs that have a narrow therapeutic index and serious concentration–dependent toxicity. TCAs fit these two characteristics. For this reason, the clinician must be alert to the changes in TCA clearance produced both by starting and stopping inducers and inhibitors. TCA plasma levels increase by starting an inhibitor and stopping an inducer, and decrease when stopping an inhibitor or starting an inducer.

Fluvoxamine and bupropion undergo extensive biotransformation, but the CYP enzymes mediating their biotransformation have not been established. That is particularly unfortunate in the case of bupropion, which is converted into three different metabolites that have longer half-lives than bupropion and hence accumulate to a greater degree than the parent drug. The relative roles of these metabolites in mediating the antidepressant efficacy and dose-dependent seizure risk of bupropion are unknown. For these reasons, bupropion fits the profile of a drug that could be affected to a clinically significant degree by the concomitant administration of a drug capable of inducing or inhibiting its metabolism. These problems are further compounded by the fact that only a modest amount of TDM research has been done with bupropion, because only the level of the parent compound was measured in most of these studies. Nonetheless, assays are commercially available to measure the parent drug and the three major metabolites, and data do exist as to what are the expected levels of each at 450 mg per day. Thus, the clinician could use TDM when coprescribing bupropion with drugs known to either induce or inhibit CYP enzymes. The dose could then be adjusted to ensure that the levels achieved approximate and do not exceed those that normally occur at 450 mg per day. Alternatively, the clinician could follow the adage of "start low and go slow" when using bupropion in combination with another drug known to inhibit

one or more CYP enzymes. For example, fluoxetine has been reported in one case to cause elevated levels of the principal metabolite, hydroxybupropion (314). In this case, this interaction was associated with psychomotor (e.g., catatonia) and behavioral (e.g., mental confusion, excitement) toxicity. Consistent with this case, patients on fluoxetine and bupropion have also experienced seizures at 50% lower doses than those on bupropion alone (498).

Specific Adverse Drug–Drug Interactions with Different Antidepressants

Tricyclic Antidepressants

Members of this class of antidepressants are likely to be involved in pharmacodynamic and CYP-mediated pharmacokinetic drug–drug interactions. The latter are of concern because of the narrow therapeutic index of TCAs.

Because of the multiple actions of TCAs (especially the tertiary amines), they have the potential to interact pharmacodynamically with a number of other medications, producing increased

- *Anticholinergic* effects (e.g., benztropine, thioridazine)
- *Antihistaminic* effects (e.g., diphenhydramine)
- *Anti-α_1-adrenergic* effects (e.g., prazosin)
- *Antiarrhythmic* effects (e.g., quinidine)

Tertiary amines, more than secondary amines, also potentiate the CNS effects of alcohol most likely as a result of their ability to block central H_1 receptors. This is an example of a drug–food interaction. Patients need to be aware of this phenomenon so that they avoid drinking while taking these medications, especially when engaged in activities that require attention and coordination.

TCAs do not inhibit any of the major CYP enzymes to any clinical degree under usual dosing conditions and thus do not cause this type of drug–drug interaction. However, TCAs are metabolized by CYP enzymes and can be the substrate of such an interaction. CYP 2D6 mediates the rate-limiting step in biotransformation of TCAs necessary for their elimination from the body. Thus, drugs that produce substantial CYP 2D6 inhibition such as bupropion, fluoxetine, and paroxetine can cause a 400% or more increase in TCA plasma levels. Because of the narrow therapeutic index of TCAs, such increases can have serious adverse consequences including death (339). TCAs should either not be used with such drugs or the dose should be kept low and adjusted by TDM. The full inhibitory effect of fluoxetine takes weeks to develop and weeks to resolve (301).

Selective Serotonin Reuptake Inhibitors

In comparison with TCAs, SSRIs cause fewer pharmacodynamic drug–drug interactions but some (i.e., fluvoxamine, fluoxetine, paroxetine) cause more CYP enzyme mediated pharmacokinetic drug–drug interactions. Unlike TCAs, SSRIs do not potentiate alcohol and perhaps even slightly antagonize its acute CNS effects. Nevertheless, there are some important adverse interactions.

The most important is the serotonin syndrome discussed earlier. Given their profound effects on central serotonin mechanisms in the brainstem, the SSRIs can interact with other central serotonin agonists to produce this syndrome (490). Although this reaction typically is mild and self-limiting once the offending agents are discontinued, it can be serious and fatalities have occurred. Because the most profound reactions have been reported when MAOIs have been added to SSRIs (263, 499), such combination therapy is contraindicated. Other agents that have been reported to produce this reaction in combination with SSRIs include the following:

- Tryptophan
- 5-Hydroxytryptophan
- Meperidine

SSRIs reduce dopamine cell firing in the substantia nigra through their effects on serotonin input to this nucleus. The net result is that they can cause generally mild extrapyramidal side effects (EPS) (500). The most common are restlessness and tremors. The same mechanism is probably responsible for their interaction with other agents that affect central motor systems. Thus, the SSRIs can potentiate the tremor seen with lithium, as well as EPS caused by antipsychotics, bupropion, and psychostimulants (376, 500).

As mentioned previously, beyond the unusually long half-life of fluoxetine and norfluoxetine, the other clinically meaningful distinction between the SSRIs is whether they produce substantial inhibition of specific CYP enzyme (Table 7-29). Fluvoxamine, fluoxetine, and paroxetine do, whereas citalopram and sertraline do not. As mentioned earlier, it is doubtful that the first three would be developed or approved for today's market because of their effects on CYP enzymes, which can cause serious and even fatal drug–drug interactions.

The clinician must also be aware of the long half-life (several days) of fluoxetine because the potential for this reaction remains present until its active metabolite, norfluoxetine, has been cleared. This can take 6 weeks or more depending on the daily dose of fluoxetine that has been used, as well as the age and health of the patient.

Venlafaxine

This antidepressant can interact with other drugs via its two mechanisms of action: serotonin and NE uptake inhibition. The former action means that the same pharmacodynamic interactions will occur with venlafaxine as with SSRIs, including the serotonin syndrome. At higher doses, venlafaxine is also prone to the same pharmacodynamic interactions as NSRIs such as secondary amine TCAs like desipramine and with newer NSRIs such reboxetine. Thus, the combination of high-dose venlafaxine plus an MAOI could produce a hypertensive crisis as well as the serotonin syndrome.

Although venlafaxine can have more interactions than SSRIs pharmacodynamically, it is comparable with citalopram and sertraline in terms of not causing CYP enzyme mediated pharmacokinetic drug–drug interactions (Table 7-29). Thus, these three antidepressants have a distinct advantage over drugs such as fluoxetine, particularly in patients who are likely to be on other medications in addition to their antidepressant.

Venlafaxine is converted by CYP 2D6 to ODV, which is subsequently cleared by CYP 3A3/4 (501). ODV has virtually the same *in vitro* pharmacology as venlafaxine. Thus, the total of venlafaxine plus ODV is believed to be the relevant concentration determining clinical effect (137). Theoretically, venlafaxine should be relatively impervious to even substantial CYP 2D6 inhibition because ODV levels would decrease proportionate to the increase in venlafaxine levels such that the total level would remain the same. In contrast, the inhibition of CYP 3A3/4 would be potentially more clinically relevant because it should decrease ODV clearance and thus increase total levels. Nevertheless, such an interaction would not be expected to do more than increase the usual dose-dependent adverse effects of venlafaxine because of its wide therapeutic index.

Nefazodone and Trazodone

The affinity of nefazodone for ACh, histamine, and α-adrenergic receptors is less than that of the tertiary amine TCAs, but slightly more than that of the SSRIs or venlafaxine, while its affinity for the histamine and the α_2-adrenergic receptors is less than that of trazodone (254, 255, 452). Thus, nefazodone should have fewer interactions with other drugs that share these or related actions than do the tertiary amine TCAs or trazodone. There have only been a few formal pharmacodynamic drug–drug interaction studies with nefazodone, but those that have been reported indicate a relatively benign profile in this regard. Nefazodone (200 and 400 mg per day for 8 days) did not potentiate the sedative-hypnotic (depressant) effects of alcohol in normal, healthy volunteers (502). Even though a direct comparison has not been done with other antidepressants, nefazodone, based on its pharmacology, would be expected to fall between the tertiary amine TCAs and trazodone on one side and the SSRIs and venlafaxine on the other in terms of potentiating the CNS effects of alcohol and sedative-hypnotics.

Because nefazodone does inhibit the 5-HT uptake pump, it has the same class warning against combined use with an MAOI. Nevertheless, there are several reasons to suspect that there may be less risk of this interaction with nefazodone than other serotonin uptake pump inhibitors. First, trazodone, an analogue of nefazodone, is one of the few antidepressants that can be used in combination with an MOAI with minimal risk of an adverse interaction. Second, the most potent action of nefazodone is 5-HT$_{2A}$ receptor blockade, rather than 5-HT uptake inhibition. Nonetheless, we recommend the conservative approach of avoiding this combination, particularly when using high doses (i.e., >450 mg per day), at which appreciable serotonin uptake inhibition is produced by nefazodone.

Because of its substantial inhibition of CYP 3A3/4, this antidepressant is prone to pharmacokinetic drug–drug interactions with substrates for this enzyme (Table 7-30). That is important because CYP 3A3/4 is responsible for approximately 50% of all known drug metabolism. Thus, there are a number of medications that either should not be used in combination with nefazodone or that must be dosed conservatively to patients on this antidepressant. Thus, nefazodone is not the antidepressant of first choice for patients who are on other medications.

Bupropion

Consistent with its most potent known mechanism of action, bupropion is an indirect dopamine agonist via its inhibition of the neuronal uptake pump for dopamine (503, 504). Hence, bupropion can potentiate the effects of other dopamine agonists. This interaction does not typically cause serious problems and may even be advantageous in specific instances such as patients with Parkinson's disease plus a depressive disorder. Because of its ability to inhibit NE uptake, bupropion would be prone to the same interactions as NSRIs such as desipramine and reboxetine.

Bupropion can be both the cause and the substrate of a CYP enzyme mediated drug–drug interaction. Few studies have been done to test the potential effects of bupropion on CYP enzymes. It is as poorly studied in this regard as TCAs and MAOIs. One study did show that bupropion at usual antidepressant doses causes substantial inhibition of CYP 2D6 comparable with that of fluoxetine and paroxetine (Bupropion package insert). Thus, bupropion should be used with care, if at all, with drugs that are principally metabolized by this enzyme. It is unknown whether bupropion inhibits other CYP enzymes to a comparable degree. Until data to the contrary are available, it would be prudent to consider that bupropion may inhibit CYP enzymes other than CYP 2D6 to a clinically meaningful degree. Thus, this antidepressant should be used cautiously in patients who are on other medications.

As previously mentioned, bupropion fits the criteria of a drug that could be the substrate of clinically meaningful pharmacokinetic drug–drug interactions. First, it has a narrow therapeutic index in terms of seizures. Second, it has a complicated metabolism leading to the production of three active metabolites, which accumulate to a greater degree than the parent compound. Unfortunately, little is known about the metabolism of bupropion beyond the fact that CYP 2B6 mediates the conversion of bupropion to hydroxybupropion. Moreover, little is known about CYP 2B6 including what drugs, if any, induce or inhibit this enzyme. Thus, bupropion should be used cautiously in patients on other medications both because it might affect them and they might affect it.

Mirtazapine

Because of its multiple receptor effects, mirtazapine, like the TCAs, can interact pharmacodynamically with a number of other medications. Some of these interactions can have beneficial consequences such as blocking some of the typical adverse effects of SSRIs and venlafaxine [nausea (5-HT$_3$ receptor blockade) and sleep disturbance (5-HT$_{2A}$ receptor blockade)]. In addition, mirtazapine is as potent as many tertiary amine TCAs at blocking the histamine receptor (505). For this reason, coadministration of mirtazapine can potentiate the sedative effects of alcohol and diazepam. This phenomenon would be expected to generalize to all BZDs as well as other sedative-hypnotic drugs. Thus, the same precautions and warnings about prescribing this drug with other sedative agents or combining with alcohol should be given to patients on mirtazapine as those on tertiary amine TCAs (mirtazapine package insert). Theoretically, mirtazapine as a result of its α_2-adrenergic receptor blockade could cause the serotonin syndrome when used in combination with SSRIs and the

serotonin syndrome and hypertensive crisis when used in combination with venlafaxine. However, mirtazapine could also treat the serotonin syndrome as a result of its blockade of 5-HT$_{2A}$, 5-HT$_{2C}$, and 5-HT$_3$ receptors. Thus, the interaction with mirtazapine and an SSRI or venlafaxine could theoretically be either beneficial or adverse depending on which action predominated. There has been a case report of serotonin syndrome when mirtazapine was used in combination with fluoxetine (506). However, there were no occurrences of the serotonin syndrome in 40 patients who were immediately switched from fluoxetine to mirtazapine in a study conducted by Preskorn and colleagues (507). Beyond the aforementioned studies, little work has been done examining the pharmacodynamic interactions of mirtazapine with other medications. Thus, the clinician should exercise caution when using this medication in combination with direct or indirect serotonin and NE agonists, as well as histamine antagonists, until more formal studies have been done or clinical experience has accumulated.

Mirtazapine has minimal potential for causing CYP enzyme mediated drug–drug interactions. This conclusion is based both on its low *in vitro* inhibitory effects on CYP enzymes and on confirmatory *in vivo* studies (501). It is also relatively protected against such an interaction because it is metabolized by several different CYP enzymes (1A2, 3A3/4, and 2D6), each contributing to a meaningful degree to its clearance. Consistent with this prediction, a study done by Wheatley and colleagues (369) showed that fluoxetine produced only minimal increases in mirtazapine plasma levels.

Monoamine Oxidase Inhibitors

MAOIs have the most serious pharmacodynamic interactions of any antidepressant class. As discussed earlier, they can cause a hypertensive crisis and the serotonin syndrome. They potentiate the hypertensive effects of most sympathomimetic amines, as well as tyramine, which is the reason for the avoidance of over-the-counter preparations containing such agents, in addition to the tyramine-free diet (508, 509). The serotonin syndrome occurs most often when MAOIs are used in combination with SSRIs and ven-lafaxine but it can also occur when MAOIs are used with tryptophan, 5-hydroxytryptophan, and some narcotic analgesics. In addition, MAOIs can also significantly potentiate the sedative and respiratory depressant effects of narcotic analgesics.

Little is known about the potential for MAOIs to interact pharmacokinetically with other drugs. Because the metabolism of selegiline is medi-ated in part by CYP 2D6 (302), fluoxetine and paroxetine could interact both pharmacodynam-ically and pharmacokinetically. The pharmacoki-netic interaction can potentiate the pharmacody-namic interaction by increasing the accumula-tion of selegiline so that it inhibits MAO-A as well as MAO-B. In this context, case reports of partial serotonin syndromes have been reported when selegiline has been used with fluoxetine (302, 510). This interaction can persist for sev-eral weeks after both drugs have been stopped because of the long half-life of fluoxetine and the irreversible inhibition of MAO produced by se-legiline. Because this interaction may present as deterioration in cognitive functioning and selegi-line is typically used in patients with Parkinson's disease, dementia may be erroneously diagnosed.

Adverse Effects Relevant to Pregnancy

A perplexing issue for clinicians is the proper level of concern when using medications in women of childbearing potential and certainly in the pregnant patient (see also Chapter 14, "The Pregnant Patient"). That is certainly true for an-tidepressants.

A fundamental concern with exposure to psy-chiatric medications during pregnancy is that these medications are by design capable of al-tering the functional activity of neurochemical modulators (e.g., the biogenic amines) in the body. Whereas these substances are primarily thought about in psychiatry relative to their role in the developed brain, they also play an im-portant chemotaxic role during in utero devel-opment of the brain and other organs. Thus, the possibility exists that exposure to such a drug in utero may cause more subtle, but still important, changes in organ development, which may not be detectable in neonates. A limited number of ani-mal studies have examined this issue in relation to antidepressants.

Although this topic is important for all classes of psychiatric medications, it may be particularly important for antidepressants, because they are the most commonly prescribed class of psychi-atric medications. Furthermore, they are dispro-portionately prescribed to women of childbear-ing potential because major depression is more likely to be diagnosed and treated in this popula-tion.

Formal human studies are limited and based on naturalistic exposure with an attempt to have a control group matched as closely as possible. However, there are inevitably differences in such groups, the most obvious and perhaps most im-portant being the reason why one group is on a medication while the other is not. In other words, the illness that led to treatment with the medica-tion (in this case a mood disorder) may itself be a risk factor for lower fetal viability, increased incidence of perinatal complications, or congeni-tal malformations including neurodevelopmental problems, as well as major structural anomalies (e.g., cleft palate, spina bifida).

Most of the studies that have been done with antidepressants are limited to TCAs and SSRIs, most likely reflecting the fact that these medica-tions are widely used (511, 512). The good news is that these studies have not detected an obvious increased risk of major structural anomalies. The cautionary note is that most of these studies as-sess the child immediately after birth and thus are insensitive to detecting neurodevelopmen-tal problems that may only emerge after longer periods of time (e.g., learning or behavioral problems).

SSRIs and Pregnancy

To illustrate this problem, studies done with flu-oxetine are reviewed here in greater detail. This SSRI is perhaps the best studied with regard to the issue of teratogenicity. The reason is related both to its widespread use in women of child-bearing potential and to the extended half-life of its active metabolite, norfluoxetine. Even though most physicians will stop medications whenever feasible in a woman who becomes pregnant, the long half-life of norfluoxetine means that it will persist in the body for many weeks after it has been discontinued. In the case of the pregnant woman, that means that her fetus will be exposed to the effects of this metabolite for a significant portion of the first trimester, even after discontinuation. Thus, the potential effects of this antidepressant on the developing fetus assumes greater importance than other shorter lived antidepressants and hence has received considerable research attention.

Several relatively large-scale naturalistic studies have examined the consequences of fluoxetine exposure during human fetal development. Chambers and colleagues (513) found no difference in the rate of spontaneous abortions or rate of major structural anomalies but did find more than a twofold increase in the incidence of three or more minor structural anomalies in neonates exposed to fluoxetine during fetal development versus controls. They also found a higher incidence of premature deliveries, lower birth weight, shorter birth length, increased rate of admission to special care nurseries, cyanosis on feeding, and jitteriness in such infants versus controls, particularly in those exposed during the last trimester. The earlier results are similar to those of Pastuszak and colleagues (514), who found no difference in the rates of major structural anomalies in neonates exposed to fluoxetine versus those exposed to TCAs or to nonteratogens. Pastuszak et al., however, also found that women exposed to fluoxetine or TCAs had twice the risk of miscarriage versus those exposed to nonteratogens. The findings of Chambers and colleagues are similar to those of Goldstein (515), who found a 13% incidence of postnatal complications in neonates exposed to fluoxetine during the last trimester.

Two preclinical studies may provide one potential mechanism for the increased incidence of postnatal complications in neonates exposed in the last trimester to fluoxetine. Stanford and Patton (516) exposed rats in utero to fluoxetine beginning on day 7 of gestation and ending on the day of birth. This exposure produced a statistically significant higher incidence of skin hematomas. This finding is consistent with the increased incidence of bruising, which can occur with fluoxetine and other SSRIs and is thought to be due to impairment in platelet clotting mechanisms secondary to the depletion of serotonin from platelets. Di Pasquale and colleagues (517) found that exposure to fluoxetine potentiated the increase in the excitatory modulation of endogenous 5-HT on the central respiratory rhythm generator in the fetal rat brainstem–spinal cord preparation. Conceivably, this effect may be relevant to respiratory complications that were reported in some human neonates in the studies by Goldstein and Chambers et al. reviewed earlier.

Prenatal exposure to fluoxetine reduced 5-HT stimulated phosphoinositide hydrolysis, whereas prenatal exposure to desipramine decreased the density of [3H]ketanserin-labeled 5-HT$_2$ receptors in 25-day-old pups (518). Similarly, in utero exposure to fluoxetine on gestational days 13 through 20 produced a significant reduction in the maximal density of hypothalamic 5-HT$_{2A/2C}$ receptors and a corresponding statistically significant reduction in 5-HT$_{2A/2C}$ receptor-mediated endocrine response (i.e., a marked and selective attenuation of adrenocorticotropin response to 2, 5-dimethoxyphenylisopropylamine) in male progeny on postnatal day 70 (519). Exposure of the mouse whole embryo in culture to either fluoxetine or sertraline inhibited the normal 5-HT–mediated proliferation of cardiac mesenchyme, endocardium, and myocardium during endocardial cushion formation (520). This effect was most pronounced when exposure began before cushion formation (embryonic day 9 in the mouse fetus). Shuey and colleagues (521) studied the effects of exposing mouse embryos to amitriptyline, fluoxetine, or sertraline (i.e., antidepressants capable of inhibiting 5-HT uptake) on 5-HT regulation of epithelial-mesenchymal interactions important for normal craniofacial morphogenesis. Such exposure produced craniofacial defects as a result of increased levels of proliferation of the subepithelial mesenchymal layers but decreased proliferation and extensive cell death in mesenchyme located five to six layers deep from the overlying epithelium. This effect was seen with all three drugs individually, consistent with their ability to inhibit 5-HT uptake and thus alter the tonic effects of 5-HT on this developmental process with the days 10 to 11 being critical in the mouse.

The clinician reviewing these findings can certainly take solace in the absence of an increased risk of spontaneous abortion or major structural malformations but not in the increased frequency of minor anomalies and postnatal complications in human neonates nor in the findings from developmental studies in rodents. Although the extrapolation of the latter to humans is uncertain, these studies do indicate that exposure can alter the important regulatory role of neurotransmitters on organogenesis, which may not be apparent in neonates in terms of major structural anomalies. These findings support the usual clinical wisdom of avoiding the use of psychiatric medications during pregnancy whenever possible. That trailing qualifier is obviously important because untreated major depression in a pregnant woman is not innocuous and may be more damaging to the fetus (e.g., suicide attempt by the mother) than treatment with antidepressants. Nevertheless, these findings raise further concern about the growing advocacy of long-term treatment with antidepressants in women of childbearing potential, particularly with a long-lived agent such as fluoxetine, which is not rapidly cleared from the body after discontinuation.

CONCLUSION

There are eight pharmacologically distinct classes of antidepressants based on their putative mechanism of action (Table 7-16). Those classes give the clinician a considerable range of options when choosing an antidepressant for a specific patient. By understanding the clinical pharmacology of these various classes as well as the individual agents comprising these classes, one can choose the antidepressant that most closely fits the needs of an individual patient in terms of safety, tolerability, and efficacy. In terms of safety, antidepressants range from those with a narrow therapeutic index (e.g., amitriptyline) to newer agents with wide therapeutic indexes. Another safety issue is drug–drug interactions, which has taken on increasing importance because so many patients take more than one medication. Again, the physician has a range of choices from those with greater risk of causing either pharmacodynamic or pharmacoki-

netic drug–drug interactions (e.g., amitriptyline and fluoxetine, respectively) to those with less risk (e.g., sertraline). Tolerability is sometimes a matter of perspective. For example, sedation and weight gain may be a problem for some patients and a benefit for others, which is why knowledge of clinical pharmacology can help optimize drug choice for a given patient. Whereas all marketed antidepressants appear to have comparable general efficacy, incomplete but growing evidence suggests that some classes may be more effective in some types of clinical depression. When a patient does not benefit in terms of efficacy from an optimal trial of one antidepressant from a given class, the clinician can switch to a class with a different mechanism of action. This course of action seems intuitively more appropriate than switching within a class.

The goal of this chapter was to organize the existing knowledge of the various antidepressants based on their clinical pharmacological class to aid the clinician in selecting the optimal treatment for a patient.

REFERENCES

1. Preskorn SH. *Outpatient management of depression: a guide for the practitioner.* 2nd ed. Caddo, OK: Professional Communications, 1999.
2. Kuhn R. The treatment of depressive states with G-22355 (imipramine hydrochloride). *Am J Psychiatry* 1958;115:459–464.
3. Crane GE. Iproniazid (Marsilid) phosphate, a therapeutic agent for mental disorders and debilitating disease. *Psychiatry Res Rep* 1957;8:142–152.
4. Kline NS. Clinical experience with iproniazid (Marsilid). *J Clin Exp Psychopathol* 1958;19[Suppl 1]:72–78.
5. Ayd FJ Jr. Drug-induced depression—fact or fallacy. *N Y J Med* 1958;58:354–356.
6. Faucett RL, Litin EM, Achor RWP. Neuropharmacologic action of rauwolfia compounds and its psychodynamic implications. *Arch Neurol Psychiatr* 1957;77:513–518.
7. Jensen K. Depression in patients treated with reserpine for arterial hypertension. *Acta Psychiatr Neurol Scand* 1959;34:195–204.
8. Lemieux G, Davignon A, Genest J. Depressive states during rauwolfia therapy for arterial hypertension. *Can Med Assoc J* 1956;74:522–526.
9. Dollerey CT, Harington M. Methyldopa in hypertension: clinical and pharmacological studies. *Lancet* 1962;i:759–763.
10. Smirk H. Hypotensive action of methyldopa. *BMJ* 1963;7:146–155.

11. Sourkes TW. The action of α-methyldopa in the brain. Br Med Bull 1965;21:66–69.

12. Schildkraut JJ. The catecholamine hypothesis of affective disorders: a review of supporting evidence. Am J Psychiatry 1965;122:509–522.

13. Bunney WE Jr, Davis JM. Norepinephrine in depressive reactions. Arch Gen Psychiatry 1965;13:483–494.

14. Coppen A, Prange AJ, Hill C, Whybrow PC, et al. Abnormalities of indolamines in affective disorders. Arch Gen Psychiatry 1972;26:474–478.

15. Lapin IP, Oxenkrug GF. Intensification of the central serotonergic processes as a possible determinant of the thymoleptic effect. Lancet 1969;i:132–136.

16. Everett GM. The dopa response potentiation test and its use in screening for antidepressant drugs. In: Garattini S, Dukes MNG, eds. Antidepressant drugs. Amsterdam: Excerpta Medica, 1967.

17. Sulser F, Bickel MH, Brodie BB. The action of desmethylimipramine in counteracting sedation and cholinergic effects of reserpine-like drugs. J Pharmacol Exp Ther 1964;144:321–330.

18. Sulser F, Owens ML, Dingell JV. In vivo modification of biochemical effects of reserpine by desipramine in the hypothalamus of the rat. Pharmacologist 1967;9:213(abst).

19. Seligman ME, Maier SF. Failure to escape traumatic shock. J Exp Psychol 1967;74:1–9.

20. Overmier JB, Seligman MEP. Effects of inescapable shock upon subsequent escape and avoidance learning. J Comp Physiol Psychol 1967;63:23–33.

21. Seligman ME. Learned helplessness. Annu Rev Med 1972;23:407–412.

22. Porsolt RD, Anton G, Blavet N, et al. Behavioral despair in rats. A new model sensitive to antidepressant treatments. Eur J Pharmacol 1979;47:379–391.

23. Porsolt RD. Behavioral despair. In: Enna SJ, Malik JB, Richelson E, eds. Antidepressants: Neurochemical, Behavioral, and Clinical Perspectives. New York: Raven Press, 1981.

24. Kent JM. SNaRIs, NaSSAs, and NaRIs: new agents for the treatment of depression. Lancet 2000;355:911–918.

25. Preskorn S. Clinical pharmacology of selective serotonin reuptake inhibitors. Caddo, OK: Professional Communications, 1996.

26. Richelson E. Biological basis of depression and therapeutic relevance. J Clin Psychiatry 1991;52[Suppl 6]:4–10.

27. Drevets WC. Neuroimaging abnormalities in the orbital and medial prefrontal cortex and amygdala in mood disorders: implications for a neural circuitry-based approach to major depression. Biol Psychiatry 2000;48(8):813–829.

28. Drevets WC, Gadde KM, Ranga K, et al. Neuroimaging studies of mood disorders. In: Charney DS, Nestler EJ, Bunney BS, eds. Neurobiology of mental illness. New York: Oxford University Press, 1999:394–418.

29. Drevets WC, Raichle ME. Reciprocal suppression of regional cerebral blood flow during emotional versus higher cognitive processes: implications for interactions between emotion and cognition. Cognition Emotion 1998;12:353–385.

30. Ongur D, Drevets WC, Price JL. Glial reduction in the subgenual prefrontal cortex in mood disorders. Proc Natl Acad Sci U S A 1998;95:13290–13295.

31. Meyer JH, Kapur S, Houle S, et al. Prefrontal cortex 5-HT$_2$ receptors in depression: An [^{18}F]setoperone PET imaging study. Am J Psychiatry 1999;156:1029–1034.

32. MacQueen G, Born L, Steiner M. The selective serotonin reuptake inhibitor sertraline: its profile and use in psychiatric disorders. 2000 (unpublished).

33. Mooney JJ, Schatzberg AF, Cole JO, et al. Urinary 3-methoxy-4-hydroxy phenylglycol and the Depression-Type Score as predictors of differential responses to antidepressants. J Clin Psychopharmacol 1991;11:339–343.

34. Janicak PG, Davis JM, Chan C, et al. Failure of urinary MHPG levels to predict treatment response in patients with unipolar depression. Am J Psychiatry 1986;143:1398–1402.

35. Davis JM, Bresnahan DB. Psychopharmacology in clinical psychiatry. In: Hales RE, Frances AJ, eds. Psychiatry update. American Psychiatric Association annual review. Vol 6. Washington, DC: American Psychiatric Press, 1987.

36. Banerjee SP, Kung LS, Riggi SJ, et al. Development of beta-adrenergic receptor subsensitivity by antidepressants. Nature 1977;268:455–456.

37. Pandey GN, Heinze WJ, Brown BD, et al. Electroconvulsive shock treatment decreases beta-adrenergic receptor sensitivity in rat brain. Nature 1979;280:234–235.

38. Pandey GN, Janicak PG, Javaid JI, et al. Increased 3H-clonidine binding in the platelets of patients with depressive and schizophrenic disorders. Psychiatry Res 1987;28:73–88.

39. Pandey GN, Pandey SC, Janicak PG, et al. Platelet serotonin-2 receptor binding sites in depression and suicide. Biol Psychiatry 1990;28:215–222.

40. Crews FJ, Smith CB. Presynaptic alpha receptor subsensitivity after long-term antidepressant treatment. Science 1978;202:322–324.

41. Siever LJ, Davis KL. Overview: toward a dysregulation hypothesis of depression. Am J Psychiatry 1985;142:1017–1031.

42. Stanley M, Mann JJ. Increased serotonin-2 binding sites in frontal cortex of suicide victims. Lancet 1983;i:214–216.

43. Pandey GN, Pandey SC, Dwivedi Y, et al. Platelet serotonin-2A receptors: a potential biological marker for suicidal behavior. Am J Psychiatry 1995;152:850–855.

44. Asberg M, Schalling D, Traskman-Bendy L, et al. Psychobiology of suicide, impulsivity and related phenomena. In: Meltzer HY, ed. Psychopharmacology: the third generation of progress. New York: Raven Press, 1987:655–668.

45. Tuomisto J, Tukiainen E. Decreased uptake of 5-hydroxytryptamine in blood platelets from depressed patients. Nature 1976;262:596–598.

46. Price LH, Charney DS, Delgado PL, et al. Serotonin function and depression: neuroendocrine and mood responses to intravenous L-tryptophan in depressed patients and healthy comparison subjects. Am J Psychiatry 1991;148:1518–1525.

47. Shopsin B, Freedman E, Gershon S. PCPA reversal of tranylcypromine effects in depressed patients. Arch Gen Psychiatry 1976;33:811–819.

48. Shopsin B, Gershon S, Goldstein M, et al. Use of synthesis inhibitors in defining a role for biogenic amines during imipramine treatment in depressed patients. Psychopharmacol Commun 1975;1:239–249.

49. Delgado PL, Charney DS, Price LH, et al. Serotonin function and the mechanism of antidepressant action: reversal of antidepressant induced remission by rapid depletion of plasma tryptophan. *Arch Gen Psychiatry* 1990;47:411–418.

50. Van Praag HM. Management of depression with serotonin precursors. *Biol Psychiatry* 1981;16:291–310.

51. Peroutka SJ, Snyder SH. Long-term antidepressant treatment decreases spiroperidol-labelled serotonin receptor binding. *Science* 1980:210;88–90.

52. Aperia B, Thoren M, Wetterberg L. Prolactin and thyrotropin in serum during ECT in patients with major depressive illness. *Acta Psychiatr Scand* 1985;72:302–308.

53. Stockmeier CA, Kellar KJ. *In vivo* regulation of the serotonin-2 receptor in rat brain. *Life Sci* 1986;38:117–127.

54. Eison MS. Azapirones: mechanism of action in anxiety and depression. *Drug Ther* 1990;Aug[Suppl]:3–8.

55. Randrup A, Munkvad I, Fog R, et al. Mania, depression and brain dopamine. In: Essman WB, Valzelli L, eds. *Current developments in psychopharmacology.* New York: Spectrum Publications, 1975:207–209.

56. Gibbons RD, Davis JM. Consistent evidence for a biological sub-type of depression characterized by low CSF monoamine levels. *Acta Psychiatr Scand* 1986;74:8–12.

57. Roy A, Karoum F, Pollack S. Marked reduction in indices of dopamine metabolism among patients with depression who attempt suicide. *Arch Gen Psychiatry* 1992;49:447–450.

58. Muscat R, Papp M, Willner P. Antidepressant-like effects of dopamine agonists in an animal model of depression. *Biol Psychiatry* 1992;31:937–946.

59. Kapur S, Mann JJ. Role of the dopaminergic system in depression. *Biol Psychiatry* 1992;32:1–17.

60. Prange AJ Jr, Wilson IC, Lynn CW, et al. L-Tryptophan in mania. *Arch Gen Psychiatry* 1974;30:56–62.

61. Stockmeier CA, Martino AM, Kellar KJ. A strong influence of serotonin axons on β-adrenergic receptors in rat brain. *Science* 1985;230:323–325.

62. Janowsky DS, El-Yousef MK, Davis JM, et al. A cholinergic-adrenergic hypothesis of mania and depression. *Lancet* 1972;2:632–635.

63. Emrich HM, Wolf R. Recent neurochemical and pharmacological aspects of the pathogenesis and therapy of affective psychoses. *Pharmacol Toxicol* 1990;66[Suppl 3]:5–12.

64. Wachtel H. The second messenger dysbalance hypothesis of affective disorders. *Pharmacopsychiatry* 1990;23:27–32.

65. Chen J, Rasenick MM. Chronic antidepressant treatment facilitates G-protein activation of adenylate cyclase without altering G protein content. *J Pharmacol Exp Ther* 1995;275:509–517.

66. Duman RS, Heninger GR, Nestler EJ. A molecular and cellular theory of depression. *Arch Gen Psychiatry* 1997;54:597–608.

67. Nibuya M, Morinobu S, Duman RS. Regulation of BDNF and trkBmRNA in rat brain by chronic electroconvulsive seizure and antidepressant drug treatments. *J Neurosci* 1995;15:7539–7547.

68. Nibuya M, Nestler EJ, Duman RS. Chronic antidepressant administration increases the expression of cAMP response element binding protein (CREB) in rat hippocampus. *J Neurosci* 1996;16:2365–2372.

69. Post RM. Molecular biology of behavior: targets for therapeutics. *Arch Gen Psychiatry* 1997;54:608.

70. Sheline YI, Wang PW, Gado MH, et al. Hippocampal atrophy in recurrent major depression. *Proc Natl Acad Sci U S A* 1996;93:3908–3913.

71. Magarinos AM, McEwen BS, Flugge G, et al. Chronic psychosocial stress causes apical dendritic atrophy of hippocampal CA3 pyramidal neurons in subordinate tree shrews. *J Neurosci* 1996;16:3534–3540.

72. Coplan JD, Andrews MW, Rosenblum LA, et al. Persistent elevations of cerebrospinal fluid concentrations of corticotropin-releasing factor in adult non-human primates exposed to early-life stressors: implications for the pathophysiology of mood and anxiety disorders. *Proc Natl Acad Sci U S A* 1996;93:1619–1623.

73. Dorus E, Pandey GN, Shaughnessy R, et al. Lithium transport across red blood cell membrane: a cell membrane abnormality in manic-depressive illness. *Science* 1979;205:932–934.

74. Halberg F. Physiological considerations underlying rhythmicity with special reference to emotional illness. In: de Ajuriaguerra JG, ed. *Cycles Biologique et Psychiatrie* Paris: Geneve & Masson, 1968.

75. Goodwin FK, Wirz-Justice A, Wehr T. Evidence that the pathophysiology of depression and the mechanism of action of antidepressant drugs involve alterations in circadian rhythms. *Adv Biochem Psychopharmacol* 1982;31:1–11.

76. Schulz H, Lund R. On the origins of early REM episodes in the sleep of depressed patients: a comparison of 3 hypotheses. *Psychiatry Res* 1985;16:65–77.

77. Wirz-Justice A, Krauchi K, Morimasa T, et al. Circadian rhythm of ^{3}H-imipramine binding in the rat suprachiasmatic nuclei. *Eur J Pharmacol* 1983;87:331–333.

78. Beedle D, Krasuski J, Janicak PG. Advances in somatic therapies: electroconvulsive therapy, repetitive transcranial magnetic stimulation, and bright light therapy. In: Janicak PG, Davis JM, Preskorn SH, et al., eds. *Principles and practice of psychopharmacotherapy update.* 2nd ed. Vol 2. Baltimore: Williams & Wilkins, 1998.

79. Skewerer RB, Duncan C, Jacobsen FM, et al. The neurobiology of seasonal affective disorder and phototherapy. *J Biol Rhythms* 1988;3:135–153.

80. Depue RA, Arbisi P, Spoont MR, et al. Dopamine functioning in the behavioral facilitation system and seasonal variation in behavior: normal population and clinical studies. In: Rosenthal NE, Blehar MC, eds. *Seasonal affective disorders and phototherapy.* New York: Guilford Press, 1989.

81. O'Rourke D, Wurtmann JJ, Brzeskinski A, et al. Treatment of seasonal affective disorder with D-fenfluramine. *Ann N Y Acad Sci* 1987;499:329–330.

82. Jacobsen FM, Sack DA, Wehr TA, et al. Neuroendocrine response to 5-hydroxytryptophan in seasonal affective disorder. *Arch Gen Psychiatry* 1987;44:1086–1091.

83. Lacoste V, Wirz-Justice A. Seasonal variation in normal subjects: an update of variables current in depression research. In: Rosenthal NE, Blehar MC, eds. *Seasonal affective disorders and phototherapy.* New York: Guilford Press, 1989.

84. Gold PW, Goodwin FK, Chrousos GP. Clinical and biochemical manifestations of depression: relation to the neurobiology of stress. Parts 1 and 2. *N Engl J Med* 1988;319:348–353 and 1988;319:413–420.

85. The American Psychiatric Association Task Force on Laboratory Tests in Psychiatry. The DST: an overview of its current status in psychiatry. *Am J Psychiatry* 1987;144:1253–1262.

86. Bartrop RW, Lazarus L, Luckhurst E, et al. Depressed lymphocyte function after bereavement. *Lancet* 1977;i:834–836.

87. Schleifer SJ, Keller SE, Camerino M, et al. Suppression of lymphocyte stimulation following bereavement. *JAMA* 1983;250:374–377.

88. Schleifer SJ, Keller SE, Bond RN, et al. Major depressive disorder and immunity: role of age, sex, severity and hospitalization. *Arch Gen Psychiatry* 1989;46:81–87.

89. Kronfol Z, Remick DG. Cytokines and the brain: implications for clinical psychiatry. *Am J Psychiatry* 2000;157:683–694.

90. Gershon ES, Berrettini W, Nurnberger J Jr, et al. Genetics of affective illness. In: Meltzer HY, ed. *Psychopharmacology: the third generation of progress.* New York: Raven Press, 1987:481–491.

91. Berretini WH, Goldin LR, Gelernter S, et al. X-chromosome markers and manic depressive illness: rejection of linkage to xq28 in nine bipolar pedigrees. *Arch Gen Psychiatry* 1990;47:366–373.

92. Post RM. Transduction of psychosocial stress into the neurobiology of recurrent affective disorder. *Am J Psychiatry* 1992;149:999–1010.

93. Angst J, Delini-Stula A, Stabl M, et al. Is a cut-off score a suitable measure of treatment outcome in short-term trials in depression? A methodological meta-analysis. *Hum Psychopharmacol* 1993;8:311–317.

94. Prien RF, Carpenter LL, Kupfer DJ. The definition and operational criteria for treatment outcome of major depressive disorder: a review of the current research literature. *Arch Gen Psychiatry* 1991;48:796–800.

95. Davis JM, Janicak PG, Wang Z, et al. The efficacy of psychotropic drugs. *Psychopharmacol Bull* 1992;28:151–155.

96. Appleton WS, Davis JM. *Practical clinical psychopharmacology.* New York: Medcomb Publishing, 1973.

97. Burt CG, Gordon WF, Holt NF, et al. Amitriptyline in depressive states: a controlled trial. *J Ment Sci* 1962;108:711–730.

98. Hordern A, Holt NF, Burt CG, et al. Amitriptyline in depressive states: phenomenology and prognostic considerations. *Br J Psychiatry* 1963;109:815–825.

99. Hasan KZ, Akhtar MI. Double blind clinical study comparing doxepin and imipramine in depression. *Curr Ther Res* 1971;13:327–336.

100. Grof P, Saxena B, Cantor R, et al. Doxepin versus amitriptyline in depression: a sequential double-blind study. *Curr Ther Res* 1974;16:470–476.

101. Linnoila M, Seppala T, Mattila M, et al. Clomipramine and doxepin in depressive neurosis: plasma levels and therapeutic response. *Arch Gen Psychiatry* 1980;37:1295–1299.

102. Rickels K, Gordon PE, Weiss CC, et al. Amitriptyline and trimipramine in neurotic depressed patients: a collaborative study. *Am J Psychiatry* 1970;127:208–218.

103. Wilson C, et al. A double-blind clinical comparison of amoxapine, imipramine and placebo in the treatment of depression. *Curr Ther Res* 1977;22:620–627.

104. Fann WE, Davis JM, Domino E, et al. *Tardive dyskinesia: research and treatment.* New York: Spectrum Medical, 1980.

105. VanDer Velde C. Maprotiline versus imipramine and placebo in neurotic depression. *J Clin Psychiatry* 1981;42:138–141.

106. Rouillon F, Phillips R, Serrurier D, et al. Rechutes de depression unipolaire et efficacite de la maprotiline. *L'Encephale* 1989;15:527–534.

107. Jukes AM. A comparison of maprotiline (Ludiomil) and placebo in the treatment of depression. *J Int Med Res* 1975;3[Suppl 2]:84–88.

108. McCallum P, Meares R. A controlled trial of maprotiline (Ludiomil) in depressed outpatients. *Med J Aust* 1975;2:392–394.

109. d'Elia G, Borg S, Hermann L, et al. Comparative clinical evaluation of lofepramine and imipramine. Psychiatric aspects. *Acta Psychiatr Scand* 1977;55:10–20.

110. Bjork K. The efficacy of zimeldine in preventing depressive episodes in recurrent major depressive disorders — a double-blind placebo-controlled study. *Acta Psychiatr Scand Suppl* 1983;68:182–189.

111. Patris M, Bouchard J-M, Bougerol T, et al. Citalopram versus fluoxetine: a double-blind, controlled, multicentre, phase III trial in patients with unipolar major depression treated in general practice. *Int Clin Psychopharmacol* 1996;11:129–136.

112. Gattaz WF, Vogel P, Kick H, et al. Moclobemide versus fluoxetine in the treatment of inpatients with major depression. *J Clin Psychopharmacol* 1995;15[Suppl 2]:35S–40S.

113. De Wilde J, Spiers R, Mertens C, et al. A double-blind, comparative, multicentre study comparing paroxetine with fluoxetine in depressed patients. *Acta Psychiatr Scand* 1993;87:141–145.

114. Clerc GE, Ruimy P, Verdeau-Paillès J. A double-blind comparison of venlafaxine and fluoxetine in patients hospitalized for major depression and melancholia. *Int Clin Psychopharmacol* 1994;9:139–143.

115. Dunner DL, Dunbar GC. Optimal dose regimen for paroxetine. *J Clin Psychiatry* 1992;53[Suppl 2]:21–26.

116. Danish University Antidepressant Group. Citalopram: clinical effect profile in comparison with clomipramine: a controlled multicenter study. *Psychopharmacology* 1986;90:131–138.

117. Danish University Antidepressant Group. Paroxetine: a selective serotonin reuptake inhibitor showing better tolerance, but weaker antidepressant effect than clomipramine in a controlled multicenter study. *J Affect Disord* 1990;18:289–299.

118. Wheatley DP, van Moffaert M, Timmerman L, et al. Mirtazapine: efficacy and tolerability in comparison with fluoxetine in patient with moderate to severe major depressive disorder. *J Clin Psychiatry* 1998;59:306–312.

119. Nelson JC, Mazure CM, Bowers MB Jr, et al. A preliminary, open study of the combination of fluoxetine and

desipramine for rapid treatment of major depression. *Arch Gen Psychiatry* 1991;48:303–307.

119a. Blier P. Possible neurobiological mechanisms underlying faster onset of antidepressant action. *J. Clin Psychiatry* 2001;62(4):7–11.

120. Weilburg JB, Rosenbaum JF, Biederman J, et al. Fluoxetine added to non-MAOI antidepressants converts nonresponders to responders: a preliminary report. *J Clin Psychiatry* 1989;50:447–449.

121. Preskorn SH. Finding the signal through the noise: the use of surrogate markers. *J Pract Psychiatry Behav Health* 1999;5:104–109.

122. Bowden CL, Schatzberg AF, Rosenbaum A, et al. Fluoxetine and desipramine in major depressive disorder. *J Clin Psychopharmacol* 1993;13:305–311.

123. Kasper S, Moller H-J, Montgomery SA, et al. Antidepressant efficacy in relation to item analysis and severity of depression: a placebo-controlled trial of fluvoxamine versus imipramine. *Int Clin Psychopharmacol* 1995;9:3–12.

124. Pande AC, Sayler ME. Severity of depression and response to fluoxetine. *Int Clin Psychopharmacol* 1993;8:243–245.

125. Feighner JP, Cohn JB, Fabre LF, et al. A study comparing paroxetine, placebo, and imipramine in depressed patients. *J Affect Disord* 1993;28:71–79.

126. Reimherr FW, Byerley WF, Ward MF, et al. Sertraline, a selective inhibitor of serotonin uptake, for the treatment of outpatients with major depressive disorder. *Psychopharmacol Bull* 1988;24:200–205.

127. Ottevanger EA. Fluvoxamine and clomipramine in depressed hospitalized patients: results from a randomized, double-blind study. *Encephale* 1995;21:317–321.

128. Arminen SL, Ikonen U, Pulkkinen P, et al. A 12-week, double-blind, multicentre study of paroxetine and imipramine in hospitalized depressed patients. *Acta Psychiatr Scand* 1994;89:382–389.

129. Beasley CM Jr, Holman SL, Potvin JH. Fluoxetine compared with imipramine in the treatment of inpatient depression: a multicenter trial. *Ann Clin Psychiatry* 1993;5:199–208.

130. Tignol J, Stoker MJ, Dunbar GC. Paroxetine in the treatment of melancholia and severe depression. *Int Clin Psychopharmacol* 1992;7:91–94.

131. Ginestet D. Fluoxetine in endogenous depression and melancholia versus clomipramine. *Int Clin Psychopharmacol* 1989;4:37–40.

132. Heiligenstein JH, Tollefson GD, Faries DE. Response patterns of depressed outpatients with and without melancholia: a double-blind, placebo-controlled trial of fluoxetine versus placebo. *J Affect Disord* 1993;30:163–173.

133. Feighner JP, Boyer WF, Meredith CH, et al. A placebo-controlled inpatient comparison of fluvoxamine maleate and imipramine in major depression. *Int Clin Psychopharmacol* 1989;4:239–244.

134. Stuppaeck CH, Geretsegger C, Whitworth AB, et al. A multicenter double-blind trial of paroxetine versus amitriptyline in depressed inpatients. *J Clin Psychopharmacol* 1994;14:241–246.

135. Fredman SJ, Fava M, Kienke AS, et al. Partial response, non-response, and relapse on SSRIs in major depression: a survey of current "next-step" practices. *J Clin Psychiatry* 2000;61:403–407.

136. Keller MB, Gelenberg AJ, Hirschfeld RMA, et al. A double-blind, randomized trial of sertraline and imipramine. *J Clin Psychiatry* 1998;59:598–607.

137. Harvey AT, Rudolph RL, Preskorn SH. Evidence of the dual mechanisms of action of venlafaxine. *Arch Gen Psychiatry* 2000;57:503–509.

138. Klamerus KJ, Maloney K, Rudolph RL, et al. Introduction of a composite parameter to the pharmacokinetics of venlafaxine and its active O-desmethyl metabolite. *J Clin Pharmacol* 1992;32:716–724.

139. Troy S, Piergies A, Lucki I, et al. Venlafaxine pharmacokinetics and pharmacodynamics. *Clin Neuropharmacol* 1992;15[Suppl 1]:324B.

140. Preskorn SH. Pharmacokinetic profile of Effexor (venlafaxine HCl). Poster displayed at the 150th Annual Meeting of the American Psychiatric Association, Philadelphia, May 21, 1994.

141. Haskins JT, Moyer JA, Muth EA, et al. DMI, WY-45,030, WY-45,881 and ciramadol inhibit locus coeruleus neuronal activity. *Eur J Pharmacol* 1985;115:139–146.

142. Guelfi JD, White C, Magni G. A randomized, double-blind comparison of venlafaxine and placebo in inpatients with major depression and melancholia. *Clin Neuropharmacol* 1992;15[Suppl 1]):323B(abst).

142a. Leon AC, Blier P, Culpepper L, et al. An ideal trial to test differential onset of antidepressant effect. *J. Clin Psychiatry* 2001;62(4):34–36.

143. Preskorn S. Antidepressant drug selection: criteria and options. *J Clin Psychiatry* 1994;55[Suppl 9A]:6–22.

144. Rudolph R, Entsuah R, Derivan A. Early clinical response in depression to venlafaxine hydrochloride. *Biol Psychiatry* 1991;29[Suppl 11]:630S(abst).

145. Rickels K, Derivan A, Rudolph RL. Venlafaxine: rapid onset of antidepressant activity. American College of Neuropsychopharmacology 29th Annual Meeting, San Juan, Puerto Rico, December 10–14, 1990:141.

146. Derivan A, Entsuah R, Rudolph R, et al. Early response to venlafaxine hydrochloride, a novel antidepressant. American Psychiatric Association 145th Annual Meeting, Washington, DC, May 2–7, 1992:82–83.

147. Venlafaxine presentation to the Food and Drug Administration Psychopharmacology Advisory Committee. Washington, DC, April 1993.

148. Baron B, Ogden A, Siegel B, et al. Rapid down regulation of adrenoceptors by co-administration of desipramine and fluoxetine. *Pharmacology* 1988;154:125–134.

148a. Stahl SM, Nierenberg AA, Gorman JM. Evidence of early onset of antidepressant effect in randomized controlled trials. *J. Clin Psychiatry* 2001;62(4):17–23.

149. Nierenberg AA, Feighner JF, Rudolph RR, et al. Venlafaxine for treatment-resistant depression. *Neuropsychopharmacology* 1994;10[Suppl 2]:85S.

150. Fontaine R, Ontiveros A, Faludi G, et al. A study of nefazodone, imipramine, and placebo in depressed outpatients. *Biol Psychiatry* 1991;29:118A.

151. Feighner JP, Pambakian R, Fowler RC, et al. A comparison of nefazodone, imipramine and placebo in patients with moderate to severe depression. *Psychopharmacol Bull* 1989;25:219–221.

152. Weise C, Fox I, Clary C, et al. Nefazodone in the treatment of outpatient major depression. *Biol Psychiatry* 1991;29:363S.

153. Yocca FD, Hyslop DK, Taylor DP. Nefazodone: a potential broad spectrum antidepressant. *Trans Am Soc Neurochem* 1985;16:115.

154. Robinson D, Roberts D, Archibald D, et al. Therapeutic dose range of nefazodone for the treatment of major depression. *J Clin Psychiatry* 1996;57[Suppl 2]:6–9.

155. Fontaine R, Ontiveros A, Elie R, et al. A double-blind comparison of nefazodone, imipramine, and placebo in major depression. *J Clin Psychiatry* 1994;55:6:234–241.

156. Nefazodone presentation to the Food and Drug Administration Psychopharmacology Advisory Committee. Washington, DC, July 1993.

157. Mendels J, Reimherr F, Marcus R, et al. A double-blind, placebo-controlled trial of two dose ranges of nefazodone in the treatment of depressed outpatients. *J Clin Psychiatry* 1995;56[Suppl 6]:30–36.

158. D'Amico M, Roberts D, Robinson D, et al. Placebo-controlled dose-ranging trial designs in phase II development of nefazodone. *Psychopharmacol Bull* 1990;26:147–150.

159. Rickels K, Schweizer E, Clary C, et al. Nefazodone and imipramine in major depression: a placebo-controlled trial. *Br J Psychiatry* 1994;164:802–805.

160. Fawcett J, Marcus R, Anton S, et al. Response of anxiety and agitation symptoms during nefazodone treatment of major depression. *J Clin Psychiatry* 1995;56[Suppl 6]:37–42.

161. Musso DL, Mehta NB, Soroko FE, et al. Synthesis and evaluation of the antidepressant activity of the enantiomers of bupropion. *Chirality* 1993:5:495–500.

162. Pandey GN, Davis JM. *Treatment with antidepressants, sensitivity of beta receptors and affective illness.* New York: Wiley, 1980.

163. Preskorn SH. Bupropion: what mechanism of action? *J Pract Psychiatry Behav Health* 2000;6:39–44.

164. Preskorn SH. Imipramine, mirtazapine, and nefazodone: multiple targets. *J Pract Psychiatry Behav Health* 2000;6:97–102.

165. Fabre LF, Brodie HK, Garver D, et al. A multicenter evaluation of bupropion versus placebo in hospitalized depressed patients. *J Clin Psychiatry* 1983;44:88–94.

166. Merideth CH, Feighner JP. The use of bupropion in hospitalized depressed patients. *J Clin Psychiatry* 1983;44:85–87.

167. Stern WC, Harto-Truax N, Bauer N. Efficacy of bupropion in tricyclic-resistant or intolerant patients. *J Clin Psychiatry* 1983;44(sec. 2):148–152.

168. Hirschfeld RM. Care of the sexually active depressed patient. *J Clin Psychiatry* 1999;60:32–35.

169. Cantwell DP. ADHD through the life span: the role of bupropion in treatment. *J Clin Psychiatry* 1998;59[Suppl 4]:92–94.

170. Jorenby DE, Leischow SJ, Nides MA, et al. A controlled trial of sustained-release bupropion, a nicotine patch, or both for smoking cessation. *N Engl J Med* 1999;340:685–691.

171. Preskorn SH. Selection of an antidepressant: mirtazapine. *J Clin Psychiatry* 1997;58[Suppl 6]:3–8.

172. Frazer A. Antidepressants. *J Clin Psychiatry* 1997;58[Suppl 6]:9–25.

173. Zivkov M, Roes KCB, Pols AB. Efficacy of Org 3770 (mirtazapine) vs. amitriptyline in patients with major depressive disorder: a meta-analysis. *Hum Psychopharmacol* 1995;10:S135–S145.

174. Fawcett JA, Barkin R. Efficacy issues with antidepressants. *J Clin Psychiatry* 1997;58[Suppl 6]:32–39.

175. Catterson M, Preskorn SH. Double-blind crossover study of mirtazapine, amitriptyline, and placebo in patients with major depression. In: New Research Program and Abstracts of the 149th annual meeting of the American Psychiatric Association, New York, May 6, 1996:NR157.

176. Wong EHF, Sonders MS, Amara SG, et al. Reboxetine: a pharmacologically potent, selective, and specific norepinephrine reuptake inhibitor. *Biol Psychiatry* 2000;47:818–829.

177. Slater SE, Gobbi G, Boucher N, et al. Effect of reboxetine on the norepinephrine reuptake processes in healthy male subjects. 40th Annual Meeting NCDEU, Boca Raton, Florida, 2000(abst).

178. Edwards DMF, Pillizzoni C, Breuel HP, et al. Pharmacokinetics of reboxetine in healthy volunteers. Single oral doses, linearity and plasma protein binding. *Biopharm Drug Dispos* 1995;16:443–460.

179. Johnstone EC. The relationship between acetylator status and inhibition of monoamine oxidase, excretion of free drug and antidepressant response in depressed patients on phenelzine. *Psychopharmacologia* 1976;46:289–294.

180. Lecrubies Y, Guelfi JD. Efficacy of reversible inhibitors of monoamine oxidase-A in various forms of depression. *Acta Psychiatr Scand Suppl* 1990;360:18–23.

181. VandenBerg CM, Blob LF, Gerrick G, et al. Blood pressure response produced by a tyramine-enriched meal following multiple dose administration of a 20 cm^2/20 mg selegiline transdermal system (STS) in healthy male volunteers. 40th Annual Meeting NCDEU, Boca Raton, Florida, 2000(abst).

182. Amsterdam JD, Bodkin A. Transdermal selegine in the treatment of patients with major depression: a double-blind placebo controlled trial. 40th Annual Meeting NCDEU, Boca Raton, Florida, 2000(abst).

183. Berwish NJ, Amsterdam JD. An overview of investigational antidepressants. *Psychosomatics* 1989;30:1–17.

184. Greenblatt M, Grosser GH, Wechsler H. Differential response of hospitalized depressed patients to somatic therapy. *Am J Psychiatry* 1964;120:935–943.

185. Quitkin F, Rifkin A, Klein DF. Monoamine oxidase inhibitors: a review of antidepressant effectiveness. *Arch Gen Psychiatry* 1979;36:749–760.

186. Rowan PR, Paykel ES, Parker RR. Phenelzine and amitriptyline: effects on symptoms of neurotic depression. *Br J Psychiatry* 1982;140:475–483.

187. Thase ME, Mallinger AG, McKnight D, et al. Treatment of imipramine-resistant recurrent depression, IV: a double-blind crossover study of tranylcypromine for anergic bipolar depression. *Am J Psychiatry* 1992;149:195–198.

188. Wheatley D. Amphetamines in general practice: their use in depression and anxiety. *Semin Psychiatry* 1969;1: 163–173.

189. Hare RH, Dominian J, Sharpe L. Phenelzine and dexamphetamine in depressive illness. *BMJ* 1962;1:9–12.

190. Overall JE, Hollister LE, Pokorny AD, et al. Drug therapy in depressions. *Clin Pharmacol Ther* 1961;3:16–22.

191. Hesbacher PT. Pemoline and methylphenidate in mildly depressed outpatients. *Clin Pharmacol Ther* 1970;11:698–710.

192. Rickels K, Ginrich RL Jr, McLaughlin W, et al. Methylphenidate in mildly depressed outpatients. *Clin Pharmacol Ther* 1972;13:595–601.

193. Robin AA, Wiseberg S. A controlled trial of methylphenidate (Ritalin) in the treatment of depressive states. *J Neurol Neurosurg Psychiatry* 1958;21:55–57.

194. Kaplitz SE. Withdrawn apathetic geriatric patients responsive to methylphenidate. *J Am Geriatr Soc* 1975;23:271–276.

195. Mendels J, Ramsey TA, Dyson WL, et al. Lithium as an antidepressant. *Arch Gen Psychiatry* 1979;36:845–846.

196. Souza FGM, Goodwin GM. Lithium treatment and prophylaxis in unipolar depression: a meta-analysis. *Br J Psychiatry* 1991;158:666–675.

197. Hollister LE, Overall JE, Shelton J, et al. Drug therapy of depression. Amitriptyline, perphenazine, and their combination in different syndromes. *Arch Gen Psychiatry* 1967;17:486–493.

198. Overall JE, Hollister LE, Meyer F, et al. Imipramine and thioridazine in depressed and schizophrenic patients. Are there specific antidepressant drugs? *JAMA* 1964;189:605–608.

199. Lesser IM. The relationship between panic disorder and depression. *J Anxiety Disord* 1988;2:2–16.

200. Lesser IM, Rubin RT, Pecknold JC, et al. Secondary depression in panic disorder and agoraphobia. I. Frequency, severity, and response to treatment. *Arch Gen Psychiatry* 1988;45:437–443.

201. Grunhaus L, Harel Y, Krugler T, et al. Major depressive disorder and panic disorder. *Clin Neuropharmacol* 1988;11:454–461.

202. Lesser IM. The treatment of panic disorders: pharmacologic aspects. *Psychiatr Ann* 1991;21:341–346.

203. Keller MB, Lavori PW, Goldenberg IM, et al. Influence of depression on the treatment of panic disorder with imipramine, alprazolam and placebo. *J Affect Disord* 1993;28:27–38.

204. Schatzberg AF, Cole JO. Benzodiazepines in depressive disorders. *Arch Gen Psychiatry* 1978;24:509–514.

205. Cassano GB, Castrogiovanni P, Conti I. Drug responses in different anxiety states under benzodiazepine treatment: some multivariate analyses for evaluation of Rating Scale for Depression scores. In: Garratini E, Mussini S, Randall LO, eds. *The benzodiazepines*. New York: Raven Press, 1973.

206. Klerman GL. The use of benzodiazepines in the treatment of depression. *Int Drug Ther Newsl* 1986;21:37–38.

207. Baldessarini RJ. Drugs and the treatment of psychiatric disorders. In: Gilman AG, Goodman LS, Gilman A, eds. *The pharmacological basis of therapeutics*. New York: Macmillan, 1980.

208. Ryan HW, Merrill FB, Scott GE, et al. Increase in suicidal thoughts and tendencies. *JAMA* 1968;203:135–137.

209. Weissman MM, Klerman GL. The chronic depressive in the community: unrecognized and poorly treated. *Compr Psychiatry* 1977;18:523–531.

210. Weisman MM, Myers JK, Thompson WD. Depression and its treatment in a US urban community. *Arch Gen Psychiatry* 1981;38:417–421.

211. Fawcett J. Targeting treatment in patients with mixed symptoms of anxiety and depression. *J Clin Psychiatry* 1990;51[Suppl 11]:40–43.

212. Rush AJ, Erman MK, Schlesser MA, et al. Alprazolam vs. amitriptyline in depressions with reduced REM latencies. *Arch Gen Psychiatry* 1985;42:1154–1159.

213. Remick RA, Fleming JAE, Buchanan RA, et al. A comparison of the safety and efficacy of alprazolam and desipramine in moderately severe depression. *Can J Psychiatry* 1985;30:597–601.

214. Feighner JP. A review of controlled studies of adinazolam mesylate in patients with major depressive disorder. *Psychopharmacol Bull* 1986;22:186–191.

215. Hicks F, Robins E, Murphy G. Comparison of adinazolam, amitriptyline, and placebo in the treatment of melancholic depression. *Psychiatry Res* 1987;23:221–227.

216. Gundlach R, Engelhardt DM, Hankoff L, et al. A double-blind outpatient study of diazepam (Valium) and placebo. *Psychopharmacologia* 1966;9:81–92.

217. McDowall A, Owen S, Robin AA. A controlled comparison of diazepam and amylobarbitone in anxiety states. *Br J Psychiatry* 1966;112:629–631.

218. Rao AV. A controlled trial with "Valium" in obsessive compulsive state. *J Ind Med Assoc* 1967;42:564–567.

219. Hall RCW, Joffe JR. Aberrant response to diazepam: a new syndrome. *Am J Psychiatry* 1972;129:738–742.

220. Lader MH, Petursson. Benzodiazepine derivatives — side effects and dangers. *Biol Psychiatry* 1981;16:1195–1201.

221. Fontaine R, Annable L, Chouinard G, et al. Bromazepam and diazepam in generalized anxiety: a placebo-controlled study with measurement of drug plasma concentrations. *J Clin Psychopharmacology* 1983;3:80–87.

222. Wilkinson CJ. Effects of diazepam (Valium) and trait anxiety on human physical aggression and emotional state. *J Behav Med* 1985;8:101–114.

223. Fontaine R, Mercier P, Beaudry P, et al. Bromazepam and lorazepam in generalized anxiety: a placebo-controlled study with measurement of drug plasma concentrations. *Acta Psychiatr Scand* 1986;74:451–458.

224. Pollack MH, Tesar GE, Rosenbaum JF, et al. Clonazepam in the treatment of panic disorder and agoraphobia: a one-year follow-up. *J Clin Psychopharmacol* 1986;47:475–476.

225. Lydiard RB, Laraia MT, Ballenger JC, et al. Emergence of depressive symptoms in patients receiving alprazolam for panic disorder. *Am J Psychiatry* 1987;144:664–665.

226. Lydiard RB, Howell EF, Laraia MT, et al. Depression in patients receiving lorazepam for panic. *Am J Psychiatry* 1989;146;629–631.

227. Goldberg SC, Ettigi P, Schulz PM, et al. Alprazolam versus imipramine in depressed out-patients with neurovegetative signs. *J Affect Disord* 1986;11:139–145.

228. Muller WEG, Rolli M, Schafer C, et al. Effects of hypericum extract (LI 60) in biochemical models of antidepressant activity. *Pharmacopsychiatry* 1997;30:102–107.

229. Nathan P. The experimental and clinical pharmacology of St. John's wort (hypericum perforatum L). *Mol Psychiatry* 1999;4:333–338.

230. Bennett DA, Jr, Phun L, Polk JF, et al. Neuropharmacology of St. John's wort (hypericum). *Ann Pharmacother* 1998;32:1201–1208.

231. Teufel-Mayer R, Gleitz J. Effects of long-term administration of hypericum extracts on the affinity and density of central serotonergic 5-HT$_{1a}$ and 5-HT$_{2a}$ receptors. *Pharmacopsychiatry* 1997;30:113–116.

232. George Washington University School of Medicine and Health Sciences, Department of Health Care Sciences. Herb-drug interactions. *Lancet* 2000;355:134–138.

233. Linde K, Ramirez G, Mulrow C, et al. St. John's wort for depression—an overview and meta-analysis of randomised clinical trials. *BMJ* 1996;313:253–258.

234. Gaster B, Holroyd J. St. John's wort for depression: a systematic review. *Arch Intern Med* 2000;160:152–156.

235. Stevinson C, Ernst E. Hypericum for depression. An update of the clinical evidence. *Eur Neuropsychopharmacol* 2000;9:501–505.

235a. Shelton RC, Keller MB, Gelenberg A, et al. Effectiveness of St. John's Wort in major depression: a randomized controlled trial. *JAMA* 2001;7:247–317.

236. Ernst E, Rand JI, Barnes J, et al. Adverse effects profile of the herbal antidepressant St. John's wort (hypericum perforatum L.). *Eur J Clin Pharmacol* 1998;54:589–594.

237. Golsch S, Vocks E, Rakoski J, et al. Reversible increase in photosensitivity to UV-B caused by St. John's wort extract. *Hautarzt* 1997;48:249–252.

238. Murray MT. *The healing power of herbs: the enlightened person's guide to the wonders of medicinal plants.* Rocklin, CA: Prima Publishing, 1995.

239. Tyler VE. *The honest herbal.* Binghamton, NY: Haworth Press, 1993.

240. Schubert H, Halama P. Depressive episode primarily unresponsive to therapy in elderly patients: efficacy of ginkgo biloba (EGb 761) in combination with antidepressants. *Geriatr Forsch* 1993;3:45–53.

241. Rosenblatt M, Mindel J. Spontaneous hyphema associated with ingestion of ginkgo biloba extract. *N Engl J Med* 1997;336:1108–1108.

242. Rowin J, Lewis SL. Spontaneous bilateral subdural hematomas associated with chronic ginkgo biloba ingestion. *Neurology* 1996;46:1775–1776.

243. Yagi M, Wada K, Sakata M, et al. Studies on the constituents of edible and medicinal plants. IV. Determination of 4-O-methylpyridoxine in serum of the patient with gin-nan food poisoning. *Yakugaku-Zasshi* 1993;113:596–599.

244. Janetzky K, Morreale AP. Probably interaction between warfarin and ginseng. *Am J Health System Pharm* 1997;54:692–693.

245. McRae S. Elevated serum digoxin levels in a patient taking digoxin and Siberian ginseng. *Can Med Assoc J* 1996;155:1237–1237.

246. D'Arcy PF. Adverse reactions and interactions with herbal medicines. Part 2. Drug interactions. *Adverse Drug React Toxicol Rev* 1993;12:147–162.

247. Weiner MA, Weiner JW. *Herbs that heal: prescription for herbal healing.* Mill Valley, CA: Quantum Books, 1994.

248. Ferreira F, Santos MS, Faro C, et al. Effects of extracts of valeriana officinalis on (^{3}H)GABA-release in synaptosomes: further evidence for the involvement of free GABA in the valerian-induced release. *Rev Portuguesa Farm* 1996;46:74–77.

249. D'Arcy PF. Adverse reactions and interactions with herbal medicines. Part 1. Adverse reactions. *Adverse Drug React Toxicol Rev* 1991;10:189–208.

250. Cui C, Yang M, Yao Z, et al. Antidepressant active constituents in the roots of morinda officinalis how. *Chung Kuo Chung Yao Tsa Chih* 1995;20:36–39, 62–63.

251. Ali B, Bashir AK, Tanira MO. The effect of rhazya stricta decne, a traditional medicinal plant, on the forced swimming test in rats. *Pharmacol Biochem Behav* 1998;59:547–550.

252. Stramentinoli G, Caho E, Alger S. The increase in SAMe concentration in rat brain after its systemic administration. *Comm Psychopharmacol* 1977;1:89–97.

253. Janicak P, Lipinski J, Davis JM, et al. Parenteral SAMe in depression: literature review and preliminary data. *Psychopharmacol Bull* 1989;25:238–242.

254. Taylor D, Carter R, Eison A, et al. Pharmacology and neurochemistry of nefazodone, a novel antidepressant drug. *J Clin Psychiatry* 1995;56[Suppl 6]:3–11.

255. Eison A, Eison M, Torrente J, et al. Nefazodone: preclinical pharmacology of a new antidepressant. *Psychopharmacol Bull* 1990;26:311–315.

256. Salazar D, Chaikin P, Swanson B, et al. The effects of nefazodone and fluoxetine on platelet serotonin uptake and whole blood serotonin. *Clin Pharmacol Ther* 1994;55:137.

257. Kavoussi RJ, Segraves RT, Hughes AR, et al. Double-blind comparison of bupropion sustained release and sertraline in depressed outpatients. *J Clin Psychiatry* 1997;58:532–537.

258. Goodnick PJ, Dominguez RA, DeVane L, et al. Bupropion slow-release response in depression: diagnosis and biochemistry. *Biol Psychiatry* 1998;44:629–632.

259. Reimherr FW, Cunningham LA, Batey SR, et al. A multicenter evaluation of the efficacy and safety of 150 and 300 mg/d sustained-release bupropion tablets versus placebo in depressed outpatients. *Clin Ther* 1998;20:505–516.

260. Pharmacia and Upjohn. Edronax. In: *ABPI compendium of data sheets and summaries of product characteristics 1998–99.* London: Datapharm Publications, 1998:997–998.

261. Nies A. Monoamine oxidase inhibitors. In: Paykel ES, ed. *Handbook of affective disorders.* New York: Guilford Press, 1982.

262. Coplan JD, Gorman JM. Detectable levels of fluoxetine metabolites after discontinuation: an unexpected serotonin syndrome. *Am J Psychiatry* 1993;150:837.

263. Feighner JP, Boyer WF, Tyler DL, et al. Adverse consequences of fluoxetine-MAOI combination therapy. *J Clin Psychiatry* 1990;51:222–225.

264. Frank E, Kupfer DJ, Perel JM, et al. Three-year outcomes for maintenance therapies in recurrent depression. *Arch Gen Psychiatry* 1990;47:1093–1099.

265. Kupfer DJ, Frank E, Perel JM, et al. Five year outcome for maintenance therapies in recurrent depression. *Arch Gen Psychiatry* 1992;49:769–773.

266. Davis JM. Overview: maintenance therapy in psychiatry. II. Affective disorders. *Am J Psychiatry* 1976;133:1–13.

267. Montgomery SA, Dufour H, Brion S, et al. The prophylactic efficacy of fluoxetine in unipolar depression. *Br J Psychiatry* 1988;153[Suppl 3]:69–76.

268. Eric L. A prospective, double-blind, comparative, multicentre study of paroxetine and placebo in preventing recurrent major depressive episodes. *Biol Psychiatry* 1991;29[Suppl 11]:254S–255S.

269. Doogan DP, Caillard V. Sertraline in the prevention of depression. *Br J Psychiatry* 1992;160:217–222.

270. Franchini L, Gasperini M, Perez J, et al. A double-blind study of long-term treatment with sertraline or fluvoxamine for prevention of highly recurrent unipolar depression. *J Clin Psychiatry* 1997;58:104–107.

271. Entsuah R, Rudolph R, Dervian A, et al. A low relapse rate confirms the long-term efficacy of venlafaxine in the treatment of major depression. Abstracts of Panels and Posters, Poster Session II. ACNP Meeting, Hawaii, December 1993:129.

272. Anton S, Robinson D, Roberts D, et al. Long-term treatment with nefazodone. *Psychopharmacol Bull* 1994;30:165–169.

273. Weihs K, Houser T, Batey S, et al. Long-term treatment of depression with buproprion sustained release. 40th Annual Meeting NCDEU, Boca Raton, Florida, 2000.

274. Bremner JD, Smith WT. Org 3770 vs. amitriptyline in the continuation treatment of depression: a placebo controlled trial. *Eur J Psychiatry* 1996;10:5–15.

275. Thase ME, Nierenberg A, Keller M, et al. Mirtazapine in relapse prevention. 40th Annual Meeting NCDEU, Boca Raton, Florida, 2000.

276. Versiani M, Mehilane L, Gaszner P, et al. Reboxetine, a unique selective NRI, prevents relapse and recurrence in long-term treatment of major depressive disorder. *J Clin Psychiatry* 1999;60:400–406.

277. Robinson D, Lerfald SC, Binnett B, et al. Continuation and maintenance treatment of major depression with the monoamine oxidase inhibitor phenelzine: a double-blind placebo-controlled study. *Psychopharmacol Bull* 1991;27:31–40.

278. Mindham RHS, Howland C, Shepherd M. An evaluation of continuation therapy with tricyclic antidepressants in depressive illness. *Psychol Med* 1973;3:5–17.

279. Georgotas A, McCue RE. Relapse of depressed patients after effective continuation therapy. *J Affect Disord* 1989;17:159–164.

280. Georgotas A, McCue RE, Cooper TB. A placebo controlled comparison of nortriptyline and phenelzine in maintenance therapy of elderly depressed patients. *Arch Gen Psychiatry* 1989;46:783–786.

281. Kane JM, Quitkin FM, Rifkin A, et al. Lithium carbonate and imipramine in the prophylaxis of unipolar and bipolar II illness. *Arch Gen Psychiatry* 1982;39:1065–1069.

282. Prien RF, Kupfer DJ, Mansky PA, et al. Drug therapy in the prevention of recurrences in unipolar and bipolar affective disorders. *Arch Gen Psychiatry* 1984;41:1096–1104.

283. Coppen A, Montgomery SA, Gupta RK, et al. A double-blind comparison of lithium carbonate and maprotiline in the prophylaxis of the affective disorders. *Br J Psychiatry* 1976;128:479–485.

284. Coppen A, Ghose K, Rama Rao VA, et al. Mianserin and lithium in the prophylaxis of depression. *Br J Psychiatry* 1978;133:206–210.

285. Bialos D, Giller E, Jatlow P, et al. Recurrence of depression after discontinuation of long-term amitriptyline treatment. *Am J Psychiatry* 1982;139:325–329.

286. Coppen A, Gupta R, Montgomery S, et al. A double blind comparison of lithium carbonate and Ludiomil in the prophylaxis of unipolar affective illness. *Pharmacopsychiatry* 1976;9:94–99.

287. Quitkin FM, Kane J, Rifkin A, et al. Lithium and imipramine in the prophylaxis of unipolar and bipolar II depression: a prospective, placebo-controlled comparison. *Psychopharmacol Bull* 1981;17:142–144.

288. Stein MK, Rickels K, Weise CC. Maintenance therapy with amitriptyline: a controlled trial. *Am J Psychiatry* 1980;137:370–371.

289. Kay DWK, Fahy Y, Garside RF. A seven-month double-blind trial of amitriptyline and diazepam in ECT-treated depressed patients. *Br J Psychiatry* 1970;117:667–671.

290. Souza FGM, Mander AJ, Goodwin GM. The efficacy of lithium in prophylaxis of unipolar depression: evidence from its discontinuation. *Br J Psychiatry* 1990;157:718–722.

291. Prien RF, Kupfer DJ. Continuation drug therapy for major depressive episodes: how long should it be maintained? *Am J Psychiatry* 1986;143:18–23.

292. American Psychiatric Association. Practice guidelines for MDD in adults. *Am J Psychiatry* 2000;157[Suppl 4]:1–45.

293. von Moltke LL, Greenblatt DJ, Grassi JM, et al. Citalopram and desmethylcitalopram *in vitro*: human cytochromes mediating transformation, and cytochrome inhibitory effects. *Biol Psychiatry* 1999;46:839–849.

294. Spigset O, Hagg S, Soderstrom E, et al. Lack of correlation between fluvoxamine clearance and CYP1A2 activity as measured by systemic caffeine clearance. *Eur J Clin Pharmacol* 1999;54:946–946.

295. Fjordside L, Jeppesen U, Eap CB, et al. The stereoselective metabolism of fluoxetine in poor and extensive metabolizers of sparteine. *Pharmacogenetics* 1999;9:55–60.

296. Coupland NJ, Bell CJ, Potokar JP. Serotonin reuptake inhibitor withdrawal. *J Clin Psychopharmacol* 1996;16:356–362.

297. Rosenbaum JF, Fava M, Hoog SL, et al. Selective serotonin reuptake inhibitor discontinuation syndrome: a randomized clinical trial. *Biol Psychiatry* 1998;44:77–87.

298. Kobayashi K, Ishizuka T, Shimada N, et al. Sertraline N-demethylation is catalyzed by multiple isoforms of human cytochrome P-450 in vitro. *Drug Metab Dispos* 1999;27:763–766.

299. Markowitz JS, DeVane CL. Rifampin-induced selective serotonin reuptake inhibitor withdrawal syndrome in a patient treated with sertraline. *J Clin Psychopharmacol* 2000;20:109–110.

300. Preskorn SH. A tale of two patients. *J Pract Psychiatry Behav Health* 1999;5:160–164.

301. Preskorn SH, Alderman J, Chung M, et al. Pharmacokinetics of desipramine coadministered with sertraline or fluoxetine. *J Clin Psychopharmacol* 1994;14:90–98.

302. Preskorn SH. A message from Titanic. *J Pract Psychiatry Behav Health* 1998;4:236–242.
303. Harvey AT, Preskorn SH. Fluoxetine pharmacokinetics and effect on CYP2C19 in young and elderly volunteers. *J Clin Psychopharmacol* 2000 *(in press)*.
304. Hartter S, Wetzel H, Hammes E, et al. Nonlinear pharmacokinetics of fluvoxamine and gender differences. *Ther Drug Monit* 1998;20:446–449.
305. Ronfeld R, Tremaine L, Wilner K. Pharmacokinetics of sertraline and its n-demethyl metabolite in elderly and young male and female volunteers. *Clin Pharmacokinet* 1997;32:22–30.
306. Preskorn SH, Burke M. Somatic therapy for major depressive disorder: selection of an antidepressant. *J Clin Psychiatry* 1992;53[Suppl 9]:5–18.
307. Feighner JP, Aden GC, Fabre LF, et al. Comparison of alprazolam, imipramine, and placebo in the treatment of depression. *JAMA* 1983;249:3057–3064.
308. Preskorn S. Pharmacokinetics of antidepressants: why and how they are relevant to treatment. *J Clin Psychiatry* 1993;54[Suppl 9]:14–34.
309. Preskorn S. Pharmacodynamics and pharmacokinetics of nefazodone. Wallingford Academy Meeting, London, April 1993.
310. Caccia S, Ballabio M, Samanin R, et al. (-)-m-Chlorophenyl-piperazine, a central 5-hydroxytryptamine agonist, is a metabolite of trazodone. *J Pharm Pharmacol* 1981;33:477–478.
311. Kahn R, Asiris G, Wetzler S, et al. Neuroendocrine evidence for serotonin receptor hypersensitivity in panic disorder. *Psychopharmacology* 1988;96:360–364.
312. Mayol R, Cole C, Luke G, et al. Characterization of the metabolites of the antidepressant drug nefazodone in human urine and plasma. *Drug Metab Dispos* 1994;22:304–311.
313. Kaul S, Shukla UA, Barbhaiya R. Nonlinear pharmacokinetics of nefazodone after escalating single and multiple oral doses. *J Clin Pharmacol* 1995;35:830–839.
314. Preskorn S. Should bupropion dosage be adjusted based upon therapeutic drug monitoring. *Psychopharmacol Bull* 1991;27:637–643.
315. Silkey B, Preskorn SH, Golbech A. Interindividual variability in steady-state plasma levels of bupropion and its major metabolites. 40th Annual Meeting NCDEU, Boca Raton, Florida, 2000.
316. Golden R, DeVane C, Laizure S, et al. Bupropion in depression: the role of metabolites in clinical outcome. *Arch Gen Psychiatry* 1985;45:145–149.
317. Winans EA, Cohen LJ. Assessing the clinical significance of drug interactions in psychiatry. *Psychiatr Ann* 1998;28:399–405.
318. Ekins S, Bravi G, Ring BJ, et al. Three-dimensional quantitative structure activity relationship analyses of substrates for CYP2B6. *J Pharmacol Exp Ther* 1999;288:21–29.
319. Timmer C, Voortman G, Delbressin L. Pharmacokinetic profile of mirtazapine. *Eur Neuropharmacol* 1996;6[Suppl 3]:41.
320. Verhoeven CHJ, Vos RME, Bogaards JJP. Characterization and inhibition of human cytochrome P450 enzymes involved in the in vitro metabolism of mirtazapine. Presentation at International Symposium on Microsomes and Drug Oxidations, Los Angeles, July 21–24, 1996.
321. Delbressin LP, Preskorn S, Horst D. Characterization and inhibition of P450 enzymes involved in the metabolism of mirtazapine. In: New Research Program and Abstracts of the 150th annual meeting of the American Psychiatric Association, San Diego, May 17–22, 1997.
322. Jannuzzo MG, Benedetti M, Duchene P. Pharmacokinetics of reboxetine in the elderly. 2nd International Symposium Meas Kinet In Vivo Drug Eff 1994;94–96(abst).
323. Fiorentini F, Poggesi I, Jannuzzo MG, et al. Pharmacokinetics of reboxetine, a new selective nonradrenaline uptake inhibitor, in patients with various degrees of hepatic and renal insufficiency. *Pharmacol Res* 1997;35:239–239.
324. Preskorn SH. To monitor or not to monitor. II: The glass is more than half full. *J Pract Psychiatry Behav Health* 1996;2:307–310.
325. Burke MJ, Preskorn SH. Therapeutic drug monitoring of antidepressants: cost implications and relevance to clinical practice. *Clin Pharmacokinet* 1999;37:147–165(abst).
326. Perry PJ, Pfohl BM, Holstad SG. The relationship between antidepressant response and tricyclic antidepressant plasma concentrations. *Clin Pharmacokinet* 1987;13:381–392.
327. Preskorn S, Weller E, Hughes C, et al. Depression in prepubertal children: DST nonsuppression predicts differential response to imipramine versus placebo. *Psychopharmacol Bull* 1987;23:128–133.
328. Preskorn SH, Jerkovich GS. Central nervous system toxicity of tricyclic antidepressants: phenomenology, course, risk factors, and role of therapeutic drug monitoring. *J Clin Psychopharmacol* 1990;10:88–94.
329. Preskorn SH. Therapeutic drug monitoring of tricyclic antidepressants: a means of avoiding toxicity. *Psychopharmacol Bull* 1989;7:237–243.
330. Preskorn SH, Othmer S, Lai C, et al. Tricyclic antidepressants and delirium. *J Clin Psychiatry* 1982;139:822–823.
331. Preskorn SH, Fast GA. Tricyclic antidepressant-induced seizures and plasma drug concentration. *J Clin Psychiatry* 1992;53:160–162.
332. Lowry MR, Dunner FJ. Seizures during tricyclic therapy. *Am J Psychiatry* 1980;127:1461–1462.
333. Tamayo M, deGatta F, Gutierrez JR, et al. High levels of tricyclic antidepressants in conventional therapy: determinant factors. *Int J Clin Pharmacol Ther Toxicol* 1988;26:495–499.
334. Petit JM, Spiker DG, Ruwitch JF, et al. Tricyclic antidepressant plasma levels and adverse effects after overdose. *Clin Pharmacol Ther* 1977;21:47–51.
335. Preskorn SH, Irwin H. Toxicity of tricyclic antidepressants: kinetics, mechanisms, intervention: a review. *Clin Psychiatry* 1982;143:151–156.
336. Vohra J, Burrows G, Hunt D, et al. The effects of toxic and therapeutic doses of tricyclic antidepressant drugs on intracardiac conduction. *Eur J Cardiol* 1975;3:219–227.
337. Rudorfer MB, Young RC. Desipramine: cardiovascular effects and plasma levels. *Am J Psychiatry* 1980;137:984–986.
338. Veith RC, Friedel RO, Bloom B, et al. Electrocardiogram changes and plasma desipramine levels

during treatment. *Clin Pharmacol Ther* 1980;27:796–802.

339. Preskorn SH, Baker B. Fatality associated with combined fluoxetine-amitriptyline therapy. *JAMA* 1997;277:682.

340. Preskorn SH. Sudden death and tricyclic antidepressants (TCA): a rare adverse event linked to high TCA plasma levels. *Nord J Psychiatry* 1993;47[Suppl 30]:49–55.

341. Preskorn SH. What happened to Tommy? *J Pract Psychiatry Behav Health* 1998;4:363–367.

342. Bjerkenstedt L, Flyckt L, Overo KF, et al. Relationship between clinical effects, serum drug concentration and serotonin uptake inhibition in depressed patients treated with citalopram. *Eur J Clin Pharmacol* 1985;28:553–557.

343. Dufour H, Bouchacourt M, Thermoz P, et al. Citalopram — a highly selective 5-HT reuptake inhibitor — in the treatment of depressed patients. *Int Clin Psychopharmacol* 1987;2:225–237.

344. Kelly M, Perry P, Holstad S, et al. Serum fluoxetine and norfluoxetine concentrations and antidepressant response. *Ther Drug Monit* 1989;11:165–170.

345. Preskorn SH, Silkey B, Beber J, et al. Antidepressant response and plasma concentrations of fluoxetine. *Ann Clin Psychiatry* 1991;3:147–151.

346. Kasper S, Dotsch M, Vieira A, et al. Plasma concentration of fluvoxamine and maprotiline in major depression: implications on therapeutic efficacy and side effects. *Eur Neuropsychopharmacol* 1992;3:13–21.

347. Laursen AL, Mikkelsen PL, Rasmussen S, et al. Paroxetine in the treatment of depression — a randomized comparison with amitriptyline. *Acta Psychiatr Scand* 1985;71:249–255.

348. Tasker TCG, Kaye CM, Zussman BD, et al. Paroxetine plasma levels: lack of correlation with efficacy or adverse events. *Acta Psychiatr Scand* 1989;80:152–155.

349. Franc J, Duncan G, Farmen R, et al. High-perfomance liquid chromatographic method for the determination of nefazodone and its metabolites in human plasma using laboratory robotics. *J Chromatogr Biomed Appl* 1991;570:129–138.

350. Maitre L, Baumann PA, Jaekel J, et al. 5-HT uptake inhibitors: psychopharmacological and neurobiochemical criteria of selectivity. In: Ho BT, Schoolar J, Usdin E, eds. *Serotonin in biological psychiatry.* New York: Raven Press, 1982:229–246.

351. Preskorn SH. Antidepressant response and plasma concentrations of bupropion. *J Clin Psychiatry* 1983;44:137–139.

352. Golden RN, DeVane CL, Laizure SC, et al. Bupropion in depression, II: the roles of metabolites in clinical outcome. *Arch Gen Psychiatry* 1988;45:145–149.

353. Ravaris CL, Nies A, Robinson DS, et al. A multiple-dose, controlled study of phenelzine in depression-anxiety states. *Arch Gen Psychiatry* 1976;33:347–350.

354. Bresnahan DB, Pandey GN, Janicak PG, et al. MAO inhibition and clinical response in depressed patients treated with phenelzine. *J Clin Psychiatry* 1990;51:47–50.

355. Janicak PG, Martis B. Strategies for treatment-resistant depression. *Depression Clinical Cornerstones* 1999;1(4):58–71.

356. McCombs JS, Nichol MB, Stimmel GL, et al. The cost of antidepressant drug therapy failure: a study of antidepressant use patterns in a Medicaid population. *J Clin Psychiatry* 1990;51[Suppl 6]:60–69.

357. Wells KB, Katon W, Rogers B, et al. Use of minor tranquilizers and antidepressant medications by depressed outpatients: results from the medical outcomes study. *Am J Psychiatry* 1994;151:694–700.

358. MacEwan WG, Remick RA. Treatment-resistant depression: a clinical perspective. *Can J Psychiatry* 1988;33:788–792.

359. Guscott R, Grof P. The clinical meaning of refractory depression: a review for the clinician. *Am J Psychiatry* 1991;148:695–704.

360. White K, Simpson G. Treatment resistant depression. *Psychiatr Ann* 1987;17:274–278.

361. Paykel ES, Van Waerkom AE. Pharmacologic treatment of resistant depression. *Psychiatr Ann* 1987;17:327–331.

362. Nemeroff CB. Augmentation regimens for depression. *J Clin Psychiatry* 1991;52[Suppl 5]:21–27.

363. Preskorn SH. The appearance of knowledge. *J Pract Psychiatry Behav Health* 1997;3:233–238.

364. Thase ME, Rush AJ. When at first you don't succeed: sequential strategies for antidepressant nonresponders. *J Clin Psychiatry* 1997;58:23–29.

365. McGrath PJ, Fava M, Stewart JW, et al. Bupropion SR for SSRI-resistant major depression. 40th Annual Meeting NCDEU, Boca Raton, Florida, 2000, Poster #10(abst).

366. Preskorn SH, Fleck R, Schroeder D. Therapeutic drug monitoring of bupropion. *Am J Psychiatry* 1990;147:1690–1690.

367. Thase ME, Zajecka J, Kornstein SG, et al. Nefazodone treatment of patients with poor response to SSRIs. 37th Annual meeting of the American College of Neuropsychopharmacology, San Juan, Puerto Rico, 1998.

368. Mischoulon D, Opitz G, Kelly K, et al. A pilot study on the effectiveness of nefazodone in depressed outpatients with or without a history of SSRI treatment failure. 40th Annual Meeting NCDEU, Boca Raton, Florida, 2000, Poster #8(abst).

369. Wheatley DP, van Moffaert M, Timmerman L, et al. Mirtazapine: efficacy and tolerability in comparison with fluoxetine in patients with moderate to severe major depression disorder. Mirtazapine-fluoxetine study group. *J. Clin Psychiatry* 1998;59(6):306–312.

370. Fava M, Dunner D, Griest J, et al. An open-label study with mirtazapine in depressed patients who are SSRI treatment failures. New Research Program Abstracts, 152nd Annual Meeting of the American Psychiatric Association, Chicago, 2000;186(abst).

371. Heninger GR, Charney DS, Sternberg DE. Lithium carbonate augmentation of anti-depressant treatment. *Arch Gen Psychiatry* 1983;40:1335–1342.

372. Nelson JC, Mazure CM. Lithium augmentation in psychotic depression refractory to combined drug treatment. *Am J Psychiatry* 1986;143:363–366.

373. Pope HG, McElroy SL, Nixon RA. Possible synergism between fluoxetine and lithium in refractory depression. *Am J Psychiatry* 1988;145:1292–1294.

374. Fava M, Rosenbaum JF, McGrath PJ, et al. Lithium and tricyclic augmentation of fluoxetine treatment for

resistant major depression: A double-blind, controlled study. *Am J Psychiatry* 1994;151:1372–1374.

375. Katona CL, Abou-Saleh MT, Harrison DA, et al. Placebo-controlled trial of lithium augmentation of fluoxetine and lofepramine. *Br J Psychiatry* 1995;166:80–86.

376. Salama AA, Shafey M. A case of severe lithium toxicity induced by combined fluoxetine and lithium carbonate [Letter]. *Am J Psychiatry* 1989;146:278.

377. Aronson R, Offman HJ, Joffe T, et al. Triiodothyronine augmentation in the treatment of refractory depression: a meta-analysis. *Arch Gen Psychiatry* 1996;53:842–848.

378. Blier P, Bergeron R. The use of pindolol to potentiate antidepressant medication. *J Clin Psychiatry* 1998;59(S5):16–23, 24–25.

379. Moreno F, Gelenberg AJ, Bachar K, et al. Pindolol augmentation of treatment-resistant depressed patients. *J Clin Psychiatry* 1997;58:437–439.

380. Perez V, Soler J, Puigdemont D, et al. A double-blind, randomized, placebo-controlled trial of pindolol augmentation in depressive patients resistant to serotonin reuptake inhibitors. *Arch Gen Psychiatry* 1999;56:375–379.

381. Berman RM, Anand A, Cappiello A, et al. The use of pindolol with fluoxetine in the treatment of major depression: final results from a double-blind, placebo-controlled trial. *Biol Psychiatry* 1999;45:1170–1177.

382. Landen M, Bjorling G, Agren H, et al. A randomized, double-blind, placebo-controlled trial of buspirone in combination with an SSRI in patients with treatment-refractory depression. *J Clin Psychiatry* 1998;59:664–668.

383. Preskorn SH. Do you believe in magic? *J Pract Psychiatry Behav Health* 1997;3:99–103.

384. Fava M. New approaches to the treatment of refractory depression. *J Clin Psychiatry* 2000;61:26–32.

385. Anton RF, Burch EA. Amoxapine versus amitriptyline combined with perphenazine in the treatment of psychotic depression. *Am J Psychiatry* 1990;147:1203–1208.

386. Post RM, Kramlinger KG. The addition of lithium to carbamazepine. Antidepressant efficacy in treatment-resistant depression. *Arch Gen Psychiatry* 1989;46:794–800.

387. Kupfer DJ, Frank E, Perel JM. The advantage of early treatment intervention in recurrent depression. *Arch Gen Psychiatry* 1989;46:771–775.

388. Rush AJ, Beck AT, Kovacs M, et al. Comparative efficacy of cognitive therapy and pharmacotherapy in the treatment of depressed outpatients. *Cognit Ther Res* 1977;1:17–37.

389. Blackburn IM, Bishop S, Glen AIM, et al. The efficacy of cognitive therapy in depression: a treatment trial using cognitive therapy and pharmacotherapy, each alone and in combination. *Br J Psychiatry* 1981;139:181–189.

390. Murphy GE, Simons AD, Wetzel RD, et al. Cognitive therapy and pharmacotherapy, singly and together in the treatment of depression. *Arch Gen Psychiatry* 1984;4:33–41.

391. Elkin I, Shea, MT, Watkins JT, et al. National Institute of Mental Health Treatment of Depression Collaborative Research Program: general effectiveness of treatments. *Arch Gen Psychiatry* 1989;46:971–982.

392. Hollon SD, DeRubeis RJ, Evans MD, et al. Cognitive-therapy and pharmacotherapy for depression: singly and in combination. *Arch Gen Psychiatry* 1992;49:774–781.

393. McKnight DL, Nelson-Gray RO, Barnhill J. Dexamethasone suppression test and response to cognitive therapy and antidepressant medication. *Behav Ther* 1992;1:99–111.

394. Blackburn IM, Moore RG. Controlled acute and follow-up trial of cognitive therapy and pharmacotherapy in outpatients with recurrent depression. *Br J Psychiatry* 1997;171:328–334.

395. Thase ME, Friedman ES, Berman SR, et al. Is cognitive behavior just a 'nonspecific' intervention for depression? A retrospective comparison of consecutive cohorts treated with cognitive behavior therapy or supportive counseling and pill placebo. *J Affect Disord* 2000;57:63–71.

396. DeRubeis RJ, Gelfand LA, Tang TZ, et al. Medications versus cognitive behavior therapy for severely depressed outpatients: mega-analysis of four randomized comparisons. *Am J Psychiatry* 1999;156:1007–1013.

397. Keller MB, McCullough JP, Klein DN, et al. A comparison of nefazodone, the cognitive behavioral analysis system of psychotherapy, and their combination for the treatment of chronic depression. *N Engl J Med* 2000;342:1462–1470.

398. Meterissian BG, Bradwejn J. Comparative studies on the efficacy of psychotherapy, pharmacotherapy, and their combination in depression: was adequate pharmacotherapy provided? *J Clin Psychopharmacol* 1989;9:334–339.

399. Klein DF. Preventing hung juries about therapy studies. *J Consult Clin Psychol* 1996;64:74–80.

400. Klerman GL, Dimascio A, Weissman M, et al. Treatment of depression by drugs and psychotherapy. *Am J Psychiatry* 1974;131:186–191.

401. Weissman MM, Klerman GL, Paykel ES, et al. Treatment effects on the social adjustment of depressed patients. *Arch Gen Psychiatry* 1974;30:771–778.

402. Klerman GL, Weissman MM, Rounsaville BJ, et al. *Interpersonal psychotherapy of depression.* New York: Basic Books, 1984.

403. Weissman MM, Jarrett RB, Rush JA. Psychotherapy and its relevance to the pharmacotherapy of major depression: a decade later (1976–1985). In: Meltzer HV, ed. *Psychopharmacology: the third generation of progress.* New York: Raven Press, 1987:1059–1069.

404. Coui L, Lipman RS, Derogatis LR, et al. Drugs and group psychotherapy in neurotic depression. *Am J Psychiatry* 1974;131:191–198.

405. Frank E, Kupfer D, Perel J, et al. Three-year outcomes for maintenance therapies in recurrent depression. *Arch Gen Psychiatry* 1990;47:1093–1099.

406. Fava GA, Rafanelli C, Grandi S, et al. Prevention of recurrent depression with cognitive behavioral therapy: preliminary findings. *Arch Gen Psychiatry* 1998;55:816–820.

407. Baldessarini R. Current status of antidepressants: clinical pharmacology and therapy. *J Clin Psychiatry* 1989;50:117–126.

408. Richelson E. Pharmacology of antidepressants in use in the United States. *J Clin Psychiatry* 1982;43:4–11.

409. Preskorn S. Tricyclic antidepressants: the whys and

hows of therapeutic drug monitoring. *J Clin Psychiatry* 1989;50[Suppl 7]:34–42.

410. Preskorn S, Irwin H. Toxicity of tricyclic antidepressants—kinetics, mechanism, intervention: a review. *J Clin Psychiatry* 1982;43:151–156.

411. Preskorn S, Fast G. Therapeutic drug monitoring for antidepressants: efficacy, safety and cost effectiveness. *J Clin Psychiatry* 1991;52:23–33.

412. Williams RB, Shertu C. Cardiac complications of tricyclic antidepressant therapy. *Ann Intern Med* 1971;74:395–398.

413. Glassman AH, Roose SP. Cardiovascular effects of tricyclic antidepressants. *Psychiatr Ann* 1987;17:340–347.

414. Roose SP, Glassman AH, Giardina EGV, et al. Nortriptyline in depressed patients with left ventricular impairment. *JAMA* 1986;256:3253–3257.

415. Giardina EGV, Bigger JT Jr, Glassman AH. Comparison between imipramine and desmethylimipramine on the electrocardiogram and left ventricular function. *Clin Pharmacol Ther* 1982;31:230.

416. Giardina EGV, Johnson LL, Vita J, Bigger JT Jr, et al. Effect of imipramine and nortriptyline on left ventricular function and blood pressure in patients treated for arrhythmias. *Am Heart J* 1985;109:992–998.

417. Muller OF, Goodman N, Bellet S. The hypotensive effect of imipramine hydrochloride in patients with cardiovascular disease. *Clin Pharmacol Ther* 1961;2:300–307.

418. Roose SP. Modern cardiovascular standards for psychotropic drugs. *Psychopharmacol Bull* 1992;28:35–43.

419. Roose SP, Glassman AH, Giardina EGV, et al. Tricyclic antidepressants in depressed patients with cardiac conduction disease. *Arch Gen Psychiatry* 1987;44:273–275.

420. Bigger JT, Giardina EGV, Perel JM, et al. Cardiac antiarrhythmic effect of imipramine hydrochloride. *N Engl J Med* 1977;296:206–208.

421. Cardiac Arrhythmia Pilot Study Investigators. Effects of encainide, flecainide, imipramine and moricizine on ventricular arrhythmias during the year after acute myocardial infarction: the CAPS. *Am J Cardiol* 1988;61:501–509.

422. Giardina EGV, Bigger JT Jr, Glassman AH, et al. The electrocardiographic and antiarrhythmic effects of imipramine hydrochloride at therapeutic plasma concentrations. *Circulation* 1979;60:1045–1052.

423. Glassman AH, Johnson LL, Giardina EGV, et al. The use of imipramine in depressed patients with congestive heart failure. *JAMA* 1983;250:1997–2001.

424. Roose SP, Glassman AH. Cardiovascular effects of TCAs in depressed patients with and without heart disease. *J Clin Psychiatry Monogr Ser* 1989;7:1–18.

425. Richelson E. Review of antidepressants in the treatment of mood disorders. In: Dunner OL. *Current Psychiatry Therapy.* 2nd ed. Philadelphia: WB Saunders, 1997:286–295.

426. Davidson J. Seizures and bupropion: a review. *J Clin Psychiatry* 1989;50:256–261.

427. Glassman AH, Davis JM. Overdose with tricyclic drugs. *Psychiatr Ann* 1987;17:410–411.

428. Callaham M, Kassel D. Epidemiology of fatal tri-

cyclic antidepressant ingestion: implications for management. *Ann Emerg Med* 1985;14:1–9.

429. Sedal L, Korman MG, Williams PO, et al. Overdose of tricyclic antidepressants; a report of two deaths and a prospective study of 24 patients. *Med J Aust* 1972;2:74–79.

430. Sunshine P, Yaffe SJ. Amitriptyline poisoning; clinical and pathological findings in a fatal case. *Am J Dis Child* 1963;106:501–506.

431. Boehnert MT, Lovejoy FH Jr. Value of the QRS duration versus the serum drug level in predicting seizures and ventricular arrhythmias after an acute overdose of tricyclic antidepressants. *N Engl J Med* 1985;313:474–479.

432. Swartz CM, Sherman A. The treatment of tricyclic antidepressant overdose with repeated charcoal. *J Clin Psychopharmacol* 1984;4:336–340.

433. Bech P. Clinical effects of selective serotonin reuptake inhibitors. In: Dahl S, Graham L, eds. *Clinical pharmacology in psychiatry. From molecular studies to clinical reality.* Berlin: Springer-Verlag, 1989:81–93.

434. Benfield P, Heel R, Lewis S. Fluoxetine: a review of its pharmacodynamic and pharmacokinetic properties and therapeutic efficacy in depressive illness. *Drugs* 1986;32:481–508.

435. Boyer W, Feighner J. An overview of fluoxetine, a new serotonin-specific antidepressant. *Mt Sinai J Med* 1989;56:136–140.

436. Rickels K, Schweizer E. Clinical overview of serotonin reuptake inhibitors. *J Clin Psychiatry* 1990;51[Suppl 12B]:9–12.

437. Stark P, Fuller R, Wong D. The pharmacologic profile of fluoxetine. *J Clin Psychiatry* 1985;46:7–13.

438. Fabre L, Scharf M, Turan M. Comparative efficacy and safety of nortriptyline and fluoxetine in the treatment of major depression: a clinical study. *J Clin Psychiatry* 1991;52[Suppl 6]:62–67.

439. Beasley CM, Dornseif BE, Pultz JA, et al. Fluoxetine versus trazodone: efficacy and activating-sedating effects. *J Clin Psychiatry* 1991;52:294–299.

440. Altamura A, Montgomery S, Wernicke J. The evidence for 20 mg a day of fluoxetine as the optimal in the treatment of depression. *Br J Psychiatry* 1988;153[Suppl 3]:109–112.

441. Teicher M, Glod C, Cole J. Emergence of intense suicidal preoccupation during fluoxetine treatment. *Am J Psychiatry* 1990;147:207–210.

442. Wirshing W, Van Putten T, Rosenberg J, et al. Fluoxetine, akathisia and suicidality: is there a causal connection [Letter]? *Arch Gen Psychiatry* 1992;49:580–581.

443. Mann J, Kapur S. The emergence of suicidal ideation and behavior during antidepressant pharmacotherapy. *Arch Gen Psychiatry* 1991;48:1027–1033.

444. Fava M, Rosenbaum J. Suicidality and fluoxetine: is there a relationship? *J Clin Psychiatry* 1991;52:108–111.

445. Nurnberg HG, Gelenberg AJ, Fava M, et al. Sildenafil for SRI associated sexual dysfunction: a three-center six weeks double blind placebo controlled study in 90 men. 40th Annual Meeting NCDEU, Boca Raton, Florida, 2000.

446. Sambunaris A, Hesselink JK, Pinder R, et al. Development of new antidepressants. *J Clin Psychiatry* 1998;58:40–53.

447. Muth EA, Moyer JA, Haskins JT, et al. Husbands GEM. Biochemical, neurophysiological, and behavioral effects of Wy-45,233 and other identified metabolites of the antidepressant venlafaxine. *Drug Dev Res* 1991;23:191–199.

448. Bolden-Watson C, Richelson E. Blockade by newly developed antidepressants of biogenic amine uptake into rat brain synaptosomes. *Life Sci* 1993;52:1023–1029.

449. Grunder G, Wetzel H, Schloer R, et al. Subchronic antidepressant treatment with venlafaxine or imipramine and effects on blood pressure: assessment by automatic 24 hour monitoring. *Pharmacopsychiatry* 1993;26:155.

450. Feighner J. The role of venlafaxine in rational antidepressant therapy. *J Clin Psychiatry* 1994;55[Suppl 9A]:62–68.

451. Fontaine R, Ontiveros A, Elie R, et al. A double-blind comparison of nefazodone, imipramine, and placebo in major depression. *J Clin Psychiatry* 1994;55:234–241.

452. Cusack B, Nelson A, Richelson E. Binding of antidepressants to human brain receptors: focus on newer generation compounds. *Psychopharmacology* 1994;114:559–565.

453. Clayton AH, McGarvey EL, Warnock J, et al. Bupropion SR as an antidote to SSRI-induced sexual dysfunction. 40th Annual Meeting NCDEU, Boca Raton, Florida, 2000.

454. Zajecka J, Dunner DL, Hirschfeld R, et al. Sexual function and satisfaction in the treatment of chronic depression with nefazodone, psychotherapy and their combination. 40th Annual Meeting NCDEU, Boca Raton, Florida, 2000.

455. Glaxo Wellcome Inc. Bupropion SR in the treatment of SSRI-induced sexual dysfunction. 40th Annual Meeting NCDEU, Boca Raton, Florida, 2000.

456. Rudorfer M, Potter W. The new generation of antidepressants. In: Extein I, ed. *Treatment of tricyclic resistant depression.* Washington, DC: American Psychiatric Press, 1989.

457. Warner M, Peabody C, Whiteford H, et al. Trazodone and priapism. *J Clin Psychiatry* 1987;48:244–245.

458. Brindley G. Pilot experiments on the actions of drugs injected into the human corpus cavernosum penis. *Br J Pharmacol* 1986;87:495–500.

459. Goldstein I, et al. Pharmacologic detumescence: the alternative to surgical shunting. *J Urol* 1986;135:308A.

460. Pantaleo-Gandais M, Chalbaud R, Charcon O, et al. Priapism evaluation and treatment. *Urology* 1984;24:345–346.

461. Preskorn S, Othmer S. Evaluation of bupropion hydrochloride: the first of a new class of atypical antidepressants. *Pharmacotherapy* 1984;4:20–34.

462. Dager S, Heritch A. A case of bupropion-associated delirium. *J Clin Psychiatry* 1990;51:307–308.

463. Golden R, James S, Sherer M. Psychosis associated with bupropion treatment. *Am J Psychiatry* 1985;142:1459–1462.

464. Liberzon I, Dequardo J, Silk K. Bupropion and delirium. *Am J Psychiatry* 1990;147:1689–1690.

465. Labbate LA, Grimes JB, Hines A, et al. Bupropion treatment of serotonin reuptake antidepressant-associated sexual dysfunction. *Ann Clin Psychiatry* 1997;9:241–245.

466. Labbate LA, Brodrick PS, Nelson RP, et al. Effects of bupropion SR on sexual functioning and nocturnal erections in healthy men. 40th Annual Meeting NCDEU, Boca Raton, Florida, 2000(abst).

467. Ashton AK, Rosen RC. Bupropion as an antidote for serotonin reuptake inhibitor-induced sexual dysfunction. *J Clin Psychiatry* 1998;59:112–115.

468. Johnston JA, Lineberry CG, Ascher JA, et al. A 102-center prospective study of seizure in association with bupropion. *J Clin Psychiatry* 1991;52:450–456.

469. Perumal A, Smith T, Suckow R, et al. Effect of plasma from patients containing bupropion and its metabolites on the uptake of norepinephrine. *Neuropharmacology* 1986;25:199–202.

470. Nelson JC. Safety and tolerability of the new antidepressants. *J Clin Psychiatry* 1997;58:26–31.

471. Bremner JD, Freeman AM, Norum D, et al. Safety of mirtazapine in overdose. *J Clin Psychiatry* 1998;59:233–235.

472. Montgomery S. Safety of mirtazapine: a review. *Int Clin Psychopharmacol* 1995;10[Suppl 4]:37–45.

473. Mucci M. Reboxetine: a review of antidepressant tolerability. *J Psychopharmacol* 1997;11:33–37.

474. Ban TA, Gaszner P, Aguglia E, et al. Clinical efficacy of reboxetine: a comparative study with desipramine, with methodological considerations. *Hum Psychopharmacol* 1998;13:S29–S39

475. Berzewski H, Van-Moffaert M, Gagiano CA. Efficacy and tolerability of reboxetine compared with imipramine in a double-blind study in patients suffering from major depressive episodes. *Eur Neuropsychopharmacol* 1997;7:S37–S47

476. Massana J. Reboxetine versus fluoxetine: an overview of efficacy and tolerability. *J Clin Psychiatry* 1998;59:8–10.

477. Robinson D, Kurtz W. Monoamine oxidase inhibiting drugs: pharmacologic and therapeutic issues. In: Meltzer H, ed. *Psychopharmacology: the third generation of progress.* New York: Raven Press, 1987.

478. Rabkin J, Quitkin F, Harrison W, et al. Adverse reactions to monoamine oxidase inhibitors. Part I. A comparative study. *J Clin Psychopharmacol* 1984;4:270–278.

479. Ravaris CL, Robinson DS, Ives JO, et al. Phenelzine and amitriptyline in the treatment of depression. A comparison of present and past studies. *Arch Gen Psychiatry* 1980;37:1075–1080.

480. Robinson D, Kayser A, Bennett B, et. al. Maintenance phenelzine treatment of major depression: an interim report. *Psychopharmacol Bull* 1986;22:553–557.

481. Holm M, Olesen F. Prescribing of psychotropic drugs in general practice. *Ugskr Laeger* 1989;151:2122–2126.

482. Preskorn SH. Do you feel lucky? *J Pract Psychiatry BehavHealth* 1998;4(1):37–40.

483. Coulehan JL, Schulberg HC, Block MR, et al. Depressive symptomatology and medical co-morbidity in a primary care clinic. *Int J Psychiatry Med* 1990;20:335–347.

484. Wolf ME, Bukowski ED, Conran J, et al. Polypharmacy: a problem of the decade of the nineties. American Psychiatric Association, 148th Annual Meeting, Miami, Florida, May 20–25, 1995:222.

485. Harvey AT, Preskorn SH. Cytochrome P450 enzymes: interpretation of their interactions with SSRIs (Part I). *J Clin Psychopharmacol* 1996;16:273–285.

486. Harvey AT, Preskorn SH. Cytochrome P450 enzymes: interpretation of their interactions with selective serotonin reuptake inhibitors (Part II). *J Clin Psychopharmacol* 1996;16:345–355.

487. Nelson DR, Kamataki T, Waxman DJ, et al. The P450 superfamily: update on new sequence, gene mapping, accession numbers, early trivial names of enzymes, and nomenclature. *DNA Cell Biol* 1993;12:1–51.

488. Nebert DW, Nelson DR, Feyereisen R. Evolution of the cytochrome P450 genes. *Xenobiotica* 1989;19:1149–1160.

489. Gonzalez FJ, Gelboin HV. Human cytochromes P450: evolution and cDNA-directed expression. *Environ Health Perspect* 1992;98:81–85.

490. Sternbach H. The serotonin syndrome. *Am J Psychiatry* 1991;148:705–713.

491. Tailor SAN, Shulman KI, Walker SE, et al. Hypertensive episode associated with phenelzine and tap beer — a reanalysis of the role of pressor amines in beer. *J Clin Psychopharmacol* 1994;14:5–14.

492. Shulman KI, Walker SE, MacKenzie S, et al. Dietary restrictions, tyramine, and the use of monoamine oxidase inhibitors. *J Clin Psychopharmacol* 1989;9:397–402.

493. Thakore J, Dinan TG, Kelleher M. Alcohol-free beer and the irreversible monoamine oxidase inhibitors. *Int Clin Psychopharmacol* 1992;7:59–60.

494. Harvey AT, Preskorn SH. Interactions of serotonin reuptake inhibitors with tricyclic antidepressants. *Arch Gen Psychiatry* 1995;52:783–784.

495. von Moltke L, Greenblatt D, Schmider J, et al. Metabolism of drugs by cytochrome P450 3A isoforms. *Clin Pharmacokinet* 1995;29[Suppl 1]:33–44.

496. Ferslew KE, Hagardorn AN, Harlan GC, et al. A fatal drug interaction between clozapine and fluoxetine. *J Forensic Sci* 1998;43:1082–1085.

497. Musshoff F, Grellner W, Madea B. Toxicologic findings in suicide with doxepin and paroxetine. *Arch Kriminol* 1999;204:28–32.

498. Rosenblatt J, Rosenblatt N. More about spontaneous postmarketing reports of bupropion related seizures. *Curr Affect Illness* 1992;11:18–20.

499. Sternbach H. Danger of MAOI therapy after fluoxetine withdrawal [Letter]. Lancet 1988;ii:850–851.

500. Ciraulo D, Shader R. Fluoxetine drug-drug interactions I: antidepressants and antipsychotics. *J Clin Psychopharmacol* 1990;10:48–50; Part II. *J Clin Psychopharmacol* 1990;10:213–217.

501. Shad MU, Preskorn SH. Antidepressants. In: Levy R, Thummel KE, Trager W, et al., eds. *Metabolic drug interactions.* Philadelphia: Lippincott Williams & Wilkins, 2000.

502. Frewer L, Lader M. The effects of nefazodone, imipramine, and placebo, alone and combined with alcohol in normal subjects. *Int Clin Psychopharmacol* 1993;8:13–20.

503. Cooper B, Hester T, Maxwell R. Behavioral and biochemical effects of the antidepressant bupropion (Wellbutrin): evidence of selective blockade of dopamine uptake *in vivo.* *J Pharmacol Exp Ther* 1980;215:127–134.

504. Ferris R, Maxwell R, Cooper B, et al. Neurochemical and neuropharmacological investigations into the mechanisms of action and bupropion hydrochloride — a new atypical antidepressant agent. In: Costa E, Racogoni B, eds. *Typical and atypical antidepressants: molecular mechanisms.* New York: Raven Press, 1982.

505. Frazer A. Antidepressants. *J Clin Psychiatry* 1997;58:9–25.

506. Benazzi F. Serotonin syndrome with mirtazapine — fluoxetine combination [Letter]. *Int J Geriatr Psychiatry* 1998;13:493–496.

507. Preskorn SH, Omo K, Shad MU. Mirtazapine treatment following fluoxetine discontinuation: the safety of an immediate switch. *Clin Ther* 2000; *(in press).*

508. McCabe B. Dietary tyramine and other pressor amines in MAOI regimens: a review. *J Am Diet Assoc* 1986;76:1059–1064.

509. Folks D. Monoamine oxidase inhibitors: reappraisal of dietary considerations. *J Clin Psychopharmacol* 1979;40:33–37.

510. Richard IH, Kurlan R, Tanner C, et al. Serotonin syndrome and the combined use of deprenyl and an antidepressant in Parkinson's disease. Neurology 1997;48:1070–1077.

511. Ramin SM, Little BB, Gilstrap LC. Psychotropics in pregnancy. In: Gilstrap LC, Little BB, eds. *Drugs and pregnancy.* New York: Elsevier, 1992:154–174.

512. Goldberg HL. Psychotropic drugs in pregnancy and lactation. *Int J Psychiatry Med* 1994;24:129–147.

513. Chambers CD, Johnson KA, Dick LM, et al. Birth outcomes in pregnant women taking fluoxetine. *N Engl J Med* 1996;335:1010–1015.

514. Pastuszak A, Schick-Boschetto B, Zuber C, et al. Pregnancy outcome following first trimester exposure to fluoxetine (Prozac). *JAMA* 1993;269:2246–2248.

515. Goldstein DJ. Effects of third trimester fluoxetine exposure on the newborn. *J Clin Psychopharmacol* 1995:15:417–420.

516. Stanford MS, Patton JH. In utero exposure to fluoxetine HCl increases hematoma frequency at birth. *Pharmacol Biochem Behav* 1993;45:959–962.

517. Di Pasquale E, Monteau R, Hilaire G. Endogenous serotonin modulates the fetal respiratory rhythm: an *in vitro* study in the rat. *Brain Res Dev* 1994:80:222–232.

518. Romero G, Toscano E, Del Rio J. Effect of prenatal exposure to antidepressants on 5-HT–stimulated phosphoinositide hydrolysis and 5-HT2 receptors in rat brain. *Gen Pharmacol* 1994;25:851–856.

519. Cabrera TM, Battaglia G. Delayed decreases in brain 5-hydroxytryptamine 2A/2C receptor density and function in male rat progeny following prenatal fluoxetine. *J Pharmacol Exp Ther* 1994;269:637–645.

520. Yavarone MS, Shuey DL, Tamir H, et al. Serotonin and cardiac morphogenesis in the mouse embryo. *Teratology* 1993;47:573–584.

521. Shuey DL, Sadler TW, Lauder JM. Serotonin as a regulator of craniofacial morphogenesis: site specific malformations following exposure to serotonin uptake inhibitors. *Teratology* 1992;46:367–378.

8

Treatment with Electroconvulsive Therapy and Other Somatic Therapies

Somatic therapies have had a long and at times dubious history in the treatment of mental disorders. Clearly, electroconvulsive therapy (ECT) has stood the test of time but has also been plagued by problems in terms of misuse, underuse, a complicated administration process, cognitive adverse effects, and a negative public image. Even so, ECT remains the most effective treatment for some of the most severely ill, medication-refractory, or medication-intolerant patients, often proving to be lifesaving (1).

Still, the development of effective, safer, and relatively cost-effective treatments is essential. In this light, although ECT continues to be the gold standard of somatic therapies, other approaches such as bright light therapy, transcranial magnetic stimulation, and vagal nerve stimulation are engendering increased interest (1, 2).

ELECTROCONVULSIVE THERAPY

ECT is the most effective treatment for more severe depressive disorders, often characterized by melancholic and/or psychotic features. Although primarily used for an acute episode, ECT may also be a useful maintenance strategy for patients with frequent relapses despite adequate pharmacotherapy.

The use of electrical stimulation to induce therapeutic seizures is the safest and most efficient form of convulsive therapy (e.g., as compared with pharmacoconvulsive therapy). In 1938, Cerletti and Bini (3) were the first to attempt this approach, and until the introduction of effective pharmacotherapy, ECT remained the primary treatment for more severe mood and psychotic episodes. Since then, however, this somatic therapy has been relegated to a secondary role, usually attempted after trials with standard psychotropics (e.g., antidepressants, antipsychotics,

lithium, and other mood stabilizers, often in multiple combinations) have proved inadequate.

Uneasiness concerning the passage of electricity through the human brain to induce seizures (a phenomenon otherwise considered pathologic) has contributed to the controversy surrounding this treatment. Thus, despite the lack of supporting documentation, some groups have continued to raise concerns about irreversible memory loss and possible brain damage after ECT (4–6). Furthermore, during its zenith, ECT was used in a wide range of cases now deemed inappropriate. Reports in the United States and the United Kingdom found that training was often inadequate and that a large proportion of facilities administered ECT improperly (7–10). Kramer (11) and the APA task force on ECT (11a) have recently presented outlines for teaching ECT that attempt to address deficits in training programs. Partly as a result of these factors, strident antipsychiatry forces have attempted to eliminate or severely curtail its use. For example, legislative restrictions were attempted in Berkeley, California, in the early 1980's and in Texas in the early 1990's. In contrast, the attitudes of professionals regarding the use of ECT are more favorable as their levels of knowledge and experience increase (12, 13).

Figure 8-1 outlines the role for ECT and possibly for other somatic interventions in the overall treatment strategy we propose throughout this book. We also believe that ECT should be considered as a first-line treatment in patients with a previous good response to ECT and in those who have been nonresponsive to or intolerant of standard pharmacotherapy in the past. Furthermore, for patients who present as high risks (e.g., acute suicidality or rapid physical deterioration), this treatment may be lifesaving. Finally, in patients who express a preference for this efficient,

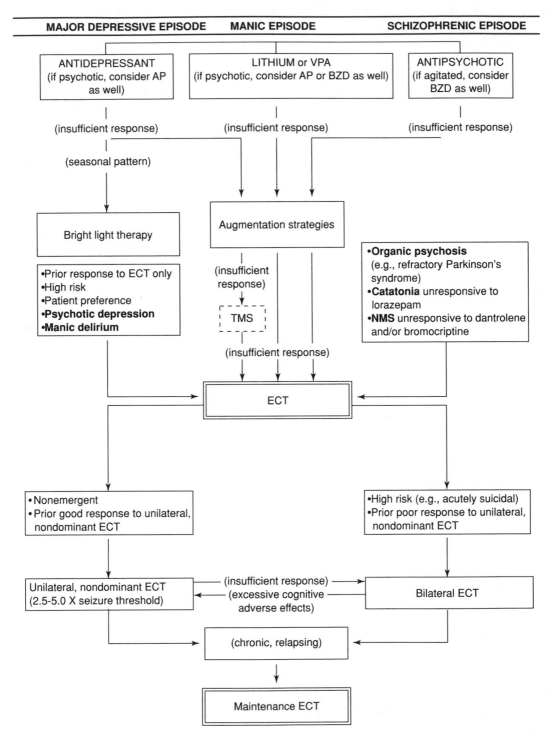

FIG. 8-1. The role of electroconvulsive therapy (ECT) and possibly of other somatic therapies in the treatment of psychiatric disorders. Adapted from Martis and Janicak, 2000.

rapidly acting, relatively short-term treatment, ECT may be an appropriate first-line therapy. For example, a report found that when compared with pharmacotherapy, ECT significantly shortened hospital lengths of stay, as well as overall cost, for patients with a major depressive disorder (14, 15).

Mechanism of Action

ECT produces improvement in the following:

- *Mood*
- *Sleep*
- *Appetite,* with associated weight gain
- *Sexual* drive
- General *interest* in the environment

Generally, theories on the mechanism of action of ECT in humans have paralleled those posited for effective mood-stabilizing pharmacotherapy, for example:

- Effect on various *neurotransmitters*
- *Antikindling* effect
- *Anticonvulsant* effect
- *Diencephalic* stimulation
- Resolution of *hemispheric dysfunction* (16)

In humans, the focus has been on pretreatment and posttreatment changes in platelets, lymphocytes, and amine metabolites in the body fluids of depressed patients (17). Although direct studies have not been possible, magnetic resonance spectroscopy allows for the noninvasive study of neurochemical changes in the human brain associated with depression and recovery, including investigations of the mechanism of action of ECT (18).

More recently, signal transduction via guanosine triphosphate-binding proteins (G-proteins) has been investigated because of the role these compounds play in transmitting extracellular signals initiated at the receptor level to a variety of intracellular effectors. Abnormalities in G-protein expression or function have been implicated in various medical and neuropsychiatric disorders, and several psychotropics are known to affect G-protein activity (19). Given their ubiquitous role in neuronal function, it is plausible that they are involved in psychiatric disorders (e.g., major depression). Existing treatments

and potential novel, site-specific drugs that target these proteins may help clarify pathophysiology, as well as the mechanism of action of various drug and somatic therapies. In this context, studies have shown that G-proteins (inhibitory and stimulatory) in mononuclear leukocytes and platelets are decreased in depression and increased in bipolar disorder (20–22). Furthermore, ECT has been shown to normalize G-protein function in both conditions (23). This normalization precedes and predicts improvement in depressed patients receiving ECT. One possibility is that ECT may stabilize dysregulated intracellular signaling, which explains why it is effective for both mania and depression. Of note, lithium and antidepressants have also been found to normalize G-protein functions (24, 25) (see Chapter 7, "Mechanism of Action").

Neurotransmitter Theories

The *amine hypothesis* of depressive mood disorders postulates a critical disruption in one or more neurotransmitters [e.g., norepinephrine or serotonin (5-HT)], culminating in a dysregulation of their activity and leading to characteristic behavioral and vegetative symptoms. Electroshock (ECS) in animals increases norepinephrine, serotonin, and dopamine synthesis in the CNS. It induces downregulation of postsynaptic β_1- and β_2-receptors in peripheral tissue (e.g., platelets), but, interestingly and differently from tricyclic antidepressants and monoamine oxidase inhibitors, appears to upregulate 5-HT_2 postsynaptic receptors (26–28). Results from both animal and human studies have been inconsistent, with potential confounds including the following:

- The use of *brain tissue in animals versus peripheral tissues in humans,* as well as the differential effects of ECS in animals versus ECT in human subjects, respectively
- A predominance of norepinephrine β_1-*receptors in the CNS* and of norepinephrine β_2-receptors in peripheral tissues
- Findings of receptor activity differences in normal young animals, with their own species-specific biochemistry and physiology, which cannot be easily generalized to baseline and

posttreatment differences in *normal humans* or *depressed patients*

A further elaboration on these theories considers the modulating interactions among several neurotransmitter systems (e.g., the *permissive hypothesis,* the *cholinergic-adrenergic balance hypothesis*). Other neurotransmitters implicated include dopamine, γ-aminobutyric acid (GABA), and endogenous opiates, all of which subserve many of the vegetative functions disrupted in depressive states. One intriguing example is the connection postulated among dopamine, GABA, and major depression, in part based on the efficacy of ECT in Parkinson's disease (see Chapter 7, "Mechanism of Action") (29–31).

Neuroendocrine Theory

Another approach considers the effects of various ligands on their receptors located in the diencephalic and mesiotemporal areas. Cell clusters in the hypothalamus coordinate the normal regulation of the vegetative functions of sleep, appetite, and sexual drive, which are typically disrupted in severe depression. In addition, the limbic area modulates many aspects of behavior and mood that are characteristically disturbed in affective disorders.

Fink and Nemeroff (32) postulated the existence of a neuropeptide, "*antidepressin,*" that is released by diencephalic stimulation and enhances hypothalamic, and perhaps limbic, function. Repeated ECT-induced seizures and the resultant increased levels of acetylcholine may promote the production of this putative peptide. In support of their theory, these authors discuss several lines of evidence. Using the analogy of the insulin-diabetes model, they note that:

- ECT enhances the production and *release of several neuropeptides* (including insulin), some of which have demonstrated transient antidepressant effects (e.g., thyrotropin-releasing hormone).
- *Vegetative* (e.g., appetite, sleep, sexual drive) and *neuroendocrine* (e.g., hypercortisolism) *dysregulation,* characteristic of severe depression and mediated by centrencephalic structures, are improved by ECT.

- ECT-induced increases in the *permeability of the blood-brain barrier* facilitate the distribution of neuropeptides throughout the CNS.

Neurophysiological Theories

Alterations in neurophysiological activity are subserved by many of the neurotransmitters discussed earlier in this section, as well as in "Mechanism of Action" in Chapter 7. After repeated seizures spaced over a given period of time (usually two to three times per week over a 3- to 5-week period), there is an increase in cerebral blood flow (primarily the result of increased systemic circulation) and an acute and sustained increase in cerebral metabolism. One of the most characteristic changes is a slowing in the electroencephalographic (EEG) pattern over a series of ECT treatments, associated with increased acetylcholine activity. Increases in amplitude and decreases in frequency appear to affect thalamocortical and diencephalic structures, which may modulate recently acquired behavior, such as psychosis or melancholic features.

EEG interictal changes are characterized by a desynchronized resting configuration, leading to high-amplitude synchronized patterns and symmetric bursts of activity characteristic of *centrencephalic seizures.* With successive treatments there is progressive slowing in the mean frequency and increases in the mean amplitude of activity, both of which seem to be necessary but not sufficient for an antidepressant effect. Within 2 to 8 weeks after a course of ECT, the EEG returns to regular rhythmic α-wave activity, comparable with baseline recordings.

ECT-induced changes in sleep architecture include decreased rapid eye movement (REM) sleep, increased stage 4 sleep, and increased total sleep time. For example, some of the authors looked at the effects of ECT on sleep architecture in a preliminary trial of five depressed patients who underwent serial sleep studies during their course of treatment. We found that all subjects improved clinically and that there was a parallel in a normalizing of all sleep parameters (e.g., total sleep time, sleep efficiency), except for REM latency. Interestingly, REM latency initially became even shorter, but then normalized by the end of the course of ECT (33). Although preliminary, we speculate that the unexpected initial decrease in REM latency might serve as a predictor of final outcome. In this context, Grunhaus et al. (34) found that sleep-onset REM periods after ECT predicted a poorer response.

The *"anticonvulsant" hypothesis* has been developed to explain the efficacy of ECT, as well as certain antiepileptic drugs. Thus, agents such as carbamazepine (CBZ) and valproate have several effects on seizure activity, including the following:

- Increasing the seizure *threshold*
- Decreasing the overall *duration* of a seizure episode
- Diminishing *neurometabolic response* to an episode
- Decreasing the phenomenon of *amygdaloid kindling*

Interestingly, ECT induces similar effects (see Chapter 10, "Mechanism of Action"). Thus, although a given ECT treatment elicits seizure activity, the net outcome is an antiseizure effect over a course of therapy. ECS is also known to diminish the phenomenon of amygdaloid kindling in animal models (35). Similarities between such neuroelectrical, stress-induced phenomena and the longitudinal course of some bipolar disorders have been noted and serve as a heuristic, nonhomologous model for understanding the development of certain mood disorders (36).

Small and colleagues (37) have promulgated the concept of *hemispheric equilibration,* which attributes efficacy to the apparent ability of ECT to restore the relative balance between right and left brain functions.

Indications and Contraindications

As noted earlier, although it is often used as a "treatment of last resort," there are situations in which ECT may be used as a first-line intervention. The American Psychiatric Association (APA) Task Force Report on ECT discusses four specific groups of patients:

- Patients who are at *high risk for suicidal behavior*
- Patients who are *rapidly deteriorating,* either physically or psychologically, or both

- Patients who have a *prior history of good response* to ECT or a poor history of response to pharmacotherapy
- Patients who *prefer* to receive this treatment rather than undergo lengthy, and possibly unsuccessful, trials of medications with their associated adverse effects (38)

Psychotic Depression

To this list, we would add *delusional* (or psychotic) depression (see also Chapters 6 and 7). Whereas some have suggested that pre-ECT nonresponse to adequate pharmacotherapy is a powerful factor for predicting nonresponse to ECT (39, 40), others have argued for its superiority over antidepressants (alone or in combination with antipsychotics) for prior drug-nonresponsive nonpsychotic or psychotic depressions (41–43). Support for this latter position comes from the discussion by Schatzberg and Rothschild (44), who separate this condition from other depressive disorders, in part because of its differential responsivity to various treatments.

One consistent finding has been that patients with psychotic depression treated with antidepressant monotherapy or even the combination of an antidepressant plus antipsychotic have a lower response rate than those depressed patients without psychotic symptoms (45). Although evidence supports an improved response when these patients undergo treatment with ECT, this apparent superiority may be related to a selection bias (46). Thus, it may be that patients with psychotic depression are more likely to receive ECT earlier in their course of illness and therefore the extent of their true drug resistance is unknown (1).

The relapse rate for psychotic versus nonpsychotic depression after a successful course of ECT has also been considered. For example, geriatric patients who had responded to either ECT or medication treatment were then followed up longitudinally (47). Those who had initially presented with psychotic features and responded to treatment subsequently demonstrated a substantially higher rate of relapse than their nonpsychotic counterparts, with maintenance tricyclic antidepressant monotherapy having limited efficacy. The overall response rate to ECT in this group of psychotic patients was 88.2% (i.e., 15 of 17), which compared favorably with the 50% response rate reported for pharmacological treatment (48). In another report on this same subject group, the response rate after 6 weeks of pharmacological treatment was only 25% versus 88.2% for patients undergoing ECT, suggesting a significant benefit in terms of rapidity of onset as well (1, 47).

In summary, it remains unclear whether ECT has differential efficacy in the psychotic versus nonpsychotic depressive subgroups, both in terms of acute response and propensity for relapse. In addition, although evidence supports superior outcomes in geriatric patients, rate and extent of recovery are not clear when comparing ECT with pharmacological treatment in this age group (1, 49).

Other Indications

In addition to depression, other indications for ECT include the following:

- *Mania* (especially manic delirium)
- *Schizophrenic* disorders (especially with "positive" symptoms)
- *Catatonia* associated with major mood disorders, schizophrenia, or organic mood disorders (e.g., systemic lupus erythematosus) (50)
- Mood disturbances secondary to an underlying *organic process*

Paradoxically, ECT is equally useful in both the acute manic and depressive phases of bipolar disorder, constituting the only truly bimodal therapy presently available. For example, in their literature review, Mukherjee et al. (51) found that ECT was associated with marked clinical improvement or remission in 80% of patients undergoing treatment for an acute manic episode. This is not the case for lithium, valproate, or CBZ, which, at best, have relatively weak acute antidepressant effects. Drug therapies may also induce a switch from a depressed to a manic phase, whereas ECT can control both phases of the illness.

In *schizophrenia,* ECT, as with antipsychotic agents, is most effective in the acutely ill patient with a more recent onset of illness. *Catatonia,* withdrawn type, characterized by immobility and an inability to interact or maintain one's basic needs (at times posing a life-threatening situation), can dramatically resolve with ECT.

Case Example: A 31-year-old man presented with unremitting psychotic symptoms and depressive periods marked by agitation and attempts at self-mutilation and physical assaults. He had been hospitalized for the past 5 years, except for a few months when he was treated as an outpatient. Previous treatment with chlorpromazine, thioridazine, loxapine, lithium, amitriptyline, and diazepam was unsuccessful. Before treatment with ECT, he was being given 120 mg per day of fluphenazine, and he continued to experience command auditory hallucinations to injure himself, persecutory and religious delusions, and increased depression and agitation. During this period, the patient bit through his lip, lacerated his scrotum, and inflicted bite wounds on his hands. The oral antipsychotic was then stopped, and the patient received 15 unilateral nondominant (UND) ECT treatments, resulting in a resolution of his agitation and self-destructive behavior. Oral fluphenazine was then resumed and switched to the decanoate form (4.0 mL every 2 weeks). The patient was placed in a work-related day program, and approximately 1 year later was doing well without rehospitalization.

Other disorders for which ECT has been reported to be helpful include the following:

- *Organic* mental disorders
- Intractable *seizures*
- *Parkinson's disease*
- *Hypopituitarism*
- *Neuroleptic malignant syndrome* (NMS)

In particular, the use of ECT during or shortly after an episode of NMS has come under scrutiny in the case report literature. A major concern has been reported fatalities associated with its use for this problem. Davis et al. (52) reviewed the world's literature, identifying approximately 1,000 NMS episodes in 755 patients. Using mortality rate as the major outcome variable, they compared patients who received nonspecific supportive treatment, specific drug treatment (i.e., dopamine agonists or dantrolene) plus supportive measures, or ECT. There was a 21% mortality rate in the nonspecific-treated group as compared with a 9.7% mortality rate in the specific drug-treated group and a 10.7% mortality rate in the ECT-treated group. Furthermore, the ECT patients who died or experienced severe adverse effects were continuing to receive concomitant high-potency antipsychotics. An analysis of the case-control data indicated that ECT was clinically effective while resulting in a similar mortality rate to that with specific drug therapies and approximately half that seen with supportive treatments. Although the specific drug-supportive therapy difference was statistically significant, the sample size in the ECT group was too small (i.e., 28) to reach statistical significance.

The APA Task Force Report on ECT supports the concept of differing levels of relative contraindications and no longer lists "absolute" restrictions for the use of ECT (38). In particular, they caution that these conditions may be associated with increased risk of morbidity and warrant special attention:

- *Space-occupying supratentorial cerebral lesions*
- A recent history of *myocardial infarction* and associated instability (less than 3 months)
- Recent *intracerebral bleeds*
- Bleeding or unstable *aneurysm* or *arteriovenous malformations*
- *Retinal detachment*
- *Pheochromocytoma*
- *American Society of Anesthesiologists* classification risk level of 4 or 5

When considering ECT in patients with any of these systemic conditions, a careful review of the risk-benefit ratio must always be conducted in conjunction with consultation from the appropriate specialists.

Efficacy

Acute Treatment

ECT is superior in efficacy when compared with placebo, sham ECT, and active drug therapy. Upon the introduction of effective pharmacother-

apy for severe depression, the relative efficacy of drug versus ECT was frequently studied. Our review of the relevant literature led to an extrapolation of the data from selected studies (primarily class I or II designs) for a quantitative analysis of the efficacy of ECT versus other treatments for an acute depressive episode (53). The comparisons with ECT included simulated (or sham) ECT, placebo, the standard tricyclic antidepressants, and the monoamine oxidase inhibitors [Tables 8-1 (54–59), 8-2 (60–63), 8-3 (56, 61–66), and 8-4 (55, 60–63)]. We also compared the relative efficacy of the bilateral (BILAT) versus the UND forms of administration [Table 8-5 (42, 67–78)]. A meta-analysis was computed on the data across all studies that met our *a priori* inclusion criteria (Tables 8-6 through 8-11).

The overall efficacy of ECT was 78%, which is significantly superior to that of tricyclic antidepressants, whose overall efficacy was 64%, as well as to placebo, simulated ECT, and the monoamine oxidase inhibitors, whose overall response rates ranged from 28% to 38%. This difference was particularly striking because many patients in the ECT-treated groups had failed previous drug trials. The adequacy of some of these, however, was questionable. Furthermore, in contrast to other reports, our analysis did not find a significant difference favoring BILAT over UND ECT (i.e., only a 7% overall difference).

Maintenance Treatment

Just as drug-treated patients require maintenance management after an adequate response for an acute episode, so do acute ECT responders. Unlike with drug-responsive patients, however, maintenance management with ECT is a more complex matter, given that most patients received ECT because of a poor response to or an intolerance of pharmacotherapy. Alternative maintenance strategies to consider in this group include the following:

- *Antidepressants* that have demonstrated at least partial benefit in the past

(*Text continues on page 345.*)

TABLE 8-1. Studies examining the efficacy of real ECT in comparison with simulated ECT

Study	Subjects and diagnosis	Experimental design	Results

Ulett G et al. (1956)	84 Inpatients
	Bipolar, depressed
	Involutional depression
	Neurotic depression
	Schizoaffective
	Other subtypes
	Schizophrenics
		Random assignment (stratified matching)
		Four groups
		Active treatment
		  ECT (21)
		  Photo. convulsion (21)
		Control
		  Subconvulsion (21)
		  I.V. anesthetic (21)
		Global ratings at weeks 4–5
			ECT > simulated-ECT
			"+" = improved; marked
			  improvement; or recovered
			"–" = slightly improved;
			  no change; worse

Brill N et al. (1959)	27 Inpatients Depressive diagnoses Bipolar, depressed Involutional Psychotic Reactive Schizoaffective 18–68 Years old	Double-blind, random assignment Real ECT groups 1. ECT alone (7) 2. ECT plus muscle relaxant (8) 3. ECT with anesthesia (3) Simulated ECT 4. Anesthesia alone (5) 5. Nitrous oxide alone (4) Doctors' Lorr scale Data combined for groups 1–3 and 4 + 5	ECT > simulated-ECT "+" = improved or recovered "–" = no change
Harris J and Robin A (1960)	12 Inpatients Depressive reactions	Double-blind, random assignment Three groups: ECT plus placebo (4) Hexobarbitone plus phenelzine (4) Hexobarbitone plus placebo (4) Global assessment 1 = No change 2 = Slight improvement 3 = Moderate improvement 4 = Great improvement	ECT > hexobarbitone plus placebo (after 2 weeks) "+" = moderate or great improvement "–" = slightly improved or no change

Study	Patient description	Methods	Results
Fahy P et al. (1963)	50 Inpatients Endogenous or involutional depression 20–60 Years old 35 females; 25 males	Blind observations and ratings by two independent raters; random assignment. Three groups: ECT (17) Imipramine 100 mg (16) Thiopentone (17) Ratings done at 3 weeks	ECT > simulated-ECT "+" = improved or recovered "−" = no change
Lambourn J and Gill D (1978)	32 Patients Depressive psychosis	Double-blind, random assignment Two groups: UND-ECT (16) UND simulated-ECT (16) (six treatments each; three times per week) Hamilton and GAS ratings	ECT = simulated-ECT "+" = 5 or more pluses on combined HAM-D and GAS scales "−" = less than 5 pluses
West E (1981)	22 Patients Primary depressive illness	Double-blind; random assignment BL ECT 40 Joules Two times per week Double waveform At least six treatments per patient All patients on 50 mg of amitriptyline Crossover if no improvement after six treatments	10/11 simulated-ECT patients crossed over to real ECT No real ECT patients crossed over to simulated-ECT "+" = no switch "−" = switched

BL, bilateral ECT; UND, unilateral nondominant ECT: "+" = responder, "−" = nonresponder (also Tables 8.6–8.10).

TABLE 8-2. Studies examining the efficacy of ECT in comparison with placebo

Study	Subjects and diagnosis	Experimental design	Results
Kiloh L et al. (1960)	81 Inpatients Endogenous or involutional depression 52 Females; 29 males	Blind ratings for patients on drugs or placebo; nonblind for ECT One of three groups, in strict rotation ECT (27) Iproniazid (26) Placebo (28) Global ratings at 3–6 weeks for placebo; or 7–10 days after last ECT	ECT > placebo "+" = greatly improved; or symptom-free "−" = worse; unchanged or slightly improved
Greenblatt M et al. (1962, 1964, personal communication)	351 Inpatients at three centers Bipolar, depressed Psychotic depression Involutional depression Schizoaffective Neurotic depression	Double-blind, except for some ECT patients; random assignment Six groups: ECT (70) Imipramine (78) Desipramine (21) Phenelzine (48) Isocarboxazid (68) Placebo (67) Global ratings on a 3-point scale: Marked improvement Moderate improvement No improvement	ECT > placebo "+" = marked or moderate improvement "−" = no improvement
Shepherd M (1965)	217 Inpatients Primary depression 40–69 Years old Females and males Patient switched to alternate treatment-nonresponders	Double-blind for medication groups; nonblind for ECT; random assignment (deteriorated patients dropped from study) Four groups: ECT (58) (4–8 treatments) Imipramine (58) Phenelzine (50) Placebo (51) Ratings for 15 symptoms; global assessment at 4 weeks	ECT > placebo "+" = good or excellent response "−" = poor or deteriorated

TABLE 8-3. Studies examining the efficacy of ECT in comparison with tricyclic antidepressants

Study	Subjects and diagnosis	Experimental design	Results
Bruce E et al. (1960)	48 Consecutive inpatients Depression	Nonblind ratings Random assignment to two groups: ECT (22) Imipramine, 225 mg (26) (three of seven IMI failures withdrawn before 4 weeks and given ECT to which they responded) Global scale at 4 weeks	ECT > imipramine "+" = good response "−" = poor response
Robin A and Harris J (1962)	31 Patients Depressed and chosen by clinician to receive ECT	Double-blind; random assignment Two groups: ECT (15) (2 times/week) plus placebo tabs Anesthetic (2 times/week) plus imipramine (16) Blind ratings with Hamilton Depression Rating Scale	ECT > imipramine "+" = marked or moderate improvement "−" = slight improvement; no improvement or withdrawn because of deterioration
Greenblatt M et al. (1962, 1964, personal communication)	351 Inpatients at three centers Bipolar, depressed Psychotic depression Involutional depression Schizoaffective Neurotic depression	Double-blind, (except for some ECT patients); random assignment Six groups: ECT (70) Imipramine (78) Desipramine (21) Phenelzine (48) Isocarboxazid (68) Placebo (67) Global ratings on a 3-point scale: Marked improvement Moderate improvement No improvement	ECT comparable to imipramine (perhaps more rapid in action) ECT > desipramine "−" = marked or moderate improvement "−" = unimproved
Fahy P et al. (1963)	50 Patients Endogenous or involutional depression 20–60 Years old 35 Females; 25 males	Blind observations and ratings by two independent raters; random assignment Three groups: ECT (17) Imipramine 100 mg (16) Thiopentone (17) Ratings done at 3 weeks	ECT comparable to imipramine "+" = improved or recovered "−" = no change

(continued)

TABLE 8-3. (Continued)

Study	Subjects and diagnosis	Experimental design	Results

Wilson I et al. (1963)	36 Inpatients
	Bipolar, depressed
	Involutional depression
	Reactive depression
	40–59 Years old; females
		Random assignment; patients blind, two raters blind (one nonblind); high interrater reliability
		Four groups:
		ECT + placebo
		  Six treatments
		  Phase I = (6)
		  Phase II = (4)
		ECT + imipramine (4)
		  Six treatments
		Imipramine
		  Phase I
		    Average daily dose = approx. 175 mg, plus anesthesia (6)
		  Phase II
		    Average daily dose = approx. 240 mg, without anesthesia (10)
		Anesthesia plus placebo (6)
		Two scales:
		Minnesota Multiphasic Personality Inventory (MMPI) Depression Scale (self-rated)
		Hamilton Depression Rating Scale
			Phase I
			  ECT slightly better than imipramine
			Phase II
			  ECT equal to imipramine
			"+" = decrease in scores on Hamilton Depression Rating Scale and MMPI depression scale
			"–" = increase in scores or no change

Shepherd M (1965)	217 Inpatients Primary depression 40–69 Years old Females and males	Random assignment; double-blind for medication groups; non-blind for ECT Four groups: ECT (58) (4–8 treatments) Imipramine (58) Phenelzine (50) Placebo (51) (deteriorated patients dropped from study) Ratings for 15 symptoms and global assessment at 4 weeks	ECT and imipramine were comparable Imipramine especially effective in men but slower onset of action; ECT especially effective in females "+" = good or excellent response "–" = poor or deteriorated

TABLE 8-4. Studies examining the efficacy of ECT in comparison with MAO inhibitors

Study	Subjects and diagnosis	Experimental design	Results
Harris J and Robin A (1960)	12 Inpatients Depressive reactions	Double-blind, random assignment Three groups: ECT plus placebo (4) Hexobarbitone plus phenelzine (4) Hexobarbitone plus placebo (4) Global assessment 1 = no change 2 = slight improvement 3 = moderate improvement 4 = great improvement	ECT > hexobarbitone plus phenelzine "+" = moderate or great improvement "−" = slightly improved or no change
Kiloh L et al. (1960)	81 Inpatients Endogenous or involutional depression 52 Females; 29 males	Blind ratings for patients on drugs or placebo; nonblind for ECT One of three groups, in strict rotation: ECT (27) Iproniazid (26) Placebo (28) Global ratings at 3–6 weeks for drugs; or 7–10 days after last ECT	ECT > iproniazid "+" = greatly improved; or symptom-free "−" = worse; unchanged or slightly improved
Greenblatt M et al. (1962, 1964, personal communication)	351 Inpatients at three centers Bipolar, depressed Psychotic depression Involutional depression Schizoaffective Neurotic depression	Double-blind, except for some ECT patients; random assignment Six groups: ECT (70) Imipramine (78) Desipramine (21) Phenelzine (48) Isocarboxazid (68) Placebo (67) Global ratings on a 3-point scale: Marked improvement Moderate improvement No improvement	ECT > MAO inhibitors "+" = marked or moderate improvement "−" = no improvement
Shepherd M (1965)	217 Inpatients Primary depressions 40–69 Years old 169 Females; 81 males	Double-blind for medication groups; nonblind for ECT; random assignment Four groups: ECT (58) (4–8 treatments) Imipramine (58) Phenelzine (50) Placebo (51) Ratings for 15 symptoms; global assessment at 4 weeks	ECT > MAO inhibitors "+" = good or excellent response "−" = poor or deteriorated

TABLE 8-5. Studies examining the effect of electrode placement on efficacy

Study	Subjects and diagnosis	Experimental design	Results

Cannicott S (1962)	50 Patients
	Depression severe enough to warrant ECT
	All females
		Double-blind; random assignment
		Two groups:
		  BL (20), mean 6.7 treatments
		  UND (30), mean 7.0 treatments
		Clinical global assessment
		  Recovered
		  Relieved
		  Unchanged
			No difference, based on clinical assessment
			"+" = recovered or relieved
			"−" = unchanged

Strain J et al. (1968)	96 Patients
	Bipolar, depressed
	Involutional psychosis
	Psychotic depression
	Depressive reaction
	Neurotic reaction
	22–82 Years old (mean age 55 years)
	Males and females
		Double-blind; random assignment
		Two groups:
		  BL (46), mean 7.5 treatments
		  UND (50), mean 8.4 treatments
		Ratings:
		  Depression Evaluation Form
		  Clyde Mood Scale (self-administered)
			No difference, based on depression rating forms
			"+" = no relapse after 1 year
			"−" = required additional treatment or hospitalization within one year

Zinkin S and Birtchnell J (1968)	44 Patients
	Depressive illness
		Double-blind; random assignment
		Two groups:
		  BL (20), mean 8.29 treatments
		  UND (24), mean 8.02 treatments
		Self-administered Depression Rating Scale
			UND showed slightly greater improvement
			"+" = decrease in score after course of ECT
			"−" = increase in score after course of ECT

Halliday A et al. (1968)	52 Patients
	Endogenous depressives; less than 1 year's duration
	<65 Years old
	Males and females
		Double-blind; random assignment
		Three groups:
		  BL (18), mean 5.5 treatments
		  UND (18), mean 5.9 treatments
		  UD (16), mean 6.2 treatments
		Ratings:
		  Hamilton Depression Rating Scale
		  Hildreth Self-Rating Scale
			UND = BL-ECT
			"+" = recovered or improved
			"−" = no change or worse

Abrams R and DeVito R (1969)	21 Patients
	Bipolar, depressed
	Neurotic depression
	22–55 Years old
	Males and females
		Double-blind; random assignment
		Two groups:
		  BL (11), six treatments
		  UNO (10), six treatments
		Hamilton Depression Rating Scale
			No difference (i.e., 80 clinical recovery in both groups)
			"+" = recovered
			"−" = not recovered

Study	Patient population	Methodology	Results
d'Elia G (1970)	59 Newly admitted patients Endogenous depression	Double-blind; random assignment Two groups: BL (29), mean 6.2 treatments UND (30), mean 7.0 treatments Cronholm-Ottosson Depression Scale	No difference between UND and BL-ECT 1 month later "+" = recovered or much improved "−" = slightly improved or unchanged
Fleminger JJ et al. (1970)	36 Patients Referred for ECT because of depression Schizophrenia and organicity ruled out	Double-blind; random assignment Three groups: BL (12) UND (12) UD (12) Self-Rating Depression Inventory (D.I.) Differences in scores after 6th treatment	All three groups comparable "+" = +5 or > "−" = < +5
Sand-Stromgren L (1973)	100 Patients Endogenous depression 61 females; 39 males	Double-blind; random assignment Two groups: BL (48), mean 8.7 treatments UND (52), mean 8.9 treatments Scale for Severity of Depression Ten weighted factors scored on a 4-point scale (0-3)	No difference in total depression score "+" = satisfactory response based on decrease in depression "−" = unsatisfactory response
Heshe J et al. (1978)	51 Patients Endogenous depression	Double-blind; random assignment Two groups: BL (24) UND (27) Clinical global evaluation of depression into: Mild Moderate Severe	BL slightly better that UND 1 week after treatments were over; no difference after 3 months "+" = definite effect, or remission "−" = no effect, or doubtful
Fraser R and Glass I (1980)	27 Elderly patients Depressive illness Mean age 73 ($\pm$6) years	Random assignment; blind independent observers Two groups: BL (15) UND (12) 4–11 treatments, based on clinical response Hamilton Depression Rating Scale	UND = BL Based on scores 3 weeks after last ECT "+" = HDRS score ≤12 "−" = HDRS score >12

(continued)

TABLE 8-5. (Continued)

Study	Subjects and diagnosis	Experimental design	Results
Sackeim H et al. (1987)	52 Patients SADS-derived, RDC diagnosis of primary major depressive disorder 18 Males; 34 females	Double-blind; random assignment Two groups: BL (27) Right Unilat (25) (low-dose titration procedure; at least 10 treatments before classified as nonresponder) Hamilton Depression Rating Scale (HDRS)	BL>UND for short-term symptom reduction "+" = at least 60% reduction in HDRS;16 total score; maintain 60% reduction for at least 1 week "-" = did not meet above criteria
Janicak P et al. (1989)	33 Patients DSM-III diagnoses: Major depression (29) BP, depressed (3) SA, depressed (1) 16 Males, 17 females	Initial assessment: all to UND (10); then double-blind, random assignment to UND or BL; 2 patients switched from UND to BL Two groups BL (13), mean 9.5 treatments UND (20), mean 9.1 treatments Hamilton Depression Rating Scale	UND = BL "+" = ≥50% reduction in HDRS "-" = <50% reduction in HDRS

BL, bilateral ECT; UD, unilateral dominant ECT; UND, unilateral nondominant ECT; BP, blood pressure; SADS, Schedule for Affective Disorders and Schizophrenia.

TABLE 8-6. Efficacy of real ECT in comparison with simulated ECT

Study	Real ECT[a]		Simulated ECT		Chi square	p value
	"+"	"−"	"+"	"−"		
Ulett G et al. (1956)	28	14	15	27	6.86	0.01
Brill N et al. (1959)	12	6	2	7	3.13	0.08
Harris J and Robin A (1960)	2	2	0	4	0.67	0.41
Fahy P et al. (1963)	12	5	8	9	1.09	.30
Lambourn J and Gill D (1978)	8	8	8	8	0.13	.72
West E (1981)	11	0	1	10	14.85	0.0001

Chi square for statistical
method of combination $= 22$
Composite p value $= 3.5 \times 10^{-6}$
Estimated difference between
real ECT and simulated ECT $= 33\%$

[a] "+" represents a responder; "−" represents a nonresponder.
Adapted from Janicak PG, Davis JM, Gibbons RD, et al. Efficacy of ECT: a meta-analysis. *Am J Psychiatry* 1985;142(3):297–302, with permission.

TABLE 8-7. Efficacy of ECT in comparison with placebo

Study	ECT		Placebo		Chi square	p value
	"+"	"−"	"+"	"−"		
Kiloh L et al. (1960)	24	3	3	25	30.56	<0.001
Greenblatt M et al. (1962, 1964)	65	5	43	24	15.19	<0.001
Shepherd M (1965)	49	14	23	37	18.10	<0.001

Chi square for statistical
method of combination $= 62$
Composite p value $= 4 \times 10^{-15}$
Estimated difference between
ECT and placebo $= 42\%$

Adapted from Janicak PG, Davis JM, Gibbons RD, et al. Efficacy of ECT: a meta-analysis. *Am J Psychiatry* 1985;142(3):297–302, with permission.

TABLE 8-8. Efficacy of ECT in comparison with tricyclic antidepressants

Study	ECT		TCAs		Chi square	p value
	"+"	"−"	"+"	"−"		
Bruce E et al. (1960)	21	1	16	10	5.96	0.01
Robin A and Harris J (1962)	12	3	3	12	8.53	0.004
Greenblatt M et al. (1962, 1964)	65	5	71	28	10.36	0.001
Fahy P et al. (1963)	12	5	10	6	0.015	0.90
Wilson I et al. (1963)	10	0	10	0	0.0002	0.99
Shepherd M (1965)	49	14	42	19	0.84	0.36

Chi square for statistical
method of combination $= 22$
Composite p value $= 3 \times 10^{-6}$
Estimated difference between
ECT and tricyclics $= 19\%$

Adapted from Janicak PG, Davis JM, Gibbons RD, et al. Efficacy of ECT: a meta-analysis. *Am J Psychiatry* 1985;142(3):297–302, with permission.

TABLE 8-9. *Efficacy of ECT in comparison with MAO inhibitors*

Study	ECT "+"	ECT "−"	MAOIs "+"	MAOIs "−"	Chi square	p value
Harris J and Robin A (1960)	2	2	0	4	0.67	0.41
Kiloh L et al. (1960)	24	3	14	12	6.38	0.01
Greenblatt M et al. (1962, 1964)	65	5	30	42	39.7	<0.001
Shepherd M (1965)	49	14	19	41	24.6	<0.001

Chi square for statistical method of combination = 75
Composite p value = 5×10^{-18}
Estimated difference between ECT and MAOIs = 46%

From Janicak PG, Davis JM, Gibbons RD, et al. Efficacy of ECT: a meta-analysis. *Am J Psychiatry* 1985;142(3):297–302, with permission.

TABLE 8-10. *Efficacy of bilateral ECT in comparison with unilateral nondominant ECT*

Study	Bilateral "+"	Bilateral "−"	Unilateral Nondominant "+"	Unilateral Nondominant "−"	Individual Chi square with yate's correction	Individual p value
Cannicott S (1962)	18	2	27	3	0.231	0.75
Strain J et al. (1968)	29	17	33	17	0.008	0.90
Halliday A et al. (1968)	17	1	13	5	1.800	0.25
Zinkin S and Birtchnell J (1968)	13	7	18	6	0.154	0.75
Abrams R and DeVito R (1969)	9	2	8	2	0.203	0.75
d'Elia G (1970)	21	8	23	7	0.006	0.90
Fleminger J et al. (1970)	10	2	7	5	1.810	0.35
Sand-Stromgren L (1973)	37	11	39	13	0.000	0.95
Fraser R and Glass I (1980)	14	1	10	2	0.042	0.90
Janicak P et al. (1989)	11	2	15	5	0.050	0.82
Heshe J et al. (1978)	24	0	20	7	5.189	0.025
Sackeim H et al. (1987)	19	8	7	18	7.704	0.006
TOTAL N	222	61	220	90		

Chi square for statistical method of combination
    Mantel-Haenszel = 4.87
    Woolf-Haldens = 2.88
Composite p value
    Mantel-Haenszel = 0.03
    Woolf-Haldens = NS
Estimated difference between Bilateral ECT and
    Unilateral Nondominant ECT = 7%

N, number; NS, not significant.

TABLE 8-11. *Statistical overview of studies comparing unilateral nondominant ECT with bilateral ECT*

	Number of studies	Number of subjects	Mantel-Haenszel Chi square	Mantel-Haenszel p value	Woolf-Haldens Chi square	Woolf-Haldens p value	Estimated difference: BILAT > UND
Studies finding no difference	10	490	0.31	NS	0.25	NS	2%
Studies finding BILAT > UND-ECT	2	103	14.2	0.0002	11.7	0.0006	32%
TOTAL RESULTS	12	593	4.87	0.03	2.88	NS	7%

- *Lithium* or lithium-antidepressant combinations, both in bipolar and unipolar disorders
- Combined *antidepressant plus antipsychotic*
- *Novel antipsychotic alone*
- *Anticonvulsants,* such as lamotrigine, valproate, or CBZ, with or without other mood stabilizers
- *Maintenance ECT,* possibly combined with a mood stabilizer, antidepressant, or antipsychotic

Although few systematic controlled data exist, open investigations support the potential value of maintenance ECT after an acute episode has remitted. This usually consists of a tapering schedule of single outpatient treatments, starting with a session every 1 to 2 weeks, and then reducing the frequency based on the patient's response. Although compliance may also be an issue with this strategy (i.e., patients are often reluctant to return as an outpatient for treatments), reports document its efficacy and safety in an otherwise chronic, relapsing depressed group (79, 80). Adding a sense of urgency to this issue are reports that patients who responded poorly to adequate *pre-ECT* pharmacotherapy may also respond poorly to ECT itself or *post-ECT* drug maintenance (40, 81).

What is clear is that without some form of effective maintenance treatment, the relapse rate is substantial (i.e., greater than 50% within the first 12 months after acute remission). Thus, prospective trials are needed to address questions such as which factors predict the likelihood of a good response to maintenance medication versus maintenance ECT and which combination strategies are best to prevent relapse after a successful acute ECT trial (1).

Special Populations

The Pregnant Patient

Certain factors slightly increase the risk of complications when ECT is administered to pregnant women, and Miller (82) has summarized the modifications in technique that can usually address these issues:

- *Raising gastric pH* before the procedure with a nonparticulate antacid such as sodium citrate,

because gastric emptying is prolonged in pregnancy
- Intubation after the first trimester with a small cuffed endotracheal tube and use of a small laryngoscope and a laryngoscope blade to reduce the risk of bleeding from attempted intubation
- *Elevation of the patient's right hip and displacement of the uterus to the left* to reduce the likelihood of aortocaval compression during the later stages of pregnancy to prevent reduction in fetal circulation
- Pretreatment with *intravenous hydration without glucose* to avoid osmotic diuresis
- *Avoidance of hyperventilation,* because this may hinder oxygen unloading from maternal to fetal hemoglobin

The author also notes that ECT may be helpful in female bipolar patients who want to plan a pregnancy and discontinue mood stabilizers to minimize risks to the fetus. In addition, ECT can be remarkably effective in cases of postpartum depression and psychosis. Indeed, given the importance of that phase of child care, it can be argued that the most rapidly effective strategy is the preferred strategy. In a related issue, Walker and Swartz (83) considered the use of ECT in high-risk pregnancies, concluding that with additional precautions (e.g., monitoring of maternal and fetal well-being) such patients can safely benefit from this therapy and significant medical and obstetric complications need not prevent its use. One example is the report of a 27-year-old pregnant patient in whom NMS developed while she was on haloperidol. Although the syndrome did not respond to dantrolene, ECT was instituted at 29 weeks and the patient's condition improved (1, 84).

The Child or Adolescent Patient

In a review, Rey and Walter (85) found no controlled trials on the use of ECT in patients 18 years of age or younger. There were 396 patients identified, 63% of whom constituted single-case reports. The data indicated the following improvement rates in this age group:

- 63% for depression
- 80% for mania

- 42% for schizophrenia
- 80% for catatonia

These response rates parallel the reports for older age groups. However, many child psychiatrists lack both knowledge and experience in this area. ECT is not part of the curriculum for most fellowships in child and adolescent psychiatry, and this topic is not even discussed in some comprehensive textbooks of child psychiatry (85, 86). As a result, ECT is a treatment of last resort, if used at all, for almost all patients in this age group.

The Elderly Patient

ECT continues to be used at a higher frequency in geriatric versus younger patients. This difference in usage probably reflects the decreased efficacy of medications seen in older patients, a lower tolerance to drug side effects, and the higher incidence of medical disorders in this age group (1).

Although ECT is a relatively costly form of treatment, one study in elderly depressed patients who responded to an acute course demonstrated that maintenance ECT *reduced the overall cost* of medical care and the relapse rate as compared with patients on maintenance medication after ECT (87). The reduced costs were evident at the 12-month follow-up, primarily through decreased hospital use. In addition, this strategy was also associated with improvements in functional status and cognition.

The Manic Patient

The manic phase of bipolar disorder is highly responsive to ECT, with a comprehensive review of this topic reporting an overall efficacy rate of 80% (51). For patients who were selected because of drug treatment resistance, the rate of response was still approximately 58%, and for patients who did not respond specifically to lithium, the response rate was 69% (88, 89). Because the seizure threshold may be lower in manic patients, the difference in efficacy between BILAT and UND electrode placement may not be as great as for patients with major depression (90–92). Finally, ECT may be particularly useful in older patients, who have decreased physio-

logical reserves and/or medical co-morbidity, in whom a prolonged episode of mania can be life-threatening and the rapidity of response to mood-stabilizing drugs insufficient (1).

Administration of Electroconvulsive Therapy

A number of improvements in the administration of ECT have enhanced its efficacy and minimized some of the more troublesome adverse effects. The improvements include the following:

- Advances in *anesthetic* techniques
- Selected stimulus *electrode placement* (e.g., UND vs. BILAT)
- Change from sinusoidal to *brief-pulse* inducing currents
- A better understanding of the role played by the *electrical stimulus* itself
- Improved assessment for the *adequacy of seizure activity*

Pre-ECT Workup

The standard pre-ECT workup should include the following:

- A complete *physical* and *neurological* examination
- Routine *hematological indices* (e.g., complete blood count) and serum *electrolytes*
- Review of cardiac status and *electrocardiogram*
- Simple *tests of cognitive function*

If deemed necessary, *spinal radiographs* (anteroposterior and lateral) to rule out spinal or other skeletal problems may be appropriate. If such x-ray studies are done before ECT, they should be repeated after ECT to document any changes that may have occurred.

Informed consent must be obtained before the administration of ECT. Often, the same severity of illness that necessitates the use of ECT also impairs a patient's capacity to consent. When the patient is unable to give adequate informed consent, the clinician and the patient's family can attempt to obtain partial conservatorship from the court allowing a family member to give substituted permission (see also Chapter 2, "Informed Consent").

Anesthesia

Anesthetic techniques that have minimized adverse effects include the use of *muscle relaxants* and, more recently, nerve stimulators to assess adequacy of relaxation, the introduction of very *rapid acting, short-duration barbiturates*, and the use of *atropinic agents* to minimize the cardiovascular response to a combination of a seizure and anesthesia (93). In addition, 100% oxygenation (adequacy monitored by a pulse oximeter) with positive-pressure ventilation can minimize related cardiac events and memory disruption.

Anesthetic Agents

The standard induction process used during ECT has included the following:

- *Anticholinergic* agents (e.g., atropine or glycopyrrolate)
- *Anesthetic* agents (e.g., methohexital)
- *Muscle relaxants* (e.g., succinylcholine)
- *β-Blockers* (when indicated) to control blood pressure and heart rate changes (e.g., esmolol or labetalol) (94, 95)

Alternative agents that may facilitate the effectiveness of ECT and enhance safety continue to be scrutinized. *Etomidate,* an alternate to methohexital, may be especially useful for geriatric patients with high seizure thresholds. A recent study showed a significant increase in seizure duration when patients were switched from methohexital to this agent (i.e., in four patients the mean seizure duration increased from 25 to 61.8 seconds) (96). Other studies, however, have not found a difference between these two agents (97, 98). A switch from methohexital to etomidate can be considered when adequate seizure duration is not obtained. Disadvantages of etomidate compared with methohexital are as follows:

- Higher *cost*
- Delayed *cognitive recovery*
- Suppression of *adrenocortical function* for 8 hours
- More *pain* on infusion (1, 99)

Although the use of *ketamine* for anesthesia induction when seizure duration is insuffi-

cient has also been recommended, recent studies did not find this agent to be helpful (100–103). Disadvantages of ketamine include the following:

- Increased *recovery time*
- Induction of *seizures in epileptic patients*
- Increase in *hypertensive response* after seizure induction

Other agents have been studied. They typically offer no significant advantage over methohexital, have additional side effects, or have an unknown effect on ECT efficacy. These agents include the following:

- Propofol
- Althesin
- Propanidid
- Fentanyl with droperidol (1, 99)

Caffeine

Use of *caffeine* has also been recommended to lower the threshold in patients who do not experience an adequate seizure (104–106). One report, however, found that caffeine appeared to produce neuronal damage in rats receiving ECS (107). Because adenosine may have neuroprotective effects, one postulated mechanism is the ability of methylxanthines (e.g., caffeine, theophylline) to block adenosine receptors. On a positive note, studies have not found a difference in cognitive disruption between patients receiving ECT with or without caffeine (108). Although the implications of the animal data for humans are not clear, and because shorter seizures may be effective in some patients, a conservative approach would be to augment with caffeine only when seizure duration is less than 20 seconds and response is inadequate (38). Alternatively, it may be appropriate to switch to BILAT electrode placement or from methohexital to etomidate when UND electrode stimulation produces inadequate seizure duration (even at maximal stimulus intensity) and response is insufficient (97, 98).

TABLE 8-12. *Bilateral versus unilateral, nondominant ECT*

BILAT-ECT	UND-ECT
• Less affected by *seizure threshold*	• May be more difficult to surpass seizure threshold
• It is *less critical* to determine seizure threshold	• *Critical to determine seizure threshold*
• High- and low-energy stimuli lead to *best response rates*	• Low-energy stimulus leads to *poorest response rate*
• Produces substantially *more cognitive* disruption, regardless of stimulus energy	• Produces *less cognitive disruption,* regardless of stimulus energy
• *Benzodiazepines* have less impact on efficacy	• *Benzodiazepines* may significantly diminish efficacy

From Beedle D, Krasuski J, Janicak PG. Advances in somatic therapies. In Janicak PG: electroconvulsive therapy, repetitive transcronial magnetic stimulation, and bright light therapy. Davis JM, Preskorn SH, Ayd FJ, eds. *Principles and Practice of Psychopharmacotherapy Update.* Vol. 2. Baltimore: Williams & Wilkins, 1998, with permission.

Electrode Placement, Energy Levels, and Treatment Frequency

In a seminal paper, Sackeim and colleagues (109) found a significant relationship between stimulus electrode placement, energy delivered, and efficacy (Table 8-12). Patients were randomly assigned to either BILAT or UND ECT. In addition, each group received either low-energy stimuli (i.e., sufficient to just surpass the seizure threshold) or high-energy stimuli (i.e., 2.5 times the energy needed to surpass the seizure threshold). The response rates, which varied dramatically even though all patients experienced generalized seizures of adequate duration, were as follows:

- 17% for UND, low energy
- 43% for UND, high energy
- 65% for BT, low energy
- 63% for BT, high energy

Furthermore, 12 of 15 patients who had not responded to low-dose UND stimulation had an 80% response rate when crossed over to high-energy BILAT stimulation. The rate of response was also faster in patients given high-energy treatments with either UND or BILAT electrode placement. Finally, approximately 1.5 more treatments were required in the low-energy versus high-energy groups (regardless of electrode placement) to obtain similar reductions in baseline depression rating scores (1).

Although BILAT treatments resulted in three times more retrograde amnesia about personal information compared with low-energy or high-energy UND treatments, it was electrode placement that significantly affected memory, with only a modest effect caused by stimulus intensity. Of note, after 2 months there were no differences in negative cognitive effects among the various groups (1).

The authors conclude that BILAT stimulus electrode placement is affected less by energy level or seizure threshold (ST) than UND placement. As a result, the efficacy of UND treatments is reduced when stimuli are at or slightly above threshold even when seizures are of adequate duration and generalization. Thus, determining the ST before the first treatment is critical for maximizing the efficacy of UND electrode placement. High-energy levels (up to 500% greater than ST) for UND placement is associated with comparable therapeutic effects when compared with BILAT-ECT at 150% greater than ST, but produced less severe and persistent cognitive disruption (110). Determining the threshold may be useful for patients receiving BILAT electrode placement as well because it may permit significantly lower dosing strategies and possibly lessen short-term cognitive changes (1).

A potential confounding issue is that patients received *benzodiazepines* during their course of ECT. In the Sackeim study (109), patients could receive up to 3 mg of lorazepam daily during the treatment course. The mean dose of lorazepam was 1.0 ($\pm$1.0) mg per day and use was similar among the four groups. In this context, a retrospective study by Jha and Stein (111) compared depressed patients receiving ECT plus benzodiazepines with depressed patients receiving ECT without benzodiazepines. Patients were matched for age, sex, diagnosis, and laterality of ECT. Although 80% of patients improved with ECT, those who received benzodiazepines with UND ECT showed a significantly poorer response ($p = 0.03$) and needed a longer hospital stay ($p = 0.02$). This effect was not seen for patients receiving BILAT-ECT plus benzodiazepines. Of interest, for patients who did not receive benzodiazepines, there was no difference between BILAT and UND treatments in this study. Others have also raised concerns about the use of benzodiazepines with ECT, usually with a UND stimulus (112–114). In our study, when UND and BILAT treatments were compared directly and benzodiazepines avoided, the response rate was not significantly different (78).

Our recommendation would be to avoid benzodiazepines, especially for patients who are receiving UND ECT. When significant tolerance, withdrawal problems, or use of long-acting benzodiazepines prevents medication discontinuance before starting ECT treatments, use of BILAT stimulus would be preferable.

The stimulus energy required to surpass the seizure threshold varies considerably among patients and cannot be estimated solely on the basis of age or gender (115). Some psychiatrists use a fixed high-stimulus dose for all patients (116). Others propose a "half-age" strategy for estimating adequate BILAT stimulation (117). Although high-energy BILAT treatments clearly maximize the likelihood of response, they also clearly maximize the negative short-term cognitive effects of ECT. Because it is not necessary for all patients to receive high-energy BILAT stimuli to respond, UND may be appropriate for certain patients if treatments are applied at adequate stimulus dosing. It is also possible that ineffective UND treatments expose patients to the risk of being labeled as ECT nonresponders, making it less likely they will be offered another course for future episodes. Thus, the cognitive risks of BILAT treatments must be balanced against the morbidity and mortality associated with a potentially less effective trial with UND ECT (1).

In this context, we would endorse the strategy of determining the seizure threshold just before the first treatment. For patients who have a low threshold, the UND technique can be undertaken with stimuli of at least 2.5 times the determined seizure threshold level. For patients who require high energy to surpass the threshold, it may be difficult to provide an adequate stimulus, primarily because of the limitations in the available ECT devices (118). In this situation, we believe the more prudent course is to start with BILAT treatments. Furthermore, because seizure threshold typically increases as treatments progress, some advocate changing patients from UND to BILAT stimulus, especially if the rate of improvement with successive treatments is less than optimal (38, 119). With this approach, one may partially attenuate the cognitive disruption while still achieving maximal efficacy (1).

Attempts to attenuate the memory dysfunction seen with BILAT ECT have led to studies of alternate bilateral electrode placements. For example, asymmetric left frontal-right frontal temporal bilateral (ABL) electrode placement has been reported to produce the same degree of efficacy while inducing fewer cognitive side effects (120).

Given the high probability of response to ECT and the potential for adverse interactions with concomitant psychotropics, we prefer to stop all medications during a course of ECT and resume drugs as indicated after completion of treatments. One exception may be the use of low doses of high-potency antipsychotics (e.g., haloperidol 2 to 5 mg per day) to control a treatment-induced acute organic syndrome or to enhance the overall benefit in certain psychotic conditions (121). Several reports have indicated that the addition of novel antipsychotics may produce a better outcome in some difficult-to-treat cases (122–126). In this context, clozapine, risperidone, and other novel agents may have inherent antidepressant or mood-stabilizing properties, perhaps as a result of their increased 5-HT_2 receptor blocking action.

Treatment Frequency

ECT administered three times per week is the conventional inpatient strategy in the United

States, whereas twice per week is more common in Europe (127). Although a three-times-per-week schedule diminishes the length of time to response, it also increases cognitive side effects (128). Studies have shown that treatments given twice per week are also effective, and even a rate of once per week can be efficacious, but response may be significantly delayed and the outcome less favorable in comparison with a two- or three-times-per-week schedule (129). *Thus, we recommend initiating treatments at a frequency of three times per week until significant improvement occurs or cognitive effects become problematic. In the latter case, we would then suggest decreasing the frequency of treatments* (1, 38).

An important related issue is the ideal frequency of *maintenance* ECT treatments (e.g., weekly, biweekly, monthly). One common clinical strategy is to taper the frequency of acute treatments to once every week for 4 weeks, then every 2 weeks, and then every 3 weeks, as clinically indicated. From a practical perspective, a monthly or bimonthly schedule would be desirable in terms of cost, convenience, risk, and side effects. Unfortunately, few data presently exist to guide clinicians as to the best interval between maintenance treatments, and this determination remains an empirical process with each patient.

Acute Mania

A second issue is the relative benefit of BILAT versus UND ECT for the treatment of acute mania. Milstein et al. (130) reported on the initial outcome of an ongoing controlled trial comparing ECT with lithium for acute mania, noting that the UND ECT patients did not respond. At that point the design was changed, and all subsequent patients assigned to the ECT group were given the BILAT administration. Final results of this study indicate that the BILAT ECT group tended to demonstrate greater improvement in comparison with lithium over an 8-week period (see Chapter 10, "Alternative Treatment Strategies: Electroconvulsive Therapy") (131). Although these data support the preferential use of BILAT over UND ECT in the treatment of acute mania, this recommendation is not accepted by all. For example, Mukherjee et al.

(91) reported no difference in efficacy with either method. Because these patients often constitute acute emergencies, starting with BILAT-ECT may maximize the chances for a rapid resolution of the manic episode.

Electrical Stimulus

Studies exploring various components of the electrical stimulus have also led to further advances. The most recent ECT devices deliver a *constant-current, brief-pulse, low-energy stimulus,* in contrast to earlier devices, which used a constant-voltage, sine wave, high-energy stimulation. These newer devices require only about one-third of the energy to elicit a grand mal seizure, thus leading to a decrease in *current density,* a critical factor that may contribute to cognitive disturbances. With the use of the brief-pulse device and UND electrode placement, there may be an increased risk for suboptimal seizure activity, including missed, abortive, or inadequate seizures. Conversely, there is the possibility of prolonged seizure activity when the threshold is maximally surpassed. Such events, defined as a continuous seizure longer than 180 seconds, can usually be aborted with 2.5 to 5.0 mg i.v. diazepam.

The best outcome may be achieved using a constant-current device with a brief-pulse stimulus sufficient to at least moderately surpass the seizure threshold, especially when using the UND placement. As noted earlier, we consider high-energy stimulation (250% to 500% of ST) and would also avoid the use of benzodiazepines, because they may diminish the efficacy of UND ECT (111). This procedure typically results in 5 to 40 J of energy being delivered. For comparison, the amount of electricity used for cardiac defibrillation or cardioversion is typically in the range of 200 to 400 J.

In this context, gender differences may be an important factor, particularly because women have a greater incidence of depression. Generally, women have lower seizure thresholds than men. Further differences in lateralization of brain function may produce differences in cognitive side effects, particularly fewer side effects with UND ECT in women (132).

Seizure Activity

The optimal seizure duration appears to be in the range of 25 to 80 seconds for a given treatment. In addition to a delivery of energy to at least moderately surpass the seizure threshold, a number of techniques may be used to achieve an adequate seizure, including the following:

- Sufficient *hydration*
- *Preinduction hyperventilation*
- Avoidance of concomitant drugs with *anticonvulsant activity*
- *Reduction in the anesthetic dose* of the most commonly used barbiturate, methohexital, or the use of alternate agents such as ketamine or etomidate
- Enhancement with intravenous *caffeine sodium benzoate* (500 to 2,000 mg) given 5 to 10 minutes before the seizure induction (106)

Adequate monitoring of seizure activity includes the use of single- or multiple-lead recordings on the *EEG* and/or the *unmodified limb* technique. This technique is achieved by applying a blood pressure cuff to an arm or a leg and inflating it above systolic levels after the anesthetic agent is administered but before the muscle relaxant is given. One then observes an unmodified seizure in this limb and counts the seconds to determine the length of a seizure episode. To ensure a generalized seizure, the ipsilateral limb should be used when applying the UND electrode placement.

Complications

Complications of ECT can be grouped under three major categories:

- *Cognitive*
- *Cardiovascular*
- *Other* effects

Cognitive Disturbances

Short-term adverse cognitive effects, which may be more severe with bilateral electrode placement, could delay or preclude an adequate trial with ECT. Strategies to circumvent this problem include the following:

- *Increasing time between treatments* (e.g., from thrice to twice or once per week)
- *Switching from BILAT to UND* electrode placement
- *Adding* low doses of either a high-potency conventional or novel *antipsychotic* to manage organic delirium (e.g., haloperidol, 1 to 2 mg per day; risperidone, 0.5 to 1 mg per day)
- Alterations in *stimulus intensity, duration, waveform,* or *path of current*

Adjunctive medications with potential memory-sparing effects have also been studied and are discussed in a review by Prudic and colleagues (133). Those agents with the most promising results include the following:

- Opioid antagonists (e.g., naloxone)
- Nootropic agents (e.g., piracetam)
- Thyroid hormone

For example, low levels of *thyroxine* (T_4) have been found in patients with significant confusion and memory problems after ECT. Furthermore, consistent with data from animal studies, 50 μg of *triiodothyronine* (T_3) given before ECT diminished amnestic effects and accelerated the antidepressant effect of ECT (134).

In addition to its anesthetic effects, *ketamine* has also demonstrated potential as a memory-sparing agent. In a recent study, rats subjected to repeated ECS developed severe deficits in learning mediated by hippocampal functioning. This effect may be influenced by long-term potentiation of hippocampal neurons during seizure activity, both spontaneous and secondary to ECS, and resolves over a 40-day period after ECS. Ketamine is a noncompetitive N-methyl-D-aspartate (NMDA) receptor-associated channel blocker that can prevent this effect if given immediately before seizure induction (see also disadvantages discussed previously) (1, 135, 136).

Although short-term memory disruptions are less pronounced with UND administration, studies that have tested patients' memory performance several weeks to months after either BILAT or UND administration generally find little difference in residual deficits with either method (78). Limited data addressing the issues of efficacy and cognitive disruption with unilateral dominant (UD) versus UND or BILAT ECT, and bifrontal versus bitemporal bilateral ECT, do not allow for definitive recommendations at this time. The authors prefer to begin with UND ECT (using the temporal-occipital or d'Elia technique) at 250% to 500% of seizure threshold if there are no mitigating factors, as noted earlier (38). If after three to five treatments the rate of response is not adequate, we then switch to bitemporal bilateral administration.

Memory disturbances typically include *anterograde amnesia* (i.e., the inability to recall newly learned material) and *retrograde amnesia* (i.e., the inability to recall previously learned material). Both types can present as deficits in either the dominant or nondominant cerebral hemispheres (i.e., verbal and nonverbal anterograde and retrograde amnesia). Some patients also complain of loss of *autobiographical memories*. It is often difficult, however, to sort out the relative contributions to memory disturbances from the induced seizures, the anesthesia, or the depressive illness itself.

The retrograde amnesia is temporally graded, in that as one goes back in time from the initiation of a course of treatments, the memory disturbance diminishes, and beyond 2 years, few or no deficits are evident. As an individual's memory recovers, the ability to recall events returns in the reverse fashion, with those memories closest to the initiation of ECT returning last. Some recall for isolated incidents shortly before or during the course of ECT may be lost permanently, because they were probably never properly stored. This can also be a complication of anesthesia.

Another important aspect to this question is the cognitive dysfunction associated with severe depression. Much of the memory effects are focused on events occurring during the illness and the period of treatment [see Abrams (94) for a detailed analysis]. Thus, many depressed patients may suffer from severe memory disturbances before their course of ECT, and paradoxically appear to improve over a course of treatment. Thus, improvement in the attention and concentration disruption often associated with severe depression is so significant, that it overrides the organic amnesia induced by the course of seizures.

Those who receive BILAT ECT tend to have more complaints about their memory subsequent to their course of treatment, perhaps representing an increased sensitivity to any type of memory lapse as a result of the greater initial disruption associated with this method. It may also represent a type of amnesia for which existing assessment scales are insufficiently sensitive. Overall, sustained memory deficits are uncommon, are rarely disabling, and are clearly outweighed by the benefits of treatment.

Cardiovascular Disturbances

In the cardiovascular system, arrhythmias and, in extreme situations, arrest may occur, usually secondary to the combination of seizure activity and anesthetic agent. The mortality rate per course of ECT treatments is in the range of 1 per 10,000 or 0.01%. This risk is less than the overall morbidity and mortality rate (i.e., 3 to 9 per 10,000) seen in severely depressed patients who go untreated or receive inadequate medication trials, and is less than the anesthetic risk for labor and delivery during childbirth. Thus, those who receive an adequate trial of ECT may actually be at a reduced risk of dying from a variety of causes.

Mortality and ECT

For example, data from the 1993 Healthcare Cost and Utilization Project (HCUP) indicate that no patients receiving ECT died during hospitalization versus 30 (0.14%) in the sample who did not receive ECT ($p < 0.0001$) (15). Legislation in Texas requires the mandatory reporting of mortality data associated with ECT, allowing for a unique opportunity to study a large population who have received this treatment. Reid and colleagues (92) reviewed all reports of ECT in Texas from September 1993 through April 1995, representing a total of 15,240 treatments. Of the patients, 88.1% were white, and 70.3% were women. Older patients received more ECT than younger patients, and only five were younger than 18 years of age. Although no deaths occurred during ongoing ECT administration, there were eight deaths within 14 days of an ECT treatment, most occurring in patients with preexisting serious medical problems. Four of the eight deaths occurred in patients aged 45 to 65 years, and the other six deaths occurred in patients older than 65 years. All were caucasian, and five were women. Two patients were receiving multiple treatments during the same anesthesia. Causes of death included the following:

- *Suicide:* No data were provided regarding whether the two patients who committed suicide were ECT responders or how many treatments they had received.
- *Accident:* One patient died as a passenger in a motor vehicle accident.
- *Myocardial infarction:* Two of the three patients who died were known to have heart disease.
- *Pulmonary embolism:* Approximately 12 hours after an ECT treatment, a patient became hypotensive and later died of a suspected pulmonary embolism.
- *Infection:* This patient refused treatment for an infection that was unrelated to ECT.

Transient elevations in blood pressure and heart rate occur with seizures, probably as a result of increased sympathetic stimulation that leads to increases in norepinephrine levels. Hypertension or increased pretreatment heart rate are strongly predictive of peak postictal change in both heart rate and blood pressure (38). Increased parasympathetic stimulation decreases the heart rate as a result of inhibition of the sinoatrial node. Stimulation of the adrenal cortex leads to increased plasma corticosteroids and stimulation of the adrenal medulla, which may also contribute to increases in blood pressure and heart rate.

Other Effects

Some patients experience *prolonged seizures,* defined as a duration greater than 120 to 180 seconds. These patients require continued oxygenation, control of ventilation, and an i.v. bolus of the anesthetic agent (20 to 40 mg methohexital) or diazepam (2.5 to 5 mg) to abort the seizure.

Patients may complain of *headaches, muscle aches,* and *nausea* associated with an individual treatment. Many also report *anticipatory anxiety* or fearfulness before receiving a treatment. This may require management with anxiolytics, but type and dose must be chosen carefully to avoid

increasing the seizure threshold, thus undermining the adequacy of therapy.

Rarely, *prolonged apnea* may occur in those susceptible because of an inability to adequately metabolize succinylcholine (i.e., increased pseudocholinesterase levels). This condition requires continued positive-pressure ventilation until the patient begins spontaneous respiration.

Conclusion

Because ECT can be highly effective, it is often counterproductive to encourage repeated, unsuccessful pharmacological trials if patients are willing to undergo this therapy. General psychiatrists who do not use ECT in their clinical practice, however, are more likely to use multiple medication trials before referral for ECT. The relative safety of ECT and its ease of administration argue against its use as a subspecialty skill. Indeed, we believe it should be regarded as a necessary skill for any general psychiatrist who works with more severely ill patients. In public sector facilities, in which ECT is frequently unavailable and staff members do not have ongoing experience with its beneficial effects, the rate of referral is predictably low and this treatment is underused (92). Thus, training should expose all psychiatry residents to the technical aspects of ECT and provide the opportunity to observe the procedure and successful response of patients to help minimize any bias [see earlier comments regarding use in younger patients (38)].

An analysis of data from the 1993 HCUP, consisting of 6.5 million computerized medical records in 913 community hospitals across 17 states, found that ECT use was greater in *older patients, caucasians,* those who were *privately insured,* and those who *lived in more affluent areas* (15). In 1993, an estimated 249,600 patients were discharged from general hospitals with a principal diagnosis of a depressive disorder. Of these patients

- 9.4% received ECT.
- 3.2% with the diagnosis of *major depression, single episode,* received ECT.
- 5.5% with the diagnosis of *major depression, single episode with psychotic features,* received ECT.

- 11.8% with the diagnosis of *major depression, recurrent with psychotic features,* received ECT.
- 0.6% with the diagnosis of *dysthymia* received ECT.
- 0.17% *18 years of age or younger* received ECT.

ECT use also varied widely by *geographic region.* For example, patients in the north central states (Minnesota, Iowa, North Dakota, South Dakota, Nebraska, and Kansas) were approximately four times more likely to receive ECT than patients in the mountain states (Montana, Idaho, Wyoming, Colorado, New Mexico, Arizona, Utah, and Nevada). These differences are supported by data from the American Psychiatric Association's Professional Activities Survey, which show that rates varied from 0.4 to 81.2 patients per 10,000 population in the 202 metropolitan areas in which ECT use was reported (138). Of note, no ECT use was reported in 115 metropolitan areas. In addition, an analysis of these data found that less than 8% of all psychiatrists in the United States provide ECT (139). Finally, depressed patients in *private, nonprofit hospitals were significantly more likely to receive ECT compared with patients in private for-profit hospitals.*

In summary, when properly administered, ECT is an effective treatment for the most severe mood and psychotic disorders encountered in clinical practice, especially those warranting hospital care. Its efficacy is even more striking given the fact that 50% of those successfully treated have previously been nonresponsive to one or more adequate courses of medication. Although primarily used for severe depression, it is also an effective antimanic therapy, and may be lifesaving in catatonic states. ECT has also been used successfully to treat special populations, other psychotic disorders, and various organic conditions, such as NMS and Parkinson's disease.

OTHER SOMATIC THERAPIES

Psychiatry, as well as medicine in general, has had many potential "therapies" promoted with much enthusiasm, only to eventually see them fall by the wayside. Although ECT has withstood both the test of time and rigorous methodological scrutiny, the same cannot be said for other somatic approaches We feel, however, that sufficient evidence exists to warrant a discussion of the potential clinical utility of bright light therapy, sleep deprivation, transcranial magnetic stimulation, and vagal nerve stimulation.

Bright Light Phototherapy

Animals exhibit a number of seasonal rhythms (e.g., body weight, hibernation, reproduction, and migration), with most species using the change in day length (i.e., photoperiod) to time seasonal events. Light has a dual role, both entraining a circadian photosensitivity rhythm and producing a photoperiodic response (e.g., gonadal growth). There is evidence that such seasonal changes are mediated by the ability of light to suppress melatonin activity. Furthermore, Lewy et al. (140) have found that sufficiently bright light (1,000 to 2,000 lux) can suppress melatonin in humans, implying that circadian (and probably annual rhythms) in humans are regulated by light just as in other mammals. The suprachiasmatic nuclei of the hypothalamus appears to function as a "master clock," coordinating a variety of circadian variables such as sleep and temperature, and circadian oscillators such as melatonin, cortisol, and thyroid-stimulating hormone (141). Extensive basic knowledge about the effects of light on seasonal rhythms in animals, in addition to the discovery that light therapy suppresses melatonin in humans, spawned a number of experiments to test the antidepressant properties of bright light, primarily for seasonal affective disorder (SAD). More recently, two large controlled trials found light therapy to be superior to placebo (142, 143). Evidence has also been published for its benefits in other conditions, including the following:

- *Nonseasonal* depression (144)
- Delayed or advanced *sleep phase* disorders (145)
- *Premenstrual* depression (146)
- *Bipolar* depression (147)

Mechanism of Action

Three major hypotheses have been advanced to explain the effects of light therapy:

- The *melatonin* hypothesis
- The *circadian rhythm phase shift* hypothesis
- The *circadian rhythm amplitude* hypothesis

The *melatonin hypothesis* postulates that winter depression is triggered by alterations in nocturnal melatonin secretion, which acts as a chemical signal of darkness. Thus, by giving light therapy before dawn or after dusk, the light period can be prolonged and secretion of melatonin can be diminished. Evidence that atenolol, which suppresses melatonin secretion, was not an effective therapy for SAD weakens this particular hypothesis (148).

The leading theory is the *circadian rhythm phase shift hypothesis*. Fall-onset seasonal affective disorder (FOSAD) is said to develop when the normal circadian rhythm phases are delayed relative to sleep because dawn comes later. Because morning light advances (whereas evening light delays) the phase position of circadian rhythms, light therapy early in the day should theoretically improve winter depression. Indeed, there is some supportive evidence for this approach; however, benefit from evening light therapy has been noted as well (149). Lewy et al. (150) have hypothesized an energizing effect to explain this phenomenon.

Human nonretinal phototransduction has been demonstrated in a study of phase shifts, providing evidence that circadian rhythms can also be adjusted by light applied to certain areas of the skin in humans (151). In this report, a 3-hour pulse of light was presented to the *popliteal region*. Body core temperature was monitored and saliva samples were collected for melatonin assay in a subset of subjects who were blind to active versus sham light stimulus. The application of light induced both phase delay and phase advance in the core nadir of body temperature and the onset of the endogenous melatonin rhythm. The basis for this effect is unclear although one possible mechanism may involve alterations in the heme molecule in red blood cells (e.g., humoral phototransduction). In this context, light is known to stimulate heme-based enzymes to form reactive gases and to cause release of nitric oxide (NO) and carbon monoxide (CO) from heme moieties. Bright light is also well known to facilitate the breakdown of unconjugated bilirubin (1, 152).

Whether nonretinal phototransduction can be used as an effective treatment for patients with depression or SAD is not known. If so, it would make dosing more convenient because it could possibly occur while patients are asleep. In addition, this observation opens the possibility of multiple pathways that may affect the biological response to environmental pacemakers such as the light-dark cycle (1).

The *circadian rhythm amplitude hypothesis* postulates that FOSAD is caused by a reduction in the amplitude of various rhythms, which are increased by light therapy. There is evidence that amplitudes of certain rhythms are abnormally low in depression, particularly in FOSAD. This hypothesis has yet to be tested under experimental conditions.

Serotonin potentiation has also been postulated as a possible mechanism, given that tryptophan depletion may reverse the antidepressant effects of light therapy (153).

Also of interest is the report by Anderson and colleagues (154) that found a reduction in the urinary output of norepinephrine and its metabolites in nine female SAD patients treated with light therapy. They concluded that the results were compatible with changes seen after antidepressant drug therapy and recommended controlled trials to confirm this preliminary finding.

Therapeutic Factors

In an attempt to shed light on the critical therapeutic components of phototherapy, investigators have also evaluated several aspects, including the following:

- Intensity
- Duration
- Timing
- Spectral qualities
- Anatomical route of administration

Studies of *light intensity* have established that bright light (BL) treatment (i.e., 2,500 lux) is superior to dim light (i.e., 300 lux or less), and Terman (155) has shown that 10,000 lux was superior to the standard of 2,500 lux. *Duration of exposure* to light also appears to be an important factor and may be inversely related to the intensity such that a half hour of 10,000 lux exposure may be as effective as 2 hours at 2,500 lux (156). The timing of treatments has been thought to be important for the beneficial effect. Thus, morning treatments appeared to be relatively more effective than evening exposure, especially in patients with hypersomnia versus those with terminal insomnia (157). Furthermore, some patients seem to respond only to morning therapy (158). In contrast, other investigators have not found the timing of light therapy to influence therapeutic outcome (148). The consideration of *spectral quality* is important because there is a potential for toxicity with long-term use of ultraviolet (UV) light. Results of preliminary studies have been mixed, with some indicating UV light was not necessary and others showing it was useful for a specific subset of depressive symptoms. This issue clearly requires further investigation to avoid, if possible, any long-term potential eye or skin complications (159). Almost all studies have used *eye exposure,* but only one study, by Wehr et al. (160), indicates that this route of administration was significantly more effective than skin exposure.

In addition, certain clinical symptoms may be more predictive of response to light therapy. For example, Terman et al. (161) found that depressed responders were characterized by more atypical symptoms such as

- Hypersomnia
- Afternoon or evening slump
- Reverse diurnal variation (worse in the evenings)
- Carbohydrate craving

Overall, the ratio of atypical to classic symptoms of depression, rather than severity per se, was the best predictor of a positive response to bright light therapy.

Acute Therapy

Fall-Onset Seasonal Affective Disorder

In modern times, the first scientific report on the benefit of *phototherapy* for FOSAD was authored by Marx in 1946 (162). Since then, there have been more than 30 controlled trials of phototherapy. Rosenthal and colleagues (163) reviewed these data and concluded that bright light was a rapid and effective treatment for FOSAD, usually achieving statistically significant differences from control treatments. Although dim light controls are technically acceptable, some patients who have read about SAD in the lay press may know they are receiving a placebo dose of light.

In reviewing the literature, Wehr and Rosenthal (164) summarized the findings for optimal phototherapy of FOSAD as follows:

- *Exposure to eyes* of diffuse visible light
- A light intensity of at least *2,500 lux*
- Initial treatment duration of at least *2 hours*
- *Daily treatment* throughout the period of risk
- Preferably *morning treatment*

Although limited, the data on drug therapy (with or without light therapy) indicate that *tricyclic antidepressants* may also benefit SAD, with agents such as imipramine reported to be comparable with phototherapy. One of the major drawbacks has been their unacceptable adverse effects. The latest generation of antidepressants such as selective serotonin reuptake inhibitors, venlafaxine, nefazodone, mirtazapine, and bupropion have become the drugs of preference, primarily because of their less troublesome side effect profiles (165) (see Chapter 7). Case report data also indicate a benefit from the *benzodiazepine* alprazolam and the *monoamine oxidase inhibitor* tranylcypromine (166, 167). Finally, the combination treatment of an *antidepressant plus phototherapy* may produce synergistic beneficial effects in patients who cannot tolerate adequate doses or who derive only partial benefit from either therapy alone (168).

Other Mood Disorders

Levitt and colleagues (169) found that augmentation with bright lights resulted in substantial improvement in seven of 10 patients who met

Research Diagnostic Criteria (RDC) for recurrent nonpsychotic treatment-resistant major depression. All had been given adequate trials with antidepressants or had relapsed after a successful course of drug therapy. Whereas five of these patients reported exacerbations of their depression in the winter months, none had experienced remissions during the summer.

Deltito and colleagues (170) studied a group of 17 non-SAD, depressed patients to test the hypothesis that bipolar spectrum, depressed patients might preferentially respond to light therapy. They randomly assigned subjects to either 400 or 2,500 lux of phototherapy (2 hours per day for 7 days) and noted that the unipolar depressed group realized an overall mild improvement, consistent with the previous literature. Somewhat surprisingly, however, the bipolar spectrum depressed patients improved dramatically on both 400 and 2,500 lux of light therapy. The authors were unsure why low-intensity light also produced a beneficial effect, but speculated that the use of the light visor in this study may have been an important factor. It is also possible that these patients might have been particularly sensitive to light exposure. They concluded that light therapy may be a safe and effective treatment for non-SAD-related, bipolar depressed patients. These findings were reaffirmed by Kripke and colleagues (171), who treated 51 major depressed and bipolar depressed patients randomly assigned to either light therapy (2,000 to 3,000 lux) or dim, red light placebo. During a 1-week treatment trial, the light therapy group showed a significantly greater improvement on global depression scores. Other reports indicate a possible role for light therapy in rapid-cycling bipolar patients (172, 173). Those with classic, endogenous, or melancholic depression, however, have not improved as much with light therapy (174).

Other Disorders

Bright light has been most studied as a treatment for SAD, and perhaps subsyndromal SAD (i.e., mild winter depression), than for other types of depression (175). As noted earlier, however, preliminary evidence indicates that phototherapy may benefit such varied conditions as the following:

- Jet lag
- Delayed sleep syndrome
- Chronobiological disorders in shift workers

For example, Lewy and Sack (176) reported on the beneficial effects of light therapy for circadian phase disorders. They recommend bright light (1 to 2 hours at 2,500 lux) be given 1 hour before bedtime in those with a phase advancement and immediately upon awakening in those who are phase delayed. Furthermore, in attempting to help patients who are blind, they report that melatonin (0.5 mg orally) can also produce beneficial phase shifts but must be administered in the opposite manner to bright light for phase-advanced or delayed conditions.

Maintenance and Prophylactic Therapy

There are virtually no controlled data addressing these issues for the treatment of SAD.

Adverse Effects

Some of the most common complaints in patients exposed to bright light therapy include the following:

- Eyestrain
- Headache
- Insomnia
- Irritability

Both bright light therapy and dawn simulation have also been associated with hypomania, which usually resolves with discontinuation of treatments. Of greater concern are some case reports of suicidal ideation with evening light exposure (177). In general, adverse effects seem more likely to occur when the light source is close to the eyes, as with head-mounted units. Damage from UV and blue light exposure on ocular structures has not been borne out (178).

Conclusion

Bright light phototherapy may be a relatively safe and effective alternative to medication, primarily for SAD (179). It may also have an additive or synergistic effect when used in combination with antidepressants for SAD, as well as other, nonseasonal, depressive disorders. One major difficulty is the inconvenience (i.e., sitting in front of a bank of lights for extended periods of time daily), but preliminary experience with portable light visors and dawn simulation may diminish this problem (180, 181).

Sleep Deprivation Therapy

There is a good rationale for associating sleep disturbances with the pathophysiology of mood disorders. Many depressed patients experience marked sleep disruption, usually insomnia, but also hypersomnia and aberrant REM activity (e.g., earlier onset, increased density). Bipolar patients often convert to mania in the early morning hours (i.e., 2 to 3 am), whereas many depressed patients feel worse in the morning, implicating a rhythmic disturbance. In this context, a striking clinical observation was that sleep deprivation produced a brief (e.g., about 24 hours) antidepressant effect (182). This phenomenon is supported by studies with varying degrees of experimental control, in addition to a substantial amount of uncontrolled evidence.

Thus, sleep deprivation may be an alternative somatic approach that holds promise for the treatment of certain depressive disorders, as well as being an aid in elucidating the biological basis of mood disorders (183). Further preliminary evidence indicates a role for sleep deprivation when used concomitantly or consecutively with antidepressants or with bright light therapy (184).

Efficacy

In 1990, Wu and Bunney (185) cited 61 open reports encompassing more than 1,700 subjects. Of those given the diagnosis of endogenous depression, 67% demonstrated improvement after sleep deprivation. Of those who were not on medication, 83% relapsed after only one night of sleep, compared with 59% of those on medication. These authors also report several patients in whom a brief nap induced a relapse. Wu and Bunney argue persuasively for the depressogenic property of sleep and how wakefulness may rapidly counteract this effect, albeit temporarily. They further postulate the possible existence of a depressive substance that is released

by sleep but metabolized during the waking period, using diurnal variation in mood as evidence for this position.

Vogel (186) reported that selective disruption of REM sleep, without interrupting slow-wave sleep, produced a gradual but sustained antidepressant effect.

Reports of hypomania or mania after sleep deprivation led Wehr and colleagues (187) to hypothesize that sleep reduction may precipitate a manic phase in bipolar patients. As all effective antidepressant therapies have been reported to precipitate a manic episode, this observation possibly strengthens the evidence for a commonality between sleep deprivation and antidepressants.

Wu and colleagues (188) have also reported on the results of a positron emission tomography (PET) scan study of 15 depressed subjects and 15 normal control subjects after a night of normal sleep and a night with sleep deprivation. The authors found evidence for overactive limbic system metabolism in a subset of depressed patients after sleep deprivation, who subsequently experienced reduced activity in this area, as well as a lessening of their depression.

Leibenluft and Wehr (189) critically reviewed the literature on the clinical application of sleep deprivation for depressive disorders, focusing on six areas: *potentiation* of antidepressant response; *hastening the onset* of response to antidepressants or mood stabilizers; *preventing recurrence* of mood cycling; as an *alternative* to antidepressants; as a *diagnostic* probe; and as a *predictor* of antidepressant or ECT response. These authors concluded that the use of sleep deprivation is counterintuitive (given that sleep disturbances typically accompany depression), that the literature to support its utility is largely uncontrolled, and that the transient and unpredictable response to this approach limits its value for most unmedicated depressed patients. They do, however, suggest that existing evidence supports the use of this modality as follows:

- As a *possible potentiation strategy* in partial drug responders
- As a technique *to hasten drug response*
- In the treatment of *premenstrual dysphoric disorder (PMDD)*

TABLE 8-13. *Transcranial magnetic stimulation critical parameters*

Parameter	Comment
Motor threshold (MT)	Lowest intensity over primary motor cortex to produce contraction of the first dorsal interosseous (FDI) or abductor pollicis brevis (APB) muscle; visual or electromyographically monitored
Stimulus coil location	Most common • Left dorsolateral prefrontal cortex (DLPFC) Less common • Right DLPFC • Vertex

Stimulus coil configuration
    Figure eight or circular shape
Stimulus pulse(s) or train
    Intensity
    Frequency (CPS or Hz)
    Duration
    Interpulse interval
	
	80%–120% of MT
	$\leq$1–20 Hz
	1 msec
	50–100 msec

Intertrain interval (ITI)	20–60 sec

From Janicak PG, Krasuski J, Beedle D, et al. Transcranial magnetic stimulation for neuropsychiatric disorders. *Psychiatr Times* 1999 (Feb):56–62.

• In *differentiating depressive pseudodementia* from primary degenerative dementia with secondary depression

Transcranial Magnetic Stimulation

A substantial proportion of depressed patients do not tolerate or respond to existing drug or somatic treatments. Transcranial magnetic stimulation (TMS) is emerging as a possible viable alternative to ECT and/or drug therapies for certain neuropsychiatric disorders (2).

The potential therapeutic effect of TMS has primarily focused on depression, with encouraging preliminary results. Advantages include efficient and cost-effective administration on an outpatient basis, and, in contrast to ECT, no anesthesia, seizure induction, or significant cognitive effects (190). Known side effects of TMS are usually benign and include discomfort at the stimulation site, muscle twitching during stimulation, and headache. Rarely, however, treatment-related seizures may occur (191). The following are important questions to resolve:

• What is the true *efficacy of TMS* for depression and possibly other neuropsychiatric conditions?

• What are the *optimal treatment parameters*?
• Where would this somatic modality fit into a *therapeutic algorithm* for depression?

In addition, the development of optimal research designs with appropriate blinding is necessary to adequately assess acute and maintenance efficacy, as well as the potential for adverse effects (192). Studies of TMS as a treatment for depression have also addressed issues such as coil location and configuration, stimulus frequency, and intensity. Varying parameters and number of treatments, however, make it difficult to compare these studies. Table 8-13 summarizes the most commonly considered parameters (193).

Coil Location and Configuration

Most studies in depression have shown that stimulation applied over the left dorsolateral prefrontal cortex is effective (194–199). Other locations at which stimulation may produce an antidepressant effect include the vertex and right prefrontal cortex (193–204). For example, low frequency (LF) -rTMS given over the *right* dorsolateral prefrontal cortex (DLPFC) may be as effective as high frequency repetitive (HF-r) TMS given over the *left* DLPFC. In addition, coil size and configuration (usually circular or figure eight) have differed in these studies and represent a potential problem in generalizing results across studies.

Stimulus Frequency

Pre-clinical work and neuroimaging suggest potential frequency-dependent effects of rTMS. Thus, higher frequencies may increase while lower frequencies may decrease brain metabolism (205). Clinically, repetitive, high frequency stimulation (i.e., >1 Hz or HF-rTMS) and repetitive, low frequency stimulation (i.e., ≤ 1 Hz or SF-rTMS) have been used.

Stimulus Intensity

Stimulus intensity is determined in relationship to each individual's motor threshold (MT), with most studies stimulating at 80% to 120% of this threshold. A review by George et al. (206) found that studies using stimulation pulses of lower intensities (e.g., 80% of MT) demonstrated only modest antidepressant effects, whereas higher intensities (e.g., 110% of MT) produced greater efficacy. Intensities greater than 120% of MT are generally avoided because of the possibility of an increased seizure risk.

Real versus Sham TMS

A persisting methodological issue is the lack of a satisfactory sham method (192). Currently, accepted sham techniques include holding the coil perpendicular or at a 45-degree angle from the scalp surface or an "active" sham (i.e., lower frequencies). These methods do not address the placebo response to a dramatically (i.e., coil over the scalp) administered "treatment" according to many researchers. Better placebo methods and designs are therefore needed to clarify the effect of real TMS. With these caveats in mind, several studies found real TMS significantly better than sham TMS (196–198, 200, 207). Padberg et al. (208) and Loo et al. (209), however, could not demonstrate a difference between real and sham TMS.

TMS for Treatment-Resistant Depression

Investigators have also assessed the efficacy of TMS in patients with drug treatment-resistant depression, albeit variably defined (194–196, 198, 204, 208–211). The generally positive results are noteworthy considering the more difficult-to-treat patients involved and clearly warrant further study. These results are also consistent with the preliminary encouraging findings in studies comparing TMS to ECT for more severely ill, often drug-resistant patients.

TMS as Augmentation to Antidepressants

Augmentation with TMS in partially responsive, depressed patients has also been investigated. In one study of 24 major depressive disorder (MDD) patients, Conca et al. (212) compared an antidepressant plus LF-rTMS (<0.17 Hz, 1.9 T, 10 sessions) with an antidepressant only. Using the Hamilton Depression Rating Scale (HDRS) as the primary outcome measure, the authors reported that the combined treatment was superior to antidepressant monotherapy.

If TMS is found to be beneficial as an augmentation strategy, an important issue is how pharmacotherapy, ECT, and TMS may complement each other in the treatment of depression. In this context, questions include whether TMS can

- *Accelerate* the onset of response
- Be an *adjunctive strategy* for treatment-resistant depression
- *Substitute* for pharmacotherapy or ECT, for at least some patients
- *Complement psychotherapies* (cognitive and interpersonal) in mild to moderate depressive episodes

A related issue is that many psychotropics are known to lower the seizure threshold. Therefore increased care is warranted when these agents are used in conjunction with TMS. However, Turnier-Shea and colleagues (213) reviewed their experience with 82 patients on various medication combinations who also received a total of 986 TMS treatments. There were no seizures reported, and the authors suggest that the concomitant use of some antidepressants and TMS should not be prohibited. Here, SF-rTMS may be preferable to HF-rTMS given that most reports of seizures involved the latter approach and because SF-rTMS may induce neuronal inhibition rather than excitation (191, 205). Imaging and EEG data in combination with clinical studies should provide more information about the effectiveness and safety of different frequencies.

TMS versus ECT

Although there are many potential methodological confounds, a crucial indicator of how TMS might be positioned in a depression treatment algorithm is its true efficacy as well as relative efficacy in comparison with ECT. In this context, preliminary reports suggest that TMS may be comparable to ECT for at least certain subgroups of depressed patients.

In an open study, Grunhaus and colleagues (214) randomly assigned 40 patients with MDD to either TMS or right UND ECT. TMS parameters were stimulation of the left DLPFC at 90% MT at 10 Hz for 2 seconds (n = 8) or 6 seconds (n = 12) for a total of 20 trains per sessions and up to 20 sessions. In the ECT group, eight patients were switched to BILAT ECT as a result of insufficient response. The authors concluded that ECT was more effective than TMS, especially for patients with MDD and psychosis. In nonpsychotic MDD, however, the therapeutic effects of TMS were similar to those of ECT. We note that antipsychotics and/or antidepressants apparently were used in the psychotic depressed group receiving ECT but not the group receiving TMS.

Presently, Janicak et al. (215) are conducting a trial of HF-rTMS versus BILAT ECT in more severely depressed patients with a crossover option if response is inadequate to the initial treatment assignment. The design initially allows for a direct comparison of these somatic therapies in a randomized, prospective, parallel design. In addition, a crossover phase allows evaluation of the alternate therapy in the event of nonresponse to the initial treatment assignment. As needed, rescue medications (e.g., anxiolytics, sedatives) are kept to a minimum. TMS parameters are stimulation with a figure eight coil over the left DLPC at 110% MT, using a frequency of 10 Hz with a figure eight coil over for 5 seconds with a 30-second intertrain interval. One thousand stimulations are

given per session for up to 20 sessions. Thus far, 14 subjects (nine men, five women) between the ages of 18 and 66 years with a *Diagnostic and Statistical Manual of Mental Disorders,* 4th ed (DSM-IV) primary diagnosis of either unipolar or bipolar depressive episode have completed the study. Overall, improvement based on the decrease from baseline HDRS scores indicate that TMS is comparable with ECT.

Finally, TMS may play a role as a combination strategy with ECT to reduce the total number of ECT treatments while achieving similar efficacy but causing fewer adverse effects (215a).

Conclusion

Preliminary results from case reports, case series, and open and increasingly better controlled trials have found TMS to be effective in the treatment of depression. TMS, antidepressants, and ECS appear to induce similar effects in animal behavioral models of depression and changes in brain neurochemical activity. These include changes in the forced swim test, increase in seizure threshold, and effects on β-noradrenergic receptor downregulation. Whereas seizures appear unnecessary to achieve clinical benefit with TMS, it is still unclear what aspects are beneficial. As noted earlier, although this modality is associated with some complications (e.g., headaches and, rarely, inadvertent seizure) relative to ECT and perhaps even pharmacotherapy under certain situations, it appears to be quite safe. Future studies of major depression should explore TMS-related issues such as the following:

- The *relative efficacy* and safety of SF-rTMS versus HF-rTMS
- As a possible *induction of early response*
- As a possible *adjunct to pharmacotherapy, ECT, or psychotherapy*
- As a *pre-ECT strategy* in selected patients
- As a *maintenance strategy*

Other issues include the use of magnetic rather than electrical stimulation to induce seizures for therapeutic purposes, and the use of TMS as a probe to clarify brain structural/functional relationships in various neuropsychiatric conditions. Figure 8-1 incorporates the potential role of TMS in a treatment algorithm for depression.

Vagus Nerve Stimulation

The vagus nerve terminates in the nucleus of the solitary tract with widespread projections, including the locus ceruleus. There are several lines of evidence that support the potential efficacy of vagus nerve stimulation (VNS) for depression, including the following:

- *Mood effects of VNS* in epileptic patients
- *Neuroimaging* data indicating VNS alters metabolism in the limbic system
- Possible mood-regulating effects of some *anticonvulsants*
- Alteration of *monoamine activity* in animals and humans (216)

VNS is delivered by the Neuro Cybernetic Prothesis System, which was approved by the FDA in 1997 for the management of refractory, partial-onset seizures. A surgical procedure is required to implant the device in the left chest wall with a lead attached to the left vagus nerve. The most frequent stimulation-related adverse effects, which rarely lead to VNS termination include the following:

- Pain
- Coughing
- Voice alteration
- Chest pain
- Nausea

Rush and colleagues (217) have published the results of a multicenter trial using VNS for treatment resistant depression. In this group of 67 nonpsychotic, depressed, treatment-resistant patients, a 10-week open trial of VNS produced a 40% to 50% reduction in baseline HDRS, CGI, and Montgomery-Ashberg Depression Rating Scale scores. Further studies are now underway.

CONCLUSION

As with TMS, we emphasize that VNS is still in the experimental stage, but preliminary positive results warrant further controlled studies to attempt replication in selected treatment resistant depression patients.

REFERENCES

1. Beedle D, Krasuski J, Janicak PG. Advances in somatic therapies: electroconvulsive therapy, repetitive transcranial magnetic stimulation, and bright light therapy. In: Janicak PG, Davis JM, Preskorn SH, et al., eds. *Principles and practice of psychopharmacotherapy. 2nd ed update,* vol 2. Baltimore: Williams & Wilkins, 1998.
2. Martis B, Janicak PG. Transcranial magnetic stimulation for major depression: therapeutic possibilities. *Int Drug Ther Newsl* 2000;35:58–71.
3. Bini L. Experimental researches on epileptic attacks induced by electric current. *Am J Psychiatry* 1938;94[May Suppl]:172–174.
4. Weiner R. Does electroconvulsive therapy cause brain damage? *Behav Brain Sci* 1984;7:1–48.
5. Coffey CE, Weiner RD, Djang WT, et al. Brain anatomic effects of electroconvulsive therapy: a prospective magnetic resonance imaging study. *Arch Gen Psychiatry* 1991;48:1013–1021.
6. Devanand DP. Does electroconvulsive therapy damage brain cells? *Semin Neurol* 1995;15:351–357.
7. Fink M. New technology in convulsive therapy: a challenge in training. *Am J Psychiatry* 1987;144:1195–1198.
8. Pippard J, Ellam L. *ECT in Great Britain, 1980: a report to the Royal College of Psychiatrists.* London: Gaskell, 1981.
9. Pippard J. Audit of electroconvulsive treatment in two National Health Service regions. *Br J Psychiatry* 1992;160:621–637.
10. Duffett R, Lelliott P. Auditing electroconvulsive therapy: the third cycle. *Br J Psychiatry* 1998;172:401–405.
11. Kramer BA. A teaching guide for electroconvulsive therapy. *Compr Psychiatry* 1999;40:327–331.
11a. American Psychiatric Association. The practice of electroconvulsive therapy: recommendations for treatment, training, and privileging, 2nd ed. Washington. D. C.: *American Psychiatric Press.* 2001.
12. Janicak PG, Mask J, Trimakas KA, et al. ECT: an assessment of mental health professionals' knowledge and attitudes. *J Clin Psychiatry* 1985;46:262–266.
13. Benbow SM. Medical students and ECT: their knowledge and attitudes. *Convuls Ther* 1990;6:32–37.
14. Markowitz J, Brown R, Sweeney J, et al. Reduced length and cost of hospital stay for major depression in patients treated with ECT. *Am J Psychiatry* 1987;144:1025–1029.
15. Olfson M, Marcus S, Sackheim HA, et al. Use of ECT for the inpatient treatment of recurrent major depression. *Am J Psychiatry* 1998;155:22–29.
16. Milstein V, Small JG, Miller MJ, et al. Mechanisms of action of ECT: schizophrenia and schizoaffective disorder. *Biol Psychiatry* 1990;27:1282–1292.
17. Leonard BE. Antidepressants: current concepts of mode of action. *Encephale* 1991;17:127–131.
18. Soares JC, Krishnan KR, Keshavan MS. Nuclear magnetic resonance spectroscopy: new insights into the pathophysiology of mood disorders. *Depression* 1996;4:14–30.
19. Manji HK. G-proteins: implications for psychiatry. *Am J Psychiatry* 1992;149:746–760.

20. Avissar S, Nechamkin Y, Roitman G, et al. Reduced G-protein functions and immunoreactive levels in mononuclear leukocytes of patients with depression. *Am J Psychiatry* 1997;154:211–217.

21. Young LT, Li PP, Kamble A, et al. Mononuclear leukocyte levels of G-proteins in depressed patients with bipolar disorder or major depressive disorder. *Am J Psychiatry* 1994;151:594–596.

22. Mitchell PB, Manji HK, Chen G, et al. High levels of G_s alpha in platelets of euthymic patients with bipolar affective disorder. *Am J Psychiatry* 1997;154:218–223.

23. Avissar S, Nechamkin Y, Roitman G, et al. Dynamics of ECT normalization of low G protein function and immunoreactivity in mononuclear leukocytes of patients with major depression. *Am J Psychiatry* 1998;155:66–671.

24. Garcia Seviella JA, Walzer C, Busquets X, et al. Density of guanine nucleotide-binding proteins in platelets of patients with major depression: increased abundance of the G alpha subunit and downregulation by antidepressant drug treatment. *Biol Psychiatry* 1997;42:704–712.

25. Li PP, Young LT, Tom YK, et al. Effects of chronic lithium and carbamazepine treatment on G-protein subunit expression in rat cerebral cortex. *Biol Psychiatry* 1993;34:162–170.

26. Pandey GN, Heinz WJ, Brown BD, et al. Electroconvulsive shock treatment decreases beta-adrenergic receptor sensitivity in rat brain. *Nature* 1979;280:234.

27. Vetulani J, Lebrecht V, Pile A. Enhancement of responsiveness of the central serotonergic system and serotonin-2 receptor density in rat frontal cortex by electroconvulsive treatment. *Eur J Pharmacol* 1981;76:81.

28. Pandey GN, Pandey SC, Isaac L, et al. Effect of electroconvulsive shock on $5HT_2$ and α_1-adrenoceptors and phosphoinositide signalling system in rat brain [Molecular Pharmacology section]. *Eur J Pharmacol* 1992;226:303–310.

29. Dysken M, Evans HM, Chan CH, et al. Improvements of depression and parkinsonism during ECT: a case study. *Neuropsychobiology* 1976;2:81–86.

30. Faber R, Trumble MR. Electroconvulsive therapy in Parkinson's disease and other movement disorders. *Movement Disord* 1991;6:293–303.

31. Moellentine C, Rummans T, Ahlskog JE, et al. Effectiveness of ECT in patients with parkinsonism. *J Neuropsychiatry Clin Neurosci* 1998;10:187–193.

32. Fink M, Nemeroff C, A neuroendocrine view of ECT. *Convuls Ther* 1989;5:296–304.

33. Lahmeyer HW, Janicak PG, Easton M, et al. ECT's effect on sleep in major depression [Abstract]. *APA New Res Abstr* 1988;NR:69.

34. Grunhaus L, Shipley JE, Eiser A, et al. Sleep-onset rapid eye movement after electroconvulsive therapy is more frequent in patients who respond less well to electroconvulsive therapy. *Biol Psychiatry* 1997;42:191–200.

35. Post RM, Ballenger JC, Uhde TW, et al. Efficacy of carbamazepine in manic-depressive illness: implications for underlying mechanisms. In: Post RM, Ballenger JC, eds. *Neurobiology of mood disorders*. Baltimore: Williams & Wilkins, 1984:777–816.

36. Post RM, Weiss SRB. Endogenous biochemical abnormalities in affective illness: therapeutic versus pathogenic. *Biol Psychiatry* 1992;32:469–484.

37. Small JG, Milstein V, Miller MS, et al. Clinical, neuropsychological and EEG evidence for mechanisms of action of ECT. *Convuls Ther* 1988;4:280–291.

38. American Psychiatric Association Task Force on ECT. *The practice of ECT: recommendations for treatment, training, and privileging.* Washington, DC: American Psychiatric Press, 2000 *(in press)*.

39. Prudic J, Sackeim H, Devanand DP. Medication resistance and clinical response to ECT. *Psychiatry Res* 1990;31:287–296.

40. Prudic J, Haskett RF, Mulsant B, et al. Resistance to antidepressant medications and short-term clinical response to ECT. *Am J Psychiatry* 1996;153:985–992.

41. Kantor S, Glassman A. Delusional depressions: natural history and response to treatment. *Br J Psychiatry* 1977;131:351–360.

42. Janicak PG, Easton MS, Comaty JE, Dowd S, Davis JM. Efficacy of ECT in psychotic and nonpsychotic depression. *Convuls Ther* 1989;5:314–320.

43. Pande AC, Grunhaus LJ, Hachett RF, Gredin JF. ECT in delusional and non-delusional depressive disorder. *J Affect Disord* 1990;19:215–219.

44. Schatzberg AF, Rothschild AJ. Psychotic (delusional) major depression: should it be included as a distinct syndrome in DSM-IV? *Am J Psychiatry* 1992;149:733–745.

45. Kocsis J, Croghan JL, Katz MM, et al. Response to treatment with antidepressants of patients with severe or moderate nonpsychotic depression and of patients with psychotic depression. *Am J Psychiatry* 1990;147:621–624.

46. Coryell W. The treatment of psychotic depression. *J Clin Psychiatry* 1998;59[Suppl]:22–27.

47. Flint AJ, Rifat SL. Two year outcome of psychotic depression in late life. *Am J Psychiatry* 1998;155:178–183.

48. Flint AJ, Rifat SL. The treatment of psychotic depression in later life: a comparison of pharmacotherapy and ECT. *Int J Geriatr Psychiatry* 1998;13:23–28.

49. Philbert RA, Richards L, Lynch CF, et al. Effect of ECT on mortality and clinical outcome in geriatric unipolar depression. *J Clin Psychiatry* 1995;56:390–394.

50. Fink M. In: Trimble M, Cummings J, eds. *Catatonia contemporary behavioral neurology.* Oxford: Butterworth-Heineman, 1997:289–309.

51. Mukherjee S, Sackheim HA, Schnur DB. Electroconvulsive therapy of acute manic episodes: a review of 50 years' experience. *Am J Psychiatry* 1994;151:169–176.

52. Davis JM, Janicak PG, Sakkas P, et al. ECT in the treatment of NMS. *Convuls Ther* 1991;7:111–120.

53. Janicak PG, Davis JM, Gibbons RD, et al. Efficacy of ECT: a meta-analysis. *Am J Psychiatry* 1985;142:297–302.

54. Ulett GA, Smith K, Gleser GC. Evaluation of convulsive and subconvulsive shock therapies utilizing a control group. *Am J Psychiatry* 1956;112:795–802.

55. Brill NQ, Crumpton E, Eiduson S, et al. Relative effectiveness of various components of ECT. *Arch Neurol Psychiatry* 1959;81:627–635.

56. Harris JA, Robin AA. A controlled trial of phenelzine in depressive reactions. *J Ment Sci* 1960;106:1432–1437.

57. Fahy P, Imlah N, Harrington J. A controlled comparison of ECT, imipramine and thiopentone sleep in depression. *J Neuropsychiatry* 1963;4:310–314.

58. Lambourn J, Gill D. A controlled comparison of simulated and real ECT. *Br J Psychiatry* 1978;133:514–519.

59. West ED. Electric convulsion therapy in depression: a double blind controlled trial. *BMJ* 1981;1:155–357.

60. Kiloh LG, Child JP, Latner GA. A controlled trial of iproniazid in the treatment of endogenous depression. *J Ment Sci* 1960;106:1139–1144.

61. Greenblatt M, Grosser GH, Wechsler H. A comparative study of selected antidepressant medications and EST? *Am J Psychiatry* 1962;119:144–153.

62. Greenblatt M, Grosser GH, Wechsler H. Differential response of hospitalized depressed patients to somatic therapy. *Am J Psychiatry* 1964;120:935–943.

63. Shepherd M. Clinical trial of the treatment of depressive illness. *BMJ* 1965;1:881–886.

64. Bruce EM, Crone N, Fitzpatrick G, et al. A comparative trial of ECT and tofranil. *Am J Psychiatry* 1960;117:76.

65. Robin AA, Harris JA. A controlled comparison of imipramine and electroplexy. *J Ment Sci* 1962;108:217–219.

66. Wilson IC, Vernon JT, Guin T, et al. A controlled study of treatments of depression. *J Neuropsychiatry* 1963;4:331–337.

67. Cannicott SM. Unilateral electroconvulsive therapy. *Postgrad Med* 1962;38:451–459.

68. Strain JJ, Brunschwig L, Duffy JP, et al. Rosenbaum AL, Bidder TG. Comparison of therapeutic effects and memory changes with bilateral and unilateral ECT. *Am J Psychiatry* 1968;125:294–304.

69. Zinkin S, Birtchnell J. Unilateral ECT: its effects on memory and its therapeutic efficacy. *Br J Psychiatry* 1968;114:973–988.

70. Halliday AM, Davison K, Browne MW, et al. A comparison of the effects on depression and memory of bilateral ECT and unilateral ECT to the dominant and non-dominant hemispheres. *Br J Psychiatry* 1968;114:997–1012.

71. Abrams R, DeVito R. Clinical efficacy of unilateral ECT. *Dis Nerv Syst* 1969;30:262–263.

72. d'Elia G. Comparison of electroconvulsive therapy with unilateral and bilateral stimulation. II. Therapeutic efficiency in endogenous depression. *Acta Psychiatr Scand Suppl* 1970;215:30–43.

73. Fleminger JJ, Horne DJ, Nair NPV, et al. Differential effects of unilateral and bilateral ECT. *Am J Psychiatry* 1970;127:430–436.

74. Sand-Stromgren L. Unilateral vs. bilateral ECT. *Acta Psychiatr Scand Suppl* 1973;240:1–65.

75. Heshe J, Roder E, Theilgaard A. Unilateral and bilateral ECT: a psychiatric and psychological study of therapeutic effect and side effects. *Acta Psychiatr Scand Suppl* 1978;275:4–181.

76. Fraser RM, Glass IB. Unilateral and bilateral ECT in elderly patients. *Acta Psychiatr Scand* 1980;62:13–31.

77. Sackeim HA, Decina P, Kanzler M, et al. Effects of electrode placement on the efficacy of titrated, low-dose ECT. *Am J Psychiatry* 1987;144:1449–1455.

78. Janicak PG, Sharma RP, Israni TH, et al. Effects of UND versus BL-ECT on memory and depression: a preliminary report. *Psychopharmacol Bull* 1991;27:353–357.

79. Clarke TB, Coffey EC, Hoffman GW, et al. Continuation therapy for depression using outpatient ECT. *Convuls Ther* 1989;5:330–337.

80. Thienhaus OS, Margletta S, Bennett JA. A study of the clinical efficacy of maintenance ECT. *J Clin Psychiatry* 1990;51:141–144.

81. Sackeim H, Prudic J, Devanand DP, et al. The impact of medication resistance and continuation pharmacotherapy on relapse following response to ECT in major depression. *J Clin Psychopharmacol* 1990;10:96–104.

82. Miller LJ. Use of electroconvulsive therapy during pregnancy. *Hosp Community Psychiatry* 1994;45:444;450.

83. Walker R, Swartz CM. Electroconvulsive therapy during high-risk pregnancy. *Gen Hosp Psychiatry* 1994;16:348–353.

84. Verwiel JM, Heinis C, Verwey B. Successful electroconvulsive therapy in a pregnant woman with neuroleptic malignant syndrome. *Ned Tijdschr Geneeskd* 1994;138:196–199.

85. Rey JM, Walter G. Half a century of ECT use in young people. *Am J Psychiatry* 1997;54:595–602.

86. Walter G, Rey JM, Starling J. Experience, knowledge and attitudes of child psychiatrists regarding electroconvulsive therapy in the young. *Aust N Z J Psychiatry* 1997;31:676–681.

87. McDonald WM, Phillips VL, Figiel GS, et al. Cost-effective maintenance treatment of resistance geriatric depression. *Psychiatr Ann* 1998;28:47–52.

88. Alexander RC, Salomon M, Ionesca-Pioggia M, et al. Convulsive therapy in the treatment of mania: McLean Hospital. *Convuls Ther* 1988;4:115–125.

89. Stromgren LS. Electroconvulsive therapy in Aarhus, Denmark in 1984: its application in nondepressive disorders. *Convuls Ther* 1989;5:227–243.

90. Mukherjee S. Mechanism of the antimanic effects of electroconvulsive therapy. *Convuls Ther* 1989;5:227–243.

91. Mukherjee S, Sakeim HA. Unilateral ECT in the treatment of manic episodes. *Convuls Ther* 1988;4:74–80.

92. Reid WH, Keller S, Leatherman M, et al. ECT in Texas 19 months of mandatory reporting. *J Clin Psychiatry* 1998;59:8–13.

93. Folk JW, Kellner CH, Beale MD, et al. Anesthesia for electroconvulsive therapy: a review. *J ECT* 2000;16:157–170.

94. Abrams R. *Electroconvulsive therapy.* New York: Oxford University Press, 1992.

95. Swartz CM. Anesthesia for ECT. *Convuls Ther* 1993;9:301–316.

96. Ilivicky H, Caroff SN, Simone AF. Etomidate during ECT for elderly seizure-resistant patients. *Am J Psychiatry* 1995;152:957–958.

97. Gran L, Bergsholm P, Bleie H. Seizure duration in unilateral electroconvulsive therapy. A comparison of the anesthetic agents etomidate and Althesin with methotrexate. *Acta Psychiatr Scand* 1984;69:472–483.

98. Kovac AL, Pardo M. A comparison between etomidate and methohexital for anesthesia in ECT. *Convuls Ther* 1992;8:118–125.

99. Bergsholm P, Swartz CM. Anesthesia in electroconvulsive therapy and alternatives to barbiturates. *Psychiatr Ann* 1996;26:709–712.

100. Staton RD, Enderle JD, Gerst JW. The electroencephalographic pattern during electroconvulsive therapy. IV. Spectral energy distributions with methohexital, innovar and ketamine anesthesias. *Clin Electroencephalogr* 1986;17:203–215.

101. Lunn RJ, Savageau MM, Beatty WW, et al. Anesthetics and electroconvulsive therapy seizure duration: implications for therapy from a rat model. *Biol Psychiatry* 1981;16:1163–1175.

102. McInnes EG, James NM. A comparison of ketamine and methohexital in electroconvulsive therapy. *Med J Aust* 1972;13:1031–1032.

103. Rasmussen KG, Jarvis MR, Zorumski CF. Ketamine anesthesia in electroconvulsive therapy. *Convuls Ther* 1996;12:217–223.

104. Kelsey MC, Grossberg GT. Safety and efficacy of caffeine-augmented ECT in elderly depressives: a retrospective study. *J Geriatr Psychiatry Neurol* 1995;8:168–172.

105. Calev A, Fink M, Petrides G, et al. Caffeine pretreatment enhances clinical efficacy and reduces cognitive effects of electroconvulsive therapy. *Convuls Ther* 1993;9:95–100.

106. Coffey CE, Figiel GS, Weiner RD, et al. Caffeine augmentation of ECT. *Am J Psychiatry* 1990;147:579–585.

107. Enns M, Peeling J, Sutherland GR. Hippocampal neurons are damaged by caffeine-augmented electroshock seizures. *Biol Psychiatry* 1996;40:642–647.

108. Shapira B, Lerer B, Gilboa D, et al. Facilitation of ECT by caffeine pretreatment. *Am J Psychiatry* 1987;144:1199–1202.

109. Sackeim HA, Prudic J, Devanand DP, et al. Effects of stimulus intensity and electrode placement on efficacy and cognitive effects of electroconvulsive therapy. *N Engl J Med* 1993;328:839–846.

110. Sackeim HA, Prudic J, Devanand DP, et al. A prospective, randomized, double-blind comparison of bilateral and right unilateral electroconvulsive therapy at different stimulus intensities. *Arch Gen Psychiatry* 2000;57:425–434.

111. Jha A, Stein G. Decreased efficacy of combined benzodiazepines and unilateral ECT in treatment of depression. *Acta Psychiatr Scand* 1996;94:101-1-4.

112. Stromgren LS, Dahl J, Fjeldborg et al. Factors influencing seizure duration and number of seizures applied in unilateral electroconvulsive therapy. Anaesthetics and benzodiazepines. *Acta Psychiatr Scand* 1980;62:158–165.

113. Pettinati HM, Stephens SM, Willis KM, et al. Evidence for less improvement in depression in patients taking benzodiazepines during unilateral ECT. *Am J Psychiatry* 1990;147:1029–1035.

114. Greenberg RM, Pettinati HM. Benzodiazepines and electroconvulsive therapy. *Convuls Ther* 1993;9:262–273.

115. Shapira B, Lidsky D, Gorfine M, et al. Electroconvulsive therapy and resistant depression: clinical implication of seizure threshold. *J Clin Psychiatry* 1996;57:32;38.

116. Farah A, McCall WV. Electroconvulsive therapy stimulus dosing: a survey of contemporary practices. *Convuls Ther* 1993;9:90–94.

117. Petrides G, Fink M. The half age stimulation strategy for ECT dosing. *Convuls Ther* 1996;12:138–146.

118. Lisanby SH, Devanand DP, Nobler MS, et al. Exceptionally high seizure threshold: ECT device limitations. *Convuls Ther* 1996;12:156–164.

119. Price TR, McAllister TW. Response of depressed patients to sequential unilateral nondominant brief-pulse and bilateral sinusoidal ECT. *J Clin Psychiatry* 1986;47:182–186.

120. Swartz CM. Asymmetric bilateral right frontotemporal left frontal stimulus electrode placement. *Neuropsychobiology* 1994;29:174–178.

121. Abraham KR, Kulhara P. The efficacy of ECT in the treatment of schizophrenia: a comparative study. *Br J Psychiatry* 1987;151:152–155.

122. Zarate CA, Tohen M, Baldassarini R. Clozapine in severe mood disorders. *J Clin Psychiatry* 1995;56:411–417.

123. Frankenburg FR, Suppes T, McLean PE. Combined clozapine and electroconvulsive therapy. *Convuls Ther* 1993;9:176–180.

124. Farah A, Beale MD, Kellner CH. Risperidone and ECT combination therapy: a case series. *Convuls Ther* 1995;11:280–282.

125. Jacobsen FM. Risperidone in the treatment of affective illness and obsessive-compulsive disorder. *J Clin Psychiatry* 1995;56:423–429.

126. Masiar SJ, Johns CA. ECT following clozapine. *Br J Psychiatry* 1991;158:135–136.

127. Lerer B, Shapira B, Calev A, et al. Antidepressant and cognitive effects of twice versus three times weekly ECT. *Am J Psychiatry* 1995;152:564–570.

128. Shapira B, Tubi N, Draxler H, et al. Cost and benefit in the choice of ECT schedule: twice a week versus three times a week ECT. *Br J Psychiatry* 1998;172:44–48.

129. Kellner CH, Monroe RR Jr, Pritchett J, et al. Weekly ECT in geriatric depression. *Convuls Ther* 1992;8:245–252.

130. Milstein V, Small JG, Klapper MH, et al. Uni- versus bilateral ECT in the treatment of mania. *Convuls Ther* 1987;3:1–9.

131. Small JG, Klapper MH, Kellams JJ, et al. ECT compared with lithium in the management of manic states. *Arch Gen Psychiatry* 1988;45:727–732.

132. Lawson JS. Gender issues in electroconvulsive therapy. *Psychiatr Ann* 1996;26:717–720.

133. Prudic JA, Sackeim HA, Spicknall K. Potential pharmacologic agents for the cognitive effects of electroconvulsive therapy. *Psychiatr Ann* 1998;28:40–46.

134. Stern RA, Nevels CT, Shelhorse ME, et al. Antidepressant and memory effects of combined thyroid hormone treatment and electroconvulsive therapy: preliminary findings. *Biol Psychiatry* 1991;30:623–627.

135. Reid IC, Stewart CA. Seizures, memory and synaptic plasticity. *Seizure* 1997;6:351–359.

136. Stewart CA, Reid IC. Ketamine prevents ECS-induced synaptic enhancement in rat hippocampus. *Neurosci Lett* 1994;178:11–14.

137. Prudic J, Sackeim HA, Decina P, et al. Acute effects of ECT on cardiovascular functioning: relations to patient and treatment variables. *Acta Psychiatr Scand* 1987;75:344–351.

138. Herman RC, Dorwart RA, Hoover CW, et al. Variation in ECT use in the United States. *Am J Psychiatry* 1998;152:869–875.

139. Herman RC, Ettner SL, Dorwart RA, et al. Characteristics of psychiatrists who perform ECT. *Am J Psychiatry* 1998;155:889–894.

140. Lewy AJ, Sack RL, Miller S, et al. Antidepressant and circadian phase-shifting effects of light. *Science* 1987;235:352–354.

141. Avery DH. The proper use of light therapy. *Dir Psychiatry* 1999;19:379–398.

142. Eastman C, Young M, Fogg L, et al. Bright light treatment of winter depression: a placebo-controlled trial. *Arch Gen Psychiatry* 1998;55:883–889.

143. Terman M, Terman JS, Ross DC. A controlled trial of timed bright light and negative air ionization for treatment of winter depression [see comments]. *Arch Gen Psychiatry* 1998;55:875–882.

144. Kripke DF. Light treatment for nonseasonal major depression: are we ready? In: Lam RW, ed. *Seasonal affective disorder and beyond: light treatment for SAD and non-SAD conditions,* 1st ed. Washington, DC: American Psychiatric Press, 1998;159–172.

145. Boulos Z. Bright light treatment for jet lag and shift work. In: Lam RW, ed. *Seasonal affective disorder and beyond: light treatment for SAD and non-SAD conditions,* 1st ed. Washington, DC: American Psychiatric Press, 1998;253–287.

146. Parry BL. Light therapy of premenstrual depression. In: Lam RW, ed. *Seasonal affective disorder and beyond: light treatment for SAD and non-SAD conditions,* 1st ed. Washington, DC: American Psychiatric Press, 1998;173–191.

147. Bauer MS. Summertime bright-light treatment of bipolar major depressive episodes. *Biol Psychiatry* 1993;33:663–665.

148. Rosenthal NE, Jacobsen FM, Sack DA, et al. Atenolol in seasonal affective disorder: a test of the melatonin hypothesis. *Am J Psychiatry* 1988;145:52–56.

149. Meesters Y, Jansen JHC, Bursma DGM, et al. Light therapy for seasonal affective disorder: the effects of timing. *Br J Psychiatry* 1995;166:607–612.

150. Lewy AJ, Sack RL, Singer CM, et al. Winter depression and the phase shift hypothesis for bright light's therapeutic effect: history, theory, and experimental evidence. *J Biol Rhythms* 1988;3:121–134.

151. Campbell S, Murphy P. Extraocular circadian phototransduction in humans. *Science* 1998;279:396–398.

152. Oren DA, Terman M. Tweaking the human circadian clock with light. *Science* 1998;279:333–334.

153. Lam RW, Zis AP, Grewal A, et al. Effects of rapid tryptophan depletion in patients with seasonal affective disorder in remission after light therapy. *Arch Gen Psychiatry* 1996;53:41–44.

154. Anderson JL, Vasile RG, Mooney JJ, et al. Changes in norepinephrine output following light therapy for fall/winter seasonal depression. *Biol Psychiatry* 1992;32:700–704.

155. Terman M. On the question of mechanism in phototherapy: considerations of clinical efficacy and epidemiology. *J Biol Rhythms* 1988;3:155–172.

156. Rosenthal NE. Diagnosis and treatment of seasonal affective disorder [Clinical Conference]. *JAMA* 1993;270:2717–2720.

157. Lewy A, Bauer V, Cutler N, et al. Morning vs evening light treatment of patients with winter depression. *Arch Gen Psychiatry* 1998;55:890–896.

158. Lam RW, Buchanan A, Mador JA, et al. Hypersomnia and morning light therapy for winter depression. *Biol Psychiatry* 1992;31:1062–1064.

159. Remé CE, Terman M. Does light therapy present an ocular hazard [Letter]? *Am J Psychiatry* 1992;149:12:1762.

160. Wehr TA, Skwerer RG, Jacobsen FM, et al. Eye versus skin phototherapy of seasonal affective disorder. *Am J Psychiatry* 1987;144:753–757.

161. Terman M, Assiera L, Terman JS, et al. Predictors of response and nonresponse to light treatment for winter depression. *Am J Psychiatry* 1996;153:1423–1429.

162. Marx H. "Hypophysäre Insuffizienz" bei Lichtmangel. *Klin Wochenschr* 1946;24/25:18–21.

163. Rosenthal NE, Sack DA, Skwerer RG, et al. Phototherapy for seasonal affective disorder. *J Biol Rhythms* 1988;3:101–120.

164. Wehr TA, Rosenthal NE. Seasonality and affective illness. *Am J Psychiatry* 1989;146:829–839.

165. Lam RW, Gorman CP, Michalon M, et al. Multicenter, placebo-controlled study of fluoxetine in seasonal affective disorder. *Am J Psychiatry* 1995;152:1765–1770.

166. Teicher MH, Glod CA. Seasonal affective disorder: rapid resolution by low-dose alprazolam. *Psychopharmacol Bull* 1990;26:197–202.

167. Dilsaver SC, Jaeckle RS. *Winter depression responds to tranylcypromine.* American College of Neuropsychopharmacology Abstracts 23rd Annual Meeting, San Juan, Puerto Rico: 1984;199.

168. Kripke DF. Light treatment for nonseasonal depression: speed, efficacy, and combined treatment. *J Affect Disord* 1998;49:109–117.

169. Levitt AJ, Joffe RT, Kennedy SH. Bright light augmentation in antidepressant nonresponders. *J Clin Psychiatry* 1991;52:336–337.

170. Deltito J, Moline M, Pollak C, et al. Effects of phototherapy on nonseasonal unipolar and bipolar depressive spectrum disorders. *J Affect Disord* 1991;23:231–237.

171. Kripke DF, Mullaney DJ, Klauber MR, et al. Controlled trial of bright light for nonseasonal major depressive disorders. *Biol Psychiatry* 1992;31:119–134.

172. Leibenluft E, Turner E, Feldman-Naim S, et al. Light therapy in patients with rapid cycling bipolar disorder: preliminary results. *Psychopharmacol Bull* 1995;31:705–710.

173. Kusumi I, Ohmori T, Kohsaka M, et al. Chronobiological approach for treatment-resistant rapid cycling affective disorders. *Biol Psychiatry* 1995;37:553–559.

174. Terman M, Amira I, Terman JS, et al. Predictors of response and nonresponse to light treatment for depression. *Am J Psychiatry* 1996;153:1423–1429.

175. Kasper S, Roger SLB, Yancey A, et al. Phototherapy in individuals with and without subsyndromal SAD. *Arch Gen Psychiatry* 1989;46:837–844.

176. Lewy AJ, Sack RL. *Chronobiologic treatments for circadian phase disorders.* Abstracts of the American College of Neuropsychopharmacology Annual Meeting, San Juan, Puerto Rico: December 1992;8.

177. Reme C, Reinboth J, Clausen M, et al. Light damage revisited: converging evidence, diverging views? *Graefe's Arch Clin Exp Ophthalmol* 1996;234: 2–11.

178. Gallin PF, Terman M, Reme CE, et al. Ophthalmologic examination of patients with seasonal affective disorder, before and after bright light therapy. *Am J Ophthalmol* 1995;119:202–210.

179. Labbate LA, Lafer B, Thibault A, et al. Side effects induced by bright light treatment for seasonal affective disorder. *J Clin Psychiatry* 1994;55:189–191.

180. Avery DH, Bolte MA, Dager SR, et al. Dawn simulation treatment of winter depression: a controlled study. *Am J Psychiatry* 1993;150:113–117.

181. Avery DH, Bolte MP, Wolfson JK, et al. Dawn simulation compared with a dim red signal in the treatment of winter depression. *Biol Psychiatry* 1994;36:181–188.

182. Pflug B, Tolle R. Disturbances of the 24-hour rhythm in endogenous depression and the treatment of endogenous depression by sleep deprivation. *Int Pharmacopsychiatry* 1971;6:187–196.

183. Wirz-Justice A, Van den Hoofdakker RH. Sleep deprivation in depression: what do we know, where do we go? *Biol Psychiatry* 1999;46:445–453.

184. Praschak-Rieder N, Willeit M, Neumeister A, et al. Therapeutic sleep deprivation and phototherapy [article in German]. *Wien Med Wochenschr* 1999;149:520–524.

185. Wu JC, Bunney WE. The biological basis of an antidepressant response to sleep deprivation and relapse: review and hypothesis. *Am J Psychiatry* 1990;147:14–21.

186. Vogel GW, Vogel F, McAbee RS, et al. Improvement of depression by REM sleep deprivation. *Arch Gen Psychiatry* 1980;37:247–253.

187. Wehr TA, Sach DA, Rosenthal NE. Sleep reduction as a final common pathway in the genesis of mania. *Am J Psychiatry* 1987;144:201–204.

188. Wu JC, Gillin JC, Buchsbaum MS, et al. Effect of sleep deprivation on brain metabolism of depressed patients. *Am J Psychiatry* 1992;149:538–543.

189. Leibenluft E, Wehr TA. Is sleep deprivation useful in the treatment of depression? *Am J Psychiatry* 1992;149:159–168.

190. Martis B, Carson V, Sharma RP, et al. Cognitive effects of repetitive transcranial magnetic stimulation on depressed patients. In: New Research Abstracts of the Annual APA meeting. Chicago, May 15, 2000, NR81: 77.

191. Wassermann EM. Risk and safety of repetitive transcranial magnetic stimulation: report and suggested guidelines from the International Workshop on the Safety of Repetitive Transcranial Magnetic Stimulation, June 5–7, 1996. *Electroencephalogr Clin Neurophysiol* 1998;108:1–16.

192. Loo CK, Taylor JL, Gandevia SC, et al. Transcranial magnetic stimulation (TMS) in controlled treatment studies: are some "sham" forms active? *Biol Psychiatry* 2000;47:325–331.

193. Janicak PG, Krasuski J, Beedle D, et al. Transcranial magnetic stimulation for neuropsychiatric disorders. *Psychiatr Times* 1999;February:56–62.

194. Figiel G, Epstein C, McDonald W, et al. The use of rapid-rate transcranial magnetic stimulation (rTMS) in refractory depressed patients. *J Neuropsychiatry Clin Neurosci* 1998;10:20–25.

195. Greer RA Repetitive Transcranial Magnetic Stimulation of the L-DLPC in depressed patients. New-research Abstracts, APA Annual Meeting. Toronto, Canada, 1998;NR301:149.

196. Nahas Z, Speer A, Molloy M, Arana G, Risch S, George M. Frequency and intensity in the antidepressant effect of left prefrontal rTMS. *Biol Psychiatry* 1998;43:94S.

197. George MS, Wassermann E, Kimbrell T, et al. Mood improvement following daily left temporal repetitive transcranial magnetic stimulation in patients with depression: a placebo-controlled crossover trial. *Am J Psychiatry* 1997;154:1752–1756.

198. Pascual-Leone A, Rubio B, Pallardo F, Catala M. Rapid-rate transcranial magnetic stimulation of left dorsolateral prefrontal cortex in drug resistant depression. *Lancet* 1996;348:233–237.

199. George MS, Wassermann E, Williams W, et al. Daily repetitive transcranial magnetic stimulation (rTMS) improves mood in depression. *Neuroreport* 1995;6: 1853–6.

200. Klein E, Kreinin I, Chistyakov A, Koren D, et al. Therapeutic efficacy of right prefrontal slow repetitive transcranial magnetic stimulation in major depression: a double-blind controlled study. *Arch Gen Psychiatry* 1999;56:315–320.

201. Catala MD, Rubio B, Pascual-Leone A. Lateralized effect of rapid-rate transcranial magnetic stimulation of the dorsolateral prefrontal cortex on depression. *Neurology* 1996;46:S28.005.

202. Feinsod M, Krenin B, Chistyakov A, et al. Preliminary evidence for a beneficial effect of low-frequency rTMS in patients with MDD and schizophrenia. *Depression Anxiety* 1998;7:65–68.

203. Kolbinger H, Hoflich G, Hufnagel A, et al. Transcranial magnetic stimulation (TMS) in the treatment of major depression-a pilot study. *Hum Psychopharmacol* 1995;10:305–310.

204. Hoflich G, Kasper S, Ruhrmann S, et al. Application of transcranial magnetic stimulation in treatment of drug resistant major depression – a report of two cases. *Hum Psychopharmacol* 1993;8:361–365.

205. Post RM, Kimbrell TA, McCann UD, et al. Repetitive transcranial magnetic stimulation as a neuropsychiatric tool: present status and future potential. *J ECT* 1999;15:39–59.

206. George MS, Nahas Z, Speer A, et al. How does TMS improve depression? Current hints about the role of intensity, frequency, location and dose. *Biol Psychiatry* 1998;43:76S.

207. Kimbrell TA, Little JT, Dunn RT, et al. Frequency dependence of antidepressant response to left prefrontal repetitive transcranial magnetic stimulation (rTMS) as a function of baseline cerebral glucose metabolism. *Biol Psychiatry* 1999;46:1603–1613.

208. Padberg F, Haag C, Zwanger P, et al. Repetitive transcranial magnetic stimulation (rTMS) in pharmacotherapy-refractory major depression: comparative study of fast, slow and sham rTMS. *Psychiatry Res* 1999;88:163–171.

209. Loo CK, Mitchell PB, Sachdev PS, et al. Double-blind controlled investigation of transcranial magnetic

stimulation in major depression. *Am J Psychiatry* 1999;156:946–948.

210. Berman RM, Narasimhan M, Sanacora G, et al. A randomized clinical trial of repetitive transcranial magnetic stimulation in the treatment of major depression. *Biol Psychiatry* 2000;47:332–337.

211. Avery D. Repetitive transcranial magnetic stimulation in the treatment of medication-resistant depression: preliminary data. *J Nerv Ment Dis* 1999;187:114–117.

212. Conca A, Koppi S, Konig P, et al. Transcranial magnetic stimulation: a novel antidepressive strategy? *Neuropsychobiology* 1996;34:204–207.

213. Turnier-Shea Y, Rybak M, Reid P, et al. Update on psychotropic medication used concurrently with transcranial magnetic stimulation. *German J Psychiatry* 1999;2:46–59.

214. Grunhaus L, Dannon PN, Schreiber S, et al. Repetitive transcranial magnetic stimulation is as effective as electroconvulsive therapy in the treatment of nondelusional major depressive disorder: an open study. *Biol Psychiatry* 2000;47:314–324.

215. Janicak PG, Martis B, Krasuski JK, et al. Repetitive transcranial magnetic stimulation versus ECT for major depression episode. In: New Research Abstracts of the Annual APA Meeting, Chicago, May 17, 2000, NR546:205.

215a. Pridmore S. Substitution of rapid transcranial magnetic stimulation treatments for electroconvulsive therapy treatments in a course of electroconvulsive therapy. *Depress Anxiety* 2000;12:118–123.

216. George MS, Sackeim HA, Rush AJ, et al. Vagus nerve stimulation: a new tool for brain research and therapy. *Biol Psychiatry* 2000;47:287–295.

217. Rush AJ, George MS, Sackeim HA, et al. Vagus nerve stimulation (VNS) for treatment-resistant depressions: a multicenter study. *Biol Psychiatry* 2000;47:276–286.

9

Indications for Mood Stabilizers

BIPOLAR DISORDER

Bipolar disorder (manic-depressive illness) represents one of the most dramatic presentations in all of medicine and simultaneously poses one of the more difficult therapeutic challenges. It is characterized by mania or hypomania, alternating irregularly or intermingling with episodes of depression; however, a small group (approximately 1%) may only experience recurrent manic episodes (i.e., unipolar mania). The estimated risk of developing a bipolar disorder is 0.5% to 1%, and the incidence of new cases per year is in the range of 0.01% for men and 0.01% to 0.03% for women (1). Bipolar spectrum can be conceived of as a continuum of more to less severe clinical presentations:

- *Bipolar I*
- *Bipolar II*
- *Cyclothymic* disorder
- *Subsyndromal* or subclinical mood disorder

If this model is embraced, it is estimated that the true risk may be in the 3% to 5% range.

Onset usually occurs by the third decade of life, but the disorder can develop later. Recent information indicates that it may be more prevalent in adolescents and children than previously believed (2).

Because the disorder consists of both manic and depressive episodes, as well as an intermingling of these mood states, it presents an organizational problem for any text. This problem occurs partly because the depressive phase is virtually identical to a unipolar depressive disorder, but also because discussion of its treatment is more complicated. Further, bipolar patients often first present with one or more depressive episodes before experiencing a manic or mixed episode. Thus, initial depressive episodes in a young adult do not necessarily dictate the diagnosis of unipolar disorder, especially with a family history of bipolarity. We emphasize that bipolar disorder requires a different approach than unipolar disorder, and its successful management, including the prevention of either phase, is best accomplished by mood stabilizers. Important evidence that distinguishes unipolar and bipolar disorders as distinct entities is their family histories (see the section "Mechanism of Action" in Chapter 10).

Although the emphasis in this chapter is on the manic phase, we underscore that the interplay between mania and depression is integral to an understanding of bipolar disorder. Thus, depression may do the following:

- *Precede* an episode of hypomania or mania
- *Intermingle* with manic symptoms during an acute exacerbation (e.g., mixed episodes)
- *Succeed* a hypomanic or manic phase
- *Occur as a distinct episode* in an intermittent and irregularly alternating pattern with hypomanic or manic episodes

These circumstances have important implications for management because drug treatment of the depressive phase may precipitate a manic episode, rapid cycling, or a more virulent course of the illness (3). Thus, if bipolar disorder is known or suspected, patients are best managed acutely, as well as for maintenance/prophylaxis, with a mood stabilizer. An antidepressant should be added only when necessary and for the shortest time frame required to alleviate the depressive symptoms.

In this chapter, we focus on mania, hypomania, and mixed episodes, referring to the depressive phase when appropriate. A more detailed discussion of the phenomenology of a depressive episode is found in Chapter 6.

Manic Syndrome

The essential feature of mania is a distinct period of an elevated, expansive, or irritable

mood accompanied by several other symptoms (4). Mania is not synonymous with euphoria or elation but is a syndrome that can occur in a wide variety of disorders and involves aberrations in mood, behavior, and thinking. Other clinical manifestations usually include the following:

• *Hyperactivity*
• Pressure of *speech*
• Flight of *ideas*
• Inflated *self-esteem*
• Decreased need for *sleep*
• *Distractibility*
• *Excessive involvement* in activities that have a high potential for painful consequences (5)

The estimated average length of an untreated acute episode is 4 to 13 months, with a range from as brief as 1 day to as long as several years (6).

Hypomania is a less severe form of its manic counterpart, typically without many of the consequences experienced during an acute, full-blown episode. Subtle indicators of hypomania may include the following:

• Increased *productivity*
• Heightened *perceptions*
• *Symptom* overlap and fluctuation
• *Altered view* of spouse, friends, others

Some have postulated a continuum from mild cognitive, perceptual, and behavioral disorganization to more severe presentations, ranging from hypomania to acute mania to manic delirium, occasionally culminating in a chronic manic state. Carlson and Goodwin (7) described the various stages of mania using this model and presented important differential diagnostic considerations at each stage (Table 9-1). This model may help to characterize the severity of an episode, as well as to guide the level of treatment intervention.

Paralleling this continuum of severity in the manic phase are the various levels of *depression*, which can range from nonpsychotic to psychotic, to delirious, to depressive stupor.

According to the *Diagnostic and Statistical Manual of Mental Disorders,* 4th ed. (DSM-IV)(8), *mixed episodes* occur when full manic and full depressive syndromes occur together.

TABLE 9-1. *Stages of mania*

Stages	Differential diagnosis
Hypomania	Idealized norm
Energetic	Substance abuse
Extroverted	Borderline disorder
Assertive	Attention deficit
	hyperactivity disorder
	General medical condition
Mania	Schizophrenia
Euphoric-grandiose	Substance abuse
	Metabolic derangement
Paranoid	Attention deficit
Irritable	hyperactivity disorder
	General medical condition
Hyperactive	
Psychotic mania	Schizophrenia
Paranoid	Substance abuse
Delusional	Metabolic derangement
Confused	General medical condition

Adapted from Carlson GA, Goodwin FK. The stages of mania: a longitudinal analysis of the manic episode. *Arch Gen Psychiatry* 1973;28:228.

Primary Symptoms of the Manic Syndrome

The *elevated mood* may be initially experienced as feeling unusually good, happy, or cheerful, and later as euphoric or elated. It often has an expansive quality, characterized by indiscriminate involvement with people and the environment. In this early period, manic patients can be playful and unaware of their changing mood, which is often recognized as excessive by those who know them well. In more severe episodes, thinking may develop into delusional notions about one's own power and self-importance.

Although an elevated mood is the prototypical symptom, the predominant disturbance may be irritability, which is most evident when the individual's goal-directed behavior is thwarted. Indeed, the clinical picture can suddenly change, with the euphoric mood quickly replaced by irritability and anger. Because these patients are acutely sensitive to criticism, they often become contentious and easily angered, even by seemingly harmless remarks. Verbal abuse is frequent, with physical violence occurring less commonly.

Goodwin and Jamison (9) summarized the incidence of typical *mood symptoms* during a manic phase from 14 studies that included 751 patients as follows:

- Irritability (80%)
- Depression (72%)
- Euphoria (71%)
- Lability (69%)
- Expansiveness (60%)

We note that the incidence of depressive symptoms occurred in about 70% of these patients, again underscoring the frequent interplay between the two mood states in bipolar disorder.

Psychomotor acceleration often accompanies the mood disturbance and is manifested by increased sociability, including efforts to renew old acquaintances, quick changes from one activity to another, and/or inappropriate increase in sexual activity. Because of inflated self-esteem, unwarranted optimism, and poor judgment, patients may engage in buying sprees, reckless driving, or foolish business investments. Such behavior may have a disorganized, flamboyant, or even bizarre quality (e.g., wearing brightly colored or strange garments or excessive, distasteful makeup). Many patients, however, can demonstrate a marked tendency to neglect themselves.

Speech can be loud, rapid, and often difficult to interrupt, frequently punctuated by jokes, puns, word play, rhymes, and witty, risqué, or droll irrelevancies. Euphoria often leads to speaking with a theatrical or dramatic flair. **As the activity level increases, associations may loosen, and speech can become totally incoherent, virtually indistinguishable from an acute schizophrenic exacerbation.** When mood is predominantly irritable, verbalizations can include complaints, hostile comments, and angry tirades.

Goodwin and Jamison (10) calculated the incidence of behavioral symptoms per episode and found the following:

- Rapid speech (98%)
- Over-talkativeness (89%)
- Hyperactivity (87%)
- Reduced sleep (81%)
- Hypersexuality (57%)
- Overspending (55%)

Although reduced sleep is often an early prodromal symptom, patients are usually brought for evaluation and treatment when their behaviors create the potential for more severe consequences (e.g., self-injurious behavior, atypical sexual behavior, significant financial indiscretions).

Associated Symptoms of the Manic Syndrome

Flight of ideas is an almost continuous flow of accelerated speech with abrupt changes from one topic to another, at times so pronounced that it becomes incomprehensible. These ideas are usually based on understandable associations, distracting stimuli, or plays on words.

Distractibility is common and characterized by rapid changes in speech or activity, resulting from a tendency to respond to irrelevant external stimuli, such as background noises or objects.

Inflated self-esteem may range from uncritical self-confidence to marked grandiosity, often reaching delusional proportions. Patients may give advice on matters for which they are untrained or about which they have no special knowledge. Despite average talents, they may unrealistically boast of extraordinary abilities (e.g., that they can compose music, write poetry, publish books, or design new inventions).

Lability of affect is characterized by rapid shifts from euphoria to anger or depression. **Depressive symptoms (e.g., tearfulness, suicidal threats, insomnia) may last moments, hours, or, more rarely, days, occasionally intermingled with or rapidly alternating with mania (e.g., mixed episode or dysphoric mania).**

A decreased need for sleep is a frequent prodromal sign and is characterized by early awakening (sometimes by several hours), a significant reduction in total sleep time, and when severe, several sleepless days with no apparent fatigue.

Psychotic symptoms, such as delusions and hallucinations, may be present in more severe episodes (both manic and depressed phases) and are usually (but not always) mood-congruent. The delusions seen in mania often have a religious, sexual, or persecutory theme. Grandiose delusions can lead to convictions about a special relationship with God or some well-known figure from the political, religious, or entertainment world. Persecutory delusions may be based on the idea that the individual is singled out because of some special relationship or attribute

(11). Hallucinations may be auditory or visual (e.g., seeing or hearing God) and usually consistent with the patient's mood (7).

Although the DSM-IV distinguishes between psychotic features that are either mood-congruent or mood-incongruent, the usefulness of this distinction remains controversial. Pope and Lipinski (12) found that "schizophrenic" symptoms were present in 20% to 50% of manic patients and that many of the delusions were mood-incongruent (i.e., delusions of persecution, catatonic symptoms, formal thought disorder, and auditory hallucinations not consistent with the mood state). In addition, Schneiderian first-rank symptoms, once thought to be pathognomonic of schizophrenia, have been reported in a significant proportion of manic cases (13, 14).

Blumenthal et al. (15) reported that psychotic features in both unipolar and bipolar disorders were indicative of an earlier age of onset and first hospitalization in comparison with their nonpsychotic counterparts. Age of onset for the first episode was found to be earlier in the bipolar group regardless of psychotic categorization. Furthermore, the authors hypothesize that delusional depressions may be related to bipolar disorder, given a higher prevalence of the latter in relatives, and postulate a predictive relationship between psychoticism and bipolarity.

TABLE 9-2. *Comparison of DSM-IV and RDC criteria for mania*

DSM-IV (1994)	RDC, 3rd ed. (1989 update)
A. Distinct period of elevated/irritable expansive mood lasting 1 week unless hospitalized	A. Distinct period of elevated or expansive irritable mood
B. At least three of the following for elevated or expansive mood, four for irritable mood:	B. At least three of the following for elevated or expansive mood, four for irritable mood:
1. Inflated self-esteem/grandiosity	1. More active than usual
2. Decreased need for sleep	2. More talkative or pressure of speech
3. More talkative or pressure of speech	3. Flight of ideas or racing thoughts
4. Flight of ideas or racing thoughts	4. Inflated self-esteem/grandiosity
5. Distractibility	5. Decreased need for sleep
6. Increased goal-directed activity/agitation	6. Distractibility
7. Excessive involvement in activities	7. Excessive involvement in activities
C. Marked impairment in social/occupational functioning or hospitalization	C. At least one of the following:
	1. Meaningful conversation not possible
	2. Serious impairment with family at home, at school, work, or socially
	3. Hospitalization (in the absence of 1 or 2)
D. Not due to direct physiologic effect of a substance or general medical condition.	D. Duration of manic features at least 1 week
	E. None of the following is present:
	1. Delusions of thought control, insertion, withdrawal, boardcasting
	2. Nonaffective hallucinations throughout the day on intermittently for 1 week
	3. Auditory hallucinations commenting or persons's thoughts/actions or two or more voices conversing with each other
	4. Had delusions/hallucinations for 1 week in absence of manic/depressive symptoms
	5. Had marked thought disorder with either blunted/inappropriate affect, delusions/ hallucinations, or grossly disorganized behavior for at least 1 week in absence of manic symptoms

DSM-IV, *Diagnostic and Statistical Manual of Mental Disorders*, 4th ed., revised; RDC, Research Diagnostic Criteria.
DSM-IV also distinguishes between psychotic features that are mood-congruent or mood-incongruent.
Adapted from Altman E, Janicak PG, Davis JM. Mania, clinical manifestations and assessment. In: Howells JG, ed. *Modern perspectives in the psychiatry of affective disorders.* New York: Brunner/Mazel, 1989;292–302.

Secondary effects of bipolar disorder can include the following:

* *Job* changes
* *Moves*
* Repetitive *marriages, divorces*
* *Bankruptcy*
* *Hypersexuality*
* Altered *self-concept* (e.g., grandiosity; low self-esteem)

Suicide

The suicide rate for bipolar disorder is estimated to be about 10%. In untreated patients, it may be as high as 25% (16, 17). Patients are at greater risk during a depressive or mixed episode of the disorder. Other important correlates include concurrent substance abuse and past suicide attempts (18).

Criteria for an Acute Manic Episode

In the United States, the Research Diagnostic Criteria (RDC) (19) and the DSM-IV (8) both provide clear inclusion and exclusion criteria for a current episode (Table 9-2). Evaluation of past episodes can be made using the Schedule for Affective Disorders and Schizophrenia—Lifetime Version (SADS-L) (20) or the Structured Clinical Interview for DSM (21). In other countries, the Present State Exam (PSE) (22) can reliably distinguish mania from other disorders. Table 9-3 reviews the various clinical presentations of primary bipolar disorder and their related DSM-IV diagnoses (23) (see also Appendices A, G, and H).

Bipolar I disorder is characterized by a history of one or more manic episodes and one or more mixed or major depressive episodes. This category can be further sub-classified as either manic, hypomanic, mixed, or depressed in presentation.

Bipolar II disorder is defined by the presence or history of at least one hypomanic episode and at least one major depressive episode, but never presenting with a full manic or mixed episode. Several recent family studies have indicated that in the American population there may be an increased risk for mania among relatives of bipolar II patients. More importantly, the highest morbid risk for bipolar II illness may occur in relatives of bipolar II rather than bipolar I or unipolar patients, suggesting that this illness breeds true in some families (24). Coryell (25) supports this position, stating that the illness appears to be phenomenologically stable over time and across generations, despite its poor diagnostic reliability.

Rapid cyclers represent a more severe, treatment-resistant subgroup that is characterized by a minimum of four episodes (i.e., hypomanic, manic, depressive, or mixed) within a 12-month period (26). Age of onset and gender may also affect rapid-cycling course of illness and response to treatment (27, 28). Bauer et al. (29) assessed hypothyroidism as a risk factor and found that, of 30 rapid-cycling patients, 23% had grade I hypothyroidism, 27% grade II, and 10% grade III. Although approximately 63% of this cohort was taking lithium carbonate or carbamazepine, the percentage of grade I hypothyroidism was significantly greater than that reported in studies of un-selected patients on long-term lithium treatment. **Their findings indicate that hypothyroidism in bipolar disorder may be a risk factor for the development of**

TABLE 9-3. *Primary bipolar disorders*

Disorder	Defining Characteristics	DSM-IV diagnosis
Bipolar I	Mania and depression	Bipolar I disorder
Bipolar II	Hypomania and depression	Bipolar II disorder
Bipolar III	Cyclothymic personality	Cyclothymic disorder
Bipolar IV	Hypomania or mania precipitated by antidepressant drugs	Substance-induced mood disorder
Bipolar V	Familial history of bipolar disorder	Major depressive disorder
Bipolar VI	Mania without depression	Mood disorder, NOS

NOS, not otherwise specified.
Adapted from Klerman G. The classification of bipolar disorders. *Psychiatr Ann* 1987;17:13–17.

rapid cycling and lends support to the hypothesis that a relative central thyroid hormonal deficiency predisposes to this course. Therefore, close attention to the early symptoms and signs of thyroid dysregulation should be a routine aspect of any evaluation.

Dysphoric mania (not listed in the DSM-IV) is characterized by "feeling out of synch" and is associated with complaints of malaise and a greater emphasis on feelings during the depressive rather than manic state. Post et al. (30) found that a high proportion of manic patients (46%) presented with marked to moderate dysphoria, as well as anger and anxiety. They also noted a positive correlation between dysphoric mania and rapid cycling. A substantial number of these episodes were correlated with two measures of severity, the peak intensity of an episode and a greater need for hospitalization, especially in female patients. Cerebrospinal fluid (CSF) norepinephrine concentrations were positively correlated with ratings of anger, depression, and anxiety during an episode. This elevation was seen, however, in other diagnostic conditions where anxiety was a major component.

Mixed manic states can be characterized as the simultaneous presence of both a depressive and manic episode, meeting full criteria for both mood syndromes (except for duration) nearly every day for at least one week. This may be a relatively common occurrence, as noted earlier in the data of Goodwin and Jamison (i.e., 71% present with euphoria and 72% with depression), as well as others (30a) (9). Krasuski and Janicak (31, 32) reviewed various models to explain the interaction between mania or hypomania and depression and noted that aggression and anxiety may be important components, in addition to dysphoria, in defining mixed states.

Cyclothymic disorder is a milder version of the classic bipolar disorder, characterized by a chronic course (i.e., 2 years or more), with swings between mild depressive and hypomanic symptoms that never reach the severity of a full manic or depressive episode. An interesting hypothesis raised by Akiskal (33) is the concept of *subclinical* or *subsyndromal mood* disorders. These conditions are often missed in cross-sectional diagnoses and are characterized by milder bipolar symptoms, often with abrupt biphasic shifts, at times precipitated by the introduction of an antidepressant. These patients have very stormy interpersonal relationships, are frequently misdiagnosed as having Axis II characterological disorders, and are recommended for long-term psychotherapy, which is usually ineffective. If these patients are properly diagnosed and managed with mood stabilizers, however, significant improvement in their overall functioning may be achieved.

Case Example: A 29-year-old woman presented for consultation on referral from a psychiatrist who had seen her in psychodynamically oriented psychotherapy for approximately 10 years. The primary difficulty was intermittent interpersonal strife with fellow workers and supervisors. Thus, although quite competent, she had switched positions frequently because of these difficulties. Her history indicated that she had never experienced a full depressive, hypomanic, or manic episode, but that these problems seemed to coincide with intermittent periods of irritability. As a result, she was placed on a trial of lithium, with therapeutic blood levels. Within several weeks of treatment initiation, her difficulties with fellow coworkers and supervisors ceased, and during 1 year of follow-up, she did not have a recurrence of these problems.

Differential Diagnosis of an Acute Manic Episode

Bipolar disorder can be divided into primary and *secondary* types, with the latter developing as a consequence of various medical conditions or substances that can alter brain function or structure. This categorization underscores the view of mania as a syndrome subsequent to various pathophysiologies.

It is important to consider explanatory precipitants in a patient with no prior history of a mood disorder. Clearly, the diagnosis of bipolar mania should not be made if the syndrome can be explained by known organic factors, which vary widely and include the following:

- Stroke
- Neoplasms
- Epilepsy
- Infections (e.g., HIV)
- Metabolic and endocrine disturbances
- Substance abuse

Therefore, a careful medical evaluation is critical and appropriate referral for consultation mandatory if an underlying organic process is suspected.

Complicated mania is an elaboration on the theme of the secondary type and is defined as "the presence of antecedent or coexisting nonaffective psychiatric disorders and/or serious medical disorders" (34). These patients can be grouped into psychiatric or medical cluster patients. The psychiatric cluster patients have had fewer prior psychiatric hospitalizations, an earlier onset of illness, and a history of prior suicide attempts. This contrasts with the medical cluster, which has a later age of onset, no prior history of suicide attempts, more organic features, and more deaths during the follow-up period.

Black et al. (34), in a retrospective, chart review, case-control study of 57 manic patients assigned to one of four treatment groups (electroconvulsive therapy, adequate or inadequate lithium therapy, or neither treatment), found complicated manics responded poorly in comparison with their uncomplicated counterparts. These authors concluded that adequate treatment was associated with recovery in the latter group, but the outcome was less clear for the complicated manics. Although there are always drawbacks to any chart review study and the small number of patients per treatment group, it does suggest consideration of alternative strategies for this subgroup (see also the section "Alternative Treatment Strategies" in Chapter 10).

Because the coexistence of substance and/or alcohol abuse disorders is much higher in bipolar patients than in the general population, their importance as comorbid factors has become increasingly recognized (35). Thus, it becomes necessary to decide whether the following is true:

- An episode of mania/depression is *drug-* or *alcohol-induced.*

- Concurrent drug or alcohol use is an attempt to *self-medicate.*
- Such activity is *unrelated to the present exacerbation.*

Further, concurrent substance abuse may do the following:

- *Complicate interpretation* of the presenting symptoms
- *Undermine* the beneficial effects of *treatment*(36)
- Adversely affect the *long-term course*

Finally, as noted earlier, comorbid substance abuse, particularly with bipolar male patients, is a strong predictor of suicide-related lethality. It is critically important to recognize these complicating disorders and aggressively intervene with appropriate clinical strategies. Referral to Alcoholics Anonymous (AA), Narcotics Anonymous (NA), and other related counseling support programs, as well as prescription of naltrexone (Revia) in the appropriate patients, may also help to diminish the risk of serious morbidity (see also the section "The Alcoholic Patient" in Chapter 14).

Schizophrenia-related disorders, such as schizophreniform disorder, can closely mimic an acute exacerbation of mania. Attention to premorbid personal and family history may help differentiate them from mood disorders. A definitive diagnosis may not be possible, however, until the course of the illness is followed for a period of time. Clinical clues include the propensity of bipolar manics (in contrast to schizophrenics) to demonstrate pressured speech, flight of ideas, grandiosity, and overinclusive thinking. Hallucinations are less common than delusions in both mania and depression, with delusions normally taking on the qualities of expansivity, hyperreligiosity, or grandiosity. Delusions are also relatively less fixed than in schizophrenia.

Schizoaffective disorder, characterized by concurrent symptoms of both schizophrenia (criterion A) and a mood disorder, meeting full criteria for a mood disorder, manic or mixed episode, can also pose a difficult diagnostic dilemma. Other criteria include a period of psychosis (2 weeks) in the absence of significant mood symptoms and

TABLE 9-4. *Mean item and total Manic Interpersonal Interaction Scale (MIIS) scores before and after clinical remission*

Item	Acutely ill	Remitted	Significance[a]
Testing of limits	8	1	$p < 0.0001$
Projection of responsibility	5	1	$p < 0.02$
Sensitivity to others' soft spots	5	1	$p < 0.01$
Attempts to divide staff	2	1	$p < 0.02$
Flattering behavior	3	1	$p < 0.002$
Ability to evoke anger	6	1	$p < 0.002$
MIIS total score	29	6	**$p < 0.002$**

[a]From paired Student's *t* test, one-tailed ($n = 5$; all numbers are rounded).
Adapted from Janowsky DS, El-Yousef M, Davis JM. Interpersonal maneuvers of manic patients. *Am J Psychiatry* 1974;131:250–254.

mood symptoms should be present for a substantial proportion of an episode. Schizoaffective probands often have family members with both affective and schizophrenic disorders.

One family study indicated that the schizoaffective-manic type tended to aggregate with classic bipolar disorder, while the schizoaffective-depressive type seemed to be more closely related to schizophrenia (37).

Other differential considerations include attention-deficit-hyperactivity disorder or more *severe characterological (or Axis II) disturbances.* For example, several of the criteria for borderline personality disorder in the DSM-IV overlap with symptoms for hypomania, including the following:

- *Impulsivity*
- *Affective* instability
- Inappropriate *anger* or *irritability*
- Unstable interpersonal *relationships*

Some patients initially diagnosed as having borderline disorder and followed longitudinally will develop periodic exacerbations in their interpersonal relationships. At times, they may even be reclassified as having either a classic bipolar disorder, a subsyndromal variant, or an atypical presentation. Peselow et al. (38) studied 66 bipolar outpatients and found that hypomania may exacerbate maladaptive personality traits, which may improve with treatment; 50%, however, continued to demonstrate at least one personality disorder, suggesting a high degree of comorbidity between bipolar illness and maladaptive person-

ality traits or disorders. Co-occurrence of personality disorders has also been associated with poorer outcome after discharge from the hospital for an acute manic episode (39).

Conversely, patients may also display certain interpersonal styles that fluctuate with the course of their illness. For example, Janowsky et al. (40) demonstrated that manic patients have a characteristic interactional style that clearly distinguishes them from schizoaffective and schizophrenic patients. Using their Manic Interpersonal Interaction Scale (MIIS) to assess changes in personality style, the authors found manic patients more likely to do the following:

- *Evoke anger* from treating personnel
- *Project responsibility* onto others
- Attempt to *divide treatment personnel* through manipulative behavior
- *Test limits*
- *Exploit* or attack others' vulnerabilities

In Table 9-4, scores on each item are presented during the manic phase and again after recovery with lithium therapy. Janowsky et al. (40) concluded that such behaviors are not attributable to premorbid personality, but rather are as characteristic of a manic episode as classic symptom changes (e.g., euphoria, flight of ideas, over-talkativeness, and grandiosity). Further, the pattern of interpersonal interactions occurred only when a patient was in a manic phase, and improved with lithium therapy.

Course of Illness

Onset

Longitudinal observations indicate that, early in the course of the illness, various phases (depressive, hypomanic, manic) are often associated with identifiable external stressors. Over time, however, patients may begin to show spontaneous fluctuations in mood, as well as increased frequency and severity of episodes.

Methods for accurately assessing the longitudinal course of mood disorders were first described by Adolph Meyer in 1951 (41). More recently, Post et al. (42) have encouraged retrospective and prospective historical graphing as an invaluable guide to the disorder's progression and response to therapy. They recommend grading episodes by three levels of severity:

- *Nonfunctional,* indicating severe depression or mania
- *Moderate severity,* reflecting impairment in work or social function
- *Mild severity*, indicating no impairment but the presence of recognized mood or behavioral alterations

The chart should also include important life events, mood, and behavior, as well as medications or other treatments. Such methods can help the clinician achieve the following:

- Supply data for *proper diagnosis*
- Plot psychological *stressors*
- Formulate *treatment* recommendations
- *Monitor* the effect of psychological and pharmacological interventions

Gender differences in the age of onset of bipolar disorder were evaluated by Sibisi (43), who used the annual U.K. "Inpatient Statistics from the Mental Health Inquiry." The cumulative inception rate was nearly equal for men and women, indicating that the liability is similar between the genders. Results such as these imply that the observed excess of middle-aged, bipolar women may be attributable to life experiences, a greater willingness to seek treatment, or other demographic factors.

Recovery Phase

It appears that a number of complications await the recovering bipolar patient after an episode of mania. For example, Lucas et al. (44) reported on a retrospective linear discriminant analysis of 100 manic episodes (1981 to 1985) during the recovery phase and found that the incidence of *subsequent depression* was 30% in the first month. Many episodes were transient, however, and did not necessarily require treatment. This phenomenon could be successfully predicted in 81% of cases in which there is a premorbid history of cyclothymia with either a personal or a family history of depression. The highly significant association between family history and postmanic depression again supports the hypothesis of a genetic basis for bipolar disorder.

Keller and colleagues (45, 46) reported the *recovery rate* in 155 bipolar I patients in an uncontrolled, naturalistic follow-up study. Patients were in the community and received different types of treatment after their index episode. They defined recovery as being either asymptomatic or manifesting only one or two symptoms of minimal severity for 8 consecutive weeks. The different types of index episode (i.e., purely manic, purely depressed, or mixed or cycling) afforded significantly different rates of recovery, such that by 8 weeks, 61% of the purely manic patients had recovered, compared with 44% of the pure depressives and only 33% of the mixed or cycling patients ($p = 0.05$). With a median follow-up of 1.5 years, these authors estimated that the probability of remaining ill for pure manics was about 7%, compared with 32% in patients who had mixed or cycling symptoms at the index episode. Pure depressed bipolar patients fell somewhere in the middle, with about a 22% probability of remaining ill. **Keller et al. (46) concluded that subtyping of episodes may be useful in terms of classifying the longitudinal course of bipolar disorders.**

Other predictors of delayed recovery by subtype included the following:

- *Purely manic*–A long duration of the index manic episode, few previous major affective

episodes, and the admitting research center
- *Purely depressed*–Longer previous episodes and earlier nonaffective psychiatric disorders
- *Mixed or cycling*–The presence of psychosis and endogenous features

Keller et al. (46) were also surprised to find that 75% of the nonrecovered patients had been treated with sustained, high levels of drug and/or somatic therapies and concluded that mixed or cycling patients have a more pernicious course and require more effective therapies. In addition, to achieve earlier remission, clinicians should begin aggressive treatment in the initial symptomatic stages, because the purely manic and depressed groups also had severe episodes despite adequate treatment (see Chapter 10 for further discussion).

Long-Term Course and Prognosis

Although biological and genetic factors are undoubtedly important, they may not explain all the variance in the course and prognosis of a bipolar disorder. Results from studies of life events and long-term course are mixed. Ellicott et al. (47), in a 2-year prospective longitudinal design, studied the effect of life stress on course of illness in 61 stable bipolar I or II outpatients. Using survival analysis, they found a significant association (i.e., 4.53 times higher risk in patients with the highest levels of stress) between life event and relapse or recurrence. Further, this observation was not explained by other potential moderating variables such as levels of medication or treatment compliance. Improvements in their design over earlier studies, which found no association between life events and episodes of illness, included the following:

- A sufficient period of *time*
- *Prospective, systematic methods* appropriate for assessing symptoms and life stresses
- Careful attention to the appropriateness of *medication* and *compliance*
- The use of *sophisticated statistical models* to evaluate the association between probability of relapse and life events

These results affirm the important impact of psychosocial factors on the course of a presumed biologically based but multifactorial disorder in which a variety of forces may play a role. Indeed, stressful life events may even alter the biology of a mood disorder. Clinically, they imply that careful attention to and reduction of stressful life events may help to attenuate or prevent subsequent episodes.

Role of Psychotic Symptoms

Rosen and colleagues (48) administered a structured interview, based on the Schedule for Affective Disorders and Schizophrenia (SADS) to 89 bipolar I patients, to compare psychotic and nonpsychotic manic patients on a number of clinical outcome and demographic variables (i.e., age, age at first treatment, and duration of illness). Overall, the psychotic manic group had a significantly poorer outcome in terms of social functioning.

Harrow et al. (49) studied the *longitudinal course of thought disorder* in 34 manic patients, comparing them with 30 schizophrenic patients, 30 nonpsychotic patients, and 34 normal control subjects. During the acute hospitalization, both manic and schizophrenic patients demonstrated severe thought disorder, which was still evident at 1-year follow-up in both the schizophrenic patients and a subsample of manics, although significantly reduced in both groups. Although they found less thought pathology at follow-up for both disorders, the trend favored manic patients, who had a more stable reduction in symptoms. In a subsequent naturalistic follow-up study, Harrow et al. (50) noted that psychosis did not predict a poorer overall outcome when compared with patients without psychosis at the index admission.

Coryell et al. (51) also conducted a *longitudinal study in patients with psychotic manic syndromes*. Fourteen patients with schizoaffective mania and 56 with psychotic mania completed a 5-year study. Mean time for recovery from the index episode for the former group was 58.6 weeks, compared with only 36.2 weeks for the latter group. Schizoaffective manics also relapsed more quickly than the psychotic group, with respective means of 44.5 versus 61.8 weeks; the differences, however, for the two groups did not persist into the second episode. Schizoaffective patients experienced more cumulative morbidity during follow-up, with the mean cumulative inpatient time double that for the psychotic manics. Mean scores on the Global Assessment Scale (GAS) were significantly worse for the schizoaffective patients, who were four times as likely to have sustained psychotic outcomes. Those with chronic subtypes of schizoaffective mania were admitted five times as often as their nonchronic counterparts, had lower GAS scores, more persistent delusions, and greater impairment in interpersonal relationships.

When combining patients from this and an earlier study, Coryell et al. (52) found that baseline variables that significantly and independently predicted a sustained delusional outcome were the following:

- *A longer duration* of the episode
- *Temporal dissociation* between psychotic features and affective syndromes
- Impaired adolescent *friendship patterns*

Subsyndromal Affective Symptoms

Fichtner and colleagues (53) followed 38 unipolar, 27 bipolar, 35 schizophrenic, and 27 other psychiatric patients for 4 years after hospital discharge, as well as 153 normal control subjects, to assess *cyclothymic mood swings* and *psychosocial adjustment*. Patients were significantly more cyclothymic at follow-up than normal control subjects, and those who demonstrated mood swings tended to have poorer posthospital outcomes than their noncycling counterparts. Although the authors commented that the presence of mood instability might reflect a greater vulnerability to persistent psychopathology, they could not distinguish significant differences among the diagnostic groups. **Monitoring for an increase in affective lability or reactivity may be useful in managing major mood disorders, as well as for predicting impending exacerbations in nonaffective psychotic disorders.**

Mortality Risk

Tohen and colleagues (54) investigated outcome by means of a 4-year follow-up study of 75 bipolar patients who had recovered from an episode of mania and found the mortality risk during this period was 4%. They noted that predictors of an unfavorable outcome included the following:

- *Poor occupational status* before the index episode
- A history of *previous episodes*
- A history of *alcoholism*
- *Psychotic features*
- Symptoms of *depression* during the index manic episode (mixed mania)
- *Male* gender
- *Interepisode affective symptoms* (perhaps a reflection of incomplete remission) at 6-month follow-up

Interventions that may improve prognosis include referrals for vocational testing and training, substance- and alcohol-abuse counseling, and aggressive management of depressive symptoms as they occur.

CONCLUSION

It is important to emphasize that the syndrome of mania has symptoms that can overlap other illnesses, including organic mood, schizoaffective, and schizophreniform disorders. In addition, there is an ongoing and intimate relationship between the manic and the depressive phases, a fact that has significant implications for diagnosis, treatment, and prognosis. The diagnosis of a bipolar disorder, manic phase, can usually be made by existing inclusion and exclusion criteria, as well as its distinctive personal and family histories. As our concept of what constitutes the syndrome of mania evolves, elaboration and refinement should help improve diagnosis, as well as assessment of response to present and future treatments for mania. Studies of the longitudinal course should clarify its clinical presentation, as well as psychosocial factors, that can alert the clinician to early, aggressive interventions to minimize the impact of this disorder.

To underscore the importance of adequate treatment for bipolar disorder, we note that it is estimated that one of every four or five untreated or inadequately treated patients commits suicide during the course of the illness, particularly during depressed or mixed episodes. Further, an increase in deaths secondary to accidents or intercurrent illnesses contributes to the greater mortality rate seen in this disorder in comparison with the general population. Unfortunately, recent epidemiological studies have indicated that only one third of bipolar patients are in active treatment despite the availability of effective therapies.

REFERENCES

1. Weissman M, Boyd J. The epidemiology of affective disorders: rate and risk factor. *Psychiatry Update* 1983;2:406–426.
2. Joyce PR. Age of onset in bipolar affective disorder and misdiagnosis as schizophrenia. *Psychol Med* 1984;14:145–149.
3. Solomon RL, Rich CL, Darko DF. Antidepressant treatment and the occurrence of mania in bipolar patients admitted for depression. *J Affect Disord* 1990;18:253–257.
4. Altman E, Janicak PG, Davis JM. Mania, clinical manifestations and assessment. In: Howells JG, ed. *Modern perspectives in the psychiatry of mood disorders.* New York: Brunner/Mazel, 1989:292–302.
5. Tyrer S, Shopsin B. Symptoms and assessment of mania. In: Paykel ES, ed. *Handbook of affective disorders.* New York: Guilford Press, 1982:2–23.
6. Goodwin FK, Jamison KR. *Manic-depressive illness.* New York: Oxford University Press, 1990:138.
7. Carlson GA, Goodwin FK. The stages of mania: a longitudinal analysis of the manic episode. *Arch Gen Psychiatry* 1973;28:221.
8. American Psychiatric Association. *Diagnostic and statistical manual of mental disorders,* 4th ed., revised. Washington, DC: American Psychiatric Press, 1994.
9. Goodwin FK, Jamison KR. *Manic-depressive illness.* New York: Oxford University Press, 1990:31.
10. Goodwin FK, Jamison KR. *Manic-depressive illness.* New York: Oxford University Press, 1990:36–37.
11. Taylor MA, Abrams R. Acute mania: clinical and genetic study of responders and nonresponders to treatments. *Arch Gen Psychiatry* 1975;32:863.
12. Pope H, Lipinski J. Differential diagnosis of schizophrenia and manic depressive illness: a reassessment of the specificity of schizophrenia symptoms in the light of current research. *Arch Gen Psychiatry* 1978;35:811–828.
13. Carpenter WT, Strauss JS, Muleh S. Are there pathognomonic symptoms in schizophrenia? An empiric investigation of Schneider's first-rank symptoms. *Arch Gen Psychiatry* 1973;28:847.
14. Taylor MA, Abrams R. The phenomenology of mania. A new look at some old patients. *Arch Gen Psychiatry* 1973;29:520.
15. Blumenthal RL, Egeland JA, Sharpe L, et al. Age of onset in bipolar and unipolar illness with and without delusions or hallucinations. *Compr Psychiatry* 1987;28:547–554.
16. Oquendo MA, Waternaux C, Brodsky B, et al. Suicidal behavior in bipolar mood disorder: clinical characteristics of attempters and nonattempters. *J Affect Disord* 2000;59:107–117.
17. Jamison KR. Suicide and bipolar disorder. *J Clin Psychiatry* 2000;61(suppl 9):47–51.
18. Goldberg JF, Garno JL, Portera L, et al. Correlates of suicidal ideation in dysphoric mania. *J Affect Disord* 1999;56:75–81.
19. Spitzer RL, Endicott J, Robins E. Use of the Research Diagnostic Criteria and the Schedule for Affective Disorders and Schizophrenia to study affective disorders. *Am J Psychiatry* 1979;136:52–56. [Revised 1989.]
20. Endicott J, Spitzer RL. A diagnostic interview: the Schedule for Affective Disorders and Schizophrenia. *Arch Gen Psychiatry* 1978;35:837. [Revised 1989.]
21. Spitzer RL, Williams JBW, Gibbon M, et al. The Structured Clinical Interview for DSM-III-R. I: history, rationale and description. *Arch Gen Psychiatry* 1992;49:624–629.
22. Wing JK, Cooper JE, Sartorius N. *Description and classification of psychiatric symptoms.* Cambridge: Cambridge University Press, 1974.
23. Klerman G. The classification of bipolar disorders. *Psychiatr Ann* 1987;17:13–17.
24. Dunner EL. Stability of bipolar II affective disorder as a diagnostic entity. *Psychiatr Ann* 1987;17:18–20.
25. Coryell W. Outcome and family studies of bipolar II depression. *Psychiatr Ann* 1987;17:28–31.
26. Dunner DL, Vijayalakshmy P, Fieve RR. Rapid cycling in manic depressive patients. *Compr Psychiatry* 1977;18:561–566.
27. Fujiwara Y, Honda T, Tanaka Y, et al. Comparison of early- and late-onset rapid cycling affective disorders: clinical course and response to pharmacotherapy. *J Clin Psychopharmacol* 1998;18:282–288.
28. Tondo L, Baldessarini RJ. Rapid cycling in women and men with bipolar manic-depressive disorders. *Am J Psychiatry* 1998;155:1434–1436.
29. Bauer MS, Whybrow PC, Winokur A. Rapid cycling bipolar affective disorder. I. Association with grade I hypothyroidism. *Arch Gen Psychiatry* 1990;47:427–432.
30. Post RM, Rubinow DR, Uhde TW, et al. Dysphoric mania: clinical and biological correlates. *Arch Gen Psychiatry* 1989;46:353–358.
30a. Cassidy F, Carroll BJ. The clinical epidemiology of pure and mixed manic episodes. *Bipolar Disorders* 2001;3:35–40.
31. Krasuski JS, Janicak PG. Mixed states: current and alternate diagnostic models. *Psychiatr Ann* 1994;24:7.
32. Krassuski JS, Janicak PG. Mixed states: issues of terminology and conceptualization. *Psychiatr Ann* 1994;24:6.
33. Akiskal HS. The milder spectrum of bipolar disorders: diagnostic, characterologic and pharmacologic aspects. *Psychiatr Ann* 1987;17:32–37.

34. Black DW, Winokur G, Bell S, et al. Complicated mania: comorbidity and immediate outcome in the treatment of mania. *Arch Gen Psychiatry* 1988;45:232–236.

35. Regier DA, Farmer ME, Rae DS, et al. Comorbidity of mental disorders with alcohol and other drug abuse. Results from the epidemiologic catchment area (ECA) study. *JAMA* 1990;264:2511–2518.

36. Weiss RD, Greenfield SF, Najavits LM, et al. Medication compliance among patients with bipolar disorder and substance abuse disorder. *J Clin Psychiatry* 1998;59:172–174.

37. Mendlewicz J, Linkowski P, Wilmotte J. Relationship between schizoaffective illness and affective disorders or schizophrenia. *J Affect Disord* 1980;2:289–302.

38. Peselow ED, Sanfilipo MP, Fieve RR. Relationship between hypomania and personality disorders before and after successful treatment. *Am J Psychiatry* 1995;152:232–238.

39. Dunayevich E, Sax KW, Keck PE Jr, et al. Twelve-month outcome in bipolar patients with and without personality disorders. *J Clin Psychiatry* 2000;61:134–139.

40. Janowsky DS, El-Yousef M, Davis JM. Interpersonal maneuvers of manic patients. *Am J Psychiatry* 1974;131:250–254.

41. Meyer A. The life chart and the obligation of specifying positive data in psychopathological diagnosis. In: Winters E, ed. *The collected papers of Adolph Meyer. Vol. 3: Medical teachings*. Baltimore: Johns Hopkins University Press, 1951;52–56.

42. Post RM, Roy-Bryne PP, Uhde TW. Graphic representation of the life course of illness in patients with affective disorder. *Am J Psychiatry* 1988;145:844–848.

43. Sibisi CDT. Sex differences in the age of onset of bipolar affective illness. *Br J Psychiatry* 1990;156:842–845.

44. Lucas CP, Rigby JC, Lucas SB. The occurrence of depression following mania: a method of predicting vulnerable cases. *Br J Psychiatry* 1989;154:705–708.

45. Keller MB. The course of manic-depressive illness. *J Clin Psychiatry* 1988;49:4–7.

46. Keller MB, Lavori PW, Coryell W, et al. Differential outcome of pure manic, mixed/cycling, and pure depressive episodes in patients with bipolar illness. *JAMA* 1986;255:3138–3142.

47. Ellicott A, Hammen C, Gitlin M, et al. Life events and the course of bipolar disorder. *Am J Psychiatry* 1990;147:1194–1198.

48. Rosen LN, Rosenthal NE, Dunner DL, et al. Social outcome compared in psychotic and nonpsychotic bipolar I patients. *J Nerv Ment Dis* 1983;171:272–275.

49. Harrow M, Grossman LS, Silverstein ML, et al. A longitudinal study of thought disorder in manic patients. *Arch Gen Psychiatry* 1986;43:781–785.

50. Harrow M, Goldberg JF, Grossman LS, et al. Outcome in manic disorders: a naturalistic follow-up study. *Arch Gen Psychiatry* 1990;47:665–671.

51. Coryell W, Keller M, Lavori P, et al. Affective syndromes, psychotic features, and prognosis. II. Mania. *Arch Gen Psychiatry* 1990;47:658–662.

52. Coryell W, Keller M, Lavori P, et al. Affective syndromes, psychotic features, and prognosis. I. Depression. *Arch Gen Psychiatry* 1990;47:651–657.

53. Fichtner CG, Grossman LS, Harrow M, et al. Cyclothymic mood swings in the course of affective disorders and schizophrenia. *Am J Psychiatry* 1989;146:1149–1154.

54. Tohen M, Waternaux CM, Tsuang M. Outcome in mania. *Arch Gen Psychiatry* 1990;47:1106–1111.

10

Treatment With Mood Stabilizers

Lithium has been used as a medicinal agent since the mid-19th century for such varied disorders as gout, diabetes, and rheumatism. With the seminal reports of Cade, and Schou et al. (1, 2) almost a century later, it emerged as the standard of treatment for bipolar disorders. John Cade, an Australian physician, serendipitously discovered this agent's antimanic properties when he injected lithium urate into guinea pigs. Mistaking toxicity for sedation in the animals, he then used it successfully in an open trial with manic patients. Mogens Schou, following up on Cade's report, was the first European to employ lithium in a series of trials using increasing degrees of methodological rigor (2–8). The term "normothymic" was proposed by Schou to describe lithium's action against both phases of a bipolar disorder, as well as its ability to prevent recurrences of unipolar depressive disorder (3).

In another serendipitous finding, Cade noted that the first patient treated with lithium relapsed when medication was withdrawn (5). From this, he inferred that lithium may also be effective for maintenance treatment. Baastrup, Schou's coworker, carried out the first definitive study of its prophylactic properties (4, 6–8). The ability of lithium to decrease the rate of recurrence in both unipolar and bipolar disorders was then confirmed in a series of studies by Hartigan and Baastrup (7–9).

Unfortunately, just as lithium had been toxic when used as a salt substitute in cardiac patients, it also caused problems when used for mania. Indeed, until its safe use was mastered, Cade is said to have banned lithium in his own hospital, regarding it as too dangerous for use in humans.

Lithium was reintroduced in the United States by Gershon in the late 1960's, and since then has remained the standard therapy for bipolar disorder (10). More recently, there has been a growing recognition that a significant proportion of pa-

tients cannot tolerate or are not adequately helped by this therapy, which has led to the reexamination and clarification of alternative monotherapy and copharmacy strategies (11).

One alternate approach has been the use of *anticonvulsants as mood stabilizers*. This approach includes such varied therapies as *electroconvulsive therapy* (ECT), *valproate* (VPA), and *carbamazepine* (CBZ), as well as several other recently introduced anticonvulsants [e.g., lamotrigine, topiramate, gabapentin]. It is of interest that some of these treatments also have a history dating back to the 1960's. For example, the first empirical investigation of CBZ was performed by Dehing in 1968 (12). While studying the behavioral effects of this anticonvulsant in epileptic patients, he noted that it had antiaggressive properties. Interestingly, lithium may also have antiaggressive properties, but its antimanic effect was discovered first. The reverse is true for CBZ, which subsequently was used for the treatment of mania by investigators in Japan (13, 14). As Schou in Europe and Gershon in the United States are credited with the introduction of lithium, Post and Ballenger (15) similarly deserve credit for introducing CBZ to the United States.

VPA was first used as a mood stabilizer by Lambert and associates in 1966 (16). Their favorable experience in a heterogeneous population of psychiatric patients was followed by several open and controlled trials in the United States and elsewhere. Indeed, this agent has now been better studied than lithium as a mood stabilizer for acute mania (17, 18).

In summary, although lithium has revolutionized the treatment of bipolar disorder, its narrow therapeutic index, numerous adverse effects, and relative ineffectiveness in a large proportion of bipolar patients has led to an expanding number of alternative approaches, including the following:

- Other *anticonvulsants* (e.g., lamotrigine, gabapentin, topiramate)
- *Novel antipsychotics (NAPs)* [e.g., clozapine, olanzapine, risperidone, quetiapine, ziprasidone, aripiprazole]
- *Calcium channel antagonists (CCAs)* (e.g., verapamil, nimodipine)
- *Cholinomimetics* (e.g., lecithin)
- *Experimental agents*(e.g., omega-3 fatty acid, tamoxifen) (19, 20)

MECHANISM OF ACTION

In the mid-1960's, Schildkraut and Bunney and Davis, independently developed the monoamine hypothesis of mood disorders. To date, a great wealth of data has been generated to test this theory (see also the section "Mechanism of Action" in Chapter 7) (21, 22). Because the early development of psychotropic agents was based on the concept that altering norepinephrine (NE) or serotonin (5-HT) activity could benefit depression or mania, it is not surprising that the action of these drugs would support the original concept. There is also a growing appreciation that receptor changes modulated by alteration in genetic expression are slower to occur, are more sustained, and may be more consistent with the time course of mood changes. Models to further clarify the underlying pathophysiology of bipolar disorder have also incorporated such factors as genetic vulnerability and cyclicity (23, 24).

As we have already noted, the history of psychiatry contains numerous preliminary findings of biological abnormalities attributed to a given diagnostic entity. Unfortunately, the great majority have not been replicated. More recently, the technology has been developed to record blood flow, biological activity, and structural changes through techniques such as functional magnetic resonance imaging (fMRI), positron emission tomography (PET), and single photon emission computerized tomography (SPECT). All of these have the potential to better "localize" pathophysiological processes. Although there will be some false starts (i.e., unreplicated findings) with these methods, we anticipate an increasing probability for meaningful replications.

Neurotransmitter and Related Hypotheses

Although the therapeutic mechanisms of various mood stabilizers are unknown, studies have concentrated on the following:

- The classic *neurotransmitters* (e.g., NE, dopamine, 5-HT, acetylcholine) implicated in affective disturbances
- *Cellular processes* involving the classic ligand-receptor interaction and beyond (e.g., G-proteins, second messenger systems)
- Subsequent *intracellular events* (e.g., protein kinase C activity)
- The *modulating interactive processes* among various neurotransmitter systems, neuromodulators, and genetic influences
- The role of *circadian rhythms*

Mood stabilizers have been shown to interact with several neurotransmitters, including the catecholaminergic, indolaminergic, cholinergic, γ-aminobutyric acid, and glutamatergic systems. Although the data are conflicting, it appears that mood stabilizers affect the pre- and the postneuronal receptors, postreceptor activity (e.g., second messenger systems) of these neurotransmitters, and a variety of intracellular targets. Still, the exact mechanisms by which they relate to the biological substrates subserving mood disorders remains unclear.

Catecholamines

Early research at our institute found that treatment with lithium decreased the β-adrenergic receptor number, consistent with the noradrenergic down-regulation hypothesis but difficult to reconcile with a complementary theory of mania (25). Lithium can also block dopamine receptor supersensitivity, and this is consistent with the postulate that mania is associated with an increased sensitivity of catecholamine receptors.

Lithium blocks the release of *thyroid hormones,* which are known to *potentiate β-noradrenergic receptor sensitivity.* This has led to the speculation that excessive thyroid activity may contribute to an episode of mania in susceptible patients, and that the antimanic effect of lithium is, at least in part, due to its antithyroid action (26). In this context, CBZ can also decrease various thyroid indices.

Another approach has been the investigation of agents such as the antihypertensive agent, clonidine, which stimulates a α_2-noradrenergic, presynaptic receptors, setting into motion a short-loop, negative-feedback system. This process culminates in a shutdown of tyrosine hydroxylase, the rate-limiting enzyme for the production of the catecholamines, thus slowing NE synthesis and release. Further, this drug acts in a rapid fashion and is highly specific for the locus ceruleus, the CNS location with the richest concentration of NE-containing neurons. As a result, it can rapidly and effectively shut down NE production.

Indolamines

Lithium may facilitate the release of 5-HT, perhaps by increasing tryptophan uptake, enhancing 5-HT release through presynaptic autoreceptors, and/or by increasing activity at postsynaptic 5-HT receptors (i.e., act as a 5-HT agonist). Some data, however, question the long-term effect of lithium on 5-HT enhancement when studied in patients, as opposed to healthy control subjects (27). Similar to lithium, clonazepam can increase 5-HT synthesis and cerebrospinal fluid (CSF) levels of its major metabolite, 5-hydroxyindoleacetic acid. Other agents known to enhance 5-HT activity by different mechanisms have also shown initial promise as potential antimanic treatments (e.g., L-tryptophan, a 5-HT precursor).

Cholinergic System

Lithium has been shown to increase red blood cell (RBC) count levels of choline, but the significance of this finding is yet to be determined (28). This activity is consistent with the cholinergic-adrenergic balance hypothesis of mood disorders, which promulgates a lack of cholinergic relative to noradrenergic activity in the manic state and the reverse in the depressed phase (29). These findings have led to the administration of drugs with cholinomimetic effects to treat acute mania. For example, a single i.v. dose of physostigmine

reversed a manic state to a depressed phase for about 1 hour (29). More recently, pilot data indicate that the anticholinesterase inhibitor, donepezil, was found effective in treatment-resistant bipolar disorder (30).

γ-Aminobutyric Acid

GABA is a major CNS inhibitory neurotransmitter, which, among other effects, may attenuate catecholaminergic systems. VPA (perhaps by inhibition of this transmitter's degradation by GABA transaminase), CBZ, and lithium have all been reported to enhance GABA activity (see also the section "Mechanism of Action" in Chapter 12).

Second Messenger Systems

Lithium's interactions with *second messenger systems*, particularly the *phosphoinositide cycle,* may deplete free inositol and alter intracellular calcium mobilization (i.e., inositol depletion hypothesis). Antagonists such as verapamil decrease calcium channel activity, diminishing intracellular Ca^{2+} concentrations, and have shown some promise as potential antimanics. Guanine nucleotide-binding proteins (G-proteins), adenylyl cyclase, and protein kinase C isoenzymes are components of signal transduction pathways that may be affected by mood stabilizers such as lithium and VPA. Lithium's effect on CNS gene expression regulation may also play an important role in this agent's ability to effect long-term mood stability (31–33).

Membrane and Cation Hypothesis

Electrolyte disturbances have been extensively studied, with disruptions in calcium and sodium activity the most consistently reported aberrations in mood disorders. In a series of studies, Dubovsky et al. (34) measured intracellular calcium ion concentrations in bipolar manic and depressed patients. They found decreases in mean concentrations in four bipolar, manic, and five bipolar, depressed, patients, in comparison with seven normothymic subjects without personal or first-degree relative histories of psychiatric disorders. Their findings were consistent with a diffuse abnormality in the mechanisms modulating intracellular calcium homeostasis. Further, this phenomenon's presence in both platelets and lymphocytes lends credence to a disruption in the cell membrane, the G-protein, or other mechanisms involved in the homeostasis of intracellular calcium ion concentrations. This may also support an extension of their findings from peripheral to neuronal tissue.

Calcium antagonists (e.g., verapamil, nimodipine) can also block dopamine, 5-HT, and endorphin activity, alter sodium activity via a sodium-calcium counter-exchange, and act as anticonvulsants. Any or all of these actions could be involved in their putative antimanic effects (35).

Cellular ionic transport mechanisms have been another line of investigation into amine neurotransmitter and neuroendocrine function in affective disturbances. Lithium and the calcium antagonists block the influx of Ca^{2+}, as well as alter intracellular calcium mobilization, thus dampening neuroelectrical activity and enhancing stabilization of neuronal membranes. Meltzer (36) postulated a specific macromolecular complex composed of at least the sodium, potassium, and calcium pumps, the ion channel, and ankyrin, which may be abnormally constituted in bipolar illness. Further elucidation of this hypothesis might help identify a specific membrane fault in bipolar disorder, as well as lead to new, more specific pharmacotherapies. For example, novel agents such as omega-3 fatty acid could possibly regulate mood stabilization in bipolar patients by inhibiting signal transduction mechanisms in neuronal membranes (19).

Neuroanatomical and Neurophysiological Hypotheses

Before the development of brain imaging techniques, *neuroanatomical correlates* were primarily related to structural lesions of the CNS. Despite the fact that abnormalities have been found in both schizophrenia and affective illness, interest in the neuropathology of mood disorders has not been as intense as for schizophrenia.

Jeste, Lohr, and Goodwin (37) reviewed the neuroanatomical studies of major mood disorders, noting that several found no difference in abnormalities between schizophrenic and mood disorders. Swayze and colleagues (38), using magnetic resonance imaging (MRI), found a nonsignificant trend for ventricular enlargement in bipolar men, whereas bipolar women did not differ significantly from normal control subjects. Dupont et al. (39) have reported on subcortical abnormalities (i.e., hyperintensities) in some bipolar patients using MRI. One study of *cerebral blood flow* (CBF), however, found no significant correlation between symptoms of mania and overall CBF (40).

One of the more consistent findings is the apparent association between secondary mania and right frontal-temporal or left parietal-occipital lesions. Such data are also consistent with neuropsychological studies pointing to a right frontal lobe disturbance in these syndromes. Taken as a whole, these results suggest a differential pathophysiological origin for structural brain abnormalities underlying bipolar disorders. If confirmed, and not simply due to epiphenomena such as drug treatment, substance abuse, or associated medical conditions (e.g., hypertension), these findings can serve as an important way to differentiate the neuroanatomical and neurophysiological mechanisms subserving schizophrenia and bipolar disorder.

Central electrophysiological measures are also partially supportive, in that *evoked response* and computer-assisted *electroencephalogram* (EEG) mapping indicate bipolar-unipolar differences, with right-sided abnormalities more common in bipolar patients. Further, P300 topographical differences have been reported between schizophrenic and psychotic manic patients (41).

The efficacy of ECT for mania is intriguing, vis-à-vis the emerging anticonvulsant strategy, because this somatic therapy has many of the same antiseizure effects as clonazepam, CBZ, and DVPX. Thus, over a course of ECT, the seizure threshold is usually raised, the duration of a given seizure episode decreases, neurometabolic response to a given seizure episode is diminished, and the phenomenon of amygdaloid kindling is attenuated. *Kindling* occurs in animals who are exposed to repeated, subthreshold electrical stimuli and eventually develop spontaneous seizures. This is particularly interesting, in that kindling in the mesolimbic structures has been analogized to the course of some bipolar disorders. Post and colleagues (42), for example, have noted similarities between the increasing intensity of response to subthreshold stimulations and eventual spontaneous seizure activity and the natural course of certain bipolar patients whose illness progressively worsens, culminating in increasing vulnerability to more frequent, non-stress-induced episodes (e.g., behavioral sensitization). In this context, Post and Weiss (43) have argued for differing pharmacosensitivity as a function of the stage of illness. By implication, different treatments (e.g., lithium, antipsychotics, anticonvulsants) may interrupt this natural course at different phases, favorably altering the disorder's progression. More recently, Ghaemi et al. (44) have postulated that interactions among second messengers, gene regulation, and synthesis of long-acting trophic factors in the context of kindling may explain how, over time, environmental stress coupled with genetic vulnerability, can lead to bipolar disorder.

Biological Rhythms Hypothesis

Chronobiological factors are important to consider, given the cyclic pattern of disturbances in bipolar disorders. Goodwin and Jamison (45) has noted that the suprachiasmatic nuclei of the hypothalamus serve as the endogenous pacemaker, temporally ordering various CNS functions. Further, they postulate this "biological clock's" organizing function may be dysregulated in bipolar disorder. Studies are hampered, however, by a dearth of longitudinal data and the masking of internal and external oscillator-driven rhythms that can alter rhythmic phase or amplitude.

One of the most consistent findings is the sleep disturbance that often precedes and may even trigger a manic phase (46). Studies on *circadian rhythms* have demonstrated that many aspects of the sleep cycle are phase-advanced in mania (i.e., occur earlier than normal), and often these patterns resemble the free-running rhythms seen in normal individuals who are removed from all time cues. In addition, there is a blunting of amplitude and a doubling of the sleep-wake cycle up to 48 hours. Lithium is known to delay the sleep-wake cycle and often slow such free-running rhythms, which in turn are partly modulated by neurotransmitters such as NE, 5-HT, and acetylcholine. Further, manipulation of the sleep-wake cycle may prevent a manic episode or be used to treat the depressive phase (e.g., sleep deprivation therapy; see also the section "Experimental Somatic Therapies" in Chapter 8).

Seasonal variation is another chronobiological rhythm that is manifested by increases in depression and suicide in spring (with smaller peaks in autumn), as opposed to mania, which increases in the summer months. These observations have led to preliminary studies on the alteration of both light and temperature as potential therapies for the two seasonal patterns of affective disturbance. The phenomenon of seasonal variation is discussed in the sections "Seasonal Affective Disorders" in Chapter 6 and "Bright Light Phototherapy" in Chapter 8.

Neuroendocrine Hypothesis

Dinan and colleagues (47) found a significant blunting of desipramine-induced growth hormone stimulation in seven drug-free bipolar patients, in comparison with seven control subjects and suggested that this phenomenon was consistent with a down-regulation of a α_2-noradrenergic receptors. Linkowski et al. (48) found elevations in nocturnal cortisol levels and an early nadir of the circadian variation. One study using the dexamethasone suppression test reported that changes in cortisol activity may be state-dependent (49). Similar phenomena have been reported for major depression and might provide an important marker to identify patients' susceptibility to clinically relevant mood fluctuations.

Lithium has several effects on the endocrine system. For example, it can interfere with the synthesis and the release of testosterone, leading to an increase in luteinizing hormone levels. The thyroid system has been most implicated in neuroendocrine theories of lithium's antimanic effects. In particular, thyroid hormones can potentiate β-NE activity, and lithium's ability to block

TABLE 10-1. *Concordance (+) and discordance (−) of mood disorder in twin pairs*

Study	Monozygotic		Dizygotic	
	(+)	(−)	(+)	(−)
Luxenburger, 1928	2	1	0	13
Rosanoff et al., 1934	16	7	11	56
Essen-Moller, 1941	2	6	0	3
Slater and Shields, 1953	4	4	7	23
Kallmann, 1954	25	2	13	42
Da Fonseca, 1959	15	6	15	24
Kringlen, 1967	2	4	0	20
Allen et al., 1974	5	10	0	34
Bertelsen et al., 1977	32	23	9	43
Total	**103 (62%)**	**63 (38%)**	**55 (18%)**	**258 (82%)**

$\chi^2 = 98.7$; $p < 0.0001$ (Mantel-Haenszel).
From Davis JM, Noll KM, Sharma R. Differential diagnosis and treatment of mania. In: Swann AC, ed. *Mania: new research treatment*. Washington, DC: American Psychiatric Press, 1986:1–58, with permission.

their release may subserve its mood-stabilizing properties (i.e., the thyroid-catecholamine receptor hypothesis) (50, 51).

Immunological Hypothesis

This line of investigation is based on evidence for a close interaction between the immune system and the CNS. For example, immunological abnormalities have been reported in relation to psychological stress in patients with psychiatric disorders such as major depression. Kronfol and House (52) studied different immune variables in manic versus schizophrenic patients and normal control subjects. In general, they found no significant differences for most measures. Results of the mitogen stimulation assays, however, revealed significant reductions in lymphocyte responsivity to the mitogens phytohemagglutin-P and concanavalin-A in bipolar patients when compared with schizophrenic patients and normal control subjects. These authors speculate that this may represent an impairment in cell-mediated immune response, as the mitogens in question stimulate mostly T cells. Potential confounds to the study include its small sample size and the effects of ongoing psychotropic drug treatment. More recently, Tsai et al. (53) reported that cell-mediated immunity activation in manic patients appeared to occur through a specific state-dependent immune response.

Genetic Hypothesis

Consistent with the dominant mode of transmission, it appears that first-degree relatives of bipolar patients have a 15% to 35% morbid risk for developing an affective disturbance. *Concordance rates* for mood disorders in twin studies demonstrate a strikingly higher incidence in monozygotic versus dizygotic twins (Table 10-1)(54). Bipolar disorder occurs more often in families with a history of this illness; similarly, unipolar disorder occurs more often in families with a history of this illness. Therefore, these two variants of affective disease appear to breed true. **In addition, bipolar patients seem to have a greater genetic loading for mood disorders than their unipolar counterparts** (55, 56). Thus, the rate of this illness in relatives of bipolar probands is 4 to 10 times greater than in unipolar proband relatives. Furthermore, even though a large proportion of bipolar proband relatives develop only unipolar symptoms, unipolar proband relatives develop predominantly unipolar symptoms.

Other disorders that are reported to be co-transmitted with bipolar, and to a lesser extent unipolar, disorders include the following:

- *Schizoaffective* disorder
- *Cyclothymic* personality
- *Hypomania* (without depression)

Another approach has been the study of *RBC/plasma lithium concentration*, which is an expression of the relationship between intracellular and extracellular levels. The lithium—sodium countertransport (an exchange diffusion process) mechanism is located in the cell membrane and determines the relative concentration of these ions (57). An abnormality in this transport function could represent an inheritable marker of susceptibility for the development of bipolar disorder (58). Clinical studies of lithium administration find that the RBC/plasma lithium ratio varies from 0.15 to 0.60 (average = 0.30) and remains constant for individuals, independent of change in symptoms (59). There is also evidence that bipolar patients have a higher mean ratio than the normal population or those with other psychiatric diagnoses, and that a greater proportion of their first-degree relatives have this elevation. This phenomenon has been demonstrated using both statistical and genetic models (60, 61).

Genetic linkage studies are particularly useful in resolving issues regarding the myriad clinical presentations, while contributing to an increased understanding of the basis for vulnerability to various mood disorders. Many studies, however, have not unequivocally established a genetic heritability for bipolar illness. For example, linkage to the genetic markers of color blindness, which is associated with a region of the X chromosome, was reported in some but not all pedigrees (62, 63). The association of bipolar disorder to chromosome 11 suggested to occur in the Amish pedigree did not replicate with a larger sample (64). A fascinating corollary to the chromosome 11 story is the nearby location of genes involved in tyrosine hydroxylase production, as well as a muscarinic cholinergic receptor gene. Similar discrepancies have plagued attempts at linkage to the HLA region of chromosome 6 (65). Recent genetic linkage data have confirmed bipolar susceptibility loci in multiple regions (i.e., polygenic inheritance of the human genome, including: 4p 16; 12q 24; 13q 32; 18p 11.2; 18q 22; 21q 11–13; and Xq 26) (66–70). Of interest, linkage studies indicate an overlap at loci 13q 32; 18p 11.2 and 22q 11–13 for susceptibility to both bipolar disorder and schizophrenia, suggesting shared genetic vulnerability and perhaps less distinction between these two disorders than our present diagnostic system indicates (71).

Conclusion

Whether any or all of these factors relate to the efficacy of mood stabilizers is still uncertain, but the final common pathway may well be the inhibition of neurotransmitter and neuroreceptor-mediated processes. What is not clear is how these drugs alter neurotransmitter function or interactions, ultimately leading to their normothymic effects. A further complication stems from the combined antimanic and antidepressant properties of at least some of these therapies (e.g., ECT, lithium), making it difficult to theorize how opposite clinical effects are mediated by biochemical changes in one direction. Table 10-2 summarizes various mechanisms of action for existing and putative mood stabilizers. This overview depicts the multiplicity of effects and overlap among agents, providing both a sense of the complexity and possible future targets for drug therapy.

MANAGEMENT OF AN ACUTE MANIC EPISODE

Bipolar disorder, particularly acute mania, can be one of the most dramatic presentations in all of medicine, posing a diagnostic and therapeutic challenge for even the most skilled clinician. Although 3 million persons in the United States are presently being treated for this disorder, it is estimated that several million more go undiagnosed, misdiagnosed, and inadequately managed.

Unfortunately, this condition is also characterized by relapses and recurrence. For example, within a year of recovery, one half will have experienced symptoms of hypomania, mania, or depression (72). Factors that may place patients at greater risk for recurrence include the following:

- Number of *previous episodes*
- Clinical *presentation* (e.g., mixed states)
- Comorbid *personality disorder* (e.g., borderline, narcissistic, histrionic)
- *Substance* or *alcohol abuse*

Although we will focus on the evidence for various pharmacological and somatic interventions of this disorder, we emphasize that without a well-conceived psychosocial rehabilitation

TABLE 10-2. Mechanisms of action of existing and putative mood stabilizers

	Ions	AEDs					Atypical APs				
	Lithium	VPA	CBZ	LTG	GBN	TOP	CLZ	RISP	OLZ	QTP	ZPD
Neurotransmitters											
NE	√(↓)		√(↓)				√	√	√	√	√
DA	√(↑)	√(↑)	√(↑)				√	√	√	√	√
5-HT	√(↑)		√(↑)						√		
GABA	√(↑)	√(↑)	√(↑)								
GLU				√(↓)	√(?)	√					
ACH	√(↑)						√		√		
Signal transduction											
G-protein-PLC	√		√(↓)								
AC (cAMP)	√(↓)		√(↓)								
Ionositol (IMP)	√(↓)		√(↓)								
cGMP	√(↓)		√(↓)								
PKC (α, ε)-marks	√(↓)	√(↓)									
GSK-3β	√(↓)										
AP-1 (fos, jun) DNA binding	√(↑)		√(↑)								
Ion channels											
Ca^{2+}	√		√	√							
Na^{2+}		√	√	√	√(↓)	√					
Cl^{+}		√	√		√(↓)						
K^{+}											
Other											
Thyroid	√(↓)		√(↓)								
Circadian rhythms	√			√							
Carbonic anhydrase inhibition						√					
Neurotropic/neuroprotective	√(?)										

AED, antiepileptic (anticonvulsant) drug; APs, antipsychotics; VPA, valproate; CBZ, carbamazepine; LTG, lamotrigine; GBN, gabapentin; TOP, topiramate; CLZ, clozapine; RISP, risperidone; OLZ, olanzapine; QTP, quetiapine; ZPD, ziprasidone.

strategy the ultimate outcome is usually compromised. Thus, an optimal treatment strategy may require the following:

- Primary *mood stabilizers* (such as lithium, VPA, CBZ); antipsychotics; antianxiety agents; or antidepressants
- A variety of *combination drug strategies*
- *Electroconvulsive therapy* (*ECT*)
- Aggressive *psychosocial therapies* (e.g., family therapy, group therapy, cognitive-behavioral therapy, and various rehabilitation programs)

Analogous to the recent progress in antidepressant and antipsychotic drug therapy development the pharmacotherapy of bipolar disorder is also experiencing major advances. Data on the efficacy of mood stabilizers for bipolar disorder focus on the following:

- Treatment of an *acute exacerbation*
- Prevention of *relapse* after an acute episode has been controlled
- Prevention of *future episodes*

We reviewed the existing literature, emphasizing the controlled trials comparing these agents with either placebo or standard treatments for acute, maintenance, and prophylactic purposes. When feasible, the results were combined using meta-analysis (see the section "Statistical Summarization of Drug Studies" in Chapter 2).

Primary Mood Stabilizers

Lithium

Indications and Contraindications

For more than 40 years, lithium has been the standard drug therapy for bipolar disorder, primarily because of the quantity and the quality of evidence supporting its role as an effective maintenance and prophylactic treatment. This latter point is a very important consideration, given the recurrent nature of this disorder. Thus, clinicians must choose the optimal strategy for acute treatment with the realization that most patients will need to continue drug therapy indefinitely. In addition, there is support for maintenance lithium's beneficial impact on the suicide rate in bipolar patients (73, 74). The author of these reports notes that the lower suicide risk associated with lithium treatment may be due to the following:

- Its *mood stabilizing* properties
- A *lower suicide risk* per se in patients who remain in treatment
- A specific *antisuicidal effect* of the lithium ion

During the depressive phase, patients will often require the addition of an antidepressant. This may further complicate their management, however, because there is the possibility of propelling patients into a manic episode, a rapid cycling course, or a more treatment-resistant phase of their illness (75, 76).

Lithium's efficacy has been established within a well-defined therapeutic blood level range for optimal benefit and minimal adverse or toxic reactions. Optimism over lithium's impact has diminished, however, because of a significant proportion of patients who are nonresponders, insufficiently responsive, or intolerant to its adverse effects. In this context, given the alarmingly high suicide rate for untreated or inadequately treated bipolar patients, the need for other effective therapies is clear. **Finally, lithium has a narrow therapeutic index and numerous side effects that limit its usefulness, especially in the context of long-term therapy.** Indeed, 75% of patients on this agent will experience adverse effects, usually involving the renal, gastrointestinal, thyroid, and/or neurological systems (77).

Lithium may also be used in the depressive phase of a bipolar disorder, alone or to augment other antidepressants, and in combination with VPA or CBZ for more treatment-resistant mania (see also Chapter 7).

Efficacy

Lithium Versus Placebo. Schou et al. (2), in a now classic study, charted the natural history of several bipolar patients and found that the introduction of lithium induced remissions, dramatically altering the course of the disorder. While some patients were also assigned to placebo, the data were not presented systematically, and therefore could not be included in our meta-analysis. Bunney et al. (78) reported on a patient treated with lithium or placebo in a longitudinal ABA design who failed to respond to placebo, improved when switched to lithium, and then relapsed when lithium was discontinued. They also described a second patient who responded to lithium after failure to respond to a long, 10-day placebo lead-in period, and again relapsed when lithium was discontinued. A subsequent report by Goodwin et al. (79) described two additional cases with an unequivocal response to lithium, four others with a probable response, one with an equivocal response, and three who deteriorated on lithium; however, there was no control group. Although not as definitive as the class I or II study designs, these naturalistic reports strongly supported lithium's efficacy (see the section "Evaluation of Drug Study Designs" in Chapter 2).

The published literature includes 107 patients evaluated in prospective random-assignment, double-blind trials that found lithium superior to placebo for the treatment of a manic episode (80–82) (Table 10-3). Maggs (80) conducted a double-blind, random-assignment, placebo-controlled, parallel trial of lithium without concomitant medications. While he found lithium clearly superior to placebo, he probably underestimated the true drug—placebo difference because he did not include the placebo nonresponding dropouts, nor did he include data that could be used in our meta-analysis. Stokes (81) also conducted a 10-day, double-blind, placebo-controlled, random-assignment trial of lithium using only a modest amount of adjunctive antipsychotics. He crossed over nonresponders every subsequent 10-day period to the opposite arm, for a total of four switches, and found lithium superior to placebo throughout the study. Again, he may have underestimated the true drug—placebo difference, however, because 10 days are often insufficient to achieve full benefit with lithium and some patients did receive

neuroleptics. In 1976, Stokes (82) used the same crossover design, this time assigning patients to high or low doses of lithium. Combining the data from his two studies, he was able to demonstrate a dose (and plasma level)—response relationship to remission. Bowden and colleagues' (83) multicenter study of the divalproex sodium (DVPX) formulation of VPA also compared lithium with placebo, significantly increasing the number of lithium-treated patients evaluated under placebo-controlled conditions (i.e., 110 patients: 74 on placebo and 36 on lithium). Marked improvement, defined as at least a 50% reduction in the manic syndrome subscale score derived from the Schedule for Affective Disorders and Schizophrenia—Change (SADS-C), occurred in 49% of the lithium group versus 25% of the placebo group ($p < 0.025$).

Lithium Versus Antipsychotics. Antipsychotics were the treatment of choice for acute mania before the introduction of lithium. Clinical experience has shown that in some cases these agents may be the only effective therapy as well as the only practical (i.e., depot preparation) treatment in noncompliant or pharmacokinetically idiosyncratic patients. Although our meta-analysis of five well-designed studies comparing neuroleptics alone with lithium alone for acute mania clearly demonstrates lithium's superior efficacy, more than 50% of those on an antipsychotic alone also responded (17, 84–88). Subsequently, Rifkin and associates (89) compared three doses of haloperidol (HPDL) for up to 6 weeks as the only treatment in 47 acutely manic patients. They found that 72% of subjects responded, excluding dropouts (most occurring in the first 2 weeks and being evenly distributed across all groups). Furthermore, 10, 30, or 80 mg/day of HPDL were equi-effective (i.e., survival analysis showed no difference among the three dosing regimens). **This is particularly noteworthy and parallels recent findings that lower doses of HPDL**

TABLE 10-3. *Lithium versus placebo: acute mania*

Number of subjects	Responders (%)		Difference (%)	χ^2	p value
	Lithium (%)	Placebo (%)			
107	54	31	23	6.0	0.01

to treat schizophrenic and schizoaffective patients are often as effective as moderate-to-high doses (90).

Lithium has been systematically compared with antipsychotics for the management of acute mania. Most believe it produces a better qualitative response, but this observation is difficult to substantiate with controlled studies. A patient once analogized this difference to an automobile engine racing out of control, describing the effect of antipsychotics as similar to applying the brakes, while lithium was similar to adjusting the carburetor (91). Lithium has a more narrowly defined range of indications, primarily benefiting bipolar disorder, but is relatively ineffective for schizophrenia, particularly the more chronic subtypes. Given its narrow spectrum of efficacy, the inclusion of groups such as schizoaffective disorder and schizophrenia in studies comparing it with antipsychotics may bias the results against lithium. Also, because antipsychotics usually have a faster onset of action, a design that allows patients to drop out early may underestimate lithium's relative efficacy.

Controlled trials. Table 10-4 summarizes the results from four of the five well-controlled, albeit small, trials comparing lithium with an antipsychotic in classic manic patients. These studies presented their data in a way that allowed for inclusion in a meta-analysis. **Each study was a well-controlled, double-blind design, finding lithium superior to an antipsychotic, and the meta-analysis of the combined studies demonstrated this difference to be highly statistically significant.**

In addition, Platman (92) studied 13 patients on lithium and 10 on chlorpromazine (CPZ), finding lithium consistently superior overall, but not statistically significant on any individual rating scale. The general state of patients on lithium was markedly superior to those on CPZ because the majority were discharged with no other treatment, whereas all of the patients on CPZ required additional concurrent drugs. Because the author did not present data on individual patients, these results could not be included in our meta-analysis, but his results are also consistent with the outcome in Table 10-4. Due to the small sample size, the results should be interpreted cautiously.

Prien et al. (93) studied 255 Veteran's Administration (VA) patients diagnosed as bipolar, manic, or schizoaffective, and assigned them to lithium or CPZ. These investigators subdivided patients into highly versus mildly agitated categories based on the Inpatient Multidimensional Psychiatric Scale, which describes patients as "exhibiting overactivity, restlessness, and/or accelerated body movement." Also, patients were categorized by the Brief Psychiatric Rating Scale (BPRS) for baseline levels of excitement, uncooperativeness, grandiosity, mannerisms, tension, and conceptual disorganization. Twenty-two percent of the lithium-treated and 14% of the CPZ-treated patients dropped out, leaving approximately 60 in each of the four groups: highly active, lithium- or CPZ-treated; and mildly active, lithium- or CPZ-treated. They found substantially more dropouts in the highly active group receiving lithium, usually due to poor

TABLE 10-4. *Lithium versus neuroleptics: acute mania*

	Lithium		Neuroleptics	
Study	Responders (number of subjects)	Nonresponders (number of subjects)	Responders (number of subjects)	Nonresponders (number of subjects)
Johnson et al., 1968, 1971	16	2	8	3
Spring et al., 1970	8	1	3	3
Takahashi et al., 1975	33	4	24	10
Shopsin et al., 1971	7	3	3	17
Total	**64 (89%)**	**10 (11%)**	**38 (54%)**	**33 (46%)**

χ^2 (Mantel-Haenszel) = 13.1; $df = 1$, $p = 0.0003$.
Adapted from Janicak PG, Newman RH, Davis JM, Advances in the treatment of mania and related disorders: a reappraisal. *Psychiatr Ann* 1992;22(2):94.

response or uncooperativeness, but the pre- and post-rating differences in all four groups were similar. An analysis of covariance found that the outcome for lithium completers did not differ from that for CPZ completers. An endpoint analysis, however, found CPZ superior to lithium in the highly active group on such measures as conceptual disorganization, psychoticism, grandiosity, and suspiciousness. There were no significant differences between the two drugs in the mildly active group. When schizoaffective patients and many of the severely disturbed patients who did not receive lithium for a sufficient duration were included, the antipsychotics were found to be superior.

Garfinkel et al. (94) compared haloperidol, lithium, and their combination for the treatment of mania, but did not present data on patients as individuals. Initially, there were seven patients in each group. By day 15, three in the lithium group, two in the HPDL group, and one in the combined drug group had dropped out. The two HPDL groups improved slightly more than the lithium monotherapy group; however, considering the small sample and the high dropout rate, we would speculate that these patients were highly disturbed and could not be managed on lithium alone for a sufficient period of time.

Braden et al. (95) did a similar study in primarily schizophrenic or schizoaffective patients, but the sample also included some affectively-ill cases (i.e., 21% met Feighner criteria for mood disorder). Of the 43 patients on lithium, 15 dropped out because they did not improve, worsened, or were unmanageable or confused. By comparison, only one of 35 treated with CPZ dropped out in the first 10 days. CPZ produced better results in the overactive group, whereas both drugs were comparable in the less active group. As with the VA study, the poor results with lithium in the overactive group may have been an artifact of insufficient duration due to the high dropout rate, or because of the inclusion of patients with a core schizophrenic illness.

Cookson et al. (96) in a random-assignment design found 10 of 12 manic patients responded to pimozide and 11 of 12 patients to CPZ. This is consistent with the observation of Post et al. (97), who, after a placebo lead-in period, found

the time course of improvement with pimozide ($n = 8$) to be similar to that with lithium ($n = 8$) or a phenothiazine ($n = 9$). Because pimozide is a more specific D_2 antagonist than CPZ, this outcome provides further support for a beneficial role with D_2 receptor blockers in the treatment of mania.

Johnstone et al. (98) performed a random-assignment, double-blind trial comparing pimozide, lithium, a combination of these two, and placebo in 120 patients with a variety of psychotic disorders (e.g., psychotic mania, psychotic depression, schizoaffective disorder, schizophreniform disorder, schizophrenia). Patients were classified as having an elevated or depressed mood or no consistent change in mood. Pimozide had a robust effect on positive symptoms across all categories (i.e., elevated mood, depressed mood, and no mood change), whereas lithium only had a modest beneficial effect ($p = 0.07$) in affectively disordered patients with an elevated mood. Heterogeneity in the diagnostic categories, however, must temper interpretation of their results.

Thus, although lithium therapy of sufficient duration may be the treatment of choice in classic milder presentations of mania, the adjunctive antipsychotics (especially the novel agents) may be preferable in conditions such as mania with psychosis and schizoaffective disorder, given their faster onset of effect and broader spectrum of activity (see the section "Alternative Treatment Strategies" later in this chapter).

Lithium Versus Anticonvulsants. A number of trials have also compared lithium to various anticonvulsant mood stabilizers such as VPA and CBZ (83, 99, 100). The results will be discussed in more detail in the sections on these specific agents. In general, lithium has been found to be comparable, but some data support better efficacy for agents such as VPA and CBZ in certain subgroups (e.g., mixed states, rapid cyclers). It is not clear, however, whether these agents have the same antisuicidal effects as lithium.

Administration of Lithium

As part of the standard prelithium workup, a thorough medical evaluation should be completed.

TABLE 10-5. *Laboratory evaluation during lithium treatment*

Prior to initiation of treatment
Renal function testing
  General screening—serum creatinine; BUN; urinalysis
  If further testing required:
    24-hour urine volume
    Creatinine clearance
    Test of renal concentrating ability
Thyroid function
  T_3, T_3RU, and T_4
  TSH
Cardiac
  ECG (if elderly or at risk for heart disease)
General (if indicated)
  CBC and differential
  Serum electrolytes
  General Chemistries

During maintenance treatment
Renal function
  Urinalysis; BUN (every 6–12 months)
  Serum creatinine (every 6–12 months when clinically indicated)
  Test of renal concentrating ability (when clinically indicated)
Thyroid function
  TSH (every 6–12 months)
  Repeat full battery with elevated TSH and/or clinical signs/symptoms

Table 10-5 lists the various laboratory tests recommended to assess overall physical status, especially renal, thyroid, hematological, and cardiac function, before initiation of treatment. In particular, the renal and the thyroid systems require a baseline assessment and periodic reevaluation with maintenance or prophylactic lithium therapy.

Because lithium has a half-life of approximately 24 hours and it takes four to five half-lives to achieve steady-state at a fixed dose, blood levels should be obtained every 5 days until an adequate therapeutic concentration is achieved or adverse effects preclude further increases. Attempts to develop dose prediction formulae to obtain therapeutic concentrations more rapidly have been promising, but they have not enjoyed widespread utilization (101–103). While premature monitoring may lead to higher than necessary dosing, more frequent measuring of levels may be warranted in patients with known sensitivity to lithium or if unexpected reactions occur. Once the initial treatment has begun, we recommend blood levels in the range of 0.8 to 1.2 mEq/L for optimal efficacy. Some patients who do not benefit from these levels may respond at slightly higher concentrations (e.g., 1.3 to 1.5 mEq/L). Conversely, a small proportion of patients who are unable to tolerate levels in the lower end of the usual therapeutic range (i.e., around 0.5 to 0.7 mEq/L) may acclimate to and benefit from concentrations as low as 0.3 to 0.4 mEq/L. Blood samples for lithium levels should be drawn 10 to 12 hours after the last dose to measure the concentration at its trough. Lithium saliva and RBC concentrations have also been promoted as more accessible or more accurate measures, respectively, but have not gained general acceptance.

Typical starting doses of lithium are 300 mg two or three times a day. The dose can vary from a low of 300 mg/day to as high as 3,000 mg/day, with the typical range between 900 and 1,800 mg/day. An individual's age, renal function, and general physical condition are important associated determining factors for the ideal dose. **Initially, dosing schedules were on a three or four times a day basis, but subsequent data indicate once or twice a day regimens may enhance compliance and minimize certain adverse effects, while not compromising efficacy.**

Lithium preparations include *lithium carbonate, sustained-release preparations,* and the liquid form, lithium citrate. The sustained-release preparations allow for a more gradual absorption of the drug, leading to blunted peak plasma levels. Because lithium has a slow onset of action, it can take weeks, and occasionally longer, to obtain an optimal clinical response. Thus, it is important to avoid a premature abandonment in those who are simply slower to respond.

Whenever possible, we prefer to treat with a mood stabilizer (e.g., lithium, VPA) alone, because of their specificity for bipolar disorder and to minimize adverse effects. This is particularly true in mild to moderately severe episodes of acute mania. In addition, if the patient can benefit from a single drug during the acute episode, this would support its benefit for maintenance and prophylactic purposes. Further, monotherapy diminishes the chance for potentially significant drug interactions and reduces cost.

Lithium Plus Other Psychotropics

From the perspective of clinical trial methodology, concurrent medications can create a dilemma for the investigator by complicating the interpretation of results. Intermediate rescue medications are often required, however, because mood stabilizers are relatively slow in their onset of action. Further, if rescue medications are avoided, this usually introduces the confound of dropouts before the experimental drug can be fully effective. When feasible, a reasonable compromise is the use of modest amounts of a benzodiazepine (BZD), such as lorazepam, only when necessary for a limited time (e.g., 7 to 10 days) into the active phase of treatment. This can reduce the number of nonresponding, highly agitated patients who may otherwise drop out of treatment; and in a trial of several weeks, the initial lorazepam effect should have dissipated by the final assessments.

There are several studies that combined lithium with other treatments such as antipsychotics, anticonvulsants (e.g., CBZ, VPA), calcium channel blockers (e.g., verapamil), or BZDs (e.g., lorazepam). Generally, in partial responders, the addition of these medications was beneficial and well tolerated.

Lithium Plus Antipsychotics. Many patients present in a very explosive, belligerent, and agitated manner, and waiting several days to weeks to gain control of an episode is not feasible. Thus, antipsychotics alone or as adjuncts are frequently required in the earliest phases of treatment, particularly with moderate to severe exacerbations, often associated with psychotic features. As a result, antipsychotics are the most commonly used adjunctive agents, because more than half of all acutely ill bipolar patients present with psychotic symptoms. In addition, many require maintenance antipsychotics to prevent frequent relapses. Antipsychotics are usually initiated in conjunction with lithium because of their more rapid impact, then carefully tapered and discontinued, when possible, after the full effect of lithium is realized.

Unfortunately, manic patients may be exposed to higher than necessary acute antipsychotic doses, perhaps because of the explosivity often associated with an exacerbation. Baldessarini et al. (104) conducted an epidemiological survey in the Boston area and found that antipsychotic dosing schedules of higher potency agents (e.g., haloperidol, fluphenazine) were three to five times greater than the CPZ dose equivalents of lower potency drugs (e.g., CPZ, thioridazine). This was consistent across a number of different diagnostic categories, including the affectively disordered patients. He postulated that the different (and at least perceived as more benign) adverse effect profile of the higher-potency drugs encouraged aggressive increases in dose to control severe, acute psychotic exacerbations.

Addressing this issue in hospitalized acutely manic patients, Janicak et al. (105) conducted a 2-week study of lithium plus random assignment to equivalent doses of CPZ or thiothixene. The dose-equivalent ratio used was 5 mg of thiothixene to 100 mg of CPZ (i.e., 1:20). During the waking hours, patients' antipsychotic doses were titrated on a 2-hour basis, so that response and adverse effects to the prior dose were the determinants for administering or holding the next dose. The aim was to compare the efficacy, side effect profiles, and optimal dose required for either antipsychotic. Our hypothesis, based on the existing empirical dose-response literature, was that the effective dose would fall between 300 and 800 mg of CPZ or a bioequivalent amount of thiothixene. After the first 4 days, patients receiving thiothixene averaged 30 mg/day and those receiving CPZ averaged 380 mg/day. By the end of the 2-week trial, the mean dose in the thiothixene-treated group was 36 mg, and the mean dose of CPZ was 480 mg (i.e., a ratio of 1:13). These amounts fell in the low to mid range of the dose-response curve previously reported. Secondly, the overall improvement was statistically significant for the entire sample when baseline values were compared with day 14, nor did clinical response differ between the two antipsychotic groups. Finally, because relatively lower doses were used, adverse effect profiles, although typical and in the expected direction (i.e., slightly

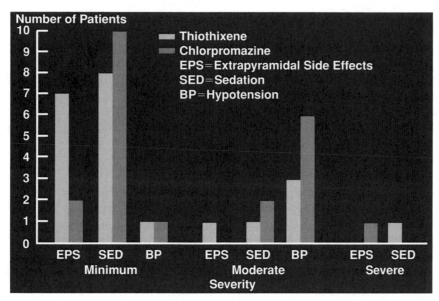

FIG. 10-1. Adverse effects of thiothixene versus chlorpromazine.

more extrapyramidal side effects for those patients receiving thiothixene and slightly more sedation and hypotension in those receiving CPZ), allowed for optimal and tolerable dosing regimens (Fig. 10-1). The blood levels of lithium (i.e., approximately 1.0 mEq/L) by the end of week 1 were adequate and almost identical for both groups. No other concomitant medications were used.

We concluded that relatively low to moderate doses of either a high- or low-potency antipsychotic were sufficient to control acutely manic patients with associated psychotic features, and at these doses, adverse effects remained in the tolerable range.

The role of *NAPs*, either as primary or adjunctive treatments, has yet to be fully explored. There have been reports that clozapine, risperidone, and olanzapine may possess thymoleptic properties (106–108). McElroy and her coworkers (109), for example, surveyed the response of 85 consecutive patients, including 14 bipolar patients with psychotic features, who received clozapine for 6 weeks. The response rates of the schizoaffective patients (both bipolar and depressed subtypes), as well as those with bipolar disorders with psychotic features, were excellent (i.e., almost 90%) and substan-

tially better than the response rate of 46% for the pure schizophrenic group. Another report concluded that the concurrent use of clozapine with VPA may result in greater efficacy and was well tolerated in most patients (110). We do not recommend the combined use of clozapine plus CBZ because of possible increased risk of bone marrow suppression. We would also avoid using clozapine plus a BZD, because this combination has been reported to cause respiratory compromise (111). Two recent controlled trials have reported a significantly greater antimanic effect for olanzapine over placebo and possible antidepressant effects for risperidone versus haloperidol in schizoaffective patients (112, 113). Other controlled trials, for agents such as risperidone, ziprasidone, and aripiprazole, are under way and will better define the role of these agents in treating mood disorders (113, 114).

Lithium Plus Benzodiazepines. Unfortunately, two retrospective chart reviews at the Connecticut Mental Health Center found that a substantial number of manic patients started on an antipsychotic while hospitalized were still on these agents 6 months after discharge and that chronic neuroleptic treatment occurred frequently in their outpatient bipolar group (115, 116). **These authors concluded that**

antipsychotic adjuncts to lithium should be reconsidered frequently and reduced whenever possible. In this context, there has been an increasing interest in adjunctive antianxiety agents for acutely manic patients to avoid concomitant antipsychotics or at least to minimize their total amount (117). The literature is generally anecdotal and parallels a similar literature of adjunctive lorazepam use in treating acute psychosis, but there have been some recent controlled trials (see the section "Management of Acute Psychosis" in Chapter 5). The most commonly studied drugs have been *lorazepam* and *clonazepam,* due to their rapidity of onset and duration of action. In addition, lorazepam can be administered intramuscularly with adequate absorption, in contrast to other BZDs. *Alprazolam* and *diazepam* have also been studied.

The major benefit of BZDs may be in diminishing some of the secondary symptoms of an acute exacerbation (e.g., insomnia, agitation, panic, and other general anxiety symptoms) that are not necessarily rapidly and specifically affected by lithium or antipsychotics. With this approach, exposure to antipsychotics may be precluded in some situations and kept to a minimum in others, thus avoiding the potential for more serious antipsychotic-induced adverse effects. Additionally, given the high comorbidity with alcohol abuse/dependence, concurrent withdrawal symptoms may also be managed with BZDs.

Relative contraindications to the use of BZDs concern patients with a history of the following:

- *Alcohol or other substance abuse* or dependency
- *Paradoxical response* to BZDs (i.e., behavioral disinhibition)
- *Known sensitivity* to this group of agents
- Acute narrow angle *glaucoma*
- *Pregnancy*

Lorazepam. Lenox et al. (118) found lorazepam and haloperidol comparable in efficacy when used as adjuncts to lithium in a double-blind study of 20 acutely manic patients. Interestingly, another report comparing lorazepam with clonazepam found a better outcome with lorazepam, using mean doses of 12 to 13 mg (119).

Clonazepam. Clonazepam is marketed primarily for petit mal variant, myoclonic, and akinetic seizures. It also has had wide psychiatric application, including the treatment of acute mania or other agitated psychotic conditions, usually in combination with lithium or antipsychotics. The literature on clonazepam's efficacy for acute mania is based on the work of Chouinard (120) and coworkers who compared this agent with placebo or standard treatments for acute mania. As noted earlier, however, another group from Montreal found that comparable doses of lorazepam were more effective than clonazepam for acute mania (119).

Typical doses of clonazepam have been in the range of 2 to 16 mg/day given on a once or twice per day schedule due to its longer half-life. A major advantage of this anticonvulsant is its relative lack of adverse effects and freedom from laboratory monitoring in comparison with CBZ and VPA. Clonazepam may be more useful when combined with lithium or CBZ rather than as a specific antimanic agent, perhaps supplanting the need for antipsychotics. In this sense, it can be viewed as a "behavioral suppressor," rather than a true "mood stabilizer" (121).

Lithium Plus Thyroid Supplementation. Treatment-resistant and rapid-cycling bipolar patients may have an increased frequency of thyroid dysfunction. Further, some patients suffer from subclinical hypothyroidism and improve with the addition of thyroid supplementation. In this context, several case reports involving this population found that high doses of the thyroid hormone levothyroxine sodium (T_4) were clinically beneficial (122–124). Kusalic (125) found that 6 of 10 rapid cyclers had hypothyroidism, based on their thyrotropin-releasing hormone stimulation tests. Further, the average number of mood episodes per year decreased by more than 75% (i.e., from 9.7 to 2.2) after thyroxine was added to the treatment regimen.

Bauer et al. (126) entered 11 rapid-cycling, treatment-refractory patients into an open trial of high-dose levothyroxine sodium, added to their previously stabilized medication regimen. The dosage of the levothyroxine was increased by 0.05 to 0.1 mg/day every 1 to 2 weeks, as tolerated, until symptoms improved or adverse effects prevented further increases. Scores on both the depressive and the manic symptom rating scales decreased significantly compared with baseline scores. These data indicate that levothyroxine, used in doses sufficient to produce supranormal circulating hormone levels, may induce remission of both depressive and manic symptoms in an otherwise refractory group of bipolar patients.

These results are complemented by a more recent report suggesting that rapid-cycling treatment nonresponders may benefit from the addition of levothyronine (127). Although these were open case reports of small sample sizes, the promising positive results warrant further study under more controlled conditions.

Valproate

VPA is available in various formulations, including DVPX (a compound composed of sodium valproate and valproic acid), dipropylacetic acid, and a closely related form, valpromide or dipropylacetamide. Reports on its benefit for the management of mood disorders date back to the mid-1960's. In the early European experience, much of the interest focused on maintenance therapy of manic-depressive disease, with patients stabilized on VPA or valpromide for up to 10 years using the drug alone or in conjunction with other psychotropics. A few investigators also studied the drug in acute mania, usually in combination with antipsychotics, and found it to be beneficial, often allowing for substantial reductions in the antipsychotic dose (128).

VPA's mechanism of action is unclear but its anticonvulsant efficacy *may* be related to the ability to increase CNS levels of GABA (Table 10-2). Due to its rapid absorption, blood levels peak in 1 to 4 hours after oral administration, and the half-life ranges from 6 to 16 hours. It is metabolized primarily through the liver and is eliminated in the urine. **VPA is highly protein-bound and usually does not saturate binding sites at serum levels below 45 to 50 μg/mL. Thus, this level would be the expected minimal threshold for its psychotropic effects.**

Indications and Contraindications

The DVPX (Depakote) formulation was the first drug since lithium to be approved and labeled by the FDA for the treatment of bipolar disorder, manic phase. This agent may also benefit some of the more lithium-resistant subtypes described earlier (see Chapter 9). Like lithium and CBZ, it does not appear to be as beneficial for the depressive phase of this illness. There are also limited data that nonresponsiveness to one anticonvulsant (e.g., CBZ) does not necessarily portend a poor response to another (e.g., DVPX) (129, 130). DVPX is contraindicated in patients with significant hepatic disease, during pregnancy, and in those with a known hypersensitivity to this agent.

Efficacy

Lambert et al. (16) first investigated VPA in a series of clinical trials including a wide variety of patients. Twelve subsequent open-design studies, representing 297 acutely ill patients, found an overall moderate-to-marked response rate to VPA of 56%. Only one study, however, met more rigorous double-blind, placebo-controlled conditions, with a total of 17 patients on VPA (131).

Brennan et al. (132) observed that six of eight manic patients responded to VPA. All then had their medication discontinued for a few days, with one relapsing but again improving upon reinstatement of VPA.

Emrich et al. (133) used a placebo lead-in period in five patients treated with VPA and found that four responded, but no subsequent placebo period was mentioned.

Although the overall response rate to VPA was 61%, a number of methodological problems complicate the interpretation of these results, including that most patients were studied under *nonblind conditions,* this agent was often used in combination with other psychotropics, plasma concentrations were usually *not monitored,* and *formal diagnostic criteria* derived from standard clinical ratings were *typically not used.*

Valproate Versus Placebo. Although there had been several small studies suggesting that this agent is effective for acute mania, in the past few years compelling clinical data have reinforced these earlier claims of benefit (132, 133). **Two class I studies have now examined the efficacy of the DVPX formulation in comparison with placebo for acute mania**.

First, in a study by Pope et al. (131), 36 previously lithium-resistant (i.e., nonresponsive and/or nontolerant) patients were treated for 3 weeks with DVPX or placebo in a random-assignment, double-blind design. DVPX was significantly more effective than placebo, with 12 of 17 patients responding to this agent, versus only six of 19 to placebo. An early high plasma level of DVPX (i.e., days 2 to 6) was found to predict response, whereas rapid cycling, predominant euphoria or dysphoria, family history of mood disorder, increased manic severity, and EEG abnormalities did not predict response (134).

Second, Bowden et al. (135) provide the strongest evidence to date for the efficacy of DVPX in acute mania from a multicenter study of 179 patients comparing this agent with placebo, with lithium as an active control. The methodology incorporated a double-blind, random-assignment, parallel design.

Marked improvement of manic symptoms occurred in the following:

* 48% of the *DVPX* group ($n = 69$)
* 49% of the *lithium* group ($n = 36$)
* 25% of the *placebo* group ($n = 74$)

Thus, both drug-treated groups experienced significantly greater benefit than achieved with placebo ($p = 0.004$ for DVPX; $p = 0.025$ for lithium). DVPX-treated patients demonstrated significantly greater improvement in elevated mood, decreased need for sleep, excessive activity, and motor hyperactivity compared with placebo-treated patients; whereas lithium-treated patients showed greater improvement in excessive activity and motor hyperactivity when compared with those on placebo. **Notably, DVPX was similarly effective in manic patients with or without a rapid-cycling course, and response to this agent was equivalent in those who were previously responsive or nonresponsive to lithium.** Supplemental chloral hydrate or lorazepam were used in the first 10 days; otherwise, there were no additional rescue medications. The definitive assessment of most patients occurred in the second and the third weeks when no adjunctive medication was used. Finally, only the lithium group had a significantly higher dropout rate due to adverse effects in comparison with those in the placebo group.

Due to these two carefully controlled trials, the evidence that DVPX is effective in acute mania is presently the best controlled data for any treatment, including lithium. We performed a meta-analysis on these two placebo-controlled trials of DVPX using the Mantel-Haenszel method for dichotomous data and the Hedges and Olkin method for continuous data (Table 10-6). Of the 175 patients evaluated, 84 were on DVPX and 91 were on placebo. As a cutoff response, we used a decrease of 7 or more points on the Mania Rating Scale. Sixty-five percent of the DVPX patients improved compared 32% on placebo ($\chi^2 = 18.3$; $p = 0.00002$). Using the continuous method, the probability that DVPX is statistically superior to placebo is 0.0004. Here the cumulative effect size is 0.55 (CI = 0.25 to 0.86). The results of the two studies are consistent withwith each other, and both meta-analysis methods demonstrate a large drug—placebo difference.

Other reports have also suggested that this agent may be helpful in subgroups often

TABLE 10-6. *Divalproex versus placebo: acute mania*[a]

Study	Number	Percent responders		Difference
		Divalproex	Placebo	
Pope et al., 1991	36	71%	29%	42%
Bowden et al., 1994	139	64%	32%	32%
Total	**175**	**65%**	**32%**	**33%**

[a] $\chi^2 = 18.3$; $df = 1$; $p = 0.00002$.

resistant to lithium. Calabrese et al. (136), for example, in a prospective longitudinal naturalistic open design, examined 101 VPA-treated *rapid-cycling* bipolar patients and found that predictors of good antimanic response included decreasing or stable episode frequencies and nonpsychotic episodes. Papatheodorou and Kutcher (137, 138), in a preliminary open trial of six bipolar *adolescents* treated with DVPX, found that five had marked improvement and one had some improvement. Deltito et al. (139) found that open treatment with DVPX monotherapy or as copharmacy was associated with marked improvement in psychopathology in a group of 31 adolescents (aged 13 to 18) suffering from mixed-presentation bipolar disorder ($n = 16$), major depression ($n = 7$), mania ($n = 4$), or psychosis not otherwise specified ($n = 4$). Other open-trial reports indicate that this agent may be effective and well tolerated in *elderly* patients, those with concurrent *substance* or *alcohol abuse,* and those with *organic mood* disorders (140–142).

Valproate Plus Antipsychotics. The best study to date addressing this issue was conducted by Muller-Oerlinghauser and colleagues (143). They compared a *neuroleptic alone* with the *combination of VPA* plus neuroleptic in a 3-week prospective, double-blind, placebo-controlled, multicenter study. A total of 136 acutely manic patients received a fixed dose of 20 mg/kg per day of VPA or placebo, in addition to a neuroleptic. They found that the mean dose of antipsychotic (in haloperidol equivalents) declined during the study in those subjects who were also receiving VPA. Based on a 50% reduction in the baseline YMS, 70% on combination therapy versus 46% on neuroleptic alone achieved this level of improvement ($p = 0.005$). Adverse events did not differ significantly between the two groups. The authors concluded that, in comparison with a neuroleptic alone, the combination treatment did the following:

- Allowed for lower *amounts* of neuroleptic.
- Produced a *more rapid remission* of symptoms.
- Produced a significantly *greater improvement* in symptoms.

Valproate Versus Lithium. The previously discussed Bowden et al. (135) study found the DVPX formulation to be comparable with lithium, which was used as a positive comparator in this placebo-controlled study. Freeman et al. (99) conducted a 3-week, double-blind, parallel-group comparison of VPA and lithium for acute mania. Both drugs demonstrated clinically significant efficacy (i.e., 9 of 14 responded to DVPX and 12 of 13 to lithium), and there was no difference in the need for rescue medications (i.e., lorazepam or chloral hydrate) between the two treatment groups. Response to VPA was associated with high pretreatment depression scores.

Valproate for Other Disorders. Data from several preliminary open trials indicate that VPA may be useful in the management of the following:

- *Panic* disorder (144)
- *Posttraumatic* stress disorder (145)
- *Personality disorder* with aggression (146)
- *Dementia* with agitation (147, 148)
- As an augmentation strategy in *schizophrenia* (148a)

Administration of Valproate

The most commonly used formulation of VPA is DVPX. DVPX is usually started at 750 to 1,000 mg on a two- or three-times-a-day schedule, with doses titrated up every few days to achieve blood levels in the range of 50 to 125 (perhaps a few up to 150) μg/mL, or until side effects prohibit further increases (149). **For most patients, an adequate trial typically requires total doses ranging from 1,000 to 2,500 mg/day.**

Several reports indicate that DVPX may also be safely administered using a loading dose strategy (150–152). For example, Keck et al. found that 20 mg/kg led to therapeutic plasma levels within 5 days. This is important, given evidence that the antimanic activity of DVPX is more likely to occur after achieving adequate serum concentrations. In this study, patients tolerated 20 mg/kg/day in divided doses for 5 days, with rapid onset of antimanic response. With increasing pressure to limit the length of hospital stays, such an accelerated response rate could represent a significant advantage. More recently, preliminary reports indicate that intravenous VPA administration may also be safely and effectively used in a loading dose strategy (153, 154).

Case Example: A 34-year-old man was hospitalized on CBZ, CPZ, lithium, and lorazepam for an acute exacerbation of mania. Despite a history of rapid cycling, he responded to an initial trial of Li_2CO_3, thiothixene, and lorazepam, but then relapsed. Increasing the thiothixene (up to 120 mg/day) was unsuccessful and poorly tolerated. The patient then improved on a regimen of loxapine (up to 250 mg/day) and clonazepam (up to 20 mg/day), but doses of each had to be reduced because of intolerable adverse effects (i.e., excessive sedation, drooling, pseudoparkinsonism), and he suffered another relapse. He again received CPZ (up to 900 mg/day) and DVPX (plasma level stabilized at 80 μg/mL), while the clonazepam was tapered slowly and discontinued. He gradually became euthymic and was able to leave the hospital after a 4-month stay, stabilized solely on CPZ (600 mg/day) and DVPX (1,250 mg/day).

VPA may also benefit the maintenance and the prophylactic phases as well, but there are only limited data in this regard, in contrast to lithium, which remains the best-studied maintenance therapy. VPA has a favorable and relatively safe side effect profile compared with other agents and can be combined with other commonly used psychotropics without significantly altering their metabolism or compromising adequacy of blood levels (155). There are also limited anecdotal data that this agent can be safe and effective in the elderly patient (156, 157).

Drug Treatment Strategy for Acute Mania

In a highly disturbed hospitalized manic patient, we prefer to supplement lithium or VPA with an adjunctive BZD, such as lorazepam, adding an antipsychotic only if necessary. Alternatively, oral loading with VPA may avoid the need for adjunctive BZD or antipsychotic. Although caution must be exercised due to the possible disin-

hibiting effects of BZDs, these agents may also attenuate withdrawal symptoms in bipolar patients who are also alcohol dependent. After a stabilization period, the adjunctive medications may then be gradually withdrawn and the patient often managed successfully with lithium or VPA only. In nonresponsive patients, assuring adequacy of the lithium or VPA dose and plasma level, as well as duration of treatment, discontinuation of concurrent antidepressants, and supplemental thyroid medication (e.g., levothyroxine, 50 to 300 mcg daily; triiodothyronine, 25 to 100 mcg daily) may all improve outcome. Neuroleptics should be used only when absolutely necessary (e.g., acute parenteral administration required) and carefully titrated upward to avoid excessive exposure. Novel antipsychotics would be our preference because they may have mood-stabilizing properties, produce fewer neurological sequelae then neuroleptics, and because there is preliminary evidence that these agents may improve response in previously treatment-refractory patients (121).

MAINTENANCE/PROPHYLAXIS

The overwhelming majority of patients who have a manic episode will have one or more recurrences. These episodes are disruptive, life-threatening, and often have a progressive deteriorating effect on the patient's capacity to cope with life's activities. Therefore, it is of critical importance that we develop effective and safe, long-term treatments. The ideal agent would be effective for both the manic and the depressed phases as an acute, maintenance, and prophylactic therapy. Unfortunately, this is not the case for any of the present agents.

Lithium

Interestingly, there are more well-controlled studies comparing lithium with placebo for maintenance and prophylactic purposes than for acute treatment. It was apparent from the earliest observations that patients relapsed when lithium was discontinued and that indefinite treatment seemed to diminish recurrences. Baastrup and Schou (158) were the first to clarify this phenomenon in a controlled, mirror-imaged trial with 88 bipolar patients, when they counted the number of episodes before and after lithium therapy. This was a large naturalistic study with objective, verifiable, and clinically important outcome measures, such as weeks in hospital or number of relapses, and a large sample size of typical, very ill patients. They found a highly significant decrease in relapses after initiation of treatment (i.e., every 60 months versus every 8 months), and that the average time in a severe episode decreased from 13 weeks per year before lithium, to 1.5 weeks per year with active treatment. Thus, lithium led to a sevenfold decrease in the number of episodes or weeks ill, representing a substantial improvement in the natural history of the disease.

Time Course of Relapse

Schou et al. (159) then studied the time course of relapse in both bipolar and unipolar patients. The plot of the natural log of the relapse rate versus time takes the form of a straight line, indicating an exponential distribution. In other words, the rate of relapse as a proportion of unrelapsed patients is fairly constant over time. Because approximately 15% receiving placebo relapsed each month (i.e., the rate constant for relapse = 0.15), the "half-life" of untreated remitted patients is approximately 4.5 months. Generalizing from the population studied, this figure gives an indication of what would happen to those not treated with lithium. Although the number of relapses is modest during the first few weeks, the cumulative number is impressive several months to years later.

Schou et al. (159) also compared the relapse rate of patients in their double-blind clinical trial with those in their naturalistic open study and found a similar rate.

A recent meta-analysis of 19 blinded, randomized, controlled trials of lithium prophylaxis by Davis et al. (160) found this agent far superior to placebo in preventing recurrence (i.e., 74% recurrence on placebo versus 29% on lithium). Further, in the mirror-image studies, there was no evidence to support relapse due to lithium withdrawal as a possible explanation for this difference (Table 10-7). Combining all controlled studies, the p value for significance $p = 10^{-133}$.

Maintenance Strategies

The maintenance properties of lithium have been verified in a large number of random-assignment, double-blind studies comparing this agent with placebo in the preventive treatment of unipolar and bipolar disorders. To summarize the bipolar studies, lithium was effective in preventing or attenuating recurrences (i.e., about 50% fewer recurrences) (Table 10-8).

Because lithium is superior to placebo in preventing a relapse once the acute episode has been controlled, duration of treatment, concurrent drug use, ideal blood levels, and method of discontinuation become critical issues.

Patients who have had more than one severe episode are probably best managed with continual, indefinite lithium prophylaxis. Even in patients who have experienced a single episode, there may be as high as a 50% chance for a recurrence within 5 months of stopping drug therapy (161). In these patients, if lithium is tolerated without breakthrough symptoms, maintenance therapy can be reevaluated in 1 to 2 years; however, there are some data that initial responders to lithium who stop treatment may trigger a more virulent phase of the disease, or may experience a recurrence less likely to benefit from the drug's reinstitution (162). For this reason, we advocate indefinite lithium therapy after one significant episode.

Because there are also some data that concurrent use of antidepressants can lead to rapid cycling in vulnerable patients, these agents may best be cautiously used on an as-needed basis or as adjuncts when there are early signs of breakthrough depressive, psychotic, or anxious symptoms. In particular, antidepressants do not prevent manic episodes, and may even precipitate them. The fact that many patients on antidepressants experience a manic phase, however, could be coincidental, rather than drug-induced. To definitively answer this question, we need to show that the number who switch to mania is higher on, as opposed to off, antidepressant therapy. Given these concerns, however, we advocate the initial use of a mood stabilizer alone to lessen the chance of a switch to mania in bipolar depressed patients. If this is insufficient, a

TABLE 10-7. Prophylactic efficacy of lithium versus placebo

Study	Study type	Diagnosis	Class	n	Relapsed on lithium (%)	Relapsed on placebo (%)	Difference (%)
Baastrup et al., 1970	U	Bipolar	i	50	0	55	55
Prien et al., 1973	U	Bipolar	i	205	43	81	38
Prien et al., 1973	U	Bipolar	i	31	50	32	42
Kane et al., 1982	U	Bipolar	i	11	25	—	46
Coppen et al., 1971	U	Bipolar	i	38	18	100	62
Melia, 1970	U	Bipolar	i	15	57	75	18
Fyrö and Petterson, 1977	U	Bipolar	i	18	0	100	100
Fieve et al., 1976	U	Bipolar	i	53	58	86	28
Cundall et al., 1972	CR	Bipolar	i	24	33	83	50
Mander et al., 1988	CR	Bipolar	i	28	0	64	64
Margo and McMahon, 1982	CC	Bipolar	iii	15	0	100	100
Persson, 1972	CC	Bipolar	iii	24	42	92	50
Small et al., 1971	DIS	Bipolar	iv	10	0	100	100
Christodouiou and Lykouras, 1982	DIS	Bipolar	iv	34	0	18	18
Hanna et al., 1972	CR	Bipolar	iii	2	0	100	100
Kane et al., 1982	U	Unipolar	i	13	29	100	71
Prien et al., 1973	U	Unipolar	i	53	63	92	29
Glen et al., 1984	U	Unipolar	i	20	45	89	44
Baastruo et al., 1970	U	Unipolar	i	34	0	88	53
Coppen et al., 1971	U	Unipolar	i	26	9	80	71
Fieve et al., 1976	U	Unipolar	i	28	57	84	7
Persson, 1972	CC	Unipolar	iii	42	29	67	38
Melia, 1970	U	Unipolar	i	3	0	100	100
Cundall et al., 1972; Christodoulou and Lykouras, 1982	COMB	Unipolar	i, iv	10	40	40	0
Hullin et al., 1972	U	Bipolar + unipolar	i	36	6	33	28
Klein et al., 1981	DIS	Bipolar + unipolar	iv	42	0	52	52
Total					**29**	**74**	**46**

U, uncrossed (parallel group); CR, crossover studies; CC, case-control studies; DIS, discontinuation studies; COMB, several small studies combined. The data for each arm were entered separately in the Mantel-Haenszel analysis.

Adapted from Davis JM, Janicak PG, Hogan DM. Mood stabilizers in the prevention of recurrent affective disorders: a meta-analysis. *Acta Psychiatr Scand* 1999;100:406–417.

TABLE 10-8. *Lithium versus placebo for bipolar disorder: maintenance treatment*

Number of subjects	Relapsed (%)		Difference (%)	χ^2	*p* value
	Lithium (%)	Placebo (%)			
739	28	76	48	151	$<10^{-34}$

mood stabilizer should be used concurrently with an antidepressant.

Alternatively, Young et al. (163) reported comparable improvement in depression in 27 bipolar patients randomly assigned under double-blind conditions to the addition of paroxetine or a second mood stabilizer. However, the combined mood stabilizer group had significantly more dropouts than the group given paroxetine plus a mood stabilizer.

Regarding optimal maintenance blood levels, Gelenberg et al. (164) found that patients maintained on standard concentrations of lithium (e.g., 0.8 to 1.0 mmol/L) had a significantly lower risk of relapse (i.e., 13%) than those on lower dose-plasma level regimens (i.e., a 38% relapse rate with levels in the range of 0.4 to 0.6 mmol/L).

Finally, data indicate that more rapid lithium discontinuation (e.g., less than 2 weeks) may decrease the time to recurrence (165).

Compliance

Unfortunately, patient noncompliance may be as high as 50% within the first year of treatment, posing a serious public health issue (166). Sensitivity to *somatic adverse effects* (especially memory problems, impaired coordination, weight gain, and tremor); *unrealistic expectations* leading to secondary depression; *cognitive* and *psychological adverse effects* on long-term lithium treatment without relapse; the positive reaction to *early euphoria* and/or hypomania; and *severity of illness* all may play a role. Further, *dual diagnosis disorders* (i.e., bipolar plus substance or alcohol abuse) are common and may contribute to more frequent exacerbations (167).

Strategies to improve compliance include the following:

- Intensive *educational efforts* at the onset of therapy

- *Dose reduction,* when feasible
- Supportive, individual, family, and when indicated, drug or alcohol abuse *counseling*
- Aggressive *intervention with early signs of relapse*

In summary, there is evidence for a higher relapse rate in patients not maintained on adequate levels of lithium, the potential for concurrent drugs (e.g., antidepressants) to exacerbate the disorder, a more rapid recurrence with abrupt discontinuation, and possible compromised future lithium responsiveness when it is stopped (43, 162). **Compliance issues remain a major factor in providing adequate long-term treatment.**

Longitudinal Course

Bipolar patients treated under typical clinical conditions may have a more difficult posthospital course than has been generally appreciated. Mander (168), for example, reported on 2745 bipolar patients initially admitted because of an episode of mania or depression, and found that lithium did not reduce the readmission rate within 3 months of discharge. As a result, he proposed that its full prophylactic effect may not occur for 6 to 12 months after the start of treatment, and that it should be reserved for long-term prophylaxis in those who have had a number of severe episodes in a defined period of time.

Harrow et al. (169) followed 73 bipolar and 66 unipolar patients in a longitudinal naturalistic design for 1.7 years after hospital discharge. Bipolar patients generally had poorer outcomes than their depressive counterparts, with more than 40% demonstrating a manic syndrome during follow-up. Surprisingly, bipolar patients complying with lithium maintenance fared no better than those who did not. The authors opine that using the "management trial" model (i.e., assessing treatment under routine clinical conditions), as opposed to the "exploratory trial" model (i.e., optimal controlled research conditions) reveals a less positive outcome for these patients. Further, lithium prophylaxis was far less effective than the 70% to 80% response rate reported in earlier trials. They conclude that a significant proportion of bipolar patients may suffer from a severe, recurrent, and pernicious disorder. Shortcomings in their design, such as inadequate monitoring of drug compliance or inadequate blood levels, however, limit the interpretability of their results.

Another way of assessing the long-term course is to monitor functional as well as symptomatic disability. In a subsequent report, Goldberg et al. (170) followed unipolar depressed and bipolar patients for up to 4.5 years. Although outcome for both groups improved over time, up to 60% of classic bipolar patients still experienced poor adjustment in one or more areas of functioning. Dion et al. (171) followed 67 classic bipolar or atypical bipolar patients in a prospective 6-month follow-up study after discharge from the hospital. Forty-four of the original 67 were interviewed at 6 months, and about one-third of the sample was found to be clearly disabled functionally, despite dramatic drops in their average symptom ratings on the BPRS, the Mania Rating Scale, and the Hamilton Depression Rating Scale. Further, in those with a previous history of more than one psychiatric admission, the rate of functional disability was closer to 50%. These investigators conclude that their findings belie the assumption that bipolar illness has a good prognosis and that appropriate rehabilitative interventions are crucial to meet the needs of these patients.

Efficacy

As noted earlier, lithium's efficacy as a maintenance therapy is one of the best-studied psychopharmacological effects. We have summarized all the placebo-controlled studies on the use of lithium to prevent relapse, including both unipolar and bipolar patients. We also performed a meta-analysis of these studies, separating out unipolar and bipolar patients (Tables 10-8 and 10-9).

Baastrup and associates (6) studied manic-depressive and recurrently depressed Danish patients who had been successfully stabilized on lithium for at least 1 year. This ensured that subjects had the type of illness that is helped by lithium, and that they could tolerate the treatment. Because it was a prospective, well-controlled, random-assignment, double-blind study (i.e., class I), potential biases were effectively eliminated. These authors demonstrated a dramatic and positive effect for lithium when compared with placebo. None of the patients who received lithium over a 5-month period relapsed, whereas 55% of the bipolar and 53% of the unipolar patients on placebo did so.

In a multihospital collaborative design, Prien and associates (172, 173) studied patients in VA, public, and private hospitals to assess a 2-year maintenance therapy program. They first examined the prophylactic value of lithium in hospitalized manic patients, and in a second study, compared prophylactic lithium, imipramine, and placebo in hospitalized depressed patients. These studies did not select known lithium responders, and therefore included many who had not previously been exposed to this therapy. Hence, there was a greater base rate of relapse in their lithium groups than in the previous Danish studies, with the relapse rate even higher in the placebo groups (i.e., almost all patients relapsed). Despite these higher absolute rates, the difference in relapse between the lithium and the placebo groups in the two VA studies was comparable with the Danish studies. In the two VA studies, whereas nearly half on lithium relapsed, almost all placebo patients (89%) did so (6, 172, 173). In Baastrup's study (6), no lithium patients relapsed, but 54% on placebo did. Similar results were obtained by

TABLE 10-9. *Lithium versus placebo for unipolar disorder: maintenance treatment*

| Number of subjects | Relapsed (%) | | Difference (%) | χ^2 | p value |
	Lithium (%)	Placebo (%)			
183	31.6	70.5	38.9	29.7	5×10^{-8}

Mendlewicz and associates (174, 175) in a study conducted in New York City. **Overall, when both the American and the European studies were combined, the drug—placebo difference was about 45%.**

Coppen et al. (176, 177) performed a collaborative study at four separate centers, randomly assigning patients to lithium or placebo for up to 2 years. This study used a slightly different design, in that patients who relapsed or became more symptomatic, short of relapse, were treated with other medications (excluding lithium) so they could remain in the study. The results were consistent with earlier findings. In the United Kingdom, Cundall and associates (178) confirmed these earlier findings in a separate study.

Our analysis also included Persson's Swedish study, which used matched patients (179). Despite some methodological flaws, we feel it was a valid study and should be counted even though it only met criteria for a class II design. Their findings were also consistent with the overall results.

Mander and Louden (180) studied 14 patients with a history of mania—by *Diagnostic and Statistical Manual of Mental Disorders,* 3rd ed. (DSM-III) criteria—who entered a randomized, double-blind, placebo-controlled, crossover trial. These patients had been stable on lithium for at least 18 months and were not taking any other psychotropics. The protocol consisted of three phases, each lasting 4 weeks. During the first phase, patients were stabilized on lithium, with adequate levels, and baseline clinical ratings were obtained. During the second and the third phases, the patients were randomized under double-blind conditions to receive an additional 4 weeks of lithium followed by 4 weeks of placebo or vice versa, so that patients acted as their own control. Relapse was defined as meeting DSM-III criteria for mania, with an increase of at least five points from baseline on the symptom checklist, and a score over 20 on the modified Manic Rating Scale. Seven patients during the placebo phase and none during the lithium phase relapsed ($p = 0.006$). The authors concluded that the recognition of withdrawal relapse will lead to better use of lithium so that its proven prophylactic advantages can be trans-

lated into improved prognosis. Further, unnecessary relapses may be prevented by counseling patients about the risks of sudden lithium discontinuation.

Using data from a National Institute of Mental Health collaborative project, Shapiro et al. (181) applied a survival analysis model to the reexamination of response to maintenance therapy in 117 patients who met Research Diagnostic Criteria for a bipolar disorder. They divided the group according to whether the index admission was for a manic or a depressive episode. Patients were stabilized in the preliminary phase and maintained on adequate doses and blood levels of lithium and imipramine for 2 months. After this, they were randomized to receive a lithium-imipramine combination ($n = 37$), lithium only ($n = 45$), or imipramine only ($n = 35$) for a 24-month study period or until relapse. These authors found that imipramine alone was a poor prophylactic treatment for bipolar disorder and that the combination therapy was the most effective strategy, not appreciably increasing the risk of relapse in either group. The most striking difference between their analysis and the earlier report of Prien et al. (182) was that the combination therapy appeared to be particularly effective after an index episode of depression, and attribute this difference in outcome to the use of the survival analysis model.

Finally, Strober et al. (183) conducted an 18-month, prospective, naturalistic follow-up study of 37 bipolar-I adolescents (i.e., 13 to 17 years old) stabilized on lithium and found a relapse rate almost three times higher in those who discontinued prophylactic lithium (92%), as compared with those who complied (38%). Further, they noted that earlier relapse in these patients predicted a greater risk of subsequent relapse; and that an early onset may be associated with a more virulent course, resistance to lithium, and the need to consider alternative mood stabilizers. Methodological problems with this study included a small sample size; lack of assessment for personality disturbances and intrafamilial environment; only a 4-week initial drug stabilization period; and lack of precision in monitoring compliance to treatment.

Bipolar Manic Versus Bipolar Depressive Phases

It is important to make a conceptual distinction between lithium's relative prophylactic effect for the manic and the depressive phases of a *bipolar disorder* and, by extension, its ability to prevent recurrent depressions in *unipolar disorder*.

In reviewing these studies, it is useful to distinguish statistical significance from magnitude of association, or effect size. A high correlation involving five subjects may be barely statistically significant, but a low correlation involving thousands of subjects may be highly significant. The percentage of patients relapsing on lithium or placebo and the difference in their relapse rates are effect sizes, whose probability of being significant is determined by both the difference in relapse rates and the sample size. Because most studies noted here had more subjects in the bipolar than in the unipolar group, statistical significance does not provide an adequate comparison of the degree of lithium prophylaxis (effect size) in each subgroup (Table 10-10).

Further, some of the studies did not report the number of manic versus depressive relapses. One exception is Coppen et al. (176, 177), who reported the mean affect morbidity score of patients receiving placebo (mean ± SD, 0.33 ± 0.05) or lithium (0.09 ± 0.05) for the manic phase, as

well as placebo (0.31 ± 0.06) or lithium (0.07 ± 0.03) for the depressive phase. Thus, this study found very similar prophylactic effects. Baastrup and associates (6) reported a comparable number of manic and depressed phase relapses in their bipolar patients. In 22 bipolar patients, 12 relapsed: six into a manic phase, five into a depressed phase, and one into a mixed phase. By contrast, Prien et al. (182) and Cundall et al. (178) found that lithium had a greater effect in preventing the manic than the depressed phase of bipolar disorder. **Overall, lithium was effective in preventing both phases of a bipolar disorder.**

Bipolar Versus Unipolar Disorder

An important body of evidence from descriptive, clinical, and genetic sources finds that bipolar disorder is a separate entity from unipolar disorder (i.e., genetically the two variants breed true; see also the section "Mechanism of Action" earlier in this chapter). When we pooled data from several studies that investigated bipolar or unipolar disorders, lithium was more effective than placebo in preventing relapse in bipolar as well as unipolar disorders (Tables 10-11 and 10-12).

Naturalistic Trials

We also reviewed a longitudinal naturalistic, collaborative study conducted in three European

TABLE 10-10. *Effectiveness of lithium in preventing recurrence of the manic versus the depressive phase of bipolar disorder*

Study	Manic phase		Depressive phase	
	Placebo	Lithium	Placebo	Lithium
Coppen et al., 1963, 1971				
Mean affect morbidity score	0.33 ± 0.05	0.09 ± 0.05	0.31 ± 0.06	0.07 ± 0.03
Baastrup et al., 1970[a]				
Number relapsed	6	10	5	10
Number not relapsed	0	28	0	28
Cundall et al., 1972				
Number relapsed	9	1	5	3
Number not relapsed	3	11	7	9
Prien et al., 1984				
Number relapsed	76	34	35	20
Number not relapsed	41	85	82	99

[a]In this study, 12 of 22 bipolars relapsed. Of the 12 patients who relapsed, relapsed to a mixed phase of bipolar illness.

Adapted from Appleton WS, Davis JM. *Practical clinical psychopharmacology*, 3rd ed. Baltimore: Williams & Wilkins, 1988:125–126.

TABLE 10-11. *Lithium maintenance versus placebo in bipolar depressed patients*

Study	Placebo	Lithium	Total
Baastrup et al., 1970			
Number relapsed	12	0	12
Number not relapsed	10	28	38
Coppen et al., 1963, 1971			
Number relapsed	21	3	24
Number not relapsed	0	14	14
Persson, 1972			
Number relapsed	11	5	16
Number not relapsed	1	7	8
Prien et al., 1984			
Number relapsed	93	47	140
Number not relapsed	24	72	96

Adapted from Appleton WS, Davis JM. *Practical clinical psychopharmacology*, 3rd ed. Baltimore: Williams & Wilkins, 1988:125–126.

countries (184–186). Although not a class I design, it does provide a large number of patients and supplements the evidence from double-blind comparisons. Investigators from Denmark, Czechoslovakia, and Switzerland used a design similar to Baastrup and Schou's classic naturalistic study (with the addition of their multinational sampling), to compare the relative effect of lithium on the course of recurrent unipolar versus bipolar disorder. As an index of prophylaxis effect, the investigators counted the number of episodes that occurred before and during lithium treatment, and used a linear regression model to provide a quantitative estimate for lithium's effect. The major independent variable was the length of time the patient was free from active disease. Lithium prevented the recurrence of both unipolar and bipolar disorder equally well.

Aagaard and Vestergaard (187) followed 133 consecutive affectively disordered patients (unipolar, bipolar, uncertain diagnosis) on lithium prophylaxis in a 2-year prospective, naturalistic design to identify predictors of outcome. The frequency of admissions before the index episode and substance abuse were the primary predictors of *nonadherence* (noncompliance), defined as stopping treatment against medical advice at least once in those 2 years. Nonresponse (defined as more than one readmission in 2 years) in compliant patients was predicted by sex (female subjects did worse), age (younger subjects did worse), and chronicity. It should be noted that lithium levels (0.5 to 0.8 mEq/L) tended to

TABLE 10-12. *Lithium maintenance versus placebo in unipolar depressed patients*

Study	Placebo	Lithium	Total
Baastrup et al., 1970			
Number relapsed	9	0	9
Number not relapsed	8	17	25
Coppen et al., 1963, 1971			
Number relapsed	12	1	13
Number not relapsed	3	10	13
Persson, 1972			
Number relapsed	14	6	20
Number not relapsed	7	15	22
Prien et al., 1984			
Number relapsed	14	13	27
Number not relapsed	2	14	16

Adapted from Appleton WS, Davis JM. *Practical clinical psychopharmacology*, 3rd ed. Baltimore: Williams & Wilkins, 1988:125–126.

be in the lower end of the therapeutic range and could have contributed to the higher relapse rate. Disappointingly, the overall response rate (63%) was poor, with a mortality rate of 15.3% (seven patients). The authors suggest that patients with a history of substance abuse should have lithium prophylaxis combined with intensive support and well-controlled management settings; and that alternative or supplementary treatment should be considered for those with frequent prior admissions and a chronic course.

Maj et al. (188) studied the long-term outcome in 79 affectively disordered patients (43 bipolar, 36 unipolar) who had been successfully managed on lithium prophylaxis for 2 years. Their goal was to prospectively monitor the course of illness for an additional 5-year period. Forty-nine completed this phase, two died (of cancer), seven were lost to follow-up, and 21 interrupted their treatment. Twenty-five patients relapsed (10 bipolar, 15 unipolar) during this period, calling into question long-term prognosis, given a favorable initial 2-year response to lithium prophylaxis. The authors discussed several other notable issues, including the following:

• Although lithium was *an effective prophylaxis in 44%* of these patients, the relapse rate was higher than that reported by earlier studies.
• There was a *decrease in morbidity* in the 5-year follow-up period, as compared with the prelithium phase.
• *Some patients,* despite adequate treatment with lithium, *relapsed after several years of successful prophylaxis,* returning to the same level of morbidity as during their prelithium period.
• Some patients developed a *persistent mild dysphoria* while on prolonged maintenance lithium.

Attitudes and Adjustment During Remission

The *correlates of attitudes toward lithium compliance* in bipolar patients were studied by Cochran and Gitlin (189). This questionnaire study was part of a larger design looking at factors in *lithium prophylaxis.* The questionnaire packets were sent to 146 patients, 48 of whom were ultimately included in the analysis. This study evaluated the usefulness of Ajzen and Fish-

bein's "Theory of Reasoned Action" to explain the relationships among lithium-related beliefs and attitudes, normative beliefs, behavioral intentions, and self-reported compliance with treatment. According to the model, lithium patients' normative beliefs (i.e., beliefs that other relevant people such as family, friends, personal psychiatrist, and lithium experts want the patient to take lithium) predict their subjective norms, which is the expectation that others want them to take lithium. Subsequently, both the subjective norm and the evaluative behavioral attitudes (i.e., positive nature of treatment) were predictive of the patients' reported intent to take lithium. This, in turn, was predictive of concurrent self-reported compliance with the medication regimen. **These results underscore the importance of the patient-physician relationship in lithium compliance.**

The possibility of an adverse effect with prophylactic lithium or some sequelae of affective illness affecting the *life satisfaction and adjustment of patients in remission* was explored by Lepkifker et al. (190). Life satisfaction scores and adjustment scores in four areas were obtained for 100 remitted patients (50 bipolar and 50 unipolar patients) matched for sex and age, a control group of 50 healthy individuals, and a control group of patients with personality disorders. Subjects rated their feelings of satisfaction in life by indicating their position on a 10-point ladder device that was based on a modification of Cantril's Self-Anchoring Striving Scale. A similar 10-point scale was used by patients to assess their levels of adjustment and overall functioning. In addition, the treating psychiatrist or therapist was asked to rate the same issues. Patients' life satisfaction and adjustment scores in the various areas investigated were significantly and positively correlated with the corresponding ratings given by the psychiatrist in the two scales of adjustment. Analysis of variance and the post hoc Duncan test were conducted on the differences obtained from the four groups for life satisfaction, currently, 5 years previously, and 5 years in the future. Unipolar and bipolar patients did not differ from healthy control subjects for current life satisfaction, but the mean rating for the other psychiatric control subjects was significantly lower than in any other group ($F = 7.92$; $p = 0.001$).

Affective patients and healthy control subjects rated life as more satisfying at present than in the past, and they also rated themselves higher than most others on scores of life satisfaction at present. The authors concluded that neither lithium as a prophylactic agent nor the affective illness interfered with either the manifest functioning or the patients' feelings of satisfaction while in remission.

Long-Term Outcome of Bipolar and Unipolar Mood Disorders

Coppen et al. (191) evaluated the status of 104 bipolar or unipolar recurrent patients after 10 years of lithium maintenance to assess mortality rate, in part because of reports indicating unusually high rates, with many deaths attributed to suicide. Compliance was very high, with only 6% discontinuing lithium therapy, and patients also received adjunctive antipsychotic and/or antidepressants when clinically indicated. No patient died of suicide during this period, in contrast to the results in lithium noncompliant patients. The authors concluded that the absence of suicide resulted from the significant reduction in morbidity achieved by the careful administration of lithium.

Schou and Weeke (192) reported on 92 Danish bipolar patients admitted between 1969 and 1983 with a first episode and who committed suicide before July 1, 1986. Information was obtained on any prophylactic or continuation treatment at the time of the suicide, and the patients were divided into seven groups (A to G), based on the type of treatment and status of their illness. It appeared that 70% of the sample were receiving the best medical and prophylactic therapy available; however, 30% may have benefited from a more effective use of the available measures. They noted that previous suicide attempts, complicating alcoholism, and a mixture of neurotic or hypochondriacal features should heighten the clinician's suspicion of a potential to commit suicide. They further recommend the following:

- That a successful course of *ECT* should be followed by at least 6 to12 months, and often a lifetime, of prophylactic drug therapy

- That *prophylactic antidepressants* should be given in full therapeutic dosages
- That *prophylactic lithium* should be considered in unipolar patients when antidepressants are unsatisfactory
- That conscientious *psychological support* should be given to improve compliance and help patients to cope with emergent problems in living

Valproate

Data on the maintenance and prophylactic effects of this agent are limited. Several open trials found that moderate to good results were obtained when VPA was used alone or in combination with lithium, although adverse effects were more significant in one combination study (193, 194). The *Physician's Desk Reference* notes that DVPX has not been evaluated in controlled clinical trials for longer than 3 weeks (195). Recently, a large randomized, placebo-controlled, blinded comparison of DVPX and lithium in the prophylaxis of bipolar episodes was completed. The study appears to support other evidence of better tolerability of DVPX than lithium. In most analyses the efficacy measures, such as time to development of a recurrent manic or depressive episode, favored both DVPX and lithium over placebo. The drug—placebo differences were greatest among patients with evidence of more severe bipolar disorder (e.g., those with one or more lifetime hospitalizations for mania). Only small and nonsignificant advantages of DVPX or lithium over placebo resulted in those patients with the mildest severity of illness. This may be due to fewer relapses than initially predicted in those mildly ill patients treated with placebo (196).

Gyulai and colleagues (197) reported the results of a large multicenter study in which 372 subjects were randomly assigned in a 2:1:1 ratio to VPA, lithium, or placebo. These researchers found equivocal evidence that VPA prevented early termination from the study due to depression when compared with placebo. In the VPA group, 6% terminated compared with 16% in the placebo group and 11% in the lithium group. The absolute number of depressive relapses and survival rates in all three groups, however, was the same.

Perhaps most crucial are data on the relative benefit of VPA in comparison with lithium for maintenance and prophylactic treatment of rapid cyclers and mixed states. In this context, Calabrese and coworkers (136) reported on a naturalistic follow-up study of 10 bipolar, rapid-cycling patients treated with VPA alone or in combination with other mood stabilizers and/or antidepressants. When VPA was used as a prophylaxis against manic episodes, psychosis predicted a poor outcome. When this agent was used as a prophylaxis against depression, more severe manic episodes predicted a positive outcome, whereas borderline personality predicted a less favorable outcome. This is an important issue to confirm, given the strong evidence supporting its acute antimanic effects (see also the section "Alternative Treatment Strategies" later in this chapter).

Conclusion

Maintenance and prophylaxis with lithium, and perhaps other mood stabilizers, favorably alters the longitudinal course of a bipolar disorder. Thus, efforts to enhance long-term compliance are a necessary part of any overall strategy. The incidence of adverse or toxic events is relatively low, and close attention to the more clinically relevant consequences can usually prevent serious sequelae (198). **An issue of critical importance for future research is the potential efficacy of alternative maintenance medication for those who fail to respond adequately to acute or long-term lithium therapy.**

It is becoming increasingly evident that prevention of relapse, as well as adequate prophylactic strategies for patients with major mood disorders, are much more complicated than was originally assumed. Factors that contribute to this situation include the following:

- *Personal* and *family histories* of psychiatric disorders
- *Type of presentation* at the index episode
- Subsequent symptomatic and functional *disability*
- *Inadequate or less than aggressive use* of combined medication and psychotherapeutic strategies
- Lack of effective drug *alternatives*

On a slightly more positive note, combination treatments, such as combined mood stabilizers or mood stabilizer plus antidepressant, may decrease relapse rates; early, aggressive intervention may shorten subsequent episodes; and newer agents, such as VPA, CBZ, or lamotrigine may benefit previously resistant subgroups of bipolar disorders. It is also encouraging that patients in good remission on lithium often view themselves favorably compared with normal control subjects on life satisfaction and adjustment measures.

It is apparent that the task of generating a systematic body of knowledge to identify prognostic indicators and successful treatment strategies for patients with major mood disorders is complicated by a multitude of issues. Results of studies investigating precipitating life events, thyroid status, lithium augmentation, diagnostic subtypes, and demographic variables have not yet led to reliable predictors. Similarly, the results of treatment studies with prophylactic and maintenance lithium therapy were also varied. It seems, however, that the overall response and mortality rates improved as compliance increased and adjunctive therapy with antipsychotics and/or antidepressants or levothyroxine was utilized. Additionally, careful attention to and reduction of stressful life events may prevent or attenuate subsequent episodes of the illness.

We have developed an approach to managing patients with bipolar disorder during the maintenance phase (Fig. 10-2). Another approach to the management of bipolar, depressed episodes is contained in Figure 10-4.

Alternative Treatment Strategies

Although lithium has been a major advance in the pharmacotherapy of severe mood disorders, a number of problems limit its usefulness, including the following:

- *Slow onset* of action in treating an acute episode
- *Diminished effectiveness* in severe manic exacerbations
- *Inadequate response*
- *Nonresponse*
- *Partial* response
- *Intolerance* to lithium

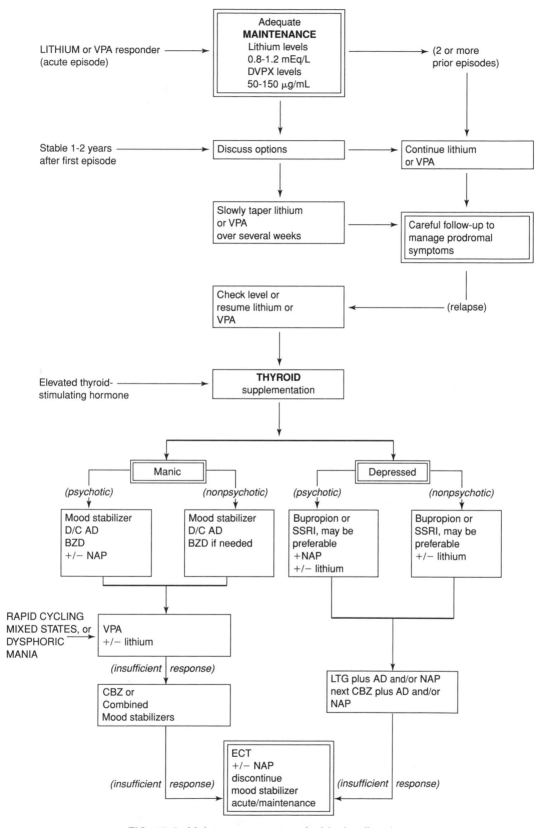

FIG. 10-2. Maintenance strategy for bipolar disorder.

- *Adverse effects*
  - Thyroid
  - Renal (e.g., excessive urination)
  - Troublesome adverse effects (e.g., mental dulling, tremor, edema, weight gain)
- *Noncompliance* (often due to adverse effects)

Further, certain subgroups of affectively disordered patients may be less likely to benefit from lithium, including the following:

- *Rapid cyclers* (5% to 20% of all bipolar patients)
- *Dysphoric, mixed,* or *complex* mania (up to 40% of all episodes)
- *More severe episodes* (e.g., with associated psychosis)
- *Schizoaffective* disorder
- *Organic* mood syndromes
- The *elderly manic patient*
- Patients with:
  - Coexisting *alcohol* or *substance abuse*
  - *Personality disorders*
  - *Mental retardation*

As a result, there are ongoing attempts to develop alternative strategies for these patients (11, 18, 121).

Because lithium has long been the standard treatment for bipolar disorder, it is often the drug of first choice. Increasingly, however, VPA has emerged as a viable alternate first-line therapy. *CBZ,* marketed as an anticonvulsant, has also been studied and used for its mood-stabilizing properties. There has never been a definitive controlled study, however, comparing the efficacy of lithium with other mood stabilizers in difficult-to-treat manic patients.

Other Anticonvulsant Drugs

Given the success of VPA and CBZ, there has been an increasing interest in clarifying whether other anticonvulsants also have mood-stabilizing properties. Clonazepam appears to have non-specific effects on hyperactivity and related anxiety features. Other anticonvulsant agents, such as *lamotrigine, gabapentin, topiramate,* and tiagabine have also been considered. Preliminary findings indicate that lamotrigine may also be beneficial for the depressed phase of bipolar dis-

order. *Phenytoin,* available since the 1940's, has rendered results that are generally (but not always) disappointing (199).

The rationale for the use of selected anticonvulsants in the treatment of bipolar disorder is based on the following factors:

- *Only partial response* or *refractoriness* to lithium
- Possible *improved efficacy for specific subtypes*
- *Noncompliance* with lithium due to intolerable adverse effects
- *Lack of antipsychotics' more serious complications,* such as tardive dyskinesia, neuroleptic malignant syndrome, other extrapyramidal reactions, or significant hypotension
- Combination strategies involving lithium, VPA, and CBZ may have beneficial *additive* or *synergistic effects* in selected patients with lithium plus VPA the most frequently used combination (200, 201)

Carbamazepine

CBZ is indicated for the management of temporal lobe epilepsy and paroxysmal pain disorders. Its anticonvulsant actions are apparently associated with the ability to reduce postsynaptic responses and to block posttetanic potentiation. The initial half-life ranges from 25 to 65 hours, but due to CBZ's ability to induce its own metabolism (i.e., autometabolism), this may be reduced to 12 to 17 hours after several weeks of treatment. Its primary psychiatric application has been as a treatment for bipolar disorder, based on the initial work of two Japanese groups in the early 1970's (13, 14). Interestingly, CBZ has a chemical structure resembling imipramine and was originally synthesized as a possible antidepressant agent.

Of note, the FDA has only approved CBZ for certain seizure and paroxysmal pain disorders, but not for the treatment of mood disorders. While the use of drugs for other than FDA-labeled indications is a common and appropriate practice, this should always be discussed with patients, as well as their families. Proper documentation includes the discussion of the rationale and the potential complications (see also the section "Informed Consent" in Chapter 2).

Our qualitative and quantitative analyses of CBZ's efficacy in acute mania, as well as for maintenance therapy, find it to be a potential alternative therapy when lithium or VPA are unsuccessful. There is also an emerging argument for its preferential use in certain lithium-resistant subtypes; however, the amount and quality of the data thus far limit any firm conclusions.

Indications and Contraindications

CBZ's spectrum of efficacy appears similar to that of lithium; however, as noted earlier, it may be superior to lithium in mixed or dysphoric mania, rapid cyclers, and more severe episodes (e.g., fulminant, aggressive, psychotic) (202). The number of patients treated with CBZ for acute mania in some form of placebo-control design is very limited. In fact, we are not aware of any double-blind, placebo-controlled, parallel design studies addressing this question (i.e., class I design).

Efficacy for Acute Treatment

Reviews of the literature comparing CBZ or oxcarbamazepine with placebo, lithium, or various antipsychotics for acute mania find a response rate approaching 70% (203, 204). One of the problems with this literature, however, is that most studies qualify for only a class III design (see also the section "Evaluation of Drug Study Designs" in Chapter 2).

As noted earlier, the first controlled empirical study of the effects of CBZ on behavior was done by Dehing (12), who described its behavioral effects in epileptic patients. He reported that it made them more active and communicative; less egocentric and stubborn; improved dysphoria, emotional lability, aggressiveness, and outbursts of rage; and had a positive effect on apathy, depression, anxiety, and hypochondriasis. He then studied its effects in a mostly nonepileptic, chronic psychiatric population that suffered from such varied disorders as dementia, psychosis, mental deficiency, and psychopathy, but not bipolar disorder. In a double-blind random-assignment design, he treated most of these patients for 1 month with placebo or CBZ. He continued the investigation after the double-blind phase on patients initially assigned to placebo and added others to the trial, for a total of 58 patients. Those receiving CBZ showed a marked improvement, in contrast to those on placebo, but there were two patients on CBZ who developed either a slight or a marked aggravation of their disorder.

Dehing qualitatively identified aggressiveness and outbursts of rage as the symptoms most helped by CBZ. It is of interest that, in addition to both VPA and lithium's mood-stabilizing effects, there is evidence they also exert an anti-aggressive effect (205). This raises the question of whether these agents act at a more fundamental level than the specific disorder being treated. Thus, like anti-inflammatory agents, they may benefit various disorders that share phenomenological and pathophysiological similarities.

Carbamazepine/Oxcarbamazepine Versus Placebo. Post and Uhde (206) studied nine manic patients using an ABA design. In our judgment, three patients had a good response to CBZ and relapsed when switched to placebo; one had an equivocal response but relapsed when CBZ was discontinued; one responded to CBZ but failed to relapse on placebo; and three neither demonstrated a clear-cut response to CBZ nor relapsed when administered placebo later. To some degree, the placebo lead-in period in the ABA design controls for the placebo effect, but with no true control group, we cannot be sure improvement was due to *cycling,* spontaneous *remission,* nonspecific effects of hospitalization, or an unrecognized *carryover medication effect.*

Emrich et al. (133) treated six patients with oxcarbamazepine, the keto derivative of CBZ. Three showed a good response, with one improving during two separate episodes. Here again, the design was a class III type, with no control group, and although the outcome was suggestive of efficacy, it is not definitive.

Goncalves and Stoll (207) studied six patients on CBZ and six on placebo; however, substantial amounts of antipsychotic augmentation were used. Virtually every placebo patient had some additional haloperidol, and two of three also received other supplemental antipsychotics. In the CBZ group, four of six received supplemental haloperidol, with none needing other antipsychotics. Despite the greater use of antipsychotics in the placebo group, the CBZ group was found statistically superior. Because significant amounts of concomitant antipsychotics were used, it is hard to draw any firm conclusion, but the outcome could be suggestive of the need for antipsychotic supplementation when CBZ is used.

Carbamazepine Versus Lithium. Other relevant evidence for CBZ comes from studies comparing it with standard treatments. Lerer et al. (208) compared CBZ with *lithium* without concomitant medication. Fourteen patients were randomly assigned to lithium and 14 to CBZ. Lithium appeared superior, with 11 patients improving, in contrast to only 4 patients improving with CBZ. A second study, by Small and colleagues (100), found CBZ and lithium comparable in efficacy in a group of 52 hospitalized, treatment-refractory manic patients. This was a double-blind randomized design that followed patients during both the acute (i.e., 8 weeks) and the maintenance phase (up to 2 years). There was a trend favoring the lithium group on the survival analysis ($p < 0.14$).

Carbamazepine Versus Antipsychotics. Because there is evidence that lithium is superior to antipsychotics in acute episodes of classic mania, it is relevant to review the data comparing CBZ with *antipsychotics.* There are four studies investigating acute mania (two with random-assignment, double-blind conditions and no concomitant drugs) (209–212). Although the two class I studies found no statistical difference between CBZ and CPZ, one found a trend favoring CBZ and the other CPZ. When a meta-analysis was done combining these two studies, the pooled data show the relative outcomes to be virtually equal. The effect size is 0.05 and the Z score 0.2, indicating that the two nonsignificant trends virtually cancel each other out. We note that the four well-controlled studies comparing lithium with antipsychotics found lithium significantly superior (Table 10-4).

Carbamazepine Plus Other Psychotropics (Open Studies). In an open study, Okuma et al. (212) added *CBZ to the previous treatment* of 107 affective, 54 schizophrenic, and 26 schizoaffective patients. Improvement was 73%, 56%,

and 62%, respectively. In an open design, Nolen (213) added *CBZ to lithium* (and, when necessary, an antipsychotic and/or antidepressant) in a small group of treatment-resistant manic patients, who then showed further improvement. Kramlinger and Post (214) added *lithium to CBZ* in seven patients with varying degrees of mania, noting that six improved and one worsened. Because there was no control group, we do not know whether the patients would have shown similar improvement had the CBZ alone been continued for a longer period of time. Indeed, one responder had been on CBZ 2 weeks, and another for 3 weeks, but the other four responders had been on treatment about a month, which is sufficient time for CBZ's effects to peak. Thus, although the data are suggestive that lithium may augment CBZ's effect, the absence of a control group and the small sample size do not allow for a definitive conclusion.

Carbamazepine Plus Antipsychotics Versus Antipsychotics Alone. Klein et al. (215) *augmented haloperidol with CBZ* in a group of newly admitted, highly destructive psychotic patients (affectively disordered or schizophrenic) and found that 19 of 23 CBZ-augmented patients improved, in contrast to 11 of 20 of the placebo-augmented. Mueller and Stoll (216) and Goncalves and Stoll (207) using random-assignment, double-blind designs in small samples of six to 10 patients per group found that the *addition of CBZ to haloperidol* also produced some increased benefit over the antipsychotic alone. Specifically, Mueller and Stoll (216) found less supplemental medication was needed when CBZ was added, and Goncalves and Stoll (207) found CBZ superior to placebo supplementation of haloperidol.

Carbamazepine Plus Antipsychotics Versus Lithium Plus Antipsychotics. Lenzi et al. (217) compared patients randomly assigned to *lithium or CBZ augmented by CPZ.* During the first week, every patient required CPZ; in the second week, 14 of 15 patients required it; and in the third week, 11 of 15 patients in each group required it. The therapeutic result of the CPZ-CBZ combination was equal to the CPZ-lithium combination, and the only difference was that patients on CBZ required less CPZ in the first week. Lusznat et al. (218) also found the

CBZ-antipsychotic combination equal to the lithium-antipsychotic combination. In studies in which most but not all patients receive two active drugs, the design clouds the effectiveness of the drug alone versus an augmentation strategy. When every patient receives a basic drug that is then supplemented with another, one can more readily determine whether the augmenting drug is helpful. All must receive the basic drug in a constant dose, however.

Efficacy for Maintenance Treatment

Although data are quite limited, Prien and Gelenberg (219) reviewed the literature on drug treatment for the prevention of recurrences in bipolar disorder, emphasizing alternative therapies to lithium, especially *CBZ,* which at that time was the most extensively studied. They felt that the strongest evidence for the prophylactic efficacy of CBZ came from other design paradigms such as the following:

• Longitudinal trials in which the test drug is *periodically discontinued* and/or *replaced by placebo*
• *Mirror-image longitudinal trials* in which the course of illness during treatment is compared with the course of illness during an equivalent time preceding the treatment
• *Long-term open trials* evaluating the test drug in patients who have failed to respond to traditional treatments or have a recent history of frequent recurrences

These investigators concluded that, before CBZ can be viewed as a long-term treatment for bipolar disorders, carefully designed prospective controlled trials with adequate sample sizes are needed to confirm its efficacy and safety and to establish its specific indications and range of clinical effects.

Eight randomized, double-blind studies compared this agent with lithium for maintenance treatment averaging 1.7 years. The sample totalled 332 patients, with both drug groups demonstrating a comparable relapse rate over this time period (Table 10-13). These studies, however, allowed concomitant medication and had other methodological problems (208, 220–225). In a related study, Stuppaek et al. (226) conducted a 5-year naturalistic follow-up of 15 unipolar depressive subjects switched from lithium to CBZ and found the rate of depression decreased from 2.11 to 0.7 depressed episodes per year. Lusznat et al. (218) studied 54 acutely manic patients who were allocated on a double-blind basis to either CBZ or lithium. The short-term effects of treatment were evaluated in an initial 6-week acute phase, and the prophylactic effects in 29 patients up to a year. Additional "rescue" medications consisted of antipsychotics, antidepressants, and sedatives. Nine of the patients in the CBZ group had a satisfactory result (i.e., did not relapse during the 12-month follow-up), compared with five in the lithium group. The authors speculated that insufficient doses may have contributed to the poor results in both treatment groups. No statistically significant differences were found,

TABLE 10-13. *Lithium versus carbamazepine: maintenance treatment*

Study	Number of subjects	Duration (years)	Relapsed (%) CBZ (%)	Lithium (%)	Difference (%)
Placidi, 1986	56	3	28	26	−2
Watkins, 1987	37	1.5	68	56	−13
Lusznat, 1988	29	1	64	80	16
Stoll, 1989	98	1	46	52	4
Cabrera, 1990	10	2	25	0	−25
Small, 1991	16	2	100	88	−13
Coxhead, 1992	28	1	46	53	7
Simhandl, 1993	58	2	59	43	−16
Total	**332**	**1.7**	**55**	**49**	**−6**

Adapted from Janicak PG, Davis JM, Preskorn SH, Ayd FJ Jr. *Principles and practice of psychopharmacotherapy,* Baltimore: Williams & Wilkins, 1993.

however, with CBZ slightly less effective than lithium for acute mania and slightly more effective as a prophylactic treatment. We would again note that the existing data do not constitute the strict demonstration of efficacy (i.e., in comparison with placebo) that is required for FDA approval (Table 10-13).

Administration of Carbamazepine

The routine pretreatment workup includes assessment of baseline *hematological* and *hepatic functions*, because these two organ systems may be adversely affected by CBZ. Once baseline medical status has been established, typical starting doses are 400 to 600 mg/day, given in divided doses. Increments of 200 mg/day can be given every 3 to 5 days until adverse effects preclude higher dosing or desired clinical response is reached. Less aggressive titration and even dose reduction may be required early in the treatment until the patient develops tolerance to its adverse effects. In terms of adequate *blood levels,* 4 to 12 μg/mL is considered the accepted therapeutic range for CBZ when used as an anticonvulsant, but an ideal blood level of CBZ as an antimanic is unknown. Preliminary data, however, find a relationship with CSF levels of CBZ's principal epoxide metabolite and clinical response. Therefore, it is desirable to titrate the dose based on clinical response and adverse effects rather than rigidly relying on plasma levels. As we discuss later, therapeutic drug monitoring of CBZ, especially during the first several weeks of therapy, is crucial due to the phenomenon of autometabolism and the potential for clinically significant drug interactions.

Case Example: A 23-year-old woman with a long history of bipolar disorder resistant to lithium monotherapy and characterized by mixed episodes and rapid cycling was hospitalized in a manic phase. She was on lithium, CBZ, and trifluoperazine, with a therapeutic lithium level but a CBZ level of only 5 μg/mL. The patient underwent a washout, during which she deteriorated, and was then placed on DVPX. Because of increasing confusion, nausea, and vomiting at therapeutic levels, she was switched back to CBZ plus low-dose trifluoperazine. She had minimal response to CBZ blood levels in the range of 6 to 10 μg/mL, but when levels were titrated up to a range of 12 to 14 μg/mL, she demonstrated marked stabilization in mood, with minimal adverse effects. When the antipsychotic was discontinued, the patient continued to do well and was discharged to outpatient follow-up.

Whereas the sequence is strongly suggestive of a beneficial effect with higher CBZ levels, we cannot rule out the possibility of a spontaneous improvement due to her history of rapid cycling.

Lamotrigine

Lamotrigine has been approved as an adjunctive treatment for partial and generalized seizures. Its mechanism of action is thought to involve inhibition of glutamate release (227, 228). Open-label, case series reports and ongoing double-blind, controlled trials have explored this agent's usefulness in both bipolar mania and depression (229, 230).

Earl et al. (231, 232) added lamotrigine to the current anticonvulsant in 326 rapid-cycling, bipolar I and II patients in an open-label design. Approximately two-thirds of the patients who were experiencing a depressive episode at the time of study entry took lamotrigine for 8 to 12 weeks. Patients experiencing a clinical response were then discontinued from other medications and randomized into a double-blind study of lamotrigine or placebo for 26 weeks of continued treatment. Because this was a severely ill population, most eventually relapsed. However, the relapse rate in patients treated with lamotrigine monotherapy was lower than the placebo group. Together with placebo-controlled data for lamotrigine in acute bipolar depression, this report suggests that lamotrigine possesses efficacy in rapid-cycling, bipolar disorder and may complement other mood stabilizers.

In a double-blind comparison of lamotrigine versus desipramine or placebo, 450 unipolar depressed patients were studied. Lamotrigine was found to be significantly better than placebo, with desipramine falling between lamotrigine and placebo in terms of efficacy.

These early trials indicate a possible bimodal therapeutic effect with lamotrigine for both the manic and depressed phases. Low starting doses and slow titration are required, however, due to the increased risk of rash (approximately 10%), of which 1% may be more severe and possibly life-threatening (233), limiting this agent's use for acute episodes.

Gabapentin

Gabapentin has been approved in the United States since 1993 for adjunctive use in the management of treatment-refractory partial epilepsy. Early evidence in open-label trials indicated possible mood-stabilizing properties (227, 234). Recent data from a placebo-controlled crossover trial, however, found no difference between gabapentin and placebo for manic or depressed episodes (235).

Topiramate

Topiramate is a recently approved anticonvulsant whose mechanism of action may be similar to that of VPA and CBZ. Topiramate in doses averaging 300 to 400 mg/day has been reported to improve mania and the course of bipolar disorder when used as an adjunct to other agents (236, 237). For example, Eads et al. (238) reported the results of an open-label trial of topiramate used as either a primary or adjunctive treatment for refractory bipolar disorder. Although about half of the patients discontinued topiramate because of side effects, those who tolerated this agent were reported to clinically improve. Forty-five subjects were diagnosed with bipolar I ($n = 27$) or bipolar II ($n = 18$) depression (239). They received open-label topiramate (mean dose = 275 mg/day; range = 100 to 400 mg), which was added to previous mood stabilizers and antidepressants, as well as other psychotropics. Nineteen patients had a full response, and only five dropped out because of failure to respond. **Of note, seven patients lost weight that they had previously gained while on lithium and VPA.**

Recently, Calabrese (240) reviewed the use of topiramate in bipolar disorder and also presented the results of two additional studies. He noted that, thus far, topiramate had been studied in 12 open clinical trials involving a total of 224 patients, mainly in manic and mixed states, and generally as an augmentation strategy. Overall, these studies reported a 50% response rate.

Topiramate was also used as monotherapy in an open-label, collaborative, pilot study conducted by three groups of experienced investigators. Eleven acutely manic patients who were nonresponsive to lithium, VPA, or their combination continue to manifest significant symptoms with a mean baseline Young Mania Rating Scales (YMS) score of 32. Five of 11 patients had a substantial response ($n = 3$) or a partial response ($n = 2$) to the introduction of monotherapy with topiramate.

Calabrese also reported on a 21-day, random-assignment, double-blind, multicenter trial involving 20 sites in the United States. Ninety-seven patients were randomized to placebo or two different doses of topiramate (i.e., 256 or 512 mg/day). Although both doses of topiramate produced a slightly greater reduction in the YMS baseline scores than placebo, the difference was not statistically significant. A dose-related, statistically significant improvement on the GAS, however, was noted for topiramate compared with placebo. Thus, the 256-mg dose produced a statistically superior improvement in comparison with placebo and the 512-mg dose almost doubled the rate of improvement over that achieved with the 256-mg dose. Although the study failed to find significant changes on the YMS scale, changes in the GAS scores were clearly significant, indicating possible efficacy for topiramate.

Tiagabine

Tiagabine is another recently approved anticonvulsant whose mechanism of action is thought to be blockade of GABA reuptake. Preliminary experience in an open-label trial of either monotherapy or augmentation therapy with this agent has not been promising (241).

Electroconvulsive Therapy

ECT is the only clearly established bimodal therapy in that it is equally effective for both the depressed and manic phases of the

disorder. Although the primary indication for ECT is a severe, unremitting, or drug-nonresponsive depressive episode, data from as early as the 1940's support its use for the treatment of acute mania, particularly manic delirium (242–244). Based on clinical experience, we would expect mania to remit rapidly with ECT, whereas lithium can take weeks. Hence, there may be a superiority for ECT over lithium in the early phases of treatment. What the final outcome would be is more problematic, but clearly, there is a need to further explore the efficacy of ECT in mania. In this light, Schnur and colleagues (245) reported on the relationship between various pretreatment symptoms and therapeutic outcome to ECT in 18 manic patients. They found that although severity of mania was not predictive, anger, irritability, and suspiciousness were more characteristic of nonresponders to ECT.

Case Example: A 28-year-old woman had been stable on lithium treatment for several years. When she became pregnant, her lithium was discontinued, and within a few weeks she was hospitalized for a severe exacerbation of mania unresponsive to CPZ in doses up to 1,200 mg/day. After a course of ECT she became euthymic and was adequately maintained on lower doses of CPZ (i.e., 50 to 100 mg/day) for the remainder of her pregnancy. The delivery and the immediate postpartum period went well, but lithium was not resumed because she opted to nurse her infant. Several weeks later, she was rehospitalized for an episode of depression, which also responded to a course of ECT. She then agreed to discontinue nursing her child and resume lithium. The patient was doing well at follow-up 1 year later.

Because the issue of informed consent is often problematic in such emergencies, a court-appointed partial conservator may be required to provide substituted permission for treatment (see the section "Informed Consent" in Chapter 2).

Efficacy

Uncontrolled studies since the mid-1970's (246, 247) have reported on ECT's comparable or superior benefit to antipsychotics or lithium. In a random assignment design, Small et al. (248) found that both the bilateral ECT (BILAT-ECT) and the lithium-treated groups improved from baseline levels. Further, at all time points the ECT-treated group showed a greater improvement, reaching statistical significance by weeks 6, 7, and 8. These patients were then followed for up to 2 years with maintenance therapy at the clinician's discretion. No differences in relapse rates, recurrence, or rehospitalization between the two groups were found. The authors concluded that BILAT-ECT was an effective and safe treatment for acute mania that could be used in patients unable to tolerate or benefit from lithium or who may pose an immediate danger to themselves because of the severity of their episode.

Small's study, however, has several methodological issues that complicate the interpretation of its results. First, most patients randomly assigned to lithium or ECT also received antipsychotics. Second, those initially assigned to receive lithium began ECT 2 to 6 weeks later, so that all had been receiving a course of ECT for 2 to 5 weeks before the final evaluation. Third, the authors note that "most of the patients who underwent ECT were also taking lithium by the fifth week and had plasma levels between 0.51 and 0.69 during weeks 4 to 8 of the study." Clearly, the most appropriate time to interpret the study would have been in the first 3 weeks, when only two of the patients receiving lithium had also received ECT and few ECT patients had begun lithium. When we looked at this period, there was no difference between the treatment groups. Again, this could be artifactual because the majority of the patients were receiving antipsychotics as well.

Mukherjee and colleagues (244) recently summarized the outcome in acute mania treated with ECT over a five-decade period. In almost 600 patients, approximately 80% demonstrated marked improvement or full remission.

Administration of Electroconvulsive Therapy

The administration of ECT to treat acute mania generally follows the same guidelines as for depression (see also Chapter 8). There is some evidence that lithium should be discontinued during a course of ECT treatments to avoid an increased risk of neurotoxicity. Some investigators indicate that bilateral (BILAT) rather than unilateral nondominant (UND) electrode placement may be the procedure of choice, but this opinion is not universal (249). A controlled trial by Milstein et al. (250) randomly assigned patients in a partially blinded design to receive lithium or ECT for an 8-week, acute treatment period. Initially, those patients assigned to the ECT group were given UND administration but did not respond. The design was then altered, and all subsequent patients were administered BILAT-ECT. Statistical and clinical comparisons were then based on the BILAT-ECT versus the lithium-treated groups, with ECT demonstrating superior efficacy over the 2-month trial period.

Complications

The central and the peripheral effects of ECT, as well as associated complications, are discussed in detail in the sections on ECT for depression (see the section "Electroconvulsive Therapy" in Chapter 8).

Experimental Therapies

Calcium Channel Antagonists

CCAs (channel blockers; influx inhibitors) have been used primarily for the treatment of cardiovascular disorders (e.g., supraventricular arrhythmias, angina, and hypertension). Agents such as verapamil exert their effects by modulating the influx of Ca^{2+} across the cell membrane, thus interfering with calcium-dependent functions. Based partly on the common effects of lithium and this class of drugs (e.g., effects on Ca^{2+} activity), the CCAs have been studied as a potential treatment for mania. Janicak et al. (251) reported the results of a 3-week, double-blind comparison of verapamil versus placebo, which did not demonstrate a beneficial effect for verapamil (up to 480 mg/day) in 33 acutely manic hospitalized patients.

Post and colleagues (252, 253) have suggested that voltage-gated calcium antagonists, such as nimodipine, may be more effective, especially in treatment-resistant and ultrarapid and ultradian

cycling patients (i.e., cycles every several weeks or hours, respectively). This is in part because such agents may penetrate the blood—brain barrier more readily than verapamil.

Efficacy

Levy and Janicak (254) recently published a review of the controlled trials using various CCAs for the treatment of bipolar disorder. Results are summarized in Table 10-14.

Verapamil Versus Placebo. Verapamil has been the most extensively studied CCA for bipolar disorder. Dubovsky (255) demonstrated a reduction of mania with verapamil in three patients, and later included four more in a random-assignment crossover study *comparing verapamil with placebo*. Unfortunately, one of the seven patients did not undergo the placebo arm of the study. Five showed a relatively dramatic response to verapamil, and the sixth a slight trend toward improvement. The patient who failed to undergo the placebo arm also showed some improvement with verapamil. Given the degree of improvement, these data suggested potential efficacy.

In a single-blind crossover design *comparing verapamil, lithium, and placebo* in 12 manic patients, Giannini et al. (256) found no difference between lithium and verapamil. The study is inconclusive, however, because it is not clear whether these patients were in an acute manic episode. If not, a month's trial is insufficient to evaluate the maintenance properties of either. The predominant symptoms, as measured by the BPRS, were mild depression, anxiety, tension, and guilt, with only a slight degree of excitement or grandiosity (i.e., ratings of 2.5 and 1.7 on a 7-point scale, respectively, at the beginning of the study), and virtually no patients had hallucinations or delusions. Although this was an AB paradigm and not a random-assignment crossover design with a control group, it did support the benefit of verapamil. Thus, patients went from mildly symptomatic to remission over a 30-day treatment period, worsened during the 10-day placebo period, and then improved again when they received lithium for 30 days.

(*Text continues on page 425*)

TABLE 10-14. CCAs for bipolar disorder: open and controlled trials–positive outcomes

Study	Diagnosis	Design	Duration	Drug and dosage	Rescue meds	Assessment	Results/comments
Nimodipine: controlled studies							
Nimodipine vs. placebo							
Pazzaglia et al., 1993	11 bipolar patients 1 unipolar patient 11 lithium refractory	DB crossover 12 patients on nimodipine	Approx. 20 weeks	Nimodipine: 90–720 mg/day	Unknown BHRS	VAS	Some response with nimodipine In rapid cyclers
Nimodipine vs. other drugs							
Pazzaglia et al., 1998[a]	23 manic patients 4 bipolar, depressed 3 BRD 30 lithium refractory	DB parallel with nimodipine B add. CBZ with 14 patients then B subst with verapamil then B subst with isradipine	<6 months	Nimodipine: 360 mg/day CBZ: 793 mg/day Verapamil: unknown Isradipine: unknown	Unknown	CGI BHRS	Some response with nimodipine Better response with addition of CBZ Better with isradipine Worse with verapamil
Verapamil: controlled studies							
Verapamil vs. placebo (crossover)							
Dose et al., 1986	8 bipolar patients with psychosis 1 lithium refractory	DB crossover: Placebo-verapamil-placebo	Unknown	Verapamil: 320–480 mg/day	1—lithium 7/8–CPZ, paraldehyde	IMPS	5/6 showed positive response to verapamil
Dubovsky et al., 1986	7 manic patients 1 lithium refractory	DB crossover: 24 days verapamil 24 days placebo No washout	Approx. 2 months	Verapamil: up to 480 mg/day	None	BPRS MSRS	Greater decrease in scores from baseline with verapamil than with placebo
Verapamil vs. lithium (crossover)							
Giannini et al., 1984	12 manic patients ? lithium refractory	DB crossover: 30 days verapamil 10 days placebo washout 30 days lithium	70 days	Verapamil: 320 mg/day Lithium: 900–1,800 mg/day	Unknown	BPRS	Verapamil and lithium "both equally effective in relieving symptoms falling in mild–moderate range"
Giannini et al., 1987	20 manic patients 0 lithium refractory	DB crossover: 180 days verapamil 180 days lithium No washout Maintenance study	1 year	Verapamil: 320 mg/day Lithium: dose to maintain Level = 0.8-1.0 mg/dL	Unknown	BPRS	Earlier response in group receiving verapamil in first 6 months Continued improvement in group receiving verapamil in second 6 months.
Verapamil vs. lithium (parallel)							
Garza-Trevino et al., 1992	20 manic patients ? lithium refractory	DB parallel: 12 patients on verapamil 8 patients on lithium	4 weeks	Verapamil: 160–320 mg/day Lithium: start 300 mg/day Adjusted up to maintain Level =0.75–15	Haloperidol Lorazepam 58% on verapamil 50% on lithium	CGI BPRS PMS	"No statistical difference between verapamil group and lithium group and both improved" significantly

Giannini et al., 1985	20 manic patients lithium refractory	DB crossover: 20 days verapamil 5 days placebo washout 20 days clonidine	45 days	Verapamil: 320 mg/day Clonidine: 17 mg/kg	Unknown	BPRS	Verapamil superior to clonidine for mania
Hoschl et al., 1989	47 manic patients 7 lithium refractory	DB parallel: 12 patients on verapamil alone 24 patients on neuroleptic and lithium 11 patients on neuroleptic	35 days	Verapamil: 120–480 mg/day Neuroleptic: equiv. 375 mg CPZ Lithium dose to Maintain Level=0.75 mmol/L	Unknown	BPRS GI	No statistically significant end-point among verapamil, lithium or neuroleptic groups
Diltiazem: open studies							
Caillard, 1985	7 manic patients ? lithium refractory	Open trial	2 weeks	Diltiazem: 120–360 mg/day	Droperidol Chloral hydrate	MSRS	Positive response in 5/7 patients receiving diltiazem
Nimodipine: open studies							
Brunet et al., 1990	6 mild–acute manic patients ? lithium refractory	Open trial	7 days	Nimodipine: 360 mg/day	Droperidol	BPRS BRMS	Improvement in symptoms between day 1 and day 7 of study in those receiving nimodipine
Verapamil: open studies							
Brotman et al., 1986	6 patients with BPD varied states ? lithium refractory	Open trial	3 weeks	Verapamil: 240–360 mg/day	1–Fluphenazine dec. 4/6—CBZ, CPZ, II	BPRS YMS	"Prompt decrease in symptoms" in 4/6 patients receiving verapamil and others
Goodnick et al., 1996	12 manic patients ? lithium refractory	Open trial ? baseline meds ? washout	14 days	Verapamil: 240–360 mg/day	Unknown	YMS	Decreased severity of symptoms in those receiving verapamil

CCAs for bipolar disorder: open and controlled trials–negative outcomes

Diltiazem: controlled studies							
Fabian et al., 1997	10 normal controls	DB crossover of diltiazem or placebo then amphetamine or placebo	<24 h	Diltiazem: 60 mg Dextroamphetamine: 20 mg	None	VAS BP CPT	Pre-treatment diltiazem doesn't attenuate manic symptons using amphetamine model
Verapamil: controlled studies (crossover) *Verapamil vs. lithium*							
Arkonac et al., 1991	15 manic patients ? lithium refractory	DB crossover 4 weeks verapamil 10 days placebo washout 4 weeks lithium	Approx. 10 weeks	Verapamil: 320 mg/day Lithium: 1200 mg/day	Unknown	BRMS	Significant decreased manic scores with lithium; significantly increased manic scores with verapamil
Verapamil: controlled studies (parallel)							
Pazzaglia et al., 1998[a]	23 manic patients 4 bipolar, depressed 3 BRD 30 lithium refractory	DB parallel with nimodipine B add. CBZ with 14 patients then B subst with verapamil then B subst with isradipine	<6 months	Average doses: nimodipine; 360 mg/day CBZ: 793 mg/day verapamil: unknown isradipine unknown	Unknown	CGI BHRS	Some response with nimodipine Better response with the addition of CBZ Worse with verapamil Better with isradipine

(continued)

TABLE 10-14 —(continued.)

Study	Diagnosis	Design	Duration	Drug and dosage	Rescue meds	Assessment	Results/comments
Verapamil: controlled studies (parallel)							
Verapamil vs. placebo Janicak et al., 1998	30 manic patients 2 mixed patients ? lithium refractory	DB parallel 15 patients on placebo 17 patients on verapamil	3 weeks	Verapamil: 480 mg/day	Chloral hydrate and lorazepam in washout tapered to zero by day 10 of DB	BPRS MRS Ham-D	No efficacy verapamil = placebo
Verapamil: vs. lithium (parallel) Walton et al., 1996	40 manic patients ? lithium refractory	SB parallel with lithium or verapamil	28 days	Verapamil: 240–360 mg/day Lithium 500–1,000 mg/day	Lorazepam used in both groups	BPRS MRS CGI GAF	Lithium is superior to to verapamil on all measures used
Verapamil: open studies Barton et al., 1987	14 manic patients 14 lithium refractory	Open trial 8 patients with acute mania	3 weeks	Verapamil 160–320 mg/day	Unknown	YMS	No positive response with verapamil
	12 CBZ refractory	4 patients with BRD 2 bipolar, depressed	18 months 2 weeks	Verapamil 240–320 mg/day Verapamil 160–320 mg/day	Varied MAO-I lithium		2/4 with mild positive response No emergence of hypomania
Lenzi et al., 1995	13 manic patients 2 mixed patients ? lithium refractory	Open trial	21 days	Verapamil: 240–400 mg/day Chlorpromazine: 50–400 mg/day	CPZ	BPRS CGI DOTES	Verapamil alone is not effective in severe mania Better response as augmentation

[a]Pazzaglia et al. (1998) study had positive outcomes with respect to nimodipine and negative outcomes with respect to verapamil.
BPD, bipolar disorder; BRD, brief reactive depression; DB, double-blind; SB, single-blind; B, blind; CBZ, carbamazepine; dec., decanoate; CPZ, chlorpromazine; MAO-I, monoamine oxidase inhibitor; BPRS, Brief Psychiatric Rating Scale; MSRS, Manic State Rating Scale; YMS, Young Mania Scale; IMPS, Inpatient Multidimensional Psychiatric Scale; GI, General Impression; BRMS, Bech Raffaelson Mania Scale; CGI, Global Clinical Impressions Scale; PMS, Patterson Mania Scale, BHRS, Bunney Hamburg Rating Scale; VAS, Visual Analogue Scale; DOTES, Dosage Record and the Treatment Emergent Symptoms Scale; GAF, Global Assessment of Functioning; CPT, Conners' Continuous Performance Test; Ham-D, Hamilton Depression Scale; MRS, Mania Rating Scale.
From Levy NA, Janicak PG. Calcium channel antagonists for the treatment of bipolar disorder. *Bipolar Disord* 2000; 2:108–119, with permission.

Dose and coworkers (257) compared *verapamil with placebo* in eight patients using an ABA design. Seven showed some degree of response, five with symptoms reemerging to a minor extent with placebo, and two showing no relapse on placebo. A concomitant antipsychotic was used in two and lithium in one.

Verapamil Versus Other Psychotropics. Garza-Trevino et al. (258) conducted a 4-week, randomized, double-blind study *comparing verapamil with lithium* for acute mania and found no clinical or statistically significant differences between the two treatments. These results are difficult to interpret, however, because data about the amount and timing of rescue medication (i.e., haloperidol, lorazepam) were not presented. Further, more patients on verapamil required these agents.

Arkonaç and his coworkers (259) investigated *verapamil in comparison with lithium* in a random-assignment, double-blind, crossover study of 15 manic patients (4 weeks of lithium or verapamil, 10 days of placebo, and then a crossover to the other agent). Subjects improved on lithium but unexpectedly worsened with verapamil. This was a well-controlled study of verapamil, but unfortunately did not confirm the previous results. Further, it is only available in abstract form, and the complete publication is needed to evaluate the study critically; its outcome, however, suggested caution in interpretation of earlier positive results.

Giannini (260) studied 24 patients in a random-assignment crossover design, finding *verapamil superior to clonidine;* however, quantitative measures of change, such as BPRS scores, were not provided.

Hoschl and Kozeny (261) reported that the degree of improvement was comparable in 12 manic patients treated with verapamil, 24 with *antipsychotics,* and 11 with *antipsychotics plus lithium.*

By contrast, a number of studies have not found verapamil monotherapy to be effective for acute mania (Table 10-14). Several case reports in the literature have not supported verapamil's potential antimanic properties. For example, Barton and Gitlin (262) found that none of eight acutely manic or hypomanic patients treated openly improved on verapamil. There are several case reports of hypomania (some monoamine oxidase inhibitor—induced) improving with verapamil. Dubovsky (255) notes that, in his experience with spontaneous mania, he has been unimpressed with verapamil in patients who had previously been unresponsive to lithium.

In a randomized, single-blind trial of 40 patients receiving lithium or verapamil, Walton et al. (263) found lithium to be superior to verapamil on all measures. Potential confounding factors included the use of lorazepam throughout the study as a rescue medication given both intravenously and orally, a 1-day washout period, and the use of antipsychotic medications on the last day of the study.

To our knowledge, the only prospective, placebo-controlled, double-blind, parallel trial to assess verapamil's efficacy in treating acute mania has been conducted at our institution. In this 3-week study, Janicak et al. (251) randomized 32 patients to placebo (15 subjects) or verapamil (17 subjects) and assessed clinical outcome using the BPRS, Hamilton Depression Rating Scale, and Mania Rating Scale. Twenty-two subjects dropped out before completing the entire study because of clinical deterioration (10 verapamil subjects and eight placebo subjects) or lack of cooperation (four verapamil subjects). Mean number of treatment days in those subjects receiving placebo and verapamil was 13.3 and 9.3, respectively. Rescue medications (chloral hydrate or lorazepam) were limited to the washout period and only during the first week of the double-blind phase. In a last observation carried forward (LOCF) analysis, no statistical difference was observed in terms of efficacy between verapamil and placebo. Verapamil did not appear to be useful as monotherapy in treating manic symptoms, inasmuch as most subjects receiving verapamil did not complete the 3-week study.

Thus, the evidence to support verapamil's efficacy in treating acute mania rests on two placebo-controlled studies with small sample sizes (i.e., fewer than eight patients), five partially controlled studies, and two open trials (Table 10-14). By contrast, one placebo-controlled study with a larger sample size (i.e., 32 patients), two partially controlled studies (i.e., with 40 and 15 patients, respectively), and two open trials had negative results (Table 10-14).

We conclude that if CCAs are effective, it may be for only a small subgroup of manic patients. Alternatively, other agents in this class (e.g., nimodipine) that pass the blood—brain barrier more readily may be better candidates to study.

Administration of Verapamil

Doses of verapamil reported to have antimanic effects have ranged from 80 mg b.i.d. to 160 mg t.i.d. Typically, the initial dose is 80 mg two or three times daily, with rapid escalation up to, but not exceeding, 480 mg/day. (Personal communication with Dubovsky and Giannini indicates some patients may require and safely tolerate doses up to 640 mg/day.) The drug is usually well tolerated, and no specific laboratory monitoring is required. Further, its lack of teratogenic potential makes this (and perhaps other CCAs) attractive alternatives to agents such as lithium, VPA, and CBZ.

Noradrenergic Agents

Clonidine

This a α_2-noradrenergic presynaptic receptor agonist is approved by the FDA as an antihypertensive. The rationale for using clonidine for mania is based on the original catecholamine hypothesis (21, 22), which postulates a *hyperfunctionality* of the noradrenergic system predisposing to mania. Because the hypothesis suggests that increases in NE neurotransmission may underlie such symptomatology, drugs that decrease central NE activity might prove to be therapeutic. Early, less well-controlled reports indicated a possible benefit for this agent, either alone or as a substitute for antipsychotics, in an acute manic exacerbation. Our own subsequent, double-blind, placebo-controlled trial, however, did not support such efficacy when clonidine was used alone for moderate-to-severe exacerbations of an acute manic episode (264). Of interest, a similar line of reasoning has also generated some equivocal data for the β-blocking agent, propranolol (265–267).

Efficacy. A number of open trials initially reported positive results with the use of clonidine for treating acute mania. For example, Jouvent et al. (268) observed improvement in three of eight bipolar patients and partial improvement in three others in an open trial with doses of clonidine ranging from 0.15 to 0.45 mg/day. But patients were also taking various concurrent drugs (i.e., droperidol, diazepam, CPZ, and lithium). A subsequent study found that three bipolar patients experienced rapid and complete remission with the addition of clonidine in doses ranging from 0.4 to 0.8 mg/day (269). Hardy et al. (270) treated 24 newly admitted acutely manic patients with doses ranging from 0.45 to 0.9 mg/day, in addition to droperidol (25 to 50 mg orally), if necessary, and some were also maintained on their previous lithium regimen. Thirteen patients showed either marked or partial improvement within 5 days of treatment. Four others, in the higher dose range (0.75 to 0.9 mg/day), did show some worsening, particularly in aggression and hostility, that improved when the drug was discontinued. Another study reported that three treatment-resistant manic patients demonstrated a rapid response with the addition of clonidine (0.2 to 0.4 mg/day) to their treatment regimens (271).

Three different, partially controlled trials for acute mania have also been reported (260, 272, 273). In the first study, 11 patients were administered clonidine in three divided doses of 17 μg/kg/day (or approximately 1.2 mg/day) under double-blind conditions. The blind consisted of telling patients and treating physicians that the capsules might or might not contain active medication, when in fact all patients received clonidine. No concurrent medications were given. After 25 days, patients showed significant reductions in their Biegel-Murphy Manic State rating scores, and all eight who discontinued the drug relapsed. Hypotension and sedation were present but tolerated. The second study was a double-blind, crossover design comparing clonidine (17 μg/kg/day) with verapamil (80 mg p.o. q.i.d.) in 20 manic male patients for two 20-day periods separated by a 5-day placebo crossover phase. Verapamil demonstrated greater antimanic properties and caused no adverse effects, in contrast to clonidine, which also produced significant hypotension. The third study had a design similar to the second, but the comparison treatment was lithium and the two treatment phases were 30 days long, separated by a 15-day placebo crossover phase. The doses of clonidine were again 17 μg/kg/day, and the lithium dose was adjusted to maintain serum levels at 1.2 mEq/L. Lithium was statistically superior to clonidine after the first 30-day period, while after the second 30 days, neither drug group was significantly better than the other, but the trend favored the lithium group. It is not clear whether these patients were in an acute exacerbation or on maintenance therapy. If the latter situation were true, the time period would be too short to adequately assess efficacy.

As noted earlier, in the only double-blind, placebo-controlled, parallel design study of clonidine, Janicak et al. (264) studied a group of acutely ill, hospitalized manic patients, many with associated psychotic features. After a washout period averaging 1 week, patients were randomly assigned to receive either clonidine or placebo for a 2-week trial. The intent was to ascertain whether clonidine alone had any inherent antimanic properties, and therefore, no other concomitant psychotropics were allowed. Unfortunately, improvement in either group was minimal and did not differ, with some patients on clonidine developing problems with rash and hypotension. Doses of clonidine were comparable with those reported in prior positive studies, averaging 0.5 mg/day.

Other possible uses, not addressed in this study, are the potential benefit of clonidine as an adjunct to lithium or anticonvulsants, possibly serving as a substitute for anxiolytics or antipsychotics, or its benefit in less severe exacerbations of mania.

Other Treatment Strategies

A number of other theoretically interesting and potentially clinically relevant treatments have also been studied, including the following:

- *Cholinomimetic agents*
- Drugs that *enhance 5-HT* functioning (e.g., precursors such as L-tryptophan)
- *Psychostimulants* (such as amphetamines or methylphenidate)
- *Atypical antipsychotics*
- *Omega-3 fatty acid*
- *Tamoxifen*

We would emphasize that, while all of these approaches are theoretically important and may possess clinical applicability, with the exception of the atypical antipsychotic olanzapine, none is presently approved by the FDA for treatment of bipolar disorder.

Cholinomimetic Agents

The beneficial effect of *precursors* (e.g., lecithin), *cholinesterase inhibitors* (e.g., physostigmine, donepezil), or *drugs with cholinomimetic effects* (e.g., bethanechol) for actue mania was discovered in part from the work of Janowsky et al. (29), leading to their *cholinergic—noradrenergic balance hypothesis*. Interestingly, lithium is also able to raise RBC choline concentrations and CNS cholinergic activity (274).

Serotonin Agents

Limited evidence indicates that the amino acid precursor of 5-HT, L-*tryptophan,* may be useful, alone or in combination with other antimanic agents to enhance overall efficacy. Contaminants in the production of this agent led to several cases of the eosinophilia myalgia syndrome (EMS) and its removal from the market for several years.

The possible antimanic effect of this 5-HT precursor was postulated based on the *permissive hypothesis* concept of diminished 5-HT activity. When oral doses of L-tryptophan (1 to 4 g) are administered, there is evidence of increased 5-HT synthesis. Three of four double-blind studies yielded positive results, holding the promise of an effective antimanic treatment (275). An advantage of this drug is its relative lack of other adverse effects.

Fenfluramine, which has serotonergic agonist properties, has also been considered, but data are lacking to support or refute any antimanic properties and concerns about cardiac effects have led to its removal from the market (276).

Psychostimulants

Anecdotal case reports and small sample size trials have shown some benefit for the use of psychostimulants to manage episodes of excitability in mania. This counterintuitive, paradoxical effect parallels their beneficial use in children with hyperactivity (277). The theoretical basis may be related to an indirect effect of these agents that leads to *enhancement of 5-HT functioning.*

Novel Antipsychotics

Early reports found clozapine to benefit some affectively disordered patients (e.g., bipolar, schizoaffective) who had previously been treatment-refractory, but improved rapidly and significantly on this agent (108, 109, 278). Further, many patients were able to sustain their early gains in psychosocial functioning over a 3-5-year period. The low incidence of EPS and TD also increased interest in potentially new indications for these agents.

The role of these agents, either as primary or adjunctive treatments for mood disorders, has yet to be fully explored (106, 108, 279–281). Theories have included the differential effects of clozapine on dopamine receptor subtypes (e.g., increased activity at the D_4 receptors, which exist in high density in the limbic system) and the greater 5-HT$_2$ to D_2 antagonism of most novel agents in comparison with neuroleptics (282). More recently, controlled trials indicate that novel antispychotics (NAPs) may play an important and perhaps unique role for more severe, psychotic, and/or refractory mood disorders (112, 283, 384).

Regarding the dopamine system, Swerdlow (285) writes that subcortical dopamine dysfunction contributes to the symptoms of mood disorders, particularly increased or decreased goal-directed behaviors and perceived changes in reinforcement. Still, the author comments that it is not enough to view such pathology in the context of too little or too much subcortical dopamine. Thus, given the complex motor,

cognitive, and affective disturbances in depression, the role of subcortical dopamine dysfunction and antidepressant action should be viewed within the context of an integrated cortico-striato-pallidothalamic circuitry.

Regarding the 5-HT system, Keck et al. (286) cite several lines of evidence to support that the thymolytic effects of clozapine (and perhaps other agents with similar properties) are mediated by the antagonism of 5-HT$_2$ receptors, including the following:

- These receptors have been implicated in the *action of standard antidepressants.*
- Most, but not all, *platelet radioligand studies* in medication-free patients with major depressive disorder have found a significant increase in the number of this receptor's binding sites compared with control subjects.
- Radioligand binding studies of the *postmortem brains* of patients with major depressive disorder who did not receive antidepressants *showed significant increases in the number of these receptors* compared with patients who had received antidepressants and normal control subjects.

In summary, the authors believe these lines of evidence support the hypersensitive-postsynaptic, serotonergic receptor theory first proposed by Aprison et al. (287).

Clozapine: Acute Clinical Trials. Owen et al. conducted an open-label, compassionate use, clozapine treatment protocol in 37 chronically psychotic patients (25 schizophrenia; 12 schizoaffective) (288). Clozapine produced a highly significant improvement in psychopathology as measured by the BPRS. Interestingly, schizoaffective patients had significantly lower total scores than their schizophrenic counterparts at the final rating.

McElroy and her coworkers (109) surveyed the response of 85 consecutive patients, including 14 *bipolar patients with psychotic features,* who received clozapine for 6 weeks. The response rates of the schizoaffective patients (both bipolar and depressed subtypes), as well as those with bipolar disorders with psychotic features, were excellent (i.e., almost 90%) and substantially better

$df = 1$, $p = 74$). We also did a meta-analysis using the Olkin-Hedges method and again olanzapine was superior to placebo with an average effect size of 0.47 (95% confidence limits 0.2–0.7, $p = 0.0003$). Both studies found the degree of superiority to be similar and the probability of significance (i.e., $p = 0.0003$) with both methods was identical. Thus, both studies found olanzapine to be superior to placebo and also replicated each other in that the degree of superiority was the same. Sedation and weight gain occurred to a significantly greater degree in the olanzapine versus placebo treated group, however, there was no difference in EPS occurrence between the groups.

Namjoshi and coworkers (297) reported the results of an extension phase study comparing olanzapine with placebo. The initial reduction achieved in YMS scores continued during this period and by the end of the extension phase reached a mean reduction of 18-points. The authors also conducted an economic analysis of the drug trial (excluding the acute treatment period) and found that the cost per month seen in the open-label extension phase (i.e., $649) was about half of that observed during the 12 months before entering the study (i.e., $1,533.)

Frazier et al. (298) also reported the results of an open trial in *children and adolescent bipolar patients* (ages 5 to 14) in which olanzapine dramatically decreased mania scores, producing a substantial overall improvement.

Tohen and coworkers (299) reported the results of a 6-week, double-blind, randomized, controlled trial augmenting standard mood stabilizers with olanzapine or placebo. *Three hundred and forty-four subjects with a manic or mixed episode* who were nonresponders to a 2-week trial of lithium or VPA were studied at 38 centers. They were then randomly assigned to 8 weeks of augmentation treatment with olanzapine or placebo. The addition of olanzapine produced a statistically superior improvement when compared with placebo augmentation ($p = 0.003$). Further, 68% of olanzapine-treated patients and 45% of placebo-treated patients achieved a 50% decrease from their baseline YMS score. Because manic and depressed symptoms coexisted in some patients, it is interesting to note that

olanzapine also produced a five-point decrease from the baseline HAM-D-21 rating scale score in comparison with a one-point decrease in the placebo group. The addition of olanzapine to lithium or VPA produced improvements in patients with and without psychotic features, but the improvement was most dramatic in those without psychotic features. Further, olanzapine produced a mean decrease of 13 points on the YMS baseline score in those with a mixed episode in comparison with a mean decrease of 7.5 points in the placebo group. Although there was no evidence of extrapyramidal side effects occurring with olanzapine, weight gain and sedation occurred more often with olanzapine augmentation.

Clozapine: Longitudinal Trials. In a naturalistic study design, Banov et al. (300) found clozapine was an effective long-term treatment in mood disorders, particularly nondepressed affective patients. After a chart review, the authors identified 193 treatment-resistant patients, including the following:

- 52 *bipolar* disorder
- 14 *unipolar* disorder
- 40 *schizophrenic* disorder
- 81 *schizoaffective* disorder
- 6 *other* disorders

After beginning clozapine, these patients were followed up for an average of 18.7 months with structured interviews conducted by raters blind to diagnosis. The affective group did as well as the comparison schizophrenic patients, with mania predicting a better outcome than depression. Further, social functioning was significantly better in the affective versus the schizophrenic group.

Zarate and his collaborators (301) conducted a systematic follow-up study, evaluating the number of hospitalizations in the 5 years before clozapine compared with the rehospitalization rate while on this agent. These authors found that monotherapy with clozapine reduced both the number of episodes and rehospitalizations in 17 previously severely ill affective patients. The yearly rate before clozapine was 0.8 ± 1.2 and after clozapine 0.4 ± 1.2, a difference that was statistically significant. Rehospitalization rates were lowest in the schizophrenic, schizoaffective bipolar, and schizoaffective depressed patients, whereas unipolar and bipolar depressed patients had the highest relapse rate.

In a review of published long-term follow-up studies, Zarate et al. (302) evaluated the benefit of clozapine in severe mood disorders and found that 71.2% ($n = 94$) of bipolar patients and 69.6% ($n = 221$) of schizoaffective patients displayed clinically significant improvement and were successfully maintained on *clozapine monotherapy* or combined treatment for periods ranging from 49 days to 4 years. Patients in manic or psychotic phases of their schizoaffective or bipolar disorder were significantly more likely to respond to clozapine than patients with schizophrenia. Although many of the studies reviewed were methodologically flawed (e.g., retrospective, nonblind, diagnostic and selection criteria not specified, not specifically designed to assess mood disorders) the combined results suggest that manic, psychotic, or mixed phases of bipolar disorder were particularly likely to respond to clozapine therapy. The authors concluded with the caveat that, because of the risk of fatal agranulocytosis, clozapine should be reserved for only those patients with a psychotic mood disorder who are considered refractory to standard treatments.

Conclusion

Figures 10-3 and 10-4 depict the recommended treatment strategies for bipolar mania and bipolar depression (11, 18, 121).

Strategy for Acute Mania

Patients presenting with mild to moderate manic symptoms should first have an adequate trial of lithium, with blood level ranges of 0.8 to 1.2 mEq/L, or VPA, with blood level ranges of 50 to 125 μg/mL. Adjunctive BZDs may be beneficial if the following occurs:

• The presentation is complicated by continued marked *agitation, insomnia, and anxiety.*
• There is concern about *adverse effects from antipsychotics.*
• *Response* is still *unsatisfactory.*

The discontinuation of concurrent antidepressants and/or the use of supplemental thyroid agents in appropriate patients may benefit those who are treatment-resistant and perhaps prevent rapid cycling.

Short-term aggressive dosing with BZDs may preclude the need for antipsychotics. Thus, lorazepam (1 to 2 mg) given every 2 to 4 hours, with doses up to 12 mg/day, has shown promise; alternatively, clonazepam may also be used.

Antipsychotics may be warranted if patients:

• Demonstrate associated *psychotic symptoms*
• Suffer from *severe agitation*
• Remain *refractory*
• Are only *partially responsive* to the primary mood stabilizer

In fact, with more moderate-to-severe episodes, a mood stabilizer alone is usually insufficient, and initial treatment often requires a concurrent antipsychotic, preferably a novel agent. In these situations, we advocate using an initial lower-dose schedule (e.g., risperidone 1 to 4 mg/day; olanzapine 2.5 to 10 mg/day). If primary mood stabilizers are ineffective or not tolerated, evidence indicates that monotherapy with agents such as olanzapine or risperidone may be effective.

VPA should be considered as the initial mood stabilizer if the following is true:

• Past treatment attempts with *lithium were unsuccessful*
• Patients demonstrate a history of *rapid cycling*
• There are symptoms of mixed or *dysphoric mania*
• An *organic mood syndrome* is suspected
• *Medical problems*, such as psoriasis, preclude the use of lithium.

This agent may be used with or without lithium, BZDs, or antipsychotics. If lithium or VPA is not effective, we would then consider a trial with CBZ.

Various combinations of mood stabilizers and antipsychotics may then be considered, always in a stepwise strategy. Although clozapine may be combined with lithium and/or VPA, we caution against the combined use of clozapine plus CBZ,

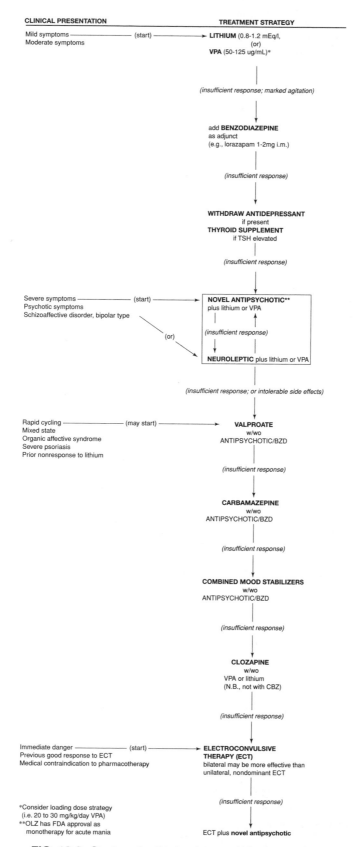

FIG. 10-3. Strategy for the treatment of bipolar mania.

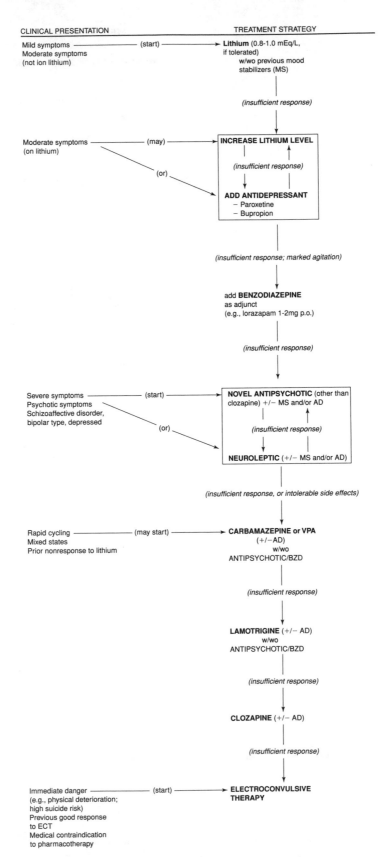

FIG. 10-4. Strategy for the treatment of bipolar depression.

than the response rate for the pure schizophrenic group (i.e., 46%).

Suppes et al. (108) successfully treated seven *treatment-refractory, psychotic, dysphoric manic patients* with clozapine. They reported that during a 3-year to 5-year follow-up, most of these patients sustained substantial gains in psychosocial function and that the six who remained on this agent were not rehospitalized. Subsequently, these same authors reported on *three rapid-cycling, nonpsychotic, bipolar patients* who also benefited from clozapine, leading the authors to opine that this drug may have mood-stabilizing properties separate from its antipsychotic effects (106). In this context, Frankenburg (289) presented a case report of a 29-year-old *bipolar man who had euthymic features and was nonpsychotic*, but had marked tremor of the jaw and severe blepharospasm. The patient had been maintained on haloperidol, fluphenazine decanoate, trihexyphenidyl, and lithium. Over 6 months, these medications were discontinued and clozapine plus lorazepam was introduced with no change in his clinical status. The author concluded that clozapine could be considered a "broad-spectrum" agent for use in patients with psychotic affective illnesses who are poorly responsive to or intolerant of standard treatment. In support, Privitera et al. (270) reported on a *rapid-cycling, bipolar II*, depressed patient whose response to clozapine was superior to that of more conventional treatments for her mood disorder.

Another report suggests that the combination of clozapine plus VPA may result in greater efficacy and was well tolerated in most patients (110). In this context, we would avoid using clozapine plus CBZ due to the possibility of further decreases in white cell counts, as well as clozapine plus a BZD, because this combination has been reported to cause respiratory compromise (111).

Risperidone: Acute Clinical Trials. Hillert et al. (107) found risperidone to have both antipsychotic and antidepressive properties in 10 patients with *schizoaffective disorder, depressed type*. These investigators prescribed 2 to 10 mg/day for 6 weeks in an open-label pilot study, and found marked improvement in

psychosis in all patients and clinically significant overall improvement in psychosis in 7 to 10 patients. Two patients required antiparkinsonian drugs; otherwise risperidone was well tolerated by the group.

Dwight et al. (291) reported their experience with risperidone in eight patients with *schizoaffective disorder* (six bipolar type; two depressive type). All six bipolar type patients showed the onset of or an increase in mania shortly after starting risperidone (mean number of treatment days = 7 ± 3; mean dose = 7 ± 1 mg/day). In this context, O'Croinin et al. (292) reported on a chronic paranoid schizophrenic patient who was admitted in an acute psychotic state unresponsive to thioridazine or CPZ. Risperidone was started (6 mg/day by day 3), but by the end of the first week she was displaying hypomanic symptoms. When risperidone was discontinued and haloperidol introduced, her hypomanic symptoms resolved.

Goodnick (293) reported on two acutely bipolar manic patients who had not responded to or could not tolerate lithium but did respond favorably to risperidone. The author also hypothesized that risperidone's ability to block 5-HT$_2$ receptors may make this agent useful for treating both mania and psychotic depression.

Sachs et al. (294) reported the results of a double-blind, randomized trial of *acute mania*. Patients were treated with risperidone, haloperidol, or placebo. Approximately 50 subjects were randomized to each group. Open lithium or VPA treatment was also used. Those patients treated with risperidone or haloperidol had a substantially greater decrease from baseline YMS scores than those on placebo (i.e., 14 for risperidone and 13 for haloperidol versus 8 points for the placebo group ($p = 0.009$). Further, 57% of the risperidone group achieved at least a 50% decrease from the YMS baseline score, compared with 38% in the placebo group. This study demonstrates that the addition of risperidone or haloperidol produced a better response than that achieved with a mood stabilizer alone.

Janicak et al. (113, 283) recently reported the results of a double-blind, randomized trial of risperidone monotherapy versus haloperidol monotherapy for controlling both psychotic and mood symptoms in 62 patients with schizoaffective disorder (bipolar or depressed subtype). These authors observed that, in comparison with haloperidol, risperidone was as follows:

- Equally effective in decreasing *manic* and *psychotic symptoms*
- *Did not worsen mania* or switch bipolar depressed or mixed subtypes into mania
- More effective for *significant depression*
- Caused *fewer extrapyramidal side effects*
- Was *better tolerated* overall

Jacobsen (295) conducted an open, prospective study to determine whether risperidone diminishes psychosis, severe agitation, or rapid cycling in patients fulfilling *Diagnostic and Statistical Manual of Mental Disorders*, 4th ed., (DSM-IV) criteria for *bipolar I, II, or major depressive disorder* who also manifested psychosis or major agitation associated with their illness. Some of those in the group fulfilled DSM-IV criteria for obsessive-compulsive disorder as well. Eighty-five percent (i.e., 17 of 20) showed complete or partial improvement after treatment. The author concluded that some affectively ill patients can benefit from treatment with risperidone, but because comparison trials were not performed, the findings do not imply that risperidone is superior to neuroleptics.

Singh and Catalan (296) successfully treated four *male psychotic manic AIDS* patients (average age, 45.8 years) with risperidone. In three patients, the Mania Rating Scale scores decreased from 43 to 8, 35 to 14, and 30 to 3 within 7 to 10 days of receiving risperidone. Although all patients had low white cell counts at presentation, there was no further clinically significant decrease during risperidone treatment and no extrapyramidal side effects were observed. The authors concluded that their preliminary observations suggest that risperidone may be effective and safe in the treatment of patients who have AIDS-related psychosis and mania.

Olanzapine: Acute Clinical Trials. Tohen et al. have published the results of two double-blind, placebo-controlled trials of *olanzapine* for the treatment of acute mania. The first study was 3 weeks in duration and included 139 patients hospitalized for an acute bipolar manic or mixed episode (112). The starting dose of olanzapine was 10 mg/day and the mean dose was 14.9 mg/day. Active drug treatment produced a statistically greater average improvement than placebo on the Young Mania Rating Scale scores whether psychosis was present or not. Further, 49% of the olanzapine treated group ($n = 70$) met the "a priori" criteria for response (i.e., a $\geq 50\%$ reduction from baseline YMS score) vs. only 24% of the placebo treated group ($n = 69$). The second study was similar in design; involved 115 patients; used a higher starting dose of olanzapine (i.e., 15 mg/day; mean dose of 16.4 mg/day); less rescue medication; and, had a 4 week treatment duration. The outcome was similar with olanzapine found statistically superior to placebo for core manic symptoms, as well as improvement in depression or those with a mixed episode (283).

Combining these two studies, there is a total of 251 patients with a 56% response rate to olanzapine versus a 33% response rate to placebo. Using the Mantle-Haenszel meta-analysis technique (see Table 10-15) on these results, olanzapine was found to be statistically superior to placebo (chi-square $= 13.1$, df $= 1$, $p = .0003$). The degree of superiority for olanzapine was the same in both studies in that there was no evidence of heterogeneity evident by the Breslow-Day Test (i.e., chi square $= 0.1$,

TABLE 10-15 *Olanzapine versus placebo: acute mania*

Study	n	Responders (%)		Difference (%)
		Olanzapine	Placebo	
Tohen et al., 1999	136	49	24	25
Tohen et al., 2000	115	65	43	22
Total	**251**	**56**	**33**	**23**[a]

[a]$\chi^2 = 13.1$; df $= 1$; $p = 0.0003$.

given the former's propensity to induce agranu-locytosis and the latter's ability to suppress bone marrow production.

Given an inadequate drug response, or in pa-tients with manic delirium who pose an imme-diate risk to themselves or others, we would consider ECT. Although BILAT stimulus elec-trode placement may be more effective than unilateral (UND) placement, this conclusion is currently only tentative, given the small num-ber of patients studied. Finally, the combined use of ECT plus an antipsychotic may benefit the most treatment-resistant patient and has not been reported to induce serious adverse events (303–306).

Strategy for Acute Bipolar Depression

The depressed phase of a bipolar disorder poses an interesting challenge. With mild to moder-ate depression, a trial with lithium alone may be sufficient and avoid exposing these patients to the potential destabilizing effects of an an-tidepressant (306a). In patients unable to bene-fit from lithium alone, an antidepressant (e.g., paroxetine, bupropion) may also be necessary on a time-limited basis. A benzodiazepine may also benefit associated anxiety or agitation. In more severe episodes (including those with psy-chotic symptoms), an antipsychotic (preferably a novel agent) may be appropriate. Alternate mood stabilizers such as carbamazepine, valproate, or lamotrigine (alone or in combination with an antidepressant) may benefit those insufficiently responsive to previous treatment approaches. In particular, lamotrigine may have substantial an-tidepressant, as well as antimanic, effects. Cloza-pine may also benefit those unresponsive to ear-lier trials with other NAPs. In those patients who pose an immediate danger, or do not benefit or cannot tolerate pharmacotherapy, ECT should be considered.

ADVERSE EFFECTS OF LITHIUM, VALPROATE, AND OTHER ANTICONVULSANTS

Since the reintroduction of lithium in the late 1960's, the treatment of bipolar disorder has been revolutionized. The recent recognition of a wider spectrum of bipolar disorder subtypes (e.g., bipolar II, rapid cycling, mixed states), some of which are less responsive to this agent, as well as a substantial proportion of patients who cannot tolerate lithium, have led to a search for alternative therapies. The most productive line of inquiry has been the study of anticonvulsant-mood stabilizers, including VPA, CBZ, and, more recently, lamotrigine, gabapentin, and top-iramate. In addition, there is growing evidence that the newer generation of antipsychotics (e.g., clozapine, risperidone, olanzapine) may have distinct mood-stabilizing properties and benefit previously treatment-refractory patients. Finally, ECT can be used for both the manic and depres-sive phases of bipolar disorder.

As with any drug or somatic therapy, each of these approaches carries the risk of adverse ef-fects, some potentially quite serious. Examples include the following:

- *Thyroid* dysregulation with lithium
- *Teratogenicity* with VPA, CBZ, and lithium
- *Hematotoxicity,* such as agranulocytosis with clozapine
- *Cognitive disruption* with lithium and ECT
- Clinically relevant *drug interations*, such as ac-celerated metabolism with CBZ

Thus, any potential strategy must carefully consider the risk-benefit ratio on an individual-ized basis, because a given patient may be partic-ularly vulnerable to certain adverse events. This section considers the potential for adverse effects associated with mood stabilizers. The goal is to help clinicians develop strategies that minimize these risks (77).

Lithium

Lithium is an alkali metal in group IA and shares many properties with similar elements such as sodium and potassium. As a compound it is rapidly absorbed and reaches peak blood levels in approximately 1 to 3 hours (6 to 8 hours with sustained release preparations), with absorption being completed in approximately 8 hours. Un-like other psychotropics, it is not protein-bound and steady-state levels are usually achieved after

TABLE 10-16 *Pharmacokinetic properties of primary mood stabilizers*

Pharmacokinetic property	Mood stabilizer		
	Lithium	Valproate	Carbamazepine
Time to reach peak concentration	1–12 hours	3–5 hours	1–5 hours
Metabolism	Renal excretion	Hepatic oxidation and conjugation	Hepatic microsomal oxidation (P450 2D6)
Half-life	20–27 hours	6–16 hours	15–30 hours initial 10–15 hours maintenance
Time to reach steady-state	4–7 days	1–3 days	2–4 days initial 4–5 days after dosage change
Protein binding	0	90–95%	70–80%
Therapeutic range	0.8–1.5 mEq/L	45–150 μg/ml (putative)	4–15 μg/mL (putative)

4 to 6 days on a fixed dose. Table 10-16 lists the pharmacokinetic properties of lithium, as well as those of the other two commonly used mood stabilizers, VPA and CBZ.

There are a number of significant complications that may develop with either acute or chronic lithium treatment and they are listed in Table 10-17. The most common systems involved are the following:

- Renal
- Gastrointestinal
- Endocrine (e.g., thyroid)
- Cardiovascular
- Central nervous
- Dermatological

Whereas renal, thyroid, cardiovascular, and toxicity-related complications pose the most potentially serious problems, careful monitoring during long-term treatment can prevent most adverse sequelae (77) (Tables 10-16 and 10-17).

Contraindications to lithium are primarily based on the presence of medical disorders involving electrolyte balance and the cardiovascular and the renal systems. Thus, patients with unstable fluid and electrolyte states, those with azotemia, or those who require diuretics must be monitored very closely. Because lithium can impair sinus node function and aggravate the sick sinus node syndrome, it should not be used in such conditions (307). When feasible, hypertensive patients on diuretics should be switched to agents such as a β-blocker so that lithium can be more safely prescribed. If lithium is used in patients on diuretics, plasma levels must be monitored more closely, and doses usually adjusted downward. Any renal disorder that impedes the filtration of lithium can lead to increased retention and possible intoxication. Although contraindicated with acute renal failure, lithium may be used in chronic, but stable, states or in patients on hemodialysis, but careful monitoring and lower doses are mandatory. Alternative drugs that are metabolized by the liver (e.g., VPA, CBZ) or ECT should be considered where appropriate. Adverse events can generally be managed by adjusting the lithium dose, adding supplements, such as L-thyroxine, in patients who develop hypothyroidism, or considering an alternative drug strategy.

In addition, special problems posed by *pregnancy* and *toxicity* must be considered.

Renal System

It is important to note that the proximal reabsorption of sodium and lithium in the kidneys is similar; therefore, states of sodium depletion, such as salt restriction, may increase retention of lithium and increase the chance for toxicity. Excretion is almost entirely through the kidneys, with a biphasic elimination half-life. The half-life of lithium varies with age, taking 18 to 20 hours in the young adult and as long as 36 hours or more in the elderly or uremic

TABLE 10-17 *Lithium: common adverse effects*

Organ system	Clinical presentation	Comments
Cardiovascular	ECG changes	T wave suppression, delayed or irregular rhythm, increase in PVCs Sick sinus node syndrome (SSNS) Myocarditis
Dermatologic	Acne Psoriasis Rashes	Worsens Treatment-refractory worsening Maculopapular and follicular
Endocrine	Hypothyroid state Hyperparathyroid state	About 5% goiter; about 4% clinically significant hypothyroidism Clinically nonsignificant
Fetus (teratogenic)	Tricuspid valve malformation Atrial septal defect	Ebstein's anomaly
Gastrointestinal	Anorexia Nausea (10–30%), Vomiting Diarrhea (5–20%)	Usually early in treatment and usually transient; may be early sign of toxicity Slow-release preparations may help
Hematological	Granulocytosis	May be useful in disorders such as Felty's syndrome, iatrogenic neutropenia. May counter Carbamazepine-induced leukopenia
Neurological	Tremor	Propranolol may help
Renal	Polyuria–polydipsia (nephrogenic diabetes insipidus)	May be an indication of morphologic changes Requires adequate hydration

patient. Conversely, someone with a high sodium intake may also require a higher dose of lithium. This creates a narrow margin of safety and requires more frequent monitoring of blood levels and precise instructions to the patient regarding changes in diet, exercise patterns, or other medications that may alter this drug's serum concentration.

Lithium's effects on renal function have engendered much interest, because it may induce certain morphological changes (e.g., interstitial fibrosis, tubular atrophy, glomerular sclerosis) in the kidneys of about 10% of patients. In a review of the literature, we concluded that, unless there are extremely toxic levels from an overdose or sustained or excessively high treatment levels, lithium's impact on the kidney usually does not translate into clinically relevant renal dysfunction (308). Of interest, Coppen (309) found no significant differences in several areas of

renal function between lithium- and nonlithium-treated patients with a history of bipolar illness. He concluded that the similarity between these two groups requires controlled studies of lithium toxicity with age- and sex-matched control subjects suffering from the same disorders, because mood disorders themselves may have adverse effects on renal morphology. There are only a few case reports demonstrating renal failure in the absence of either acute or sustained lithium toxicity (310, 311). Hetmar et al. (312) concluded that lithium-related impairment in renal function (i.e., tubular and glomerular) is related to age, episodes of toxicity, preexisting renal disease, and treatment schedule (i.e., multiple vs. single daily doses) rather than duration of therapy. **In summary, although morphological changes occur secondary to chronic lithium exposure, we believe clinically relevant nephrotoxicity is unlikely.**

At one time, sustained-release preparations were thought to reduce renal toxicity, but more recent evidence has cast doubt on this assumption (313). A patient on long-term maintenance lithium should have renal function monitored periodically (i.e., every 12 months) with a urinalysis, BUN, and creatinine. If abnormal, a more intensive evaluation should include 24-hour urine osmolality and creatinine clearance. It is advisable to reduce maintenance lithium to optimal minimal dose-blood levels and, if possible, to avoid concomitant antipsychotics, which may enhance toxicity. **Some data support the use of a once-a-day dose schedule to minimize peak lithium concentrations over a 24-hour period** (314).

The syndrome of *polyuria-polydipsia* occurs in up to 60% of lithium patients, leading some to abandon an otherwise effective treatment. Lithium is also the most common cause of nephrogenic diabetes insipidus, which results from the drug's inhibitory effects on the cAMP-dependent action of antidiuretic hormone (ADH) on renal distal tubules (77, 315). Diabetes insipidus occurs in 12% to 20% of patients treated with lithium, usually resulting in urine volumes in excess of 3000 mL/24-hour. These symptoms may imply kidney damage and should be prevented or corrected when possible (316, 317). Strategies to manage this complication include the following:

- Adequate *fluid replacement*
- *Dose* or *schedule adjustments* (e.g., reduce dose or switch to a single daily dose schedule)
- *Potassium* supplementation (10 to 20 mEq/L/day)
- The use of *diuretics,* such as a thiazide or amiloride, with careful attention paid to lithium and potassium levels (318, 319)
- *Switching preparations* from a standard to a sustained-release form, or vice versa
- Possible use of *indomethacin*, with required lithium dose reduction (320, 321)

The *nephrotic syndrome*, characterized clinically by proteinuria, is a rare and idiosyncratic reaction to lithium. As with other uncommon adverse effects, the issue of causation versus coincidence must be considered. Treatment includes cessation of the drug and, when necessary, corticosteroids such as prednisone (322).

In summary:

- *Renal complications* are common but not usually serious.
- *Polyuria/polydipsia* may compromise quality of life and compliance.
- *Amiloride* and *indomethacin* are the most effective therapies for polyuria/polydipsia and syndrome of inappropriate ADH, respectively (77).

Gastrointestinal System

The most frequent early complaints involve this organ system. Nausea, which typically occurs shortly after a dose, can be controlled by taking the drug with meals, and although sustained-release preparations can also help in this regard, they may lead to diarrhea because of the unabsorbed drug's local irritation to the bowel.

Endocrine System

Lithium appears to exert its primary antithyroid effect by preventing the release of thyroid hormones (e.g., T_3, thyroxine) (323). In addition, this agent inhibits iodine uptake into the thyroid gland and the iodination of tyrosine. Although it has several antithyroid effects, significant clinical sequelae are relatively few. It is estimated that approximately 5% of patients taking lithium for 18 months or more will develop hypothyroidism or diffuse nontender goiter, with female patients at much greater risk (324). Further, 3% develop a benign, diffuse nontoxic goiter, and mild increases in thyroid-stimulating hormone (TSH) may be found in up to 23% of patients. Those at greater risk include the following:

- The *elderly*
- *Women*
- Those with a prior *history of thyroid disease*
- Patients taking other *medications that may interfere with thyroid function*

Therefore, extra precaution should be exercised in patients with preexisting thyroid disease or those taking other drugs that may interfere with thyroid function (e.g., CBZ, phenytoin, ketoconazole). During maintenance therapy, physiological monitoring at baseline and on at least a yearly basis is generally recommended (e.g., TSH, T_3, T_4, T_3-resin uptake, free thyroxin index), but careful attention to early signs and symptoms of hypofunction (e.g., weight gain, cold intolerance, hair loss) may be more productive. Thyroid-stimulating hormone is sensitive to early thyroid changes and, if elevated, should prompt treatment with thyroid supplements to avoid goiter or hypothyroidism.

Ironically, this adverse effect may at times be heralded by the onset of depression and can be mistaken for a recurrence of the original disorder. An early warning may be an increase in thyroid-stimulating hormone levels at or slightly above the upper limits of normal. Further, this situation may render a patient less responsive to lithium and/or precipitate a phase of rapid cycling (325, 326). If it is necessary to continue lithium despite clinical hypothyroidism, thyroid supplements should be instituted, with T_3 (starting dose of 25 μg/day) or T_4 (starting dose of 50 μg/day). Doses may be gradually increased every few weeks until the patient is euthyroid. When necessary, stopping lithium and switching to another mood-stabilizing agent will usually result in prompt reversal of hypothyroidism.

The effect of long-term lithium prophylaxis (up to 22 years) on thyroid function was examined by ultrasonic evaluation in 100 bipolar and unipolar patients by Perrild et al. (327). Goiter was more common in those patients on lithium for 1 to 5 years (40%), as well as in those on treatment for more than 10 years (50%), when compared with those who had never received lithium previously (i.e., 16%). Smoking also appeared to contribute significantly to goiter and thyroid size. Subclinical or overt hypothyroidism was found in 4% and 21% of patients (mostly women) treated with lithium for 1 to 5 years or for more than 10 years, respectively. Interestingly, more than half had no signs of autoimmune thyroid disease, indicating a direct effect by lithium on the thyroid gland. The authors noted that earlier reported discrepancies in the frequency of goiter (i.e., 3.6% to 48%) may be due to reliance on palpation only, an inaccurate and irreproducible method of assessment.

In summary:

- *Thyroid dysfunction is common* with lithium therapy.
- *Routine monitoring* of thyroid function tests is necessary.
- *Thyroid supplementation* is appropriate if clinically significant complications occur.

Cardiovascular System

The effects of lithium on the cardiovascular system are usually tolerated at both therapeutic and toxic plasma levels. Common changes include the following:

- *T wave* flattening or inversion
- *U waves*
- *Conduction delays,* such as first-degree atrioventricular block

As noted earlier, lithium is contraindicated in patients with unstable congestive heart failure or the sick sinus node syndrome (307, 328). In older patients or those with prior cardiac histories, a pretreatment ECG should be obtained. Except for the potential adverse interactions with diuretics, the concomitant use of other cardiac drugs is generally safe. Because verapamil may lower serum levels of lithium, however, more careful monitoring may be required to assure continued therapeutic effects (329). Some data also indicate that verapamil may predispose to lithium neurotoxicity. Conversely, increased lithium levels leading to toxicity has occurred with methyldopa and enalapril. When antihypertensive therapy is necessary, β-blockers are a reasonable choice when lithium is coadministered.

Central Nervous System

Tremor, a frequent complaint, is the benign essential type and can usually be managed with propranolol (30 to 240 mg) in divided doses (330).

TABLE 10-18 *Lithium: other common adverse effects*

Adverse effect	Estimated incidence	Comments
Edema	10–15%	Primarily ankles and feet Transient or intermittent Secondary to effects on sodium/carbohydrate metabolism Caution about diuretics and sodium restriction to avoid lithium toxicity
Weight gain	Approximately 75%	Mean = 4 kg 2% over 20 kg 20% over 10 kg Worse with antidepressants or antipsychotics
Tremor	10–65%	Dose-related Worse with antidepressants or antipsychotics Men > women Incidence greater with increasing age Reduce dose or use β-blocker
Psychological complaints	Approximately 10%	Often leads to noncompliance with treatment
Poor concentration/memory		May be early sign of toxicity
Fatigue/weakness		May mimic depressive phase of disorder
Diminished sex drive		Check for hypothyroidism
"Grayness of life" or mental dulling		Patients may miss the euphoria or "high"

Metoprolol may be preferred for patients with bronchospastic disease. Some reports suggest that neurological sequelae secondary to lithium use may be underrecognized (331, 332) and reversed when lithium is discontinued or an agent such as VPA is substituted. Indeed, the authors of one study (331) found that 9 of 10 measures of *cognition, creativity, and fine motor performance* improved significantly when patients were taken off lithium, shedding further light on its potential for deleterious CNS effects. We would note, however, that there is also evidence that enduring neuropsychological deficits may be part of a more chronic, severe bipolar disorder (333). Although not usually posing a serious threat, CNS effects are potentially significant in terms of compliance (Table 10-18).

CNS adverse effects can be the result of toxic serum levels, which may result from accidental or intentional patient ingestion of lithium doses exceeding clinical needs (334). Patients with organic brain impairment are also at increased risk of neurotoxicity. Toxicity may also be caused by reduced clearance of lithium from the body, resulting from dehydration, sodium depletion, the concomitant use of diuretics and nonsteroidal anti-inflammatory drugs (NSAIDs), or renal disorders. An EEG during toxic states may show diffuse slow waves in the range of 5 to 7 cps. The severity of acute lithium toxicity (e.g., with an overdose) can be assessed by the level of neurological impairment (Table 10-19). The basis for neurotoxicity when lithium was combined with such therapies as haloperidol, verapamil, and ECT is uncertain. Thus, it would be preferable to avoid such combinations. When necessary, however, the lowest effective dose of any agent should be used.

Because no antidote is available, *treatment is supportive*. A patient's condition should be monitored closely, including fluid intake and output, mental status, and serum levels of lithium, creatinine, and electrolytes. Patients with normal renal function should be able to clear lithium unassisted. If necessary, attempts should be made to remove excess lithium from the body by *gastric lavage* and *emesis*.

In summary:

- *Cognitive effects* and *tremor* are common.
- *Neurotoxicity* occurs with excessive doses/levels.

TABLE 10-19 *Effects of lithium toxicity*

Mild (1.5–2.0 mEq/L)	Moderate (2.0–2.5 mEq/L)	Severe (>2.5 mEq/L)
Listlessness	Coarse tremors	Altered consciousness
Nausea	Confusion or delirium	Choreoathetosis
Diarrhea	Ataxia	Seizures
Slurred speech		Coma and death

From Janicak PG, Munson LG. Practical management of adverse effects associated with mood stabilizers. In: Balon R, ed. *Adverse effects of mood stabilizers: practical management of the side effects of psychotropic drugs.* New York: Marcel Dekker, 1999: 119–143, with permission.

- Treatment may involve *supportive measures, dialysis,* and *β-blockers* for tremors.

Other Adverse Effects

Patients also experience miscellaneous complications such as the following:

- *Edema*
- *Weight gain*
- *Psychological complaints* (332, 333, 335, 336)

Although most of these adverse effects can be readily managed by the tincture of time, dose adjustment, or alternative preparations, they may precipitate noncompliance in patients particularly sensitive to such complications. *Edema* is probably related to secondary sodium retention and is usually more troublesome than significant. Weight gain is common with lithium. On average, patients will gain about 9 pounds during therapy with this agent, but larger gains often occur, especially when this agent is combined with antidepressants and/or antipsychotics. Because this problem can occur with the three most commonly used mood stabilizers, an aggressive weight management program should always be started at the initiation of treatment. Patients on lithium should also be cautioned about self-medicating with diuretics to manage weight gain.

Dermatological Effects

Early in the course of lithium therapy, exacerbations of *psoriasis and acneiform eruptions* as well as other skin reactions may occur. Possible mechanisms have included lithium's ability to decrease cAMP as well as to increase the number and activity of polymorphonuclear leukocytes. Those with a predisposition to skin disorders are most at risk for this complication, with women more likely than men to experience a dermatological reaction to lithium. These problems may clear spontaneously or may require lithium dose reduction, appropriate dermatological intervention, or lithium discontinuation (77).

Perinatal Complications

When clinically possible, lithium treatment should be discontinued during pregnancy and nursing (see also the section "The Pregnant Patient" in Chapter 14). Prophylactic lithium is often given to female bipolar patients of childbearing age, but there are questions about potential teratogenicity, with the greatest concern centering on the possibility of cardiac malformations (e.g., Ebstein's anomaly, a tricuspid valve malformation), especially with exposure earlier in the first trimester. A prospective study of first trimester exposure to lithium by Jacobsen et al. (337), however, found no differences in overall teratogenesis between pregnant women on lithium and a matched control group not exposed to this agent.

Schou (338) has reviewed and summarized five important questions in this area, including the following:

- The risk of *malformations* in the unborn child
- The potential for *later developmental anomalies*
- Changes in lithium *pharmacokinetics during pregnancy*
- The possibility of lithium exerting *"other effects"* during pregnancy

• The inadvisability of lithium therapy if the mother is *breastfeeding* her newborn

Because of the possible slightly increased risk of cardiovascular malformation, Schou suggests that fertile women treated with lithium should use contraceptive methods and that the drug be stopped before a planned pregnancy or immediately upon recognition of an unplanned pregnancy. In a woman known to experience severe exacerbations on discontinuation of lithium, however, the risk-benefit ratio of continuing lithium must be carefully weighed, especially in light of the more recent data of Jacobsen and colleagues (337). Unfortunately, potential alternative treatments such as CBZ and VPA also have teratogenic potential, particularly neural tube defects (339).

Considering the potential interaction between pregnancy and the course of a bipolar disorder, Schou (340) notes that one study found the following:

• *A decrease in hospital admission frequency* for bipolar patients during pregnancy (i.e., about three-quarters normal rate)
• An *eightfold increase* in admissions during the first month postpartum
• *Twice the admission rate* between the *second and twelfth month postpartum*

Finally, when given in large doses, lithium may increase the risk of fetal macrosomia, premature delivery, and perinatal mortality (based on unpublished data on 241 infants).

Newborn infants of mothers on lithium have also shown transient CNS depression and reduced feeding activity, as well as goiter and hypothyroidism, which generally resolve spontaneously a few months postpartum. Because lithium can produce goiter in the newborn, the thyroid status of the mother should be carefully monitored during pregnancy. Lithium plasma concentrations one-tenth to one-half of the mother's have been found in nursing infants, and this fact must be balanced by an increasing awareness of the beneficial mental and physical effects of nursing for both mother and child.

The issue of later "behavioral teratogenesis" was studied in 60 "lithium" children (whose mothers took lithium when pregnant) as compared with 57 normal siblings. Reassuringly, the incidence of anomalous developmental disorders was essentially equal (340).

The renal clearance of lithium can be altered during the various phases of pregnancy, usually requiring the following:

• *Increased doses* late in pregnancy
• The *cessation* of lithium 2 to 3 days before delivery
• *Restarting* lithium a few days postpartum at an appropriately lowered dose

The issue of the risks posed by a father on lithium therapy at the time of conception has yet to be adequately addressed.

In considering whether to maintain patients on lithium during pregnancy, the clinician must take into account the risks of an exacerbation of bipolar disorder to both mother and fetus. Although it would be ideal to avoid lithium therapy, at least during the first trimester, when critical organogenesis is occurring, this may not be possible.

During pregnancy, *serum lithium levels need to be carefully monitored*. The 50% to 100% increase in glomerular filtration rate (GFR) that normally occurs in the third trimester will proportionally lower lithium levels due to its increased clearance. Thus, dosage may need to be increased to maintain a therapeutic range (341). Because the GFR and lithium clearance quickly return to normal after delivery, it may be wise to stop the drug shortly before delivery and restart a few days after delivery at a lower dose. In summary:

• Lithium carries a low risk of *teratogenicity*.
• The *changing physiology during pregnancy* can alter lithium levels.
• *Nursing* should be avoided if a patient is on lithium.

Toxicity

Lithium toxicity (chronic, subacute, or acute) can be secondary to any factor that reduces body clearance, or secondary to acute or sustained elevated doses (and therefore plasma levels) (342). The degree of toxicity can be classified as follows:

- *Early signs*—ataxia, dysarthria, lack of coordination (343)
- *Mild*—usually occurring in the range of 1.5 to 2.0 mEq/L and most often characterized by listlessness, nausea, slurring of speech, diarrhea, and coarse tremors
- *Moderate*—usually occurring in the range of 2.0 to 2.5 mEq/L and most often characterized by coarse tremors and other CNS reactions, confusion or delirium, and pronounced ataxia
- *Severe*—beginning with levels at 2.5 to 3.0 mEq/L and above, most often characterized by significant alterations in consciousness, spontaneous attacks of hyperextension of the extremities, choreoathetosis, seizures, coma, or death (Table 10-19)

The EEG will often show diffuse slow-wave activity in the 5 to 7 cps range. The more severe episodes usually occur in patients who accidentally or purposely overdose on lithium, and this may lead to other medical complications, such as pulmonary edema, pneumonia, and cardiac arrhythmias.

With an acute overdose, treatment includes discontinuation of lithium and use of various supportive measures, because no antidote is available. Initial steps recommended by Ayd (334) include the following:

- *Serum measurements* of lithium, creatinine, electrolytes, and plasma osmolality
- *Gastric lavage*
- *Monitoring of fluid* intake and output
- Obtaining a history about the *timing* and *amount* of lithium taken
- A *neurological exam,* including a mental status examination and a baseline EEG

With normal renal function, all that may be necessary is watchful waiting, careful monitoring of the clinical status, and repeated serum lithium determinations.

The goal is to remove lithium from the system and correct any electrolyte imbalance. Emesis or gastric lavage is often helpful, with forced diuresis, peritoneal dialysis, and hemodialysis used only in more moderate to severe cases (e.g., levels exceeding 2.5 mEq/L). Generally, the outcome even with severe lithium toxicity is recovery; however, there is the possibility of irreversible neurological or renal damage in a small percentage of patients. When death occurs, it is usually secondary to circulatory or respiratory collapse.

Drug Interactions

There are several clinically significant drug interactions with lithium, including the following:

- Many *NSAIDs* (indomethacin, phenylbutazone, sulindac, naproxen, diclofenac, ibuprofen) can raise lithium levels.
- *Thiazide diuretics* can raise lithium levels.
- *Indapamide,* a nonthiazide sulfonamide diuretic, can raise lithium levels.
- *Certain antibiotics* (e.g., oral tetracyclines) may diminish lithium's clearance through the kidneys, leading to increases in plasma levels and possible intoxication (344, 345) (Table 10-20).
- *Other drugs, such as verapamil, caffeine, theophylline, osmotic diuretics, carbonic anhydrase inhibitors,* or aminophylline, can increase lithium excretion, possibly dropping plasma levels below the therapeutic threshold

TABLE 10-20 *Lithium drug interactions*

Drugs that may **increase** lithium levels	Drugs that may **decrease** lithium levels
NSAIDs: ibuprofen, indomethacin, naproxen	Calicum antagonists: verapamil
Thiazide diuretics: hydrochlorothiazide	Xanthines: caffeine, theophylline
Nonthiazide diuretics: indapamide	Osmotic diuretics: mannitol
Antibiotics: tetracyclines	Carbonic anhydrase inhibitors: acetazolamide

From Janicak PG, Munson LG. Practical management of adverse effects associated with mood stabilizers. In: Balon R, ed. *Adverse effects of mood stabilizers: practical management of the side effects of psychotropic drugs.* New York: Marcel Dekker, 1999: 119–143, with permission.

TABLE 10-21 *Lithium: neurotoxicity*

Cerebellar symptoms are the most common neurologic sequelae (including tremors, cogwheeling, drowsiness, confusion, disorientation, muscle fasciculation, ataxia, extrapyramidal side effects, and seizures)
Risk factors include:
  Fever
  Major surgery
  Renal failure
  Low food/salt intake
  Age
  Acute overdose
Concurrent medications that may predispose:
  Neuroleptics
  Carbamazepine
  Calcium channel blockers
  Diuretics
  Methyldopa
May correspond more closely to cerebrospinal fluid lithium levels

---

(329). Further, if doses are increased to compensate for this effect, care must be taken to readjust the lithium downward when these concomitant agents are reduced or discontinued.

Analgesics, such as *aspirin* or *acetaminophen,* and *furosemide,* a loop diuretic, are better choices because they apparently do not interfere with lithium's reabsorption.

Neurotoxic reactions have been periodically reported with lithium alone or in combination with *antipsychotics, CBZ, verapamil,* or *methyldopa,* with the elderly probably at much greater risk for such events (Table 10-21). Although such drug combinations are often necessary and usually well tolerated, common clinical sense dictates that only the minimally effective doses be prescribed. It is also advised that patients carry or wear some form of identification indicating that they are receiving lithium treatment.

The question of increased neurotoxic reactions with the combination of lithium and an antipsychotic (especially haloperidol) has been vigorously debated since the report of Cohen and Cohen (346–349). Possible explanations have included the following:

- The use of *increased doses* of high potency antipsychotics

- *Toxic blood levels* of lithium
- *An additive* or *synergistic effect* with the combination, thus increasing the chances of neurotoxicity
- Misdiagnosed *neuroleptic malignant syndrome*

Whereas this combination is usually administered safely, using the lowest effective doses of neuroleptic, as well as of lithium, is the best strategy.

Valproate

VPA, as well as other anticonvulsants, has proven efficacious in the treatment of bipolar disorder. Although these medications tend to share many common side effects, other adverse effects are drug-specific. Rarely, these side effects may be life-threatening, but all may contribute to patient noncompliance and treatment failure. *Gastrointestinal discomfort, sedation, dizziness,* and *incoordination* often occur with the initiation of therapy and may be minimized or avoided by starting at low doses and increasing them slowly. Other more serious side effects, such as *hepatotoxicity, hematopoietic suppression, pancreatitis,* and *severe skin reactions,* may occur at any time and are more specifically linked to a particular medication. Before initiating therapy, baseline laboratory tests should be obtained, particularly a complete blood count with differential, electrolyte panels, and liver function tests. Results may help in choice of treatment agent and warn the physician of areas that may require more careful monitoring (77).

Specific adverse effects of VPA involve several systems, and include the following:

- Hepatic
- Gastrointestinal
- Pancreatic
- Weight gain
- Neurological
- Dermatological (Tables 10-22 to 10-24)

Hepatic

VPA is metabolized in the liver and may cause mild, transient elevations in serum transaminases

TABLE 10-22 *Anticonvuisants: adverse effects*

Clonazepam	Carbamazepine	Valproate
Gastrointestinal upset	Gastrointestinal upset	Gastrointestinal upset
Nausea	Nausea	Nausea
Vomiting	Vomiting	Vomiting
Diarrhea	Anorexia	Diarrhea
Sedation	Sedation	Sedation
Ataxia	Ataxia/clumsiness	
Tremor	Dizziness	Tremor
	Blurred vision/diplopia	
Weight loss/gain		Weight gain/loss
Alopecia		Transient alopecia
Polydipsia/polyuria	Inappropriate antidiuretic hormone syndrome	Edema

Note: Adverse reactions are usually dose-related and subside with time. It is recommended to begin with low doses and gradually increase as clinically indicated to avoid premature discontinuation of medication trial.

TABLE 10-23 *Anticonvulsants: behavioral and cognitive effects*

Clonazepam	Carbamazepine	Valproate
Lethargy	Lethargy	
	Impaired task performance	Impaired task performance
Behavioral disinhibition		
Irritability	Irritability	Hyperactivity
	Dysomnia	
Aggression		Aggression
Depression	Depression	Depression
Confusion	Confusion	Psychosis
Sexual dysfunction		

TABLE 10-24 *Anticonvulsants: idiosyncratic effects*

Clonazepam	Carbamazepine	Valproate
Elevated SGOT, SGPT, alkaline phosphatase	Elevated SGOT, SGPT, alkaline phosphatase	Elevated LDH/SGOT, SGPT
	Hepatic failure	Hepatotoxicity or failure (1/40,000) Reye-like syndrome
	Pancreatitis	Pancreatitis
Anemia	Aplastic anemia/agranulocytosis	
Leukopenia	Leukopenia	
Thrombocytopenia	Thrombocytopenia	Thrombocytopenia
Eosinophilia		
	Cardiovascular	
	CHF	
	Edema	
	AV block	
Rash	Rash	Rash
	Allergic dermatitis	Allergic dermatitis
	Stevens-Johnson syndrome (severe form of erythema multiforme)	
	Lyell's syndrome	

AV, atrioventricular; CHF, congestive heart failure; LDH, lactic dehydrogenase; SGOT, serum glutamic oxaloacetic transaminase; SGPT, serum glutamate pyruvate transaminase.

and lactate dehydrogenase. These elevations usually appear early in therapy, are dose-dependent, and resolve spontaneously. Laboratory abnormalities may be noted in 20% to 40% of patients and do not predispose to the development of more serious hepatic injury. VPA can also interfere with the conversion of ammonia to urea and result in hyperammonemia in approximately 20% of patients. This is usually asymptomatic but infrequently may cause lethargy (77, 350).

Serious hepatotoxicity is possible but rare. Hepatic failure occurs in only one in 40,000 cases and appears to be an idiosyncratic reaction that is not dose-related. Children under the age of 2, especially those receiving anticonvulsant polypharmacy, with mental retardation, and/or with poor nutritional status have been shown to be at greatest risk (351, 352). To our knowledge, no cases of hepatic failure have been reported in adults with bipolar disorder who were receiving VPA monotherapy, but liver failure has been reported in older children and in a mentally retarded adult with epilepsy taking VPA alone (77, 352, 353).

The appearance of laboratory abnormalities does not require cessation of treatment; however, if enzyme levels do not stabilize or return to normal, VPA should be discontinued and an alternate mood-stabilizing agent such as lithium used in its place. Liver function tests should be monitored more often during the first several weeks of therapy and every 6 to 12 months afterward. Routine liver function testing probably does not significantly prevent the occurrence of these unpredictable drug effects. Therefore, patients should be cautioned to immediately report symptoms of possible early hepatotoxicity such as easy bruising, decreased appetite, malaise, jaundice, and periorbital or dependent edema. In summary:

- Elevation of *liver enzymes* is common.
- Serious *hepatotoxicity* is rare.
- Patients should be *educated about early symptoms* so as to detect hepatotoxicity as quickly as possible (77).

Gastrointestinal

Nausea, appetite loss, and vomiting were frequent with earlier formulations of VPA but are less common with the *enteric coated formulations*. When these symptoms occur, taking the medication with food is often helpful (354).

Pancreatic

Reports of life-threatening pancreatitis have occurred in children and adults on this agent. While rare, elevated serum amylase levels are usually confirmatory. Some have been hemorrhagic and led to a rapid decline after initial symptoms, culminating in death. Cases have occurred both shortly after initiation of VPA, as well as after years of exposure. Therefore, it is important to educate patients and their families about the earliest symptoms, including the following:

- Abnormal pain
- Nausea and/or vomiting
- Anorexia

Prompt medical evaluation should be sought if these symptoms occur, and VPA discontinued if pancreatitis is the basis.

Weight Gain

Substantial weight gain has been reported in 7% to 57% on VPA of patients and often leads to noncompliance. Patients should be warned about this and advised to initiate an aggressive *weight management program* from the outset of treatment, since there are no specific remedies short of discontinuing the drug.

Neurological

Sedation is frequent but usually subsides over time. If present, *tremors* usually appear early, are dose-related, and are present at rest and worsen with action or positioning (77).

Strategies to prevent tremor include using the lowest possible dose; switching to the sprinkle formation, which minimizes peak and trough serum levels; or the addition of a β-blocker (e.g., *propranolol* or *metoprolol*), which reduce the amplitude of tremors without affecting their frequency. About 50% to 70% will experience full symptomatic control with a β-blocker; however, prolonged use may cause fatigue, weight gain, diarrhea, impotence, and depression (355). Typical doses of propranolol to control tremor are 120 to 240 mg in divided doses. Doses as high as 320 mg/day, however, may be required (356). Doses of 100 to 200 mg/day of metoprolol are also effective. Relative contraindications to the use of these agents include heart failure, second- or third-degree atrioventricular block, asthma, and insulin-dependent diabetes mellitus (77).

Alprazolam may also relieve tremor at doses of 0.75 to 3 mg/day (357). Because chronic use can lead to habituation or dependence, alprazolam is best used episodically for patients who require only intermittent tremor reduction to prevent social embarrassment or occupational interference. Methazolamide, a carbonic anhydrase inhibitor, has been reported to reduce hand tremor (at doses of 50 to 300 mg/day) in several open studies (358, 359). A controlled trial, however, could not confirm the efficacy of this agent in the treatment of tremor but did report that side effects such as paresthesias, sedation, headache, and gastrointestinal symptoms were common (77, 356).

Dermatological

Hair loss (alopecia) has been reported in up to 4% of patients. It is often transient and may be attenuated with selenium (50 μg/day) and/or zinc sulfate (50 mg/day).

Pregnancy

Women of childbearing age exposed to this agent should be counseled as to its *possible teratogenic effects*. One percent to 2% of fetuses exposed to VPA in the first trimester have developed neural tube defects and 1% spina bifida (77, 361–363).

Because of these potential complications, appropriate contraception should be used if treatment with VPA is begun. In addition, all women of childbearing age given VPA should also take *folate* (1 mg/day). VPA should be discontinued if pregnancy occurs and *ultrasonography* used to assess fetal development (362, 363).

While a recent review concluded that there is evidence of neuroendocrine perturbations with VPA, it was also noted that well-controlled monotherapy studies are limited. Given the apparent increased incidence of polycystic ovarian syndrome (PCOS) associated with VPA therapy and uncertainty about the mechanism (e.g., weight gain, interference with steroid metabolism), further study is warranted and clinicians should carefully monitor female patients on this agent for increased testosterone levels. Other strategies to minimize the risk of this complication include the following:

- Maintenance of *normal weight*
- Monitoring of *serum lipid profiles*
- Monitoring of *hemoglobin A1C*
- Monitoring of *menstrual cycle*
- *Hormonal contraception,* which may prevent development of PCOS (77, 364)

Toxicity

Coma and death may occur with an acute overdose of this agent (365). Following attempts to remove any remaining drug with gastric lavage, other interventions may include these:

- Hemodialysis
- Hemoperfusion
- Naloxone (77, 366, 367)

Drug Interactions

Drug interactions with VPA occur primarily because of its protein-binding capacity and impact on drug metabolism. Since this agent is more than 90% protein-bound, it competes for the same binding sites as other highly protein-bound drugs (e.g., aspirin, phenytoin). Free serum concentrations of displaced drugs are then increased and the pharmacologically active unbound drug may cause toxicity, even when total serum levels are in the accepted range. Thus, when VPA is used with drugs that are also significantly protein bound, measuring free drug levels and adjusting doses accordingly may avoid adverse events (77).

VPA is also a nonspecific but weak inhibitor of the CYP-450 enzyme system, causing serum levels of other hepatically metabolized drugs to be increased. For example, concomitant use of VPA with diazepam, ethosuximide, or phenobarbital can increase the levels of these latter drugs. VPA may also cause an elevation in serum levels of CBZ's epoxide metabolite, possibly inducing toxicity. Usually, however, these changes are not clinically significant (367).

Carbamazepine

CBZ's molecular structure is similar to imipramine. It is primarily metabolized by the liver and, like lithium, has a narrow therapeutic index, predisposing to toxicity with elevated serum levels.

Like most anticonvulsants, CBZ may cause adverse side effects involving multiple organ systems, and include the following:

- Neurological
- Hepatic
- Hematological
- Dermatological
- Cardiovascular

Neurological

Various CNS adverse effects have been reported with CBZ and include sedation, dizziness, ataxia/clumsiness, blurred vision/diplopia, and impaired task performance. Although uncommon, fatal CBZ toxicity does occur. CBZ overdose is characterized by neurological symptoms such as diplopia, dysarthria, ataxia, vertigo, nystagmus, and coma. Infrequently, cyclic coma with biphasic fluctuations of consciousness, seizures, respiratory depression, cardiac conduction defects, and the need for artificial ventilation may occur. Plasma levels are only moderately correlated to severity, but as noted earlier, more than 15 μg/ml in children or 20 μg/ml in adults should be considered serious. Charcoal hemoperfusion or gastric lavage with activated charcoal has been used in such cases,

whereas benefit from plasmapheresis is controversial (77, 114, 368).

Hepatic

CBZ can cause a mild, transient increase in *serum transaminases* and alkaline phosphatase levels. They usually do not exceed 1.5 times normal levels and subside with ongoing treatment. If liver function tests (LFTs) increase two to three times normal levels, hepatotoxicity may result. With prolonged CBZ therapy, a syndrome resembling a mild viral hepatitis may occur; but usually improves after drug discontinuation.

Because CBZ is metabolized via the liver, this constitutes a relative contraindication in patients with hepatic dysfunction. Therefore, LFTs should be obtained before initiating CBZ therapy and monitored regularly every 6 to 12 months. Sustained LFT levels usually warrant the withdrawal of CBZ.

Hematological

CBZ should not be used when there is a history of drug-induced hematological reactions; bone marrow suppression; hypersensitivity to this agent or other tricyclics; and/or hepatic dysfunction.

Leukopenia (i.e., WBC count less than 3,000/mm^3) has been reported in up to 10% of patients treated with this agent. It is usually benign and self-limited, tending to occur during the first month of drug exposure (77, 369).

More serious hematopoietic suppression can occur and, as noted earlier, CBZ is contraindicated with a prior history of bone marrow suppression. Aplastic anemia has been reported to occur in one out of 125,000 cases. Agranulocytosis may also rarely occur. Of some comfort, Tohen et al. (370) reported no serious hematological dyscrasias in more than 2,000 patients receiving either CBZ or VPA.

While such reactions typically appear during the first 6 months of therapy, they can occur at any time, requiring ongoing monitoring of the hematological system. Patients without impaired hematological function can usually tolerate moderate decreases in WBC counts. Discontinuation of CBZ is recommended when total WBC counts drop below 3,000/mm^3 or the neutrophil count drops below 1,500/mm^3 (371).

Because the onset of bone marrow suppression may be insidious, it is prudent to instruct patients to monitor themselves for the appearance of fever, malaise, sore throat, petechiae, or other evidence of possible hematological dysfunction rather than simply relying on periodic laboratory surveillance. In cases of suspected bone marrow involvement, medication should be discontinued immediately and medical intervention sought promptly. For these reasons, we would discourage the combined use of CBZ and clozapine.

Dermatological

CBZ can cause morbilliform rashes which may also produce intense pruritus, usually within the first 6 weeks of therapy. Approximately 10% of patients develop a rash but do not usually require cessation of the drug. The involvement of the mucous membranes, fever, or other constitutional symptoms may indicate the development of *Stevens-Johnson* or *Lydell* syndromes. These rashes are rare but potentially life-threatening, occurring in less than one out of 50,000 patients. Their appearance requires immediate cessation of CBZ and prompt medical intervention.

Cardiovascular

Rarely, CBZ can cause *depression of atrioventricular conduction* and ventricular automaticity. This is secondary to the drugs membrane—depressant effects, similar to those of quinidine and procainamide (372). Thus, patients with significant, preexisting atrioventricular conduction disturbances should not receive CBZ (77).

Because CBZ can cause hyponatremia, it should be used cautiously in patients on a salt-restricted diet (373). Hyponatremia is rarely clinically significant when sodium values are above 125 mmol/L. Low sodium levels, as well as concomitant diuretic and lithium users, may predispose to the development of the syndrome of inappropriate ADH. Since CBZ enhances the effects of ADH, it can lead to impairment of free water clearance from the body. Older patients are at higher risk and should be closely monitored for this adverse effect which can be managed by dose reduction of CBZ. More severe cases, however, usually require switching to another agent (77).

Pregnancy

There is an increased risk of *craniofacial defects*, *spina bifida*, and *developmental delay* in children whose mothers received CBZ while pregnant. Thus, women of childbearing age should avoid this agent. If not practical, contraception should be diligently used to avoid pregnancy. In this context, dose adjustment of oral hormonal drugs may be necessary, since CBZ may accelerate their metabolism and compromise contraceptive effectiveness.

Toxicity

An acute overdose of CBZ can produce significant neurological symptoms. Diplopia may be a useful clinical indicator of developing toxicity, since severity is not necessarily correlated with plasma levels. Life-threatening seizures and coma may occur when levels exceed 20 to 25 μg/ml. Lower levels can produce drowsiness, ataxia, blurred vision, dysarthria, choreiform movements, or behavioral changes (374–375). *Gastric lavage, hemoperfusion,* and *plasmapheresis* may be beneficial, especially in more serious cases (77, 376).

Other common adverse effects associated with CBZ are listed in Tables 10-22 to 10-24.

Drug Interactions

CBZ stimulates the CYP-450 enzyme system, increasing clearance of concomitantly prescribed drugs also metabolized by this system (377). Thus, the dose of these medications may need to be increased to maintain efficacy (372). Levels of CBZ may also be influenced by other hepatically metabolized, co-prescribed drugs. VPA, isonicotine, hydrazine, and erythromycin are some of the agents that can increase CBZ levels, while agents such as

TABLE 10-25 *Carbamazepine drug interactions*

Drugs decreased by CBZ	Drugs increasing CBZ	Drugs decreasing CBZ
Haloperidol	Verapamil	Phenytoin
Oral contraceptives	Imipramine	Barbiturates
Theophylline	Erythromycin	Primidone
Warfarin	Fluoxetine	Folic acid
Folic acid	Isoniazid	
Doxycycline	Nicotinamide	
	Cimetidine	
	Diltiazem	

CBZ, carbamazepine.
From Janicak PG, Munson LG. Practical management of adverse effects associated with mood stabilizers. In: Balon R, ed. *Adverse effects of mood stabilizers: practical management of the side effects of psychotropic drugs.* New York: Marcel Dekker, 1999: 119–143, with permission.

phenytoin and primidone can lower them. Table 10-25 summarizes the potentially clinically significant interactions between CBZ and other commonly co-prescribed medications (379, 380).

CBZ-induced decreases in serum levels of oral contraceptives (OCs), theophylline, warfarin, and antipsychotics are also potentially clinical relevant (381, 382).

As noted above, OC failure may lead to accidental pregnancy and exposure of the developing fetus to potentially teratogenic properties of CBZ (383). Therefore, OC levels should be closely monitored and patients should notify their physician of spotting, an indicator of OC failure. Prothrombin time and the International Normalized Ratio (INR) should be monitored when patients are on warfarin and CBZ concomitantly. Patients stabilized on an antipsychotic may decompensate when CBZ is added. This may necessitate an increase in the antipsychotic dose and is one indication for TDM of antipsychotic drug levels (384). Conversely, when CBZ is discontinued, the dose of these other agents may need to be lowered to avoid toxicity. In summary:

• CBZ *potently induces* of the CYP-450 microsomal enzyme system.

• *Levels of other drugs that are substrates of this system should be monitored* with the addition or deletion of CBZ.
• CBZ may also *accelerate its own metabolism,* requiring dose increases to maintain efficacy.

Newer Anticonvulsants

Although earlier reports found that gabapentin, lamotrigine, topiramate, and tiagabine may possess mood-stabilizing properties, this has not been confirmed. These agents may also cause gastric upset, drowsiness, and mild neurological symptoms. Rash may occur early in treatment, with lamotrigine posing the greatest risk (385). Dermatological emergencies (e.g., Stevens-Johnson or Lydell's syndrome) are associated with any anticonvulsant but occur more frequently when lamotrigine and VPA are used concurrently (386). This may be due to the inhibitory action of VPA on lamotrigine metabolism. Therefore, when possible, this combination should be avoided.

The most common adverse effects reported with topiramate include sedation, difficulty concentrating, inattention, confusion, and language difficulties. Although weight loss is listed as an adverse event, this may be a distinct advantage for this agent, given the problem of weight gain associated with other commonly used mood stabilizers and antipsychotics (236, 237).

All anticonvulsants (with the exception of gabapentin) are potentially teratogenic and should be used only when necessary and with increased caution in women of childbearing age. A recent review by Chaudron and Jefferson (387) indicates that all mood stabilizers have been found in breast milk and may produce adverse effects in the nursing infant. Gabapentin and lamotrigine do not exhibit significant protein binding, nor do they affect hepatic metabolism. This minimizes the potential of adverse drug interactions. Because gabapentin is eliminated via the kidneys, it should be avoided in patients with compromised renal function. Conversely, it may be an appropriate choice for those with hepatic dysfunction (77).

ADVERSE EFFECTS OF OTHER DRUGS

Antipsychotics

These agents possess an adverse effect profile that poses significant and potentially serious complications (see also the section "Adverse Effects" in Chapter 5). In particular, patients suffering from mood disorders and associated psychosis who are exposed to neuroleptics may be at greater risk for *tardive dyskinesia* and perhaps the *neuroleptic malignant syndrome* (388). Although lower potency agents are likely to induce less severe *extrapyramidal reactions,* they are more likely to produce significant *anticholinergic effects, excessive sedation,* and *orthostasis,* as well as a mental dulling, which many consider a major impediment to compliance. As noted earlier, the lithium-high-potency neuroleptic combination has also been associated with an increased risk for neurotoxic reactions, but debate continues as to the most critical factors involved with this complication.

Preliminary reports indicate that the new generation of antipsychotics (e.g., clozapine, risperidone, olanzapine, quetiapine) may possess mood-stabilizing properties separate and distinct from their antipsychotic effects (106, 107, 114). Although these agents are generally more benign than the neuroleptics, the life-threatening risk associated with clozapine-induced agranulocytosis must always be considered.

Benzodiazepines

Significant adverse effects include *excessive drowsiness, ataxia, possible withdrawal syndrome* with abrupt discontinuation, and complaints of *behavioral* and *dysphoric mood* changes (see also Chapter 12). Common adverse drug interactions include the potentiation of alcohol and other sedative-hypnotics. One issue of concern, especially with outpatients, is the large percentage of bipolar patients who abuse these drugs (see Tables 10-17 to 10-25 for comparison with lithium, as well as other non-BZD anticonvulsants) (167). Conversely, BZDs used in the management of acute mania may also attenuate concurrent symptoms of alcohol withdrawal in these patients.

Calcium Channel Blockers

The most common adverse effects are *hypotension* and *bradycardia,* which are usually easily managed unless there is preexisting heart disease. Dubovsky et al. (389) reported severe cardiotoxicity when verapamil was combined with lithium in two elderly patients. One had a profound bradycardia with a heart rate of 36 beats/minute; another, who had a sinus bradycardia and atrioventricular ectopy, developed an acute myocardial infarction and died.

Other reported potentially significant drug interactions include the combination of verapamil or nifedipine with CBZ, which, at times, can lead to toxicity secondary to increases in CBZ levels, and neurotoxic reactions when verapamil or diltiazem is combined with lithium.

Clonidine

The most common adverse effects with clonidine are *hypotension, dry mouth, drowsiness,* and *dermatological reactions.* These are usually mild, but hypotensive effects may be significant in normotensive manic patients. Higher doses (e.g., 0.8 to 1.2 mg) have also been reported to induce a *paradoxical excitement* in some patients (270).

CONCLUSION

Bipolar disorder is often difficult to diagnose and difficult to treat. Various pharmacological strategies have been proposed and rigorously tested as potential mood stabilizers. Whereas the adverse effects of most of these agents are typically mild and readily managed, the increasing number of potential drug therapies for bipolar disorder must necessarily complicate the issue of adverse effects and drug interactions. Of particular importance are problems associated with the following:

- The *hepatic* system
- The *hematopoietic* system
- The *thyroid* gland
- *Pregnancy*

Balancing the potential benefits of this increasing array of drug therapies with their potential risks will continue to challenge clinicians working with such patients.

REFERENCES

1. Cade JFJ. Lithium salts in the treatment of psychotic excitement. *Med J Aust* 1949;36:349–352.
2. Schou M, Juel-Neilson N, Stromgren E, et al. The treatment of manic psychosis by the administration of lithium salts. *J Neurol Neurosurg Psychiatry* 1954;17:250–260.
3. Schou M. Normothymotics, "mood normalizers": are lithium and the imipramine drugs specific for affective disorders? *Br J Psychiatry* 1963;109:803–804.
4. Baastrup PC, Schou M. Prophylactic lithium. *Lancet* 1968;1:1419–1422.
5. Cade JFJ. The story of lithium. In: Ayd FJ Jr, Blackwell B, eds. *Discoveries in biological psychiatry.* Philadelphia: JB Lippincott, 1970:218–229.
6. Baastrup P, Poulsen KS, Schou M, et al. Prophylactic lithium: double-blind discontinuation in manic-depressive and recurrent-depressive disorders. *Lancet* 1970;2:326–330.
7. Baastrup PC. The use of lithium in manic-depressive psychosis. *Compr Psychiatry* 1964;5:396–408.
8. Baastrup PC. Lithium-behandling of mani-depressiv psykose: en psykoseforebyggende behandlingsmade (Lithium treatment of manic-depressive psychosis: a procedure for preventing psychotic relapses). *Nordisk Psykiatrisk Tiddskrift* 1966;20:441–450.
9. Hartigan GP. The use of lithium salts in affective disorders. *Br J Psychiatry* 1963;109:810–814.
10. Gershon S, Yuwiler A. Lithium ion: a specific psychopharmacological approach to the treatment of mania. *J Neuropsychiatry* 1960;1:229–241.
11. Janicak PG, Winans E. The use of copharmacy in the treatment of acute mania. *Dir Psychiatry* 1998;18:1–15.
12. Dehing J. Studies on the psychotropic action of tegretol. *Acta Neurol Belg* 1968;68:895–905.
13. Takezaki H, Hanaoka M. The use of carbamazepine (Tegretol) in the control of manic-depressive psychosis and other manic, depressive states [Japanese]. *Sheishin-Igaku* 1971;13:173–183.
14. Okuma T, Kishimoto A, Inoue K, et al. Anti-manic and prophylactic effects of carbamazepine on manic-depressive psychosis. *Folia Psychiatr Neurol Jpn* 1973;27:283–297.
15. Post RM, Ballenger JC, Reus VI, et al. Effects of carbamazepine in mania and depression. Presented at the Scientific Proceedings of the 131st Annual Meeting of the American Psychiatric Association, Atlanta, May 1978.
16. Lambert PA, Cavaz G, Barselli S, et al. Action neuropsychotrope d'un novel anti-epeliptique: le depamide. *Ann Med Psychol* 1966;1:707–710.
17. Janicak PG, Newman R, Davis JM. Advances in the treatment of mania and related disorders: a reappraisal. *Psychiatr Ann* 1992;22:92–103.
18. Janicak PG, Davis JM, Ayd FJ Jr, et al. Advances in the pharmacotherapy of bipolar disorder. In: Janicak PG, ed. *Principles and practice of psychopharmacotherapy update.* Baltimore: Williams & Wilkins, 1995:1(3).
19. Stoll AL, Severus E, Freeman MP, et al. Omega-3 fatty acids in bipolar disorder. *Arch Gen Psychiatry* 1999;56:407–412.
20. Manji HK, Lenox RH. Protein kinase C signaling in the brain: molecular transduction of mood stabilization in the treatment of manic-depressive illness. *Biol Psychiatry* 1999;46:1328–1351.
21. Schildkraut JJ. The catecholamine hypothesis of affective disorders (a review of supporting evidence). *Am J Psychiatry* 1965;122:509–522.
22. Bunney WE Jr, Davis JM. Norepinephrine in depressive reactions. *Arch Gen Psychiatry* 1965;13:483–494.
23. Akiskal HS. Mood disorders: introduction and overview. In: Sadock BJ, Sadock VA, eds. *Kaplan & Sadock's comprehensive textbook of psychiatry. Vol. 1,* 7th ed. Philadelphia: Lippincott Williams & Wilkins, 2000:1284–1298.
24. Kelsoe JR. Mood disorders: genetics. In: Sadock BJ, Sadock VA, eds. *Kaplan & Sadock's comprehensive textbook of psychiatry. Vol. 1,* 7th ed. Philadelphia: Lippincott Williams & Wilkins, 2000:1308–1318.
25. Pandey G, Davis JM. Treatment with antidepressants and down regulation of beta-adrenergic receptors. *Drug Dev Res* 1983;3:393–406.
26. Lee S, Chow CC, Wing YK, et al. Thyroid function and psychiatric morbidity in patients with manic disorder receiving lithium therapy. *J Clin Psychopharmacol* 2000;20:204–209.
27. Price LH, Charney DS, Delgado PL, et al. Lithium treatment and serotonergic function. *Arch Gen Psychiatry* 1989;46:13–19.
28. Hanin I, Mallinger AG, Kopp V, et al. Mechanism of lithium-induced elevation in red blood cell choline content: an *in vitro* analysis. *Commun Psychopharmacol* 1980;4:345–355.
29. Janowsky D, El Yousef MK, Davis JM, et al. A cholinergic-adrenergic hypothesis of mania and depression. *Lancet* 1972;2(778):632–635.
30. Burt T, Sachs G, Demopulos C. Donepezil in treatment-resistant bipolar disorder. *Biol Psychiatry* 1999;45:959–964.
31. Manji HK, Potter WZ, Lenox RH. Signal transduction pathways: molecular targets for lithium's actions. *Arch Gen Psychiatry* 1995;52:531–543.
32. Moore GJ, Bebchuk JM, Parrish JK, et al. Temporal dissociation between lithium-induced changes in frontal lobe myo-inositol and clinical response in manic-depressive illness. *Am J Psychiatry* 1999;156:1902–1908.
33. Ikonomov OC, Manji HK. Molecular mechanisms underlying mood stabilization in manic depressive illness: the phenotype challenge. *Am J Psychiatry* 1999;156:1506–1514.
34. Dubovsky SL, Murphy J, Thomas M, et al. Abnormal intracellular calcium ion concentration in platelets and lymphocytes of bipolar patients. *Am J Psychiatry* 1992;149:118–120.
35. Levy NA, Janicak PG. Calcium channel antagonists for the treatment of bipolar disorder. *Bipolar Disord* 2000;2:108–119.
36. Meltzer HL. Is there a specific membrane defect in bipolar disorders? *Biol Psychiatry* 1991;30:1071–1074.

37. Jeste DV, Lohr JB, Goodwin FK. Neuroanatomical studies of major affective disorders. A review and suggestions for further research. *Br J Psychiatry* 1988;153:444–459.

38. Swayze VW, Andreasen NC, Alliger RJ, et al. Structural brain abnormalities in bipolar affective disorder: ventricular enlargement and focal signal hyperintensities. *Arch Gen Psychiatry* 1990;47:1054–1059.

39. Dupont RM, Jernigan TL, Butler N, et al. Subcortical abnormalities detected in bipolar affective disorder using magnetic resonance imaging. Clinical and neuropsychological significance. *Arch Gen Psychiatry* 1990;47:55–59.

40. Silfverskiold P, Risberg J. Regional cerebral blood flow in depression and mania. *Arch Gen Psychiatry* 1989;46:253–259.

41. Salisbury DF, Sheraton ME, McCurley RW. P300 topography differs in schizophrenia and manic psychosis. *Biol Psychiatry* 1999;45:98–106.

42. Post RN, Roy-Byrne PP, Uhde TW. Graphic representation of the life course of illness in patients with affective disorder. *Am J Psychiatry* 1988;145:844–848.

43. Post RM, Weiss SRB. Sensitization, kindling, and anticonvulsants in mania. *J Clin Psychiatry* 1989;50(Suppl 12):23–30.

44. Ghaemi SN, Boiman EE, Goodwin FK. Kindling and second messengers: an approach to the neurobiology of recurrence in bipolar disorder. *Biol Psychiatry* 1999;45:137–144.

45. Goodwin FK, Jamison KR. *Manic depressive illness.* New York: Oxford University Press, 1990.

46. Hudson JI, Lipinski JF, Keck PE, et al. Polysomnographic characteristics of young manic patients. Comparison with unipolar depressed patients and normal control subjects. *Arch Gen Psychiatry* 1992;49:378–383.

47. Dinan TG, Yatham LM, O'Keane V, et al. Blunting of noradrenergic-stimulated growth hormone release in mania. *Am J Psychiatry* 1991;148:936–938.

48. Linkowski P, Kerkhofs M, Onderbergen AV, et al. The 24-hour profile of cortisol, prolactin, and growth hormone secretion in mania. *Arch Gen Psychiatry* 1994;51:616–624.

49. Cassidy F, Ritchie JC, Carroll BJ. Plasma dexamethasone concentration and cortisol response during manic episodes. *Biol Psychiatry* 1998;43:747–754.

50. Whybrow PC, Prange AJ. A hypothesis of thyroid-catecholamine-receptor interaction: its relevance to affective illness. *Arch Gen Psychiatry* 1981;38:106–113.

51. Joffe RT, Roy-Byrne PP, Udhe TW, et al. Thyroid function and affective illness: a reappraisal. *Biol Psychiatry* 1984;19:1685–1691.

52. Kronfol Z, House DJ. Immune function in mania. *Biol Psychiatry* 1988;24:341–343.

53. Tsai S, Chen K, Yang Y, et al. Activation of cell-mediated immunity in bipolar mania. *Biol Psychiatry* 1999;45:989–994.

54. Davis JM, Noll KM, Sharma R. Differential diagnosis and treatment of mania. In: Swann AC, ed. *Mania: new research and treatment.* Washington, DC: American Psychiatric Press, 1986:1–58.

55. Mendlewicz J, Fieve RR, Rainer JD, et al. Manic-depressive illness: a comparative study of patients with and without a family history. *Br J Psychiatry* 1972;120:523–530.

56. Mendlewicz J, Rainer JD. Adoption study supporting genetic transmission in manic-depressive illness. *Nature* 1977;268:327–329.

57. Dorus E, Paney GN, Davis JM. Genetic determinant of lithium ion distribution. *Arch Gen Psychiatry* 1975;32:1097–1102.

58. Dorus E, Pandey GN, Shaughnessy R, et al. Lithium abnormality across red cell membrane: a cell membrane abnormality in manic-depressive illness. *Science* 1979;205:932–934.

59. Garver DL, Hitzemann R, Hirschowitz J. Lithium ratio *in vitro. Arch Gen Psychiatry* 1984;41:497–505.

60. Dorus E, Cox NJ, Gibbons RD, et al. Lithium ion transport and affective disorders within families of bipolar patients. *Arch Gen Psychiatry* 1983;40:545–552.

61. Gibbons RD, Dorus E, Ostrow DG, et al. Mixture distributions in psychiatric research. *Biol Psychiatry* 1984;19:935–961.

62. Risch N, Baron M. X-linkage and genetic heterogeneity in bipolar-related major affective illness: reanalysis of linkage data. *Ann Hum Genet* 1982;46:153–166.

63. Baron M, Risch N, Hamburger R, et al. Genetic linkage between X-chromosome markers and bipolar affective disorders. *Nature* 1987;326:289–292.

64. Kelsoe JR, Ginns EI, Egeland JA, et al. Re-evaluation of the linkage relationship between chromosome 11p loci and the gene for bipolar affective disorder in the Old Order Amish. *Nature* 1989;342:238–242.

65. Turner WJ, King S. Two genetically distinct forms of bipolar affective disorder. *Biol Psychiatry* 1981;16:417–439.

66. Berretini W. Diagnostic and genetic issues of depression and bipolar illness. *Pharmacotherapy* 1995;15:695–755.

67. deBruyn A, Souesy D, Mendelbaum K, et al. Linkage analysis of families with bipolar illness and chromosome 18 markers. *Biol Psychiatry* 1996;39:679–688.

68. Vallada H, Craddock N, Vasques L, et al. Linkage studies in bipolar affective disorder with markers on chromosome 21. *J Affect Disord* 1996;41:217–221.

69. Berrettini WH, Ferraro TN, Goldin LR, et al. A linkage study of bipolar illness . *Arch Gen Psychiatry* 1997;54:27–35.

70. Gershon ES. Bipolar illness and schizophrenia in oligogenic diseases: implications for the future. *Biol Psychiatry* 2000;47:240–244.

71. Berrettini WH. Susceptibility loci for bipolar disorder: overlap with inherited vulnerability to schizophrenia. *Biol Psychiatry* 2000;47:245–251.

72. Solomon DA, Keitner GI, Miller IW, et al. Course of illness and maintenance treatments for patients with bipolar disorder. *J Clin Psychiatry* 1995;56:5–13.

73. Nilsson A. Lithium therapy and suicide risk. *J Clin Psychiatry* 1999;60(suppl 2): 85–88.

74. Tondo L, Baldessarini RJ. Reduced suicide risk during lithium maintenance treatment. *J Clin Psychiatry* 2000;61(suppl 9):97–104.

75. Hurowitz GI, Liebowitz MR. Antidepressant-induced rapid cycling: six case reports . *J Clin Psychopharmacol* 1993;13:52–56.

76. Altshuler LL, Post RM, Leverich GS, et al. Antidepressant induced mania and cycle acceleration: a controversy revisited. *Am J Psychiatry* 1995;152:1130–1138.

77. Janicak PG, Munson LG. Practical management of adverse effects associated with mood stabilizers. In: Balon R, ed. *Adverse effects of mood stabilizers: practical management of the side effects of psychotropic drugs.* New York: Marcel Dekker, 1999:119–143.

78. Bunney WE, Goodwin FK, Davis JM, et al. A behavioral-biochemical study of lithium treatment. *Am J Psychiatry* 1968;125:499–512.

79. Goodwin FK, Murphy DL, Bunney WE. Lithium. *Lancet* 1969;79:212–213.

80. Maggs R. Treatment of manic illness with lithium carbonate. *Br J Psychiatry* 1963;109:562–565.

81. Stokes PE, Stoll PM, Shamoian CH. Efficacy of lithium as acute treatment of manic-depressive illness. *Lancet* 1971;1:1319–1325.

82. Stokes P, Kocsis J, Arcuni O. Relationship of lithium chloride dose to treatment response in acute mania. *Arch Gen Psychiatry* 1976;33:1080–1085.

83. Bowden CL, Brugger AM, Swann AC, et al. Efficacy of divalproex vs lithium and placebo in the treatment of mania. *JAMA* 1994;271:918–924.

84. Johnson G, Gershon S, Hekimian LJ. Controlled evaluation of lithium and chlorpromazine in the treatment of manic states: an interim report. *Compr Psychiatry* 1968;9:563.

85. Johnson G, Gershon S, Burdock EI. Comparative effects of lithium and chlorpromazine in the treatment of acute manic states. *Br J Psychiatry* 1971; 119:267.

86. Spring G, Schweid D, Gray L. A double-blind comparison of lithium and chlorpromazine in the treatment of manic states. *Am J Psychiatry* 1970;126:1306–1310.

87. Takahashi R, Sakuma A, Itoh K. Comparison of efficacy of lithium carbonate and chlorpromazine in mania. *Arch Gen Psychiatry* 1975;32:1310–1318.

88. Shopsin B, Kim SS, Gershon S. A controlled study of lithium vs. chlorpromazine in acute schizophrenia. *Br J Psychiatry* 1971;119:435–440.

89. Rifkin A, Doddi, S, Karajgi B, et al. Dosage of haloperidol for mania. *Br J Psychiatry* 1994;165:113–116.

90. Janicak PG, Javaid JI, Sharma RP, et al. A two-phase double-blind randomized study of three haloperidol palsma levels for acute psychosis with management of initial non-responders. *Acta Psychiatr Scand* 1997;95:343–350.

91. Schou M. *Lithium treatment of manic-depressive illness: a practical guide,* 3rd ed. Basel, Switzerland: Karger, 1986.

92. Platman SR. A comparison of lithium carbonate and chlorpromazine in mania. *Am J Psychiatry* 1970;127:351–353.

93. Prien RF, Caffey EM, Klett CJ. Comparison of lithium carbonate and chlorpromazine in the treatment of mania. *Arch Gen Psychiatry* 1972,26:146–153.

94. Garfinkel PE, Stancer HC, Persad E. A comparison of haloperidol, lithium carbonate, and their combination in the treatment of mania. *J Affect Disord* 1980;2:279–288.

95. Braden W, Fink EB, Qualls CB, et al. Lithium and chlorpromazine in psychotic inpatients. *Psychiatry Res* 1982;7:69–81.

96. Cookson J, Silverstone T, Wells B. Double-blind comparative clinical trial of pimozide and chlorpromazine in mania. *Acta Psychiatr Scand* 1981;64:381–397.

97. Post RM, Jimerson DC, Bunney WE, et al. Dopamine and mania: behavioral and biochemical effects of the dopamine receptor blocker pimozide. *Psychopharmacology* 1980;67:297–305.

98. Johnstone EC, Crow TJ, Frith CD, et al. The Northwick Park "functional" psychosis study: diagnosis and treatment response. *Lancet* 1988;2:119–125.

99. Freeman TW, Clothier JL, Pazzaglia P, et al. A double-blind comparison of valproate and lithium in the treatment of acute mania. *Am J Psychiatry* 1992;149:108–111.

100. Small JG, Klapper MH, Milstein V, et al. Carbamazepine compared with lithium in the treatment of mania. *Arch Gen Psychiatry* 1991;48:915–921.

101. Zetin M, Garber D, De Antonio M, et al. Prediction of lithium dose: a mathematical alternative to the test-dose method. *J Clin Psychiatry* 1986;47:175–178.

102. Markoff RA, King M Jr. Does lithium dose prediction improve treatment efficiency? Prospective evaluation of a mathematical method. *J Clin Psychopharmacol* 1992;12:305–308.

103. Terao T, Okuno K, Okuno T, et al. A simple and more accurate equation to predict daily lithium dose. *J Clin Psychopharmacol* 1999;19:336–340.

104. Baldessarini RJ, Katz B, Cotton P. Dissimilar dosing with high potency and low potency neuroleptics. *Am J Psychiatry* 1984;141:748–752.

105. Janicak PG, Bresnahan DB, Sharma RP, et al. A comparison of thiothixene with chlorpromazine in the treatment of mania. *J Clin Psychopharmacol* 1988;8:33–37.

106. Suppes T, Phillips KA, Judd CR. Clozapine treatment of nonpsychotic rapid cycling bipolar disorder: a report of three cases. *Biol Psychiatry* 1994;36:338–340.

107. Hillert A, Maier W, Wetzel H, et al. Risperidone in the treatment of disorders with a combined psychotic and depressive syndrome—a functional approach. *Pharmacopsychiatry* 1992;25:213–217.

108. Suppes T, McElroy SL, Gilbert J, et al. Clozapine in the treatment of dysphoric mania. *Biol Psychiatry* 1992;32:270–280.

109. McElroy SL, Dessain EC, Pope HG, et al. Clozapine in the treatment of psychotic mood disorders, schizoaffective disorder, and schizophrenia. *J Clin Psychiatry* 1991;52:411–414.

110. Kando JC, Tohen M, Castillo J, et al. Concurrent use of clozapine and valproate in affective and psychotic disorders. *J Clin Psychiatry* 1994;55:255–257.

111. Sassim N, Grohmann R. Adverse drug reactions with clozapine and simultaneous application of benzodiazepines. *Pharmacopsychiatry* 1988;21:306–307.

112. Tohen M, Sanzer TM, McElroy SL, et al. Olanzapine versus placebo in the treatment of acute mania. *Am J Psychiatry* 1999;156:702–709.

113. Janicak PG, Verma M, Martis B. Antipsychotics in the treatment of mood disorders: part I. *Int Drug Ther Newsl* 1999;34:73–80.

114. Janicak PG, Verma M, Martis B. Antipsychotics in the treatment of mood disorders: part II. *Int Drug Ther Newsl* 1999;34:81–88.

115. Sernyak MJ, Johnson R, Griffin R, et al. Neuroleptic exposure following inpatient treatment of acute mania with lithium and neuroleptic. *Am J Psychiatry* 1994;151:133–135.

116. Sernyak MJ, Godleski LS, Griffin RA, et al. Chronic neuroleptic exposure in bipolar outpatients. *J Clin Psychiatry* 1997;58:193–195.

117. Easton M, Janicak P. The use of benzodiazepines in psychotic disorders: a review of the literature. *Psychiatr Ann* 1990;20:535–544.

118. Lenox RH, Newhouse PA, Creelman WL, et al. Adjunctive treatment of manic agitation with lorazepam versus haloperidol: a double-blind study. *J Clin Psychiatry* 1992;53:47–52.

119. Bradwejn J, Shriqui C, Koszycki D, et al. Double-blind comparison of the effects of clonazepam and lorazepam in acute mania. *J Clin Psychopharmacol* 1990;10:403–408.

120. Chouinard G. Clonazepam in the acute and maintenance treatment of bipolar affective disorder. *J Clin Psychiatry* 1987;48(Suppl 10):29–36.

121. Janicak PG. Copharmacy strategies for bipolar disorder. *Psychiatr Ann* 1998;28:357–363.

122. Joffe R, Levitt A, Bagby M, et al. Predictors of response to lithium and triiodothyronine augmentation of antidepressants in tricyclic non-responders. *Br J Psychiatry* 1993;163:574–578.

123. Garbutt J, Mayo J, Gillette G, et al. Lithium potentiation of tricyclic antidepressants following lack of T3 potentiation. *Am J Psychiatry* 1986;143:1038–1039.

124. Schöpf J, Lemarchand T. Lithium addition in endogenous depressions resistant to tricyclic antidepressants or related drugs: relation to the status of the pituitarythyroid axis. *Pharmacopsychiatry* 1994;27:198–201.

125. Kusalic M. Grade II and grade III hypothyroidism in rapid-cycling bipolar patients. *Neuropsychobiology* 1992;25:177–181.

126. Bauer MS, Whybrow PC. Rapid cycling bipolar affective disorder. II. Treatment of refractory rapid cycling with high-dose levothyroxine: a preliminary study. *Arch Gen Psychiatry* 1990;47:435–440.

127. Afflelou S, Auriacombe M, Cazenave M, et al. Administration of high dose levothyroxine in treatment of rapid cycling bipolar disorders. Review of the literature and initial therapeutic apropos of 6 cases. *Encephale* 1997;23:207–217.

128. Ballenger JC. The use of anticonvulsants in manic-depressive illness. *J Clin Psychiatry* 1988;49(Suppl 11):21–25.

129. Post RM. Introduction: emerging perspectives on valproate in affective disorders. *J Clin Psychiatry* 1989;50(Suppl 3):3–9.

130. Post RM, Berrettini W, Uhde TW. Selective response to the anticonvulsant carbamazepine in manic-depressive illness: a case study. *J Clin Psychopharmacol* 1984;4:178–185.

131. Pope HG Jr, McElroy SL, Keck PE, et al. A placebo-controlled study of valproate in mania. *Arch Gen Psychiatry* 1991;48:62–68.

132. Brennan MJW, Sandyk R, Borsook D. Use of sodium valproate in the management of affective disorders: basic and clinical aspects. In: Emrich HM, Okuma T, Muller AA, eds. *Anticonvulsants in affective disorders.* Amsterdam: Excerpta Medica, 1984:56–65.

133. Emrich HM, Dose M, Zerssen DV. The use of sodium valproate, carbamazepine, and oxcarbazepine in patients with affective disorders. *J Affect Disord* 1985;8:243–250.

134. McElroy SL, Keck PE, Pope HG, et al. Correlates of antimanic response to valproate. *Psychopharmacol Bull* 1991;27:127–133.

135. Bowden CL, Brugger AM, Swann AC, et al. Efficacy of divalproex vs lithium and placebo in the treatment of mania. *JAMA* 1994;271:918–924.

136. Calabrese JR, Woyshville MJ, Kimmel SE, et al. Predictors of valproate response in bipolar rapid cycling. *J Clin Psychopharmacol* 1993;13:280–283.

137. Papatheodorou G, Kutcher SP. Divalproex sodium treatment in late adolescent and young adult acute mania. *Psychopharmacol Bull* 1993;29:213–219.

138. Papatheodorou G, Kutcher SP, Katic M, et al. The efficacy and safety of divalproex sodium in the treatment of acute mania in adolescents and young adults: an open clinical trial. *J Clin Psychopharmacol* 1995;15:110–116.

139. Deltito JA, Levitan J, Damore J, et al. Naturalistic experience with the use of divalproex sodium on an inpatient unit for adolescent psychiatric patients. *Acta Psychiatr Scand* 1998;97:236–240.

140. Risinger RC, Risby ED, Risch SC. Safety and efficacy of divalproex sodium in elderly bipolar patients [Letter]. *J Clin Psychiatry* 1994;55:215.

141. Stoll AL, Banov M, Kollerener M, et al. Neurologic factors predict a favorable valproate response in bipolar and schizoaffective disorders. *J Clin Psychopharmacol* 1994;14:311–313.

142. Rosenthal RN, Perkel C, Singh P, et al. A pilot open randomized trial of valproate and phenobarbital in the treatment of acute alcohol withdrawal. *Am J Addict* 1998;7:189–197.

143. Muller-Oerlinghausen B, Retzow A, Henn FA, et al. Valproate as an adjunct to neuroleptic medication for the treatment of acute episodes of mania: a prospective, randomized, double-blind, placebo-controlled, multicenter study. *J Clin Psychopharmacol* 2000;20:195–203.

144. Baetz M, Bowen RC. Efficacy of divalproex sodium in patients with panic disorder and mood instability who have not responded to conventional therapy. *Can J Psychiatry* 1998;43:73–77.

145. Clark RD, Canive JM, Calais LA, et al. Divalproex in posttraumatic stress disorder: an open-label clinical trial. *J Trauma Stress* 1999;12:395–401.

146. Kavoussi RJ, Coccaro EF. Divalproex sodium for impulsive aggressive behavior in patients with personality disorder. *J Clin Psychiatry* 1998;59:676–680.

147. Herrmann N. Valproic acid treatment of agitation in dementia. *Can J Psychiatry* 1998;43:69–72.

148. Narayan M, Nelson JC. Treatment of dementia with behavioral disturbance using divalproex or a combination of divalproex and a neuroleptic. *J Clin Psychiatry* 1997;58:351–354.

148a. Wassef AA, Hafiz NG, Hampton D, Malloy M. DVPX sodium augmentation of haloperidol in hospitalized patients with schizophrenia: clinical and economic implications. *J Clin Psychopharmacol* 2001;21:21–26.

149. Bowden CL, Janicak PG, Orsulak P, et al. Relationship of serum valporate concentration to response in mania. *Am J Psychiatry* 1996;153:765–770.

150. Keck PE, McElroy SL, Tugrul KC, et al. Valproate oral loading in the treatment of acute mania. *J Clin Psychiatry* 1993;54:305–308.

151. Hirschfeld RM, Allen MH, McEvoy JP, et al. Safety and tolerability of oral loading divalproex sodium in acutely manic bipolar patients. *J Clin Psychiatry* 1999;60:815–818.

152. Martinez JM, Russell JM, Hirschfeld RM. Tolerability of oral loading of divalproex sodium in the treatment of acute mania. *Depress Anxiety* 1998;7:83–86.

153. Norton JW, Quarles E. Intravenous valproate in neuropsychiatry. *Pharmacotherapy* 2000;20:88–92.

154. Grunze H, Erfurth A, Amann B, et al. Intravenous valproate loading in acutely manic and depressed bipolar I patients. *J Clin Psychopharmacol* 1999;19:303–309.

155. Wassef A, Watson DJ, Morrison P, et al. Neuroleptic-valproic acid combination in treatment of psychotic symptoms: a three-case report. *J Clin Psychopharmacol* 1989;9:45–48.

156. McFarland BH, Miller MR, Straumfjord AA. Valproate use in the older manic patient. *J Clin Psychiatry* 1990;51:479–481.

157. Chen ST, Altshuler LL, Melnyk KA, et al. Efficacy of lithium vs. valproate in the treatment of mania in the elderly: a retrospective study. *J Clin Psychiatry* 1999;60:181–186.

158. Baastrup P, Schou M. Lithium as a prophylactic agent. *Arch Gen Psychiatry* 1967;16:162–172.

159. Schou M, Thomsen K, Baastrup PC. Studies on the course of recurrent endogenous affective disorders. *Int Pharmacopsychiatry* 1970;5:100–106.

160. Davis JM, Janicak PG, Hogan DM. Mood stabilizers in the prevention of recurrent affective disorders: a meta-analysis. *Acta Psychiatr Scand* 1999;100:406–417.

161. Suppes T, Baldessarini RJ, Faedda GL, et al. Risk of recurrence following discontinuation of lithium treatment in bipolar disorder. *Arch Gen Psychiatry* 1991;48:1082–1088.

162. Post RM, Leverich GS, Altshuler L, et al. Lithium-discontinuation refractoriness: preliminary observations. *Am J Psychiatry* 1992;149:1727–1729.

163. Young LT, Joffe RT, Robb JC, et al. Double-blind comparison of addition of a second mood stabilizer versus an antidepressant to an initial mood stabilizer for treatment of patients with bipolar depression. *Am J Psychiatry* 2000;157:124–126.

164. Gelenberg AJ, Kane JM, Keller MB, et al. Comparison of standard and low levels of lithium for maintenance treatment of bipolar disorder. *N Engl J Med* 1989;321:1489–1493.

165. Faedda GL, Tondo L, Baldessarini RJ, et al. Outcome after rapid vs. gradual discontinuation of lithium treatment in bipolar disorders. *Arch Gen Psychiatry* 1993;50:448–455.

166. Shaw E. Lithium noncompliance. *Psychiatr Ann* 1986;16:583–587.

167. Regier DA, Farmer ME, Rae DS, et al. Comorbidity of mental disorders with alcohol and other drug abuse. Results from the epidemiologic catchment area (ECA) study. *JAMA* 1990;264:2511–2518.

168. Mander AJ. Use of lithium and early relapse in manic-depressive illness. *Acta Psychiatr Scand* 1988;78:198–200.

169. Harrow M, Goldberg JF, Grossman LS, et al. Outcome in manic disorders. A naturalistic follow-up study. *Arch Gen Psychiatry* 1990;47:665–671.

170. Goldberg JF, Harrow M, Grossman LS. Course and outcome in bipolar affective disorder: a longitudinal follow-up study. *Am J Psychiatry* 1995;152:379–384.

171. Dion GL, Tohen M, Anthony WA, et al. Symptoms and functioning of patients with bipolar disorder six months after hospitalization. *Hosp Commun Psychiatry* 1988;39:652–657.

172. Prien RF, Caffey EM Jr, Klett CJ. Prophylactic efficacy of lithium carbonate in manic-depressive illness. *Arch Gen Psychiatry* 1973;28:337–341.

173. Prien RF, Caffey EM Jr, Klett CJ. Factors associated with lithium responses in the prophylactic treatment of bipolar manic-depressive illness. *Arch Gen Psychiatry* 1974;31:189–192.

174. Mendlewicz J, Fieve R, Stallone F. Relationship between effectiveness of lithium therapy and family history. *Am J Psychiatry* 1973;130:1011–1013.

175. Stallone F, Shelley E, Mendlewicz J, et al. The use of lithium in affective disorders: III. A double-blind study of prophylaxis in bipolar illness. *Am J Psychiatry* 1973;130:1006–1010.

176. Coppen A, Noguera R, Bailey J, et al. Prophylactic lithium in affective disorders. *Lancet* 1971;2:275–279.

177. Coppen A, Peet M, Bailey J, et al. Double-blind and open prospective studies of lithium prophylaxis in affective disorders. *Psychiatr Neurol Neurochir* 1963;76:500–510.

178. Cundall RL, Brooks PW, Murray LG. A controlled evaluation of lithium prophylaxis in affective disorders. *Psychol Med* 1972;2:308–311.

179. Persson G. Lithium prophylaxis in affective disorders: an open trial with matched controls. *Acta Psychiatr Scand* 1972;48:462–479.

180. Mander AJ, Louden JB. Rapid recurrence of mania following abrupt discontinuation of lithium. *Lancet* 1988;2:15–17.

181. Shapiro DR, Quitkin FM, Fleiss JL. Response to maintenance therapy in bipolar illness. *Arch Gen Psychiatry* 1989;46:401–405.

182. Prien RF, Kupfer DJ, Mansky PA, et al. Drug therapy in the prevention of recurrences in unipolar and bipolar affective disorders. Report of the NIMH Collaborative Study Group comparing lithium carbonate, imipramine, and a lithium carbonate-imipramine combination. *Arch Gen Psychiatry* 1984;41:1096–1104.

183. Strober M, Morrell W, Lampert C, et al. Relapse following discontinuation of lithium maintenance therapy in adolescents with Bipolar I illness: a naturalistic study. *Am J Psychiatry* 1990;147:457–461.

184. Angst J, Weiss P, Grof P, et al. Lithium prophylaxis in recurrent affective disorders. *Br J Psychiatry* 1970;116:604–614.

185. Schou M, Baastrup PC, Grof P, et al. Pharmacological and clinical problems of lithium prophylaxis. *Br J Psychiatry* 1970;116:615–619.

186. Grof P, Schou M, Angst J, et al. Methodological problems of prophylactic trials in recurrent affective disorders. *Br J Psychiatry* 1970;116:599–603.

187. Aagaard J, Vestergaard P. Predictors of outcome prophylactic lithium treatment: a 2-year prospective study. *J Affect Disord* 1990;18:259–266.

188. Maj M, Pirozzi R, Kemali D. Long-term outcome of lithium prophylaxis in patients initially classified as complete responders. *Psychopharmacology* 1989;98:535–538.

189. Cochran SD, Gitlin MJ. Attitudinal correlates of lithium compliance in bipolar affective disorders. *J Nerv Ment Dis* 1988;176:457–467.

190. Lepkifker E, Horesh N, Floru S. Life satisfaction and adjustment in lithium-treated affective patients in remission. *Acta Psychiatr Scand* 1988;78:391–395.

191. Coppen A, Standish-Barry H, Bailey J, et al. Long-term lithium and mortality. *Lancet* 1990;335:1347.

192. Schou M, Weeke A. Did manic depressive patients who committed suicide receive prophylactic or continuation treatment at the time? *Br J Psychiatry* 1988;153:324–327.

193. Prien RF, Potter WZ. NIMH workshop report on treatment of bipolar disorder. *Psychopharmacol Bull* 1990; 26:409–427.

194. Solomon DA, Ryan CE, Keitner GI, et al. A pilot study of lithium carbonate plus divalproex sodium for the continuation and maintenance treatment of patients with bipolar I disorder. *J Clin Psychiatry* 1997;58:95–99.

195. *Physicians' desk reference,* 51st ed. Montvale, NJ: Medical Economics, 1997:417.

196. Bowden CL, Calabrese JR, McElroy SL, et al. A randomized, placebo-controlled 12-month trial of divalproex and lithium of outpatients with bipolar I disorder. Divalproex Maintenance Study Group. *Arch Gen Psychiatry* 2000;57:481–489.

197. Gyulai L, Bowden CL, Calabrese JR, et al. Efficacy of divalproex in the prevention of depression in patients with bipolar I disorder over a 12-month period. Presented at the American Psychiatric Association Annual Meeting, Chicago, May 13–18, 2000.

198. Schou M. Lithium prophylaxis: myths and realities. *Am J Psychiatry* 1989;146:573–576.

199. Mishory A, Yaroslavsky Y, Bersudsky Y, et al. Phenytoin as an antimanic antoconvulsant: a controlled study. *Am J Psychiatry* 2000;157:463–465.

200. Ketter TA, Pazzaglia PJ, Post RM. Synergy of carbamazepine and valproic acid in affective illness: case report and review of the literature. *J Clin Psychopharmacol* 1992;12:276–281.

201. Freeman MP, Stoll AL. Mood stabilizer combinations: a review of safety and efficacy. *Am J Psychiatry* 1998;155:12–21.

202. Post RM. Non-lithium treatment for bipolar disorder. *J Clin Psychiatry* 1990;51(Suppl 8):9–16.

203. Post RM. Alternatives to lithium for bipolar affective illness. In: Tasman A, Goldfinger S, Kaufman C, eds. *American Psychiatric Press review of psychiatry. Vol 9.* Washington, DC: APA Press, 1990:170–202.

204. Chou JCY. Recent advances in the treatment of acute mania. *J Clin Psychopharmacol* 1990;11:3–21.

205. Lindenmayer J-P, Kotsaftis A. Use of sodium valproate in violent and aggressive behaviors: a critical review. *J Clin Psychiatry* 2000;61:123–128.

206. Post RM, Uhde TW. Carbamazepine in bipolar illness. *Psychopharmacol Bull* 1985;21:10–17.

207. Goncalves N, Stoll KD. Carbamazepin bei manischen Syndromen. *Nervenarzt* 1985;56:43–47.

208. Lerer B, Moore M, Meyendorff E, et al. Carbamazepine versus lithium in mania: a double-blind study. *J Clin Psychiatry* 1987;48:89–93.

209. Okuma T, Inanaga K, Otsuki S, et al. Comparison of the antimanic efficacy of carbamazepine and chlorpromazine: a double-blind controlled study. *Psychopharmacology* 1979;66:211–217.

210. Grossi E, Sacchetti E, Vita A, et al. Carbamazepine versus chlorpromazine in mania: a double-blind trial. In: Emrich HM, Okuma T, Muller AA, eds. *Anticonvulsants in affective disorders.* Amsterdam: Excerpta Medica, 1984:177–187.

211. Sethi BB, Tiwari SC. Carbamazepine in affective disorders. In: Emrich HM, Okuma T, Muller AA, eds. *Anticonvulsants in affective disorders.* Amsterdam: Excerpta Medica, 1984:167–177.

212. Okuma T, Yamashita I, Takahashi R, et al. A double-blind study of adjunctive carbamazepine versus placebo on excited states of schizophrenia and schizoaffective disorder. *Acta Psychiatr Scand* 1989;80:250–259.

213. Nolen WA. Carbamazepine: an alternative in lithium-resistant bipolar disorder. In: Emrich HM, Okuma T, Muller AA, eds. *Anticonvulsants in affective disorders.* Amsterdam: Excerpta Medica, 1984;132–138.

214. Kramlinger KG, Post RM. Adding lithium carbonate to carbamazepine: antimanic efficacy in treatment-resistant mania. *Acta Psychiatr Scand* 1989;79:378–385.

215. Klein E, Bental E, Lerer B, et al. Carbamazepine and haloperidol versus placebo and haloperidol in excited psychoses. *Arch Gen Psychiatry* 1984;41:165–170.

216. Mueller AA, Stoll KD. Carbamazepine and oxcarbazepine in the treatment of manic syndromes: studies in Germany. In: Emrich HM, Okuma T, Muller AA, eds. *Anticonvulsants in affective disorders.* Amsterdam: Excerpta Medica, 1984:139–147.

217. Lenzi A, Grossi E, Massimetti G, et al. Use of carbamazepine in acute psychosis: a controlled study. *J Int Med Res* 1986;14:78–84.

218. Lusznat RM, Murphy DP, Nunn CMH. Carbamazepine vs. lithium in the treatment and prophylaxis of mania. *Br J Psychiatry* 1988;153:198–204.

219. Prien RF, Gelenberg AJ. Alternatives to lithium for preventive treatment of bipolar disorder. *Am J Psychiatry* 1989;146:840–848.

220. Placidi GF, Lenzi A, Lazzerini F, et al. The comparative efficacy and safety of carbamezepine versus lithium: a randomized, double-blind 3-year trial in 83 patients. *J Clin Psychiatry* 1986;47:490–494.

221. Watkins SE, Callender K, Thomas DR, et al. The effect of carbamazepine and lithium on remission from affective illness. *Br J Psychiatry* 1987;150:180–182.

222. Stoll KD, Goncalves N, Krober HL, et al. Use of carbamazepine in affective illness. In: Lerer B, Gershon S, eds. *New directions in affective disorders.* New York: Springer-Verlag, 1989:540–544.

223. Cabrera JF, Muhlbauer HD, Schley J, et al. Long-term randomized clinical trial on oxcarbamazepine vs. lithium in bipolar and schizoaffective disorders: preliminary results. *Pharmacopsychiatry* 1986;19:282–283.

224. Coxhead N, Silverstone T, Cookson J. Carbamazepine versus lithium in the prophylaxis of bipolar affective disorder. *Acta Psychiatr Scand* 1992;85:114–118.

225. Simhandl C, Denk E, Thau. The comparative efficacy of carbamazepine low and high serum level and lithium carbonate in the prophylaxis of affective disorders. *J Affect Disord* 1993;28:221–231.

226. Stuppaek C, Barnas C, Schwitzer J, et al. The role of carbamazepine in the prophylaxis of unipolar depression. *Neuropsychobiology* 1993;27:154–157.

227. Keck PE Jr, McElroy SL, Strakowski SM. Anticonvulsants and antipsychotics in the treatment of bipolar disorder. *J Clin Psychiatry* 1998;59(suppl 6): 74–81.

228. Anand A, Charney DS, Oren DA. Attenuation of the neuropsychiatric effects of ketamine with lamotrigine. Support for hyperglutamatergic effects of *N*-methyl-D-aspartate receptor antagonists. *Arch Gen Psychiatry* 2000;57:270–276.

229. Suppes T, Brown ES, McElroy SL, et al. Lamotrigine for the treatment of bipolar disorder: a clinical case series. *J Affect Disord* 1999;53:95–98.

230. Calabrese JR, Bowden CL, Sachs GS, et al. A double-blind placebo-controlled study of lamotrigine monotherapy in outpatients with bipolar I depression. *J Clin Psychiatry* 1999;60:79–88.

231. Earl NL, Greene P, Ascher J, et al. Mood stabilization with lamotrigine in rapid-cycling bipolar disorder. Presented at the American Psychiatric Association Annual Meeting, Chicago, May 13–18, 2000.

232. Greene P, Earl NL, Monaghan E, et al. Mood stabilization with lamotrigine in rapid-cycling bipolar disorder: a double-blind, placebo-controlled study. Presented at the American Psychiatric Association Annual Meeting, Chicago, May 13–18, 2000.

233. Wong IC, Mawer GE, Sander JW. Factors influencing the incidence of lamotrigine-related skin rash. *Ann Pharmacother* 1999;33:1037–1042.

234. McElroy SL, Soutullo CA, Keck PE Jr, et al. A pilot trial of adjunctive gabapentin in the treatment of bipolar disorder. *Ann Clin Psychiatry* 1997;9:99–103.

235. Frye MA, Ketter TA, Leverich GS, et al. The increasing use of polypharmacotherapy for refractory mood disorders: 22 years of study. *J Clin Psychiatry* 2000;61: 9–15.

236. Marcotte D. Use of topiramate, a new anti-epileptic as a mood stabilizer. *J Affect Disord* 1998;50:245–251.

237. Glauser TA. Topiramate. *Epilepsia* 1999;40(suppl 5):S71–S80.

238. Eads LA, Kramer T, Wooten G. Use of topiramate as a mood stabilizer. Presented at the American Psychiatric Association Annual Meeting, Chicago, May 13–18, 2000.

239. Hussain M, Chaudhry Z. Treatment of bipolar depression with topiramate [Abstract]. Presented at the XI World Congress of Psychiatry, Hamburg, Germany, August 6–11, 1999; [free communication] 41–45, 58.

240. Calabrese JR. Update on the use of topiramate in bipolar disorder. Presented at the American Psychiatric Association 2000 Annual Meeting, Chicago, May 13–18, 2000.

241. Grunze H, Erfuth A, Marcuse A, et al. Tiagabine appears not to be efficacious in the treatment of acute mania. *J Clin Psychiatry* 1999;60:759–762.

242. Rennie TAC. Manic-depressive disease: prognosis following shock treatment. *Psychiatr Q* 1943;17:642–654.

243. Thorpe FT. Intensive electrical convulsive therapy in acute mania. *J Mental Sci* 1947;93:89–92.

244. Mukherjee S, Sackeim HA, Schnur DB. Electroconvulsive therapy of acute manic episodes: a review of 50 years' experience. *Am J Psychiatry* 1994;151:169–176.

245. Schnur DB, Mukherjee S, Sackeim HA, et al. Symptomatic predictors of ECT response in medication-nonresponsive manic patients. *J Clin Psychiatry* 1992;53:63–66.

246. McCabe MS. ECT in the treatment of mania: a controlled study. *Am J Psychiatry* 1976;133:688–691.

247. Black DW, Winokur G, Nasrallah H. Treatment of mania: a naturalistic study of ECT versus lithium in 438 patients. *J Clin Psychiatry* 1987;48:132–139.

248. Small JG, Klapper MH, Kellams JJ, et al. ECT compared with lithium in the management of manic states. *Arch Gen Psychiatry* 1988;45:727–732.

249. Mukherjee S, Sackeim HA, Lee C. Unilateral ECT in the treatment of manic episodes. *Convuls Ther* 1988;4:74–80.

250. Milstein V, Small JG, Klapper MH, et al. Uni- versus bilateral ECT in the treatment of mania. *Convuls Ther* 1987;3:1–9.

251. Janicak PG, Sharma RP, Pandey G, et al. Verapamil for the treatment of acute mania: a double-blind, placebo-controlled trial. *Am J Psychiatry* 1998;155:972–973.

252. Post RM, Ketter TA, Pazzaglia PJ, et al. Receptor, ion channel, and neuropeptide targets for drug development: implications from the anticonvulsant model. *Am Coll Neuropsychopharmacol Abstr Panels Posters* 1992;Dec:9.

253. Pazzaglia PJ, Post RM, Ketter TA, et al. Nimodipine monotherapy and carbamazepine augmentation in patients with refractory recurrent affective illness. *J Clin Psychopharmacol* 1998;18:404–413.

254. Levy NA, Janicak PG. Calcium channel antagonists for the treatment of bipolar disorder. *Bipolar Disord* 2000;2:108–119.

255. Dubovsky SL, Franks RD, Allen S, et al. Calcium antagonists in mania: a double-blind study of verapamil. *Psychiatry Res* 1986;18:309–320.

256. Giannini AJ, Houser WL, Loiselle RH, et al. Antimanic effects of verapamil. *Am J Psychiatry* 1984;141:1602–1603.

257. Dose M, Emrich HM, Cording-Tommel C, et al. Use of calcium antagonists in mania. *Psychoneuroendocrinology* 1986;11:241–243.

258. Garza-Trevino ES, Overall JE, Hollister LE. Verapamil versus lithium in acute mania. *Am J Psychiatry* 1992;149:121–122.

259. Arkonaç O, Kantarci E, Eradamlar N, et al. Verapamil vs. lithium in acute manics. *Biol Psychiatry* 1991;29:376S.

260. Giannini AJ, Loiselle RH, Price WA, et al. Comparison of antimanic efficacy of clonidine and verapamil. *J Clin Pharmacol* 1985;25:307–308.

261. Hoschl C, Kozeny J. Verapamil in affective disorders: a controlled, double-blind study. *Biol Psychiatry* 1989;25:128–140.

262. Barton BM, Gitlin MJ. Verapamil in treatment-resistant mania: an open trial. *J Clin Psychopharmacol* 1987;7:101–103.

263. Walton S, Berk M, Brook S. Superiority of lithium over verapamil in mania: a randomized, controlled, single-blind trial. *J Clin Psychiatry* 1996;57:543–546.

264. Janicak PG, Sharma RP, Easton M, et al. A double-blind, placebo-controlled trial of clonidine in the treatment of acute mania. *Psychopharmacol Bull* 1989;25:243–245.

265. von Zerssen D. Beta-adrenergic blocking agents in the treatment of psychoses. A report on 17 cases. *Adv Clin Pharmacol* 1976;12:105–114.

266. Emrich HM, von Zerssen D, Müller H-J, et al. Action of propranolol in mania: comparison of effects of the d- and the l-stereoisomer. *Pharmakopsychiatry* 1979;12:295–304.

267. Möller H-J, von Zerssen D, Emrich HM, et al. Action of D-propranolol in manic psychoses. *Arch Psychiatry Neurol Sci* 1979;227:301–317.

268. Jouvent R, Lecrubier Y, Puesh AJ, et al. Antimanic effect of clonidine. *Am J Psychiatry* 1980;137:1275–1276.

269. Zubenko GS, Cohen BM, Lipinski JF, et al. Clonidine in the treatment of mania and mixed bipolar disorder. *Am J Psychiatry* 1984;141:1617–1618.

270. Hardy C, Lecrubier Y, Widlocker D. Efficacy of clonidine in 24 patients with acute mania. *Am J Psychiatry* 1986;143:1450–1453.

271. Maguire J, Singh AN. Clonidine: an effective antimanic agent? *Br J Psychiatry* 1987;150:863–864.

272. Giannini AJ, Extein I, Gold MS, et al. Clonidine in mania. *Drug Dev Res* 1983;3:101–103.

273. Giannini AJ, Pascarzi GA, Loiselle RH, et al. Comparison of clonidine and lithium in the treatment of mania. *Am J Psychiatry* 1986;143:1608–1609.

274. Stoll AL, Cohen BM, Hanin I. Erythrocyte choline concentrations in psychiatric disorders. *Biol Psychiatry* 1991;29:309–320.

275. Chouinard G, Young SN, Annable L. A controlled clinical trial of L-tryptophan in acute mania. *Biol Psychiatry* 1985;20:546–557.

276. Pearce JB. Fenfluramine in mania. *Lancet* 1973;1:427.

277. Chiarello RJ, Cole JO. The use of psychostimulants in general psychiatry. *Arch Gen Psychiatry* 1987;44:286–295.

278. Green AL, Zalma A, Berman I, et al. Clozapine following ECT: a two-step treatment. *J Clin Psychiatry* 1994;55:388–390.

279. Tohen M, Zarate CA Jr, Centorrino F, et al. Risperidone in the treatment of manics. *J Clin Psychiatry* 1996;57:249–253.

280. Ghaemi SN, Sachs GS, Baldassano CF, et al. Acute treatment of bipolar disorder with adjunctive risperidone in outpatients. *Can J Psychiatry* 1997;42:196–199.

281. Rothschild AJ, Bates KS, Boehringer KL, et al. Olanzapine response in psychotic depression. *J Clin Psychiatry* 1999;60:116–118.

282. Van Tol HHM, Bunzow JB, Guan H-C, et al. Cloning of the gene for a human dopamine D_4 receptor with high affinity for the antipsychotic clozapine [Letter]. *Nature* 1991;350:610–614.

283. Janicak PG, Keck PE Jr, Davis JM, et al. A double-blind, randomized, prospective evaluation of the efficacy and safety of risperidone versus haloperidol in the treatment of schizoaffective disorder (in press).

284. Tohen M, Jacobs TG, Grundy SL, et al. A double-blind, placebo-controlled study of olanzapine in patients with acute bipolar mania. *Arch Gen Psychiatry* 2000;57:841–849.

285. Swerdlow NR. Dopamine and depression: circuitous logic? *Biol Psychiatry* 1993;33:757–758.

286. Keck PE, McElroy SL, Strakowski SM, et al. Pharmacological treatment of schizoaffective disorders. *Psychopharmacology* 1994;114:529–538.

287. Aprison MH, Takahashi R, Tachiki K. Hypersensitive serotonergic receptors involved in clinical depression: a theory. In: Halver B, Aprison MH, eds. *Neuropharmacology and behavior.* New York: Plenum, 1978:23–48.

288. Owen RR, Beake BJ, Marby D, et al. Response to clozapine in chronic psychotic patients. *Psychopharmacol Bull* 1989;25:253–256.

289. Frankenburg FR. Clozapine and bipolar disorder [Letter]. *J Clin Psychopharmacol* 1993;13:289–290.

290. Privitera MR, Lamberti JS, Maharaj J. Clozapine in bipolar depressed patients [Letter]. *Am J Psychiatry* 1993;150:986.

291. Dwight MM, Keck PE Jr, Stanton SP, et al. Antidepressant activity and mania associated with risperidone treatment of schizoaffective disorder. *Lancet* 1994;344:554–555.

292. O'Croinin F, Zibin T, Holt L. Hypomania associated with risperidone [Letter]. *Br J Psychiatry* 1995; 2:51.

293. Goodnick PJ. Risperidone treatment of refractory acute mania [Letter]. *J Clin Psychiatry* 1995;56:431–432.

294. Sachs G, Bowden C, Chou J, et al. Risperidone versus placebo as combination therapy to mood stabilizers in the treatment of the manic phase of bipolar disorder: focus on efficacy. Presented at the American Psychiatric Association Annual Meeting, Chicago, May 13–18, 2000.

295. Jacobsen FM. Risperidone in the treatment of affective illness and obsessive-compulsive disorder. *J Clin Psychiatry* 1995;56:423–429.

296. Singh AN, Catalan J. Risperidone in HIV-related manic psychosis. *Lancet* 1994;344:1029–1030.

297. Namjoshi MA, Risser RC, Feldman PD, et al. Clinical, humanistic, and economic outcomes associated with long-term treatment of mania with olanzapine. Presented at the American Psychiatric Association Annual Meeting, Chicago, May 13–18, 2000.

298. Frazier JA, Biederman J, Jacobs TG, et al. Olanzapine in the treatment of bipolar disorder in juveniles. Presented at the American Psychiatric Association Annual Meeting, Chicago, May 13–18, 2000.

299. Tohen M, Roy Chengappa KN, Suppes TR, et al. Efficacy of olanzapine added to valproate or lithium in the treatment of bipolar I disorder. Presented at the American Psychiatric Association Annual Meeting, Chicago, May 13–18, 2000.

300. Banov MD, Zarate CA, Tohen M, et al. Clozapine therapy in refractory affective disorders: polarity predicts response in longterm follow-up. *J Clin Psychiatry* 1994;55:295–300.

301. Zarate CA, Tohen M, Banov MD, et al. Is clozapine a mood stabilizer? *J Clin Psychiatry* 1995;56:108–112.

302. Zarate CA, Tohen M, Baldessarini RJ. Clozapine in severe mood disorders. *J Clin Psychiatry* 1995;56:411–417.

303. Chanpattana W, Chakrabhand MLS, Kongsakon R, et al. Short-term effect of combined ECT and neuroleptic therapy in treatment-resistant schizophrenia. *J ECT* 1999;15:129–139.

304. Frankenburg FR, Suppes T, McLean PE. Combined clozapine and electroconvulsive therapy. *Convuls Ther* 1993;9:176–180.

305. Farah A, Beale MD, Kellner CH. Risperidone and ECT combination therapy: a case series. *Convuls Ther* 1995;11:280–282.

306. Kupchik M, Spivak B, Mester R, et al. Combined electroconvulsive-clozapine therapy. *Clin Neuropharmacol* 2000;23:14–16.

307. Mitchell JE, Mackenzie TB. Cardiac effects of lithium therapy in man: a review. *J Clin Psychiatry* 1982;43:47–51.

307a. Preda A, MacLean RW, Mazure CM, et al. Antidepressant-associated mania and psychosis resulting in psychiatric admissions. *J Clin Psychiatry* 2001;62:30–33.

308. Janicak PG, Davis JM. Clinical usage of lithium in mania. In: Burrows GD, Norman TR, Davies B, eds. *Antimanics, anticonvulsants and other drugs in psychiatry.* Amsterdam: Elsevier Science Publishers, 1987: 21–34.

309. Coppen A, Bishop ME, Bailey JE, et al. Renal function in lithium and non-lithium treated patients with affective disorders. *Acta Psychiatr Scand* 1980;62:343–355.

310. Ausiello DA. Case records of the Massachusetts General Hospital—Case 17-1981. *N Engl J Med* 1981;304:1025–1032.

311. Rafaelson OJ, Bolwig TG, Ladefuged J, et al. Kidney function and morphology in long-term lithium treatment. In: Cooper TB, Gershon S, Kline NS, et al., eds. *Lithium controversies and unresolved issues.* Oxford, England: Excerpta Medica, 1979:578–583.

312. Hetmar O, Bolwig TG, Brun C, et al. Lithium: long-term effects on the kidney: I. Renal function in retrospect. *Acta Psychiatr Scand* 1986;73:574–581.

313. Gitlin M. Lithium and the kidney: an updated review. *Drug Saf* 1999;20:231–243.

314. Bowen RC, Grof P, Grof E. Less frequent lithium administration and lower urine volume. *Am J Psychiatry* 1991;148:189–192.

315. Baraban JM, Worley PF, Snyder SH. Second messenger systems and psychoactive drug action: focus on the phosphoinositide system and lithium. *Am J Psychiatry* 1989;146:1251–1260.

316. Lee RV, Jampol LM, Brown WV. Nephrogenic diabetes insipidus and lithium intoxication: complication of lithium carbonate therapy. *N Engl J Med* 1971;284:93–94.

317. Rosten MD, Forest JN. Treatment of severe lithium-induced polyuria with amiloride. *Am J Psychiatry* 1986;143:1563–1568.

318. Billings PR. Amiloride in the treatment of lithium induced diabetes insipidus (letter). *N Engl J Med* 1985;312:1575–1576.

319. Cogan E, Abramow M. Amiloride in the treatment of lithium-induced diabetes insipidus [Letter]. *N Engl J Med* 1985;312:1576.

320. Jefferson JW, Greist JH, Ackerman DL, et al. *Lithium encyclopedia for clinical practice,* 2nd ed. Washington, DC: American Psychiatric Press, 1987.

321. Grindlinger GA, Boylan MJ. Amelioration by indomethacin of lithium discontinuation. *Crit Care Med* 1987;15:538–539.

322. Wood IK, Parmelee DX, Foreman JW. Lithium-induced nephrotic syndrome. *Am J Psychiatry* 1989;146:84–87.

323. Shopsin B. Effects of lithium on thyroid function; a review. *Dis Nerv Sys* 1970;31:237–244.

324. Jefferson JW. Lithium carbonate-induced hypothyroidism. Its many faces. *JAMA* 1979;242:271–272.

325. Bauer M, Whybrow P. The effect of changing thyroid function on cyclic affective illness in a human subject. *Am J Psychiatry* 1986;143:633–636.

326. Frye MA, Denicoff KD, Bryan AL, et al. Association between lower serum free T4 and greater mood instability and depression in lithium-maintained bipolar patients. *Am J Psychiatry* 1999;156:1909–1914.

327. Perrild H, Hegedüs L, Baastrup PC, et al. Thyroid function and ultrasonically determined thyroid size in patients receiving long-term lithium treatment. *Am J Psychiatry* 1990;147:1518–1521.

328. Rosenquist M, Bergfeldt H, Aili H, et al. Sinus node dysfunction during long-term lithium treatment. *Br Heart J* 1993;70:371–375.

329. Weinrauch LA, Beloh S, d'Elia JA. Decreased lithium during verapamil therapy. *Am Heart J* 1984;108:1378–1380.

330. Koller WC. Diagnosis and treatment of tremors: symposium on movement disorders. *Neurol Clin* 1984;2:499–501.

331. Kocsis JH, Shaw E, Stokes PE, et al. Neuropsychologic effects of lithium discontinuation . *J Clin Psychopharmacol* 1993;13:268–275.

332. Stoll AL, Locke CA, Vuckovic A, et al. Lithium-associated cognitive and functional deficits reduced by a switch to divalproex sodium: a case series. *J Clin Psychiatry* 1996;57:356–359.

333. McKay AP, Tarbuck AF, Shapleske J, et al. Neuropsychological function in manic-depressive psychosis evidence for persistent deficits in patients with chronic, severe illness. *Br J Psychiatry* 1995;167: 51–57.

334. Ayd FJ. Acute self poisoning with lithium. *Int Drug Ther Newsl* 1988;23:1–2.

335. Vestergaard P, Poulstrup I, Schou M. Prospective studies on a lithium cohort. 3. Tremor, weight gain, diarrhea, psychological complaints. *Acta Psychiatr Scand* 1988;78:434–441.

336. Garland EJ, Remick RA, Zis AP. Weight gain with antidepressants and lithium. *J Clin Psychopharmacol* 1988;8:323–330.

337. Jacobsen SJ, Jones K, Johnson K, et al. Prospective multicentre study of pregnancy outcome after lithium exposure during first trimester. *Lancet* 1992;339:530–533.

338. Schou M. Lithium treatment during pregnancy, delivery, and lactation: an update. *J Clin Psychiatry* 1990;51:410–412.

339. Rosa FW. Spina bifida in infants of women treated with carbamazepine during pregnancy. *N Engl J Med* 1991;324:674–677.

340. Schou M. What happened later to the lithium babies? *Acta Psychiatr Scand* 1976;54:193–197.

341. Scott JR, DiSaia PJ, Hammond CB, et al. *Danforth's obstetrics and gynecology.* Philadelphia: Lippincott, 1994;381–382.

342. Simard M, Gumbiner B, Lee A, et al. Lithium carbonate intoxication. *Arch Intern Med* 1989;149:36–46.

343. Colgate R. The ranking of therapeutic and toxic side effects of lithium carbonate. *Psychiatr Bull* 1992;16:473–475.

344. Ragheb M. The clinical significance of lithium—nonsteroidal anti-inflammatory drug interactions. *J Clin Psychopharamacol* 1990;10:350–354.

345. Gelenberg AJ. Lithium and antibiotics. *Biol Ther Psychiatry* 1985;8:46.

346. Kahn EM, Schulz SC, Perel JM, et al. Change in haloperidol level due to carbamazepine—a complicating factor in combined medication for schizophrenia. *J Clin Psychopharmacol* 1990;10:54–57.

347. Cohen WJ, Cohen NH. Lithium carbonate, haloperidol and irreversible brain damage. *JAMA* 1974;230:1283–1287.

348. Karki SD, Holden JMC. Combined use of haloperidol and lithium. *Psychiatr Ann* 1990;20:154–161.

349. Goldney RD, Spence ND. Safety of the combination of lithium and neuroleptic drugs. *Am J Psychiatry* 1986;143:882–884.

350. Kulick SK, Kramer DA. Hyperammonemia do to valproate as a cause of lethargy in a postictal patient. *Ann Emerg Med* 1993;22:610.

351. Dreifuss FE, Santilli N, Langer DH, et al. Valproic acid hepatic fatalities: a retrospective review. *Neurology* 1987;37:379–385.

352. Dreifuss FE, Langer DH, Moline KA, et al. Valproic acid hepatic fatalities. II. U.S. experience since 1984. *Neurology* 1989;39:201–207.

353. Konig SA, Siemes H, Blaker F, et al. Severe hepatotoxicity during valproate therapy: an update and report of eight new fatalities. *Epilepsia* 1994;35:1005–1015.

354. Wilder BJ, Karas BJ, Penry JK, et al. Gastrointestinal tolerance of divalproex sodium. *Neurology* 1983;33:808–811.

355. Calzetti S, Findley IJ, Perucca E, et al. The response of essential tremor to propranolol: evaluation of clinical variables governing its efficacy on prolonged administration . *J Neurol Neurosurg Psychiatr* y 1873;46:393–398.

356. Jefferson D, Marsden CD. Metoprolol in essential tremor. *Lancet* 1980;1:427.

357. Huber SJ, Paulson GW. Efficacy of alprazolam for essential tremor. *Neurology* 1988;38:241–243.

358. Muenter MD, Daube JR, Caviness JN, et al. Treatment of essential tremor with methazolamide. *Mayo Clin Proc* 1991;66:991–997.

359. Busenbark K, Pahwa R, Hubble J, et al. The effect of acetazolamide on essential tremor: an open label trial. *Neurology* 1992;42:1394–1395.

360. Busenbark K, Pahwa R, Hubble J, et al. Double-blind controlled study of methazolamide in the treatment of essential tremor. *Neurology* 1993;43:1045–1047.

361. Jeavons PM. Sodium valproate and neural tube defects. *Lancet* 1982;2:1282–1283.

362. Miller LJ. Psychiatric medications during pregnancy: understanding and minimizing risks. *Psychiatr Ann* 1994;24:69–75.

363. Centers for Disease Control. Valproate: a new cause of birth defects - report from Italy and follow-up from France. *MMWR* 1983;32:438–439.

364. Chappell KA, Markowitz JS, Jackson CW. Is valproate pharmacotherapy associated with polycystic ovaries? *Ann Pharmacother* 1999;33:1211–1216.

365. Schnabel R, Rainbeck B, Janssen F. Fatal intoxication with sodium valproate. *Lancet* 1984;2:221–222.

366. Mortensen PB, Hansen HE, Pedersen B, et al. Acute valproate intoxication: biochemical investigations and haemodialysis treatment. *Int J Clin Pharmacol Ther Toxicol* 1983;21:64–68.

367. Stelman GS, Woerpel RW, Sherard ES. Treatment of accidental sodium valproate overdose with an opiate antagonist [Letter]. Ann Neurol 1979;6:274.

368. Masland RL. Carbamazepine: neurotoxicity. In: Woodbury DM, Perry JK, Pippinger CE, eds. *Antiepileptic drugs.* New York: Raven Press, 1982: 521–531.

369. Hart RG, Easton JD. Carbamazepine and hematological monitoring. *Ann Neurol* 1982;11:309–312.

370. Tohen M, Castillo J, Baldessarini RJ, et al. Blood dyscrasias with carbamazepine and valproate: a pharmacoepidemiological study of 2,228 patients at risk. *Am J Psychiatry* 1995;152:413–418.

371. Joffe RT, Post RM, Roy-Byrne PP, et al. Hematological effects of carbamazepine in patients with affective illness. *Am J Psychiatry* 1985;142:1196–1199.

372. Beermann B, Hedhag O. Depressive effects of carbamazepine on idioventricular rhythm in man. *Br Med J* 1978;2:171–172.

373. Soelberg SP, Hammer M. Effects of long-term carbamazepine treatment on water metabolism and plasma vasopressin concentrations. *Eur J Clin Pharmacol* 1984;26:719–722.

374. Hojer J, Malmlund HO, Berg A. Clinical features in 28 consecutive cases of laboratory confirmed massive poisoning with carbamazepine along. *Clin Toxicol* 1993;31:449–488.

375. Tidballs J. Acute toxic reaction to carbamazepine. *Pediatr Pharmacol Ther* 1992;121:295–299.

376. Kale P, Thompson P, Provenzaro R, et al. Evaluation of plasmapheresis in the treatment of acute overdose of carbamazepine. *Ann Pharmacother* 1993;24:866–870.

377. Janicak PG, Davis JM. Pharmacokinetics and drug interactions. In: Sadock BJ, Sadock VA, eds. *Kaplan & Sadock's comprehensive textbook of psychiatry. Vol. 2,* 7th ed. Philadelphia: Lippincott Williams & Wilkins, 2000:2250–2259.

378. Pollock BG. Recent developments in drug metabolism of relevance to psychiatrists. *Harvard Rev Psychiatry* 1994;2:204–213.

379. Baciewicz AM. Carbamazepine drug interactions. *Ther Drug Monitor* 1986;8:305–317.

380. Bertilsson L, Tomson T. Clinical pharmacokinetics and pharmacological effects of carbamazepine and carbamazepine-10,11-epoxide. *Clin Pharmacokinet* 1986;11:177–198.
381. Jonkman JH, Upton RA. Pharmacokinetic drug interaction with theophylline. *Clin Pharmacokinet* 1985;9:309–334.
382. Hansen JM, Siersback-Nielsen K, Skovsted L. Carbamazepine induced acceleration of diphenylhydantoin and warfarin metabolism in man. *Clin Pharmacol Ther* 1979;20:519–525.
383. Coulam CB, Annegers JF. Do anti-convulsants reduce the efficacy of oral contraceptives? *Epilepsia* 1979;20:519–525.
384. Arana GW, Goff DC, Freedman H, et al. Does carbamazepine- induced reduction of plasma haloperidol-levels worsen psychotic symptoms? *Am J Psychiatry* 1986;143:650–651.
385. Richens A. Safety of lamotrigine. *Epilepsia* 1994;35(suppl):537–540.
386. Schlumberger E, Chavez F, Palacios L, et al. Lamotrigine in treatment of 120 children with epilepsy. *Epilepsia* 1994;35:359–367.
387. Chaudron LH, Jefferson JW. Mood stabilizers during breastfeeding: a review. *J Clin Psychiatry* 2000;61:79–90.
388. Wolf ME, De Wolfe AS, Ryan JJ, et al. Vulnerability to tardive dyskinesia. *J Clin Psychiatry* 1985;46:367–368.
389. Dubovsky SL, Franks RD, Allen S. Verapamil: a new antimanic drug with potential interactions with lithium. *J Clin Psychiatry* 1987;48:371–372.

11

Indications for Antianxiety and Sedative-Hypnotic Agents

GENERALIZED ANXIETY DISORDER

Anxiety is characterized by fear and apprehension that may or may not be associated with a clearly identifiable stimulus. Anxiety is a common reaction to significant life stress, is seen in conjunction with almost every psychiatric disorder, and is a common component of numerous organic disorders as well (e.g., hyperthyroidism, hypoglycemia, pheochromocytoma, complex partial seizures, pulmonary disorders, acute myocardial infarction, caffeine intoxication, various substances of abuse). Anxiety is almost invariably accompanied by physical symptoms such as the following:

- Tachycardia, palpitations, chest tightness, diaphoresis
- Breathing difficulties
- Nausea, diarrhea, intestinal cramping
- Dry mouth

According to the Epidemiologic Catchment Area (ECA) Study (1990), anxiety disorders are the most prevalent psychiatric conditions in the United States (1–6). Of the 11 categories listed in the *Diagnostic and Statistical Manual of Mental Disorders,* 4th ed. (DSM-IV) (7), generalized anxiety disorder (GAD) may be the most commonly diagnosed, although its true incidence may actually be lower than that of phobic and obsessive-compulsive disorders (see also Appendices A, I, J, K, L, P, and R).

Before 1980, the term "anxiety neurosis" was used to describe a syndrome that included both chronic generalized anxiety and panic attacks. GAD and panic were first listed as discrete diagnoses in the DSM-III, in part because of observed differences in their response to available drug treatments (i.e., the former to benzodiazepines, the latter to antidepressants; for a more

detailed discussion of panic disorder, see Chapter 13).

To differentiate it from transient anxiety, the DSM-IV defines GAD as excessive anxiety or worry (i.e., apprehensive expectation, in contrast to DSM-III-R, which included unrealistic worries) occurring more days than not for at least 6 months or longer about a number of events or activities (such as work or school performance). A requirement that the person must find it difficult to control the worry has been added. In addition, Criterion C now has a six-item set that is simpler, more reliable, and more coherent than the 18-item set in DSM-III-R. Hence, now the patient must have at least three or more of the following symptoms:

- Restlessness
- Easy fatigability
- Difficulty concentrating
- Irritability
- Muscle tension
- Disturbed sleep

GAD may be diagnosed along with another Axis I disorder (including another anxiety disorder) provided that the GAD symptoms are present at least sometimes without symptoms of the other disorder and that the anxiety is not focused on the symptoms of the other disorder.

Few long-term follow-up studies of GAD have been conducted, but available evidence indicates it may last for many years, with waxing and waning symptoms, often complicated by other, intercurrent physical or psychiatric disorders (8, 9). Although a DSM-IV—derived diagnosis requires an anxiety duration of at least 6 months, clinicians frequently encounter very symptomatic patients who do not meet this criterion (10, 11). Thus, in addition to formalized diagnostic criteria, clinical judgment and experience are critical in deciding when anxiety is a discrete disorder requiring primary treatment and when it is a manifestation of another disorder.

This crucial differential diagnosis requires that clinicians know that GAD and other anxiety disorders are lifelong, biologically based, and often crippling conditions that can cause moderate to severe suffering and handicap an otherwise healthy person, and can usually be confirmed by a careful history. Freud emphasized these facts when he wrote: "The expectation that every neurotic phenomenon can be cured may, I suspect, be derived from the layman's belief that the neuroses are something quite unnecessary which have no right whatsoever to exist. Whereas in fact they are severe, constitutionally fixed illnesses, which rarely restrict themselves to only a few attacks but persist as a rule over long periods or throughout life" (12).

Differential psychiatric diagnosis includes the following:

- *Substance-induced* disorders (such as caffeine intoxication)
- *Adjustment* disorder with anxious mood (characterized by lack of full symptom criteria for GAD and the presence of a recognized psychosocial stressor)
- *Psychotic, eating,* or *mood* disorders in which anxiety is related to the underlying condition

PHOBIC DISORDERS

All of these disorders are characterized by disabling anxiety (at times also associated with panic attacks) and avoidance because of exposure to the following:

- Places or situations *from which one cannot readily escape*
- A *specific feared object* or *situation* (e.g., heights)
- Certain types of *social* or *performance situations*

Agoraphobia

Agoraphobia (literally, fear of the marketplace) is the dread of being in places or situations from which escape might be difficult. This condition also includes worry about suddenly developing embarrassing or incapacitating panic-like symptoms (e.g., loss of bladder control, dizziness) for which help might not be available. The agoraphobic patient often does the following:

- *Restricts travel*
- *Needs a companion* when away from home
- *Endures intense anxiety* when confronted with a feared situation

Agoraphobia may accompany panic disorder, but ECA data indicate that the majority of agoraphobic patients either fail to meet lifetime criteria for panic disorder or have no history of panic symptoms (3). Questions about this diagnosis, however, have been raised (i.e., many with agoraphobia without history of panic disorder were found to have specific phobic disorders) (13, 14).

Social Phobia

Social phobia is the persistent fear of being judged by others and/or of embarrassing oneself in public (e.g., of being unable to answer questions in social situations, of choking when eating in front of others). This condition is also referred to as **social anxiety disorder.** Exposure to the feared situation provokes an immediate anxiety response. As a result, the phobic situation is preferably avoided or endured with intense anxiety, and, secondarily, anticipatory avoidant behavior can interfere with occupational or social functioning (but need not be incapacitating), or there is marked distress about having the fear. Typically, the person is aware of the excessive and/or unreasonable nature of these concerns. The diagnosis is not made if one simply avoids social situations that normally provoke some distress, such as public speaking. If an Axis III or another Axis I disorder is present, social phobia is diagnosed only if the fear is unrelated to these conditions.

Formerly one of the least studied of the major psychiatric disorders, social phobia has become the object of increasing research, the results of which are filling in previous gaps in our knowledge concerning definition, prevalence, etiology, pathophysiology, assessment, and treatment (15, 16). Differential diagnosis includes the following:

- *Separation* anxiety disorder
- *Avoidant personality* disorder, characterized by marked anxiety and avoidance of most social situations
- *GAD*
- *Specific phobia,* characterized by fear of a specific object or situation other than fear of social embarrassment or humiliation
- *Panic* disorder with agoraphobia characterized by avoidance of certain social situations because of fear of having a panic attack (see Chapter 13)
- *Performance* anxiety

Specific Phobia

Formerly called "simple phobia," specific phobia is a marked, excessive, or unreasonable and persistent fear of a specific object or situation (e.g., snakes, heights, thunderstorms). Exposure to the phobic stimulus provokes immediate and intense anxiety that the individual recognizes as excessive or unreasonable. The degree of impairment frequently depends on whether the feared object or situation is commonly encountered or can be easily avoided. The diagnosis should only be made if avoidant behavior interferes with the person's normal routine, social activities, or relationships, or if there is marked distress about having the fear. Differential diagnosis may include the following:

- *Major depression* with social withdrawal
- *Panic* disorder with agoraphobia
- *Social phobia*
- *Psychosis*, characterized by avoidance behavior in response to delusions
- *Posttraumatic stress* disorder characterized by avoidance of stimuli associated with the trauma
- *Obsessive-compulsive* disorder characterized by avoidance of situations associated with dirt or contamination

PSYCHOLOGICAL FACTORS AFFECTING A MEDICAL CONDITION

Psychological factors affecting a medical condition were formerly referred to as "psy-chosomatic" (DSM-I) or "psychophysiological" (DSM-II) disorders. **The diagnosis is made when psychologically meaningful environmental stimuli are temporally related to the initiation or exacerbation of a physical condition with demonstrable organic pathology (e.g, rheumatoid arthritis) or a known pathophysiological process (e.g., migraine)** (7). Further, the condition should not meet criteria for somatoform disorders, which are characterized by physical symptoms suggesting medical disease, but for which no demonstrable pathology or known pathophysiological process can be found.

SLEEP DISORDERS

The sleep disorders are categorized into primary disorders (i.e., dyssomnias and parasomnias), those related to another mental disorder, those related to a general medical disorder, and those that are substance induced. Like anxiety, disturbances of sleep affect nearly all of us at one time or another. Also like anxiety, disordered sleep may present as follows:

- A *transient phenomenon* that may or may not be related to an identifiable stimulus
- *Secondary* to numerous medical and/or psychiatric conditions
- A *primary*, discrete disorder

The International Classification of Sleep Disorders lists 88 types, with insomnia the most prominent symptom for many of these (17). Chronic insomnia is the most common sleep problem for which patients consult practitioners (18) and usually reflects psychological/behavioral disturbances (19). Differences in treatment recommendations support the distinction between DSM-IV and the International Classification for Sleep Disorders (20). The DSM-IV divides primary disorders into two major groups: the *dyssomnias* (in which the predominant disturbance is the amount, quality, or timing of sleep) and the *parasomnias* (in which the predominant disturbance is an abnormal event occurring during sleep) (7).

Dyssomnias

Primary Insomnia

Primary insomnia is characterized by difficulty initiating or maintaining sleep or by not feeling rested after an apparently adequate amount of sleep for at least 1 month. Further, it causes significant stress or impairment in various areas of functioning. This condition may represent a lifelong pattern of poor sleep habits, or it may develop as a result of distressing events, but then persist after the stressor resolves. It is characterized by excessive daytime worry about being able to fall or stay asleep. Anxiety tends to perpetuate a vicious cycle of sleeplessness that is aggravated by worry about sleeplessness. Patients with primary insomnia, however, may fall asleep when they are not trying and may experience little or no difficulty sleeping away from their normal environment. The diagnosis is made only if this condition is not symptomatic of another mental disorder or known organic factor.

Secondary insomnia related to a known organic factor may occur in conjunction with a physical illness (but not the person's emotional reaction to the illness), psychoactive substance abuse, or certain medications. Secondary insomnia may also be related to another mental disorder.

Primary Hypersomnia

These disorders are characterized by excessive daytime sleepiness for at least 1 month. The *daytime sleepiness* (falling asleep easily and unintentionally) is not accounted for by an inadequate amount of nighttime sleep. Another criteria is the presence of hypersomnia nearly every day for at least 1 month or episodically for longer periods of time, resulting in occupational or social impairment.

As with the insomnia disorders, hypersomnias may be categorized as primary, as secondary to another mental disorder (e.g., mood disorders, schizophrenia, somatoform disorder, borderline personality disorder), or as secondary to a known organic factor such as the following:

- Psychoactive *substance abuse*
- Prolonged use of *medications* with sleep-inducing properties, such as sedatives or antihypertensives
- Sleep *apnea*, sleep *myoclonus*
- *Restless legs* syndrome
- *Narcolepsy*
- *Kleine-Levin* syndrome
- *Epilepsy*
- *Hypothyroidism*
- *Hypoglycemia*
- *Multiple sclerosis*
- *Organic* mental disorders

The diagnosis is not made if hypersomnia occurs only during the course of a circadian-rhythm sleep disorder.

Narcolepsy is a relatively uncommon condition that may be either idiopathic or, more rarely, secondary to organic brain damage. It is characterized by irresistible attacks of refreshing sleep lasting from 30 s to 20 min and the accelerated appearance of rapid eye movement (REM) sleep, usually within 10 min of sleep onset. Additional symptoms may include cataplexy (brief weakness in isolated muscle groups or paralysis of almost all skeletal muscles) triggered by intense emotion, with or without a concomitant sleep attack; sleep paralysis; and hypnagogic or hypnopompic hallucinations. The roughly 30% of narcoleptic patients who have hallucinatory experiences also have a higher than expected rate of associated psychotic disorders. A polysomnographic diagnosis of narcolepsy requires sleep latencies of less than 10 min on the multiple sleep latency test, as well as the presence of multiple sleep-onset REM periods in the absence of other sleep pathologies (such as sleep apnea, nocturnal myoclonus, circadian rhythm disorders, or acute drug withdrawal). These criteria have been shown to be stable and highly reliable traits of narcolepsy (21).

Breathing-related sleep disorder is a potentially life-threatening abnormal respiratory condition. It includes cessation of both nasal and oral air flow (apnea), which in some patients may last up to 2 min. **The most prominent sign is loud snoring.** This disorder can also include hypopneas and hypoventilation. There are three forms of breathing-related sleep disorders:

- *Obstructive sleep apnea* involving blockage of the oropharynx
- *Central sleep apnea* involving lack of diaphragmatic effort
- *Central alveolar hypoventilation,* which most commonly occurs in very overweight individuals

Typical complications include insomnia and excessive daytime sleepiness due to frequent nighttime awakenings. Sleep electroencephalogram (EEG) reveals absent or decreased slow-wave sleep, and, in some patients, early-onset REM sleep. If untreated, long-term effects of sleep apnea include increased incidence of hypertension; vascular events (e.g., myocardial infarction, stroke); poor work performance; increased risk of traffic accidents; and stress in personal relationships (22, 23).

Circadian Rhythm Sleep Disorder

This disorder occurs when there is a mismatch between the normal rest—activity schedule for a person's environment and the person's circadian sleep—wake pattern. There are four subtypes:

- Delayed *sleep phase* type
- *Jet lag* type
- *Shift work* type
- *Unspecified*

Transient disturbances may occur as a result of rapid time zone changes (as in transoceanic flights) or staying up late for a few days. Diagnosis of a sleep—wake schedule disorder, however, is made only if complaints meet criteria for an insomnia or a hypersomnia disorder. These disorders often improve when the person is able to resume a normal sleep—wake pattern.

Parasomnias

This group of disorders is characterized by the occurrence of an abnormal event during sleep, specific sleep stages, or the threshold between sleep and wakefulness. These conditions usually involve complaints focused on the abnormal occurrence itself rather than any effect it might have on sleep. Parasomnias include the following:

- *Nightmare* disorder
- *Sleep terror* disorder
- *Sleepwalking* disorder

Nightmare Disorder

Formerly known as "dream anxiety disorder," this condition involves vivid dreams, often characterized by recurring themes of threats to survival, security, or self-esteem. Because the dreams are most likely to occur during REM sleep, autonomic agitation is minimal during the dream but may occur upon awakening. The repeated awakenings associated with the dreams, as well as the dreams themselves, are accompanied by significant anxiety and difficulty returning to sleep. Upon awakening, however, the person is alert, fully oriented, and able to give a detailed account of the dream. The diagnosis is not made if the dreams are attributable to a known organic factor, such as a medication or general medical condition. One example is the abrupt withdrawal from REM-suppressant agents (e.g., tricyclic antidepressants) that may result in REM rebound and associated nightmares.

Sleep Terror Disorder

Sleep terror disorder (also known as "pavor nocturnus") is characterized by recurrent episodes of abrupt awakening from sleep in the first third of the major sleep episode, usually during nonrapid eye movement (NREM) periods that are characterized by EEG delta-wave activity. The episode can be dramatic and is likely to begin with a panicky scream. The person often sits up in bed exhibiting signs of intense anxiety and autonomic arousal (e.g., tachycardia, rapid breathing and pulse, dilated pupils, sweating, etc.) and may be confused, disoriented, and unresponsive to comforting gestures. Patients may describe a sense of terror and fragmentary images, but are usually unable to recount a complete dream. Interestingly, morning amnesia for the episode usually occurs. An organic factor (e.g., brain tumor, epileptic seizures during sleep) responsible for these disturbances precludes the diagnosis of sleep terror disorder.

Sleepwalking Disorder

Sleepwalking disorder (or somnambulism) is characterized by episodes of complex behaviors that initially include sitting up and performing perseverative moments (e.g., picking at the sheet, as well as getting out of bed and moving around). Like sleep terror, this disorder usually occurs during non-REM sleep in association with EEG delta-wave activity. This disorder often proceeds to such activities as leaving the bed, walking, dressing, and opening or closing windows and doors. During an episode, the person usually has a blank stare, is unresponsive to others, and is very difficult to awaken. With the exception of a brief period of confusion or disorientation, no impairment of mental activity or behavior occurs upon awakening, although amnesia for the episode is typical. The diagnosis is not made if an organic factor such as epilepsy is responsible for the disturbance. Differential diagnosis includes psychogenic fugue and sleep drunkenness.

CONCLUSION

Anxiety disorders substantially diminish one's quality of life and ability to function (24). In the attempt to manage anxiety-related phenomena, as well as sleep disturbances, various treatments (both drug and nondrug) have been used over the course of history. Today, our understanding of the basis for such conditions is becoming more refined, allowing identification of differentiating qualities that will ultimately dictate more specific and effective remedies as discussed in Chapter 12.

REFERENCES

1. Myers JR, Weissman MM, Tischler GL, et al. Six month prevalence of psychiatric disorders in three communities. *Arch Gen Psychiatry* 1984;41:959–970.
2. Robins LN, Helzer JE, Weissman MM, et al. Lifetime prevalence of specific psychiatric disorders in three sites. *Arch Gen Psychiatry* 1984;41:949–958.
3. Regier DA, Narron WE, Rae DS. The epidemiology of anxiety disorders: the Epidemiologic Catchment Area (ECA) experience. *J Psychiatr Res* 1990;24(Suppl 2):3–14.
4. Regier DA, Farmer ME, Rae DS, et al. Comorbidity of mental disorders with alcohol and other drug abuse. *JAMA* 1990;264:2511–2518.
5. Blazer D, Hughes D, George U. Stressful life events and the onset of generalized anxiety syndrome. *Am J Psychiatry* 1987;144:1178–1183.
6. Helzer JE, Robins LN, McEvoy L. Post-traumatic stress disorder in the general population: findings of the Epidemiologic Catchment Area Survey. *N Engl J Med* 1987;317:1630–1634.
7. American Psychiatric Association. *Diagnostic and statistical manual of mental disorders,* 4th ed., revised. Washington, DC: American Psychiatric Association, 1994.
8. Rickels K, Schweizer E. The clinical course and long-term management of generalized anxiety disorder. *J Clin Psychopharmacol* 1990;10:101s–110s.
9. Mahe V, Balogh A. Long-term pharmacological treatment of generalized anxiety disorder. *Int Clin Psychopharmacol* 2000;15:99–100.
10. Barlow DH, Blanchard EB, Vermilyea JA, et al. Generalized anxiety and generalized anxiety disorder: description and reconceptualization. *Am J Psychiatry* 1986;143:40–44.
11. Maier W, Gansicke M, Freyberger HJ, et al. Generalized anxiety disorder (ICD-10) in primary care from a cross-cultural perspective: a valid diagnostic entity? *Acta Psychiatr Scand* 2000;101:29–36.
12. Freud S. *Introductory lectures on psychoanalysis.* New York: Norton, 1977.
13. Goisman RM, Warshaw MG, Steketee GS, et al. DSM-IV and the disappearance of agoraphobia without a history of panic disorder: new data on a controversial diagnosis. *Am J Psychiatry* 1995;152:1438–1443.
14. Wittchen HU, Reed V, Kessler RC. The relationship of agoraphobia in a community sample of adolescents and young adults. *Arch Gen Psychiatry* 1998;55:1017–1024.
15. Lieb R, Wittchen H-U, Höfler M, et al. Parental psychopathology, parenting styles, and the risk of social phobia in offspring. *Arch Gen Psychiatry* 2000;57:859–866.
16. Nutt DJ, Bell CJ, Malizia AL. Brain mechanisms of social anxiety disorder. *J Clin Psychiatry* 1998;59(17):4–9.
17. Diagnostic Classification Steering Committee. *International classification of sleep disorders: diagnostic and coding manual.* Rochester, MN: American Sleep Disorders Association, 1990.
18. Chesson A Jr, Hartse K, Anderson WM, et al. An American Academy of Sleep Medicine report. Standards of Practice Committee of the American Academy of Sleep Medicine. *Sleep* 2000;23:237–241.
19. Vgontas AN, Kales A. Sleep and its disorders. *Annu Rev Med* 1999;50:387–400.
20. Buysse DJ, Reynolds CF III, Kupfer DJ, et al. Effects of diagnosis on treatment recommendations in chronic insomnia–a report from the APA/NIMH DSM-IV field trial. *Sleep* 1997;20:542–552.

21. Rosenthal L, Krestevska S, Murlidhar A, et al. Reliability of sleep onset REM periods in narcolepsy. *Sleep Res* 1992;21:254.
22. Nieto FJ, Young TB, Link BK, et al. Association of sleep-disordered breathing, sleep apnea, and hypertension in a large community-based study. *JAMA* 2000;283:1829–1836.

23. Peppard PE, Young T, Palta M, et al. Prospective study of the association between sleep-disordered breathing and hypertension. *N Engl J Med* 2000;342:1378–1384.
24. Mendlowicz MV, Stein MB. Quality of life in individuals with anxiety disorders. *Am J Psychiatry* 2000;157:669–682.

12

Treatment With Antianxiety and Sedative-Hypnotic Agents

From time immemorial, human beings have sought ways to achieve surcease from subjectively distressing and disabling anxiety, as well as to counteract debilitating insomnia. Early recorded history documents that the anxiolytic and soporific effects of alcohol were discovered centuries ago, and ever since people have imbibed to ease anxiety, tension, and agitation, and lull them into a somnolent state. It was not until the 19th century, however, that chemists synthesized the bromides and the barbiturates, thereby inaugurating an era of relentless attempts to manufacture safer and more effective alternatives.

Humanity's centuries-old, avid search for substances that would relieve these conditions has resulted in a progression from alcohol to opiates to the synthesis of bromides and barbiturates. Each of these, however, shares treatment-limiting and potentially life-threatening disadvantages, including the following:

- Rapid development of *tolerance* to their therapeutic effects
- Serious *adverse effects*
- High risk of *dependence*
- Significant *withdrawal effects*
- *Lethality* in overdose

Meprobamate (a bis-carbamate ester), first marketed in the early 1950's, was originally considered an improvement over the barbiturates, but soon was recognized to have essentially the same liabilities as its predecessors.

The benzodiazepines (BZDs), which were introduced nearly 40 years ago, were hailed as a breakthrough because they have fewer of the drawbacks of prior anxiolytics and sedative-hypnotics, are effective in a range of disorders, and are safe in combination with most drugs (except other sedatives), as well as alone in overdose, and are generally mild in terms of side effects. **For these reasons, BZDs quickly became, and remain, among the most widely prescribed drugs worldwide.**

More recently, non-BZD anxiolytics, such as buspirone, and nonbarbiturate, non-BZD hypnotics, such as zolpidem and zaleplon, have been developed. The more recent anxiolytics and hypnotics offer equal efficacy, fewer serious adverse effects, and less risk of a fatal consequence due to accidental or intentional overdose. Unfortunately, these compounds have not entirely eliminated the hazards of tolerance, dependency, and withdrawal syndromes, although they do have a lower abuse potential than their predecessors.

In addition to buspirone and the non-barbituate, non-BZP hypnotics, selective serotonin reuptake inhibitors (SSRIs), venlafaxine, and other new antidepressants all represent attempts to achieve anxiolytic and hypnotic effects seen with the BZDs, while avoiding their unwanted properties.

These assets, however, do not justify cavalierly dispensing these newer agents, which must also be prescribed judiciously. Failure to monitor their usage may endanger the patient, invite governmental restrictions, and possibly become the basis for a malpractice suit or the revocation of one's medical license. For these reasons, it is imperative for clinicians to become knowledgeable about the basic pharmacology of these drugs, along with their appropriate clinical indications, dosages, and duration of usage. **Most importantly, the appropriate clinical indications, as well as their limitations, must receive as much attention as their assets.**

Nevertheless, BZDs have been the subject of a debate that tends to center on issues related to overuse, misuse, and abuse. Indeed, many BZD-treated patients, their families, and their physicians now wonder whether one should be

TABLE 12-1. *Medical users versus nonmedical users and/or abuses of benzodiazepine (BZD)*

Medical users	Nonmedical users and/or abusers
Are more likely to be females over age 50.	Are more likely to be males between the ages of 20 and 35.
Take a BZD prescribed and supervised by a physician for a recognized medical indication.	Take a BZD that may or may not have been obtained from a physician, but not for a recognized medical indication; self-administer the drug without physician supervision for "kicks" or to "get high."
Usually take the prescribed dose or less.	Usually take doses in excess of established therapeutic doses.
Take only the BZD.	Usually abuse a number of drugs. Abuse BZDs infrequently compared to other drugs. BZDs frequently abused with a wide variety of other drugs such as alcohol, illegal drugs (marijuana, cocaine), and controlled prescription drugs (methadone).
Do not usually develop tolerance and a need to progressively escalate the dose.	Often quickly develop tolerance and have to escalate the dose to obtain the desired effect.
Dislike BZD sedative effects.	Like and seek BZD sedative effects.
Prefer a placebo to a BZD.	Prefer a BZD to a placebo.
Seldom take more than diazepam, 40 mg/day, or its equivalent.	Frequently take diazepam, 80–120+ mg/day, or its equivalent.
Seldom at high risk of a severe withdrawl reaction.	Often at high risk of a severe withdrawal reaction.
Do not constitute a serious medical or social problem.	Constitute a serious medical and/or social problem.
Usually do not obtain a BZD from a "script doctor" who sells prescriptions for a fee.	Usually obtain a BZD from a "script doctor" or some other illegal source.

considered an abuser after taking these drugs for longer than a few weeks. Thus, recent reviews generally support earlier conclusions that even long-term therapeutic use is rarely accompanied by inappropriate drug-taking or drug-seeking behavior (e.g., high and sustained dosage escalation; trying to obtain the drug from several physicians or illicitly) (2–8). An international study of expert judgment on the therapeutic dose dependence and abuse liability of BZDs in the long-term treatment of anxiety disorders led to the conclusion that although the BZDs pose a higher risk of dependence than most potential substitutes, they have a lower risk than older sedatives and recognized drugs of abuse (9). Although this may be correct, there appears to be a clear distinction between BZD abusers and therapeutic-dose users. Almost exclusively, the former are reported to also abuse other prescription or street drugs, or alcohol; take BZDs in large doses for euphoriant effects or to potentiate other (usually il-

licit street) drugs; and prefer drugs other than BZDs when available. In contrast, patients who take a BZD continuously for more than 4 to 6 weeks may become dependent on the drug, but the vast majority:

- Do not drink more than *social amounts of alcohol.*
- Do not have a history of *dependence* on other drugs.
- Do not *abuse* BZDs.
- Do not take more than the *prescribed* dosage.
- Usually attempt to *reduce dosage* to avoid "addiction."
- Are able to *successfully withdraw* from BZDs without resorting to another dependence-inducing drug (Table 12-1).

These distinctions are important because the advantages and the disadvantages of the therapeutic use of BZDs should not be confused with their abuse.

BZD: MECHANISM OF ACTION

In 1977, BZD receptors were identified when it became possible to map their location within the CNS. They were found to be intimately related to γ-aminobutyric acid (GABA), the most prevalent inhibitory neurotransmitter system in the brain, which acts in the following locations:

- *Stellate inhibitory interneurons* in the cortex
- *Striatal afferents* to globus pallidus and substantia nigra
- *Purkinje cells* in the cerebellum

Further, the recognition sites for GABA receptors were found to be coupled to chloride ion channels. When GABA binds to its receptors, these channels open and allow chloride ions to flow into the neuron, making it more resistant to excitation. GABA exerts its actions at two physiologically and pharmacologically distinct classes of receptors, $GABA_A$ and $GABA_B$. $GABA_B$ receptors are insensitive to BZDs or barbiturates; however, these drugs do bind to a site on $GABA_A$ receptors, which are linked to, but distinct from, the GABA recognition site. BZDs enhance the affinity of the recognition site for GABA, ultimately potentiating its inhibitory action. Barbiturates apparently interact with sites directly related to the chloride ion channel, prolonging the duration of its opening by as much as four- to fivefold. Some evidence indicates that alcohol's effects are also due in part to enhancement of $GABA_A$ receptor function (10).

Recently, Low et al. (11) found that a specific, $GABA_A$ receptor subunit may mediate the therapeutic effects of the BZDs. Thus, in mice, a knock-in point mutation for the α_2 versus α_3 subunit rendered diazepam ineffective for its anxiolytic effects. This indicates that the efficacy of BZDs is mediated by α_2 $GABA_A$ receptors.

Pharmacology

All BZDs are not the same, because differences in chemical structure profoundly influence the milligram potency, duration of action, and type and frequency of side effects (Table 12-2). This variety makes it possible to select a specific BZD most likely to benefit the individual patient while minimizing the risks.

BZDs facilitate GABA-mediated transmission, thus acting as an indirect $GABA_A$ agonist. There are two BZD receptor subtypes in the brain, BZ_1 (type 1 or omega$_1$) and BZ_2 (type 2 or omega$_2$). A peripheral BZD receptor (omega$_3$) is very abundant in peripheral tissues. There are also three types of ligands:

- *Agonists* (e.g., diazepam), which are anxiolytic and anticonvulsant
- *Antagonists* (e.g., flumazenil), which are neutral
- *Inverse agonists* (e.g., FG 7142), which are anxiogenic and proconvulsant

TABLE 12-2. *Benzodiazepine differences*

Factors	Short-acting	Long-acting
Potency	High	Low
Daily dosage frequency	Q 4–6 h	B.I.D. or once daily
Interdose anxiety	Frequent	Rare
Accumulation	Little or none	Common
Hypnotic hangover effects	None or mild	Mild-to-moderate
Rebound anxiety	Frequent	Infrequent
Dependency risk	High	Low
Onset withdrawal symptoms	1–3 days	4–7 days
Duration withdrawal symptoms	2–5 days	8–5 days
Withdrawal severity	Severe	Mild-to-moderate
Paradoxical effects	Frequent	Infrequent
Anterograde amnesia	Frequent	Infrequent
I.M. administration	Rapid absorption	Slow absorption
I.V. risk	Low	High with rapid injection
Active metabolites	None or few	Many

There is a high density of BZD receptors within the amygdala, suggesting it is an important site for the actions of anxiolytic drugs.

In one study, an inverse agonist was administered to human subjects producing anxiety, terror, cold sweats, tremor, agitation, fear of impending death, and "intense inner strain" (12). BZD antagonists apparently lack intrinsic activity, but may have both agonist and inverse agonist effects (13). For example, they are reported to reverse the increased anxiety that may occur after withdrawal of chronic BZD or alcohol use, and to reverse BZD-caused amnestic effects (14–17).

These and other findings related to manipulation of the BZD-GABA-receptor complex indicate it is an important substrate in the neurobiological regulation of anxiety. Other systems also may play a role, however, including the noradrenergic and serotonergic systems, as well as a number of peptides and hormones (10).

Major Subgroups

BZDs belong to one of three major subgroups:

- *1,4-BZDs*–contain nitrogen atoms at positions 1 and 4 in the diazepine ring. This grouping accounts for most therapeutically important agents (e.g., bromazepam, chlordiazepoxide, clonazepam, clorazepate, diazepam, flunitrazepam, flurazepam, lorazepam, lormetazepam, midazolam, nitrazepam, oxazepam, prazepam, quazepam, temazepam)
- *1,5-BZDs* –contain nitrogen atoms at positions 1 and 5 in the diazepine ring (e.g., clobazam)
- *Tricyclic BZDs* –often consist of the 1, 4-BZD nucleus with an additional ring fused at positions 1 and 2 (e.g., alprazolam, adinazolam, loprazolam, and triazolam)

In addition, another group of diazepines features replacement of the fused benzene ring with other heteroaromatic systems such as thieno or pyrazolo. Most compounds of this type are under investigation (e.g., brotizolam, a thienodiazepine). Because pharmacological effects are comparable with the BZDs, both groups of diazepines are considered "BZDs" from a clinical standpoint.

TREATMENT OF GENERALIZED ANXIETY DISORDER

Although other drugs exert anxiolytic effects, the BZDs are the drugs most commonly used in the treatment of generalized anxiety disorder (GAD) and thus are the primary focus of this chapter. Alternative treatment strategies, as well as disorders in which BZDs have demonstrated little or no efficacy, are also discussed. Figure 12-1 gives an overview of the differential diagnoses and related treatment strategies for various anxiety disorders.

Acute Treatment

Several well-controlled studies have examined the efficacy of BZDs in the acute treatment of GAD. Almost all indicate that these anxiolytics quickly reduce symptoms in many patients, with most improvement occurring in the first week of treatment (18). Nevertheless, they may not be universally effective, with some investigators finding no difference between BZDs and placebo (19). Overall, Rickels (20) reported that about 35% of patients show marked improvement, 40% show moderate improvement, and 25% remain unchanged.

Patients most likely to respond to a BZD have been reported to have these characteristics:

- *Acute, severe* anxiety
- Precipitating *stresses*
- *Low level of depression* or interpersonal problems
- *No previous treatment* or a good response to earlier treatment
- Expectation of *recovery*
- Desire to use *medication*
- Awareness that symptoms are *psychological*
- Some improvement in the *first treatment week* (21, 22)

Many of these patients derive benefit from short-term BZD therapy only. In one study, 50% of those treated with diazepam (15 to 40 mg/day) for 6 weeks maintained their improvement during subsequent placebo therapy for an additional 18 weeks (23). In another study, 70%

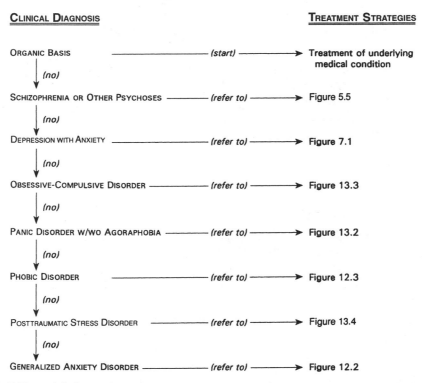

FIG. 12-1. Differential diagnosis of various anxiety-related disorders and treatment strategies (see specified figures in this and other chapters).

treated for 4 weeks with either lorazepam or clorazepate maintained improvement during 2 weeks on placebo (24). Even the chronically anxious may benefit from brief (4 to 6 weeks) treatment (25). In many cases, although discontinuation of medication may eventually lead to a reemergence of anxiety, symptoms may not always be continuous, be functionally significant, or cause patients to seek further treatment (26).

Ideally, BZD treatment of acute anxiety, GAD, and other anxiety-related disorders should be with the lowest possible dose for the shortest possible time (27). Doses should be flexible rather than arbitrary and taken intermittently at a time of increased symptoms rather than on a fixed daily schedule. In general, 1 to 7 days of BZD treatment are recommended for a reaction to an acute situational stress, although 1 to 6 weeks of treatment may be needed for short-term anxiety due to specific life events (28).

Long-Term Treatment

Anxiety disorders are often lifelong, biologically based, and frequently crippling disorders that can cause moderate to severe suffering and handicap an otherwise healthy person. Freud emphasized these facts about anxiety disorders when he wrote: "The expectation that every neurotic phenomenon can be cured may, I suspect, be derived from the layman's belief that the neuroses are something quite unnecessary which have no right whatever to exist. Whereas in fact they are severe, constitutionally fixed illnesses, which rarely restrict themselves to only a few attacks but persist as a rule over long periods or throughout life" (29).

Because these disorders are chronic, long-term treatment is usually required to achieve optimal benefit. Even when long-term BZD therapy is appropriate, however, periodic reassessment of its efficacy, safety, and necessity is good medical practice. This lessens any risk of protracted BZD therapy. In this context, there are data indicating that the following is true:

- *Long-term users* account for the bulk of anxiolytic (and hypnotic) BZDs sold in the United States (and probably worldwide).
- About 80% of hypnotics sold are consumed by individuals reporting daily use of *4 months or longer.*
- The number of *long-term users* of anxiolytic (and hypnotic users) has increased in recent years, even though the efficacy of long-term use has not been established (30).

Unfortunately, although needed, effective, and reasonably safe, long-term BZD therapy for anxiety disorders has had various problems associated with it, especially in the elderly, including the following:

- Excessive daytime *drowsiness*
- *Cognitive impairment* and confusion
- *Psychomotor impairment* and a risk of falls
- *Paradoxical reactions,* depression
- *Intoxication* even on therapeutic dosages
- *Amnestic* syndromes
- *Respiratory* problems
- *Abuse* and dependence
- Breakthrough *withdrawal* reactions

Thus, clinical judgment plays a major role in the decision to continue BZD anxiolytic treatment beyond 4 to 6 weeks. Although long-term administration may maintain initial improvement, further gains are unlikely (31). To lessen the likelihood of adverse effects and withdrawal phenomena, many U.S. investigators now recommend limiting BZD use to 4 months or fewer, and British guidelines are even more stringent, indicating use should not exceed 2 to 4 weeks (14). The chronic nature of anxiety disorders and the frequency of eventual relapse after treatment discontinuation, however, suggest that in some patients long-term treatment may be indicated (23, 26, 28).

Unfortunately, only limited controlled data exist on the efficacy of chronic BZD administration. In one double-blind study, the effectiveness of continuous treatment with diazepam (15 to 40 mg/day) for up to 22 weeks was assessed in chronically anxious subjects diagnosed

according to the *Diagnostic and Statistical Manual,* 3rd ed., (DSM-III) (33). Half of all patients switched to placebo experienced a slow return of their original symptoms, indicating diazepam continues to be effective for at least 22 weeks. In a study involving clorazepate, investigators also found continuing efficacy for up to 6 months (34). Although no controlled studies have been conducted on the efficacy of BZD therapy beyond 6 months' duration, the fact that long-term therapeutic use is rarely accompanied by dosage escalation suggests anxiolytic efficacy is retained even after prolonged use (1–5, 35). Evidence indicates, however, that an unknown number of patients are long-term BZD users not because of the drug's therapeutic efficacy but because they have become dependent on the therapeutic doses that they take to preclude the occurrence of subjectively distressing discontinuance syndrome symptoms.

As Griffiths has cogently observed: "While it is true that the majority of people who use benzodiazepines do so for relatively short periods of time (1 month), the majority of the drug dispensed is consumed by chronic long-term users under conditions in which efficacy has not been established and there are no generally accepted medical recommendations for use" (30). In support of this position, Griffiths cites a rigorous 1990 survey of the general population in the United States showing that 25% of past-year users of anxiolytics (primarily BZDs) reported daily use of 12 months or greater (36). Further, many long-term users continue to report high levels of baseline anxiety or "psychic distress" (2, 35, 37–42). This may represent the following:

- *Undertreatment*
- *Partial responsiveness* that would worsen without treatment
- Presence of symptoms *more responsive to a different class* of drug (e.g., an antidepressant)
- Development of some degree of *tolerance* to the anxiolytic effect of the BZD
- Development of a *chronic state of withdrawal*

In two studies, Rickels and coinvestigators (41, 42) found that baseline measures taken before BZD discontinuation showed significant anxiety and depressive symptomatology despite long-term drug therapy. In addition, patients who successfully completed either abrupt or gradual drug withdrawal achieved lower anxiety and depression levels than they had while receiving medication. This finding is not unexpected because this process selects patients with a good prognosis.

In her study of 50 consecutive patients attempting withdrawal from BZDs taken for 1 to 22 years, Ashton (40) reported that all had a variety of anxiety and/or depressive symptoms, which had been gradually increasing over several years despite continuous BZD use. Several (number not given) had also received unsuccessful behavioral therapy, and 10 had become agoraphobic. Twelve had undergone extensive gastroenterological or neurological investigations for which various treatments had been ineffective. Ashton notes that it is arguable whether these patients would have developed their symptoms without BZD treatment; however, their symptoms:

- Were *not present* prior to initiation of the BZD.
- Were *not amenable* to other treatments during BZD use.
- Largely *disappeared* when the BZD was discontinued.

A more recent study of the extent and appropriateness of BZD use in an elderly community confirmed that the prevalence and incidence of hypnotic use are strongly associated with increasing age. This study showed a high proportion of long-term users (61% to 70%), as well as high continued use (52%) among new users. Many of the long-term users were concurrently depressed. The findings of this study led to the conclusion that many older people still use BZDs contrary to official guidelines with regard to their mental health. These findings also add to the weight of opinion that persistent and long-term BZD use should be discouraged (43).

Conclusion

The diagnosis of all patients on long-term BZD therapy should be reassessed on a regular, intermittent basis because the high rate of comorbidity for GAD with other psychiatric disorders suggests that an alternative approach (such as an antidepressant or BZD discontinuation) may be more appropriate in certain patients. In addition,

the following offer the best means of avoiding the dependence or withdrawal symptoms associated with long-term use:

- Regular treatment *monitoring*
- *U*se of the *lowest possible dosages* compatible with achieving the desired therapeutic effect
- Use of *intermittent* and *flexible dosing schedules* rather than a fixed regimen
- *Gradual dosage reduction*

Summarizing their study of 119 long-term BZD users, Rickels et al. (35) reported, "One hard-learned lesson is that [they] are in need of much more intensive psychiatric and social support than other anxious or depressed patients." Nevertheless, some patients' quality of life may depend on long-term, therapeutic use of a BZD (44). Although periodic attempts to discontinue the medication should be made to determine whether return of anxiety represents a withdrawal reaction or reemergence of the original disorder, categorical withholding of BZDs may do more harm than good. For example, some may turn to more dangerous drugs in an effort to obtain relief, while others may seek a more permanent solution through suicide.

Alternative Treatment Strategies

In some patients, careful listening, astute questioning, and appropriate advice may be the best form of intervention. This contributes immensely to the patient–physician relationship, which is a powerful treatment tool. Bereavement-induced acute anxiety and insomnia should not be considered a disorder requiring drug therapy, although such patients may benefit from grief counseling and/or very brief use of a BZD if the disturbance is severe. Some psychotherapies have been reported effective to teach techniques for coping with and reducing anxiety. If drug therapy is indicated, non-BZDs, such as buspirone and various antidepressants, may be useful alternatives.

Buspirone

Buspirone is an azapirone anxiolytic that acts as a partial 5-HT$_{1A}$ agonist. In contrast to the BZDs, this agent has no immediate effect on the

TABLE 12-3. *Buspirone versus placebo or a benzodiazepine for generalized anxiety disorder*

Responders (%)		n	Responders (%)		n	Difference (%)
75	Buspirone	106	23	Placebo	111	52[a]
31	Buspirone	531	29	Benzodiazepine	290	02[b]

[a]$\chi^2 = 58; df = 1; p < 10^{-13}$.
[b]$\chi^2 = 2.3; df = 1; p = NS$.

anxiety seen in patients undergoing medical procedures (e.g., endoscopy, cardioversion). Further, it cannot be given parenterally, because the drug is not available in an i.v. or i.m. formulation. Buspirone does not produce disinhibition euphoria and even in high doses has not been found to have antipsychotic activity.

The absence of adverse effects of the BZD type and its lack of abuse potential are major advantages. The lack of sedative properties may be very important, because many dislike this feeling and find it interferes with various activities, such as problem solving, driving, and overall work function.

While buspirone does not interact with brain BZD receptors, it has been shown to be superior to placebo and as effective as BZDs for GAD (45–48) (Table 12-3). In a long-term follow-up study of chronic GAD patients who participated in a 6-month trial comparing clorazepate and buspirone, Rickels and Schweizer (33) found a nonsignificant trend for former buspirone-treated patients to report less anxiety than former clorazepate-treated patients. In addition, whereas 65% of the former clorazepate-treated group were still taking anxiolytic medication at 40-month follow-up, no former buspirone patient was taking a psychotropic.

The side-effect profile of buspirone is different from BZDs in that there is:

- No *sedation*
- No *memory* or psychomotor impairment
- No interaction with *alcohol*
- No *abuse* potential
- No *disinhibition* phenomenon (49)

Buspirone differs clinically in four important ways from the BZDs:

- *It is only useful when taken regularly for several weeks, because it has no immediate effect after a single tablet and is not helpful in treating an acute episode.* Many patients who have taken BZDs expect relief after a single tablet, but buspirone cannot be used on such a prn basis.
- It has demonstrated *antidepressant properties* in double-blind studies.
- It has *not been shown effective for panic attacks* in several small studies.
- It *does not block BZD withdrawal symptoms.* This is often a critical consideration because many patients have previously been on or are presently taking a BZD.

Clinical studies have also found that anxious patients treated for up to 12 months are able to stop treatment abruptly without withdrawal symptoms (34, 50).

Buspirone has a slower onset of anxiolytic action (1 to 2 weeks) than the BZDs, however, and requires t.i.d. dosing. Increased antianxiety effects have been observed in some patients treated concurrently with low doses of buspirone and a BZD (51). Although this agent may not be as effective in patients who have previously used a BZD, some can be successfully switched (52). A recent assessment of the impact of prior BZD use on response to buspirone showed that patient attrition was significantly higher in the recent BZD treatment group than in the remote and no prior BZD groups. Lack of efficacy was given as the primary reason by patients who were receiving buspirone. Also in the buspirone group, adverse events occurred more frequently in the recent BZD treatment group than in the remote BZD treatment group and no prior BZD treatment groups (53). In such cases, a 2-week to 4-week period of concurrent use before BZD tapering may help preclude the return of anxiety.

We think that buspirone may be the drug of choice for many patients with GAD who have not

TABLE 12-4. Clinical differences between buspirone and the benzodiazepines

	Buspirone	Benzo-diazepines
Acute effect on anxiety	$-^a$	$+^b$
Acute effect on psychotic agitation	0	+
Anticonvulsant effects	0	+
Chronic effect on anxiety	+	+
Effect on depression	+	0^c
Effect on acute panic attack	0	Alprazolam
Augment selective serotonin reuptake inhibitor for obsessive-compulsive disorder	+	0
Sedation	0	+
Potentiate alcohol	0	+
Disinhibition euphoria	0	+
Potential for abuse	0	+
Alleviate benzodiazepine withdrawal syndrome	0	+
Available i.v. or i.m.	0	+

^{a}Not studied.

^{b}+, present; 0, absent.

^{c}Most benzodiazepines do not have an antidepressant effect, with the possible exception of alprazolam.

taken BZDs previously. Buspirone may also have an advantage in patients who have problems with BZD withdrawal symptoms. Increased antianxiety effects have been observed in some patients treated concurrently with low doses of buspirone and a BZD (Table 12-4). Further, buspirone may be indicated in individuals with GAD with histories of chemical dependency who have failed or who could not tolerate antidepressants (54).

Venlafaxine

In the 1990s, evidence accumulated indicating that the latest generation of antidepressants were effective in a range of anxiety disorders, including GAD. Of these new antidepressants, venlafaxine, especially its extended-release formulation (Ven XR), was documented to be efficacious in outpatients with GAD without associated major depression. These data came from clinical trials conducted by expert clinical psychopharmacologists with broad experience in the assessment of psychotropic medications for anx-

iety disorders. The first of these trials (55) compared the efficacy of Ven XR with buspirone. The second trial (56) results also supported the efficacy of Ven XR in nondepressed outpatients with GAD. Following these confirmations of the efficacy of Ven XR in the short-term treatment of GAD patients without major depressive disorder, a third study was conducted to ascertain the long-term efficacy of Ven XR (57). This third study was a 6-month randomized controlled trial which found that Ven XR was safe and effective in a similar population of GAD patients. The 251 patients in this trial, conducted in 14 outpatient settings, were randomly assigned to receive either Ven XR at 75 to 225 mg/day or placebo titrated clinically for 28 weeks. At the conclusion of this study, 67% of the Ven XR patients but only 33% of the placebo patients were rated much or very much improved. Rating measures showed statistically significant ($p < 0.001$) differences from week 1 or 2 through week 28 in favor of Ven XR. Nausea, somnolence, and dry mouth were the most frequent patient-reported adverse events. This study was the first placebo-controlled demonstration of the long-term efficacy of any drug class in treating outpatients with *Diagnostic and Statistical Manual*, 4th ed., (DSM-IV)—diagnosed GAD. **These results indicate that Ven XR is an effective, rapidly acting, safe, once-daily agent for long-term treatment of GAD.**

Imipramine and Amitriptyline

Two studies have indicated that the tricyclic antidepressant (TCA) imipramine may be as effective as BZDs in the treatment of GAD (58, 59). No studies longer than 8 weeks' duration have been conducted, however, and imipramine's onset of anxiolytic action may be even slower than that of buspirone. Although adverse effects also may limit usefulness, its lack of dependence liability may make it an appropriate alternative in chronically anxious patients who also suffer from panic and depression.

The other tertiary TCA that has dual serotonergic-noradrenergic effects, amitriptyline, like imipramine, appears to be consistently effective in anxiety disorders. Newer antidepressants such as mirtazapine, nefazodone, paroxetine, and venlafaxine may also benefit patients with anxiety disorder (60–63).

β-Blockers and Antihistamines

Despite very limited efficacy in most anxious patients, β-blockers may be useful for highly somatic individuals, such as those with performance anxiety. Antihistamines are quite sedating, have little dependence potential, and are generally safe in terms of other complications, except their anticholinergic effects, which are common. We would note that reports of diphenhydramine abuse should lead to judicious prescribing of this antihistamine with close monitoring for signs of misuse.

Numerous clinical trials have also attested to the anxiolytic efficacy of hydroxyzine. Controlled trials have confirmed its efficacy and safety at a fixed dose of 50 mg in GAD (64). In a double-blind, parallel-group, multicenter study in France and Great Britain, a total of 244 patients with GAD were allocated randomly to treatment with hydroxyzine (12.5 mg t.i.d.), buspirone 5 mg morning and midday and 10 mg in the evening, or placebo. The results showed both hydroxyzine and buspirone to be more efficacious than placebo, indicating that hydroxyzine can be a useful treatment for GAD (65).

Abecarnil

The partial BZD agonist, abecarnil, has also been found to be useful as a safe, effective, short-term treatment for GAD (66–68).

Natural Remedies

Kava Kava (piper methysticum) is a member of the pepper tree family and for centuries has been a part of cultural traditions in the South Pacific islands, where it is used to induce a sense of tranquillity and to enhance sociability. It has had an integral role in a variety of social and therapeutic settings. Today, kava is rapidly becoming a popular herb in Europe, where it is used medicinally as a treatment for stress and anxiety, and recreationally in kava bars, which are also cropping up in the United States. Findings from extensive an-

imal testing suggest that kava has the following characteristics:

- It may be an *anxiolytic.*
- The development of *tolerance and withdrawal would be unlikely* at therapeutic doses.
- It may work through inhibition of sodium or calcium channels, having an *antiglutaminergic effect* (69).

Kava my also potentiate 5-HT$_{1A}$ agonist drugs, thereby suggesting either a direct or indirect serotonergic mechanism of action. Effects on GABA$_A$ and NMDA are unclear.

Major controlled clinical trials of kava in anxiety disorders support the likelihood that it may be of benefit in treating these disorders (70–75). Early onset of action was noted in two of three placebo-controlled trials, and effects of the drug have been noted on several scales. Kava is generally well-tolerated at doses of 210 to 240 mg/kl (kavalactones) daily, without the accompaniment of sedation or other adverse effects. Treatment for up to 6 months was examined in one study with the finding that the drug did not lose its effectiveness over time relative to placebo; however, studies of the safety and efficacy of long-term use of kava are needed. While recreational use of the herb is spreading, clinicians should be aware that consumption might result in an alcohol intoxication-like state in doses higher than those recommended. As with other medications and herbs, use in pregnant women and women who are nursing is not recommended.

Conclusion

It is not yet clear how useful, or how detrimental, chronic BZD therapy may be for patients with GAD. Whenever possible, BZD discontinuation (using a gradual tapering schedule) should be attempted to clarify persistence of anxiety or the existence of masked drug-induced adverse effects. Alternative strategies include the following:

- *Nondrug* interventions
- The azapirone *buspirone*

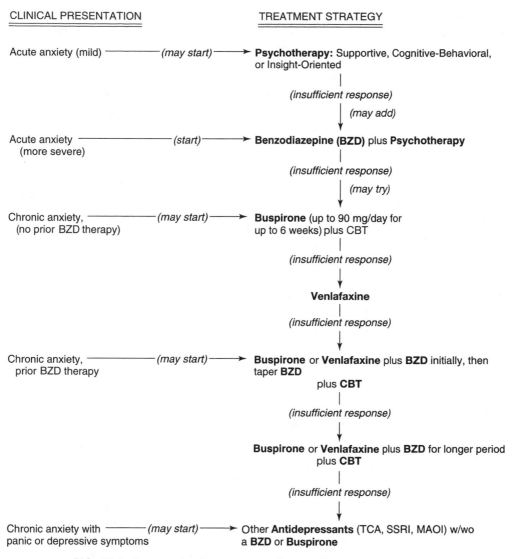

FIG. 12-2. Strategy for the treatment of generalized anxiety disorder.

- ADs such as *venlafaxine*
- *β-Blockers* or *antihistamines* in selected cases
- Possibly *kava*

Figure 12-2 summarizes the strategy we would recommend for the management of acute or chronic generalized anxiety.

TREATMENT OF PHOBIC DISORDERS

All of these disorders are characterized by disabling anxiety (at times also associated with panic attacks) and avoidance behavior because of exposure to the following:

- Places or situations from which one *cannot readily escape*
- A *specific feared object* or situation (e.g., heights)
- Certain types of *social* or *performance* situations

Agoraphobia

Agoraphobia may be associated with or without panic disorders (see also the section "Panic

Disorder" in Chapter 13). Inasmuch as most drug treatment studies have involved agoraphobic patients with panic disorder, there is relatively little evidence to suggest any agent is more than minimally effective for agoraphobia alone. *In vivo* exposure therapy, however, may be very useful in those willing to tolerate the distress associated with confronting the feared situation (76, 77).

Social Phobia

Although behavioral treatments for social phobia have been well studied, there are very limited data on its pharmacological management. *β-Blockers* (propranolol, atenolol) have been recommended, but available evidence indicates their effect may be no different than that of placebo (78). In a controlled study, the *monoamine oxidase inhibitor* (MAOI) phenelzine has been shown to be more effective than placebo (78, 79). Anecdotal reports have also described efficacy with *alprazolam, clonidine, and fluoxetine,* but systematic data are lacking (80–83).

A preliminary investigation has shown that sertraline therapy can be an effective treatment for social phobia. In this study, 80% were considered responders with all measures of social anxiety and avoidance, depression, and social functioning showing a statistically significant change from baseline to endpoint (84). Versiani's review of the literature led to a ranking of drug efficacy for social phobia: classic MAOIs > SSRIs > BZDs > RIMAs (84a).

Specific Phobia

Available evidence indicates that *systematic desensitization and in vivo exposure* are the most effective treatment methods available. Pharmacological treatment has not been well investigated, but studies involving antidepressants suggest that TCAs and MAOIs are ineffective (85–87). In addition, three studies suggest that sedative-hypnotic anxiolytics may undermine the behavioral treatment of specific phobias (88–90). In another study, volunteers with animal phobias were exposed to their phobic object 1.5 hours after administration of either tolamolol, diazepam, or placebo in a double-blind crossover

design. Tolamolol abolished the stress-induced tachycardia but had no beneficial behavioral or subjective effects (91).

Conclusion

Limited data exist to support drug management in phobic disorders. Behavioral techniques, especially for specific phobic conditions, are currently the treatment of choice. MAOIs, SSRIs, clonidine, and alprazolam may benefit some patients. Figure 12-3 summarizes the management strategy we would recommend.

TREATMENT OF SLEEP DISORDERS

DSM-IV (92) divides sleep disorders into three categories:

- *Primary* sleep disorders
  - Dyssomnias
  - Parasomnias
- Sleep disorders *related to another mental disorder*
- *Other* sleep disorders

Dyssomnias consist of problems associated with the amount, quality or timing of sleep, whereas *parasomnias* involve pathological, behavioral, or psychological events that occur with sleep, specific sleep stages, or sleep-wake transitions (see also Chapter 11). The other two categories usually require treatment of the mental or physical condition that has created the sleep disturbance. For all categories, the short-term use of hypnotics may play a role.

Treatment Principles

BZDs may offer temporary symptomatic relief for transient and short-term insomnia. They generally are not recommended as a long-term primary treatment for chronic insomnia or in patients with sleep apnea. Several of these agents are currently marketed in the United States or elsewhere for use as hypnotics (Table 12-5), but other BZDs can also serve the same purpose.

To administer any hypnotic rationally, effectively, and safely, clinicians should be familiar with the principles of appropriate prescribing

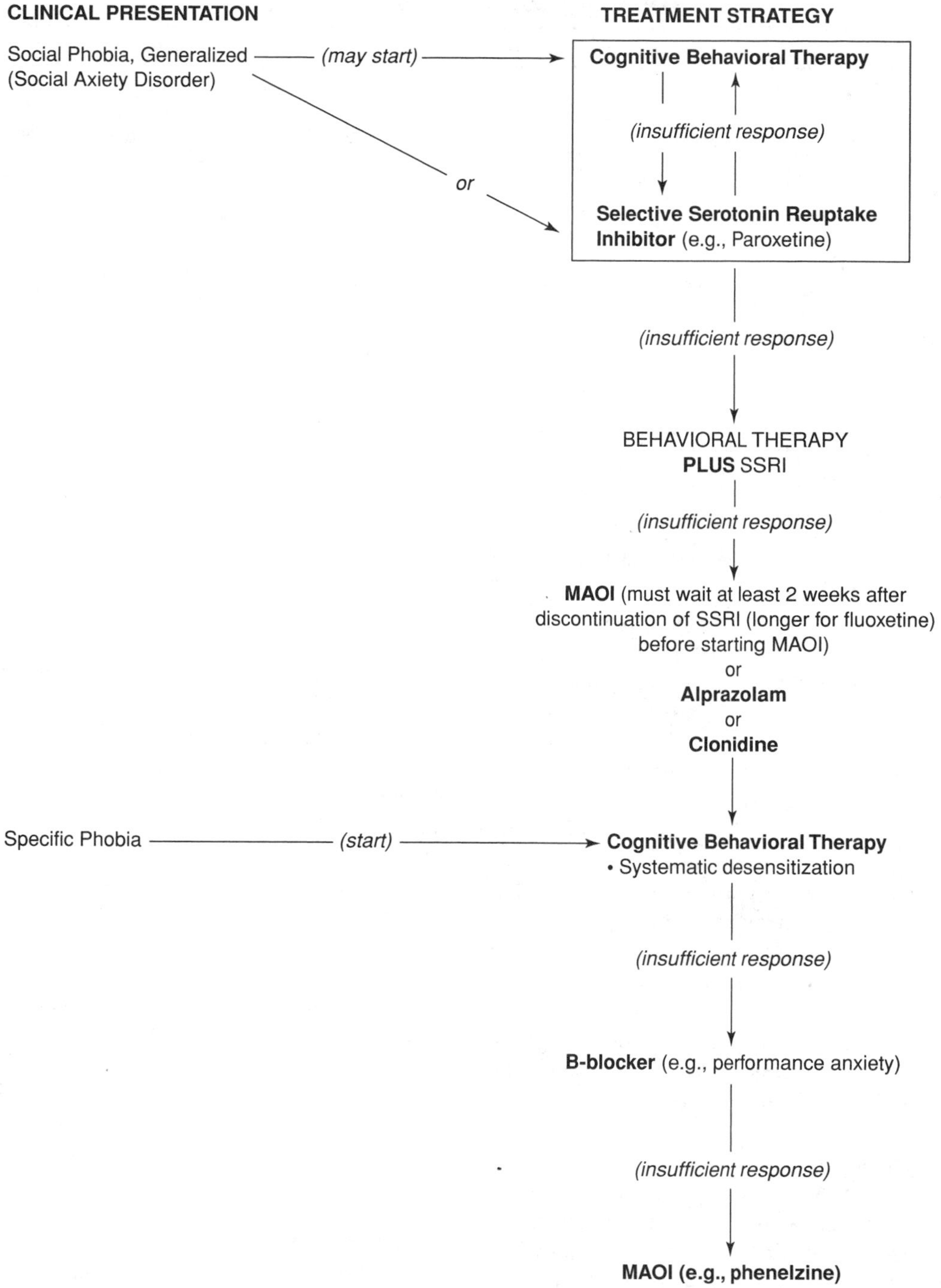

CLINICAL PRESENTATION   **TREATMENT STRATEGY**

Social Phobia, Generalized ——— *(may start)* ———→ **Cognitive Behavioral Therapy**
(Social Axiety Disorder)

(insufficient response)

or

Selective Serotonin Reuptake Inhibitor (e.g., Paroxetine)

(insufficient response)

BEHAVIORAL THERAPY **PLUS** SSRI

(insufficient response)

MAOI (must wait at least 2 weeks after discontinuation of SSRI (longer for fluoxetine) before starting MAOI)
or
Alprazolam
or
Clonidine

Specific Phobia ——————— *(start)* ——————→ **Cognitive Behavioral Therapy**
• Systematic desensitization

(insufficient response)

B-blocker (e.g., performance anxiety)

(insufficient response)

MAOI (e.g., phenelzine)

FIG. 12-3. Strategy for the treatment of phobic disorders.

(Table 12-6), as well as the pharmacology of the specific hypnotic.

Similar to the BZD anxiolytics, BZD hypnotics can be classified by their elimina- tion half-life into those that are long-acting, those that are intermediate-acting, and those that are short-acting (Table 12-5). The *Physician's Desk Reference* (PDR) (93) aptly calls

TABLE 12-5. *Benzodiazepine hypnotics*

Drug	Half-life (hours)	Metabolites
Long-acting		
Flunitrazepam[a]	19–22	None
Flurazepam	72–150	Several, including *N*-desalkylflurazepam
Medazepam[a]	65	*N*-desmethyldiazepam
Nitrazepam	18–34	None
Quazepam	72–150	*N*-desalkylflurazepam
Intermediate-acting		
Estazolam	15–18	None
Lormetazepam[a]	9	None
Temazepam	8–38	None
Short-acting		
Brotizolam[a]	3–6	None
Midazolam	1.5–3.5	None
Triazolam	2–5	None

[a] Not available in the U.S.

attention to the postulated relationship between the elimination rate of hypnotics and their profile of common untoward effects. It points out that the type and duration of hypnotic effects and the profile of unwanted effects during the administration of hypnotic drugs may be influenced by the biological half-life of the administered drug and any active metabolites formed. When half-lives are long, parent compound or metabolites may accumulate during periods of nightly administration and may impair cognitive and/or motor performance during waking hours. The possibility of interaction with other psychoactive drugs or alcohol is also enhanced. In contrast, if half-lives (including half-lives of active metabolites) are short, parent compound and metabolites are cleared before the next dose is ingested and carryover effects related to excessive sedation or CNS depression should be minimal or absent.

Because *long-acting* BZD hypnotics have persistent activity extending well into the next day, they can be useful for the treatment of nocturnal awakenings and late-onset insomnia (early morning awakening), especially if there is a daytime anxiety component. These, with their elimination half-life, include the following:

- Flunitrazepam (20 to 30 hours)
- Nitrazepam (15 to 38 hours)
- Medazepam (65 hours)

- Flurazepam (72 to 150 hours)
- Quazepam (72 to 150 hours)

The long half-lives of flurazepam and quazepam are due to their metabolite desalkylflurazepam.

Short- to intermediate-acting BZD hypnotics may have some residual effects the next day due to accumulation on daily ingestion. These, with their elimination half-life, include the following:

- Estazolam (15 to 18 hours)
- Lormetazepam (10 to 12 hours)
- Temazepam (8 to 12 hours)

Ultrashort-acting BZD hypnotics have a rapid fall in plasma level due either to a sustained distribution phase or to a rapid elimination. They are most useful in the treatment of early-onset insomnias (delayed sleep onset). The various drugs within this group have different rates of decline of plasma levels and therefore may sustain sleep to varying degrees. Generally, because of their short duration of action, rapidly eliminated BZD hypnotics do not have next-day residual effects, because they do not accumulate with daily usage. These, with their elimination half-life, include the following:

- Midazolam (1.5 to 3.5 hours)
- Triazolam (1.5 to 5 hours)
- Brotizolam (3 to 6 hours)

TABLE 12-6. *Principles of hypnotic prescribing*

1. Since sleep disturbance may be symptomatic of an underlying physical or psychiatric disorder, *a hypnotic should* be prescribed only after the patient has been carefully evaluated.
2. All hypnotics should be *prescribed only for short-term management* (7–10 nights) of insomnia. There is consensus in the United State among pharmaceutical manufacturers, the FDA, and the medical community that hypnotics should be used on a short-term basis.
3. Because insomnia is often transient and intermittent, *prolonged administration* of a hypnotic is generally considered to be *neither necessary nor recommended*.
4. For patients who have taken a hypnotic for 2 weeks, *reassessment to determine whether there is a continuing need should be done before prescribing another course of the hypnotic*.
5. The failure of insomnia to remit after 2 weeks of treatment suggests that it is due to a *medical or psychiatric disorder*, which should be diagnosed and treated.
6. Worsening of insomnia or the emergence of new abnormalities of thinking or behavior also may be due to an *unrecognized psychiatric or physical disorder*.
7. *Do not prescribe quantities exceeding a 1-month supply*.
8. Although not absolutely contraindicated, a hypnotic should be prescribed for patients with a history of alcohol or substance abuse or who have a marked personality disorder *only for short-term treatment and only under strict medical supervision*.
9. Before prescribing a hypnotic, clinicians should *fully inform the patient of the drug's risks and benefits*, and that treatment will be short term, and that refills will be limited. A patient information leaflet on the selected hypnotic should be given to, and reviewed with, the patient.
10. The patient should be made fully cognizant of the *safe use of prescribed hypnotics* (e.g., caution when operating machinery; avoidance of alcohol).
11. If retreatment becomes necessary, after drug-free intervals of 1 or more weeks, *it should only be done after another evaluation of the patient*.
12. For all patients, the risk of *psychological or physical dependence* on a hypnotic should be minimized by prescribing the least amount of the drug for the shortest period of time feasible. This is especially important for the elderly.
13. A hypnotic should not be prescribed for insomnia in the presence of *pain* unless insomnia persists after pain is controlled with analgesics.
14. Before prescribing a hypnotic, a comprehensive prescription and over-the-counter *drug history should be taken* from the patient to avert any adverse drug–drug interaction.
15. All patients with a *history of seizures* should be warned not to abruptly stop hypnotic therapy, regardless of their concomitant anticonvulsant drug regimen.
16. Because hypnotics may cause *cognitive impairment and respiratory depression*, a hypnotic should be carefully prescribed for patients with any pulmonary disease, chronic obstructive pulmonary disease (COPD), sleep apnea, and dementia.

Some short-acting BZDs (e.g., midazolam and triazolam) are ultrarapidly eliminated and their effect on sleep duration may be so short that patients may awaken earlier then they desire. Brotizolam, in contrast, has a half-life of around 5 hours that places it in the middle of the range of activity of the rapidly eliminated hypnotics. Thus, brotizolam may not only induce sleep quickly but also sustain sleep without residual effects the next day and without accumulation on repeated ingestion.

Some hypnotics have a short half-life and no active metabolites. During nightly use for an extended period, pharmacodynamic tolerance or adaptation to some effects may develop. If the drug has a short elimination half-life, it is possible that a relative deficiency of the parent compound or its active metabolites (i.e., in relationship to the receptor site) may occur at some point in the interval between each night's use. This sequence of events may account for two clinical findings reported to occur after several weeks of nightly use of rapidly eliminated hypnotics: increased wakefulness during the last third of the night and the appearance of increased signs of daytime anxiety.

If given in a large enough dose, any BZD may have hypnotic effects. In this context, anxiolytic BZDs such as clorazepate, diazepam, and lorazepam are often used as hypnotics

TABLE 12-7. *Sleep disruption in the elderly: considerations*

1. As health deteriorates with age, sleep becomes poorer.
2. True age-related sleep deterioration occurs after age 75 years.
3. Somatic and psychiatric diseases, unfavorable habits, and lifestyle factors increase a propensity to insomnia in the elderly
4. Cardiac disease and stroke, cancer, painful conditions, respiratory disorders, and nocturnal polyuria often disturb sleep.
5. Dementia and depression are often associated with sleep disturbances.
6. In view of the above, attempts to improve sleep should first be focused on elimination of somatic and psychiatric symptoms as far as possible and on modification of lifestyle factors that may affect sleep quality.
7. Although many hypnotic drugs are not suitable for long-term use, they can be used in elderly patients with severe disease and poor quality of life, providing that careful individualization of therapy and monitoring are done, along with appropriate selection of the hypnotic.

Adapted from Asplund R. Sleep disorders in the elderly. *Drugs Aging* 1999;14:91–103.

when anxiety is a prominent symptom associated with insomnia. Clorazepate is a prodrug for *N*-desmethyldiazepam, a slowly eliminated metabolite, which makes clorazepate appropriate for this clinical indication. Desmethyldiazepam has useful hypnotic activity and produces a steady anxiolytic effect through the next day. A single 15 or 22.5 mg bedtime dose is usually effective. Diazepam and its active metabolite, desmethyldiazepam, also are slowly eliminated, tend to accumulate, and tend to have a daytime anxiolytic effect with repeated ingestion. A single 5 or 10 mg bedtime dose is usually effective.

Benzodiazepine Hypnotics

Table 12-7 lists considerations regarding sleep disruption in the elderly, and Table 12-8 lists considerations regarding BZD hypnotics in this population.

Short-Term Treatment

Sleep onset latency generally is improved (i.e., shortened) with all BZD hypnotics, although this may vary considerably with individual patients. Those with relatively rapid onset of hypnotic activity include flurazepam, diazepam,

TABLE 12-8. *Benzodiazepine hypnotics for the elderly: considerations*

1. The most important factors to be considered when choosing a benzodiazepine hypnotic from among those available are their pharmacokinetic properties.
2. Microsomal oxidation may be compromised in the elderly, which may prolong the half-life and increase accumulation of long-acting hypnotics such as flurazepam.
3. Because the metabolic breakdown of hypnotics may be diminished in the elderly, the initial benzodiazepine dose for elderly patients should be one-third that recommended for younger patients.
4. Long-acting benzodiazepines are relatively contraindicated for elderly patients because they increase the risk of impaired cognitive function, falls, and hip fractures.
5. Flurazepam has the highest increase of risk for falls in the elderly.
6. There are no studies regarding the long-term effectiveness of benzodiazepine hypnotics for sleep disorders in the elderly.
7. Triazolam can cause rebound insomnia and anterograde amnesia.
8. The performance-impairing effects of triazolam are dose dependent and functionally coupled to its sleep-inducing properties.
9. Sedative-hypnotics should be used with caution in the elderly because they increase the risk of falling and hip fractures.
10. Chronic use of benzodiazepine has resulted in tolerance, abuse, and physical, as well as psychological, dependence.
11. A patient needing a hypnotic for more than several weeks should have drug-free periods to reduce the risk of dependence.

and chlorazepate. Somewhat slower onset occurs with triazolam, estazolam, quazepam, alprazolam, lorazepam, chlordiazepoxide, clonazepam, and temazepam in the newer formulations. Early observations that temazepam was ineffective in improving sleep onset latency may be the result of the formulation initially used in the United States, which was slowly absorbed (94–96). Reformulation, however, has improved this agent's absorption rate and onset of hypnotic activity (97) (see also Chapter 3). In contrast, oxazepam, halazepam, and prazepam tend to have a delayed onset, requiring administration at least 30 to 60 min before bedtime (98).

Long-acting BZDs usually maintain sleep throughout the night and tend to decrease daytime anxiety, whereas short-acting drugs may result in early morning awakening.

Long-acting compounds, such as quazepam and flurazepam, have been shown in sleep laboratory studies to maintain their hypnotic efficacy when given nightly for 4 weeks, although they were somewhat less effective toward the end of this period (99–106). One study reported that estazolam, with an intermediated half-life, retained its hypnotic efficacy for up to 6 weeks (107). Although triazolam in the 0.5 mg dose has been studied extensively and findings indicate a high degree of initial efficacy, some evidence indicates that the shorter-acting, high-potency BZDs such as triazolam and lorazepam may lose their sleep-promoting property within 3 to 14 days of continuous use (102, 108–114).

Whether hypnotic efficacy is retained with lower recommended doses of many BZDs is unclear. The efficacy of lower doses of triazolam (0.25 and 0.125 mg) has not been well established (112, 115–119). Flurazepam (15 mg) may be effective for 1 week but not for 2 weeks (119–121). Temazepam (15 mg) was reported effective for 2 weeks in one study but not in another (95, 123). Estazolam (1.0 and 2.0 mg) has been reported effective for 1 week, but longer term efficacy with the lower dose has not been reported (124).

Long-Term Treatment

No studies have demonstrated the hypnotic efficacy of BZDs beyond 12 weeks. Further, in studies involving a parallel placebo group, there was no difference between active medication and placebo after 2 to 3 weeks of treatment (115, 121, 125).

A sleep laboratory study involving middle-aged and elderly chronic insomniacs indicated that tolerance develops with continuous use. Thus, Schneider-Helmert (126) investigated the effects of continuous, long-term BZD use (6 months to years) in dosages ranging from 0.25 mg/day to twice the recommended dose. Compared with drug-free insomniacs, BZD users were found to have loss of hypnotic effectiveness and substantial suppression of delta and rapid eye movement (REM) sleep. Abrupt drug discontinuation resulted in recovery from this suppression with no increase in insomnia. Although drugs with short, intermediate, and long half-lives were all represented, only small differences were found among BZDs. Subjectively perceived hypnotic efficacy was not confirmed by objective measurement (i.e., those on BZDs showed a 72-minute overestimation of sleep and upon drug withdrawal a 61-minute overestimation of sleep onset latency). Schneider-Helmert concluded that long-term users' overestimation of sleep while taking a BZD coupled with awareness of their sleep disturbance on discontinuation may explain why such patients develop "low-dose dependence." Citing the findings of Lucki et al. that with continuous use there were still BZD-impaired memory functions shortly after taking the drug, Schneider-Helmert also speculated that overestimation of time spent sleeping may be the result of drug-induced anterograde amnesia (127).

Estazolam

Estazolam is a 1, 4-triazolobenzodiazepine hypnotic indicated for the short-term management of insomnia characterized by difficulty falling asleep, frequent nocturnal awakenings, or early morning awakenings. This drug depresses limbic and subcortical levels of the brain and potentiates the effect of GABA on its receptor, which increases inhibition and blocks cortical and limbic arousal. It is rapidly and completely absorbed through the gastrointestinal tract in 1 to 3 hours.

Peak plasma levels occur within 2 hours. Estazolam is 93% plasma protein bound and extensively metabolized in the liver. Elimination half-life ranges from 15 to 18 hours. Estazolam is highly lipid soluble.

Because insomnia is often transient and intermittent, the prolonged administration of estazolam is generally neither necessary nor recommended. Caution should be exercised in prescribing this hypnotic for elderly or debilitated patients, as well as for those with impaired renal or hepatic function, because of increased sensitivity or reduced capacity to metabolize and eliminate the drug. The recommended initial dose is 1 mg, but some may need a 2 mg dose. For the elderly, a 0.5 or 1 mg dose is appropriate.

Estazolam potentiates the CNS depressant effects of phenothiazines, narcotics, antihistamines, MAOIs, barbiturates, alcohol, general anesthetics, and TCAs. Use with cimetidine, disulfiram, oral contraceptives, and isoniazid may diminish hepatic metabolism and result in increased plasma concentrations of estazolam and increased CNS depressant effects. Heavy smoking (more than 20 cigarettes/day) accelerates estazolam's clearance. Theophylline antagonizes estazolam's pharmacological effects.

Quazepam

Quazepam is a 1, 4-BZD hypnotic that acts on the limbic system and thalamus of the CNS by binding to BZD receptors responsible for sleep. It is well absorbed from the gastrointestinal tract, with peak plasma levels of about 15 ng/mL within 2 hours. Steady-state plasma levels appear after 7 days of once-daily administration. The drug is more than 95% bound to plasma proteins. Mean elimination half-life of the parent drug and 2-oxoquazepam is 39 hours, while the other metabolite, desalkylflurazepam, has a half-life of 73 hours. The elimination half-lives of the parent drug and of 2-oxoquazepam are the same in elderly patients, but the elimination half-life of desalkylflurazepam in the elderly is twice that in young adults. Quazepam is available in unscored 7.5 and 15 mg strength tablets.

For healthy adults, quazepam therapy is best initiated with a 15 mg dose. In some patients, because of individual variations in response, the dose may be reduced to 7.5 mg. Elderly and debilitated patients should be started on 7.5 mg.

Use with alcohol, CNS depressants, antihistamines, opiate analgesics, and other BZDs increases CNS depression. **Quazepam is a pregnancy-risk category X drug, and breastfeeding while taking it is not recommended.**

Temazepam

This BZD sedative-hypnotic depresses the CNS at the limbic and subcortical levels of the brain. It potentiates the effect of GABA on its receptor, which increases inhibition and blocks cortical and limbic arousal. Temazepam is well absorbed through the gastrointestinal tract, with peak plasma levels in 1 to 3 hours. Onset of action occurs at 30 to 60 min. Temazepam is 98% protein bound, and its half-life ranges from 8 to 12 hours.

Compared with other BZD hypnotics, temazepam is less lipid soluble and hence should be administered about 1 hour before retiring, during which time patients would be well advised to use nonpharmacological measures to induce relaxation (128).

Temazepam is rarely beneficial in patients with psychoses and may induce paradoxical reactions. It may exacerbate myasthenia gravis, Parkinson's disease, and chronic obstructive pulmonary disease. Temazepam may decrease plasma levels of haloperidol.

Abuse of gelatin-filled temazepam capsules in the United Kingdom was so extensive in Britain that the U.K. health authorities removed this formulation from the market. All other formulations of temazepam are still available in the United Kingdom (129, 130).

Triazolam

Triazolam is a triazolobenzodiazepine sedative-hypnotic that depresses the CNS at the limbic and subcortical levels of the brain. It potentiates the effect of GABA on its receptor, which increases inhibition and blocks cortical and limbic arousal. It is well absorbed through the gastrointestinal tract with peak levels in 1 to 2 hours. Onset of action occurs at 15 to 30 minutes. Triazolam is

90% protein bound, with an elimination half-life of 1.5 to 5 hours.

Triazolam potentiates the CNS depressant effects of phenothiazines, narcotics, antihistamines, MAOIs, barbiturates, alcohol, general anesthetics, and antidepressants. Use with cimetidine and disulfiram may increase triazolam's plasma concentration.

Nefazodone substantially decreases the clearance rate for triazolam, which results in a 400% increase in triazolam's serum levels (131). *Erythromycin* can also interfere with the metabolism of triazolam, resulting in decreased clearance and increased plasma levels, possibly causing toxicity. Troleandomycin and other *macrolide antibiotics*, such as clarithromycin, flurithromycin, josamycin, midecamycin, or roxithromycin, also may inhibit triazolam's metabolism (132). The coadministration of *itraconazole* and triazolam can produce a marked elevation of triazolam plasma levels associated with statistically significant impairment of psychomotor tests and a prolongation of other effects (e.g., amnesia, lethargy, and confusion) for hours after awakening (133).

Triazolam can reach dangerous concentrations when administered to patients on systemic therapy with *ketoconazole*, which may result in statistically significant alterations in psychomotor test performance. In one study, when healthy volunteers were given low doses of triazolam (a single 0.25 mg dose) combined with ketoconazole, peak plasma concentrations rose threefold, and elimination half-life increased six- to sevenfold. Most volunteers experienced several hours of amnesia and felt tired and confused the next morning, 17 hours after the triazolam dose (133, 134). A second study comparing placebo with triazolam in healthy volunteers also taking ketoconazole produced findings comparable with the first study. In this second study, ketoconazole prolonged triazolam's half-life and reduced its clearance by about ninefold, while increasing impairment on neuropsychological performance (135).

In high doses, triazolam (e.g., 0.5 to 1.0 mg) may cause a syndrome of severe anxiety, paranoia, hyperacusis, altered smell and taste, and paraesthesia. Increased daytime anxiety typically occurs between doses of triazolam when it is used regularly as a hypnotic. These symptoms may be withdrawal effects because of triazolam's rapid elimination rate (see also Chapter 14).

Alternative Drug Treatments

Zopiclone

This non-BZD hypnotic, *cyclopyrrolone*, is indicated for short-term management of insomnia. Zopiclone has a BZD-like profile, a short half-life of 3.5 to 6.5 hours, no active metabolites, minimal rebound effects, and less abuse potential than BZDs. The usual therapeutic dose is oral 7.5 mg administered 30 to 60 minutes before bedtime. Zopiclone has a well-documented capacity to reduce sleep latency, improve quality and duration of sleep, and reduce the frequency of nighttime awakenings. In clinical trials, 7.5 mg doses of zopiclone have been found to be as effective as triazolam 0.5 mg, temazepam 20 mg, flurazepam 15-30 mg, and nitrazepam 5 to 10 mg for the short-term treatment of insomnia (136).

Zopiclone is relatively well tolerated (137). The most common adverse reaction is taste alteration. A postmarketing analysis of 10,000 cases revealed that zopiclone has a relatively low incidence of side effects (about 8%) (138). Like BZDs, zopiclone has a dose-related "hangover" effect (139). Rebound insomnia has occurred after short-term use (5 to 14 days) but does not appear to be as severe, even after abrupt withdrawal (140, 141). Abuse, tolerance, and physical and psychological dependence have been reported with zopiclone (142). Zopiclone has been shown to be as effective a hypnotic as triazolam in the elderly (143). More comparisons with short to medium half-life BZDs for the treatment of insomnia are needed to show that zopiclone has an advantage over the BZDs.

Zolpidem

This non-BZD hypnotic of the *imidazopyridine* class has no muscle relaxant, anxiolytic, or anticonvulsant effects at sedative doses. It is rapidly absorbed after oral administration, reaching peak blood levels in about 2.2 hours, and is highly bound to plasma protein. Elimination half-life is 2.4 hours in adults and 2.9 hours in the

TABLE 12-9. *A comparison of zolpidem and triazolam*

Zolpidem	Triazolam
Rapidly absorbed, reaching maximum serum concentration in 2 hours.	Rapidly absorbed, reaching maximum serum concentration in <2 hours.
Elimination half-life ranges from 2.4 to 2.9 hours.	*Elimination half-life* ranges from 1.5 to 5 hours.
Metabolites inactive.	Metabolites inactive.
Schedule IV drug.	Schedule IV drug.
Does not increase daytime sleepiness.	*May increase* daytime sleepiness.
No rebound insomnia.	*Rebound* insomnia.
Efficacy *maintained up to 6 months.*	Efficacy *diminishes after 2 weeks.*
May impair cognitive function.	May impair cognitive function.
May produce withdrawal symptoms.	*Does produce* withdrawal symptoms.

elderly. Its duration of action is 6 to 8 hours. It has no active metabolite. Its usual starting dose for adults is oral 10 mg immediately before bedtime, and its maximal dose is 20 mg. In the elderly, the starting dose is 5 mg immediately before bedtime. Zolpidem was well tolerated and improved sleep patterns in two patients with dementia and severe nighttime wandering and appears to be useful for restoring normal sleep patterns in elderly patients (144). Compared with older hypnotic drugs, zolpidem has similar sleep-enhancing properties, but is less likely to affect sleep architecture. Zolpidem has a more pronounced effect on sleep stages 3 and 4 than triazolam. A comparison of zolpidem and triazolam is summarized in Table 12-9. Zolpidem appears to be well tolerated in adults and in the elderly when administered in accordance with prescribing instructions. This drug does not appear to impair memory (145). The available data indicate that when zolpidem is administered according to instructions, the risk of abuse or dependence is minimal. Zolpidem has no or minimal rebound effects and less abuse potential than BZDs (146–148).

There is a need for more comparisons with short to medium half-life BZDs for the treatment of insomnia to show that zolpidem has any advantages over the BZDs. One placebo-controlled, randomized polysomnographic study of 24 patients with chronic insomnia found that zolpidem (10 mg) was comparable with triazolam (0.5 mg) and superior to placebo in enhancing sleep efficacy. Further, rebound insomnia occurred during the posttreatment, 3-day withdrawal phase in the triazolam group, but not in the zolpidem or the placebo groups (149).

Depressed individuals effectively treated with SSRIs often report persistent insomnia and require adjunctive sleep-promoting therapy. A study of the efficacy of zolpidem in this patient population showed that a dose of 10 mg was effectively and safely coadministered with an SSRI, resulting in improved self-rated sleep, daytime functioning, and well-being (150).

Adverse Effects

Several *psychotic reactions* to zolpidem have been reported–two cases of amnestic psychotic reaction and a psychotic reaction with hallucinations in an anorectic patient (151). Zolpidem 5 mg was prescribed for a 34-year-old woman with chronic insomnia. Twenty minutes after taking the recommended adult dose (10 mg), she experienced feelings of objects in her environment. She then slept uneventfully and recalled the unusual experience in the morning. Zolpidem may also cause transient *cognitive* and *behavioral problems* similar to those of BZDs (152).

Most of the drugs associated with *sleepwalking* and *night terrors* induce an increase of slow-wave sleep. Zolpidem increases delta sleep, and this effect is dependent on the age of the subject (i.e., it is observed in young adults). Drug-induced sleepwalking may need a combination of events in order to occur, such as a past history of sleepwalking, a medication increasing delta sleep, and a precipitating external or internal (such as a full bladder) stimulus (153, 154).

Case Example: Zolpidem was abused by a 33-year-old man who had been prescribed 10 mg/day for insomnia associated with depression. The patient took 30 mg and noticed improvement of depressive symptoms. With continued escalated doses (up to 150 to 280 mg/day), *tolerance* developed. He occasionally noticed signs of intoxication with severe ataxia after doses of 80 to 100 mg but never experienced the more common side effects of high-dose zolpidem. Dose reduction caused depressive mood recurrence with apathy and drug-craving. A *grand mal* seizure after ingesting 60 to 80 mg resolved without supportive measures (155).

Zaleplon

This newest non-BZD hypnotic is a *pyrazolopyrimidine* derivative with a full agonist activity on central BZD receptors B2 type. It is an effective hypnotic for the short-term treatment of insomnia. Because of its very short half-life (almost an hour), it may be useful for patients experiencing difficulty falling asleep and in those who wake up at night and who have trouble falling back to sleep. Zaleplon is rapidly absorbed after oral administration and its mean, apparent elimination half-life is similar to that obtained after i.v. infusion. Zaleplon is extensively metabolized in the liver by aldehyde oxidase, and to a lesser extent by CYP3A4. This drug is excreted in the urine (156).

Zaleplon's onset time, time to maximal drug effect, and duration of action are shorter than with triazolam. Hence, despite its non-BZD structure and unique BZD receptor binding profile, its behavioral pharmacological profile is similar to that of triazolam (157). Like zolpidem, zaleplon in recommended doses decreases sleep latency with minimal effect on sleep stages. Thus, it differs from BZDs, which prolong the first two stages of sleep and shorten stages 3 and 4 REM sleep (158).

A comparison of the duration of the residual hypnotic and sedative effects of zaleplon with those of zolpidem and placebo following nocturnal administration at various times before morning awakening demonstrated that zaleplon 10 mg is free of residual hypnotic or sedative effects when administered as little as 2 hours before waking in normal subjects. Zolpidem's residual effects were still apparent on objective assessments up to 5 hours after nocturnal administration, longer than has been reported from studies involving daytime administration (159).

A comparison of the residual effects of zaleplon (10 or 20 mg), triazolam (0.25 mg), and placebo on memory, learning, and psychomotor performance in healthy adults was conducted. Behavioral, cognitive, and psychomotor evaluations were performed before bedtime and after awakening at 1.25 hours (peak plasma concentration) and 8.25 hours after administration. The 10 mg dose of zaleplon produced no significant changes versus placebo in postdose psychometric tests, including Immediate and Delayed Word Recall, Paired Associates Learning, Digit Span, Digit Substitution, and Divided Attention Tests. Zaleplon 20 mg (twice the therapeutic dose) showed effects similar to those produced by the usual doses of zolpidem and triazolam. These results indicate that the recommended 10 mg dose of zaleplon does not significantly impair cognitive or psychomotor skills (160).

A study evaluated the relationship of dose, plasma concentration, and time to the pharmacodynamics of zaleplon and zolpidem found that the kinetics of these drugs were not significantly related to dose. However, zaleplon had more rapid elimination and higher apparent oral clearance. On a number of measures, 20 mg of zaleplon was comparable with 10 mg of zolpidem. Dynamic effects of both drugs were significantly related to plasma concentration. The results of this study led to the conclusion that the BZD agonist effects of zaleplon and zolpidem were dose and concentration dependent and that at the usual clinically effective hypnotic dose (10 mg of either drug), agonist effects of zolpidem exceeded those of zaleplon (161).

The data on zaleplon to date indicate that it has some advantages over other hypnotics, including a favorable safety profile, as indicated by the absence of rebound insomnia and withdrawal symptoms when zaleplon is discontinued (162). In addition, when taken by a nursing mother, zaleplon is transferred through breast milk to her infant in such very small quantities that this is unlikely to be important (163).

A 10 mg bedtime dose of zaleplon is usually effective. A few patients may require a 20 mg dose. A 5 mg dose is safer and effective for elderly and debilitated patients or for those with hepatic impairment. A 5 mg dose is also preferable and safer for patients taking cimetidine, which increases zaleplon's serum concentration by almost 85%.

Other Classes of Drugs

Sedative antidepressants, such as amitriptyline, doxepin, or trazodone, in low doses, have hypnotic efficacy and may be less likely to evoke the adverse effects associated with higher doses.

Antihistamines, such as diphenhydramine and doxylamine, may be effective for up to 1 week, but controlled data on longer use are lacking (164, 165). These drugs may produce excessive anticholinergic adverse effects. Doxylamine is potentially hazardous for the elderly, impairing vision, delaying urination, impeding gastrointestinal movement resulting in constipation, or obstipation, and intestinal blockage. The anticholinergic effects of antihistamines can also cause impairment of cognitive function and delirium. Hence, judicious prescribing of these drugs in the elderly is warranted.

Barbiturates and *barbiturate-like drugs,* such as chloral hydrate, although effective hypnotics, are considered far less safe than BZDs in terms of tolerance, interaction with alcohol, and lethality in overdose. Therefore, their use is not generally recommended.

Natural Remedies

Melatonin

Although melatonin may be helpful in the alleviation of jet lag and improving accommodation to schedule changes in shift work, we would caution that it is not approved by the Federal Drug Administration (FDA), which requires more definitive evidence of effectiveness and safety than is currently available. Hence, there is little control over type of manufacture, relative purity or accuracy of dosage, safety, and potential long-term side effects. For example, a study of random samples of over-the-counter melatonin revealed unknown substances. All three melatonin samples contained several contaminants presumably introduced during the manufacturing process (166, 167).

Garfinkel et al. (168) conducted an investigation of melatonin's effects on sleep quality in 12 elderly subjects with insomnia [seven men, five women; mean age, 76 years (range, 68 to 93 years; standard deviation (SD), ±8 years)]. These authors used a randomized, double-blind, crossover design with 2 mg controlled-release melatonin or a placebo taken 2 hours before desired bedtime every night for 3 weeks. After a 1-week washout, the subjects then received 3 weeks' treatment with the other preparation. Compared with placebo, the controlled-release melatonin improved the sleep quality of these elderly subjects and was well tolerated. Further, 2 months' treatment with 2 mg of controlled-release melatonin in these relatively healthy elderly subjects was much more effective than 1 week of treatment (168).

In another study, melatonin (0.3 mg) or placebo were given half an hour before bedtime on 3 consecutive nights to nine elderly insomniacs (age, 51 to 70 years) complaining of prolonged sleep latency, multiple nocturnal awakenings, or early morning awakening (169). Core body temperature and motor activity were monitored every morning, and a sleep questionnaire was administered for each night. Melatonin greatly reduced movements during the night, hastened sleep onset, decreased awakenings at night, and improved the perception of sleep quality without increased morning sleepiness. Further, this dose of melatonin had no effect on core body temperature.

Andrade et al. (169a) conducted a placebo-controlled, double-blind study, which found that a mean stable dose of 5.4 mg of melatonin was helpful for initial insomnia in medically-ill patients for whom standard sedative-hypnotics may be problematic.

Melatonin may play a role in the treatment of some insomnia disorders. However, optimal dose and timing of administration need to be established. The effect of oral doses (0.3 or 1.0 mg) given at 6, 8, or 9 pm were measured polysomnographically. Either dose given at any of the three timepoints decreased sleep onset latency and latency to stage 2 sleep. Melatonin did not suppress REM sleep or delay its onset. Neither dose of melatonin induced "hangover" effects. The results of this study add to the evidence that nocturnal melatonin secretion may be involved in physiological sleep onset and that exogenous melatonin may be useful in treatment of insomnia (170).

A placebo-controlled, double-blind, crossover design study to assess the sleep-promoting effects of three melatonin replacement delivery strategies in a group of patients with age-related, sleep-maintenance insomnia was conducted. A high physiological dose of immediate-release melatonin was given 30 minutes before bedtime, a controlled-release dose was given 30 minutes before bedtime, and an immediate-release dose was given 4 hours after bedtime. All three treatments shortened latency to persistent sleep, demonstrating that high physiological doses of melatonin can promote sleep in this population. Melatonin, however, was not effective in sustaining sleep, nor did treatment improve total sleep time, sleep efficiency, or wake after sleep onset. Finally, melatonin did not improve subjective reports of nighttime sleep and daytime alertness (171).

The body clock is on an approximate 24-hour schedule. Bright light (i.e., sunlight) in the morning regulates the clock, keeping it on a 24-hour schedule. Based on the timing of the bright light (presumably at sunrise), melatonin is released about 14 hours later. With transmeridinal jet travel, destination time is shifted many time zones, but the body clock remains on the home time zone, and as a result, the traveler feels tired and experiences a poorer mental performance (jet lag). Because bright light and melatonin help readjust the body clock, their judicious use can help reduce jet lag (172, 173).

To some degree, you can reset the body clock before you leave for eastern travel by getting up early with artificial bright light and then going to bed earlier. Alternatively, Arendt (173) recommends late afternoon melatonin for 2 days before departure and after destination arrival melatonin for 4 days. For western travel, one can go to bed late and sleep later. Arendt does not recommend morning melatonin as pretravel medication because it can cause sleepiness, but does recommend 4 days of evening melatonin at destination. For more exact timing, the reader is referred to Lewy et al. (172), who provide detailed nomograms and a logical explanation of the timing of rhythm shifts.

There are several double-blind studies that support melatonin administration. For example, rapid deployment aviation groups sent to the Middle East demonstrated longer sleep duration and better test performance on melatonin than did the placebo group (174, 175). Arendt (173), who has had extensive experience with both controlled and uncontrolled studies, summarized the overall experience in 386 subjects, showing a 60% reduction in jet lag for eastern travel and a 40% reduction for western travel.

In conclusion, as Chase and Gidal (176) have commented, although some evidence indicates that melatonin may have modest efficacy, especially in insomnia, jet lag, and sleep disorders in neurologically impaired patients, adequate long-term studies examining both efficacy and toxicity are lacking. In addition, further studies evaluating dose-response relationships and drug interactions are warranted.

Valerian

This herbal product has a long history of use throughout the world as a sedative, hypnotic, and anxiolytic (177). Similar to the BZDs, extracts of valerian appear to have an affinity for GABA receptors, probably because of the relatively high content of GABA that has been documented as a constituent of valerian (178). Human clinical studies confirm a mild sedative effect. Valerian doses of 400 to 900 mg in humans have been shown to improve the quality of sleep and to reduce sleep latency without producing a "hangover." An interaction of valerian with melatonin-binding sites may contribute to its sedative properties, as may its potential to inhibit the reuptake of and/or stimulate GABA release from nerve terminals. High doses of valerian may have anticonvulsant and spasmolytic effects. Valerian also has some anxiolytic and mild antidepressant properties that may contribute to its usefulness as a treatment for BZD withdrawal (179). Several studies suggest that valerian is at least as effective as small doses of barbiturates and BZDs. No evidence indicates that valerian is a more efficacious treatment than existing hypnotics or other treatments for insomnia. Finally, valerian's promotion of "natural" sleep occurs after several weeks of use, which makes it unsuitable for the acute treatment of insomnia and/or as an alternative for BZD and non-BZD hypnotics.

Side effects include hepatotoxic effects, although the offending preparation often contained a mixture of ingredients and possibly adulterants or contaminants. Insufficient information exists to recommend valerian in pregnancy and during lactation, although no reports have shown teratogenicity. One study reported a possibly hazardous interaction between valerian root and fluoxetine (179a).

Alternative Nondrug Treatments

Alternate nondrug treatments include stimulus control, progressive muscle relaxation, paradoxical intention, biofeedback, sleep restriction, multicomponent cognitive behavior therapy (179b), sleep hygiene education, imagery training, and cognitive therapy. Practice parameters for these nonpharmacological therapies have been formulated by the American Academy of Sleep Medicine (180, 181). Only stimulus control, progressive muscle relaxation, paradoxical intention, sleep restriction, biofeedback, and multicomponent cognitive-behavior therapy, however, meet the American Psychological Association criteria for probable efficacious treatments (182).

Sleep Hygiene Techniques

Appropriate sleep hygiene techniques should always be considered and, when possible, used in lieu of pharmacotherapy. When medication is given, such nonpharmacological approaches may significantly decrease the amount and duration of drug exposure. Sleep therapies include the following:

- Stimulus control
- Sleep restriction
- Relaxation techniques
- Paradoxical intention
- Sleep hygiene education

Stimulus control attempts to decrease sleep-incompatible behavior and to regulate the sleep-wake schedule. It incorporates a series of instructions such as going to bed only when sleepy; using the bedroom only for sleep or sex; leaving the bedroom if unable to fall asleep within 15 to 20 minutes and returning again only when feeling sleepy; always arising at the same time each morning, regardless of the amount of sleep; and never taking naps.

Sleep restriction attempts to decrease the amount of time spent in bed versus the actual amount of time spent sleeping. The goal is to achieve a window of sleep efficiency between 80% and 90%. Thus, if above or below this range, one would increase or decrease time in bed by 15 to 20 minutes.

Relaxation techniques can address increased arousal, which can be somatic, cognitive, or both. Somatic arousal is usually modified by muscle relaxation and/or biofeedback, whereas increased cognitive arousal can be moderated by attention-focusing procedures, such as imagery training or meditation.

Paradoxical intention focuses on staying awake as a means of diminishing performance anxiety.

Sleep hygiene education emphasizes alterations in lifestyle, such as the following:

- Improved *health practices* (e.g., diet, exercise, avoiding substance use)
- Alteration of *environmental factors* (e.g., lighting, noise, temperature)

In addition to supplying basic information about changes that occur in sleep patterns over the life cycle, patients should be encouraged to do the following:

- *Reduce* or *avoid* the use of alcohol, nicotine, caffeine, or hypnotics (including over-the-counter preparations)
- Avoid daytime *naps*.
- Get regular *exercise*.
- Go to bed and wake up at the *same time* every day.
- Use the bedroom *only for sleep or sex* (not for reading, watching television, or working).

If sleep onset does not occur within 30 minutes, patients should get out of bed and not return until they are sleepy.

Behavioral Therapies

Although several behavioral approaches have been investigated, including biofeedback, progressive relaxation, hypnosis, and others, results have been mixed and there is little consensus regarding their use. Marin et al. (182) reviewed this literature and performed a meta-analysis of the efficacy of psychological interventions. **After reviewing 59 treatment outcome studies involving more than 2, 000 patients, these authors concluded that stimulus control and sleep restriction were the most effective therapeutic procedures.** Furthermore, clinical improvements were well maintained at an average follow-up of 6 months, documenting that nonpharmacological interventions produced reliable and durable changes in sleep latency and time awake after sleep onset in individuals with chronic insomnia.

Sleep Deprivation

Noting that chronic insomniacs often underestimate their actual sleep time, Spielman et al. (183) conducted a study in which subjects initially were allowed to stay in bed only as long as their own estimate of time spent asleep. Results indicated that the mild sleep deprivation produced tended to improve sleep onset latency and efficiency.

Conclusion

The BZDs will usually shorten sleep onset latency with brief (1-week to 2-week) periods of treatment, and the use of longer acting agents (e.g., flurazepam) tends to avoid rebound insomnia. Lower dose strategies may also be effective for some patients, requiring only 1 to 2 weeks of therapy. No studies have demonstrated hypnotic efficacy beyond 3 months. Alternative strategies that may be effective for chronic insomnia include the use of sleep hygiene techniques and/or low doses of sedating antidepressants, such as trazodone. Figure 12-4 outlines the treatment strategy we would recommend.

PHARMACOKINETICS

It is sometimes said that all BZDs are essentially the same, with no major differences among them. This is misleading, however, because variations in chemical structure and pharmacokinetics profoundly influence the following:

- *Potency*
- *Onset* and *duration* of clinical activity
- Type and frequency of *adverse effects* after both single and multiple doses
- *Withdrawal* phenomena

These differences often make it possible to select a specific drug most likely to benefit an individual patient, while minimizing the risk.

Lipid Solubility

The more lipid-soluble the BZD, the more readily it passes from the plasma through the lipophilic blood-brain barrier and, thus, the more rapid its onset of action. BZDs can be subdivided on the basis of lipophilicity–a factor that plays an important role in absorption. Midazolam, quazepam, and diazepam are among the more lipophilic of the BZDs. Because increasing lipophilicity also increases the rate of redistribution from blood and brain into adipose tissue, BZDs that are less lipophilic may have more persistent brain concentrations due to reduced peripheral distribution (97, 184).

Absorption

BZDs with rapid absorption produce a more rapid onset of clinical activity than those with slower absorption. BZDs given orally differ in their speed of absorption from the gastrointestinal tract. For example, absorption time is 0.5 hours for clorazepate, 1 hours for diazepam, 1.3 hours for triazolam, 2 hours for alprazolam and lorazepam, 2 to 3 hours for oxazepam, and 3.6 hours for flurazepam. Absorption, however, may be influenced by the presence or absence of food in the gastrointestinal tract. Thus, patients who take a BZD hypnotic with a bedtime snack may experience a slower onset of hypnotic activity than if the same drug were taken several hours after a meal.

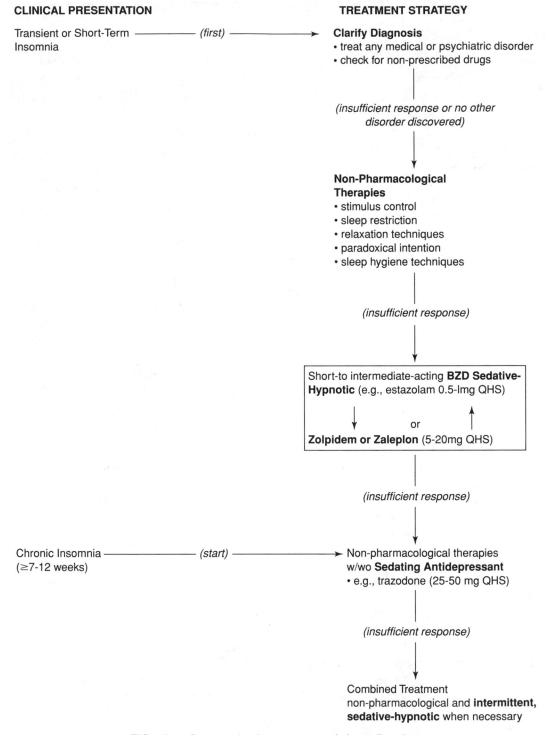

FIG. 12-4. Strategy for the treatment of sleep disorders.

Protein Binding

BZDs also differ in their plasma protein binding capacity. The percentage of unbound oxazepam is 0.2% to 0.3%, diazepam 0% to 2%, of chlordiazepoxide 3% to 8%, and of lorazepam 7% to 12%.

Metabolism and Elimination

BZDs biotransformed by hepatic oxidation have relatively long half-lives and usually have active metabolites (Table 12-10). Those biotransformed by glucuronide conjugation have relatively short half-lives and no active metabolites. Only a few BZDs (e.g., clonazepam) are biotransformed by nitro reduction. Although oxidized BZDs and their metabolites may be more likely to accumulate due to age, liver disease, or concomitant use of estrogens or cimetidine, clinical data substantiating this theory are incomplete.

Biotransformation

Based on metabolic profile, BZDs can be divided into three groups:

- Those *biotransformed by oxidative metabolism in the liver,* primarily *N*-demethylation or hydroxylation (e.g., adinazolam, chlordiazepoxide, clobazam, diazepam, flunitrazepam, and medazepam), often yield pharmacologically active metabolites that must undergo further metabolic steps before excretion.

- Unlike oxidized BZDs, *conjugated BZDs* (e.g., lorazepam, lormetazepam, oxazepam, and temazepam) do not have active metabolites. Only the parent compounds account for clinical activity.
- BZDs that undergo a *high first-pass effect* before reaching the systemic circulation (e.g., brotizolam, clotiazepam, midazolam, and triazolam) may have short-lived but active metabolites.

The first category of BZDs is more likely to be influenced by such factors as old age, liver disease, or coadministration of other drugs that may stimulate or impair hepatic oxidizing capacity. Another difference is that these BZDs tend to have longer elimination half-lives than agents that are conjugated directly.

Based on elimination half-life, BZDs can again be divided into three groups:

- *Ultrashort-acting* (less than 5 hours), such as midazolam, triazolam, and brotizolam
- *Short-to-intermediate acting* (6 to 12 hours), such as oxazepam, bromazepam, lorazepam, loprazolam, temazepam, estazolam, lormetazepam, and alprazolam
- *Long-acting* (more than 12 hours), such as flunitrazepam, clobazam, flurazepam, clorazepate, ketazolam, chlordiazepoxide, and diazepam

Onset and duration of BZD clinical activity are not necessarily related to elimination half-life. When given in single doses, BZDs with

TABLE 12-10. *Benzodiazepine anxiolytics*

Name (proprietary name)	Metabolism	Half-life including metabolites	Lipid solubility	Active metabolites
Alprazolam (Xanax)	Oxidation	8–15	Moderate	No
Bromazepam[a]	Oxidation	20–30	Low	No
Chlordiazepoxide (Librium)	Oxidation	10–20	Moderate	Yes
Clobazam[a]	Oxidation	20–30	Moderate	Yes
Clorazepate (Tranxene)	Oxidation	40–100	—	Yes
Diazepam (Valium)	Oxidation	20–70	High	Yes
Halazepam (Paxipam)	Oxidation	40–100	Low	Yes
Lorazepam (Ativan)	Conjugation	10–20	Moderate	No
Oxazepam (Serax)	Conjugation	5–15	Moderate	No
Prazepam (Centrax)	Oxidation	40–100	Low	Yes

[a]Not available in the United States.

long half-lives may have a shorter duration of action than BZDs with shorter half-lives because of extensive distribution. During multiple dosing, however, BZDs with longer half-lives accumulate slowly, and after termination of treatment disappear slowly, whereas BZDs with short half-lives have minimal accumulation and disappear rapidly when treatment stops (185).

Potency

BZDs differ considerably in potency, which refers to the milligram dose needed to produce a given clinical effect. These differences are in part due to differences in receptor site affinity. If given in the appropriate dose, any BZD may exert anxiolytic, hypnotic, or anticonvulsant effects. For example, anxiolytic BZDs, such as clorazepate and diazepam, are often used as hypnotics when anxiety is a prominent symptom associated with insomnia.

Drug Interactions

With the important exception of additive effects when combined with other CNS depressants, including alcohol, BZDs interact with very few drugs. Disulfiram (see the section "The Alcoholic Patient" in Chapter 14) and cimetidine may increase BZD blood levels, and diazepam may increase blood levels of digoxin and phenytoin. Antacids may reduce the clinical effects of clorazepate by hindering its biotransformation to desmethyldiazepam. Coadministration of a BZD and another drug known to induce seizures may possibly increase seizure risk, especially if the BZD is abruptly withdrawn. Furthermore, as noted earlier, important interactions have been reported among nefazodone, erythromycin, troleandomycin, and other macrolide antibiotics, as well as itraconazole. In each case, metabolism is inhibited, and triazolam levels can increase significantly.

Conclusion

As reviewed and emphasized in Chapter 3, the physical and the pharmacokinetic properties of various psychotropics, including the BZDs, often have clinically relevant implications. This realization can serve to enhance efficacy and/or minimize adverse effects. Thus, while ignorance of these properties may put patients at unnecessary risk, a working knowledge of these issues can often produce an ideal clinical outcome.

ADVERSE EFFECTS OF ANXIOLYTICS

Relative to other psychotropics, acute BZD treatment is associated with fewer unwanted effects. **Sedation is usually the most prominent initial complication, subsiding in about a week as anxiolytic action emerges** (186). Confusion, ataxia, excitement, agitation, transient hypotension, vertigo, and gastrointestinal distress may also occur in a small number of patients.

Behavioral Disinhibition

A possible association between the clinical use of a BZD and aggressive behavior was reported not long after chlordiazepoxide first became available for prescription (187). Since then, numerous case reports and studies have suggested that some BZD-treated patients experience increased hostility and aggressiveness, ranging from feelings to overt behavior. One literature review found that the phenomenon is difficult to characterize because it may include various manifestations, including the following:

- Hostility
- Aggressiveness
- Rage reactions
- Paroxysmal excitement
- Irritability
- Behavioral dyscontrol (188)

Nevertheless, the reviewers reported that no variable (e.g., pretreatment hostility, severity of anxiety, length of treatment, dose) was consistently predictive of hostility and aggressiveness. In addition, patients with a history of character disorder, aggressive behavior, or substance abuse are not more likely to experience aggressive dyscontrol during BZD treatment; and indeed, there are numerous reports of such patients experiencing no adverse consequences (189, 190). **Based on BZD efficacy studies that reported adverse effects, the reviewers estimated the incidence of aggressive dyscontrol to be less** than 1%–comparable with that of placebo. The incidence of overt rage reactions appears to be even lower. A comparison of the frequency of behavioral disinhibition due to alprazolam, clonazepam, or no BZD in an inpatient population has been published recently (191). The authors reported that these types of behaviors did not differ among the three groups and that disinhibition may not be an important clinical issue.

Overdose

Fatalities due to acute BZD overdose alone are extremely rare. Nevertheless, fatal overdoses with triazolam in the elderly have been reported (192, 193). Even with ingestion of massive doses, recovery appears to be rapid and without serious complications or aftereffects (194–197). Combined ingestion of BZDs with other CNS depressants (alcohol, barbiturates, narcotics, or TCAs), however, may result in severe CNS and respiratory depression or hypotension. Severity of symptoms appears to depend more on the type and quantity of the other drugs than on the BZD plasma level (194–196).

Few overdoses with alprazolam alone have been reported. However, one fatality due to alprazolam intoxication has been published, along with a description of the distribution of alprazolam and an active metabolite α-hydroxyalprazolam in tissues obtained at autopsy (198).

Psychomotor Impairment

Numerous studies of acute or chronic dosing in normal volunteers and anxious patients indicate that BZDs may impair certain types of psychomotor functioning, such as coordination and sustained attention. These studies have produced conflicting results, however, particularly in anxious subjects or those on chronic dosing. Some patients have exhibited few or no decrements, and it has been postulated that by reducing anxiety (which itself can impair functioning), a BZD may paradoxically improve performance. Several studies have found, however, that drivers taking a BZD are at increased risk for a serious automobile accident (199–202). In

addition, the combination of therapeutic doses of a BZD and even a small amount of alcohol may produce significant psychomotor decrements that are greater than would be expected with either substance alone (i.e., a synergistic effect).

Cognitive Impairment

It has been known for almost three decades that even single doses of BZDs impair cognitive function. It also has been demonstrated that psychological impairment occurs in normal subjects and after short courses of treatment in anxious patients (203). In a study designed to establish whether ability is impaired in long-term BZD users, as well as to determine the nature and extent of any deficit, investigators assessed a wide range of cognitive functions using a battery of neuropsychological tests (204). They found that patients taking high therapeutic doses for long periods of time performed poorly on tasks involving visuospatial ability and sustained attention, implying that these individuals may not be functioning well in everyday life. Test results also indicated that subjects were not aware of their reduced ability. This is consistent with clinical evidence provided by patients who, after discontinuing a BZD, often report improved concentration and increased sensory perception and who only realized their functioning had been below par after stopping the drug (205).

Case Example: A 44-year-old man, who worked as a tenured graduate school professor, after several years of analytically oriented psychotherapy, became dissatisfied with the persistence of his GAD symptoms. He persuaded his therapist to prescribe an anxiolytic for him, beginning with diazepam, 2 mg twice daily. Because of only minimal relief the diazepam dose was increased first to 5 mg b.i.d. and ultimately to 10 mg t.i.d. This daily dose effectively alleviated the patient's more distressing GAD symptoms. For the next year and a half, the patient took between 25 and 35 mg daily, as he attempted to adjust the dose commensurate with his perceived need to be symptom-controlled. During this time, his wife observed that he seemed "slowed down" at times, even though he worked regularly and was otherwise "the same as ever, only less anxious." His therapist, who saw him once monthly during this period, also thought that he was less anxious and improved and "doing well" on his maintenance diazepam regimen. The therapist's monitoring of the patient's diazepam prescriptions and refills did not suggest any overuse of this drug.

The therapist, patient, and family were all surprised when school officials informed the patient of student complaints about a decline in his teaching performance. The patient indignantly challenged these allegations, insisting that he was not aware of any change in his teaching. On the insistence of school officials, however, the patient saw a second psychiatrist in consultation. Although the patient did not seem "drugged, " various performance tests were ordered. These disclosed some cognitive impairment that the psychologist considered drug-induced. A tapered discontinuation of diazepam over a 3-month period to a maintenance dose of 5 mg b.i.d. resulted in a marked change in the patient. He became more alert and more active, and his teaching more dynamic and effective. His family was pleased with the transformation to his "old self." The patient acknowledged the change in himself but continued to insist that he was unaware of the adverse drug-induced effects on his cognitive functions.

Similar findings were reported in a study of elderly patients, in whom the onset of cognitive impairment was often insidious, became evident only after years of treatment, and improved with drug discontinuation (206). In a study comparing chronic pain patients receiving no medication, narcotics alone, or BZDs alone, the last group was significantly more likely to exhibit signs of cognitive impairment and concomitant EEG changes than those treated with narcotics (207).

Imaging Studies

The demonstration of structural brain abnormalities in conjunction with cognitive impairment in those who have abused alcohol for prolonged periods prompted Ron (208) and Lader et al. (209) to ascertain whether this could be true in long-term BZD users, some of whom had de-

tectable cognitive impairment during drug withdrawal. Brain computerized tomography (CT) scans were done on 20 patients, none of whom abused alcohol or took other drugs but were receiving or had recently discontinued long-term (2 to 20 years) BZD treatment. Their scans were then compared with those of age- and sex-matched normal control subjects, as well as with chronic alcoholics. In some of the BZD patients the mean ventricular to brain ratio measured by planimetry was increased over the mean values of the control subjects, although it was less than that in the alcoholics. There was no significant relationship between computed tomography (CT) scan appearance and age, or the duration of BZD therapy.

Schmauss and Krieg (210) subsequently confirmed these findings in 17 BZD-dependent inpatients who reported no history of other types of chemical dependency, including abuse of alcohol. Brain CT scans before drug withdrawal revealed a significantly higher ventricular to brain ratio (VBR) in those dependent on high and low doses compared with matched control subjects. Further, the mean VBR was significantly higher in the high- than in the low-dose-dependent patients, suggesting a dose-dependent effect. Neither age nor duration of use accounted for the observed differences in the VBR values.

Uhde and Kellner (211) reported a positive correlation between duration of BZD exposure and VBR in their study of panic patients, 19 of whom reported being treated with a BZD for a mean of 3.6 years (range, 0.5 to 12 years). Noting that 70% of their sample was composed of subjects with fewer than 2.5 years of BZD treatment, they speculated that the lack of association between VBR and duration of BZD use in the Lader et al. study might be related to exclusion of subjects within the lower range of drug exposure.

The clinical significance of these CT scan alterations is unknown, and it is important to note that two similar studies found no statistically significant differences between the CT scans of long-term BZD users and matched control subjects (212, 213). Poser et al. (212) did find, however, that patients with combined BZD—alcohol dependence showed some degree of cerebral atrophy. Uhde and Kellner (211) also observed that the apparent association between VBR and duration of BZD exposure may be secondary to alcohol consumption, because long-term BZD users also may be more frequent users, but not necessarily abusers, of alcohol.

Withdrawal Phenomena

All BZDs have the capacity to produce dependence and, thus, evoke withdrawal symptoms. Although some studies have found little or no evidence, there is now a large body of data indicating that continuous use of a BZD, even at therapeutic doses, will result in withdrawal symptoms in some patients (214, 215). **It also has been reasonably well-established that the longer a BZD is taken, even in therapeutic doses, the greater the likelihood of withdrawal reactions when it is discontinued, especially abruptly** (3). The most commonly reported withdrawal symptoms include the following:

- Various *gastrointestinal* symptoms
- *Diaphoresis*
- *Tremor, lethargy, dizziness, headaches*
- *Increased acuity* for sound and smell
- *Restlessness,* insomnia, irritability, anxiety
- *Tinnitus*
- Feelings of *depersonalization*

These are usually described as mild in intensity and fairly short in duration (i.e., a few days to a few weeks). None is considered life-threatening or permanently debilitating and, with the exception of the relatively rare occurrence of seizures, delirium, and/or psychosis, all are thought to be readily managed.

In some patients, however, discontinuation, whether abrupt or gradual, may evoke highly distressing symptoms, including the following:

- Severe and prolonged *depression* (40, 216)
- *Hallucinations* (40, 217–219)
- Protracted *tinnitus* (217–220)
- Opisthotonos, choreoathetosis, myoclonus, and bizarre *involuntary muscular movements* (221–223)
- *Delirium* with catatonic features (224)
- *Panic* and agoraphobia (40, 217, 225)

There are also reports indicating that in some patients withdrawal may be painful and protracted, possibly lasting 6 months to 1 year (40, 217, 226). Ashton (217), noting that her withdrawal patients were usually frightened, often in intense pain, and genuinely prostrated, stated, "The severity and duration of the illness are easily underestimated by medical and nursing staff, who tend to dismiss the symptoms as neurotic." Chouinard (227) has observed that rebound anxiety can be so severe the patient believes he or she is going to die.

Withdrawal symptoms are *unlikely to occur after only 3 to 4 months of continuous use of a BZD*. Early indications of dependence have been noted, however, with reports of withdrawal symptoms after only 6 weeks of continuous use, particularly with the short-acting agents such as alprazolam (23, 24, 228–232).

Evidence also supports a clinically significant rebound-withdrawal phenomena between doses of alprazolam, sometimes referred to as "interdose" or "breakthrough" symptoms (233, 234). Mellor and Jain (218) raised the possibility that some long-term diazepam users may be subject to a similar phenomenon:

> Patients receiving long-term diazepam treatment who complain of episodes of anxiety may be suffering from intermittent withdrawal symptoms. Characteristically, such patients have reduced their dose of diazepam after being symptom-free for a period. A week or so later their condition apparently recurs, so the previous dose is resumed, and they obtain relief. Sometimes the dose of the drug has not changed, yet the symptoms reappear, causing the dose to be raised until they disappear (218).

Benzodiazepine Discontinuance Syndrome

Meaningful BZD discontinuance symptoms usually only occur when BZD treatment is abruptly terminated. This syndrome is first manifested by rebound symptoms that resemble the symptoms for which the BZD was prescribed, except that rebound symptoms are more severe and emerge soon after discontinuation. Rebound anxiety and insomnia are clearly established as possible consequences to the discontinuation of BZDs, particularly those having a short half-life (235, 236). The duration of the rebound syndrome is short, usually lasting only a few days after the drug is discontinued, and it may be followed by a recurrence of symptoms. It does not imply the existence of physical dependence (24, 231, 237). **Rebound anxiety and insomnia are the most common discontinuance symptoms. Although often severe and almost always uncomfortable, they usually disappear rapidly (i.e., at between a day or two, to 1 to 2 weeks). To avoid these distressing effects, users often restarted the medication, leading to long-term BZD use and dependence.**

Rebound symptoms usually are followed by recurrence symptoms, which may persist until effective treatment is prescribed. In contrast to rebound and recurrence symptoms, withdrawal symptoms are subjective and objective events that did not exist prior to the use of the BZD. These tend to appear after rebound and recurrence symptoms, but not necessarily. Common discontinuance symptoms include insomnia, restlessness, irritability, unsteadiness, flu-like symptoms, hyperacusis, anxiety, and depression. Uncommon symptoms are tinnitus, seizures, and psychosis, which rarely may be life-threatening (238).

Withdrawal seizures originally were thought to occur only when high BZD doses were abruptly stopped, but now there is evidence that seizures may follow abrupt discontinuance of therapeutic doses of a BZD, especially short half-life BZDs. One report (239) discusses five cases of seizures after withdrawal of flunitrazepam, lorazepam, or triazolam. Both abrupt cessation of BZD intake and use of high doses seemed to be critical for the appearance of seizures. Shorter elimination half-life and higher potency might also contribute to the seizures observed in these patients. **Seizures are virtually unknown when a BZD is gradually discontinued**.

Protracted Benzodiazepine Withdrawal Syndrome

True BZD withdrawal symptoms usually resolve spontaneously and may be completely gone in 4 to 12 weeks. However, 10% to 15% of chronic BZD users develop a *protracted withdrawal syndrome* that may last for months or years. **It is thought that this syndrome reflects the slow reversal of receptor changes in the brain induced by the BZD.** In a few patients, somatic symptoms persist for years in the absence of psychopathological signs of anxiety or hysteria, suggesting a pharmacological causation. The protracted phase of BZD withdrawal emerges from the acute phase and is characterized by the following:

- *Gradually* declining symptoms
- Punctuated by *wave-like* recurrences
- Interspersed with *periods of normalcy*

Recovery may not be complete, and long-lasting symptoms may include anxiety, insomnia, depression, various sensory and motor phenomena, and gastrointestinal disturbances (217).

Management of protracted BZD withdrawal is a therapeutic challenge that must be met as promptly as possible. Otherwise, the discomforting symptoms of this condition may compel the patient to seek relief by resuming BZD consumption. For this reason and because protracted BZD withdrawal often is not responsive to non-BZD pharmacotherapy or to various psychotherapeutic or psychological regimens, intravenous administration of the *BZD antagonist flumazenil* has been used to treat a few patients with protracted BZD withdrawal (240). Despite flumazenil's short half-life (1 hour), benefits lasted a few hours to several days. Improvement was observed in some longstanding BZD withdrawal symptoms, including clouded thinking, tiredness, muscular symptoms, and perceptual symptoms (e.g., "pins and needles" feeling, pain, subjective sensations of body distortion). When present, mood symptoms also improved. Side effects typically were mild or absent (241).

Benzodiazepine Postwithdrawal Syndrome

While similar to the protracted withdrawal syndrome, the BZD postwithdrawal syndrome (BPWS) refers to symptoms reported by patients who:

- Have been withdrawn from *chronic BZD therapy*

- Have experienced *typical withdrawal symptoms*
- Then experienced the *postwithdrawal syndrome,* which reportedly can last for many months after the final molecule of the BZD has disappeared from the body (242)

According to Peter Tyrer,

There is considerable overlap between the symptoms of the post-withdrawal syndrome and the actual withdrawal reaction, but the symptoms of post-withdrawal are much more like those of clinical anxiety; feelings of tension and threat, and bodily feelings such as unsteadiness, shaking, palpitations and gastrointestinal symptoms are prominent. Symptoms that develop as secondary complications of anxiety, such as agoraphobia, may also be present. There is reasonable clinical evidence for BPWS, but it is not known for how long the symptoms last. There is also no good pharmacological explanation of the phenomenon. During BPWS patients are more susceptible to stressful stimuli and continue to need support. If patients do take a BZD at this time, this may not necessarily lead to continued dependence. Nevertheless, there is obviously some risk in restarting BZDs and other psychological methods of relieving anxiety, particularly cognitive approaches, are preferable (243).

Until the early 1990's, only a few physicians (primarily British) reported on BPWS. There is disagreement about whether symptoms persisting beyond 6 months after total BZD discontinuation are directly attributable to drug therapy. Are these persistent symptoms due to a neurosis, a personality disorder, or malingering, and not to BZD therapy? Presently, there is no definitive answer to this question, and more research is needed to ascertain whether BPWS is attributable to factors unrelated to BZD therapy. Until this is done, these are the known salient factors related to the BPWS:

- BZD dependence and withdrawal have received *increasing attention* in the media and medical literature since 1979.
- Initially, attention was given primarily to only the withdrawal syndrome that occurs after 4 to 6 weeks' exposure to a BZD, the symptoms of which begin within 2 to 5 days of stopping the BZD and persist for several weeks

before resolving. This is categorized as the *immediate withdrawal syndrome,* the majority of the symptoms of which overlap with those of normal anxiety. Some symptoms (particularly gross disturbances of perception of light, sound, and taste; epileptic seizures; and confusional symptoms) are almost unequivocally those of withdrawal rather than relapse of anxiety.
- BPWS arises after withdrawal has been completed and, according to some patients, *may persist for many years.*
- BPWS can *continue sometimes even when BZD therapy has been reinstituted.*
- There is considerable overlap of the symptoms of BPWS and the actual withdrawal reaction, but *the symptoms of postwithdrawal are much more like those of clinical anxiety.* Feelings of tension and threat, and bodily feelings, (e.g., unsteadiness, shaking, palpitations, and gastrointestinal symptoms) are prominent.
- Symptoms that develop as *secondary complications of anxiety,* such as panic attacks and agoraphobia, may develop in BPWS.
- It is not currently known *how long BPWS lasts.*
- If patients with BPWS take a BZD, this does not necessarily lead to continued *dependence.*
- *Cognitive therapy* is considered to be the treatment of choice.

Persistent Benzodiazepine Dependence Syndrome

Persistent BZD dependence syndrome (PBDS) is a physiological state that is not pathological but the normal consequence of the pharmacological effects of BZDs prescribed for therapeutic objectives. It does not produce irreversible physical or psychiatric harm, and it is the Achilles' heel of long-term BZD therapy. This alleged syndrome has been described only in anecdotal reports, with patients typically reporting "withdrawal" symptoms not present during or before BZD treatment that persist for many months or years after treatment is stopped. Table 12-11 illustrates the major differences between persistent PBDS and BPWS.

Shader and Greenblatt (237) have stated that there is no reliable evidence to support the

TABLE 12-11. *Comparison of PBDS and BPWS*

Factors	PBDS	BPWS
Incidence	Occurs in *10-15%* of long-term BZD users on BZD dose reduction or discontinuation	*Unknown*, but patients insist it is common
Onset	*Shortly after dose reduction* (hours or days) or discontinuation of BZD	*Usually weeks* after BZD discontinuation and as soon as immediate withdrawal symptoms subside
Causative BZD	*Any BZD*, but *shorter-acting* BZDs (e.g., lorazepam and alpra zolam) are most common	*Any BZD*, but *shorter-acting* BZDs (e.g., lorazepam and alpra zolam) are most common
Duration	*While BZD is taken*	Currently unknown. *May persist for years after BZD discontinuation*
Symptoms	Much more like those of *clinical anxiety*	Those of an *anxiety disorder*
Preferred Therapy	*Cognitive psychotherapy*	*Cognitive psychotherapy*

PBDS, persistent benzodiazepine dependence syndrome; BPWS, benzodiazepine post withdrawal syndrome; BZD, benzodiazepine.

Comments:

These two conditions are similar in many respects. The major difference clinically is that PBDS exists as long as the patient takes a benzodiazepine continuously and may be a predecessor of BPWS.

BPWS arises *only after* BZD discontinuation. It may or may not be preceded by PBDS. It is always preceded by immediate BZD withdrawal symptoms. It evolves almost as imperceptibly as the unfolding of a flower, with symptoms gradually becoming more manifest as the immediate withdrawal symptoms subside.

Both PBDS and BPWS occur in patients with avoidant personalities and in those with a more chronic anxiety or depressive disorder. The symptoms of both are thought to arise from the anxiety disorder and/or the personality of the person. Both the anxiety and the personality disorder existed *before* treatment with the BZD.

The symptoms of PBDS are caused in part by the pharmacological actions of the BZD, and in part by the patient's reaction to the abstinence symptoms evoked by dosage reduction or BZD discontinuation. The symptoms experienced during BPWS are attributable largely to the personality of the patient or any preceding psychiatric disorder.

existence of PBDS. Experimental neuropharmacological studies document that all side effects of BZDs, whether behavioral or neurochemical, disappear within several days or weeks after the drug is eliminated. The weight of evidence indicates that any new symptoms that persist for more than 2 months after the last dose of a BZD either are a part of the premorbid condition or have appeared by coincidence or as a consequence of the natural history of the underlying illness.

Assuming its existence, this disorder may occur in certain patients who have been taking therapeutic (or higher) doses of a BZD for more than 2 months. Indeed, the longer the patient has consumed a BZD, the greater the likelihood of this syndrome, which has two components:

- A *physiological dependency* due to cellular adaptation to the presence of the BZD
- A *psychological dependency* on BZD ingestion

The former component is a physiological state that continues undisturbed until the BZD dosage is sharply reduced and its plasma level begins to fall, following which there is a cellular response to the absence of the prior level of BZD. This abstinence response can be minimized by gradual withdrawal of the BZD.

A BZD's pharmacokinetics may play a role in the occurrence, in part accounting for the increase in its incidence after the advent of short-acting BZD anxiolytics and hypnotics (e.g., lorazepam, alprazolam, and triazolam).

The second component of the PBDS is a psychological dependency that occurs in a segment of long-term BZD users. In many patients, psychological dependence precedes physiological dependence and in most it exists independent of any coexisting physiological dependency. Psychological dependency may be responsible for continued BZD use resulting in the development of physiological dependency, because psychological dependency is a symptom of an underlying anxiety or mixed anxiety-depressive neurosis or a personality disorder that preexisted

BZD administration and for which therapy was originally prescribed. Patients with this underlying disorder are typically anxious, phobic, and obsessively sensitive to somatic and emotional changes. Many are agoraphobic and suffer from anticipatory anxiety. They fear the anxiety and subjective distress they believe will recur in the absence of whatever they consider protects them from their anxiety-generated symptoms. When such patients are treated with a BZD that provides a modicum of relief from their anxiety, they quickly develop a fear of being without it.

When the very short-acting anxiolytic, alprazolam, became available, some patients treated with it developed *clock-watching* **in response to their experiencing** *interdose anxiety*. To them, such action was necessary to know when to take the next dose of alprazolam to preclude interdose anxiety. Thus, patients treated their psychological dependency by repeated alprazolam dosing, thereby inducing physiological dependency. This example of the genesis of PBDS illustrates how a patient's neurosis or personality disorder can be responsible first for psychological dependency and then for physiological dependency. This phenomenon has increased in frequency with the advent of short-acting and ultrashort-acting BZD anxiolytics and hypnotics.

PBDS can occur in patients taking any BZD, but is least likely to occur in patients treated with a long-acting BZD. Usually persistent dependence on these BZDs does not develop unless the patient has a moderately severe neurosis or personality disorder that is his or her motivation for long-term BZD therapy. In these patients, anticipatory anxiety makes them vulnerable to overreacting to the idea or occurrence of dosage reduction. Hence, even before the BZD dose is reduced, these patients experience somatic and/or psychic distress that is generated by the thought of being without their usual BZD dosage.

This is not an unusual phenomenon. It has been observed in patients who have become psychologically dependent on an inactive placebo, as well as in patients psychologically dependent on medicines not known to cause physiological dependency and withdrawal symptoms. Another example of psychological dependency on a BZD is the patient who allays anxiety about being without a pill by carrying it at all times, comforted by the knowledge that a tablet is at hand in case of need. Such patients may become acutely anxious whenever the pill has been lost or left at home.

The types of anxious personalities cited above develop PBDS not because of any inherent toxic effect of the BZD but because of their psychological disorder. A characteristic symptom of a PBDS is the rapid onset of discomfort whenever the patient thinks he or she will be without the BZD or that its dose is being lowered. Such patients can be uneventfully withdrawn from the BZD by very gradual dosage taper, which is difficult to accomplish without the patient's knowledge and cooperation. Withdrawing such patients from a BZD requires recognition of their personality disorder and the need for its treatment before drug discontinuation is initiated.

In summary, no more than one third of all patients treated with a BZD for longer than 2 months develop PBDS. The other two thirds may develop a physical dependency on the BZD, but neither dosage reduction nor gradual tapering evokes the anxiety symptoms manifested by PBDS patients. Hence, it is the patient's personality disorder or underlying anxiety disorder and not physical dependency on the BZD that is responsible.

Therapeutic Dose Dependence

It is extremely difficult to state precisely when BZD therapeutic dose dependence was first recognized. In the first 15 years, the BZD field was dominated by intermediate- and long-acting 1, 4-BZDs, chiefly chlordiazepoxide and diazepam. A minority of patients were treated continuously with these drugs for longer than 1 year; the majority were treated for less than a few months. Most patients were prescribed low therapeutic doses (e.g., 15 to 40 mg chlordiazepoxide/day; 10 to 20 mg diazepam/day), not all of which was taken regularly by all patients.

Because BZD dependency is related to daily dosage and duration of exposure (i.e., the higher the daily dose and the longer the duration of use the greater the risk of dependency), and not all patients appeared to become dependent on therapeutic doses regardless of duration of usage, the occurrence and recognition of therapeutic dose dependence were minimized. Furthermore, chlordiazepoxide and diazepam have pharmacologically active metabolites that protect against abstinence symptoms, which are the only proof of dependence.

Although there were occasional anecdotal reports or "signals" that BZD therapeutic dose dependency was occurring, these were not attention-getting, and prescribers doubted the occurrence of this phenomenon or dismissed it as infrequent and not clinically significant. During the late 1960's, there was an increasing concern about the extensive American consumption of BZDs, not because of a widespread occurrence of recognized dependency and withdrawal symptoms, but mainly on the presumption that such extensive usage meant addiction with its unfavorable connotations. There were advocates for control of all BZDs and sedative-hypnotics. An editorial in the *Journal of the American Medical Association* on dependence and withdrawal concluded that physicians can do thek following:

- Can *allay* fear of *BZDs* by publicizing the truth about these drugs
- Can *minimize risk of BZD dependence* by:
- Restricting prescriptions to *valid clinical indications*
- Prescribing the *lowest doses* possible
- *Limiting refills*
- *Carefully monitoring* the patient's condition, especially those patients with histories of alcohol or drug abuse
- *Should obviate the risk of moderate to severe withdrawal reactions by gradual discontinuation* of use of these drugs in all patients with known or suspected long-term, heavy BZD use (2)

When the high-potency, short-acting BZD lorazepam was marketed in the United States in 1978, prescriptions escalated rapidly, and many patients were taken off their longer-acting BZDs and given lorazepam. Within 2 years, physicians had become aware of two distinct groups among lorazepam-treated patients. One exhibited what appeared to be a recurrence of the anxiety disorder for which the prior BZD had been prescribed. These patients actually were dependent on the therapeutic doses of the BZD they took before lorazepam, and their symptoms were due

to abstinence from the prior BZD despite taking lorazepam. The second group consisted of individuals who complained of interdose anxiety that was relieved by shortening the interval between doses of lorazepam. These breakthrough symptoms were not considered indicators of dependence, but of insufficient anxiolytic lorazepam dosage. Other patients developed withdrawal symptoms when lorazepam was abruptly discontinued after months of treatment with therapeutic doses.

Most physicians felt these symptoms were a reflection of the patient's anxiety disorder and not a manifestation of dependence. Their opinions were reinforced when resumption of lorazepam therapy resulted in symptom amelioration, suggesting recontrol of the patient's anxiety disorder. Rarely were these patients considered dependent, mainly because they had not escalated lorazepam dosage, or manifested any signs or symptoms of drug-seeking behavior. They appeared to be typical medical users of prescribed medication.

Discontinuing Treatment

Short-Term Treatment

Although gradual discontinuation is generally thought to lessen the occurrence and/or intensity of withdrawal symptoms, rebound-withdrawal phenomena may still occur with slow tapering, even in patients who have taken a BZD for only a few weeks. **Rickels et al. (24), reporting on a study of clorazepate and lorazepam, warned physicians not to mistakenly attribute a substantial return of symptoms that occurs early after BZD discontinuation as a recurrence of original symptoms necessitating further treatment.** These authors added, "Such guidelines are important for clinical practice because the few patients who experience rebound anxiety after only weeks of therapy and who resume medication needlessly may represent the very patients who become chronic users."

Long-Term Treatment

As noted earlier, abrupt discontinuation of long-term use of therapeutic doses is likely to result in withdrawal symptoms (244). In a study of the effects of *abrupt* discontinuation of short and long half-life BZDs in long-term users, Rickels et al. found the following:

- A withdrawal syndrome *occurred in the majority* of patients.
- The withdrawal syndrome *occurred earlier and was more severe for short half-life* (alprazolam, lorazepam) than for long half-life drugs (diazepam, clorazepate).
- *Factors contributing* to greater withdrawal severity included short half-life, higher daily dose, greater state and trait psychopathology, and lower educational level.
- Only 73% of long half-life and 43% of short half-life BZD-treated patients were *able to remain drug-free for 1 week*.
- At 5 weeks, only 45% of long half-life and 38% of short half-life BZD-treated patients were still *drug-free* (41).

Although gradual dose reduction may ameliorate the intensity of withdrawal symptoms after long-term therapeutic use of BZDs, mild-to-moderate symptoms are still likely to occur. In a companion study to the one just cited, the same group of investigators reported that almost 90% of short and long half-life BZD-treated patients experienced some withdrawal symptoms despite *gradual* dosage taper (25% per week) (42). They also reported the following:

- Thirty-two percent of long half-life and 42% of short half-life BZD-patients were *unable to tolerate taper* and either continued or resumed daily drug use.
- Unlike the abrupt discontinuation study, *severity and time course of withdrawal symptoms were similar* for both short and long half-life agents.
- Factors contributing to greater withdrawal severity included female sex, higher Eysenck *neuroticism,* and higher alcohol intake.
- At 5 weeks, 56% of long half-life and 53% of short half-life BZD-treated patients were still *BZD-free*.

These findings indicate that, despite the likelihood of withdrawal symptoms with both abrupt and gradual discontinuation, gradual taper may lessen the incidence and intensity of symptoms, particularly in patients taking a short half-life compound.

Nevertheless, gradual withdrawal may still be difficult. Schweizer et al. (42) found that although the initial 50% dose reduction was characterized by minimal withdrawal severity and could be accomplished fairly rapidly, the majority of symptoms occurred during the last half of the tapering process. Tyrer (245) made a similar observation, stating that "withdrawal symptoms may develop only when patients have reduced to what many clinicians would regard as subtherapeutic doses, and the difficulty that patients have in withdrawing from this dose cannot be explained only by psychological dependence." Schweizer et al. (42) also concluded that dose reduction of 25% per week may be too rapid for many long-term users. In their study, 51% of patients were unable to tolerate that schedule and required an even more gradual taper.

With most BZDs, the rate of reduction may be fairly rapid down to about 50% of the original dose. Subsequent decreases should be slower (e.g., 10% to 20% of the new dose at 3-day to 5-day intervals). For patients who become increasingly anxious as their dose is being decreased, **use of a plateau period** in which no further tapering occurs may allow them to relax, adjust to the lower dose, and then resume the gradual discontinuation process. Plateau periods also allow clinicians to assess whether anxiety that emerges during dose reduction is due to withdrawal or a recurrence of an underlying anxiety disorder. Withdrawal anxiety lessens over time, whereas symptoms of an anxiety disorder worsen.

As noted earlier, alprazolam requires a very extended and gradual taper (234, 246, 247). The package insert suggests that "the daily dose be decreased not more than 0.5 mg every 3 days." According to this recommendation, if a patient has been treated with alprazolam 10 mg daily (a dose not uncommon for severe panic disorders), it would take at least 60 days to wean the patient off alprazolam. Some long-term alprazolam users, however, may require 0.25 mg decrements as far apart as every 4 to 7 days. Following this schedule, the patient taking alprazolam 10 mg daily would require up to 6 months to discontinue the drug (see Fig. 13-1, in Chapter 13, for a suggested tapering schedule).

Lorazepam, also reported difficult to discontinue in some patients, has been associated with higher dropout rates and more severe withdrawal phenomena than longer-acting BZDs (248, 249). Ashton (30) noted that patients taking lorazepam experienced drug craving (feeling they could not get through the day without their tablets) before being switched to diazepam for BZD discontinuation.

Other than slow taper, no consistently effective treatment to alleviate withdrawal symptoms has been reported. Although several compounds have been studied (e.g., β-blockers, clonidine, carbamazepine, abercamil, ondansetron), results have been contradictory (250). **Carbamazepine, however, may be useful in seizure-prone patients** (251). Valproate (VPA) has also been reported to benefit patients undergoing BZD discontinuation after long-term dependence (252), which may be related to VPA's potential anxiolytic properties, its ability to alleviate withdrawal phenomena, or both. The azaspirone anxiolytic buspirone has been reported ineffective in suppressing withdrawal symptoms, particularly in long-term BZD users (253, 254). Hydroxyzine has also been found beneficial in treating patients for lorazepam withdrawal (255).

Among the recently evaluated treatments for BZD withdrawal are anticonvulsants (carbamazepine and VPA) (256), melatonin (257), and ondansetron (258). Of these, odansetron had no significant effects on severity of withdrawal symptoms; melatonin was found to effectively facilitate discontinuation of BZD therapy while maintaining good sleep; and carbamazepine and VPA may be beneficial in the management of BZD discontinuation but not in decreasing the severity of BZD withdrawal (259, 260).

To manage withdrawal insomnia, we recommend the supplemental use of hypnotics such as zolpidem or a sedating antidepressant such as trazodone. Rickels et al. recommend the supplemental use of hypnotics such as diphenhydramine, doxylamine, or chloral hydrate or a sedating TCA such as doxepin (259). These investigators also recommend that chronic BZD users with evidence of depression or panic be treated with adequate doses of an appropriate antidepressant, a management technique that may help patients succeed in discontinuation.

Guidelines for Benzodiazepine Discontinuation

Until recently few guidelines were available to help physicians determine whether continued BZD use is appropriate and, if not, how to prevent BZD discontinuation syndromes (e.g., PBDS and the immediate withdrawal syndrome). Rickels (261) and his colleagues suggest tapering schedules, emphasizing the need to treat the patient's underlying psychopathology.

A composite of other suggested approaches to discontinuing a BZD include the following:

- Considering the *pattern of use* for the individual (versus abuse)
- Balancing therapeutic *risk* and *benefit* (burden of anxiety disorder)
- Forming a *therapeutic alliance,* giving positive support that medication will be decreased slowly to avoid rebound anxiety and relapse of the underlying anxiety disorder and withdrawal symptoms
- *Gradually reducing the dose* (depending on the pharmacokinetics) with the slowest reduction in the final few weeks and observing for delayed discontinuation symptoms (2 to 4 weeks or longer) with long-acting BZDs
- Reassuring that with gradual tapering the *symptoms are likely to be brief and manageable* (if no drug or alcohol abuse)
- Considering the need, if any, for *alternative treatments* (e.g., psychotherapy, behavioral therapy, or alternative medications)
- Reassuring that the *discontinuation syndrome is the nature of the psychophysiological process* and not the fault of the patient or the doctor

Importance of Tapering

Since the late 1960's, it has been known that the risk of developing dependence on any BZD is dose- and time-related. The higher the BZD dose, and the longer it is taken, the greater the risk of dependence and the greater the risk of intense withdrawal symptoms after abrupt discontinuation. Protracted use of low therapeutic doses of a BZD may result not only in dependence but also in withdrawal symptoms, the severity of which may also increase the longer the drug is consumed.

It also has been known that the risk of abstinence symptoms can be lessened by graduated dosage reduction or tapered discontinuation. **Tapering is necessary for patients who have taken a BZD for more than 4 months, especially those who have taken a potent, short-acting BZD such as alprazolam.** Abstinence symptoms may be avoided or minimized by very gradual taper, over many months, coupled with psychological support and/or cognitive psychotherapy. For some, tapering can be accomplished as an outpatient procedure; for others, it can only be achieved in a hospital. Those who have been taking high doses or have a history of seizures or psychotic episodes during previous attempts at withdrawal generally should be hospitalized. Tapering is particularly important in any patient with a history of seizures from any cause.

Gradual tapering may not avert the discomforts and hazards of BZD withdrawal. Aside from suggestions that it may be worth substituting a long-acting BZD for a short-acting BZD, until the 1980's little was written on the management of BZD withdrawal. Since 1980, researchers have been investigating possible pharmacotherapies that with gradual tapering may lessen abstinence symptoms and shorten the withdrawal syndrome, including the following:

- Propranolol (262)
- Clonidine (263)
- Carbamazepine or valproate (252, 264)

Extensive experience with gradual tapering from protracted BZD therapy indicates that it is effective within 6 to 9 months, with few patients needing tapering beyond 12 months. There is no general agreement on the optimal tapering schedules. Instead, tapering should be titrated against the patient's withdrawal symptoms and ability to tolerate them. Before, during, and after tapering, patients need and should have the support of physicians, relatives, and friends. Tapered withdrawal can be uncomfortable, and without support, patients are tempted to resume BZD use.

Seizures

Although rare, seizures may occur after the abrupt discontinuation of both high and therapeutic doses of any BZD. Some researchers have suggested that short-acting drugs are associated with increased seizure risk when compared with longer-acting compounds, but this is difficult to evaluate due to the relatively small number of published case reports and inherent problems in assessing anecdotal data. A review of the reports on lorazepam and oxazepam, however, found that in almost all cases patients had stopped the drug abruptly and that at least one (and often more than one) of the following factors was present:

- *High dose*
- *Extended duration* of use (4 months to years)
- Concomitant or immediately subsequent ingestion of *other drugs associated with seizure induction*
- *History of seizures* (265)

Published case reports on alprazolam show a slightly different profile (266–269). Four patients had taken the drug for 4.5 months or less; one had also taken chlorpromazine and trazodone; and a fifth patient had taken alprazolam (3 mg/day for 26 weeks) and phenelzine (45 mg/day for 13 weeks), abruptly stopping both. **According to the FDA's Spontaneous Adverse Event Reporting System, more seizures have been reported with alprazolam than with all other BZDs combined** (270). The next highest incidence was reported for lorazepam. The FDA report stated the following:

- Most alprazolam seizures were in connection with *high-dose therapy.*
- Dose-duration data suggest occurrence at therapeutic doses with *chronic therapy* and a *shortened time* until risk when higher doses are used.

- Although some seizures occurred during stable alprazolam therapy, they often occurred when a *concomitant drug* that may also lower the seizure threshold was given, such as maprotiline.
- With intentional taper, most seizures occurred *at or near the end.*

According to the report, reasons for excess seizure reports for alprazolam may include specific drug effect, higher degree of manufacturer surveillance, and higher doses used. This last issue may be due to this agent's reported efficacy and increasing use in panic disorder, which usually requires higher doses for longer periods.

One recent report also detailed three cases of convulsive status epilepticus after abrupt discontinuation of long-term use of 25 mg *lorazepam* in one patient and more than 20 mg *flunitrazepam* in two patients. These patients were nonepileptics and free of other high-risk factors for seizure (271).

Conclusion

All patients should be instructed to adhere to their physician's gradual discontinuation program and not be swayed by well-meaning but ill-informed friends or relatives who may urge a "cold turkey" approach. The clinician also must recognize the particular susceptibilities of each patient and be willing to provide reassurance, encouragement,

and information about symptoms, both in the early stages of discontinuation and for a prolonged follow-up period. As Farid and Bulto (272) have observed, "Patients who have been on these drugs for longer periods need more sensitive handling, and with some of them it may take months if not years to wean them off their benzodiazepines. The difficulty we face is not long-term prescribing of benzodiazepines but rather too quick a reduction of the prescribed dose with little other form of help being offered."

ADVERSE EFFECTS OF SEDATIVE-HYPNOTICS

Miscellaneous adverse effects reported with the various BZD hypnotics are listed in Table 12-12.

Sedation and Central Nervous System Depression

Although some studies have reported that sleep-deprived people are impaired in their daytime functioning, others have found that in patients with chronic insomnia, sleep loss is actually slight, excessive daytime sleepiness is rare, and daytime performance is normal (273–277). Whether BZDs enhance daytime performance by reducing loss of sleep is in fact unknown. Many studies, however, indicate that they impair rather than improve next-day performance, and a review of those studies using performance and

TABLE 12-12. *Miscellaneous adverse effects reported with benzodiazepine hypnotics*

Estazolam	Flurazepam	Quazepam	Temazepam	Triazolam
Hypokinesia	Headache	Headache	Gastrointestinal disturbances	Headache
Headache	Paresthesias	Fatigue	Sleep disturbances	Paresthesias
Asthenia	Dizziness	Dry mouth	Visual disturbances	Visual disturbances
Nausea	Tinnitus	Dyspepsia	Weakness	Tinnitus
Nervousness	Bad taste in mouth		Lack of concentration	Gastrointestinal disturbances
Dizziness				
Lethargy	Dry mouth		Loss of equilibrium	
Dysphoria	Gastrointestinal disturbances		Falling	
	Sleep disturbances			
	Dermatologic problems			

vigilance tests concluded that BZDs with short half-lives induce longer-lasting impairment than those with long half-lives, perhaps due to the latter's more extensive distribution (278). **In general, the adverse effects of BZD hypnotics are dose-dependent, with higher doses tending to produce more symptoms than lower doses** (101, 279–284).

BZDs with active metabolites and slow elimination, such as diazepam, flurazepam, and quazepam, are well known for producing unwanted daytime sedation (111, 285, 286). Nevertheless, other studies have found no or inconsistent residual impairment with lower doses of flurazepam and quazepam (101, 284–290). Some evidence indicates that quazepam (15 or 30 mg) may have a lower potential than the same dosages of flurazepam for producing daytime somnolence and residual impairment (284). Excessive daytime CNS depression, however, may occur with all BZDs, including those with short and intermediate half-lives (111, 279, 291). In a review of 45 double-blind, controlled trials, CNS depression (drowsiness, dizziness, fatigue, lightheadedness, and incoordination) was the most frequent adverse effect of triazolam, occurring in 14.2% of patients receiving 0.25 mg and in 19.5% of those receiving 0.5 mg (279). CNS effects also may be frequent with temazepam and estazolam (107, 292–295).

Central Nervous System Stimulation

With short-acting agents, such as triazolam, numerous reports have detailed increased daytime anxiety and early morning insomnia (108, 112, 296–302). Because these are the opposite of the intended therapeutic effect, they may not be attributed to the drug and may actually reinforce its use. CNS stimulation has been reported in 2.8% of patients given 30 mg flurazepam (279).

Behavioral Effects

Short-term use of triazolam has been associated with serious behavioral adverse effects, including the following:

- Confusion
- Psychotic-like symptoms
- Disinhibition
- Amnesia (108, 111, 112, 299, 303–310)

Memory impairment or periods of amnesia and automatic behavior have been reported with single doses of triazolam the day after its nighttime use (311–315). Amnesia has been reported with lorazepam and other BZDs, but appears to be considerably more problematic with triazolam (291, 316–322). In a recent controlled study, for example, triazolam produced a 40% rate of next-day memory impairment or amnesia, although no episodes occurred with temazepam (315). Although behavioral adverse effects also have been reported for temazepam, FDA statistics indicate that for hostility reactions reported on 329 drugs, triazolam ranked first (310, 323). Analysis of individual cases reported to the FDA's Spontaneous Adverse Event Reporting System for such symptoms as amnesia, confusion, bizarre behavior, agitation, and hallucinations found that rates for triazolam were 22-99 times higher than those for temazepam (324). Even when reports involving triazolam dosages above 0.5 mg or other contributing factors were excluded, reporting rates for triazolam were still 4 to 26 times greater. These results could, however, be partly due to the publicity in the media regarding this phenomenon.

Case Example: A 56-year-old man, who worked as an engineer, consulted his family physician because of progressive fatigue of 3 months' duration. Aside from moderate obesity (176 pounds) and slight hypertension (145/90), the physical examination was negative. Urinalysis detected 2+ glycosuria. Blood chemistries were normal except for 285 blood glucose level. Further workup confirmed early adult-onset diabetes. After being informed of his diagnosis, the patient developed distressing middle insomnia and a worsening of his fatigue. His physician advised a tropical vacation and prescribed triazolam (0.25 mg) at bedtime. On the first night of his vacation, the patient took his first dose and retired early. Two days later he "woke up, " that is, "I became aware of myself and my surroundings but I couldn't remember what I had done since I arrived in the Bahamas and took that sleeping pill."

Frightened by his amnesia, the patient returned home worried that he might have a more serious problem than "just diabetes." He told his physician that he was afraid of "losing my mind." A complete physical, neurological, and psychiatric evaluation only confirmed the patient's diabetes. He was therefore diagnosed as having a triazolam-induced anterograde amnesia. The patient was reassured that he had an iatrogenic reaction and advised not to take triazolam.

Discontinuing Treatment

Rebound Insomnia

Even after relatively short periods of administration, discontinuation of short and intermediate half-life BZDs, such as triazolam and temazepam, may result in marked worsening of sleep, even worse than baseline levels (i.e., rebound insomnia), although this does not seem to occur with zolpidem (95, 102, 103, 109, 110, 113, 285, 297, 316, 325–337). Gradual dose reduction may attenuate the incidence of rebound, and with flurazepam and quazepam, little sleep disturbance occurs, even after abrupt drug withdrawal (99–106, 280, 338–341).

Differences in the development of tolerance and the occurrence of rebound insomnia have been well established with rapidly versus slowly eliminated BZD hypnotics. A meta-analysis of sleep laboratory studies has recently shown that tolerance with intermediate and long-term use clearly developed with triazolam but only marginally with midazolam and zolpidem. Rebound insomnia on the first withdrawal night was intense with triazolam and mild with zolpidem. The data led to the conclusion that differences exist among the rapidly eliminated hypnotics with respect to tolerance and rebound insomnia. This conclusion suggests that, in addition to short elimination half-life, other pharmacological properties are implicated in the mechanisms underlying these side effects (342).

Although one study of long-term BZD hypnotic use found no increase in insomnia after abrupt discontinuation of a variety of BZDs, a withdrawal syndrome consisting of inability to fall asleep and disruption of sleep may occur (126, 327, 343). Time of onset may vary according to the drug's rate of elimination (244).

Syncope and Inflammatory Reactions

Triazolobenzodiazepines differ from other BZDs in being potent and specific inhibitors of the binding of platelet-activating factor (PAF) to its receptor (344). Noting that initial reports of serious adverse effects associated with triazolam included blistering of hands, feet, and tongue, some authors have speculated that effects on PAF mechanisms may account for the higher incidence of certain unusual withdrawal symptoms noted with these drugs (345, 346). These authors state that disturbance of PAF (a potent hypotensive agent) mechanisms could explain the association of triazolam with syncope, and added this problem to the U.S. package insert for 1990. In addition, they counted all adverse reactions suggesting inflammation or altered micropermeability reported to the FDA's Spontaneous Adverse Event Reporting System since the introduction of temazepam, flurazepam, and triazolam. Reactions including pharyngitis, glossitis, vasculitis, asthma, and facial edema totaled 31 for temazepam, 78 for flurazepam, and 673 for triazolam.

Seizures and Psychotic Reactions

Seizures have been reported after withdrawal of high doses of triazolam or relatively low doses combined with alcohol (347–349). The FDA has reported "a signal of an association" for withdrawal seizures associated with triazolam (350). In a chart review of 150 consecutive patients withdrawn from BZDs, three of 25 triazolam patients experienced seizures, compared with two of 125 given other BZDs (351). Psychosis with delirium also has been reported after discontinuation of high triazolam doses (352).

CONCLUSION

Although the BZD hypnotics are a significant advance over their predecessors in terms of safety, they also carry their own risks (7). In particular, the shorter-acting agents may predispose patients to such complications as rebound anxiety, insomnia, amnesia, paradoxical disinhibition, and seizures with abrupt discontinuation. Coupled with the evidence that long-term benefit beyond 12 weeks is unproven, careful, time-limited, intermittent prescribing is the only reasonable management strategy. Newer agents such as zolpidem and zaleplon may be less problematic, but more experience is needed.

REFERENCES

1. Mitler MM. Nonselective and selective benzodiazepine receptor agonists–where are we today? *Sleep* 2000;23(suppl 1):S39–S47.
2. Ayd FJ Jr. Benzodiazepines: dependence and withdrawal. *JAMA* 1979;242:1401–1402.
3. Woods JH, Katz JL, Winger G. Abuse liability of benzodiazepines. *Pharmacol Rev* 1987;39:251–413.
4. American Psychiatric Association. *Benzodiazepine dependence, toxicity, and abuse*. Washington, DC: American Psychiatric Association, 1990.
5. Uhlenhuth EH, DeWit H, Balter MB, et al. Risks and benefits of long-term benzodiazepine use. *J Clin Psychopharmacol* 1988;8:161–167.
6. Garvey MJ, Tollefson GD. Prevalence of misuse of prescribed benzodiazepines in patients with primary anxiety disorder or major depression. *Am J Psychiatry* 1986;143:1601–1603.
7. Gelenberg AJ, ed. The use of benzodiazepine hypnotics: a scientific examination of the clinical controversy. *J Clin Psychiatry* 1992;53(suppl):1–87.
8. Fraser AD. Use and abuse of the benzodiazepines. *Ther Drug Monit* 1998;20:481–489.
9. Uhlenhuth EH, Balter MB, Ban TA, et al. International study of expert judgment on therapeutic use of benzodiazepines and other psychotherapeutic medications: IV. Therapeutic dose dependence and abuse liability of benzodiazepines in the long-term treatment of anxiety disorders. *J Clin Psychopharmacol* 1999;19(suppl 2):23S–29S.
10. Zorumski CF, Isenberg KE. Insights into the structure and function of GABA-benzodiazepine receptors: ion channels and psychiatry. *Am J Psychiatry* 1991;148:162–163.
11. Low K, Cristani F, Keist R, et al. Molecular and neuronal substrate for the selective attenuation of anxiety. *Science* 2000;290:131–138.
12. Dorow R, Horowski R, Paschelke G, et al. Severe anxiety induced by FG-7142, a beta-carboline ligand for benzodiazepine receptors. *Lancet* 1983;2:98–99.
13. Handley SL. New directions in benzodiazepine research. *Curr Opin Psychiatry* 1989;2:59–62.
14. File SE. Chronic diazepam treatment: effect of dose on development of tolerance and incidence of withdrawal in an animal test of anxiety. *Hum Psychopharmacol* 1989;4:59–63.
15. File SE, Zharkovsky A, Hitchcott PK. Effects of nitrendepine, chlordiazepoxide, flumazenil and baclofen on the increased anxiety resulting from alcohol withdrawal. *Prog Neuropsychopharmacol Biol Psychiatry* 1992;16:87–93.
16. Dorow R, Berenberg D, Duka T, et al. Amnestic effects of lormetazepam and their reversal by the benzodiazepine antagonist Ro 15-1788. *Psychopharmacology* 1987;93:507–514.
17. Gentil V, Gorenstein C, Camargo CHP, et al. Effects of flunitrazepam on memory and their reversal by two antagonists. *J Clin Psychopharmacol* 1989;9:191–197.
18. Downing RW, Rickels K. Early treatment response in anxious outpatients treated with diazepam. *Acta Psychiatr Scand* 1985;72:522–528.
19. Meibach RC, Dunner D, Wilson LG, et al. Comparative efficacy of propranolol, chlordiazepoxide, and placebo in the treatment of anxiety. A double-blind trial. *J Clin Psychiatry* 1987;48:355–358.
20. Rickels K. Use of antianxiety agents in anxious outpatients. *Psychopharmacology* 1978;58:1–17.
21. Rickels K. Benzodiazepines in the treatment of anxiety. In: Usdin E, Skolnick P, Tallman JF, et al., eds. *Pharmacology of benzodiazepines*. London: Macmillan, 1982:37–44.
22. Dubovsky SL. Generalized anxiety disorder: new concepts and psychopharmacologic therapies. *J Clin Psychiatry* 1990;51(suppl 1):3–10.
23. Rickels K, Case G, Downing RW, et al. Long-term diazepam therapy and clinical outcome. *JAMA* 1983;250:767–771.
24. Rickels K, Fox IL, Greenblatt DJ. Clorazepate and lorazepam: clinical improvement and rebound anxiety. *Am J Psychiatry* 1988;145:312–317.
25. Rickels K, Case WG, Downing RS, et al. Indications and contraindications for chronic anxiolytic treatment: is there tolerance to the anxiolytic effect? In: Kemali D, Racagni G, eds. *Chronic treatments in neuropsychiatry*. New York: Raven Press, 1985:193–204.
26. Rickels K, Case G, Downing R, et al. One-year follow-up of anxious patients treated with diazepam. *J Clin Psychopharmacol* 1986;6:32–36.
27. Lader MH. Limitations on the use of benzodiazepines in anxiety and insomnia: are they justified? *Eur Neuropsychopharmacol* 1999;9(suppl 6):S399–S405.
28. Rickels K, Case WG, Diamond L. Relapse after short-term drug therapy in neurotic outpatients. *Int Pharmacopsychiatry* 1980;15:186–192.
29. Freud S. *Introductory lectures on psychoanalysis*. New York: Norton, 1977.
30. Griffiths RR. Commentary on review by Woods and Winger. Benzodiazepines: long-term use among patients is a concern and abuse among polydrug abusers is not trivial. *Psychopharmacology* 1995;118:116–117.
31. Rickels K. Antianxiety therapy: potential value of long-term treatment. *J Clin Psychiatry* 1987;48:7–11.
32. Committee on Safety of Medicines. *Benzodiazepines, dependence and withdrawal symptoms*. Number 21, January 1988.
33. Rickels K, Schweizer E. The clinical course and long-term management of generalized anxiety disorder. *J Clin Psychopharmacol* 1990;10(suppl):101s–110's.
34. Rickels K. Buspirone, clorazepate and withdrawal. Presented at the Annual Meeting of the American Psychiatric Association, Dallas, 1985.
35. Rickels K, Case WG, Schweizer EE, et al. Low-dose dependence in chronic benzodiazepine users: a preliminary report on 119 patients. *Psychopharmacol Bull* 1986;22:407–415.

36. Balter MB, Uhlenhuth EH. New epidemiologic findings about insomnia and its treatment. *J Clin Psychiatry* 1991;52(suppl 12):34–39.

37. Rodrigo EK, King MB, Williams P. Health of long-term benzodiazepine users. *Br Med J* 1988;296:603–606.

38. Mellinger GD, Balter MB, Uhlenhuth EH. Prevalence and correlates of the long-term use of anxiolytics. *JAMA* 1984;251:375–379.

39. Le Goc I, Feline A, Frebault D, et al. Caracteristiques de la consommation de benzodiazepines chez des patients hospitalises dans un service de medicine interne. *Encephale* 1985;2:1–6.

40. Ashton H. Benzodiazepine withdrawal: outcome in 50 patients. *Br J Addict* 1987;82:665–671.

41. Rickels K, Schweizer E, Case WG, et al. Long-term therapeutic use of benzodiazepines. I. Effects of abrupt discontinuation. *Arch Gen Psychiatry* 1990;47:899–907.

42. Schweizer E, Rickels K, Case WG, et al. Long-term therapeutic use of benzodiazepines. II. Effects of gradual taper. *Arch Gen Psychiatry* 1990;47:908–915.

43. Taylor C, McCracken CF, Wilson KC, et al. Extent and appropriateness of benzodiazepine use. Results from an elderly urban community. *Br J Psychiatry* 1998;173:433–438.

44. Markowitz JS, Weissman MH, Ouellette R, et al. Quality of life in panic disorder. *Arch Gen Psychiatry* 1989;46:984–992.

45. Goldberg HL, Finnerty RJ. The comparative efficacy of buspirone and diazepam in the treatment of anxiety. *Am J Psychiatry* 1979;136:1184–1187.

46. Kastenholz KV, Crimson ML. Buspirone, a novel non-benzodiazepine anxiolytic. *Clin Pharm* 1984;3:600–607.

47. Rickels K, Weisman K, Norstad N, et al. Buspirone and diazepam in anxiety: a controlled study. *J Clin Psychiatry* 1982;43:81–86.

48. Sussman N. Treatment of anxiety with buspirone. *Psychiatr Ann* 1987;17:114–120.

49. Lucki I, Rickels K, Giesecki MA, et al. Differential effects of the anxiolytic drugs diazepam and buspirone on memory function. *Br J Clin Pharmacol* 1987;23:207–211.

50. Goa KL, Ward A. Buspirone: a preliminary review of its pharmacological properties and therapeutic efficacy as an anxiolytic. *Drugs* 1986;32:114–129.

51. Sussman N, Chou CY. Current issues in benzodiazepine use for anxiety disorders. *Psychiatr Ann* 1988;18:139–205.

52. Schweitzer E, Rickels K. Failure of buspirone to manage benzodiazepine withdrawal. *Am J Psychiatry* 1986;258:204–205.

53. DeMartinis N, Ryan M, Rickels K, et al. Prior benzodiazepine use and buspirone response in the treatment of generalized anxiety disorder. *J Clin Psychiatry* 2000;61:91–94.

54. Roerig JL. Diagnosis and management of generalized anxiety disorder. *J Am Pharm Assoc* 1999;39:811–821.

55. Davidson JR, DuPont RI, Hedges D, et al. Efficacy, safety and tolerability of venlafaxine extended release and buspirone in outpatients with generalized anxiety disorder. *J Clin Psychiatry* 1999;60:528–535.

56. Rickels K, Pollack MH, Sheehan DV, et al. Efficacy of extended-release venlafaxine in nondepressed outpatients with generalized anxiety disorder. *Am J Psychiatry* 2000;157:968–974.

57. Gelenberg AJ, Lydiard RB, Rudolph RL, et al. Efficacy of venlafaxine extended-release capsules in nondepressed outpatients with generalized anxiety disorder: a 6-month randomized controlled trial. *JAMA* 2000;283:3082–3088.

58. Kahn RJ, McNair DM, Lipman RS, et al. Imipramine and chlordiazepoxide in depressive and anxiety disorders: 2. Efficacy in anxious outpatients. *Arch Gen Psychiatry* 1986;43:79–85.

59. Rickels K, Downing RW, Schweizer E. Antidepressants in generalized anxiety disorder. Presented at the Annual Meeting of the American Psychiatric Association, Chicago, May 1987.

60. Feighner JP. Overview of antidepressants currently used to treat anxiety disorders. *J Clin Psychiatry* 1999;60(suppl 22):18–22.

61. Goodnick PJ, Puig A, DeVane CL, et al. Mirtazapine in major depression with comorbid generalized anxiety disorder. *J Clin Psychiatry* 1999;60:446–448.

62. Hedges DW, Reimherr FW, Strong RE, et al. An open trial of nefazodone in adult patients with generalized anxiety disorder. *Psychopharmacol Bull* 1996;32:671–676.

63. Rocca P, Fonzo V, Scotta M, et al. Paroxetine efficacy in the treatment of generalized anxiety disorder. *Acta Psychiatr Scand* 1997;95:444–450.

64. Ferreri M, Hantouche EG. Recent clinical trials of hydroxyzine in generalized anxiety disorder. *Acta Psychiatr Scand Suppl* 1998;393:102–108.

65. Lader M, Scotto JC. A multicentre double-blind comparison of hydroxyzine, buspirone and placebo in patients with generalized anxiety disorder. *J Psychopharmacol (Berl)* 1998;139:402–406.

66. Rickels K, DeMartinis N, Aufdembrinke B. Double-blind, placebo-controlled trial of abecarnil in the treatment of patients with generalized anxiety disorder. *J Clin Psychopharmacol* 2000;20:12–18.

67. Lydiard RB, Ballenger JC, Rickels K. A double-blind evaluation of the safety and efficacy of abecarnil, alprazolam, and placebo in outpatients with generalized anxiety disorder. Abecarnil Work Group. *J Clin Psychiatry* 1997;58(suppl 11):11–18.

68. Pollack MH, Worthington JJ, Manfro GG, et al. Abecarnil for the treatment of generalized anxiety disorder: a placebo-controlled comparison of two dosage ranges of abecarnil and buspirone. *J Clin Psychiatry* 1997;58(suppl 11):19–23.

69. Ayd FJ Jr. Psychiatry and herbal remedies. *Int Drug Ther Newsl* 2000:28–32.

70. Lechmann E, Kinzler E, Friedemann J. Efficacy of a special kava extract (Piper methysticum) in patients with states of anxiety, tension and excitedness of non-mental origin. A double-blind placebo-controlled study of four weeks' treatment. *Phytomedicine* 1996;2:113–119.

71. Warnecke G. Psychosomatische dysfuncktion en im weiblichen klimakterium. Klinishe wirksamkeit und vertraglichkeit van kava-extract WS 1490. *Fortschr Med* 1991;109:119–122.

72. Volz HP, Kieser M. Kava-kava extract WS 1490 versus placebo in anxiety disorders-a randomized placebo-

controlled 25-week outpatient trial. *Pharmacopsychiatry* 1997;30:1–5.

73. Lindenberg D, Pitule-Schodel H. D, L-Kava in comparison with oxazepam in anxiety disorders. A double-blind study of clinical effectiveness. *Fortschr Med* 1990;108:49–50, 53-54.

74. Woelke H, et al. Behandlung von Angst-Patienten. *Z Allg Med* 1993;69:271–277.

75. Singh NN, Ellis CR, Singh YN. A double-blind, placebo-controlled study of the effects of kava (Kavatrol ^{TM}) on daily stress and anxiety in adults. Presented at the Third Annual Alternative Therapies Symposium, San Diego, April 1–4, 1998.

76. Marks I, O'Sullivan G. Drugs and psychological treatments for agoraphobia/panic and obsessive-compulsive disorders: a review. *Br J Psychiatry* 1988;153:650–658.

77. Noyes R, Chaudry DR, Domingo DV. Pharmacologic treatment of phobic disorders. *J Clin Psychiatry* 1986;47:445–452.

78. Liebowitz MR, Gorman JM, Fyer AJ, et al. Pharmacotherapy of social phobia: an interim report of a placebo-controlled comparison of phenelzine and atenolol. *J Clin Psychiatry* 1988;49:252–258.

79. Liebowitz MR, Fyer AJ, Gorman JM, et al. Phenelzine in social phobia. *J Clin Psychopharmacol* 1986;6:93–98.

80. Lydiard RB, Laraia MT, Howell EF, et al. Alprazolam in social phobia. *J Clin Psychiatry* 1988;49:17–19.

81. Goldstein S. Treatment of social phobia with clonidine. *Biol Psychiatry* 1987;22:369–372.

82. Sternbach H. Fluoxetine treatment of social phobia. *J Affect Disord* 1987;13:183–192.

83. Schneier FR, Chin SJ, Hollander E, et al. Fluoxetine in social phobia. *J Clin Psychopharmacol* 1992;12:62–64.

84. Van Amerigen M, Mancini C, Streiner D. Sertraline in social phobia. *J Affect Disord* 1994;31:141–145.

84a. Versiani M. A review of 19 double-blind, placebo-controlled studies in social anxiety disorder (social phobia). *World J Biol Psychiatry* 2000;1:27–33.

85. Zitrin CM, Klein DF, Woerner MG, et al. Treatment of phobias. I: Comparison of imipramine hydrochloride and placebo. *Arch Gen Psychiatry* 1983;40:125–138.

86. Ballenger JC, Sheehan DV, Jacobson G. Antidepressant treatment of severe phobic anxiety. Presented at the Annual Meeting of the American Psychiatric Association, Toronto, May 1977.

87. Sheehan DV, Ballenger JC, Jacobsen G. Treatment of endogenous anxiety with phobic, hysterical, and hypochondriacal symptoms. *Arch Gen Psychiatry* 1980;37:51–59.

88. Cameron OG, Liepman MR, Curtis GC, et al. Ethanol retards desensitization of simple phobias in non-alcoholics. *Br J Psychiatry* 1987;150:845–849.

89. Marks IM. *Cure and care of neuroses: theory and practice of behavioral psychotherapy.* New York: Wiley, 1981.

90. Hunt D, Adams R, Egan K, et al. Opioids: mediators of fear or mania. *Biol Psychiatry* 1988;23:426–428.

91. Bernadt MW, Silverstone T, Singleton W. β-Adrenergic blockers in phobic disorder. *Br J Psychiatry* 1980;137:452–457.

92. American Psychiatric Association. *Diagnostic and statistical manual of mental disorders,* 4th ed. Washington, DC: American Psychiatric Press, 1994.

93. *Physicians' desk reference.* Montvale, NJ: Medical Economics Co.

94. Mitler MM. Evaluation of temazepam as a hypnotic. *Pharmacotherapy* 1981;1:3–13.

95. Bixler EO, Kales A, Soldatos CR, et al. Effectiveness of temazepam with short-, intermediate-, and long-term use: sleep laboratory evaluation. *J Clin Pharmacol* 1978;18:110–118.

96. Mitler MM, Seidel WF, van den Hoed J, et al. Comparative efficacy of temazepam: a long-term sleep laboratory evaluation. *Br J Clin Pharmacol* 1979;8:63s–68s.

97. Greenblatt DJ. Benzodiazepine hypnotics: sorting the pharmacokinetic facts. *J Clin Psychiatry* 1991; 52(suppl 9):4–10.

98. Gillin JC, Byerley WF. The diagnosis and management of insomnia. *N Engl J Med* 1990;322:239–248.

99. Dement WC, Carskadon MA, Mitler MM, et al. Prolonged use of flurazepam: a sleep laboratory study. *Behav Med* 1978;5:25–31.

100. Kales A, Bixler EO, Scharf M, et al. Sleep laboratory studies of flurazepam: a model for evaluating hypnotic drugs. *Clin Pharmacol Ther* 1976;19:576–583.

101. Kales A, Bixler EO, Soldatos CR, et al. Quazepam and flurazepam: long-term use and extended withdrawal. *Clin Pharmacol Ther* 1982;32:781–788.

102. Mamelak M, Csima A, Price V. A comparative 25-night sleep laboratory study on the effects of quazepam and triazolam on the sleep of chronic insomniacs. *J Clin Pharmacol* 1984;24:65–75.

103. Oswald L, Adam K, Borrow S, et al. The effects of two hypnotics on sleep, subjective feelings and skilled performance. In: Passouant P, Oswald I, eds. *Pharmacology of the states of alertness.* Elmsford, NY: Pergamon Press, 1979;51–63.

104. Kales A, Allen C, Scharf MB, et al. Hypnotic drugs and their effectiveness. All night EEG studies of insomniac subjects. *Arch Gen Psychiatry* 1970;23:226–232.

105. Kales A, Kales JD, Bixler EO, et al. Effectiveness of hypnotic drugs with prolonged use: flurazepam and pentobarbital. *Clin Pharmacol Ther* 1975;18:356–363.

106. Kales J, Kales A, Bixler EO, et al. Effects of placebo and flurazepam on sleep patterns in insomniac subjects. *Clin Pharmacol Ther* 1971;12:691–697.

107. Lamphere J, Roehrs T, Zorick F, et al. Chronic hypnotic efficacy of estazolam. *Drugs Exp Clin Res* 1986;12:687–691.

108. Kales A, Kales JD, Bixler EO, et al. Hypnotic efficacy of triazolam: sleep laboratory evaluation of intermediate-term effectiveness. *J Clin Pharmacol* 1976;16:399–406.

109. Kales A, Bixler EO, Soldatos CR, et al. Dose-response studies of lormetazepam: efficacy, side effects, and rebound insomnia. *J Clin Pharmacol* 1982;22:520–530.

110. Kales A, Soldatos CR, Bixler EO, et al. Midazolam: dose-response studies of effectiveness and rebound insomnia. *Pharmacology* 1983;26:138–149.

111. Kales A, Soldatos CR, Vela-Bueno A. Clinical comparison of benzodiazepine hypnotics with short and long elimination of half-lives. In: Smith DE, Wesson DR, eds. *The benzodiazepines. Current standards for medical practice.* Lancaster, U.K.: MTP Press, 1986.

112. Kales A, Bixler EO, Vela-Bueno A, et al. Comparison of short and long half-life benzodiazepine hypnotics: triazolam and quazepam. *Clin Pharmacol Ther* 1986;40:378–386.

113. Kales A, Bixler EO, Vela-Bueno A, et al. Alprazolam: effects on sleep and withdrawal phenomena. *J Clin Pharmacol* 1987;27:508–515.

114. Committee on the Review of Medicines. Systematic review of the benzodiazepines. *Br Med J* 1980;280:910–912.

115. Roth T, Kramer M, Lutz T. The effects of triazolam (0.25 mg) on the sleep of insomnia subjects. *Drugs Exp Clin Res* 1977;1:279–285.

116. Mamelak M, Csima A, Price V. The effects of a single night's dosing with triazolam on sleep the following night. *J Clin Pharmacol* 1990;30:549–555.

117. Fernandez Guardiola A, Jurado JL. The effect of triazolam on insomniac patients using a laboratory sleep evaluation. *Curr Ther Res* 1981;29:950–958.

118. Seidel W, Cohen SA, Bliwise NG, et al. Dose-related effects of triazolam on a circadian rhythm insomnia. *Clin Pharmacol Ther* 1986;40:314–320.

119. O'Donnell VM, Balkin TJ, Andrade JR, et al. Effects of triazolam on performance and sleep in a model of transient insomnia. *Hum Perform* 1988;1:145–160.

120. Roehrs T, Zorick F, Kaffeman M, et al. Flurazepam for short-term treatment of complaints of insomnia. *J Clin Pharmacol* 1982;22:290–296.

121. Mamelak M, Adele C, Buck L, et al. A comparative study of the effects of brotizolam and flurazepam on sleep and performance in the elderly. *J Clin Psychopharmacol* 1989;9:260–267.

122. Bonnet MH. Effect of sleep disruption on sleep, performance, and mood. *Sleep* 1985;8:11–19.

123. Kales A, Bixler EO, Soldatos CR, et al. Quazepam and temazepam: effects of short- and intermediate-term use and withdrawal. *Clin Pharmacol Ther* 1986;39:345–352.

124. Pierce MW, Shu VS. Efficacy of estazolam: the United States clinical experience. *Am J Med* 1990;88(suppl 3A):6s–11s.

125. Kripke DF, Hauri P, Roth T. Sleep evaluation in chronic insomnia during short- and long-term use of two benzodiazepines, flurazepam and midazolam. *Sleep Res* 1987;16:99.

126. Schneider-Helmert D. Why low-dose benzodiazepine-dependent insomniacs can't escape their sleeping pills. *Acta Psychiatr Scand* 1988;78:706–711.

127. Lucki I, Rickels K, Geller AM. Chronic use of benzodiazepines and psychomotor and cognitive test performance. *Psychopharmacology* 1986;88:416–433.

128. Monane M. Insomnia in the elderly. *J Clin Psychiatry* 1992;53(suppl):23–28.

129. Anonymous. Gelatin-filled temazepam capsules. *Lancet* 1995;346:303.

130. Carnwath T. Temazepam tablets as drugs of misuse. *Br Med J* 1993;307:385–386.

131. Green DS, Dockens RC, Salazar DE, et al. Coadministration of nefazodone and benzodiazepines. I: pharmacokinetic assessment [Abstract]. *Clin Pharmacol Ther* 1994;55:141.

132. Warot D, Bergougnan L, Lamiable D, et al. Troleandomycin-triazolam interaction in healthy volunteers: pharmacokinetic and psychometric evaluation. *Eur J Clin Pharmacol* 1987;32:389–393.

133. Varhe A, Olkkola KT, Neuvonen PJ. Oral triazolam is potentially hazardous to patients receiving systemic antimycotics ketoconazole or itraconazole. *Clin Pharmacol Ther* 1994;56:601–607.

134. Shader RI. Question the experts. *J Clin Psychopharmacol* 1994;14:293.

135. Greenblatt DJ, von Moltke LL, Harmatz JS, et al. Interaction of triazolam and ketoconazole. *Lancet* 1995;345:191.

136. Kim YJ. Review of zopiclone. *Pharm News* 1991;20:1–9.

137. Hajak G. A comparative assessment of the risks and benefits of zopiclone: a review of 15 years' clinical experience. *Drug Safety* 1999;21:457–469.

138. Delahaye C, Ferrand B, Pieddeloup C, et al. Post marketing surveillance of zopiclone: interim analysis on the first 10,000 cases in a clinical study in general practice. *Int Clin Psychopharmacol* 1990;5(suppl 2):131–138.

139. Lader M, Denney SC. A double-blind study to establish the residual effects of zopiclone on performance in healthy volunteers. *Pharmacology* 1983;27(suppl 2):98–108.

140. Prinz PN, Vitiello MV. Geriatrics. Sleep disorders and aging. *N Engl J Med* 1990;323:520–526.

141. Bianchi M, Musch B. Zopiclone discontinuation: review of 25 studies assessing withdrawal and rebound phenomena. *Int Clin Psychopharmacol* 1990;5(suppl 2):139–145.

142. Luty S, Sellman D. Imovane–a benzodiazepine in disguise. *Aust NZ J Med* 1993;106:293.

143. Mouret J, Ruel D, Maillard F, et al. Zopiclone versus triazolam in insomniac geriatric patients: a specific increase in delta sleep with zopiclone. *Int Clin Psychopharmacol* 1990;5(suppl 2):47–55.

144. Shelton PS, Hocking LB. Zolpidem for dementia-related insomnia and nighttime wandering. *Ann Pharmacother* 1997;31:319–322.

145. Frattola L, Maggioni M, Cesana B, et al. Double-blind comparison of zolpidem 20 mg versus funitrazepam 2 mg in insomniac patients. *Drugs Exp Clin Res* 1990;16:371–376.

146. Thome J, Ruchsow M, Rosler M, et al. [Zolpidem dependence and depression in the elderly.] *Psychiatr Prax* 1995;22:165–166.

147. Darcourt G, Pringuey D, Salliere D, et al. The safety and tolerability of zolpidem–an update. *J Psychopharmacol* 1999;13:81–93.

148. DeClerck A, Smits M. Zolpidem, a valuable alternative to benzodiazepine hypnotics for chronic insomnia. *J Int Med Res* 1999;27:253–263.

149. Monti JM, Attali P, Monti D, et al. Zolpidem and rebound insomnia–a double-blind, controlled polysomnographic study in chronic insomniac patients. *Pharmacopsychiatry* 1994;27:166–175.

150. Asnis GM, Chakraburtty A, DuBoff EA, et al. Zolpidem for persistent insomnia in SSRI-treated depressed patients. *J Clin Psychiatry* 1999;60:668–676.

151. Ansseau M, Pichot W, Hansenne M, et al. Psychotic reactions to zolpidem. *Lancet* 1992;339:809.

152. Pies R. Dose-related sensory distortions with zolpidem. *J Clin Psychiatry* 1995;56:35–36.

153. Iruela LM. Zolpidem and sleepwalking. *J Clin Psychopharmacol* 1995;15:223.

154. Mendelson WB. Sleepwalking associated with zolpidem [Letter]. *J Clin Psychopharmacol* 1994;14:150.
155. Gericke CA, Ludolph AC. Chronic abuse of zolpidem. *JAMA* 1994;272:1721–1722.
156. Rosen AS, Fournie P, Darwish M, et al. Zaleplon pharmacokinetics and absolute bioavailability. *Biopharm Drug Depos* 1999;20:171–175.
157. Rush CR, Frey JM, Griffiths RR. Zaleplon and triazolam in humans: acute behavioral effects and abuse potential. *Psychopharmacology* 1999;145:39–51.
158. Wagner J, Wagner ML, Hening WA. Beyond benzodiazepines: alternative pharmacologic agents for the treatment of insomnia. *Ann Pharmacother* 1998;32:680–691.
159. Danjou P, Paty I, Fruncillo R, et al. A comparison of the residual effects of zaleplon and zolpidem following administration 5 to 2 hours before awakening. *Br J Clin Pharmacol* 1999;48:367–374.
160. Troy SM, Lucki I, Unruh MA, et al. Comparison of the effects of zaleplon, zolpidem, and triazolam on memory, learning, and psychomotor performance. *J Clin Psychopharmacol* 2000;20:328–337.
161. Greenblatt DJ, Harmatz JS, von Moltke LL, et al. Comparative kinetics and dynamics of zaleplon, zolpidem, and placebo. *Clin Pharmacol Ther* 1998;64:553–561.
162. Elie R, Ruther E, Farr I, et al. Sleep latency is shortened during 4 weeks of treatment with zaleplon, a novel benzodiazepine hypnotic. Zaleplon Clinical Study Group. *J Clin Psychiatry* 1999;60:536–544.
163. Darwish M, Martin PT, Cevallos WH, et al. Rapid disappearance of zaleplon from breast milk after oral administration to lactating women. *J Clin Pharmacol* 1999;39:670–674.
164. Rickels K, Morris RJ, Newman H, et al. Diphenhydramine in insomniac family practice patients: a double-blind study. *J Clin Pharmacol* 1983;23:235–242.
165. Rickels K, Ginsberg J, Morris RJ, et al. Doxylamine succinate in insomniac family practice patients: a double-blind study. *Curr Ther Res* 1984;35:532–540.
166. Lamberg L. Melatonin potentially useful but safety, efficacy remain uncertain. *JAMA* 1996;276:1011–1014.
167. Williamson BL, Tomlinson AJ, Naylor S, et al. Contaminants in commercial preparations of melatonin [Letter]. *Mayo Clin Proc* 1997;72:1094–1095.
168. Garfinkel D, Laudon M, Nof D, et al. Improvement of sleep quality in elderly people by controlled-release melatonin. *Lancet* 1995;346:541–554.
169. Wurtman RJ, Zhdanova IV. Improvement of sleep quality by melatonin. *Lancet* 1995;346:1491.
169a. Andrade C, Srihari BS, Reddy KP, et al. Melatonin in medically ill patients with insomnia: a double-blind, placebo-controlled study. *J Clin Psychiatry* 2001;62:41–45.
170. Zhdanova IV, Wurtman RJ, Lynch HJ, et al. Sleep-inducing effect of low doses of melatonin ingested in the evening. *Clin Pharmacol Ther* 1995;57:552–558.
171. Hughes RJ, Sack RL, Lewy AJ. The role of melatonin and circadian phase in age-related sleep-maintenance insomnia: assessment in a clinical trial of melatonin replacement. *Sleep* 1998;21:52–68.
172. Lewy AJ, Sack RL, Blood ML, et al. Melatonin marks circadian phase position and resets the endogenous circadian pacemaker in humans. *Ciba Found Symp* 1995;183:303–321.
173. Arendt J. Discussion of melatonin marks circadian phase position and resets the endogenous circadian pacemaker in humans. *Ciba Found Symp* 1995;183:317–318.
174. Petrie K, Dawson AG, Thompson L, et al. A double-blind trial of melatonin as a treatment for jet lag in international cabin crew. *Biol Psychiatry* 1993;33:526–530.
175. Comperatore CA, Lieberman HR, Kirby AW, et al. Melatonin efficacy in aviation missions requiring rapid deployment and night operations. *Aviat Space Environ Med* 1996;67:520–524.
176. Chase JF, Gidal BE. Melatonin: therapeutic use in sleep disorders. *Ann Pharmacother* 1997;10:1218–1226.
177. Ayd FJ Jr. Psychiatry and herbal remedies. *Int Drug Ther Newsl* 2000;17–18.
178. Bodesheim U, Holz J. Isolation and receptor binding properties of alkaloidsand ligands from Valeriana officinalis. *Pharmazie* 1997;52:386–391.
179. Rasmussen P. A role for phytotherapy in the treatment of benzodiazepine and opiate drug withdrawal. *Eur J Herbal Med* 1997;3:11–21.
179a. Yager J, Siegfried SL, DiMatteo TL. Use of alternative remedies by psychiatric patients: illustrative vignettes and a discussion of the issues. *Am J Psychiatry* 1999;156:1432–1438.
179b. Edinger JD, Wohlgemuth WK, Radtke RA, et al. Cognitive behavioral therapy for treatment of chronic primary insomnia: a randomized controlled trial. *JAMA* 2001;285:517.
180. Chesson AL Jr, Anderson WM, Littner M, et al. Practice parameters for the nonpharmacologic treatment of chronic insomnia. An American Academy of Sleep Medicine report. Standards of Practice Committee of the American Academy of Sleep Medicine. *Sleep* 1999;22:1128–1133.
181. Marin CM, Hauri PJ, Espie CA, et al. Nonpharmacologic treatment of chronic insomnia. An American Academy of Sleep Medicine review. *Sleep* 1999;22:1134–1156.
182. Marin C, Culbert JP, Schwartz SM. Non-pharmacological intervention for insomnia. A meta-analysis of treatment efficacy. *Am J Psychiatry* 1994;151:1172–1180.
183. Spielman AJ, Saskin P, Thorpy MJ. Treatment of chronic insomnia by restriction of time in bed. *Sleep* 1987;10:45–56.
184. Greenblatt DJ, Shader RI, Abernethy DR. Current status of benzodiazepines (1). *N Engl J Med* 1983;309:354–358.
185. Greenblatt DJ, Shader RI. Pharmacokinetics of antianxiety agents. In: Meltzer HY, ed. *Psychopharmacology: the third generation of progress.* New York: Raven Press, 1987:1377–1386.
186. File SE, Pellow S. Behavioral pharmacology of minor tranquilizers. *Pharmacol Ther* 1987;35:265–290.
187. Ingram IM, Timbury GC. Side effects of librium. *Lancet* 1960;2:766.
188. Dietch JT, Jennings RK. Aggressive dyscontrol in patients treated with benzodiazepines. *J Clin Psychiatry* 1988;49:184–188.
189. Lion JR. Benzodiazepines in the treatment of aggressive patients. *J Clin Psychiatry* 1979;40:70–71.
190. Kalina RK. Diazepam: its role in the prison setting. *Dis Nerv Syst* 1964;25:101–107.

191. Rothschild AJ, Shindul-Rothschild JA, Viguera A, et al. Comparison of the frequency of behavioral disinhibition on alprazolam, clonazepam, or no benzodiazepine in hospitalized psychiatric patients. *J Clin Psychopharmacol* 2000;20:7–11.

192. Sunter JP, Bal TS, Cowan WK. Three cases of triazolam poisoning. *Br Med J* 1988;297:719.

193. O'Dowd JJ, Spragg PP, Routledge PA. Fatal triazolam poisoning. *Br Med J* 1988;297:1048.

194. Greenblatt DJ, Allen MD, Noel BJ, et al. Special article: acute overdosage with benzodiazepine derivatives. *Clin Pharmacol Ther* 1977;21:497.

195. Jatlow P, Dobular K, Bailey D. Serum diazepam concentrations in overdose. Their significance. *Am J Clin Pathol* 1979;72:571–577.

196. Divoll M, Greenblatt DJ, Lacasse Y, et al. Benzodiazepine overdosage: plasma concentrations and clinical outcome. *Psychopharmacology(Berl)* 1981;73:381–383.

197. Greenblatt DJ, Woo E, Allen MD, et al. Rapid recovery from massive diazepam overdose. *JAMA* 1978;240:1872–1874.

198. Jenkins AJ, Levine B, Locke JL, et al. A fatality due to alprazolam intoxication. *J Anal Toxicol* 1997;21:218–220.

199. Bo O, Hafner O, Langard O, et al. Ethanol and diazepam as causative agents in road accidents. In: Iraelstam S, Lambert S, eds. *Alcohol, drugs, and traffic safety*. Toronto: Addiction Research Foundation of Ontario, 1975.

200. Skegg DCG, Richards SM, Doll R. Minor tranquilizers and road accidents. *Br Med J* 1979;1:917–919.

201. Warren R. Drugs detected in fatally injured drivers in the province of Ontario. In: Goldberg L, ed. *Alcohol, drugs, and traffic safety. Vol. 1.* Stockholm: Almquist and Wiksell, 1981.

202. O'Hanlon JF, Haak TW, Blaauw GJ, et al. Diazepam impairs lateral position control in highway driving. *Science* 1982;217:79–81.

203. McNair DM. Anti-anxiety drugs and human performance. *Arch Gen Psychiatry* 1973;29:609–617.

204. Golombok S, Moodley P, Lader M. Cognitive impairment in long-term benzodiazepine users. *Psychol Med* 1988;18:365–374.

205. Petursson H, Gudjonsson GH, Lader MH. Psychosomatic performance during withdrawal from long-term benzodiazepine treatment. *Psychopharmacology* 1983;81:345–349.

206. Larson E, Kukull WA, Buchner D, et al. Adverse drug reactions associated with global cognitive impairment in elderly persons. *Ann Intern Med* 1987;107:169–173.

207. Hendler N, Cimini C, Ma T, et al. A comparison of cognitive impairment due to benzodiazepines and to narcotics. *Am J Psychiatry* 1980;137:828-830.

208. Ron M. *The alcoholic brain: CT scan and psychological findings. Psychological medicine monographs (supplement 3).* Cambridge: Cambridge University Press, 1983.

209. Lader MH, Ron M, Petursson H. Computed axial brain tomography in long-term benzodiazepine users. *Psychol Med* 1984;14:203–206.

210. Schmauss C, Krieg JC. Enlargement of cerebrospinal fluid spaces in long-term benzodiazepine users. *Psychol Med* 1987;17:869–873.

211. Uhde TW, Kellner CH. Cerebral ventricular size in panic disorder. *J Affect Disord* 1987;12:175–178.

212. Poser W, Poser S, Roscher D, et al. Do benzodiazepines cause cerebral atrophy [Letter]. *Lancet* 1983;1:715.

213. Perera KMH, Powell T, Jenner FA. Computerized axial tomographic studies following long-term use of benzodiazepines. *Psychol Med* 1987;17:775–777.

214. Bowden CL, Fisher JG. Safety and efficacy of long-term diazepam therapy. *South Med J* 1980;73:1581–1584.

215. Laughren TP, Battey Y, Greenblatt DJ, et al. A controlled trial of diazepam withdrawal in chronically anxious outpatients. *Acta Psychiatr Scand* 1982;65:171–179.

216. Olajide D, Lader M. Depression following withdrawal from long-term benzodiazepine use: a report of four cases. *Psychol Med* 1984;14:937–940.

217. Ashton H. Benzodiazepine withdrawal: an unfinished story. *Br Med J* 1984;288:1135–1140.

218. Mellor CS, Jain VK. Diazepam withdrawal syndrome. Its prolonged and changing nature. *Can Med Assoc J* 1982;127:1093–1096.

219. Schmauss C, Apelt S, Emrich HM. Characterization of benzodiazepine withdrawal in high- and low-dose dependent psychiatric inpatients. *Brain Res Bull* 1987;19:393–400.

220. Busto U, Fornazzari L, Naranjo CA. Protracted tinnitus after discontinuation of long-term therapeutic use of benzodiazepines. *J Clin Psychopharmacol* 1988;5:359–362.

221. Speirs CJ, Navey FL, Brooks DJ, et al. Opisthotonos and benzodiazepine withdrawal in the elderly. *Lancet* 1986;2:1101.

222. O'Flaherty S, Evans M, Epps A, et al. Choreoathetosis and clonazepam [Letter]. *Med J Aust* 1985;142:453.

223. Rapport DJ, Covington EG. Motor phenomena in benzodiazepine withdrawal. *Hosp Community Psychiatry* 1989;40:1277–1279.

224. Hauser P, Devinsky O, De Bellis M, et al. Benzodiazepine withdrawal delirium with catatonic features. Occurrence in patients with partial seizure disorder. *Arch Neurol* 1989;46:696–699.

225. Arana GW, Epstein S, Molloy M, et al. Carbamazepine-induced reduction of plasma alprazolam concentrations: a clinical case report. *J Clin Psychiatry* 1988;49:448–449.

226. Higgitt AC, Lader MH, Fonagy P. Clinical management of benzodiazepine dependence. *Br Med J* 1985;291:688–690.

227. Chouinard G. Additional comments on benzodiazepine withdrawal. *Can Med Assoc J* 1988;139:119–120.

228. Murphy SM, Owen RT, Tyrer PJ. Withdrawal symptoms after six weeks' treatment with diazepam [Letter]. *Lancet* 1984;2:1389.

229. Pecknold JC, McClure DJ, Fleury D, et al. Benzodiazepine withdrawal effects. *Prog Neuropsychopharmacol Biol Psychiatry* 1982;6:517–522.

230. Power KG, Jerrom DWA, Simpson RJ, et al. Controlled study of withdrawal symptoms and rebound anxiety after six-week course of diazepam for generalized anxiety. *Br Med J* 1985;290:1246–1248.

231. Fontaine R, Chouinard G, Annable L. Rebound anxiety in anxious patients after abrupt withdrawal

of benzodiazepine treatment. *Am J Psychiatry* 1984;141:848–852.

232. Wells BG, Evans RL, Ereshefsky L, et al. Clinical outcome and adverse effect profile associated with concurrent administration of alprazolam and imipramine. *J Clin Psychiatry* 1988;49:394–399.

233. Herman JB, Rosenbaum JF, Brotman AW. The alprazolam to clonazepam switch for the treatment of panic disorder. *J Clin Psychopharmacol* 1987;7:175–178.

234. Rashid K, Patrissi G, Cook B. Multiple serious symptom formation with alprazolam. Presented at the Annual Meeting of the American Psychiatric Association, Montreal, 1988.

235. Johnson LD, O'Malley PM, Bachman JG. *National survey results on drug use from the monitoring the future study, 1975–1993.* NIDA, NIH Publication No. 94-3804. USDHHS. Washington, DC: U.S. Government Printing Office, 1994.

236. de Wit H, Griffiths RR. Testing the abuse liability of anxiolytic and hypnotic drugs. *Drug Alcohol Depend* 1991;28:83–111.

237. Shader RI, Greenblatt DJ. Use of benzodiazepines in anxiety disorders. *N Engl J Med* 1993;328:1398–1405.

238. Salzman C. Behavioral side effects of benzodiazepines. In: Kane JM, Lieberman JA, eds. *Adverse effects of psychotropic drugs.* New York: Guilford Press, 1992;139–152.

239. Martinez-Cano H, Vela-Bueno A, de Iceta M, et al. Benzodiazepine withdrawal syndrome seizures. *Pharmacopsychiatry* 1995;28:257–262.

240. Saxon L, Hjemdahl P, Hiltunen AJ, et al. Effects of flumazenil in the treatment of benzodiazepine withdrawal: a double-blind pilot study. *Psychopharmacology (Berl)* 1997;131:153–160.

241. Lader M, Morton S. Benzodiazepine withdrawal syndrome. *Br J Psychiatry* 1991;158:435–436.

242. Higgitt A, Fonagy P, Toone B, et al. The prolonged benzodiazepine withdrawal syndrome: anxiety or hysteria? *Acta Psychiatr Scand* 1990;82:165–168.

243. Tyrer P. The benzodiazepine post-withdrawal syndrome. *Stress Med* 1991;7:1–2.

244. Busto V, Sellers EM, Naranjo CA, et al. Withdrawal reaction after long-term therapeutic use of benzodiazepines. *N Engl J Med* 1986;315:854–859.

245. Tyrer P. Dependence as a limiting factor in the clinical use of minor tranquilisers. *Pharmacol Ther* 1988;36:173–188.

246. Mellman TA, Uhde TW. Withdrawal syndrome with gradual tapering of alprazolam. *Am J Psychiatry* 1986;143:1464–1466.

247. Ayd FJ Jr. Benzodiazepine prescribing. *Int Drug Ther Newsl* 1989;24:41–42.

248. Kemper N, Poser W, Poser S. Benzodiazepinabhaengigkeit. *Dtsch Med Wochenschr* 1980;105:1707–1712.

249. Tyrer PJ, Seivewright N. Identification and management of benzodiazepine dependence. *Postgrad Med* 1984;60:41–44.

250. Pinna G, Galici R, Schneider HH, et al. Alprazolam dependence prevented by substituting with the beta-carboline abecarnil. *Proc Natl Acad Sci USA* 1997;94:2719–2723.

251. Rickels K, Case WG, Schweizer E. Withdrawal from benzodiazepines. In: Hindmarch I, Beaumont G, Brandon S, et al., eds. *Benzodiazepines: current concepts–biological, clinical and social perspectives.* West Sussex, U.K.: John Wiley & Sons, 1990:199–210.

252. Apelt S, Emrich HM. Sodium valproate in benzodiazepine withdrawal . *Am J Psychiatry* 1990;147:950–951.

253. Schweizer E, Rickels K. Failure of buspirone to manage benzodiazepine withdrawal. *Am J Psychiatry* 1986;143:1590–1592.

254. Jerkovich GS, Preskorn SH. Failure of buspirone to protect against lorazepam withdrawal symptoms [Letter]. *JAMA* 1987;258:204–205.

255. Lemoine P, Touchon J, Billardon M. Comparison of 6 different methods for lorazepam withdrawal. A controlled study, hydroxyzine versus placebo. *Encephale* 1997;23:290–299.

256. Pages KP, Ries RK. Use of anticonvulsants in benzodiazepine withdrawal. *Am J Addict* 1998;7:198–204.

257. Garfinkel D, Zisapel N, Wainstein J, et al. Facilitation of benzodiazepine discontinuation by melatonin: a new clinical approach. *Arch Intern Med* 1999;159:2456–2460.

258. Romach MK, Kaplan HL, Busto EU, et al. A controlled trial of ondansetron, a 5-HT$_3$ antagonist, in benzodiazepine discontinuation. *J Clin Psychopharmacol* 1998;18:121–131.

259. Rickels K, DeMartinis N, Rynn M, et al. Pharmacologic strategies for discontinuing benzodiazepine treatment. *J Clin Psychopharmacol* 1999;19:12S–16S.

260. Rickels K, Schweizer E, Garcia Espana F, et al. Trazodone and valproate in patients discontinuing long-term benzodiazepine therapy: effects on withdrawal symptoms and taper outcome. *Psychopharmacology (Berl)* 1999;141:1–5.

261. Rickels K, Case WG, Schweizer E, et al. Benzodiazepine dependence: management of discontinuation. *Psychopharmacol Bull* 1990;26:63–68.

262. Tyrer P, Rutherford D, Huggett T. Benzodiazepine withdrawal symptoms and propranolol. *Lancet* 1981;1:520–522.

263. Keshavan MS, Crammer JL. Clonidine in benzodiazepine withdrawal. *Lancet* 1985;1:1325–1326.

264. Schweitzer E, Rickels K, Case WG, et al. Carbamazepine treatment in patients discontinuing long-term benzodiazepine therapy: effects on withdrawal severity and outcome. *Arch Gen Psychiatry* 1991;48:448–452.

265. Ayd FJ Jr. Oxazepam: update 1989. *Int Clin Psychopharmacol* 1990;5:1–15.

266. Breier A, Charney DS, Nelson CJ. Seizures induced by abrupt discontinuation of alprazolam. *Am J Psychiatry* 1984;141:1606–1607.

267. Levy AB. Delirium and seizures due to abrupt alprazolam withdrawal: case report. *J Clin Psychiatry* 1984;45:38–39.

268. Noyes R, Perry PJ, Crowe RR, et al. Single case study: seizures following the withdrawal of alprazolam. *J Nerv Ment Dis* 1986;174:50–52.

269. Naylor MW, Grunhaus L, Cameron O. Single case study: myoclonic seizures after abrupt withdrawal from phenelzine and alprazolam. *J Nerv Ment Dis* 1987;175:111–114.

270. Department of Health and Human Services, Public Health Service, Food and Drug Administration

Center for Drugs and Biologics. *Seizures associated with alprazolam.* DHHS, 1986.

271. Gatzonis SD, Angelopoulos EK, Daskalopoulou EG, et al. Convulsive status epilepticus following abrupt high-dose benzodiazepine discontinuation. *Drug Alcohol Depend* 2000;59:95–97.

272. Farid BT, Bulto M. Benzodiazepine prescribing [Letter]. *Lancet* 1989;2:917.

273. Linnoila M, Erwin CW, Logue PE. Efficacy and side effects of flurazepam and a combination of amobarbital and secobarbital in insomniac patients. *J Clin Pharmacol* 1980;20:117–123.

274. Balter MB, Uhlenhuth EH. The beneficial and adverse effects of hypnotics. *J Clin Psychiatry* 1991;52(suppl 7):16–23.

275. Hindmarch I. Residual effects of hypnotics: an update. *J Clin Psychiatry* 1991;52(suppl 7):14–15.

276. Church MW, Johnson LC. Mood and performance of poor sleepers during repeated use of flurazepam. *Psychopharmacology* 1979;61:309–316.

277. Members of the Consensus Panel, Freedman DX (panel chairman). Drugs and insomnia. The use of medications to promote sleep. *JAMA* 1984;251:2410–2414.

278. Kaolega S. Benzodiazepines and vigilance performance: a review. *Psychopharmacology* 1989;91:143–156.

279. Greenblatt DJ, Shader RI, Divoll M, et al. Adverse reactions to triazolam, flurazepam, and placebo in controlled clinical trials. *J Clin Psychiatry* 1984;45:192–195.

280. Greenblatt DJ, Divoll M, Harmatz JS, et al. Kinetics and clinical effects of flurazepam in young and elderly noninsomniacs. *Clin Pharmacol Ther* 1981;30:475–486.

281. Salkind MR, Silverstone T. A clinical and psychometric evaluation of flurazepam. *Br J Clin Pharmacol* 1975;2:223–226.

282. Johnson L, Chernik D. Sedative hypnotics and human performance. *Psychopharmacology (Berl)* 1982;72:101–113.

283. Greenblatt DJ, Divoll M, Abernethy DR, et al. Benzodiazepine kinetics: implications for therapeutics and pharmacogeriatrics. *Drug Metab Rev* 1983;14:251–292.

284. Dement WC. Objective measurements of daytime sleepiness and performance comparing quazepam with flurazepam in two adult populations using the multiple sleep latency test. *J Clin Psychiatry* 1991;52(suppl 9):31–37.

285. Mitler MM, Seidel WF, van den Hoed J, et al. Comparative hypnotic effects of flurazepam, triazolam, and placebo. A long-term simultaneous nighttime and daytime study. *J Clin Psychopharmacol* 1984;4:2–13.

286. Bliwise D, Seidel WF, Karacan I, et al. Daytime sleepiness as a criterion in hypnotic medication trials: comparison of triazolam and flurazepam. *Sleep* 1983;6:156–165.

287. Ellinwood E, Linnoila M, Marsh G. Plasma concentrations in chronic insomniacs of flurazepam and midazolam during fourteen-day use and their relationship to therapeutic effects and next-day performance and mood. *J Clin Psychopharmacol* 1990;10(suppl):68s–75s.

288. Nikaido AM, Ellinwood EH. Comparison of the effects of quazepam and triazolam on cognitive-neuromotor performance. *Psychopharmacology* 1987;92:459–464.

289. Wickstrom E, Godtlibssen OB. The effects of quazepam, triazolam, flunitrazepam and placebo, alone and in combination with ethanol, on daytime sleep, memory, mood and performance. *Hum Psychopharmacol* 1988;3:101–110.

290. Lee A, Lader M. Tolerance and rebound during and after short-term administration of quazepam, triazolam and placebo to healthy volunteers. *Int J Clin Psychopharmacol* 1988;3:31–47.

291. Bixler EO, Kales A, Brubaker BH, et al. Adverse reactions to benzodiazepine hypnotics: spontaneous reporting systems. *Pharmacology* 1987;35:286–300.

292. Heel RC, Brogden RN, Speight TM, et al. Temazepam: a review of its pharmacological properties and therapeutic efficacy as an hypnotic. *Drugs* 1981;21:321–340.

293. Walsh JK, Targum SD, Pegram V, et al. A multi-center clinical investigation of estazolam: short-term efficacy. *Curr Ther Res* 1984;36:866–874.

294. Dominguez RO, Goldstein BJ, Jacobson AF, et al. Comparative efficacy of estazolam, flurazepam, and placebo in outpatients with insomnia. *J Clin Psychiatry* 1986;47:362–365.

295. Scharf MB, Roth PB, Dominguez RA, et al. Estazolam and flurazepam: a multi-center, placebo-controlled comparative study in outpatients with insomnia. *J Clin Pharmacol* 1990;40:461–467.

296. Morgan K, Oswald I. Anxiety caused by a short-life hypnotic. *Br Med J* 1982;284:942.

297. Kales A, Soldatos CR, Bixler EO, et al. Early morning insomnia with rapidly eliminated benzodiazepines. *Science* 1983;220:95–97.

298. Carskadon MA, Seidel WF, Greenblatt DJ, et al. Daytime carryover of triazolam and flurazepam in elderly insomniacs. *Sleep* 1982;5:361–371.

299. Tan TL, Bixler EO, Kales A, et al. Early morning insomnia, daytime anxiety, and organic mental disorder associated with triazolam. *J Fam Pract* 1985;20:592–594.

300. Adam K, Oswald I. Can a rapidly eliminated hypnotic cause daytime anxiety? *Pharmacopsychiatry* 1989;22:115–119.

301. Moon CAL, Ankier SI, Hayes G. Early morning insomnia and daytime anxiety–a multicentre general practice study comparing loprazolam and triazolam. *Br J Clin Pract* 1985;Sept:352–358.

302. DeTullio PL, Kirking DM, Zacardelli DK, et al. Evaluation of long-term triazolam use in an ambulatory veterans administration medical center population. *Ann Pharmacother* 1989;23:290–293.

303. Poitras R. A propos d'épisodes d'amnesies anterogrades associes a l'utilisation du triazolam. *Union Med Can* 1980;109:427–429.

304. Shader RI, Greenblatt DJ. Triazolam and anterograde amnesia: all is not well in the Z-zone [Editorial]. *J Clin Psychopharmacol* 1983;3:273.

305. Huff JS, Plunkett HG. Anterograde amnesia following triazolam use by two emergency room physicians. *J Emerg Med* 1989;7:153–155.

306. Einarson TR, Yoder ES. Triazolam psychosis–a syndrome? *Drug Intell Clin Pharmacol* 1982;16:330.

307. Schogt B, Cohn D. Paranoid symptoms associated with triazolam. *Can J Psychiatry* 1985;30:462–463.
308. Soldatos CR, Sakkas PN, Bergiannaki JD, et al. Behavioural side effects of triazolam in psychiatric inpatients: report of five cases. *Drug Intell Clin Pharmacol* 1986;20:294–297.
309. Kirk T, Roache JD, Griffiths RR. Dose-response evaluation of the amnestic effects of triazolam and pentobarbital in normal subjects. *J Clin Psychopharmacol* 1990;10:161–168.
310. Regestein QR, Reich P. Agitation observed during treatment with newer hypnotic drugs. *J Clin Psychiatry* 1985;46:280–283.
311. Morris HH, Estes ML. Traveler's amnesia: transient global amnesia secondary to triazolam. *JAMA* 1987;258:945–946.
312. Morris HH, Estes ML. In reply [Letter]. *JAMA* 1988;259:351–352.
313. Bixler EO, Kales A, Manfredi RL, et al. Triazolam-induced brain impairment: frequent memory disturbances. *Eur J Clin Pharmacol* 1989;36:A171.
314. Kales A, Vgontzas AN. Not all benzodiazepines are alike. In: Stefanis CN, Rabavilas AD, Soldatos CR, eds. *Psychiatry: a world perspective. Vol. 3.* Amsterdam: Elsevier Science, 1990;379–384.
315. Bixler EO, Kales A, Manfredi RL, et al. Next-day memory impairment with triazolam use. *Lancet* 1991;337:827–831.
316. Kales A, Bixler EO, Soldatos CR, et al. Lorazepam: effects on sleep and withdrawal phenomena. *Pharmacology* 1986;32:121–130.
317. Healy M, Pickens R, Meisch R, et al. Effects of clorazepate, diazepam, lorazepam, and placebo on human memory. *J Clin Psychiatry* 1983;44:436–439.
318. Lister RG, File SE. The nature of lorazepam-induced amnesia. *Psychopharmacology* 1984;83:183–187.
319. Mac DS, Kumar R, Goodwin DW. Anterograde amnesia with oral lorazepam. *J Clin Psychiatry* 1985;46:137–138.
320. Sandyk R. Transient global amnesia induced by lorazepam. *Clin Neuropharmacol* 1985;8:297-298.
321. Lister RG. The amnesic action of benzodiazepines in man. *Neurosci Biobehav Rev* 1985;9:87–94.
322. Roth T, Hartse KM, Saab PG, et al. The effects of flurazepam, lorazepam, and triazolam on sleep and memory. *Psychopharmacology* 1980;70:231–237.
323. Kowley G, Springen K, Iarovice D, et al. Sweet dreams or a nightmare? *Newsweek* 1991(Aug 19):38–44.
324. Wysowski DK, Barash D. Adverse behavioral reactions attributed to triazolam in the Food and Drug Administration's Spontaneous Reporting System. *Arch Intern Med* 1991;151:2003–2008.
325. Adam K, Oswald I, Shapiro C. Effects of loprazolam and of triazolam on sleep and overnight urinary cortisol. *Psychopharmacology (Berl)* 1984;82:389–394.
326. Bixler EO, Kales A, Soldatos CR, et al. Flunitrazepam. An investigational hypnotic drug: sleep laboratory evaluations. *J Clin Pharmacol* 1977;17:569–578.
327. Kales A, Soldatos CR, Bixler EO, et al. Rebound insomnia and rebound anxiety: a review. *Pharmacology* 1983;26:121–137.
328. Scharf MB, Bixler EO, Kales A, et al. Long-term sleep laboratory evaluation of flunitrazepam. *Pharmacology* 1979;19:173–181.

329. Mamelak M, Csima A, Price V. The effects of brotizolam on the sleep of chronic insomniacs. *Br J Clin Pharmacol* 1983;16(suppl):377–382.
330. Monti JM. Sleep laboratory and clinical studies of the effects of triazolam, flunitrazepam and flurazepam in insomniac patients. *Methods Find Exp Clin Pharmacol* 1981;3:303–326.
331. Monti JM, Debellis J, Gratadoux E, et al. Sleep laboratory study of the effects of midazolam in insomniac patients. *Eur J Clin Pharmacol* 1982;21:479–484.
332. Roth T, Kramer M, Lutz T. Intermediate use of triazolam: a sleep laboratory study. *J Int Med Res* 1976;4: 59–62.
333. Scharf MB, Kales A, Bixler EO, et al. Lorazepam–efficacy, side effects and rebound phenomena. *Clin Pharmacol Ther* 1982;31:175–179.
334. Vela-Bueno A, Oliveros JC, Dobladez-Blanco B, et al. Brotizolam: a sleep laboratory evaluation. *Eur J Clin Pharmacol* 1983;25:53–56.
335. Vogel GW, Thurmond A, Gibbons P, et al. The effect of triazolam on the sleep of insomniacs. *Psychopharmacology* 1975;41:65–69.
336. Vogel GW, Barker K, Gibbons P, et al. A comparison of the effects of flurazepam 30 mg and triazolam 0.5 mg on the sleep of insomniacs. *Psychopharmacology* 1987;47:81–86.
337. Gillin JC, Spinweber CH, Johnson LC. Rebound insomnia: a critical review. *J Clin Psychopharmacol* 1989;9:161–172.
338. Greenblatt DJ, Harmatz JS, Zinny MA, et al. Effect of gradual withdrawal on the rebound sleep disorder after discontinuation of triazolam. *N Engl J Med* 1987;317:722–728.
339. Bliwise D, Seidel W, Greenblatt DJ, et al. Nighttime and daytime efficacy of flurazepam and oxazepam in chronic insomnia. *Am J Psychiatry* 1984;141:191–195.
340. Mendelson WB, Weingartner H, Greenblatt DJ, et al. A clinical study of flurazepam. *Sleep* 1982;5:350–360.
341. Berlin RM, Conell LJ. Withdrawal symptoms after long-term treatment with therapeutic doses of flurazepam: a case report. *Am J Psychiatry* 1983;140:488–490.
342. Soldatos CR, Dikeos DG, Whitehead A. Tolerance and rebound insomnia with rapidly eliminated hypnotics: a meta-analysis of sleep laboratory studies. *Int Clin Psychopharmacol* 1999;14:287–303.
343. Lagier G. Troubles possible apres arret d'un traitement prolonge par les benzodiazepines chez l'homme (toxicomanies exclues). *Therapie* 1985;40:51–57.
344. Kornecki E, Lenox RH, Hardwick DH, et al. Interactions of the alkyl-ether-phospholipid, platelet activating factor (PAF) with platelets, neural cells, and the psychotropic drugs triazolobenzodiazepines. *Adv Exp Med Biol* 1987;221:477–488.
345. van der Kroef C. Het Halcion-syndroom-een iatrogene epidemie in Nederland. *Tijdschr Alcohol Drugs* 1982;8:156–162.
346. Adam K, Oswald I. Possible mechanism for adverse reactions to triazolam [Letter]. *Lancet* 1991;338:1157.
347. Tien Y, Gujavarty KS. Seizure following withdrawal from triazolam. *Am J Psychiatry* 1985;142:1516–1517.

348. Schneider LS, Syapin PJ, Pawluczyk S. Seizures following triazolam withdrawal despite benzodiazepine treatment. *J Clin Psychiatry* 1987;48:418–419.
349. Laplane D, Baulac M, Lacombley L. Convulsions douze heures apres la prise d'une benzodiazepine a demi-vie courte. *Presse Med* 1988;17:439.
350. Anello C. Adverse behavior reactions attributed to triazolam in the FDA's Spontaneous Reporting System. Presented at the Pharmacological Drugs Advisory Committee Meeting, Washington, DC, September 1989.
351. Martinez-Cano H, Vela-Bueno A. Triazolam [Letter]. *Lancet* 1991;337:1483.
352. Heritch AJ, Capwell R, Roy-Byrne PP. A case of psychosis and delirium following withdrawal from triazolam. *J Clin Psychiatry* 1987;48:168–169.

13

Assessment and Treatment of Other Disorders

PANIC DISORDER

Clinical Presentation

In 1964, Klein (1) described a syndrome characterized by:

- Sudden, spontaneous, unexpected feelings of *terror and anxiety*
- The *autonomic* equivalence of anxiety
- The *desire to flee* the situation and to return to a safe place
- A *phobic avoidance* of the places where such attacks occur

These symptoms typically occur in public places, such as supermarkets, restaurants, elevators, and crowded stores. Indeed, individuals may develop three disorders:

- The *panic attack* itself
- Secondary *anticipatory anxiety* that they will have another episode in certain places
- A *phobic avoidance* of the feared situation

Most individuals have many of the symptoms during an attack, but not necessarily every possible symptom. There is also a group (perhaps 25%) who have these attacks without the subjective sense of anxiety or who experience insufficient symptoms to meet diagnostic criteria (i.e., limited symptom attacks). These individuals may have a rapid heartbeat, diaphoresis, and tremors, without feeling acutely anxious. This last point is important because these patients often develop the physiological symptoms of anxiety in public places or in unexpected or unprovoked situations. Although it may be in a public place, they are not under any specific stress nor in a highly emotional situation. When it occurs for the first time, patients frequently seek help in an emergency room or from a family physician. Typically, after a medical workup, they are told that there is nothing wrong with them except stress. What is interesting is that the attacks occur in nonstress-ful situations, so the psychiatric stress-diathesis model is not appropriate. Clearly, the explanation given by the medical personnel is incorrect, because it is inconsistent with what has happened to the patient. Thus, the patient often assumes the existence of a medical condition that has gone unrecognized.

This syndrome often develops in patients in their twenties, and some, with the more severe form, rarely leave home for periods of many years, or until they are effectively treated by medication, cognitive behavior therapy, or other behavior/psychological therapies. **Family studies of panic disorder (PD) find an increased occurrence of attacks in first-degree relatives** (2).

A serious complication of PD is the abuse of sedatives and alcohol through attempts at self-medication. In several studies, those who did well on antidepressants did not return to alcohol or drug abuse, but those in the control groups, not maintained on medication, often returned to a level of drug abuse that eventually necessitated rehospitalization. **Another complication is the risk of suicide, which may be as high in patients with PD as in those suffering from a major depressive disorder** (3–6).

Mitral Valve Prolapse Syndrome

Mitral valve prolapse syndrome occurs more frequently in patients with PD than in control subjects, but there is also a high incidence in the general population. It is often referred to as the click-murmur or Reed Barlow syndrome and is characterized by a nonejection click with or without a late-systolic, high-pitched heart murmur, best heard at the apex. The syndrome also includes such symptoms as cardiac awareness, atypical chest pain, palpitations, shortness of breath, weakness, fatigue, and dizziness, as well as musculoskeletal abnormalities (e.g., a double-jointed pectus excavatum, kyphoscoliosis, straight back, and a tall-thin body habitus).

Patients with symptomatic, mitral valve prolapse often excrete elevated urinary epinephrine and norepinephrine. The diagnosis can be confirmed by echocardiography.

DaCosta's Syndrome

Irritable heart, cardiac neurosis, or DaCosta's syndrome, has been described since the Civil War. It is manifested by cardiac symptoms and autonomic adrenergic predominance (excess levels of or supersensitivity to peripheral catecholamines). Lactate-induced panic attacks in patients are also correlated with elevated epinephrine excretion in comparison with normal control subjects.

How PD, mitral valve prolapse, DaCosta's syndrome, and a hyperadrenergic predominance might relate to each other is unknown at this time.

Provocative Tests for Panic Disorder

In 1951, Cohen and White (7) observed that abnormally high lactic acids levels developed after running in patients suffering from what they called "effort syndrome." This led Pitts and McClure (8) to show that lactate infusions can precipitate anxiety attacks in patients with PD, but not in control subjects. Furthermore, Kelly and colleagues (9) observed that effective drug treatment resulted in a cessation of lactate-induced panic attacks. In contrast, unsuccessful treatment did not prevent reinfusion-produced panic attacks. Liebowitz et al. (10) also noted that these patients often responded to lactate with a panic attack, but reinfusion after successful drug treatment failed to reproduce such episodes. Panic attacks have also been induced by such diverse compounds as CO_2, isoproterenol, meta-chlorophenyl piperizine (mCPP), and flumazenil. The various mechanisms by which these agents produce symptoms provide fertile ground for elucidating the biological basis of PD (11).

Drug Therapy for Panic Disorder

In the past decade, there has been an important change in the pharmacotherapy of anxiety disorders involving the increasing use of antidepres-

sants. Thus, benzodiazepines (BZDs) have been steadily replaced by these agents for a variety of anxiety disorders. Currently, the selective serotonin reuptake inhibitors (SSRIs) are viewed as the first choice for obsessive-compulsive disorder (OCD) and PD. Recently, the Food and Drug Administration (FDA) approved venlafaxine XR (Effexor XR) for the treatment of generalized anxiety disorder (GAD), paroxetine for the treatment of social anxiety disorder, and sertraline for PD. Accumulating clinical evidence indicates that nefazodone and mirtazapine are also effective therapies for GAD. Furthermore, venlafaxine, nefazodone, and mirtazapine may also be beneficial therapies for PD, social phobias, and posttraumatic stress disorder (PTSD).

Like GAD, PD with or without phobic avoidance is a chronic, debilitating illness (12–16). Although there is little consensus about the most effective drug treatments, options include the following:

- Selected *BZDs*
- *Antidepressants*
  - SSRIs
  - Tricyclics antidepressants (TCAs)
  - Irreversible monoamine oxidase inhibitors (MAOIs)
  - Reversible monoamine oxidase inhibitors (RIMAs)
  - Venlafaxine, nefazodone, mirtazapine

All of the drugs listed are recognized as drugs that may benefit patients with PD. In addition, behavioral and cognitive therapy, alone or in combination with pharmacotherapy, can be effective antipanic therapies.

Although drugs often prevent the panic attack, they may not alter the anticipatory anxiety. Thus, patients continue to expect the attacks, not realizing that with drug treatment they usually will not recur. Patients may insist that there is no improvement in their condition because they have not gone to public places to test the benefit of the medication. After medication has effectively blocked the panic attack, patients must then learn that they may never have another episode. Thus, drug response can dissociate the syndrome into its two pathological, psychophysiological processes: panic attack and

TABLE 13-1. *Benzodiazepines for panic disorder*

Benzodiazepine	Advantages	Disadvantages
Alprazolam/lorazepam	Rapid onset action, most useful for initial stages of panic disorder treatment Good tolerance Efficacy against anticipatory anxiety	Higher doses required than those effective for generalized anxiety disorder Dose-related sedation Risk of developing tolerance and dependency Interdose rebound reaction Risk of severe withdrawal reaction Need for multiple daily doses
Clonazepam	Can be easily discontinued, compared with shorter-acting benzodiazepines	Slow onset of antipanic action Risk of treatment-emergent depression

anticipatory anxiety. Psychological treatment is sometimes useful for overcoming the anticipatory anxiety and for helping patients return to the situations in which attacks were experienced.

Benzodiazepines

Until the 1980s, the BZDs were considered ineffective in the treatment of PD. Early controlled studies with the triazolobenzodiazepine *alprazolam,* however, demonstrated its antipanic properties. To achieve this benefit, this agent must often be given in higher doses (4 to 10 mg per day) than when given as an anxiolytic. Although alprazolam usually produces its therapeutic effect during the first week, antidepressants may take several weeks.

Another high-potency BZD, *clonazepam,* also has been shown to be effective. In addition, there is evidence that higher than usual doses of *diazepam, lorazepam, bromazepam,* or *clobazam* may also block panic attacks (17).

Rapid onset of action and favorable side effect profiles are advantages that some BZDs have in comparison with TCAs, MAOIs, SSRIs, and other antipanic drug therapies. Not all patients respond to therapy with BZDs, however. Also, BZDs lack therapeutic efficacy in treating patients with major depression, a frequent complication of PD. Furthermore, abrupt discontinuation of BZDs produces withdrawal symptoms (see Chapter 12). Nevertheless, familiarity with the assets and liabilities of each BZD pre-

scribed for PD enhances the art of antipanic pharmacotherapy and its efficacy. The latter is important because, compared with other antipanic drugs, BZDs have advantages for PD therapy that are offset by their disadvantages as listed in Table 13-1 (18).

In the past decade, the use of BZDs for antipanic therapy has declined. This decline is in part attributable to the growing awareness of the disadvantages of BZDs, especially the risk of dependency and abuse.

Alprazolam

Short-Term Efficacy. Although at least one study found no difference between alprazolam and placebo, several short-term studies have reported that alprazolam reduces the frequency and intensity of panic attacks (19–27) (Table 13-2). In phase I of a cross-national collaborative study, including approximately 500 patients at eight sites, alprazolam was superior to placebo at the end of week 1 in improving spontaneous and situational panic attacks, anxiety, and secondary disability (23). At week 4, 50% of alprazolam patients and 28% of placebo patients were free of panic attacks. At week 8, however, 50% of those on placebo were also free of panic attacks, compared with 59% of those receiving alprazolam. These data reflect group efficacy and not individual responses over time. Furthermore, there was considerable variability and, at times, instability of response in individual patients. Explanations

TABLE 13-2. *Alprazolam versus placebo: treatment of panic disorder*

Number of studies	Number of subjects	Responders (%)		Difference (%)	Chi square	*p* value
		Alprazolam (%)	Placebo (%)			
7	1,486	72	45	26	122.7	2×10^{-28}

offered for the high rate of placebo response in this and other studies include:

- The possible *surreptitious use* of antianxiety and antidepressant medication (a reality that should not be ignored)
- Consistently normal *dexamethasone suppression tests*
- *Lower anxiety ratings* at the start of treatment
- *Behavioral benefits* derived from inclusion in the study (28–30)

Alprazolam was also compared with imipramine and placebo in a sample of 1,168 randomly assigned subjects in the Cross-National Collaborative Panic Study, Phase Two. This study was conducted at 12 centers and assessed clinical change over 8 weeks of double-blind treatment. Improvement occurred with alprazolam by weeks 1 and 2 and with imipramine by week 4. By the end of week 8, the effects of the two active drugs were similar and both were superior to placebo for most outcome measures (31).

Long-Term Efficacy. **The question of whether there is long-term benefit with alprazolam remains largely unanswered.** Although improvement appears to be sustained in many patients as long as the medication is continued, several researchers have reported high rates of relapse, within 14 months after the drug is discontinued (32–34).

Nagy et al. (35) did a 2.5-year follow-up study of 60 patients with PD or agoraphobia with panic attacks who completed a 4-month combined drug and behavioral group treatment program and were discharged on a regimen of alprazolam. These authors found that the short-term improvement on alprazolam and behavior therapy was maintained during alprazolam maintenance, indicating that tolerance to alprazolam did not develop. Furthermore, many patients who

decreased or discontinued the drug also sustained improvement. The ability to discontinue alprazolam was associated with lower initial frequency of panic attacks. Those patients receiving non-pharmacological therapy in the follow-up period tended to have greater symptom severity. Finally, current or past depression was related to greater illness severity, episodes of depression after treatment were common, and depression was not prevented by low-dose alprazolam plus behavioral therapy. Because of the naturalistic design of the study and the use of both pharmacological and nonpharmacological interventions, the investigators cautioned that their results did not differentiate among the relative contributions of alprazolam, behavioral therapy, or their combination.

Dose. **Because of its relatively short duration of effect (2 to 6 hours), alprazolam must be given in divided doses, as frequently as four to five times daily.** In the treatment of PD, effective doses range from 2 to 10 mg per day, which is considerably higher than those recommended for GAD. One acute fixed-dose study found that approximately 60% of patients respond to 2 mg and 75% respond to 6 mg. In another study, 6 mg was also more effective than 2 mg (36, 37).

Some evidence indicates that patients maintained on alprazolam therapy may require lower doses than those used initially. As noted earlier, Nagy et al. (35) found that many patients sustained their improvement with lower dosages, and others have reported similar findings (32, 38). By contrast, Rashid et al. (39) found an increase in alprazolam dose over time.

Adverse Effects. Sedation, ataxia, and *fatigue* are the most common adverse effects reported with acute use of alprazolam in PD (39). Although tolerance to the sedative effect may develop within a few days of treatment initiation, this adaptation may be only partial. At weeks 4 and 8 in the Cross-National Collaborative study, many patients still showed signs of sedation (48% and 39%, respectively), ataxia (25% and 16%, respectively), and fatigue (19% and 16%, respectively) (23).

In an open study of outpatients who took alprazolam for a mean of 13.3 months, Rashid et al. (39) reported the occurrence of the following symptoms:

- Bone or joint *stiffness* or lancinating pain
- Excessive *lacrimation* without accompanying affect
- Tightness *in the intercostal muscles*
- Labored *respirations* or air hunger
- Frequent *changes in accommodation*; visual clouding
- Brief bursts of *profuse sweating* unrelated to exertion
- Rapidly alternating *mood swings*

Some of the symptoms were withdrawal-like, occurring within a 4-hour time frame of any given dose. Other "interdose" symptoms, including irritability and increased anxiety and panic, also have been reported with alprazolam (40). The use of alprazolam in PD patients has been associated with the following:

- The emergence of *depressive symptoms,* a phenomenon also reported with clonazepam and lorazepam (34, 35, 41–43)
- *Aggressive behavior* and assaultiveness in patients with and without histories of major depression (40, 44)
- Possible increased incidence of *behavioral dyscontrol* (45)

Although emergence of behavioral dyscontrol has been reported with a variety of BZDs and appears to be idiosyncratic, a question raised in recent years is whether there is an increased incidence with alprazolam. Rosenbaum et al. (46) described extreme anger or hostility in 8 of 80 private practice patients, one of whom had a history of aggressive behavior. Gardner and Cowdry (47) reported that 7 of 12 patients with borderline personality disorder and histories of dyscontrol who were given alprazolam (1 to 6 mg per day) had serious recurrent episodes of dyscontrol. Finally, FDA statistics indicate that alprazo-

TABLE 13-3. *Symptoms reported with discontinuation of alprazolam treatment for panic disorder*

Confusion
Clouded sensorium
Heightened sensory perception
Dysosmnia
Paresthesias
Muscle cramps, twitch, tension
Blurred vision
Diarrhea
Decreased appetite
Weight loss
Malaise
Weakness
Tachycardia
Dizziness
Light-headedness
Faintness
Excessive sweating
Deprssion
Irritability
Increased plasma cortisol levels
Headache
Motor restlessness

lam ranks second (behind triazolam) for hostility reactions reported in 329 drugs (48).

Discontinuation Effects. **As noted in Chapter 12, alprazolam requires an extended and very gradual taper, even when given for only a few weeks.** Despite very slow dosage reduction, however, a substantial number of patients may experience worsening of symptoms, including severe rebound panic and increased anxiety (32, 34, 49–52). Other reported symptoms are listed in Table 13-3. In some patients, symptoms may not occur in the initial phases of taper but appear when the dose reaches lower levels (49, 50, 53). Withdrawal symptoms have been reported to last as long as 4 weeks, although in many patients they subside within 1 to 2 weeks (34, 49). Abrupt taper or sudden discontinuation may increase the risk of delirium and seizures (54–56). A guide to properly tapering alprazolam is provided in Figure 13-1 (57, 58).

Clonazepam

Short-Term Efficacy. Since its approval by the FDA in the mid-1990's, clonazepam has been

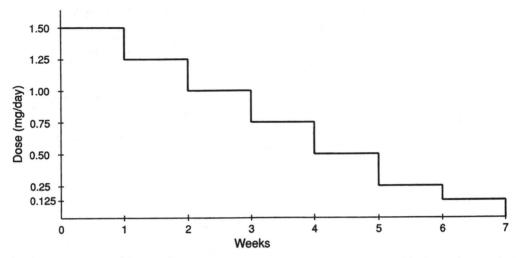

FIG. 13-1. Suggested alprazolam tapering schedule. To discontinue therapy with alprazolam, patients who have been taking more than 2.0 mg per day should reduce their daily dose by not more than 0.5 mg, and they should maintain that daily dose for 1 week before further reduction. When the total daily dose is reduced to 2.0 mg or when a patient is taking less than 2.0 mg per day, the daily dose should be reduced by not more than 0.25 mg per day each week until complete discontinuation is achieved.

used successfully to treat PD with agoraphobia. This drug has several advantages over other BZDs and can be considered a first-line agent for PD (59).

Several open trials have reported significant improvement or remission of panic attacks in patients given clonazepam (60–66). One double-blind, placebo-controlled study comparing the efficacy of alprazolam, clonazepam, and placebo found both drugs superior to placebo and comparable with each other (67). Because favorable response to clonazepam usually occurs early in treatment, lack of initial improvement may predict treatment failure (42, 61, 68). Interdose and morning rebound anxiety have not been reported. Clonazepam is not approved by the FDA for panic attacks, and because there are only a few controlled studies, there is only limited knowledge about its efficacy for this indication.

Long-Term Efficacy. Clonazepam has been shown to be effective for long-term use to manage PD or agoraphobia with panic attacks. In a 1-year follow-up study of clonazepam for PD or agoraphobia with panic attacks, Pollack et al. (42) reported that 18 of 20 (90%) patients, many

of whom had failed to respond to or tolerate other BZDs or antidepressants, maintained a good response. One patient was in complete remission at 44 weeks and remained well even off medication at 56 weeks. Tolerance to therapeutic efficacy did not appear to develop, although 40% required a dose increase (from 0.25 to 4.5 mg) to maintain initial improvement. Interestingly, 10 patients (50%) had discontinued clonazepam at follow-up because of adverse effects, inadequate response, or preference for a previously used treatment.

Dose. Effective daily doses of clonazepam have ranged from 0.25 to 9 mg. A review of open trials disclosed that most patients were maintained on 2 to 3 mg per day (68). In the comparison between alprazolam and clonazepam, average therapeutic doses were 5.2 and 2.4 mg per day, respectively (67). Because of its long half-life, clonazepam may be given twice daily, in the morning and at bedtime. Initially, lower doses should be given in the morning to allow for the development of tolerance to this agent's significant sedative effect.

Switching from Alprazolam. Research comparing clonazepam and alprazolam showed that panic was equally well controlled with both agents. In an open trial, Herman et al. (69) recruited 48 PD patients successfully treated with alprazolam but distressed by interdose or morning rebound. Using a standard protocol, 41 patients completed a transition to clonazepam treatment, and 39 continued on this drug for a mean duration of 40 weeks at an average dose of 1.5 mg per day (range, 0.125 to 3 mg per day). Two patients reported mild sedation but did not discontinue the medication. Although two others rated clonazepam as "worse" than alprazolam and switched back successfully to the latter, 34 rated clonazepam as better, and five considered it the same as alprazolam.

Adverse Effects. Sedation is the most prominent initial effect of clonazepam, usually subsiding in 2 to 3 days, but may persist in some patients. Other reported effects include the following:

- Ataxia
- Irritability
- Nausea
- Dysthymia

In their long-term follow-up study, Pollack et al. (42) found that five patients had stopped clonazepam because of adverse effects (dysthymia, one; irritability, two; nausea and sedation, two) and that four patients required dose reductions because of adverse effects (predominantly sedation).

Like alprazolam, clonazepam may cause treatment-emergent *depression* in some patients. Pollack et al. (42) also reported that only 10% of their patients who remained on clonazepam had a history of depression, although 47% lost to follow-up and 30% who eventually required alternate treatment had histories of dysthymia or depression. Of 31 patients without a prior history of affective illness, depression developed in three on low daily dosages (0.75, 1.5, and 2 mg), one was switched to alprazolam, and the others responded to the addition of desipramine or imipramine. These investigators recommend that, until further data are available, PD patients with chronic or concurrent depression should not be given clonazepam alone and that those in

whom depression develops during clonazepam therapy should have their dose lowered or an adjunctive antidepressant added.

Some evidence indicates that clonazepam may induce depression more often than alprazolam. In a review of 177 patients given clonazepam and a matched number given alprazolam, Cohen and Rosenbaum (70) reported that depression developed in 5.5% of the clonazepam patients compared with only 0.7% of those on alprazolam.

An earlier review found a high incidence of aggressive dyscontrol in neurological patients given clonazepam, most of whom were children (71), an observation that has led to speculation that this agent may be associated with an increased incidence of aggressivity in psychiatric patients. In this context, there have been reports of irritability in 2 of 50 panic patients and threatening or assaultive behavior in 4 of 13 schizophrenic patients on clonazepam (42, 72). Other investigators using this drug in patients with PD, however, have not reported such adverse effects (60, 63).

Discontinuation Effects. **There has been speculation that the longer duration of action of clonazepam may provide better protection against withdrawal symptoms and rapid reemergence of panic.** Limited data, however, are available on specific discontinuation effects associated with this treatment for PD, although mild rebound anxiety has been observed (63). A number of patients with a variety of psychiatric disorders have been switched successfully from high daily doses of alprazolam to clonazepam (73, 74). Subsequent gradual discontinuation of the latter produced no major withdrawal phenomena, although two patients experienced mild reemergence of panic symptoms that subsided with small dose increases. These symptoms did not recur during further dose tapering and discontinuation. Like all other BZDs, clonazepam should be reduced gradually, because abrupt cessation may lead to withdrawal symptoms ranging from mild to severe (75, 76).

Two studies have also compared discontinuation effects in PD patients given either alprazolam or diazepam. Burrows et al. (53) reported severe difficulties in 20% to 30% of patients discontinuing either drug, with those on diazepam having slightly more difficulty than those on alprazolam. Roy-Byrne et al. (50) found greater increases in anxiety 1 week after abrupt discontinuation of medication in patients taking alprazolam compared with those taking diazepam. Although there were no significant differences in frequency of panic attacks during drug taper, at discontinuation, the frequency of increased panic attacks was 50% higher in the alprazolam than in the diazepam group and three times greater in the diazepam versus placebo group.

Clonazepam has been shown to be effective for long-term therapy without development of tolerance as manifested by dose escalation or worsening of clinical status (77). Daily doses of 1 to 2 mg offer the best balance of therapeutic benefit and tolerability (78).

Discontinuation during and after slow tapering has been shown to be well tolerated (79). A slow discontinuation of clonazepam usually results in a benign withdrawal course. Withdrawal from higher doses, particularly rapid withdrawal, however, can be associated with more severe discontinuation symptoms (80).

Other Benzodiazepines

There is some evidence that higher than usual doses of lower potency BZDs may also be effective in treating PD (17, 25, 43, 81–84). For example, studies comparing alprazolam with lorazepam or diazepam indicate approximately equal efficacy (25, 43, 84, 85). In addition, there is evidence that higher than usual doses of diazepam, lorazepam, bromazepam, or clobazam may also block panic attacks.

Conclusion

Many patients may require long-term, indefinite BZD therapy for their PD. Fortunately, most naturalistic follow-up studies indicate an absence of tolerance to the antipanic-antiphobic effects of these drugs. Indeed, many patients appear to derive comparable efficacy at lower maintenance doses of BZDs (86). If discontinuation is appropriate or necessary, a gradual tapering and careful evaluation of withdrawal symptoms versus reemergence of the disorder itself is required (see also Chapter 12). Discontinuation is probably easier with a longer acting, high-potency BZDs (87).

Antidepressants

In 1962, Klein and Fink (88) reported that imipramine blocked panic attacks but had only a minor effect on phobic avoidance or anticipatory anxiety. This clinical observation has been validated by approximately 15 double-blind studies, and TCAs have since been studied for their antipanic efficacy. Although many TCAs are effective antipanic agents, they differ in safety and efficacy, a fact that mandates fitting the drug to the individual patient based on the known advantages and potential adverse effects of each TCA (Table 13-4).

Subsequent research and extensive clinical experience have provided evidence that antidepressants are safe and effective therapies for PD. This efficacy is particularly true for PD patients with co-morbid depression. As more data accumulate, it is evident that SSRIs and other new antidepressants are preferable to the TCAs, primarily because the latter have fewer side effects and are better tolerated than the TCAs.

TABLE 13-4. *Tricyclic antidepressants for panic disorder*

Advantages	Disadvantages
Well studied, with established acute and prophylactic efficacy	Slow onset of antipanic effects
Beneficial for co-morbid depression	Initial stimulant effects
	Sedative and anticholinergic effects
	Cardiac effects—palpitations, dizziness, orthostatic hypotension
	Weight gain
	Need for split (at least twice daily) doses

TABLE 13-5. *Tricyclic antidepressant versus placebo: treatment of panic disorder*

Number of studies	Number of subjects	Responders (%) TCA (%)	Placebo (%)	Difference (%)	Chi square	*p* value
7	1,072	72	51	21	51.4	7×10^{-13}

TABLE 13-6. *Selective serotonin reuptake inhibitor versus placebo: treatment of panic disorder*

Number of studies	Number of subjects	Responders (%) SRI (%)	Placebo (%)	Difference (%)	Chi square	*p* value
4	148	80	30	50	35.5	3×10^{-9}

Results from studies comparing TCAs, SSRIs, and MAOIs with placebo in the treatment of PD are summarized in Tables 13-5, 13-6, and 13-7. The results of studies comparing alprazolam or SSRIs with standard TCAs are summarized in Tables 13-8 and 13-9. All drugs were superior to placebo, although no significant differences in efficacy were noted among them.

Tricyclics

Imipramine has been the most widely studied TCA for the treatment of PD and agoraphobia, with excellent data to show that it is an effective antipanic agent (89, 90). Other TCAs reported to have therapeutic efficacy in PD include the following:

- Desipramine
- Nortriptyline
- Amitriptyline
- Doxepin (91–93)

Most studies comparing imipramine and alprazolam indicate that both drugs produce a comparable reduction of symptoms, although onset of action is considerably slower with a TCA, requiring 2 weeks to as long as 12 weeks (21, 24, 26, 37, 85, 92).

In addition to producing anticholinergic effects and hypotension, TCAs may actually worsen the patient's condition early in treatment by increasing anxiety, jitteriness, and dysphoria (93). For example, clomipramine causes jitteriness more than any other psychopharmacological treatment for PD. Very early

TABLE 13-7. *Monoamine oxidase inhibitor versus placebo: treatment of panic disorder*

Number of studies	Number of subjects	Responders (%) MAOI (%)	Placebo (%)	Difference (%)	Chi square	*p* value
3	92	90	34	56	29.3	6×10^{-8}

TABLE 13-8. *Alprazolam versus tricyclic antidepressant: treatment of panic disorder*

Number of studies	Number of subjects	Responders (%) Alprazolam (%)	TCA (%)	Difference (%)	Chi square	*p* value
3	868	71	68	3	0.5	NS

TABLE 13-9. *Selective serotonin reuptake inhibitor versus tricyclic antidepressant: treatment of panic disorder*

Number of studies	Number of subjects	Responders (%)		Difference (%)	Chi square	p value
		SRI (%)	TCA (%)			
3	133	73	63	10	1.3	NS

in the clinical evaluation of imipramine, the first TCA to be tested for antipanic efficacy, it was observed that some patients (approximately 25%) initially react to imipramine with feelings of restlessness, autonomic symptoms (sweating and flushing), and increased anxiety and apprehension. These psychological and physical symptoms generated unwanted subjective distress that constitute a "jitteriness reaction," which prompted some patients to discontinue imipramine. This phenomenon has also been reported with the SSRIs. Ultimately, this reaction was proven to be dose-dependent, and it could be averted by starting with a low dose (e.g., 10 to 25 mg) of imipramine, followed by gradual increments of 10 mg. Later it was found that imipramine therapy in doses of 150 to 250 mg per day for PD with agoraphobia produced a marked response rate of approximately 75% (when it was the sole or main treatment), making it the standard TCA pharmacotherapy for PD.

Alprazolam has been shown to be effective in alleviating the jitteriness syndrome (94). A patient's inability to tolerate these adverse effects may be the most important treatment-limiting factor with these drugs. Alternatively, short-term combination with another BZD may be helpful until the full impact of the antidepressant is realized.

Data on recurrence of PD after antidepressant discontinuation are sparse and inconsistent, in part because of varying definitions of relapse. Existing controlled and open trials note that patients do relapse after discontinuance. For example, Sheehan and Paji (95) found that most of their PD patients had a recurrence when medication was stopped. Recent studies also confirm that therapeutic gains are lost in many instances when treatment is stopped after short-term med-

ication or cognitive- behavioral therapy (CBT) (96). Rates have ranged from less than 33% to more than 90% (21, 89, 93, 97–102). An evaluation of long-term outcome of PD at a mean of 5.3 years following a controlled trial that included antidepressants and behavioral counseling found that complete recovery can occur even after many years of severe illness in a substantial proportion of patients who receive both antidepressants and behavioral counseling in the acute stage of treatment (103).

In this context, Gittleman-Klein and Klein (104) conducted a double-blind, placebo-controlled study of 35 nonpsychotic, school-phobic children. They found a good response in all children given imipramine but in only 21% of those on placebo. Because PD patients often experienced separation anxiety as children, this suggests that some cases of school phobia may be the childhood equivalent of PD, for which imipramine is effective.

Selective Serotonin Reuptake Inhibitors

All SSRIs have an antipanic effect. Their advantages are limited adverse effects and lack of toxicity. **Because of more acceptable adverse effect profiles, the SSRIs are usually the drugs of choice.** Several studies consistently indicate that SSRIs such as fluoxetine, sertraline, paroxetine, fluvoxamine, as well as agents such as clomipramine and trazodone, all possess antipanic efficacy, although the last may be less effective than imipramine (24, 105–109).

Fluoxetine, paroxetine, fluvoxamine, and citalopram, as well as clomipramine, have been shown in placebo-controlled, double-blind studies to be safe and effective antipanic drugs for short- term PD therapy. Evidence also is accumulating to suggest that these drugs may be effective for long-term panic treatment, but more data are needed to confirm this.

Paroxetine was the first SSRI approved for the treatment of PD with or without agoraphobia. Oral doses of 10 to 60 mg per day significantly reduce the frequency of panic attacks, and long-term therapy has been shown to be efficacious for the symptoms of PD (110). Long-term paroxetine therapy has also been shown not only to maintain efficacy but also to produce continued improvement. This is an important asset for antipanic pharmacotherapy in a chronic illness subject to relapse (111).

The lag time for the antipanic onset may be longer than when paroxetine is used as an antidepressant (112). The good tolerability of paroxetine, including lack of dependence and relative safety in overdose, often makes this SSRI a preferred initial choice for treatment of PD.

SSRIs sometimes cause an initial jitteriness similar to that noted with initial imipramine therapy for PD. This may be more common with SSRIs than with other currently available non-TCA antidepressant therapies for PD. Just as low initial imipramine doses avert this reaction, initiating SSRI therapies with one fourth to one half the usual starting antidepressant dose followed by gradual increments with low doses can avert this reaction. This syndrome can also be blocked by add-on, low-dose, as-needed BZD therapy (e.g., alprazolam or lorazepam).

Available evidence suggests that due to this better tolerability, SSRIs are the best choice for patients with PD (113). SSRIs also offer benefits of ease of dosing and no safety or dependence problems. This contrasts with the poor tolerance associated with TCAs and with dependence problems associated with BZDs (114). In addition, because of the longer half-life, fluoxetine at doses ranging from 10 to 60 mg administered once *weekly* appears to be an effective maintenance treatment for patients with PD whose successful initial treatment was with *daily* fluoxetine (115).

Monoamine Oxidase Inhibitors

At about the same time that imipramine was being studied in the United States, investigators in England noted that some patients with hysteria responded positively to MAOIs. Subsequently, researchers in England and Canada showed MAOIs to be superior to placebo in hysteria with phobic symptoms, a subcategorization that may be similar to that described by Klein.

It is well-established that the MAOIs available in the United States (e.g., phenelzine, tranylcypromine) are effective antipanic and antiphobic agents. Of these, phenelzine has been the most extensively studied. As with the other nonselective MAOIs, however, it also carries the risk of hypertensive and hyperpyrexic reactions (see also Chapter 5).

One Type B MAOI (i.e., selegiline) has a low propensity to cause hypertensive and hyperpyrexic reactions, but there is scant information on its use for PD. On the other hand, among the selective and reversible inhibitors of monoamine oxidase A (RIMAs) such as brofaromine, some may be as effective as phenelzine without posing the same risks.

Although clinical experience indicates *tranylcypromine* may be an effective antipanic agent, there are no controlled trials confirming this observation. *Phenelzine,* however, has been found to be very effective in both open and controlled designs (21, 116, 117). Onset of action is similar to that of other antidepressants, and although adverse effects tend to be less troublesome than with tricyclics, dietary restrictions may limit the usefulness of MAOIs in some patients. Unfortunately, the relapse rate may be comparable to that seen with BZDs and TCAs. For example, Kelly et al., in a follow-up of 246 patients, found that 50% who had discontinued MAOIs relapsed within 1 year (118).

Other Drug Therapies

Valproate

An emerging database supports the use of anticonvulsants (particularly valproate) for the treatment of patients with PD, including those with co-morbid alcohol abuse and treatment- refractory PD (119–121). At least a 50% reduction in panic attacks and at least a 40% complete remission were noted in these trials. For example, in two placebo-controlled trials, there was a trend favoring valproate over placebo in reducing the number of spontaneous panic attacks and the duration of these attacks (122). The dosage of valproate in these studies was comparable to that recommended for bipolar treatment (123). Valproate has also been shown to be useful in the treatment of PD patients with concomitant mood instability who have not responded to conventional therapy (124). Given this agent's potential effect on the γ-aminobutyric acid (GABA) neurotransmitter system, its use alone or in combination with other GABA-ergic agents (e.g., clonazepam) may be particularly helpful in treatment-resistant PDs (125). Ongoing controlled investigations should soon clarify the value of this drug for PD.

Preliminary evidence also supports the efficacy of gabapentin in the treatment of PD (125a).

Olanzapine

There has been a report of two patients with treatment-resistant PD who responded to treatment with olanzapine added to ongoing treatment with clonazepam (2 mg per day), ketazolam (30 mg per day), and venlafaxine (150 mg per day). The first patient was started on 7.5 mg at bedtime, and 2 weeks later he was much calmer and sleeping well. Olanzapine was increased to 12.5 mg per day, and venlafaxine was replaced with nefazodone up to 60 mg per day. Over the next few weeks, he improved progressively and clonazepam and ketazolam were discontinued. After 4 months, he was free from panic attacks and left his home alone. The second patient had 10 mg olanzapine daily added to ongoing treatment with 75 mg per day amitriptyline and 10 mg per day diazepam. After 2.5 months, she was being given olanzapine and had started going out on her own (126).

Nondrug Therapies for Panic Disorder

Nondrug approaches found to be beneficial include the following:

- Exposure therapy
- Cognitive therapy
- Applied relaxation (127–130)

According to Marks (127), however, nonexposure therapies usually fail to achieve reliable fear reduction. Although exposure may produce intense temporary discomfort, gains usually begin within a few hours of treatment; however, several weeks or months may be required to obtain maximal benefit. Long-term effect has been reported to range from 4 to 8 years, even with drug discontinuation (131). Cognitive behavioral therapy (CBT) is well documented in the usual clinical setting, even in the hands of therapists without formal competence. Group therapy is a feasible arrangement, and the results from group treatment are comparable to those of individual approaches (133). A recent evaluation of the effect of combining CBT and pharmacotherapy in the treatment of OCD led to the conclusion that either CBT or medication alone is more effective than no treatment. The authors also concluded that combination of CBT and medication seems to potentiate treatment efficacy; they found it more clinically beneficial to introduce CBT after a period of medication rather than to start both therapies simultaneously (134).

Combination Therapies

Although several studies have found that the combination of *imipramine and behavioral therapy* may be superior to either treatment alone, no studies have specifically examined the effects of combining the *behavioral techniques with BZDs* (132–138). In a review of the literature, however, Wardle found that diazepam was superior to placebo in three of four studies in which patients also received exposure therapy (139). Combined treatment with BZDs and CBT may be advantageous for some patients, but it must be carefully designed to avoid potential problems (140).

The question of combining a *tricyclic with a BZD* also has not been formally studied. Nevertheless, to help patients achieve the rapid results associated with BZD treatment while avoiding the possibility of dependence and severe rebound that may occur on discontinuation, some recommend initiating treatment with low doses of a BZD and imipramine. The BZD is then gradually tapered and withdrawn when imipramine reaches therapeutic levels (141).

An evaluation of the combination of moclobemide and CBT in patients with PD with agoraphobia disclosed that the combination of moclobemide with CBT did not yield significantly better short-term results than CBT with placebo (142). Group CBT has also been found to be effective for patients failing to respond to pharmacotherapy for PD (143). Finally, in a 12-week placebo-controlled study comparing the relative efficacy of paroxetine, clomipramine, and cognitive therapy in PD with or without agoraphobia, paroxetine and clomipramine were consistently superior to placebo, whereas cognitive therapy was superior on only a few measures (144).

Conclusion

PD and its related symptoms can be quite disabling. The recognition that specific drug therapies can effectively block the panic episodes has brought new found hope for thousands of patients. Optimal outcome, however, often requires the addition of various behavioral techniques to manage all related components of the disorder (e.g., panic attack, anticipatory anxiety, phobic avoidance).

Appendices I and J summarize the diagnostic criteria and Figure 13-2 summarizes a therapeutic strategy consistent with the data reviewed in this section. **The concurrent use of drug plus behavioral therapy seems to offer the best chance for improvement in the majority of patients.**

OBSESSIVE-COMPULSIVE DISORDER

Obsessions **are persistent anxiety-provoking ideas, thoughts, impulses, or images that are recognized as originating internally.** They are experienced as intrusive and senseless, prompting the patient to ignore, suppress, or neutralize them. Typical obsessive themes include the following:

- Contamination
- Aggression
- Safety or harm
- Sex
- Religious scrupulosity
- Somatic fears
- An excessive need for symmetry or exactness

If another illness is present, the diagnosis of OCD requires that the content of the obsessions be unrelated to the focus of the other disorder.

Compulsions **are repetitive, purposeful, intentional behaviors performed in response to an obsession, typically according to certain rules or in a stereotyped fashion.** These behaviors are designed to neutralize obsessions, but again, the individual recognizes them as unreasonable or excessive. Typical compulsive behaviors include the following:

- Cleaning
- Washing
- Checking
- Excessive ordering and arranging
- Counting
- Repeating
- Collecting

An additional requirement for the diagnosis of OCD relates to the severity dimension. Thus, symptoms should cause marked distress, be time consuming (often taking up to several hours per day), and interfere significantly with normal functioning. Because patients do not necessarily volunteer their symptoms, screening questions such as, "Do you wash your hands over and over?" "Do you have to check things repeatedly?" "Do you have thoughts that distress you and cannot get rid of?" may be necessary (149).

Epidemiology

OCD, once thought to be very rare, was found to have a lifetime prevalence of 2.5% by an National Institute of Mental Health (NIMH) Epidemiologic Catchment Area study (150). Other epidemiological surveys, such as in Edmonton, Canada, have found a similar prevalence (i.e., 3.0%) (151). A two-stage survey in adolescents first used a preliminary screening of more than 5,000 high school students with an OCD inventory and then a personal semistructured interview by a team of 13 skilled clinicians. Corrected for age of incidence, this study also yielded figures (i.e., 1.9% ± 0.7%), similar to those in adult populations, further validating the earlier studies (152). Approximately half of OCD patients have their onset before age 21 years (mean age

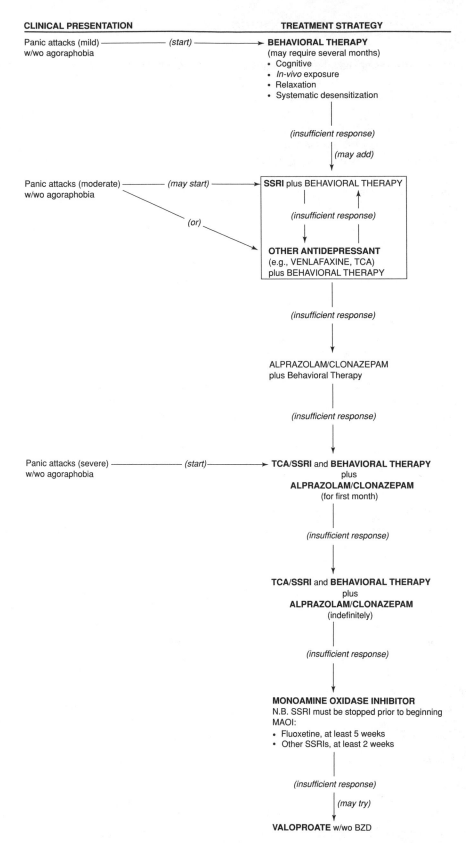

CLINICAL PRESENTATION

Panic attacks (mild) ———————— *(start)* ————————→ **BEHAVIORAL THERAPY**
w/wo agoraphobia

TREATMENT STRATEGY

BEHAVIORAL THERAPY
(may require several months)
• Cognitive
• *In-vivo* exposure
• Relaxation
• Systematic desensitization

(insufficient response)

(may add)

Panic attacks (moderate) ———————— *(may start)* ————————→ **SSRI** plus BEHAVIORAL THERAPY
w/wo agoraphobia

(or)

(insufficient response)

OTHER ANTIDEPRESSANT
(e.g., VENLAFAXINE, TCA)
plus BEHAVIORAL THERAPY

(insufficient response)

ALPRAZOLAM/CLONAZEPAM
plus Behavioral Therapy

(insufficient response)

Panic attacks (severe) ———————— *(start)* ————————→ **TCA/SSRI** and **BEHAVIORAL THERAPY**
w/wo agoraphobia   plus
                                                              ALPRAZOLAM/CLONAZEPAM
                                                              (for first month)

(insufficient response)

TCA/SSRI and **BEHAVIORAL THERAPY**
plus
ALPRAZOLAM/CLONAZEPAM
(indefinitely)

(insufficient response)

MONOAMINE OXIDASE INHIBITOR
N.B. SSRI must be stopped prior to beginning
MAOI:
• Fluoxetine, at least 5 weeks
• Other SSRIs, at least 2 weeks

(insufficient response)

(may try)

VALOPROATE w/wo BZD

FIG. 13-2. Treatment strategy for panic disorder with or without agoraphobia.

19.8 years ± 1.9 years). In general, onset is in childhood, adolescence, or young adulthood, and although the disorder fluctuates somewhat, it usually persists throughout life (153). Less than 10% of cases become progressive, with the adult manifestation essentially being identical to that in childhood, with only the content of the symptoms changing (154).

Rasmussen and Eisen (149) have suggested three underlying psychological dysfunctions:

- An abnormality of *risk assessment*
- A pathological *doubt*
- A need for *certainty* or *perfection*

Cross-cultural studies show that OCD occurs in many different groups and is essentially identical, although the content may differ slightly. For example, the Saudis, with their religious association of body washing and prayers, are often obsessed about these issues. By contrast, Hindus are more concerned about cleanliness, because it plays a prominent role in their religion (155).

Co-morbid Disorders

A substantial number of OCD patients, as many as 50%, also have associated major depression. Many also have some symptoms of depression, whether it be feeling sad, hopeless, or inadequate, having sleep disturbances, or having other changing vital functions. This disorder, however, starts at a younger age than depression (i.e., approximately half of OCD patients are first seen before age 21 years). There is also a somewhat higher incidence of *phobias, PD,* and *alcohol abuse* with OCD than in the general population. Similarly, Eisen and colleagues (156) found that 7.8% (6 of 77) of their patients met *Diagnostic and Statistical Manual of Mental Disorders,* 3rd ed., revised (DSM-III-R) criteria for both OCD and *schizophrenia* or *schizoaffective disorder.*

The association with Gilles de la Tourette's disorder is particularly important. Although only a few OCD patients have tics, the prevalence is much higher than in the general population. Conversely, obsessive-compulsive symptoms are common in Tourette's patients. Thus, there is a clear association between Tourette's disorder and

OCD. Tourette's is familial, and most likely genetically transmitted (157). Less is known about the heritability of OCD, but there is some suggestion that it is, at least in part, genetically determined (158–160).

Several large studies have investigated the prevalence of both Tourette's disorder and OCD in index cases having Tourette's disease (161, 162). In the cases of Tourette's disorder with OCD symptoms, the age-corrected ratio is 18%, with relatives having Tourette's disorder, chronic tics, or OCD (10%). In relatives of patients that have Tourette's symptoms only, 17% have either Tourette's disorder or chronic tic disorder and 14% have OCD. Thus, the incidence of OCD in relatives is identical in index cases of those with Tourette's disorder with OCD and index cases of Tourette's disorder only. Finally, follow-up studies find that Tourette's disorder develops in a significant percentage of children with OCD (163).

A great many OCD patients have movement disorders, and, conversely, a wide variety of movement disorders also include OCD symptoms, such as the following:

- Sydenham's chorea
- Postencephalitic Parkinson's disease
- Huntington's disease (164)

Occasionally, OCD is also associated with *organic brain syndromes, epilepsy,* and other *disorders of the basal ganglia.*

Differential Diagnosis of Obsessive-Compulsive Disorder

Although the full spectrum of OCD is not known, having effective drugs means that atypical presentations can be treated. If improvement with these drugs occurs, this supports the proposition that the variant is a manifestation of OCD (165). Several disorders may be variants of OCD, and similarities to this condition include their obsessional quality, familial patterns, and responsiveness to similar drug therapies (166). They may include

- *Trichotillomania* (or hair pulling)
- *Nail biting*
- *Bowel* or *bladder obsessions*

- *Pathological jealousy*
- *Dysmorphophobia* (i.e., obsession that a body part is disfigured)
- *Cancer phobias*
- *Self-mutilation* (e.g., picking at one's face) (167–172)

Because many of these disorders have overlapping symptoms and respond to the same treatments, the concept of an obsessive-compulsive spectrum disorder (OCSD) has been proposed (173). These disorders are characterized by obsessive thoughts or preoccupation with body appearance, bodily sensations, body weight, or body illness, or by stereotyped, ritualistic, or driven behaviors, such as tics, hair pulling, sexual compulsions, pathological gambling, or other impulsive-type disorders. The following conditions have been frequently classified as OCSD:

- *Body dysmorphic* disorder
- *Anorexia nervosa, bulimia nervosa, binge-eating* disorder
- *Autism*
- *Tourette's* syndrome
- *Prader-Willi* syndrome
- *Trichotillomania,* onychophagia
- *Kleptomania,* compulsive buying
- *Paraphilias* (174)

OCSD has been responsive to drugs such as the SSRIs (175).

Schizophrenia

Although many *schizophrenic patients* demonstrate obsessive-compulsive symptoms, this problem has received little systematic investigation. There are conflicting case reports of patients with obsessive-compulsive symptoms who failed to benefit when given an antiobsessional drug in addition to an antipsychotic, and other cases in which this strategy was beneficial (176). There are also reports of certain repetitive behaviors that mimic OCD that are benefited by the addition of clomipramine (177–179). Schulz has proposed the term "schizo-obsessive" to describe this clinical presentation (180).

Personality Disorders

One study of 17 OCD patients on medication found that nine of the 10 responders no longer met criteria for the diagnosis of a personality disorder, whereas five of the seven nonresponders continued to meet criteria. These data imply that some personality disorders may be secondary to a primary diagnosis of OCD (181).

Anxiety Disorders

Some obsessions or compulsions may masquerade as a specific phobia or agoraphobia; conversely, anxiety about OCD symptoms may mimic a panic attack. Alternatively, it is possible that the co-morbidity is real and has some significance other than definitional.

There are clear biological distinctions between OCD and PD. For example, panic attacks are produced by CO_2 inhalation, lactate infusion, yohimbine administration, psychostimulants, isoproterenol, and mCPP. By contrast, none of these agents except mCPP exacerbates obsessions or compulsions. Furthermore, OCD is benefited most by clomipramine or SSRIs, whereas panic attacks are helped by a variety of antidepressants (e.g., TCAs, SSRIs, MAOIs).

Biological Correlates of Obsessive-Compulsive Disorder

Genetics

OCD tends to run in families. A study of the NIMH cohort of 70 children with OCD found that 25% of fathers and 9% of mothers had the disorder, and, in general, there was an increased familial occurrence in first-degree relatives of OCD patients (152). In addition, studies of twins find that two of three monozygotic twins are concordant for OCD (182).

As noted earlier, there is also a genetic association between OCD and Tourette's disorder, with many Tourette's patients experiencing OCD symptoms (183–185). Tourette's disorder is thought to be an autosomal dominant disease, and although it has not been localized as yet, studies are actively in process, with at least 50% of the autosomal genome excluded as the locus (186, 187).

Neuropsychiatric Disorders

As noted earlier, several neurological disorders that involve the basal ganglia (e.g., caudate nucleus, globus pallidus, putamen) also manifest OCD symptoms (188). They include such varied conditions as

• Huntington's disease
• Choreoacanthocytosis
• Sydenham's chorea
• Postencephalitic parkinsonism

Imaging Studies

A small number of OCD patients have been evaluated with functional (e.g., positron emission tomography [PET] and single photon emission computed tomography [SPECT]) or structural imaging (e.g., magnetic resonance imaging [MRI] and computed tomography [CT]). Thus far, there are indications that an abnormality might be located near the head of the caudate nucleus, the globus pallidus, or the orbital frontal area. This finding is consistent with a basal ganglia or frontal cortical-subcortical circuit disorder (189, 190).

Neurotransmitters

Two lines of evidence implicate the serotonin system. First, it has a significant role at several sites in the circuitry connecting the frontal cortical and the basal ganglia locations. Second, agents that benefit OCD have potent serotonin effects (e.g., clomipramine, SSRIs).

Animal Models

There are also some animal models of OCD, including the following

• Lick *granuloma*: Several studies show that large dogs who lick their forepaws repetitively, producing a severe lesion, are benefited by clomipramine or fluoxetine, but not desipramine (191).
• *Feather picking* in parrots and a similar disorder in monkeys are also helped by clomipramine (192, 193).

Drug Treatment of Obsessive-Compulsive Disorder

Most antidepressants block serotonin (5-HT) or norepinephrine uptake. Only a few, however, are highly potent or selective blockers of 5-HT uptake. Earlier, amitriptyline was considered a potent serotonin uptake inhibitor; however, it proved to have only a modest effect in comparison with some of the newer agents (e.g., clomipramine, fluoxetine, sertraline, paroxetine, and fluvoxamine). Although clomipramine is a well-studied drug for OCD, its active metabolite, desmethylclomipramine, also inhibits norepinephrine uptake. Therefore, *in vivo,* clomipramine affects both amine systems, making it a distinct high-potency SRI, but not serotonin- specific. By contrast, fluoxetine, sertraline, paroxetine, fluvoxamine, and citalopram have negligible norepinephrine-blocking properties, making them both highly potent and highly specific for serotonin.

The fact that clomipramine benefits OCD whereas other standard tricyclics and MAOIs are relatively ineffective suggests that only SRIs have the necessary properties to be effective. This argument was countered by Marks et al. (194), who suggested that some OCD patients are depressed and that antidepressants primarily helped the mood disorder, only secondarily improving OCD. Because of this controversy, it is important to demonstrate that SRIs are specifically effective in OCD, and this is best accomplished by placebo-controlled trials. A second question relates to their specificity, which can be demonstrated by comparing these agents with conventional antidepressants. If the SRIs are found to be more effective, this would have implications for the biological basis of OCD, as well as the mechanism of action of these "antiobsessive" agents.

Goodman has opined that "the backbone of pharmacologic treatment for OCD is a 10- to 12-week trial with an SRI in adequate doses. In most cases, treatment should be initiated with an SSRI because of the superior safety, tolerability, and equivalent efficacy of this class of drugs compared with clomipramine" (195). Fluoxetine, sertraline, fluvoxamine, and paroxetine have, in separate multicenter trials, demonstrated efficacy and tolerability in the treatment of OCD (196). Citalopram, a recently marketed SSRI, also should be effective in the treatment of OCD (197).

Meta-analysis of Serotonin Reuptake Inhibitors for Obsessive-Compulsive Disorder

The primary question for this meta-analysis was whether the high-potency SRIs are differentially effective in OCD. Because we cannot argue for greater efficacy of SRIs over placebo if they are only shown to be superior to standard antidepressants (because we do not know whether any antidepressant would be more effective than placebo), we also performed meta-analyses of those studies comparing individual SRIs (i.e., clomipramine, fluvoxamine), as well as all SRIs, with placebo. Indeed, there are several published double-blind, random-assignment studies comparing high-potency SRIs with placebo or standard antidepressants, including the following comparative agents:

- Placebo
- Desipramine
- Imipramine
- Nortriptyline
- Doxepin
- Amitriptyline
- Clorgyline (198–217)

Ideally, the rating assessment used for our analyses should be predetermined so as not to introduce a bias; however, these studies used a variety of instruments to evaluate efficacy. This created an issue concerning which instrument should be chosen for entry into the meta-analysis. A quantitative rating scale designed specifically to assess obsessive-compulsive symptoms would be the instrument of choice, so we rank-ordered those available, starting with the Yale-Brown Obsessive-Compulsive Rating Scale (YBOCS). This hierarchy was then applied in each study to choose the best scales available. When more than one scale was used, we also performed separate analyses for each to control for the possibility that investigators chose the rating assessment with the biggest drug—drug or drug—placebo difference. We entered the results into a computer program developed for meta-analyses of crossed designs (218).

Serotonin Reuptake Inhibitors Versus Placebo

The meta-analysis of all studies comparing clomipramine or SRIs with placebo for the treatment of OCD found that the active drug produced a better result in every trial. We then calculated the effect size and the statistical significance for *clomipramine* alone and *fluvoxamine* alone. Their results showed a highly significant effect for both drugs (Tables 13-10 and 13-11). There were also several studies with *sertraline, fluoxetine,* and *paroxetine* that demonstrated similar results (219–226).

TABLE 13-10. *Clomipramine versus placebo for obsessive-compulsive disorder*

	Number of studies	Effect size	Variance	Z	*p* value
Measure 1	9	1.26	0.007	14.8	10^{-49}
Measure 2	9	1.17	0.007	14.3	10^{-46}

TABLE 13-11. *Selective serotonin reuptake inhibitors versus placebo for obsessive-compulsive disorder*

Drug	Number of studies	Effect size	Variance	Z	*p* value
Fluoxetine	2	.43	.01	4.43	0.000005
Fluvoxamine	6	.58	.01	5.2	10^{-7}
Paroxetine	1	.52	.01	3.9	0.000005
Sertaline	4	.52	.01	5.8	10^{-9}

TABLE 13-12. *Clomipramine versus standard antidepressants (not SSRIs) for obsessive-compulsive disorder*

	Number of studies	Effect size	Variance	Z	pvalue
Measure 1	10	0.79	0.01	7.6	10^{-14}
Measure 2	10	0.70	0.009	7.2	10^{-12}

TABLE 13-13. *Selective serotonin reuptake inhibitors versus clomipramine for obsessive-compulsive disorder*

Drug	Number of studies	Effect size	Z	pvalue
Fluoxetine	2	−.27	1.3	NS
Fluvoxamine	3	.10	.6	NS
Sertraline	1	.32	2.0	.04

Serotonin Reuptake Inhibitors Versus Standard Antidepressants

Also of interest was the comparison of clomipramine with other standard non-SRI antidepressants. When clomipramine was considered in the meta-analysis, the effect sizes were essentially unchanged (i.e., 0.79 and 0.70; Z scores = 7.6 and 7.2; probabilities of 10^{-14} and 10^{-12}). These results were highly homogeneous, with the effect sizes consistent over all studies (Table 13-12).

Whether we considered clomipramine alone or with any of the SSRIs, the evidence clearly found them to be more effective than standard antidepressants. Given this evidence, we believe that first-line drug therapy should include at least three separate trials with different SRIs, and one of them should be clomipramine.

Effect size is not an absolute measure but a relative measure against a comparator. It is our view that the large effect size seen in the early trials may be, in part, because the enrolled patients had no prior drug therapy or history of nonresponse, because there was no alternative drug treatment. When many patients undergo successful treatment, others may not volunteer for a subsequent trial, leaving a more resistant population for study. Because the SSRIs are safer than clomipramine, it is important to know whether the latter is more effective to justify its greater risk. Three studies (Table 13-13) found

fluvoxamine equal to clomipramine: two found fluoxetine equal to clomipramine; one showed sertraline superior to clomipramine, probably because of the high dropout rate related to side effects with clomipramine. Although more data are needed, it seems that all the high-potency SSRIs are equally effective, and therefore, we recommend starting with the SSRIs for reasons of safety and ease of use.

Another interesting development is the growing clinical literature on the use of SSRIs in body dysmorphic disorder, which may be part of the OCD spectrum. Also of interest are positive clinical reports with these agents in the treatment of pathological gambling, sexual compulsions, kleptomania, and compulsive buying.

Augmentation Strategies for Obsessive-Compulsive Disorder

Monodrug treatment can reduce the severity of OCD by up to 67% but typically does not completely eliminate the disorder. Combination with other adjunctive therapies (e.g., drugs or psychotherapy) can produce a qualitatively better change.

Drug Augmentation

Every case report suggested that adding *lithium* to the SRIs was beneficial, so several controlled studies compared lithium supplementation with clomipramine, and one added lithium or placebo to fluvoxamine (227). Neither study provided evidence that adjunctive lithium was helpful. *Inositol* augmentation of an SSRI in treatment-refractory patients also did not lead to significant improvement in the majority of cases (228). A series of patients with OCD, trichotillomania, and Tourette's syndrome who were refractory to treatment with SSRIs were given *risperidone* augmentation. In a number of cases, this proved clinically effective, but some patients experienced adverse effects (229). The results of an open-label trial suggest that *olanzapine* may also be effective in augmenting ongoing SSRI treatment for a portion of OCD patients refractory to SSRI monotherapy (230).

Another study of nine treatment-resistant patients (despite vigorous treatment with clomipramine plus lithium) found that three patients responded to the addition of *trazodone*, relapsed when trazodone was discontinued, and responded again when it was readministered (231). A small, double-blind study comparing trazodone with placebo in 21 patients, however, found no difference in therapeutic benefit between this agent and placebo (232).

Fenfluramine augmentation of SRIs in one open study benefited six of seven patients (233). Many patients have both Tourette's and OCD symptoms, and one case study found that *pimozide* helped Tourette's symptoms, whereas *fluvoxamine* helped the OCD symptoms, suggesting some specificity for each symptom (234). In a naturalistic study of Tourette's with associated OCD, adjunctive *fluoxetine* produced 81% improvement in the complicating OCD symptoms (235).

Some evidence indicates that *buspirone* may be helpful in OCD, with one small study finding buspirone alone equieffective to clomipramine (236). Preliminary data also indicate that buspirone may be an effective augmentation of the SRIs.

In one series of nine patients who received open *antipsychotic* augmentation of fluvoxamine (with or without lithium), those who had co-morbid tic disorder or schizotypal personality disorder were further benefited. In another nine patients who did not have either of these disorders, only two were helped by antipsychotic augmentation (237).

There is also some evidence to support trials with *clonazepam* (as an augmentor or alone) or MAOIs for treatment-resistant OCD (238).

Nondrug Augmentation

Concurrent with the introduction of clomipramine in 1966, Meyer (239) first reported on the benefit of behavioral therapy for OCD. Thus, while studies were finding the SRIs possessed antiobsessive properties above and beyond their antidepressant effects, a parallel literature also developed demonstrating the efficacy of behavioral techniques for OCD, especially prolonged (i.e., at least 20 hours) *in vivo* exposure and response prevention (240). Furthermore, and in contrast to the high relapse rate with drug discontinuation, a substantial number of patients continue to demonstrate benefit months to years after behavioral interventions (241, 242). Limited therapist contact time allowing patients the independence to develop and implement their own programs also seems to be a more cost-effective approach (203). **In general, pure obsessives are less responsive, whereas compulsive behaviors are more responsive to behavioral interventions.**

No psychotherapy other than CBT has been demonstrated in multiple randomized, controlled trials to be helpful for OCD. Furthermore, Simpson and Kozak, in their review of exposure and ritual prevention (EX/RP) and cognitive therapy (CT) in the treatment of OCD patients (age 18 years and older), concluded that no convincing evidence exists that any particular set of cognitive procedures is as good or better than potential EX/RP (243). These authors also contend that, to date, EX/RP "is the most helpful psychosocial treatment for OCD and may be one of the best ways to augment SSRI pharmacotherapy; however, EX/RP does have important limitations: in most patients treatment can manage, but not obliterate OCD."

Because significant OCD symptoms often remain or recur, even when there is substantial

improvement with a specific therapy, a combined complementary approach seems to be the optimal strategy for most patients.

Maintenance Drug Therapy for Obsessive-Compulsive Disorder

Clear clinical evidence indicates that most patients relapse if SRIs are discontinued. For example, in a random assignment study in which placebo was substituted for clomipramine, 16 of 18 patients relapsed on placebo by week 7 (241). A second, 2-month study of patients maintained on clomipramine found that only two relapsed and nine remained well, whereas eight relapsed and only one remained well when desipramine was substituted (244).

Conclusion

In controlled trials, SRIs are better than placebo. All studies found these agents consistently and significantly more effective than standard antidepressants; but each had a small sample size, and the results were not striking. Because of the consistency across studies, however, our meta-analysis with clomipramine was highly statistically significant.

This observation is a rare phenomenon in pharmacology. Meta-analyses of studies comparing various standard antidepressants for major depressive disorder reveal that all are equally efficacious (see Chapter 7). Similarly, meta-analyses of studies comparing antipsychotics find all equally efficacious for psychotic disorders (see Chapter 5). It is unusual to find a subclass of drugs more efficacious than others in the same class. Hence, if some antidepressants are clearly more effective than other antidepressants in OCD, it is truly noteworthy.

In addition to finding that the SRIs are more effective than standard antidepressants, the results are also homogeneous, in that the degree to which these drugs outperform their earlier generation counterparts remains consistent across all studies. The question of an even more selective efficacy for clomipramine over the SSRIs, however, remains unanswered because of a paucity of well-designed studies. Those reported,

however, found no significant difference in efficacy (245). Because clomipramine is not a pure serotonergic drug (i.e., it also inhibits norepinephrine uptake by virtue of an active metabolite), its mechanism of antiobsessive action remains uncertain. Studies designed to address these questions may shed light on a specific biochemical dysfunction or possible aberrant interactions among different neurotransmitterin systems.

More recently, Canadian investigators (246) examined the efficacy and tolerability of clomipramine compared with the SSRIs in OCD therapy. Based on the results of their findings, these authors concluded that recently expressed opinions that clomipramine should be used to treat OCD after two to three failed SSRI trials are not supported by research evidence. They concluded that both clomipramine and the SSRIs may be used as first-line treatment.

Two other observations help to differentiate the antiobsessive effects of SRIs from their antidepressive effects, as well as address the concerns raised by Dr. Marks (194, 203). The first is provided by the differential rate of improvement for these agents for depression versus for OCD. Generally, the rate of improvement in depression is rapid, the largest change occurring in the first few weeks and decreasing dramatically by the fourth to sixth week, because most patients are then recovered. The rate of improvement with these agents for OCD, however, is much slower (taking approximately twice as long), suggesting a different mechanism of action.

The second observation concerns mechanism of action and stems from subgroup analyses. In the collaborative studies of Ciba-Geigy, patients were selected for OCD without depression and the total improvement was compared with those who had OCD with depression. There was no difference in the antiobsessive effects of these agents in either group. This analysis treated associated depression as a discontinuous variable (i.e., present or absent). An alternative method is to correlate the degree of coexisting depression to improvement in OCD. When this was done, no correlation was evident. Returning to Dr. Marks' hypothesis, if serotonin agents improved OCD as a secondary effect to their antidepressive properties, there should be a high correlation between improvement in a coexisting depression and obsessive symptoms.

Based on our results, we conclude that SRIs are more effective than placebo or other standard antidepressants in the treatment of OCD, although equieffective to standard antidepressants for depression. Our review distinguished the antiobsessive properties from the antidepressant properties of these agents.

Appendices I and J summarize the diagnostic criteria and Figure 13-3 summarizes the treatment strategy we would suggest given the evidence thus far. **The concurrent use of drug plus behavioral therapy seems to offer the best chance for improvement in most patients.** Finally, in those most severely affected (i.e., manifest an unremitting course despite several adequate trials of drug and behavioral therapies), psychosurgical intervention may offer the only viable chance for relief of this disabling disorder (247, 248). If a patient is refractory to standard drug and behavioral therapies, then neurosurgery should be considered. This is true especially for patients whose quality of life is extremely poor as a result of impairment caused by OCD (248a, 248b). Stereotactic psychosurgery that selectively severs fiber connections between the orbitofrontal cortex and the dorsomedial and related thalamic nuclei may ameliorate OCD symptoms (248c, 248d). In Russia, cingulotomy for OCD is permitted only in patients with the following criteria:

- *Clinicopsychopathological* permissibility (duration of disease, resistance to medication, psychopathological status)
- *Physiological* permissibility (the presence of a brain target, defining the psychopathological status)
- *Technical* permissibility (the availability of proper stereotactic, imaging, electrophysiological, and other apparatus necessary to carry out the surgical treatment) (249)

Swedish investigators conducted a prospective, long-term study of personality traits in patients with intractable obsessional illness treated by capsulotomy. These authors found that the incidence of adverse personality changes after capsulotomy is low and does not increase with time (250). German investigators have reported that ventromedial frontal leukotomy performed during the 1970's should be restricted as a treatment of last resort for severe and refractory OCD but not obsessive personality disorder (251).

TRICHOTILLOMANIA

Trichotillomania, listed in the DSM-IV under "Impulse Control Disorders Not Elsewhere Classified" (252), is characterized by impulses to pull out one's hair, often involving multiple sites (scalp, eyebrows, and eyelashes commonly; pubic, axillary, chest, and rectal areas less commonly) (253). Some clinicians have proposed that this condition is a variant of OCD, based on similarities in phenomenology, family history, and response to treatment. Originally thought to occur more frequently in females, it has become evident that it may affect males just as often. Many victims of this disorder have histories beginning in childhood and refractoriness to all attempted remedies. Co-morbidity of trichotillomania with mood, anxiety, substance abuse, and eating disorders is also common (254). Others have noted that trichotillomania may also coexist with mental retardation and psychotic disorders (see Appendix Q).

MAOIs, TCAs, lithium, clomipramine (alone or with topical steroids), fluoxetine, and fluvoxamine may reduce the frequency and intensity of this disorder (210, 226, 255–261); however, controlled trials are needed to conclusively establish efficacy. Relapse after initial improvement has also been reported, however. Data also indicate that both trichotillomania and OCD may respond to venlafaxine (262, 263). For children, such treatments should be reserved for only those with the more severe, refractory forms.

In addition, behavioral and pharmacological co-treatment can offer substantial clinical benefit for trichotillomania, in both hair pulling symptoms and ancillary measures of functioning (264) (Fig. 13-3).

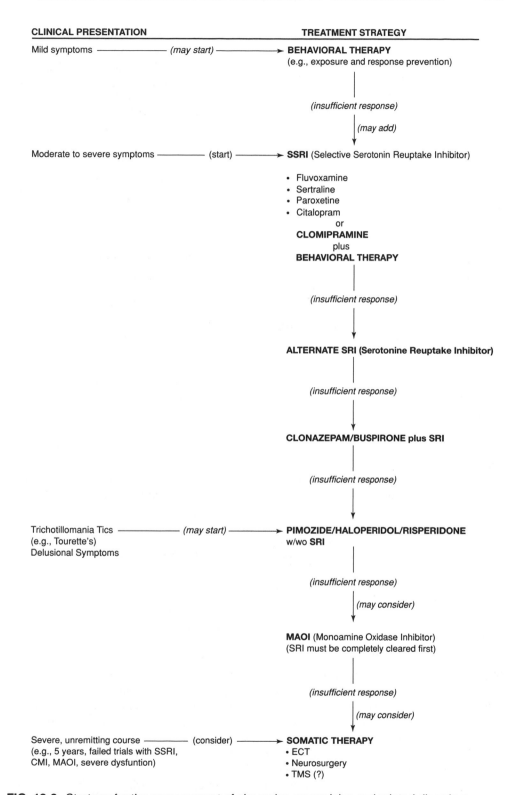

FIG. 13-3. Strategy for the management of obsessive-compulsive and related disorders.

POSTTRAUMATIC STRESS DISORDER

PTSD is attributable to an unusual experience that would be very stressful for almost anyone (e.g., serious threat to life or physical integrity or involvement of the person or a loved one in a major catastrophe, such as a serious traffic accident) (265). This largely environmental- induced disorder has been frequently observed in combat veterans with a history of exposure to overwhelming stress (266). The patient re-experiences the traumatic event by

- Intrusive *recollections* (e.g., flashbacks, nightmares)
- *Dreams*
- Acting or feeling as if the traumatic event was *recurring*
- Intense *psychological distress* on exposure to events that symbolize or resemble the traumatic event
- *Hyperarousal*
- *Emotional numbing*

Other manifestations of the disorder include persistent avoidance of stimuli associated with the trauma and symptoms of increased arousal, neither of which were present before the incident. To qualify for this diagnosis, a symptomatic period of at least 1 month is required (see Appendices I and J).

Co-morbidity is frequent. For example, Shore et al. (267) found that among their patients with PTSD, 28% also had GAD, 29% had depression, 12% had phobias, and 10% had alcohol abuse problems.

Drug Therapy for Posttraumatic Stress Disorder

Nearly every category of psychoactive drug has been prescribed for patients with PTSD. Clinical experience has verified the findings of controlled studies, namely that most of the drugs that are effective for PTSD are also useful for both major depression and PD. In particular, symptoms associated with hyperarousal or reexperiencing of the traumatic incident are benefited by drug therapies (268). This is true not only for the TCAs (i.e., amitriptyline, imipramine, desipramine, and doxepin) and MAOIs (particularly phenelzine), but also perhaps for BZDs (e.g., alprazolam), lithium, carbamazepine, valproate, buspirone, fluoxetine, propranolol, and clonidine (269). Because there is a lack of comparative data suggesting any superior efficacy for any particular drug, the selection for a patient with PTSD must be individualized and based on consideration of the drug's half-life, adverse effect profile, and any co-morbidity with the PTSD.

Pharmacological Treatment Options

Tricyclic Antidepressants

Two placebo-controlled trials found that TCAs were beneficial for PTSD. An 8-week study of amitriptyline (50 to 300 mg per day) versus placebo was conducted in male combat veterans with PTSD. Amitriptyline was found to be more effective than placebo (i.e., a 50% response rate for amitriptyline and a 17% response rate for placebo) (270). In another 8-week, placebo-controlled study, imipramine (50 to 300 mg per day) was compared with placebo in 60 Vietnam veterans with PTSD. The results (as indicated by various rating scales) also showed that there was a greater symptom reduction in the imipramine-versus placebo-treated patients (271).

Selective Serotonin Reuptake Inhibitors

There have been four placebo-controlled studies and three open-label controlled studies of SSRIs in PTSD.

In a controlled trial, fluoxetine 40 mg per day was shown to be superior to placebo for both PTSD and depressive symptoms (272). Since then, fluoxetine, despite the high placebo response rate, was found superior to placebo in a randomized, double-blind study in measures of PTSD, disability, and vulnerability to stress. In this study, 85% of the fluoxetine versus 62% of the placebo patients were very much or much improved (273).

In a 12-week trial involving nearly 200 adult outpatients with PTSD, preliminary data showed a significantly larger decrease in the Clinician-Administered PTSD Scale (CAPS) total score for sertraline (43%) than for placebo (31%). Sertraline also was shown to have positive effects on quality of life (274). In addition, sertraline has been shown to be effective in the treatment of PTSD with co-morbid alcoholism (275).

A 12-week open-label study of paroxetine in 19 civilians with PTSD found this agent to be efficacious for PTSD. The results also showed that people who had been exposed to any kind of childhood trauma were less likely to respond to therapy (276).

In a 10-week open-label study, fluvoxamine (10 to 250 mg per day) in 10 combat veterans with chronic PTSD was also shown to be effective and well tolerated (277).

Data from unpublished, uncontrolled studies indicate favorable responses to SSRIs within 8 to 12 weeks in patients with chronic PTSD. The time to onset of therapeutic response in these patients is similar to that seen in patients with major depression.

Presently, most experts recommend the SSRIs as a first-line medication for PTSD despite their troublesome adverse effects. These drugs can alleviate PTSD symptom clusters, anxiety, and depression, as well as dissociative symptoms, as shown in an open-label trial by Marshall et al. (276).

Other Antidepressants

Other Serotonergic Antidepressants. In recent years, new antidepressants with serotonergic actions have also been shown to benefit patients with chronic PTSD, many of whom had been treatment refractory. These drugs include venlafaxine (278), mirtazapine (279), and nefazodone (280).

Bupropion. Preliminary data from an investigation of bupropion in the treatment of male combat veterans with PTSD indicate that this agent may produce significant improvement in hyperarousal symptoms but no significant change in intrusivenes, avoidance, and total CAPS scores. Bupropion decreased depressive symptoms and most patients reported global improvement, although PTSD symptoms remained mostly unchanged (281).

Trazodone. Preliminary data suggest that trazodone may be effective in reducing the three primary symptom clusters of PTSD. These findings, however, need to be confirmed in a double-blind, placebo-controlled, larger sample size study (282).

Monoamine Oxidase Inhibitors

Phenelzine. The efficacy of both reversible and irreversible MAOIs for the treatment of PTSD has been studied in controlled trials. Phenelzine has been shown to be superior to placebo and imipramine in patients with chronic PTSD who had a very low placebo response (271, 283). Thus, we believe phenelzine is worth trying for patients who can adhere to dietary and medicinal restrictions.

Brofaromine. Although no reversible selective MAOIs are available in the United States, brofaromine has been evaluated in two controlled trials (284, 285). The outcomes were mixed, with no evidence of efficacy in one of these trials (284). In the other study, however, a subgroup of patients (50%) who had had PTSD for at least 1 year responded favorably (285).

Moclobemide. Moclobemide is a reversible, selective, MAO-A inhibitor currently available in other countries but not in the United States. An open-label study in 20 patients with PTSD suggested that moclobemide was effective at the end of 12 weeks of treatment, with 11 patients no longer meeting criteria for PTSD (286). Controlled, double-blind studies should be conducted to confirm these findings.

Benzodiazepines

Currently, no data indicate that BZDs are effective as a primary treatment for PTSD. Most authors recommend that, if prescribed, these agents should be used in combination with other effective treatments, primarily to address refractory hyperarousal symptoms. As always, potential for problems with dependence and withdrawal should be carefully considered.

Mood Stabilizers

The outcomes reported in open trials and case reports suggest that agents such as lithium, carbamazepine, and valproate may be useful in treating PTSD (287–289). The effective doses of these drugs for PTSD are those usually recommended for treatment of bipolar disorder. These mood stabilizers appear to benefit affective dysregulation, irritability, hostility, intrusive symptoms, depression, anxiety, and hyperarousal (288). For example, a 12-week double-blind, placebo- controlled trial of lamotrigine (up to a maximum dose of 500 mg per day, if tolerated) was conducted in 15 patients with PTSD. Patients receiving active treatment had a response rate twice as high (50%) as that for patients on placebo. Because lamotrigine can cause serious skin rashes, a slow-dose escalation is required for this drug, which then may be slow to act (290, 291).

Atypical Antipsychotics

Recent case reports have suggested that atypical antipsychotics may also benefit patients with PTSD. For example, low doses of risperidone in combination with an antidepressant or mood stabilizer were reported effective for nightmares and flashbacks in patients with treatment- refractory PTSD (292). Both clozapine and olanzapine have also been reported to reduce PTSD symptoms in patients with a co-morbid psychotic disorder (293, 294). Finally, olanzapine added to fluoxetine resulted in significant improvement of hyperarousal symptoms in a patient with treatment-refractory PTSD caused by severe childhood physical and sexual abuse (295).

Combined Pharmacotherapy and Psychotherapy

As with other anxiety-related disorders, there is growing support for the treatment of PTSD with combined pharmacotherapy and psychotherapy. Thus, data indicate that:

• Pharmacotherapy may facilitate engagement and trauma-focused psychotherapy.
• Psychotherapy may help patients ambivalent about pharmacotherapy.

• Co-treatment may help patients fearful of becoming addicted or developing a lifelong dependency on pharmacotherapy.

Acute Stress Disorder

This is a new category that involves a person who has been exposed to a traumatic event that he or she experienced, witnessed, or was confronted with involving actual or threatened death or serious injury, or a threat to the physical integrity of self or others. Furthermore, the person's response involves intense fear, helplessness, or horror. DSM-IV criteria also include the following:

• Having three or more *dissociative symptoms* while experiencing or after experiencing the traumatic event
• Persistently *experiencing the traumatic event* in one of several ways (e.g., recurrent images, flashbacks)
• *Avoidance of cues* that evoke recollections of the trauma
• *Intense anxiety symptoms,* sleep disruption, irritability, impaired concentration, excessive alertness, startle response, or motor restlessness
• Significant *psychosocial* and *psychological dysfunction*
• *Symptom duration* from 2 days to 4 weeks, with onset within 4 weeks of the trauma

Furthermore, the disturbance is not due to physiological effects of a drug of abuse, medication, or general medical condition, is not better accounted for by brief psychotic disorder, and is not merely an exacerbation of a preexisting Axis I or Axis II disorder (252). This diagnostic category, however, has provoked considerable discussion about its validity and inclusion in DSM-IV (296–301).

DISSOCIATIVE DISORDERS

Formerly known as hysterical neuroses of the dissociative type, dissociative disorders are currently classified into five categories by the DSM-IV:

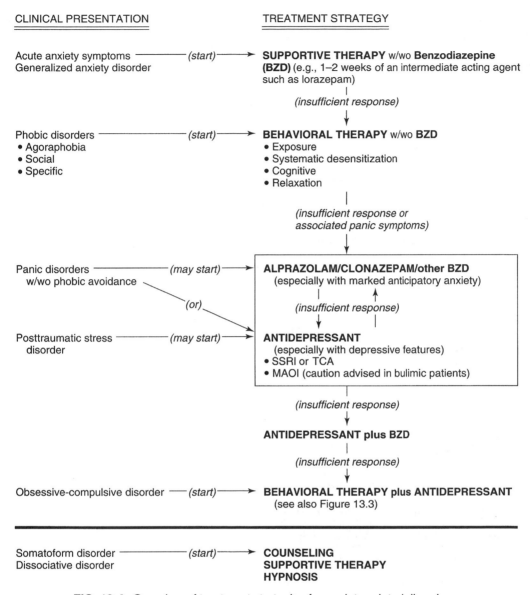

FIG. 13-4. Overview of treatment strategies for anxiety-related disorders.

* *Amnesia*
* *Fugue*
* *Dissociative identity* disorder
* *Depersonalization* disorder
* *Dissociative* disorder not otherwise specified (302) (see also Appendices I and L)

Psychotherapy, with emphasis on the strength of the therapeutic alliance, has been used more often than drugs for such patients, with hyp-

notherapy specifically used as an intervention for multiple personality (dissociative identity) disorder (303, 304). In The Netherlands, individual psychotherapy and adjunctive anxiolytic or antidepressant medications are the most widely endorsed treatment modalities (305).

Despite their common occurrence, there is a paucity of data on the pharmacotherapy of these disorders, with most drug interventions based on symptom manifestation, thus:

- *Anxiolytics* are used for associated anxiety.
- *Antidepressants* are used for associated depression.
- *Antipsychotics* are used for any underlying psychosis (e.g., schizophrenia).

Generally, pharmacotherapy is low-dose and short-term, prescribed only as long as necessary to alleviate acutely distressing symptoms. Further complicating matters, these patients are often noncompliant and often overreact to the usual pharmacological effects of these drugs. **In short, they are usually not good candidates for psychopharmacotherapy and seldom derive more than limited symptomatic benefit.**

CONCLUSION

Appendices I, J, K, and L summarize the diagnostic criteria, and Figure 13-4 gives an overview of our recommended approach to the management of several anxiety-related disorders.

REFERENCES

1. Klein DF. Delineation of two drug-responsive anxiety syndromes. *Psychopharmacologia* 1964;5:397–408.
2. Carey G, Gottesman II. Twin and family studies of anxiety, phobic and obsessive disorders. In: Klein DF, Rabkin J, eds. *Anxiety: new research and changing concepts.* New York: Raven Press, 1981.
3. Weissman MM, Klerman GL, Markowitz JS, et al. Suicidal ideation and suicide attempts in panic disorder and attacks. *N Engl J Med* 1989;321:1209–1214.
4. Johnson J, Weissman MM, Klerman GL. Panic disorder, comorbidity, and suicide attempts. *Arch Gen Psychiatry* 1990;47:805–808.
5. Fawcett J. Suicide risk factors in depressive disorders and in panic disorder. *J Clin Psychiatry* 1992;5[3, Suppl]:9–13.
6. Lepine JP, Chignon JM, Teherani MS. Suicide attempts in patients with panic disorder. *Arch Gen Psychiatry* 1993;50:144–149.
7. Cohen M, White P. Life situations, emotions and neurocirculatory asthenia. *Psychosom Med* 1951;13:335–357.
8. Pitts FN, McClure JN. Lactate metabolism in anxiety neurosis. *N Engl J Med* 1967;277:132–136.
9. Kelly D, Mitchell-Heggs N, Sherman D. Anxiety and the effects of sodium lactate assessed clinically and physiologically. *Br J Psychiatry* 1971;119:129–141.
10. Liebowitz MR, Gorman JM, Fyer A, et al. Lactate provocation of panic attacks. II. Biochemical and physiologic findings. *Arch Gen Psychiatry* 1985;42:709–719.
11. Nutt D, Lawson C. Panic attacks. A neurochemical overview of models and mechanisms. *Br J Psychiatry* 1992;160:165–178.
12. Coryell W, Noyes R, Clancy J. Panic disorder and primary unipolar depression. A comparison of background and outcome. *J Affect Disord* 1983;5:311–317.
13. Uhde TW, Boulenger JP, Roy-Byrne PP, et al. Longitudinal course of panic disorder: clinical and biological considerations. *Prog Neuropsychopharmacol Biol Psychiatry* 1985;9:39–51.
14. Breier A, Charney DS, Heninger GR. Agoraphobia with panic attacks: development, diagnostic stability and course of illness. *Arch Gen Psychiatry* 1986;43:1029–1036.
15. Markowitz JS, Weissman MM, Ouellette R, et al. Quality of life in panic disorder. *Arch Gen Psychiatry* 1989;46:984–992.
16. Weissman MM. Impact of panic disorder on the quality of life. Presented at the Annual Meeting of the American Psychiatric Association, New York, May 1990.
17. Judd FK, Norman TR, Burrows GD. Pharmacotherapy of panic disorder. *Int Rev Psychiatry* 1990;2:287–298.
18. American Psychiatric Association. Practice guidelines for the treatment of patients with panic disorder. *Am J Psychiatry* 1998;155[Suppl]:1–34.
19. Klosko JS, Barlow DH, Tassinari RB, et al. Alprazolam vs. cognitive behavior therapy for panic disorder: a preliminary report. In: Hand I, Witchen HU, eds. *Panic and phobias.* New York: Springer Verlag, 1988: 54–65.
20. Chouinard G, Annable L, Fontaine R, et al. Alprazolam in the treatment of generalized anxiety and panic disorders: a double-blind, placebo-controlled study. *Psychopharmacology* 1982;77:229–233.
21. Sheehan DV, Claycomb JB, Surnam OS. Monoamine oxidase inhibitors and alprazolam in the treatment of panic disorder and agoraphobia. *Psychiatr Clin North Am* 1985;8:49–62.
22. Sheehan DV, Coleman JH, Greenblatt DJ, et al. Some biochemical correlates of panic attacks with agoraphobia and their response to a new treatment. *J Clin Psychopharmacol* 1984;4:66–75.
23. Charney DS, Heninger GR. Noradrenergic function and the mechanism of action of antianxiety treatment. I. The effect of long-term alprazolam treatment. *Arch Gen Psychiatry* 1985;42:458–467.
24. Charney DS, Woods SW, Goodman WK, et al. Drug treatment of panic disorder: the comparative efficacy of imipramine, alprazolam, and trazodone. *J Clin Psychiatry* 1986;47:580–586.
25. Dunner DL, Ishiki D, Avery DH, et al. Effect of alprazolam and diazepam on anxiety and panic attacks and panic disorder: a controlled study. *J Clin Psychiatry* 1986;47:458–460.
26. Rizley R, Kahn RJ, McNair DM, et al. A comparison of alprazolam and imipramine in the treatment of agoraphobia and panic disorder. *Psychopharmacol Bull* 1986;22:167–172.
27. Ballenger JC, Burrows GD, DuPont RL, et al. Alprazolam in panic disorder and agoraphobia: results from a multicenter trial. I. Efficacy in short-term treatment. *Arch Gen Psychiatry* 1988;45:413–422.
28. Clark DB, Taylor CB, Roth WT, et al. Surreptitious drug use by patients in a panic disorder study. *Am J Psychiatry* 1990;147:507–509.

29. Coryell W, Noyes R. Placebo response in panic disorder. *Am J Psychiatry* 1988;145:1138–1140.

30. Marks IM, De Albuquerque A, Cottraux J, et al. The "efficacy" of alprazolam in panic disorder and agoraphobia: a critique of recent reports. *Arch Gen Psychiatry* 1989;46:668670.

31. Cross-National Collaborative Panic Study, Second Phase Investigators. Drug treatment of panic disorder. Comparative efficacy of alprazolam, imipramine, and placebo. *Br J Psychiatry* 1992;160:191–202.

32. DuPont RL, Pecknold JC. Alprazolam withdrawal in panic disorder patients. Presented at the Annual Meeting of the American Psychiatric Association, Dallas, Texas, May 1985.

33. Sheehan DV. One-year follow-up of patients with panic disorder and withdrawal from long-term antipanic medications. In: Program and abstracts of the Panic Disorder Biological Research Workshop, April 16, 1986, Washington, DC, p. 35.

34. Fyer AJ, Liebowitz MR, Gorman JM, et al. Discontinuation of alprazolam in panic patients. *Am J Psychiatry* 1987;144:303–308.

35. Nagy LM, Krystal JH, Woods SW, et al. Clinical and medication outcome after short-term alprazolam and behavioral group treatment in panic disorder. *Arch Gen Psychiatry* 1989;46:993–999.

36. Ballenger JC, Lydiard RB, Lesser IM, et al. Acute fixed dose alprazolam study in panic disorder patients. Presented at the Pharmacology/Pharmacokinetic Studies Workshop at the Panic Disorder Biological Research Workshop, Washington, DC, April 1986.

37. Uhlenhuth EH, Matuzas W, Glass RM, et al. Response of panic disorder to fixed doses of alprazolam or imipramine. *J Affect Disord* 1989;17:261–270.

38. Sheehan DV. Benzodiazepines in panic disorder and agoraphobia. *J Affect Disord* 1987;13:169–181.

39. Rashid K, Patrisi G, Cook B. Multiple serious symptom formation with alprazolam. Presented at the Annual Meeting of the American Psychiatric Association, Montreal, May 1988.

40. Noyes R, DuPont RL, Pecknold JC, et al. Alprazolam in panic disorder and agoraphobia: results of a multicenter trial. II. Patient acceptance, side effects, and safety. *Arch Gen Psychiatry* 1988;45:423–428.

41. Lydiard BR, Laraia MT, Ballenger JC, et al: Emergence of depressive symptoms in patients receiving alprazolam for panic disorder. *Am J Psychiatry* 1987;144:664–665.

42. Pollack MH, Tesar GE, Rosenbaum JF, et al. Clonazepam in the treatment of panic disorder and agoraphobia: a one-year follow-up. *J Clin Psychopharmacol* 1986;6:302–304.

43. Charney DS, Woods SW, Goodman WK, et al. The efficacy of lorazepam in panic disorders. Presented at the Annual Meeting of the American Psychiatric Association, Chicago, May 1987.

44. Pyke RE, Kraus M. Alprazolam in the treatment of panic attack patients with and without major depression. *J Clin Psychiatry* 1988;49:66–68.

45. Bond AJ, Curran HV, Bruce MS, et al. Behavioural aggression in panic disorder after 8 weeks' treatment with alprazolam. *J Affect Disord* 1995;35:117–123.

46. Rosenbaum JE, Woods SW, Groves JE, et al. Emergence of hostility during alprazolam treatment. *Am J Psychiatry* 1984;141:792–793.

47. Gardner DL, Cowdry RW. Alprazolam-induced dyscontrol in borderline personality disorder. *Am J Psychiatry* 1985;142:98–100.

48. Kowley G, Springen K, Iarovice D, et al. Sweet dreams or a nightmare? *Newsweek* 1991;(Aug 19):38–44.

49. Pecknold JC, Swinson RP, Kuch K, et al. Alprazolam in panic disorder and agoraphobia: results from a multicenter trial. III. Discontinuation effects. *Arch Gen Psychiatry* 1988;45:429–436.

50. Roy-Byrne PP, Dager SR, Cowley DS, et al. Relapse and rebound following discontinuation of benzodiazepine treatment of panic attacks: alprazolam versus diazepam. *Am J Psychiatry* 1989;146:860–865.

51. Mellman TA, Uhde TW. Withdrawal syndrome with gradual tapering of alprazolam. *Am J Psychiatry* 1986;143:1464–1466.

52. Rickels K, Schweizer E, Weiss S, et al. Maintenance drug treatment for panic disorder. II. Short- and long-term outcome after drug taper. *Arch Gen Psychiatry* 1993;50:61–68.

53. Burrows GD, Norman TR, Judd FK, et al. Short-acting versus long-acting benzodiazepines: discontinuation effects in panic disorders. *J Psychiatr Res* 1990;24[Suppl 2]:65–72.

54. Levy AB. Delirium and seizures due to abrupt alprazolam withdrawal: case report. *J Clin Psychiatry* 1984;45:38–39.

55. Noyes R Jr, Chaudhry DR, Domingo DV. Pharmacologic treatment of phobic disorders. *J Clin Psychiatry* 1986;47:455–452.

56. Brown JL, Hauge KJ. A review of alprazolam withdrawal. *Drug Intell Clin Pharm* 1986;20:837–884.

57. Rickels K, Schweizer E. Panic disorder: long-term pharmacotherapy and discontinuation. *J Clin Psychopharmacol* 1998;18[Suppl 2]:12S–18S.

58. Bruce TJ, Spiegel DA, Hegel MT. Cognitive-behavioral therapy helps prevent relapse and recurrence of panic disorder following alprazolam discontinuation: a long-term follow-up of the Peoria and Dartmouth studies. *J Consult Clin Psychol* 1999;67:151–156.

59. Davidson JR. Use of benzodiazepines in panic disorder. *J Clin Psychiatry* 1997;58[Suppl 2]: 26–28.

60. Spier SA, Tesar GE, Rosenbaum JF, et al. Treatment of panic disorder and agoraphobia with clonazepam. *J Clin Psychiatry* 1986;47:238–242.

61. Tesar GE, Rosenbaum JF. Successful use of clonazepam in patients with treatment resistant panic. *J Nerv Ment Dis* 1986;174:477–482.

62. Fontaine R, Chouinard G. Antipanic effect of clonazepam. *Am J Psychiatry* 1984;141:149.

63. Fontaine R. Clonazepam for panic disorders and agitation. *Psychosomatics* 1985;26[Suppl 12]:13–16.

64. Beaudry P, Fontaine R, Chouinard G, et al. Clonazepam in the treatment of patients with recurrent panic attacks. *J Clin Psychiatry* 1986;47:83–85.

65. Beckett A, Fishman SM, Rosenbaum JF. Clonazepam blockade of spontaneous and CO_2 inhalation-provoked panic in a patient with panic disorder. *J Clin Psychiatry* 1986;47:475–476.

66. Judd FK, Burrows GD. Clonazepam in the treatment of panic disorder [Letter]. *Med J Aust* 1986;145:59.

67. Tesar GE, Rosenbaum JE, Pollack MH, et al. Clonazepam versus alprazolam in the treatment of panic disorder: interim analysis of data from a prospective,

double-blind, placebo-controlled trial. *J Clin Psychiatry* 1987;48[Suppl]:16–19.

68. Pollack MH, Rosenbaum JE, Tesar GE, et al. Clonazepam in the treatment of panic disorder and agoraphobia. *Psychopharmacol Bull* 1987;23:141–144.

69. Herman JB, Rosenbaum JF, Brotman AW. The alprazolam to clonazepam switch for the treatment of panic disorder. *J Clin Psychopharmacol* 1987;7:175–178.

70. Cohen LS, Rosenbaum JF. Clonazepam: new uses and potential problems. *J Clin Psychiatry* 1987;48[Suppl 10]:50–55.

71. Browne TR. Clonazepam. *N Engl J Med* 1978; 299:812–816.

72. Karson CN, Weinberger DR, Bigelow L, et al. Clonazepam treatment of chronic schizophrenia: negative results in a double-blind, placebo-controlled trial. *Am J Psychiatry* 1982;139:1627–1628.

73. Albeck JH. Withdrawal and detoxification from benzodiazepine dependence: a potential role for clonazepam. *J Clin Psychiatry* 1987;48[Suppl 10]:43–48.

74. Patterson JF. Withdrawal from alprazolam dependency using clonazepam: clinical observations. *J Clin Psychiatry* 1990;5[Suppl 5]:47–49.

75. Jaffe R, Gibson E. Clonazepam withdrawal psychosis [Letter]. *J Clin Psychopharmacol* 1986;6:193.

76. Ghadirian AM, Gauthier S, Wong T. Convulsions in patients abruptly withdrawn from clonazepam while receiving neuroleptic medication [Letter]. *Am J Psychiatry* 1987;144:686.

77. Worthington JJ III, Pollack MH, Otto MW, et al. Long-term experience with clonazepam in patients with a primary diagnosis of panic disorder. *Psychopharmacol Bull* 1998;34:199–205.

78. Rosenbaum JF, Moroz G, Bowden CL. Clonazepam in the treatment of panic disorder with or without agoraphobia: a dose-response study of efficacy, safety, and discontinuance. Clonazepam Panic Disorder Dose-Response Study Group. *J Clin Psychopharmacol* 1997;17:390–400.

79. Moroz G, Rosenbaum JF. Efficacy, safety, and gradual discontinuation of clonazepam in panic disorder: a placebo-controlled, multicenter study using optimized doses. *J Clin Psychiatry* 1999;60:604–612.

80. Davidson JR, Moroz G. Pivotal studies of clonazepam in panic disorder. *Psychopharmacol Bull* 1998;34: 169–174.

81. Noyes R Jr, Anderson DJ, Clancy J, et al. Diazepam and propranolol in panic disorder and agoraphobia. *Arch Gen Psychiatry* 1984;41:287–292.

82. Rickels K, Schweizer EE. Benzodiazepines for treatment of panic attacks: a new look. *Psychopharmacol Bull* 1986;22:93–99.

83. Howell EF, Laraia M, Ballenger JC, et al. Lorazepam treatment of panic disorder. Presented at the Annual Meeting of the American Psychiatric Association, Chicago, May 1987.

84. Schweizer E, Fox I, Case WG, Rickels K. Alprazolam versus lorazepam in the treatment of panic disorder. Presented at the Annual NCDEU Meeting, Key Biscayne, Florida, May 1987.

85. Ballenger JC, Howell EF, Laraia MT, et al. Comparison of four medications in panic disorder. Presented at the Annual Meeting of the American Psychiatric Association, Chicago, May 1987.

86. Davidson JRT. Continuation treatment of panic disorder with high-potency benzodiazepines. *J Clin Psychiatry* 1990;51[Suppl 12A]:31–37.

87. Pollack MH. Long-term management of panic disorder. *J Clin Psychiatry* 1990;51[Suppl 5]:11–13.

88. Klein DF, Fink M. Psychiatric reaction patterns to imipramine. *Am J Psychiatry* 1962;119:432–438.

89. Lydiard RB, Ballenger JC. Antidepressants in panic disorder and agoraphobia. *J Affect Disord* 1987;13:153–168.

90. Liebowitz MR. Antidepressants in panic disorders. *Br J Psychiatry* 1989;155[Suppl 6]:46–52.

91. Lydiard RB. Desipramine in agoraphobia with panic attacks: an open, fixed-dose study. *J Clin Psychopharmacol* 1987;7:258–260.

92. Schweizer E, Rickels K, Weiss S, et al. Maintenance drug treatment of panic disorder. I. Results of a prospective, placebo-controlled comparison of alprazolam and imipramine. *Arch Gen Psychiatry* 1993;50:51–60.

93. Noyes R, Garvey MJ, Cook BL, et al. Problems with tricyclic antidepressant use in patients with panic disorder or agoraphobia: results of a naturalistic follow-up study. *J Clin Psychiatry* 1989;50:163–169.

94. Amsterdam JD, Hornig-Rohan M, Maislin G. Efficacy of alprazolam in reducing fluoxetine-induced jitteriness in patients with major depression. *J Clin Psychiatry* 1994;55:394–400.

95. Sheehan DV, Paji BA. Panic disorder. In: Dunner DL, ed. *Current psychiatric therapy.* Philadelphia: WB Saunders, 1992:275–282.

96. Liebowitz MR. Panic disorder in chronic illness. *J Clin Psychiatry* 1997;58[Suppl 13]:5–8.

97. Zitrin CM, Klein DF, Woerner MG, et al. Treatment of phobias: I. Comparison of imipramine hydrochloride and placebo. *Arch Gen Psychiatry* 1983;40:125–138.

98. Fyer AJ, Liebowitz MR, Gorman JM, et al. Comparative discontinuation of alprazolam and imipramine in panic patients. Presented at the Annual Meeting of the ACNP, San Juan, Puerto Rico, December 1988.

99. Mavissakalian M, Michelson L. Two-year follow-up of exposure and imipramine treatment of agoraphobia. *Am J Psychiatry* 1986;143:1106–1112.

100. Zitrin CM, Juliano M, Kahan M. Five-year relapse rate after phobia treatment. Presented at the Annual Meeting of the American Psychiatric Association, Chicago, May 1987.

101. Cohen SD, Monteiro W, Marks IM. Two-year follow-up of agoraphobics after exposure and imipramine. *Br J Psychiatry* 1984;144:276–281.

102. Mavissakalian M, Perel JM. Protective effects of imipramine maintenance treatment in panic disorder with agoraphobia. *Am J Psychiatry* 1992;149:1053–1057.

103. O'Rourke D, Fahy TJ, Brophy J, et al. The Galway Study of Panic Disorder. III. Outcome at 5 to 6 years. *Br J Psychiatry* 1996;168:462–469.

104. Gittleman-Klein R, Klein DF. Controlled imipramine treatment of school phobia. *Arch Gen Psychiatry* 1971;25:204–207.

105. Gorman JM, Liebowitz MR, Fyer AJ, et al. An open trial of fluoxetine in the treatment of panic attacks. *J Clin Psychopharmacol* 1987;7:329–332.

106. Schneier FR, Liebowitz MR, Davies SO, et al. Fluoxetine in panic disorder. *J Clin Psychopharmacol* 1990;10:119–121.

107. Den Boer JA, Westenberg HGM, Kamerbeek WDJ, et al. Effect of serotonin uptake inhibitors in anxiety disorders: a double-blind comparison of clomipramine and fluvoxamine. *Int Clin Psychopharmacol* 1987;2: 21–32.

108. Mavissakalian M, Perel J, Bowler K, et al. Trazodone in the treatment of panic disorder and agoraphobia with panic attacks. *Am J Psychiatry* 1987;144:785–787.

109. Black DW, Wesner R, Bowers W, et al. A comparison of fluvoxamine, cognitive therapy, and placebo in the treatment of panic disorder. *Arch Gen Psychiatry* 1993;50:44–50.

110. Foster RH, Goa KL. Paroxetine: a review of its pharmacology and therapeutic potential in the management of panic disorder. *CNS Drugs* 1997;8:163–188.

111. Lecrubier Y, Judge R. Long-term evaluation of paroxetine, clomipramine and placebo in panic disorder. *Acta Psychiatr Scand* 1997;95:153–160.

112. Bougerol T, Farisse J. Pharmacological treatment of panic disorder. *Encephale* 1996;22[Special Issue 5]: 46–53.

113. Baldwin DS, Birtwistle J. The side effect burden associated with drug treatment of panic disorder. *J Clin Psychiatry* 1998;59[Suppl 8]:39–44.

114. Davidson JR. The long-term treatment of panic disorder. *J Clin Psychiatry* 1998;59[Suppl 8]:17–21.

115. Emmanuel NP, Ware MR, Brawman-Mintzer O, et al. Once-weekly dosing of fluoxetine in the maintenance of remission in panic disorder. *J Clin Psychiatry* 1999;60:299–301.

116. Lydiard RB, Ballenger JC. Panic-related disorders: evidence for the efficacy of the antidepressants. *J Anxiety Disord* 1988;2:77–94.

117. Buigues J, Vallejo J. Therapeutic response to phenelzine in patients with panic disorder and agoraphobia with panic attacks. *J Clin Psychiatry* 1987;48:55–59.

118. Kelly D, Guirguis W, Frommer E, et al. Treatment of phobic states with antidepressants. A retrospective study of 246 patients. *Br J Psychiatry* 1970;116:387–398.

119. Lum M, Fontaine R, Elie R, et al. Probable interaction of sodium divalproex with benzodiazepines. *Prog Neuropsychopharmacol Biol Psychiatry* 1991;15:269–273.

120. Primeau F, Fontaine R, Beauclair L. Valproic acid and panic disorder. *Can J Psychiatry* 1990;35:248–250.

121. Roy-Byrne PP, Ward NG, Donnelly PJ. Valproate in anxiety and withdrawal syndromes. *J Clin Psychiatry* 1989;50[Suppl 3]: 44–48.

122. Zajecka J, et al. Efficacy of valproic acid vs placebo in the treatment of panic disorder. *Psychopharmacol Bull* 1994;30:735.

123. Ayd FJ Jr. Panic disorder/divalproex. In: *Lexicon of psychiatry, neurology, and the neurosciences,* 2nd ed. Philadelphia: Lippincott Williams & Wilkins, 2000.

124. Baetz M, et al. Efficacy of divalproex sodium in patients with panic disorder and mood instability who have not responded to conventional therapy. *Can J Psychiatry* 1998;43:73–77.

125. Ontiveros A, Fontaine R. Sodium valproate and clonazepam for treatment-resistant panic disorder. *J Psychiatr Neurosci* 1992;17:78–80.

125a. Pande AC, Pollack MH, Crockatt J, et al. Placebo-controlled study of gabapentin treatment of panic disorder. *J Clin Psychopharmacol* 2000;20(4):467–71.

126. Etxebeste M, Aragues E, Malo P, et al. Olanzapine and panic attacks [Letter]. *Am J Psychiatry* 2000;157:659–660.

127. Marks IM. *Fears, phobias and rituals.* New York: Oxford University Press, 1987.

128. Barlow DH. *Anxiety and its disorders: the nature and treatment of anxiety and panic.* New York: Guilford Press, 1988.

129. Clum GA, Borden JW. Etiology and treatment of panic disorders. *Prog Behav Modif* 1989;24:192–222.

130. Beck AT, Emery G. *Anxiety disorders and phobias: a cognitive perspective.* New York: Basic Books, 1985.

131. Ost LG. Applied relaxation: description for a coping technique and review of controlled studies. *Behav Res Ther* 1987;25:397–409.

132. Marks I, O'Sullivan G. Drugs and psychological treatments for agoraphobia/panic and obsessive-compulsive disorders. *Br J Psychiatry* 1988;153:650–658.

133. Martinsen EW, Olsen T, Tonset E, et al. Cognitive-behavioral group therapy for panic disorder in the general clinical setting: a naturalistic study with 1-year follow-up. *J Clin Psychiatry* 1998;59:437–442.

134. O'Connor K, Todorov C, Robillard S, et al. Cognitive-behavior therapy and medication in the treatment of obsessive-compulsive disorder: a controlled study. *Can J Psychiatry* 1999;44:64-71.

135. Mavissakalian M, Michelson L, Dealy RS. Pharmacological treatment of agoraphobia: imipramine versus imipramine with programmed practice. *Br J Psychiatry* 1983;143:348–355.

136. Telch MJ, Agras WS, Taylor CB, et al. Combined pharmacological and behavioral treatment of agoraphobia. *Behav Res Ther* 1985;23:325–335.

137. Mavissakalian M, Michelson L. Agoraphobia: relative and combined effectiveness of therapist-assisted in vivo exposure and imipramine. *J Clin Psychiatry* 1986;47:117–122.

138. Klein DF, Ross DC, Cohen P. Panic and avoidance in agoraphobia: application of path analysis to treatment studies. *Arch Gen Psychiatry* 1987;44:377–385.

139. Wardle J. Behavioral therapy and benzodiazepines: allies or antagonists? *Br J Psychiatry* 1990;156:163–168.

140. Spiegel DA, Bruce TJ. Benzodiazepines and exposure-based cognitive behavior therapies for panic disorder: conclusions from combined treatment trials. *Am J Psychiatry* 1997;154:773–781.

141. Sargent M. NIMH Report: panic disorder. *Hosp Community Psychiatry* 1990;41:621–623.

142. Loerch B, Graf-Morgenstern M, Hautzineger M, et al. Randomised placebo-controlled trial of moclobemide, cognitive-behavioral therapy and their combination in panic disorder with agoraphobia. *Br J Psychiatry* 1999;174:205–212.

143. Otto MW, Pollack MH, Penava SJ, et al. Group cognitive-behavior therapy for patients failing to respond to pharmacotherapy for panic disorder: a clinical case series. *Behav Res Ther* 1999;37:763–770.

144. Bakker A, van Dyck R, Spinhoven P, et al. Paroxetine, clomipramine, and cognitive therapy in the treatment of panic disorder. *J Clin Psychiatry* 1999;60:831–838.

145–148. [Reserved]

149. Rasmussen SA, Eisen JL. The epidemiology and differential diagnosis of obsessive compulsive disorder. *J Clin Psychiatry* 1992;53[Suppl 4]:4–10.

150. Karno M, Golding JM, Sorenson SB, et al. The epidemiology of obsessive-compulsive disorder in five US communities. *Arch Gen Psychiatry* 1988;45:1094–1099.

151. Bland RC, Orn H, Newman SC. Lifetime prevalence of psychiatric disorders in Edmonton. *Acta Psychiatr Scand* 1988;77[Suppl 338]:24–32.

152. Flament MF, Whitaker A, Rapoport JL, et al. Obsessive compulsive disorder in adolescence: an epidemiological study. *J Am Acad Child Adolesc Psychiatry* 1988;27:764–771.

153. Rasmussen SA. Obsessive-compulsive disorder in dermatologic practice. *J Am Acad Dermatol* 1985;13:965–967.

154. Goodwin DW, Guze SB, Robins E. Follow-up studies in obsessional neurosis. *Arch Gen Psychiatry* 1969;20:182–187.

155. Mahgoub OM, Abdel-Hafeiz HB. Pattern of obsessive-compulsive disorder in eastern Saudi Arabia. *Br J Psychiatry* 1991;158:840–842.

156. Eisen JL, Beer DA, Pato MT, et al. Obsessive compulsive disorder in patients with schizophrenia or schizoaffective disorder. *Am J Psychiatry* 1997;154:271–273.

157. Comings DE, Comings BG. Hereditary agoraphobia and obsessive-compulsive behavior in relatives of patients with Giles de la Tourette's syndrome. *Br J Psychiatry* 1987;15:195-199.

158. Pauls DL, Leckman JF. The inheritance of Gilles de la Tourette's syndrome and associated behaviors: evidence for autosomal dominant transmission. *N Engl J Med* 1986;315:993–997.

159. Nestadt G, Samuels J, Riddle M, et al. A family study of obsessive-compulsive disorder. *Arch Gen Psychiatry* 2000;57;358–363.

160. Pauls DL, Alsobrook JP II. The inheritance of obsessive-compulsive disorder. *Child Adolesc Psychiatr Clin N Am* 1999;8:481–496.

161. Pauls DL, Raymond CL, Stevenson JM, Leckman JF. A family study of Gilles de la Tourette Syndrome. *Am J Hum Genet* 1991;48:154–156.

162. Shapiro AK, Shapiro E. Evaluation of the reported association of obsessive compulsive symptoms or disorders with Tourette's disorder. *Compr Psychiatry* 1992;23:152–165.

163. Rapoport JL, Swedo SE, Guze BH, et al. Childhood obsessive compulsive disorder. *J Clin Psychiatry* 1992;53[Suppl 4]:11–16.

164. Cummings JL, Cunningham K. Obsessive-compulsive disorder in Huntington's disease. *Biol Psychiatry* 1992;31:263–270.

165. Fallon BA, Liebowitz MR, Hollander E, et al. The pharmacotherapy of moral or religious scrupulosity. *J Clin Psychiatry* 1990;51:517–521.

166. Ratnasuriya RH, Marks IM, Forshaw DM, et al. Obsessive slowness revisited. *Br J Psychiatry* 1991;159:273–274.

167. Stein DJ, Hollander E. Dermatology and conditions related to obsessive-compulsive disorder. *J Am Acad Dermatol* 1992;26:237–242.

168. Fishbain DA, Goldberg M. Fluoxetine for obsessive fear of loss of control of malodorous flatulence. *Psychosomatics* 1991;32:105–107.

169. Epstein S, Jenike MA. Disabling urinary obsessions: an uncommon variant of obsessive-compulsive disorder. *Psychosomatics* 1990;31:450–452.

170. Jenike MA, Vitagliano HL, Rabinowitz J, et al. Bowel obsessions responsive to tricyclic antidepressants in four patients. *Am J Psychiatry* 1987;144:1347–1348.

171. Lane RD. Successful fluoxetine treatment of pathologic jealousy. *J Clin Psychiatry* 1990;51:345–346.

172. Viswanathan R, Paradis C. Treatment of cancer phobia with fluoxetine [Letter]. *Am J Psychiatry* 1991;148:1090.

173. Hollander E. Obsessive-compulsive spectrum disorders: an overview. *Psychiatr Ann* 1993;23:355–358.

174. Goodman WK, et al. Fluvoxamine in the treatment of obsessive-compulsive disorder and related conditions. *J Clin Psychiatry* 1997;58[Suppl 5]:32–49.

175. Hollander E. Treatment of obsessive-compulsive spectrum disorders with SSRIs. *Br J Psychiatry* 1998;35[Suppl]:7–12.

176. Poyurovsky M, Isakov V, Hromnikov S, et al. Fluvoxamine treatment of obsessive-compulsive symptoms in schizophrenic patients: an add-on open study. *Int Clin Psychopharmacol* 1999;14:95–100.

177. Pulman J, Yassa R, Ananth J. Clomipramine treatment of repetitive behavior. *Can J Psychiatry* 1984;29:254–255.

178. Zohar J, Kaplan Z, Benjamin J. Clomipramine treatment of obsessive compulsive symptomatology in schizophrenic patients. *J Clin Psychiatry* 1993;54:385–388.

179. Berman I, Sapur BL, Chang HHS, et al. Treatment of obsessive-compulsive symptoms in schizophrenic patients with clomipramine. *J Clin Psychopharmacol* 1995;15:206–210.

180. Schulz SC. The low-dose neuroleptics in the treatment of "schizo-obsessive" patients. *Am J Psychiatry* 1986;143:1318–1319.

181. Ricciardi JN, Baer L, Jenike MA, et al. Changes in DSM-III-R Axis II diagnoses following treatment of obsessive-compulsive disorder. *Am J Psychiatry* 1992;149:829–831.

182. Lenane M, Swedo SE, Rapoport JL. Rates of obsessive compulsive disorder for first-degree relatives of patients with trichotillomania. *J Child Psychol Psychiatry* 1992;33:925–933.

183. Frankel M, Cummings JL, Robertson MM, et al. Obsessions and compulsions in Gilles de la Tourette's syndrome. *Neurology* 1986;36:378–382.

184. Grad LR, Pelcovitz D, Olson M, et al. Obsessive-compulsive symptomatology in children with Tourette's syndrome. *J Am Acad Child Adolesc Psychiatry* 1987;26:69–73.

185. Robertson MM. The Gilles de la Tourette syndrome and obsessional disorder. *Int Clin Psychopharmacol* 1991;6[Suppl 3]:69–84.

186. Pakstis AJ, Heutink P, Pauls DL, et al. Progress in the search for genetic linkage with Tourette syndrome: an exclusion map covering more than 50% of the autosomal genome. *Am J Hum Genet* 1991;48:281–294.

187. The Tourette Syndrome Association International Consortium for Genetics. A complete genome screen in sib pairs affected by Gilles de la Tourette syndrome. *Am J Hum Genet* 1999;65:1428–1436.

188. George MS, Melvin JA, Kellner CH. Obsessive-compulsive symptoms in neurologic disease: a review. *Behav Neurol* 1992;5:3–10.

189. Baxter LR Jr, Schwartz JM, Guze BH, et al. PET imaging in obsessive-compulsive disorder with and without depression. *J Clin Psychiatry* 1990;51[Suppl 4]:61–69.

190. Rapoport JL. Recent advances in obsessive-compulsive disorder. *Neuropsychopharmacology* 1991;5:1–10.

191. Rapoport JL, Ryland DH, Kriete M. Drug treatment of canine acral lick. An animal model of obsessive-compulsive disorder. *Arch Gen Psychiatry* 1992;49:517–521.

192. Roskopf WJ, Woerpel RW, Reed-Blake S, et al. Feather picking in psittacine birds. In: Proceedings of the Association of Avian Veterinarians, Miami, June 16–22, 1986.

193. Levine BS. Psychogenic feather-picking. *Avian/Exotic Pract* 1984;1:23–25.

194. Marks IM, Stern RS, Mawson D, et al. Clomipramine and exposure for obsessive-compulsive rituals: I. *Br J Psychiatry* 1980;136:1–25.

195. Goodman WK. Obsessive-compulsive disorder: diagnosis and treatment. *J Clin Psychiatry* 1999;60[Suppl 18]:27–32.

196. Pigott TA, Seay SM. A review of the efficacy of selective serotonin reuptake inhibitors in obsessive-compulsive disorder. *J Clin Psychiatry* 1999;60:101–106.

197. Pato MT. Beyond depression: citalopram for obsessive-compulsive disorder. *Int Clin Psychopharmacol* 1999;14[Suppl 2]:S19–S26.

198. Thoren P, Asberg M, Cronholm B, et al. Clomipramine treatment of obsessive-compulsive disorder 1. A controlled clinical trial. *Arch Gen Psychiatry* 1980;37:1281–1285.

199. Bick PA, Hackett E, Chouinard G. Multicenter placebo controlled study of sertraline in obsessive-compulsive disorder. *Arch Gen Psychiatry* 1989;46:23–28.

200. Flament MF, Rapoport JL, Berg CJ, et al. Clomipramine treatment of childhood obsessive compulsive disorder: a double-blind controlled study. *Arch Gen Psychiatry* 1985;42:977–983.

201. Goodman WK, Price LH, Rasmussen SA, et al. Efficacy of fluvoxamine in obsessive-compulsive disorder. *Arch Gen Psychiatry* 1989;46:36–44.

202. Karabanow O. Double-blind controlled study in phobias and obsessions. *J Int Med Res* 1977;5[Suppl 5]:42–48.

203. Marks IM, Lelliott P, Basoglu M, et al. Clomipramine, self-exposure and therapist-aided exposure for obsessive-compulsive rituals. I. *Br J Psychiatry* 1988;152:522–534.

204. Montgomery SA. Clomipramine in obsessional neurosis: a placebo controlled trial. *Pharm Med* 1980;1:189–192.

205. Perse TL, Greist JH, Jefferson JW, et al. Fluvoxamine treatment of obsessive-compulsive disorder. *Am J Psychiatry* 1987;144:1543–1548.

206. Ciba-Geigy Multi-Center Drug Trial Data, Protocol 59.

207. Ciba-Geigy Multi-Center Drug Trial Data, Protocol 61.

208. Goodman WK, Price LH, Delgado PL, et al. Specificity of serotonin reuptake inhibitors in the treatment of obsessive-compulsive disorder. *Arch Gen Psychiatry* 1990;47:577–585.

209. Leonard HL, Swedo SE, Rapoport JL, et al. Treatment of obsessive-compulsive disorder with clomipramine and desipramine in children and adolescents. *Arch Gen Psychiatry* 1989;46:1088–1092.

210. Swedo SE, Leonard HL, Rapoport JL, et al. A double-blind comparison of clomipramine and desipramine in the treatment of trichotillomania (hair pulling). *N Engl J Med* 1989;321:497–501.

211. Zohar J, Mueller EA, Insel TR, et al. Serotonergic responsivity in obsessive-compulsive disorder. Comparison of patients and healthy controls. *Arch Gen Psychiatry* 1987;44:946–951.

212. Lei BS. Crossover therapy. *Chin J Neurol Psychiatry* 1986;19:275–278.

213. Mavissakalian M, Michelson L. Tricyclic antidepressants in obsessive-compulsive disorder. Anti-obsessional or anti-depressant agents. *J Nerv Ment Dis* 1983;171:301–306.

214. Volavka J, Neziroglu F, Yaryura-Tobias JA. Clomipramine and imipramine in obsessive-compulsive disorder. *Psychiatry Res* 1985;14:83–91.

215. Cui YH. Double-blind trial of clomipramine vs doxepine. *Chin J Neurol Psychiatry* 1986;19:279–281.

216. Ananth J, Pecknold JC, Van Den Steen N, et al. Double-blind comparative study of clomipramine and amitriptyline in obsessive neurosis. *Prog Neuropsychopharmacol Biol Psychiatry* 1981;5:257–262.

217. Insel TR, Murphy DL, Cohen RM, et al. Obsessive-compulsive disorder: a double-blind trial of clomipramine and clorgyline. *Arch Gen Psychiatry* 1983;40:605–612.

218. Gibbons RD, Hedeker DR, Davis JM. Estimation of effect size from a series of experiments involving paired comparisons. *J Educ Stat* 1993;18:271–279.

219. Chouinard G, Goodman W, Greist J, et al. Results of a double-blind placebo controlled trial of a new serotonin uptake inhibitor, sertraline, in the treatment of obsessive-compulsive disorder. *Psychopharmacol Bull* 1990;26:279–284.

220. Fineberg N. Refining treatment approaches in obsessive-compulsive disorder. *Int Clin Psychopharmacol* 1996;11[Suppl 5]:13–22.

221. Freeman CPL, Trimble MR, Deakin JFW, et al. Fluvoxamine versus clomipramine in the treatment of obsessive compulsive disorder: a multicenter, randomized, double-blind, parallel group comparison. *J Clin Psychiatry* 1994;55:301–305.

222. Koran LM, McElroy SL, Davidson JRT, et al. Fluvoxamine versus clomipramine for obsessive-compulsive disorder: a double-blind comparison. *J Clin Psychopharmacol* 1996;16:121–129.

223. Greist J, Chouinard G, DuBoff E, et al. Double-blind parallel comparison of three dosages of sertraline and placebo in outpatients with obsessive-compulsive disorder. *Arch Gen Psychiatry* 1995;52:289–295.

224. Wood A, Tollefson GD, Birkett M. Pharmacotherapy of obsessive compulsive disorder–experience with fluoxetine. *Int Clin Psychopharmacol* 1993;8:301–306.

225. Pigott TA, Pato MT, Bernstein SE, et al. Controlled comparisons of clomipramine and fluoxetine in the treatment of obsessive-compulsive disorder. *Arch Gen Psychiatry* 1990;47:926–932.

226. Turner SM, Jacob RG, Beidel DC, et al. Fluoxetine treatment of obsessive-compulsive disorder. *J Clin Psychopharmacol* 1985;5:207–212.

227. McDougle CJ, Goodman WK, Price LH. Lithium augmentation in fluvoxamine-refractory obsessive compulsive disorder. American College Neuropsychopharmacol Panels and Posters, 28th Annual Meeting, Maui, Hawaii, December 12–15, 1989:176.

228. Seedat S, Stein DJ. Inositol augmentation of serotonin reuptake inhibitors in treatment-refractory obsessive-compulsive disorder: an open trial. *Int Clin Psychopharmacol* 1999;14:353–356.

229. Stein DJ, Bouwer C, Hawkridge S, et al. Risperidone augmentation of serotonin reuptake inhibitors in obsessive-compulsive and related disorders. *J Clin Psychiatry* 1997;58:119–122.

230. Weiss EL, Potenza MN, McDougle CJ, et al. Olanzapine addition in obsessive-compulsive disorder refractory to selective serotonin reuptake inhibitors: an open-label case series. *J Clin Psychiatry* 1999;60:524–527.

231. Hermesh H, Aizenberg D, Munitz H. Trazodone treatment in clomipramine-resistant OCD. *Clin Neuropharmacol* 1990;13:322–328.

232. Pigott TA, L'Heureux F, Rubenstein CS, et al. A double-blind, placebo controlled study of trazodone in patients with OCD. *J Clin Psychiatry* 1992;12:156–162.

233. Hollander E, DeCaria CM, Schneier FR, et al. Fenfluramine augmentation of serotonin reuptake blockade antiobsessional treatment. *J Clin Psychiatry* 1990;51:119–123.

234. Delgado PL, Goodman WK, Price LH, et al. Fluvoxamine/pimozide treatment of concurrent Tourette's and obsessive-compulsive disorder. *Br J Psychiatry* 1990;157:762–765.

235. Como PG, Kurlan R. An open-label trial of fluoxetine for obsessive-compulsive disorder in Gilles de la Tourette's syndrome. *Neurology* 1991;41:872–874.

236. Pato MT, Pigott TA, Hill JL, et al. Controlled comparison of buspirone and clomipramine in obsessive-compulsive disorder. *Am J Psychiatry* 1991;148:127–129.

237. McDougle CJ, Goodman WK, Price LH, et al. Neuroleptic addition in fluvoxamine-refractory OCD. *Am J Psychiatry* 1990;147:652–654.

238. Jenike MA, Rauch SL. Managing the patient with treatment resistant obsessive-compulsive disorder: current strategies. *J Clin Psychiatry* 1994;55[Suppl 3]:11–17.

239. Meyer V. Modification of expectations in cases with obsessional rituals. *Behav Res Ther* 1966;4:273–280.

240. Greist JH. An integrated approach to treatment of obsessive compulsive disorder. *J Clin Psychiatry* 1992;53[Suppl 4]:38–41.

241. Pato M, Zohar-Kadouch R, Zohar J, et al. Return of symptoms after discontinuation of clomipramine in patients with obsessive-compulsive disorder. *Am J Psychiatry* 1988;145:1521–1525.

242. Pato MT, Murphy DL, De Vane CL. Sustained plasma concentrations of fluoxetine and/or norfluoxetine four and eight weeks after fluoxetine discontinuation. *J Clin Psychopharmacol* 1991;11:224–225.

243. Simpson HB, Kozak M. Cognitive-behavioral therapy for obsessive-compulsive disorder. *J Psychiatr Pract* 2000;6:59–68.

244. Leonard HL, Swedo SE, Lenane MC, et al. A double-blind desipramine substitution during long-term clomipramine treatment in children and adolescents with obsessive-compulsive disorder. *Arch Gen Psychiatry* 1991;48:922–927.

245. Piggott TA, Pato MT, Bernstein SE, et al. A controlled comparison of clomipramine and fluoxetine in the treatment of obsessive-compulsive disorder. 28th Annual Meeting of the American College of Neuropsychopharmacology, Abstracts of Panels and Posters, Maui, Hawaii, December 12–15, 1989:173.

246. Todorov C, Freeston MH, Borgeat F. On the pharmacotherapy of obsessive-compulsive disorder: is a consensus possible? *Can J Psychiatry* 2000;45:257–262.

247. Birley JLT. Modified frontal leucotomy: a review of 106 cases. *Br J Psychiatry* 1964;110:211–221.

248. Sykes M, Tredgold R. Restricted orbital undercutting. A study of its effects on 350 patients over the ten years 1951–1960. *Br J Psychiatry* 1964;110:609–640.

248a. Baer L, Rauch SL, Ballantine HT, et al. Cingulotomy for intractable obsessive compulsive disorder: prospective long-term follow-up of 18 patients. *Arch Gen Psychiatry* 1995;52:384–392.

248b. Spangler CR, Corgrove CR, Ballantine HT, et al. Magnetic resonance image-guided stereotaxic cingulotomy for intractable psychiatric disease. *Neurosurgery* 1998;38:1071–1076.

248c. Zohar J, Sasson Y, Hendler T, et al. Contemplating neurosurgery for refractory OCD. The perspective of the referring psychiatrist. Presented at the 20th CINP meeting, Melbourne, Australia, June 1996.

248d. Rapoport JL, Inoff-Germain G. Medical surgical treatment of obsessive-compulsive disorder. *Neurol Clin* 1997;15:421–428.

249. Korzenev AV, Shoustin VA, Anichkov AD, et al. Differential approach to psychosurgery of obsessive disorders. *Stereotact Funct Neurosurg* 1997;68:226–230.

250. Mindus P, Edman G, Andreewitch S. A prospective, long-term study of personality traits in patients with intractable obsessional illness treated by capsulotomy. *Acta Psychiatr Scand* 1999;99:40–50.

251. Irle E, Exner C, Thielen K, et al. Obsessive-compulsive disorder and ventromedial frontal lesions: clinical and neuropsychological findings. *Am J Psychiatry* 1998;155:255–263.

252. American Psychiatric Association. *Diagnostic and statistical manual of mental disorders,* 4th ed. Washington, DC: American Psychiatric Press, 1994.

253. Ayd FJ Jr. Trichotillomania. In: *Lexicon of psychiatry, neurology, and the neurosciences,* 2nd ed. Philadelphia: Lippincott Williams & Wilkins, 2000.

254. Rapoport JL. *The boy who couldn't stop washing.* New York: Dutton, 1989.

255. Christenson GA, Mackenzie TB, Mitchell JE. Characteristics of 60 adult chronic hair pullers. *Am J Psychiatry* 1991;148:365–370.

256. Freeman CP, Hampson M. Fluoxetine as a treatment for bulimia nervosa. *Int J Obes* 1987;II[Suppl 3]:171–174.

257. Eras GG, Pope GH, Levine LR. Fluoxetine in bulimia nervosa, double-blind study. Presented at the Annual Meeting of the American Psychiatric Association, Philadelphia, May 1989.

258. George MS, Brewerton TD, Cochrane C. Trichotillomania (hair pulling) [Letter]. *N Engl J Med* 1990;322:470–471.

259. Jenike MA. Trichotillomania (hair pulling) [Letter]. *N Engl J Med* 1990;322:472.

260. Stanley MA, et al. Fluvoxamine treatment of trichotillomania. *J Clin Psychopharmacol* 1997;17:278–283.

261. Christenson GA, Popkin MK, Mackenzie TB, et al. Lithium treatment of chronic hair pulling. *J Clin Psychiatry* 1991;52:116–120.

262. Rauch SL, O'Sullivan RL, Jenike MA. Open treatment of OCD with venlafaxine: an open series of ten cases. *J Clin Psychopharmacol* 1996;16:81–83.

263. O'Sullivan RL, Keuthen NJ, Rodriguez D, et al. Venlafaxine treatment of trichotillomania: an open series of ten cases. Presented at the Annual Meeting of the American Psychiatric Association, San Diego, 1997.

264. Keuthen NJ, et al. Retrospective review of treatment outcome for 63 patients with trichotillomania. *Am J Psychiatry* 1998;155:560–561.

265. Epstein RS. Posttraumatic stress disorder: a review of diagnostic and treatment issues. *Psychiatr Ann* 1989;19:556–563.

266. Helzer JE, Robins LN, McEvoy L. Post-traumatic stress disorder in the general population. Findings of the Epidemiologic Catchment Area Survey. *N Engl J Med* 1987;317:1630–1634.

267. Shore JH, Vollner WM, Tatum EL. Community patterns of post-traumatic stress disorder. *J Nerv Ment Dis* 1989;177:681–685.

268. Silver JM, Sandberg DP, Hales RE. New approaches in the pharmacotherapy of posttraumatic stress disorder. *J Clin Psychiatry* 1990;51[Suppl 10]:33–38.

269. Davidson J. Drug therapy of post traumatic stress disorder. *Br J Psychiatry* 1992;160:309–314.

270. Davidson JRT, Kudler H, Smith R, et al. Treatment of posttraumatic stress disorder with amitriptyline and placebo. *Arch Gen Psychiatry* 1990;47:259–266.

271. Kosten TR, Frank JB, Dan E, et al. Pharmacotherapy for posttraumatic stress disorder using phenelzine or imipramine. *J Nerv Ment Dis* 1991;179:366–370.

272. van der Kolk BA, Dreyfuss D, Michaels M, et al. Fluoxetine in posttraumatic stress disorder. *J Clin Psychiatry* 1994;55:517–522.

273. Connor KM, Sutherland SM, Tupler LA, et al. Fluoxetine in post-traumatic stress disorder: randomised, double-blind study. *Br J Psychiatry* 1999;175:17–22.

274. Baker D, Brady K, Goldstein S, et al. Double-blind flexible dose multicenter study of sertraline and placebo in outpatients with post-traumatic stress disorder. *Eur Neuropsychopharmacol* 1998;8[Suppl 2]:261.

275. Brady KT, Sonne SC, Roberts JM. Sertraline treatment of comorbid posttraumatic stress disorder and alcohol dependence. *J Clin Psychiatry* 1995;56:502–505.

276. Marshall RD, Schneier FR, Fallon BA, et al. An open trial of paroxetine in patients with noncombat-related, chronic posttraumatic stress disorder. *J Clin Psychopharmacol* 1998;18:10–18.

277. Marmar CR, Schoenfeld F, Weiss DS, et al. Open trial of fluvoxamine treatment for combat-related posttraumatic stress disorder. *J Clin Psychiatry* 1996;57[Suppl 8]:66–70.

278. Hamner MB, Frueh BC. Response to venlafaxine in a previously antidepressant treatment-resistant combat veteran with post-traumatic stress disorder. *Int Clin Psychopharmacol* 1998;13:233–234.

279. Connor KM, Davidson JR, Weisler RH, et al. A pilot study of mirtazapine in post-traumatic stress disorder. *Int Clin Psychopharmacol* 1999;14:29–31.

280. Hidalgo R, Hertzberg MJ, Mellman T, et al. Nefazodone in post-traumatic stress disorder: results from six open-label trials. *Int Clin Psychopharmacol* 1999;14:61–68.

281. Canive JM, Clark RD, Calais LA, et al. Bupropion treatment in veterans with posttraumatic stress disorder: an open study. *J Clin Psychopharmacol* 1998;18:379–383.

282. Hertzberg MA, Feldman ME, Beckham JC, et al. Trial of trazodone for posttraumatic stres disorder using a multiple baseline group design. *J Clin Psychopharmacol* 1996;16:294–298.

283. Frank JB, Kosten TR, Giller EL Jr. A randomized clinical trial of phenelzine and imipramine for posttraumatic stress disorder. *Am J Psychiatry* 1988;145:1289–1291.

284. Baker DG, Diamond BI, Gillette G, et al. A double-blind randomized, placebo-controlled, multi-center study of brofaromine in the treatment of post-traumatic stress disorder. *Psychopharmacology (Berl)* 1995;122:386–389.

285. Katz RJ, Lott MH, Arbus P, et al. Pharmacotherapy of post-traumatic stress disorder with a novel psychotropic. *Anxiety* 1994;1:169–174.

286. Neal LA, Shapland W, Fox C. An open trial of moclobemide in the treatment of post-traumatic stress disorder. *Int Clin Psychopharmacol* 1997;12:231–237.

287. Forster PL, Schoenfeld FB, Marmar CR, et al. Lithium for irritability in post-traumatic stress disorder. *J Trauma Stress* 1995;8:143–149.

288. Ford N. The use of anticonvulsants in posttraumatic stress disorder: case study and overview. *J Trauma Stress* 1996;9:857–863.

289. Fesler FA. Valproate in combat-related posttraumatic stress disorder. *J Clin Psychiatry* 1991;52:361–364.

290. Hertzberg MA, Butterfield MI, Feldman ME, et al. A preliminary study of lamotrigine for the treatment of posttraumatic stress disorder. *Biol Psychiatry* 1999;45:1226–1229.

291. Davidson JRT. Pharmacotherapy of posttraumatic stress disorder: treatment options, long-term follow up, and predictors of outcome. *J Clin Psychiatry* 2000;61[Suppl 5]:52–56.

292. Leyba CM, Wampler TP. Risperidone in PTSD [Letter]. *Psychiatr Serv* 1998;49:245–246.

293. Hamner MB. Clozapine treatment for a veteran with comorbid psychosis and PTSD [Letter]. *Am J Psychiatry* 1996;153:841.

294. Israyelit L. Schizoaffective disorder and PTSD successfully treated with olanzapine and supportive psychotherapy. *Psychiatr Ann* 1998;28:424–426.

295. Burton JK, Marshall RD. Categorizing fear: the role of trauma in a clinical formulation. *Am J Psychiatry* 1999;156:761–766.

296. Harvey AG, Bryant RA. Dissociative symptoms in acute stress disorder. *J Trauma Stress* 1999;12:673–680.

297. Marshall RD, Spitzer R, Liebowitz MR. Review and critique of the new DSM-IV diagnosis of acute stress disorder. *Am J Psychiatry* 1999;156:1677–1685.

298. Bryant RA, Sackville T, Dang ST, et al. Treating acute stress disorder: an evaluation of cognitive behavior therapy and supportive counseling techniques. *Am J Psychiatry* 1999;156:1780–1786.

299. Harvey AG, Bryant RA. The relationship between acute stress disorder and posttraumatic stress disorder: a 2-year prospective evaluation. *J Consult Clin Psychol* 1999;67:985–988.

300. Classen C, Koopman C, Hales R, et al. Acute stress disorder as a predictor of posttraumatic stress disorder. *Am J Psychiatry* 1998;155:620–624.

301. Bryant RA, Harvey AG. Acute stress disorder: a crit-ical review of diagnostic issues. *Clin Psychol Rev* 1997;17:757–773.

302. Nemiah JC. Dissociative disorders (hysterical neuroses, dissociative type). In: Kaplan HI, Sadock BJ, eds. *Comprehensive textbook of psychiatry,* 5th ed, Vol 1. Baltimore: Williams & Wilkins, 1989:1028–1024.

303. Kluft RP. An overview of the psychotherapy of dissociative identity disorder. *Am J Psychother* 1999;53:289–319.

304. Powell RA, Gee TL. The effects of hypnosis on dissociative identity disorder: a reexamination of the evidence. *Can J Psychiatry* 1999;44:914–916.

305. Sno HN, Schalken HF. Dissociative identity disorder: diagnosis and treatment in the Netherlands. *Eur Psychiatry* 1999;14:270–277.

14

Assessment and Treatment of Special Populations

This chapter clarifies the clinical assessment and drug treatment issues raised by patients whose symptoms occur in the context of specialized circumstances. Thus, this last chapter covers two major topics:

- Special diagnostic and treatment issues raised during the *life cycle*
- *Medical conditions* complicating psychiatric assessment and drug therapy

Special life cycle issues concern the following:

- The pregnant patient
- The child and the adolescent patient
- The personality-disordered patient
- The elderly patient
- The dying patient

Complicating medical issues can occur in the following:

- The alcoholic patient
- The human immunodeficiency virus (HIV)-infected patient
- The eating-disordered patient

Because volumes have been published for most of these populations, we do not provide a comprehensive review of each of these issues. Instead, we underscore how complications related to each of these specialized groups may alter the clinician's approach to diagnosis and treatment. Such circumstances are always considered in the context of changes in the risk—benefit ratio posed by these patients.

THE PREGNANT PATIENT

No other area of psychiatry raises the anxiety of a treating clinician more than the drug management of the pregnant patient. The risk—benefit ratio must be considered from several important perspectives:

- Decreased or increased likelihood of *conceiving*
- The risk of *spontaneous abortion* or *premature labor*
- The risk of toxicity or withdrawal symptoms to the *fetus* and *neonate*
- The risk to the *pregnant mother* as a result of her altered physiology
- The risk of *breastfeeding* while on a psychotropic
- The risk of various *postpartum disorders*
- The risk of *morphological teratogenicity*
- The risk of future *behavioral teratogenicity* in the young newborn
- The risk to the mother or fetus from an *untreated or inadequately managed mental disorder* (1)

These issues are growing in importance because of the increasing number of pregnancies in women with more severe and chronic mental disorders (2, 3), and because studies indicate that 50% to 65% of pregnancies in the United States are not planned (4) and up to one third of women receive psychotropics during pregnancy (5). For example, women are at risk for substantial mood dysregulation during the perinatal period, including the following:

- Clustering of mood and anxiety disorders during the *childbearing* years
- *A depression prevalence* during pregnancy comparable to the nongravid state
- *Bipolar disorder,* which is often destabilized during this period
- *Postpartum* mood dysregulation, particularly in patients with a prior history of mood disorder

Thus, the need for antidepressants, anxiolytics, mood stabilizers, or other psychotropics may be even greater during this period (6).

Effects on brain morphogenesis may not be apparent for several years. Because psychotropics target the brain, this fact should be of concern. Furthermore, drugs such as amphetamines and barbiturates have been found to adversely affect the development of laboratory animals. Thus, it is important to weigh both known and potential risks of psychotropics against the risks of untreated symptoms.

Drug Therapy During the Perinatal Period

If psychotropics are to be used during the perinatal period, medication with the lowest possible risk should be considered (e.g., FDA risk categories in Table 14-1). In this context, a series of excellent reviews have been recently published (6–8) to help guide clinicians in the most appropriate management of these patients.

TABLE 14-1. *Food and drug administration risk categories*

Category	Interpretation
A	Controlled studies show no risk. Adequate, well-controlled studies in pregnant women have failed to demonstrate risk to the fetus.
B	No evidence of risk in humans. Either animal findings show risk, but human findings do not or, if no adequate human studies have been done, animal findings are negative.
C	Risk cannot be ruled out. Human studies are lacking, and animal studies are either positive for fetal risk or lacking as well. However, potential benefits may justify potential risk.
D	Positive evidence of risk. Investigational or postmarketing data show risk to the fetus. Nevertheless, potential benefits may outweigh risks.
X	Contraindicated in pregnancy. Studies in animals or humans or investigational or postmarketing reports have shown fetal risks that clearly outweigh any possible benefit to the patient.

Antipsychotics

The issue of antipsychotics during pregnancy warrants careful scrutiny, given the apparent increasing birth rate in patients with psychotic disorders and the need for chronic drug therapy to maintain optimal functioning (9). Although the literature is unclear regarding the potential for both abnormal fetal developmental and later behavioral teratogenicity, it is clear that many patients will require antipsychotic therapy during pregnancy. Miller (2, 3) has provided specific clinical guidelines:

- *Avoidance of low-potency phenothiozine antipsychotics,* if possible, during the period of highest risk for teratogenicity (i.e., 4 to 10 weeks after conception)
- *Tapering of antipsychotics,* if possible, 2 weeks before the estimated date of confinement (EDC) to minimize withdrawal effects in the neonate
- Use of *higher potency agents* (e.g., haloperidol) to minimize sedation, orthostasis, gastrointestinal slowing, tachycardia, and morphological teratogenicity
- *Avoidance of clozapine if possible,* although other novel antipsychotics (e.g., risperidone, olanzapine) have not been studied as long
- Immediate discontinuation of the antipsychotic and the use of bromocriptine when needed to manage symptoms if a *neuroleptic malignant syndrome* develops
- Resumption of the antipsychotic immediately *postpartum* in chronically psychotic women to minimize development of a postpartum episode
- *Avoidance of routine prophylaxis with antiparkinsonian agents,* including benztropine, diphenhydramine, and amantadine, all of which have been associated with congenital anomalies. Calcium supplementation may be a useful alternative (10), and propranolol or atenolol may be used for akathisia if cardiovascular status is stable (7).

Antidepressants

Serious depression develops in approximately 10% of pregnant women (11). Most data on teratogenicity involve the tricyclic antidepressants (i.e., desipramine, imipramine, nortriptyline, amitriptyline) and the SSRIs. Thus far, no major deficits have been identified; however, neonatal toxicity and withdrawal symptoms have been reported. Monoamine oxidase inhibitors (MAOIs) are known animal teratogens, but the lack of human data limits any conclusions. The selective serotonin reuptake inhibitor (SSRI) fluoxetine has been implicated as posing a greater risk for perinatal adverse and withdrawal effects usually seen in adults but not for major fetal anomalies (12). Insufficient experience also precludes any firm suggestions about bupropion, trazodone, venlafaxine, nefazodone, or mirtazapine. Clinical guidelines for the management of depression during pregnancy include the following:

- *Nondrug approaches* (e.g., cognitive-behavioral therapy) are always preferable when effective.
- If necessary, *agents that have been better studied and have fewer side effects* should be given preference (e.g., fluoxetine).
- *Nortriptyline* and *desipramine* may be the tricyclic antidepressants (TCAs) of choice, given their extensive assessment during pregnancy and well-known therapeutic concentrations, which should be monitored.
- If an antidepressant is withdrawn during pregnancy, it should be *gradually tapered* to avoid maternal or fetal withdrawal syndromes.
- If clinically possible, *drug tapering or dose reduction should begin 3 weeks before the EDC* (7).
- Those with a prior history may be more susceptible to *postpartum depression,* and maintenance antidepressant therapy should be carefully considered.

Mood Stabilizers

Bipolar disorder is a recurring illness whose course is even more complicated during pregnancy. Furthermore, most effective drug therapies [e.g., lithium, valproate, carbamazepine (CBZ)] carry significant pharmacokinetic, physiological, and teratogenic risks. The effects of lithium during the first trimester on the developing fetal heart (i.e., Ebstein's anomaly) have been well publicized, but it appears to be a weak cardiovascular teratogen (13). Dosing requirements usually increase during pregnancy but should be decreased (e.g., 50%) during labor because of the large fluid loss, which may then cause lithium toxicity. Detailed discussion of these issues can be found in Chapter 10, "Adverse Effects of Lithium and Valproate." Whereas teratogenicity has been well documented for either valproate (VPA) or CBZ alone, their combined use may be particularly detrimental (14, 15).

The following are clinical strategies to minimize the risks to mother and fetus, either from drug-induced anomalies or the potential ravages of the disease process:

- There should be frank discussion about *family planning*.
- The *risk–benefit* ratio should be carefully weighed when contemplating whether to initiate, continue, or withdraw drug therapy.
- Consider *alternative therapies* when feasible, such as antipsychotics or electroconvulsive therapy (ECT) modified for pregnancy.
- If lithium is necessary during the first trimester, *sonography* can help evaluate the presence and severity of such anomalies as Epstein's tricuspid valve defect.
- Lithium should be given in *smaller, divided doses* to avoid higher peak plasma levels.
- If the patient is exposed to VPA or CBZ, the presence of *neural tube defects* should be evaluated (e.g., serum alpha protein, amniocentesis, ultrasound), especially if they are used together.
- If anticonvulsants are used, daily *folate* (1 mg per day) may decrease the risk of neural tube defects and *vitamin K* (20 mg per day) may prevent drug-induced bleeding.
- The increased risk of a postpartum episode with bipolar disorder warrants the *resumption of medication soon after delivery*.

Antianxiety Agents

The experience of pregnancy itself is often anxiety provoking, and symptoms sufficient to warrant drug therapy are common in this group (16). Although this discussion primarily focuses on the benzodiazepines (BZDs), antidepressants and buspirone may also be used for women of childbearing age with certain anxiety-related disorders. Perhaps the best-documented adverse effect of the BZDs is a neonatal withdrawal syndrome, which has been reported to occur with several of the agents (e.g., diazepam, alprazolam, and triazolam). In addition, there is a weak positive relationship between diazepam exposure and oral clefts (17).

Clinical issues and approaches should include the following:

- Alternative, *nondrug management* of anxiety (e.g., behavioral therapies, relaxation techniques, psychotherapy, or cessation of stimulants such as caffeine whenever possible)
- If a BZD is necessary, possible use of *lorazepam* because of its possible lower accumulation in fetal tissue; **avoidance of diazepam until after the tenth week of gestation to avoid oral defects**
- *Gradual tapering of a BZD* before delivery to minimize any neonatal withdrawal phenomena
- Avoidance of *diphenhydramine* because of both fetal teratogenic and withdrawal complications (18)
- Reversal of fetal or neonatal toxicity with *flumazenil* (19)

Premenstrual Dysphoric Disorder

A related issue is premenstrual dysphoric disorder (PMDD), which affects 3% to 8% of women in their reproductive years. Unlike the much milder and more prevalent premenstrual syndrome (PMS), PMDD is characterized by the following symptoms:

- Persistent *irritability* or marked anger
- Tension, marked *anxiety*
- *Dysphoria,* hopelessness, self-deprecation
- *Mood lability,* fatigue, decreased energy
- *Dyssomnia*
- *Appetite* fluctuations
- Feelings of being *out of control*
- Other *physical symptoms*

Furthermore, these symptoms have a significant impact on a woman's interpersonal relations and general lifestyle and usually require the help of a mental health professional. Typically, at least five symptoms have been present in most menstrual cycles within the previous year, usually during the last week of the luteal phase, begin to remit within a few days after the onset of the follicular phase, and are absent during the week after menses (20).

Pharmacological management of this disorder has focused on several different classes of agents:

- Lithium
- Alprazolam
- Various antidepressants (21)

Although trials with lithium have been disappointing, evidence indicates that alprazolam (0.75 to 4 mg per day) during the luteal phase in women with a well-defined symptomatic period can be helpful (22–26).

The majority of positive studies have found that later generation antidepressants, especially those with strong serotonergic effects, are effective and may have a more rapid onset of action when used for PMDD (27). Thus, studies with SSRIs (e.g., fluoxetine, sertraline), nefazodone, venlafaxine, and clomipramine have all shown promise. In several studies, luteal phase dosing has been as effective or more effective than continuous dosing in women with PMDD.

Nursing

Although breastfeeding is desirable for a variety of reasons (e.g., decreased infections, lower mortality rates), certain issues should be considered when psychotropic use is contemplated, including the following:

- *Risks* associated with continued *breastfeeding*
- *Risks* associated with *stopping medication*
- *Lowest* effective *dose*
- *Possibility of weaning* if the neonate has adverse effects and sustained drug plasma levels

Conclusion

In summary, although it is always preferable to avoid psychotropics during pregnancy, many factors must be weighed before making the best decision for both the mother and the fetus.

Because there are very few clear and absolute contraindications to the use of these agents during pregnancy, a carefully informed decision involving the patient, her family, and the physician is the only rational approach.

PMDD is an important related disorder affecting a substantial proportion of women during their reproductive years. Promising drug therapies are emerging. In addition, nondrug approaches such as exercise, relaxation training, calcium supplementation, increased complex carbohydrate consumption, and cognitive-behavioral therapy may also be helpful (28).

THE CHILD AND ADOLESCENT PATIENT

Arguably, no area in clinical psychopharmacology has greater potential benefits for effective treatment than child and adolescent psychiatry. The data on which to form treatment decisions, however, is limited (Table 14-2).

This situation is true for virtually all areas of pediatric clinical pharmacology. Of prescription drugs marketed in the United States, 80% are not approved by the FDA for use in children (29). The situation has changed little in the past 20 years. In 1973, 78% of the 2,000 prescription medications listed in the *Physician's Desk Reference* had labeling with proscription against their use in children. The same was true in 1992. Of the 53 new drugs approved in 1996, 37 were approved for the treatment of conditions that occur in children as well as adults, yet 30 of these drugs were approved only for adults.

The psychiatrist prescribing medications for child and adolescent patients will likely take little comfort in the fact that he or she is no worse off than his or her colleagues in other areas of pediatric medicine. These psychiatrists are faced with the conundrum of either depriving children of potentially effective medication treatment or prescribing such medication "off label" and without optimal information on dosing, efficacy, and safety in children and adolescents.

The irony is that early and effective treatment intervention in a disease process often lessens its long-term sequelae. Unrecog-

nized or ineffectively treated childhood and adolescent psychiatric conditions are likely to have profound and lifelong effects on the patient's psychosocial development. They can interfere with the development of self-esteem, with family and peer relationships, with school performance, and, later, in the workplace. The consequences are likely to persist even after the resolution of the acute episode, profoundly affecting further psychosocial adjustment (30). Inadequate treatment of pediatric psychiatric disorders may lead to

- Persistent poor *self-image*
- Poor *interpersonal relationships*
- Chronic *underachievement*
- *Dropping out* of school
- *Substance abuse*
- *Legal* problems

Over the past decade, there has been a growing awareness on the part of the government, the medical profession, the pharmaceutical industry, and the public about the importance of having empirical data on which to base medication treatment decisions for children and adolescents. Both the National Institute of Mental Health (NIMH) and the FDA have taken steps to increase the amount of information available on the optimal treatment of children and adolescents with medications. At the request of the director of NIMH, the Institute of Medicine formed a committee to assess the status of research in mental disorders affecting children and adolescents. The resulting report, "Research on Children and Adolescents with Mental, Behavioral, and Developmental Disorders," led to a 5-year plan to stimulate a wide range of clinical research including clinical psychopharmacology and to develop young investigators in this area (31, 32). During the same time frame, the American Academy of Pediatrics issued its "Guidelines for the Ethical Conduct of Studies to Evaluate Drugs in Pediatric Populations" (35). To encourage research, the FDA in the late 1990's offered 6 months of patent extension to manufacturers of selected approved drugs if they conducted appropriate studies in children and adolescents. This approach meant that a

TABLE 14-2. Scientific knowledge in pediatric psychopharmacology versus frequency of use: a mismatch?

Category	Indication	Levels of supporting data[a]				Estimated frequency of use	
		Short-term efficacy	Long-term efficacy	Short-term safety	Long-term safety	Rank in descending order (NAMCS)	Rank in descending order (NDTIS)
Stimulants	ADHD	A	B	A	A	1	1
SSRIs	Major depression	B	C	A	C		
	OCD	A	C	A	C	2	2
	Anxiety disorders	C	C	C	C		
Central adrenergic agonists	Tourette's disorder	B	C	B	C	3	4
Valproate and carbamazepine	ADHD	C	C	C	C		
	Bipolar disorders	C	C	A[b]	A[b]	4	7
	Aggressive conduct	C	C	A	A[b]		
TCAs	Major depression	C	C	B	B	5	3
	ADHD	B	C	B	B	5	3
BZDs	Anxiety disorders	C	C	B	C	6	6
Antipsychotics	Schizophrenia; Other psychoses	B	C	C	B	7	5
	Tourette's disorder	A	C	B	B		
Lithium	Bipolar disorder	B	C	B	C	8	8
	Aggression	B	C	C	C		

NAMCS, National Ambulatory Medical Care Survey; NDTIS, National Disease and Therapeutic Index Survey; SSRI, selective serotonin reuptake inhibitor; TCA, tricyclic antidepressant; ADHD, attention-deficit hyperactivity disorder; OCD, obsessive-compulsive disorder; BZD, benzodiazepine.

[a]A = adequate data to inform prescribing practices; for efficacy and short-term safety: ≥ 2 randomized controlled trials (RCTs) in youth; for long-term safety: epidemiological evidence and/or minimal adverse incident report to the Food and Drug Administration. **B** = for efficacy and short-term safety: 1 RCT in youth or mixed results from ≥ 2 RCTs. **C** = adult-based controlled data in the absence of appropriate trials in children.

[b]Safety data based on studies of children with seizure disorder.

Reproduced with permission from Jensen PS, Bhatara VS, Vitiello B, et al. Psychoactive medication prescribing practices for U.S. children: gaps between research and clinical practice. *J Am Acad Child Adolesc Psychiatry* 1999; 38:557–565.

company could more than recoup the cost of the study by the additional revenue generated during the extended period of patent protection. To put this matter in perspective, 6 months of additional patent protection is worth $100 million if the drug has annual sales of $200 million.

As a result of these efforts, more research is under way in child and adolescent clinical psychopharmacology than ever before. The full impact of this increased research activity will take several years to be realized owing to the lag time between initiating and completing a research program in clinical psychopharmacology. The first information to come to light will be on the pharmacokinetics of newly approved drugs in children and adolescents simply because such studies are faster to complete than are clinical trials for efficacy, safety, and tolerability. Such pharmacokinetic data can aid the determination of the optimal dose and dosing schedule for the efficacy/safety trials (34–36).

Treatment Issues

There are some important differences in the physician–patient relationship when the patient is a child or unemancipated adolescent. First, the child psychiatric patient often is brought to the clinician because someone else (e.g., parent, teacher) is concerned or annoyed by the child's behavior. Thus, the patient may be a passive, if not reluctant, participant in treatment. Second, there is a greater possibility with children than with adults that a beneficial medication may have deleterious effects on growth and development. Therefore, clinicians need to consider the following questions carefully before initiating treatment:

- Does the child or adolescent have a disorder or syndrome of a type and of *sufficient severity to warrant medication?*
- Do the *needs and desires of the child or adolescent and the parent conflict* or are they in synchrony?
- What is the patient's *social and family situation* and how will it influence treatment outcome?

- Will the parent or guardian be able to *assist with the administration and monitoring of the medication*?
- What *other forms of treatment* may be needed (e.g., education about the condition and about better behavioral management techniques, family therapy, or individual psychotherapy)?
- *What does the patient think* about his or her condition, the need for treatment, and the specific treatment being recommended?
- How will the treatment *affect the patient's self-concept and relations* with others?
- How is the patient doing *in school* and why? (If there have been any significant changes in level of functioning, then the time course and magnitude of the changes should be carefully assessed.)
- Have *all the options been reasonably discussed* and their relative merits and liabilities weighed?
- What *outcome parameters* will be used to document the potential beneficial and adverse effects of the medication?
- Is the *addition of a second or third medication necessary* (e.g., if the first treatment fails, should it be discontinued rather than resorting to polypharmacy)?

Pharmacokinetic Issues

Ideally, drug doses in children and adolescents should be based on systematic studies in this age group. As outlined earlier, more work in this area is under way now than ever before. Although the pharmacokinetic data will be an important step forward, optimal dosing should also be based on efficacy and safety studies in these populations. Children may also be more sensitive to the beneficial or adverse effects of specific medications. **Until such data are available, optimal dosing in children and adolescents will be difficult and will, by necessity, be based on extrapolations from adult data.** Hence, the guiding principle remains to start low and go slow, aiming for the lowest effective dose. Although the concentration-response curves for efficacy and safety may be different in children

TABLE 14-3. *Developmental patterns for specific drug-metabolizing enzymes*

Cytochrome P450	Development pattern
	Phase I enzymes
1A2	Adult level reached by 4 months but exceeded by age 1–2 years. Decline to adult levels by the conclusion of puberty. Gender differences are possible during puberty.
2C9, 2C19	Adult activity reached by 6 months but exceeded by 1.5 to 1.8 times by age 3–4 years. Decline to adult levels by conclusion of puberty.
2D6	Adult levels obtained by 3–5 years of age.
3A4	Adult levels reached by 6–12 months but then exceeded by 1–4 years of age. Decline to adult levels by the conclusion of puberty.
	Phase II enzymes
NAT2	Adult activity present by 1–3 years of age.
TPMT	Adult activity achieved by 7–9 years of age.
UGT	Adult activity by 6–18 months of age.
ST	May exceed adult levels during early childhood.

NAT2, *N*-acetyltransferase-2; TPMT, thiopurine methyltransferase; UGT, glucoronosyltransferase; ST, sulfotransferase.

and adolescents than in adults, the prescriber can use therapeutic drug monitoring (TDM) for at least some newer medications to determine whether the patient is achieving a concentration that has proven to be both effective and safe in adults (see Chapter 3).

There are a number of pharmacokinetic differences between children and adolescent in comparison with adults. These differences frequently lead to the need for higher doses on a milligram-per-kilogram basis to achieve the same drug concentrations in adults on the usually effective adult doses. These differences are summarized in the following paragraphs.

Most psychotropic medications are highly lipophilic. The percentage of total body fat, which is a reservoir for these lipid-soluble compounds, increases during the first year of life and then decreases until the prepubertal increase (30). Thus, children at different ages have different volumes of deep storage, which can affect the overall residual time a drug remains in the body after its discontinuation.

The acquisition of adult levels of both cytochrome P450 (CYP) and phase II drug-metabolizing enzymes is enzyme- and isoform-specific (37). Recent research has shown that the traditional view of a locked-step progression of drug-metabolizing capacity is overly simplistic. Still, some generalizations can be made

(Table 14-3). The activity of most drug-metabolizing enzymes is absent in the fetus but rapidly increases over the first years of life such that toddlers and older children have levels of several, but not all, drug-metabolizing enzymes exceeding those of adults. These levels decline from that point until "usual" adult levels are achieved by the conclusion of puberty. Developmental changes over the first 2 decades of life in the activity of specific CYP enzymes is reflected in the increase and then decrease in theophylline clearance (1A2), the decline in the clearance of phenytoin (2C9/10, 2C19), and the decrease in the ratio of carbamazepine-10,11-epoxide to CBZ (3A3/4) (38, 39). Further details are provided in Table 14-3.

The rate of drug metabolism is also, in part, dependent on liver mass. Relative to body weight, the liver of a toddler is 40% to 50% greater and that of a 6-year-old child is 30% greater than that of an adult (30). That difference in size is another reason that children tend to clear drugs more rapidly than adults and frequently need higher doses on a milligram-per-kilogram basis to achieve the same plasma levels and clinical effect.

By 1 year of age, glomerular filtration rate and renal tubular mechanisms for secretion have reached adult levels; however, fluid intake may be greater in children. **Thus, lithium has a shorter**

half-life and more rapid renal clearance in children as compared with adults (40).

Nevertheless, the interindividual differences in the clearance of psychiatric medications are as great in children and adolescents as in adults, which should not be surprising. For example, genetically determined differences in CYP 2D6 function are expressed at birth. Hence, 5% to 10% of children and adolescents of northern European origin are deficient in CYP 2D6 activity and will develop four to six times higher levels of drugs that are predominantly metabolized by this isoenzyme than individuals with a functional copy.

Of all psychiatric medications, the psychostimulants have been the best studied in terms of their pharmacokinetics in children and adolescents (Table 14-4). Next have been studies of antidepressants, while few studies have been done on the pharmacokinetics of antipsychotics and anxiolytics in this age range.

As discussed in Chapter 3, TDM can be used to assess the ability of patients to clear a drug. Using these results, the prescriber can adjust the dose to achieve adult concentrations. Still, this approach is only an approximation of what might be optimal for a child or adolescent patient. These patients may be either more or less sensitive to either the beneficial or adverse effects of the drug and thus might need a concentration either higher or lower than that needed in adults to achieve an optimal response. Nevertheless, TDM results can serve as a reasonable reference point in the absence of more definitive efficacy and safety data in children and adolescents. Using TDM as a frame of reference, the prescriber should carefully adjust the dose based on clinical assessment of safety and efficacy. It may also be prudent to divide the daily doses more frequently than is done in adults to avoid excessively high peak plasma drug concentrations, which may be associated with increased tolerability and safety problems.

Treatment of Attention Deficit Hyperactivity Disorder in Children and Adolescents

Attention deficit hyperactivity disorder (ADHD) is one of the best studied and most effectively treated of all disorders in medicine. The data supporting its validity are more compelling than for many nonpsychiatric medical conditions (41, 42). A quarter-century of published treatment studies and clinical experience document the short-term effectiveness of pharmacological management (43).

Hyperactivity in children was first described clinically in 1902 and the first report of treatment with a stimulant was in 1937 (44). *Hyperactivity was the initial focus but recently the importance of attentional problems and impulsivity has also been recognized, as reflected in Diagnostic and Statistical Manual, 4th ed (DSM-IV) criteria* (45). These criteria require an enduring symptom pattern that has resulted in functional impairment.

The increased recognition of the importance of attentional problems and impulsivity has led to increased diagnosis of the condition. For example, girls are being given the diagnosis more frequently than they have in the past (46).

TABLE 14-4. *Psychostimulants used to treat attention deficit disorder in children and adolescents*

Feature	Methylphenidate	Pemoline	Dextroamphetamine
Elimination half-life	2–3[a]	2–12	6–7
Time to peak plasma concentration (T_{max})	1–3	1–5	3–4
Onset of behavioral effect	1	3–4 wk	1
Duration of behavioral effect	3–4	Not available	4
Daily dose range			
mg/kg/d	0.6–1.7	0.5–3.0	0.3–1.25
mg/d	10–60	37.5–112.5	5–40

[a]All time values are given in hours unless otherwise noted.

Community surveys across geographically, racially, and socioeconomically diverse populations have generally yielded prevalence rates of 2% to 6% of school-aged children, although rates as high as 12% to 16% have been found in some populations (41). ADHD accounts for at least 10% of behavioral problems seen in general pediatric settings and up to 50% in child psychiatric settings (47).

There is perhaps as much support for a biochemical basis of ADHD as there is for any of the common psychiatric disorders. Up to a 92% concordance rate has been found in monozygotic twins and a 33% rate in dizygotic twins (48, 49). Abnormalities have also been documented with magnetic resonance imaging (MRI), single photon emission computed tomography (SPECT), and neurophysiological studies, including heart rate deceleration, electroencephalogram amplitude of response to stimulation, and habituation on evoked response (50).

Up to 65% of children with ADHD have one or more "co-morbid" psychiatric disorders (51). These co-morbid conditions include the following:

- *Oppositional* disorder (up to 40%)
- *Conduct* disorder (up to 20%)
- *Mood* disorders (up to 20%)
- *Tics* or *Tourette's* syndrome (approximately 7%) (52)

Parenthetically, 60% of patients with Tourette's syndrome have ADHD. Learning disorders (especially reading) and subnormal intelligence are also increased in patients with ADHD and vice versa (53, 54).

On average, symptom severity diminishes by 50% every 5 years between the ages of 10 and 25 years (55, 56). Hyperactivity declines more quickly than impulsivity or inattentiveness. However, symptoms of the condition persist into adulthood in many cases. The strongest predictors of symptomatic persistence are psychiatric co-morbidity, particularly with conduct or bipolar disorder and a family history of ADHD or substance abuse (57). A prospective study followed up a cohort of patients older than 16 years old with persistent ADHD symptoms and an age-matched control group and found an 11-fold increase in ongoing ADHD symptoms, a nine-fold increase in antisocial personality disorder, and a four-fold increase in substance abuse (58).

The relationship between ADHD and substance abuse disorders is complex. There is no increased risk of substance abuse in ADHD patients relative to age-matched control subjects younger than 14 years old (41). Persistence of significant ADHD symptoms beyond 16 years of age coupled with both a family history of ADHD and substance abuse are significant risk factors for subsequent substance abuse. These patients frequently have co-morbid conduct or bipolar disorder.

The improved recognition of ADHD and its response to treatment has led to a dramatic increase in methylphenidate production and use in the United States. This increase has gained media attention and raised concerns about overdiagnosis or misdiagnosis, as well as the possibility of stimulant abuse (diversion of prescription methylphenidate or other stimulants). However, the available evidence does not support these concerns (41).

In children and adolescents, the decision to medicate is based on problems with inattention, impulsivity, and hyperactivity that are persistent and sufficiently severe to cause functional impairment at school, at home, and with peers. Before treatment with psychostimulants is instituted, other treatable causes should be ruled out and behavioral interventions considered. To maximize the likelihood of successful treatment with psychostimulants, parents or guardians should be involved in the treatment plan, including monitoring the administration of the medication, learning new disciplinary techniques, and participating in the patient's follow-up appointments (42).

As in the treatment of other psychiatric disorders, psychosocial interventions play an important role in the treatment of ADHD (59). These interventions can occur in four ways relative to medications:

- *Before* (particularly in mild cases)
- *Concurrently* in cases in which family issues are particularly significant or when such

approaches have been implemented before the referral for medication management

- *After response to medication has been achieved* but problematic behavioral problems remain
- When multiple *medication trials have failed*

Education for both patient and family is as important as formal behavioral therapy. Its goal should be that all are equipped with the information they need to be active participants in treatment.

Ideally, assessment measures would be incorporated into the treatment plan to assess baseline symptoms and response to treatment. Such measures include the Clinical Global Impression (CGI) scale, the ten-item Conners' Global Index for parents (Conners-P) and Teachers (Conners-T) (60), and the SNAP (Swanson, Nolan, and Pelham) rating scale (61). The latter has also been used in surveys of school-aged children (62). The results have been used to produce age-adjusted cutoffs that distinguish normal from abnormal degrees of inattentiveness and hyperactive/impulsive behavior. Thus, this scale can also be used to aid in documentation of the diagnosis as well as to monitor response to treatment.

Psychostimulants

This group of medications has been studied for the treatment of hyperactivity or ADHD since 1936 and has consistently shown robust efficacy in more than 150 randomized clinical trials (RCTs) of school-aged children. There are more than 3,000 citations and 250 reviews of stimulant treatment (63–65). Robust short-term stimulant-related improvement in ADHD has been reported in 161 controlled RCTs, including five preschool, 140 school-age, seven adolescent, and nine adult studies (66). There were 133 trials with methylphenidate, 22 with dextroamphetamines, and six with pemoline. In addition, two studies found treatment with mixed amphetamine salts to be superior to placebo (67, 68). **Claims that the effects of psychostimulants in children are paradoxical and do not apply to adults are spurious.** Moderate doses of these agents improve attention, concentration, and overall cognitive functioning in adults just as they do in children. Only at higher doses do psychostimulants cause distractibility and increased psychomotor activity in both children and adults, although the dose needed to produce these symptoms in children may be higher. This appears to be a difference in sensitivity, because by 3 years of age, children are similar to adults in terms of absorption, distribution, metabolism, elimination, and protein binding of these drugs (69).

Methylphenidate

This agent is the most widely used and best-studied medication for this condition. A meta-analysis of five studies that directly compared methylphenidate and dextroamphetamine found that 38% of ADHD children responded equally well to either of these medications, whereas the majority of the remaining children had a good response to one but not the other (43). However, there were no clinically useful predictors of which stimulant would work best in which child. This fact has led to the practice of always trying a second type of stimulant if the first does not work (70). Methylphenidate is generally given in divided doses (e.g., in the morning before school and again at lunch time) consistent with its half-life (Table 14-4). This short half-life allows plasma levels to decrease before bedtime, accounting for why insomnia is not more problematic.

The short half-life of methylphenidate can also be a disadvantage in specific patients because of an end-of-dose rebound in dysfunctional behavior. There can also be problems with the child taking the medication at school. For these reasons, a sustained-release version of methylphenidate has been developed, but there are several limitations with this product, including the following:

- Its *pharmacokinetics* are less reliable.
- *Onset of action* is frequently delayed.
- *Overall effectiveness* is less and more variable from day to day.
- *Rapid* and *high plasma drug concentrations* can result if a child chews the sustained-release capsule rather than swallowing it (71).

More recently, a new oral, osmotic, extended-release formulation of methylphenidate (Concerta), with both an immediate and continuous release component, has been approved by the FDA (72). When taken once daily, it results in plasma levels similar to those achieved with a three-times-a-day schedule of the immediate-release formulation. In addition, serum concentrations appear to fluctuate less. The additional cost, however, is significant.

Amphetamines

Amphetamines also have a longer half-life than methylphenidate, but not as long as pemoline (Table 14-4). Proponents of these agents cite the longer half-life as one of the reasons that amphetamines are better agents for the treatment of ADHD. Most clinicians use methylphenidate first but there is growing use of dextroamphetamine. This agent is clearly a useful alternative because as many as 20% of children who respond poorly to one psychostimulant respond well to another. Dextroamphetamine is also less expensive, but is frequently not covered by medical assistance programs. Concerns have also been raised about its abuse potential and the possibility of the child's medication being diverted to the illicit drug market. These concerns have led to underutilization of amphetamines.

Pemoline

Pemoline has been associated with 13 cases of hepatic failure since 1975. These cases have principally occurred in children younger than 10 years of age who were taking at least one other drug in addition to pemoline. Although rare, these cases have raised considerable debate as to whether pemoline has a role in the treatment of ADHD. If pemoline is used, liver function tests are recommended at baseline and then every 2 weeks. The efficacy of pemoline is based on a double-blind study involving both a placebo and active (methylphenidate) comparison treatment arm (73). Nevertheless, the magnitude of its effect is generally not as great as that of either methylphenidate or amphetamine. In addition, the time of onset of activity is appreciably delayed when compared with other agents.

The half-life of pemoline is longer than that of either methylphenidate or dextroamphetamine (Table 14-4), which increases further with chronic dosing (73). For these reasons, pemoline may be given once a day to some children and may have a role in patients for whom the effects of methylphenidate do not persist long enough for optimal control of distractibility and hyperactivity. Nevertheless, the longer duration of activity is not consistent for all children. For this reason, the duration of activity of pemoline must be individually assessed to determine whether this possible advantage is occurring. Some clinicians also believe that pemoline has less abuse potential than either methylphenidate or amphetamine.

The starting dose of pemoline for children weighing less than 35 kg is 37.5 mg in the morning; for heavier children, the starting doses is 56.25 mg. Each week the dose can be escalated in 18.75-mg increments to a maximum of 112.5 and 150 mg in lighter and heavier children, respectively (74).

The effective drug treatment of ADHD does more than simply reduce the child's activity level and increase the attention span, although these effects may be central to the overall improvement (75). Research has also documented improvement in off-task behavior, as well as in arithmetic and language tasks (71). There is usually an increase in positive social behavior in school, improved teacher-child interactions, and a more positive relationship between the mother and the child (76–78).

Long-Term Psychostimulant Therapy

As summarized earlier, the initial clinical trials with psychostimulants documented their acute efficacy. Because this condition is chronic, an important question is whether this efficacy is maintained over a longer treatment interval. Several studies have shown continued beneficial effects of stimulants over periods ranging from 12 to 24 months (79, 80). In the Multi-Modality Treatment study (MTA) of ADHD, 85% of 579 children were given stimulant medication for

14 months (81, 82). The group that received extensive medication management (i.e., careful dose adjustment, three-times-a-day dosing, and regular follow-up) had superior outcome compared with children with medication given according to usual community clinical practice. The beneficial effects of the psychostimulants remained robust for longer than 14 months.

Given the longitudinal course of this disorder, the next question is whether the benefits of psychostimulants persist into adolescence and even into adulthood. To date, little has been done to assess the effectiveness of psychostimulants in adolescence. One study of 13- to 18-year-old patients found two different doses of methylphenidate (mean = 15 and 31 mg per day) to be effective when compared with that of placebo (83). The results fit a dose–response curve, with the higher dose being superior to the lower dose, and both doses being superior to placebo, based on rating scores by parents and teachers. The design was not ideal, however, because the majority of patients were on methylphenidate at the time of referral to the study. Thus, the population may have been biased in terms of drug responsiveness. On the other hand, the outcome provides support for continuing methylphenidate in adolescents who responded as children and yet remain sufficiently symptomatic to warrant continued treatment.

Evidence also indicates that effective treatment during childhood leads to better ultimate outcome as adults. A follow-up study compared the status of children who received at least 3 years of continuous methylphenidate treatment with a group who were diagnosed before psychostimulant availability (84). The former had less subsequent psychiatric treatment, had fewer car accidents, led more independent lives, had achieved a higher educational level, and demonstrated less aggression than the never-medicated group. The drug-treated group also reported a more positive view of their childhood, higher self-esteem, and better social skills. These findings were also supported by Loney and colleagues (85), who reported that children with ADHD who were given psychostimulants for 6 months or longer did better in terms of better parent ratings and had fewer problems with alcohol and drug abuse than those who were not given psychostimulants.

Inasmuch as these studies were retrospective, the possibility always exists that the ability of the child and the family to stay in treatment was a more critical variable than medication. The available evidence, however, suggests that effective treatment of ADHD may have long-lasting effects on the psychosocial adjustment of the patient. In a related follow-up study, conduct disorders in adolescents almost exclusively occurred in those who retained features of ADHD (86). **Conceivably, effective intervention early in childhood may alter the course, decreasing the likelihood of development of conduct disorder as an adolescent and antisocial personality disorder with its various complications (e.g., alcohol and drug abuse, criminality) as an adult.**

These intriguing findings underscore the fact that drug therapy does not occur in a vacuum. Effective treatment of psychiatric disorders regardless of the patient's age can significantly affect the ability to interact and master one's environment successfully. It also affects the way others perceive the patient and, thus, affects their social relationships. Drug therapy can augment and be augmented by education about the illness and its treatment as well as by more formal psychotherapy, when necessary. The findings with ADHD simply underscore this point, because there are similar findings with childhood depressive disorder (87).

Adverse Effects of Psychostimulants

In the MTA study of 579 children given psychostimulant medication for 14 months, the percentage of families reporting adverse effects in their child were as follows: 88 (36%) none, 122 (50%) mild, 28 (11%) moderate, and seven (3%) severe (85).

The most common adverse effects of psychostimulants include the following:

- Anorexia
- Weight loss
- Irritability
- Insomnia
- Abdominal pain

These effects are usually self-limited, often disappearing after 2 to 3 weeks. Less common but more serious adverse effects include the following:

- Increased *blood pressure*
- *Tachycardia*
- Precipitation of a *tic-like movement* disorder
- *Nightmares*
- Hypersensitivity *rash*
- *Hepatotoxicity,* as manifested by elevated liver function tests
- *Psychotic symptoms*

Blood pressure and heart rate should be monitored at each visit during the dose titration phase to permit early detection of adverse effects. To minimize the risk of development of movement disorders or psychotic symptoms, psychostimulants should be used cautiously in any patient with a history of tics or psychotic symptoms, or with a family history of Tourette's syndrome or schizophrenia. Nevertheless, studies have shown that psychostimulants are effective in treating ADHD in patients with co-morbid Tourette's syndrome and that they do not exacerbate tics in the majority of such patients (88, 89). Furthermore, no evidence indicates that psychostimulants can lower the seizure threshold or cause seizures.

As mentioned earlier, the emerging consensus is that the growth spurt in adolescence after psychostimulant discontinuation compensates for any earlier effect on growth velocity. Thus, eventual height is not compromised. What is less clear is whether this compensatory growth spurt would hold true for those continued on psychostimulants through adolescence. Hence, clinicians have an increased responsibility to determine whether a medication has had a positive effect and should continue it during adolescence only when such an effect has been satisfactorily documented.

Even when a positive effect has been documented, children are typically given a holiday off the psychostimulant during summer months when demands on their attention, concentration, and activity levels are fewer. The goal is to give the patient as long a holiday off the medication as possible. It should be at least 2 weeks so the clinician can determine whether the child needs to have the medication reinstituted during the next school year. When the continued need for the medication is equivocal, a holiday off the medication during the school year is also warranted.

These medications are often discontinued when the child reaches puberty. One reason for this practice is that adolescents may be more likely to abuse psychostimulants. There is also the aforementioned issue about the potential developmental effects (e.g., growth spurt) of continuing psychostimulants during adolescence. For both of these reasons, clinical data supporting their necessity must be even more substantial. If the patient relapses to a significant extent, then the clinician may consider reinstituting medication based on documented beneficial effects of methylphenidate in adolescents. In such instances, the clinician must be mindful of the possibility of abuse and monitor growth and development closely.

Antidepressants

A number of studies indicate that some but not all antidepressants are effective in ADHD. Spencer and colleagues (66) found 29 studies (involving 1,016 patients) that supported the efficacy of TCAs in the treatment of ADHD. Desipramine is the TCA with the most efficacy data. *Desipramine,* based on a meta-analysis of five randomized trials involving 170 ADHD patients had efficacy (i.e., effect size) comparable with that of methylphenidate (90, 91). However, desipramine produced a higher rate of adverse effects compared with psychostimulants. Moreover, several sudden, unexpected deaths have been reported in children on desipramine (92, 93). Although there are reasons to question whether desipramine had a role in these deaths, these reports have raised considerable concern among child and adolescent psychiatrists and have limited the use of this medication in this population. Some more limited evidence supports the efficacy of either *imipramine or nortriptyline* for ADHD (94–97).

Three randomized clinical trials support the efficacy of *bupropion* in ADHD. The first used doses up to 6 mg/kg (98); the other two used doses of 100 to 300 mg per day in equally divided daily doses spaced at least 6 hours apart (99, 100). The concern with bupropion is its seizure risk, which requires that its daily dose stay below 450 mg per day in adults (i.e., approximately 6.5 mg/kg). Virtually no work has been done to determine the plasma concentrations of bupropion and its three active metabolites in children and adolescents. Hence, it is unknown whether a limit of 6.5 mg per kg is also appropriate for children. No data exist as to whether children are more or less sensitive to bupropion in terms of seizure risk at the same drug concentration. Also, little is known about pharmacokinetic drug–drug interactions that could reduce the clearance of bupropion. For these reasons, cautious dosing is advised when prescribing bupropion for children on other medications that can reduce oxidative drug metabolism (see Chapters 3 and 7 for more details).

Other Agents

A number of clinical trials have found clonidine to be superior to placebo in treating ADHD (101–104). However, these studies were generally not as methodologically rigorous as those with either psychostimulants or antidepressants. *Clonidine* has been used as monodrug therapy and in combination with methylphenidate. Hunt (101) did a crossover study of clonidine alone, methylphenidate alone, and the combination in 25 children with ADHD and conduct disorder. The combination was reported to be superior to either agent alone in reducing parent ratings of conduct problems. However, the combination has never been tested in children with ADHD alone for the core symptoms of hyperactivity, inattention, and impulsivity. There is also concern about the safety of this combination because there have been four deaths in children (105). However, there were enough complicating factors present in each of these cases that no conclusions could be drawn about the role of methylphenidate and clonidine in these deaths. **For these reasons, the use of clonidine for the treatment of ADHD should be tried only after trials of more than one psychostimulant and after an antidepressant trial.**

Limited data are also available on the efficacy of *guanfacine* in ADHD. First, there were several open-label trials that had promising results (106–108). Recently, a double-blind study found guanfacine to be superior to placebo; however, the effect size was about half that traditionally found with psychostimulants (109).

Treatment of Major Depressive Disorder in Children and Adolescents

Major depressive disorder (MDD) can occur in children as young as 6 years of age. The diagnosis is based on the same criteria as in adults. These patients typically have a high familial loading for psychiatric disorders (110), with more than 70% of mothers having MDD, either pure or complicated by the presence of other psychiatric syndromes. Fathers, however, are more likely to have alcohol abuse or dependence, as opposed to MDD. Given this familial pattern, it is not surprising that many children and adolescents with MDD frequently also meet criteria for other psychiatric syndromes, particularly conduct and oppositional disorder (110).

Despite the diagnostic challenges that remain in trying to understand the nature of MDD in children and adolescents, advances in its treatment has progressed considerably since the last edition of this textbook. Over this interval, selective serotonin reuptake inhibitors (SSRIs) have superseded TCAs as the treatment of first choice based both on efficacy and safety considerations. As in adults, specific psychotherapies (cognitive therapy, cognitive-behavioral therapy, and interpersonal therapy) may be as effective as antidepressant medication, at least in mild to moderate depression in children and adolescents (111, 112). Also, evidence indicates that depression in children and adolescents may be more influenced than is depression in adults by psychosocial variables such as peers and family, as well as other environmental factors (113).

The latter factor may account in part for the higher placebo response, particularly in many of the earlier antidepressant trials in children and adolescents. For example, Puig-Antich and colleagues (114) reported more than a 68% placebo response, whereas others have found similar rates. One reason for the high "placebo" response rate in these earlier studies may be the degree of psychosocial treatment that these patients received. Most of these studies involved several weeks of hospitalization, which was more feasible in the 1980's than it is now. Such hospitalizations removed the patient from what often was a chaotic home life, and these patients typically received intensive individual, group, and milieu psychotherapy. Generally, such intensive psychotherapy services were not available in more recent trials of the newer antidepressants, and consistent with this fact are the lower placebo response rates. Thus, the newer antidepressants may not actually be more effective than the TCAs. Instead, the difference may be that the placebo treatment in the more recent studies was less effective than the "placebo" treatment of the older studies, permitting more recent studies to detect a drug–placebo difference in efficacy.

The high placebo response rate found in children and adolescents with MDD may also be due to the heterogeneous nature of the disorder in this population. Hughes and colleagues (115) found that children and adolescents with major depression plus concomitant conduct or oppositional disorder had a higher response rate to placebo than to imipramine. Nevertheless, an empirical trial of an antidepressant, particularly the safer newer antidepressants, may still be warranted in such patients.

Selective Serotonin Reuptake Inhibitors

From 1996 to 1997, 792,000 prescriptions for SSRIs were written to treat depression in children and adolescents between 6 and 18 years of age, primarily because of the safety of these medications compared with TCAs and because of growing evidence of their efficacy (116, 117).

The first double-blind study of *fluoxetine* failed to show a difference in response rates but suffered from a high "placebo" or nonspecific treatment response rate (118). Emslie and colleagues (119) subsequently demonstrated the superiority of an SSRI over placebo in both children and adolescents aged 7 to 17 years. Their study involved 48 subjects randomized to drug and 48 to placebo. Using the "intent to treat" sample, 27 (56%) of those receiving fluoxetine responded versus 16 (33%) on placebo, with response defined as a clinical global scale rating of "much" or "very much" improved ($p < 0.05$). However, no significant differences were observed in terms of complete remission, defined as a score of 28 or less on the Children's Depression Rating Scale. Remission occurred in 31% of fluoxetine-treated cases versus 23% of placebo-treated cases. Furthermore, there was no difference in response and remission rates between subjects 12 years and younger (n = 48) versus subjects 13 years or older (n = 48).

Since the study by Emslie and colleagues, there has also been a positive, double-blind, placebo-controlled study with *paroxetine* (120), and *sertraline* has also shown promise in an open-label trial in adolescents with major depression (121).

Tricyclic Antidepressants

As mentioned earlier, the clinical trials with TCAs in children and adolescents with MDD have generally been disappointing (120, 122, 123). In addition, these medications have a less favorable adverse effect profile and thus higher patient attrition rates during the acute treatment phase compared with newer antidepressants. They also have a lower therapeutic index (i.e., difference between therapeutic and toxic dose; see Chapter 7).

Despite these challenges, two positive, double-blind, placebo-controlled studies have shown TCAs to be superior to placebo in children suffering from major depression (124, 125). In the study by Kashani and colleagues, there were only nine subjects in each treatment group, the maximal dose of *amitriptyline* used was low (1.5 mg/kg per day), and the statistical results were modest ($p < 0.05$, based on a one-tail t-test, presuming drug would be superior to placebo). In the double-blind, placebo-controlled study by Preskorn and colleagues (126), the group sample sizes were somewhat larger (n = 15 per cell). The *imipramine* dose was adjusted based on TDM to ensure that the patient achieved plasma levels that had previously been found safe and effective. Imipramine was superior to placebo through the first 3 weeks of treatment ($p < 0.05$, based on a two-tail t-test); however, the response rates in the imipramine and placebo groups were not different by the end of 6 weeks.

Kramer and Feiguine (127) conducted the first double-blind study of amitriptyline in adolescents with major depression. At the end of 6 weeks, all subjects had improved and the only difference was a lower score on the Depression Adjective Checklist in the group receiving the TCA versus the control subjects. Geller and colleagues (128) were unable to find a difference in efficacy between *nortriptyline* and placebo. Kutcher and colleagues (129) randomly assigned 60 adolescent subjects to either *desipramine* (up to 200 mg per day) or placebo and found a 48% response rate on drug versus 35% on placebo.

Other Antidepressants

The first studies of *venlafaxine* and *nefazodone* in both children and adolescents examined pharmacokinetics, safety, and tolerability of these agents (35, 36). As expected, the clearance was modestly more rapid in children and adolescents for both of these medications when compared with clearance in adults, but the difference was not sufficient to warrant a significant change in the milligram per kilogram daily dose. These studies should be followed up by appropriately designed efficacy studies.

Continuation Treatment

There are no studies to guide how long antidepressants should be continued in children and adolescents once a response has been achieved. A naturalistic study by Emslie and colleagues (130) of 70 children and adolescents with MDD revealed that 98% recovered from their index episodes of MDD within 1 year of their initial evaluation. More than 80% received antidepressants, but the nature of the treatment was determined by the individual clinician rather than dictated by a treatment protocol. More than 60%

of these patients had at least one recurrence during a 1- to 5-year follow-up period. Of those with a recurrence, 47% occurred within 1 year of their recovery and 70% within 2 years. These results are consistent with earlier studies indicating that 54% to 72% of children and adolescents with MDD have a recurrent episode when followed up for 3 to 8 years (130, 131). Until studies are done, it would seem prudent to follow the same continuation and maintenance treatment guidelines for children and adolescents as for adults with MDD (see Chapter 7).

Adverse Effects of Antidepressants

The adverse effects of SSRIs, venlafaxine, and nefazodone in children and adolescents are comparable with those in adults (see Chapter 7) and have been documented in both clinical trials and practice (35, 36, 119–121, 123). As in adults, isolated case reports have described behavioral activation in children and adolescents given SSRIs (133, 134). The significance of such reports in terms of a causal link to the drug is difficult because of their rare and anecdotal nature and because the patients are at increased risk for such behavioral disturbances relative to the general population as a result of their underlying psychiatric disorder.

The adverse effects of TCAs are also similar to those reported in adults (see Chapter 7). The secondary amine TCAs (e.g., desipramine, nortriptyline) are generally as well tolerated as newer antidepressants. Increased blood pressure may be more likely to occur in children than in adults but hypertension per se is rare (135). The most common cardiovascular effect is mild tachycardia. Despite their generally favorable adverse effect profile, secondary amine TCAs can cause serious toxicity in children and adolescents just as in adults when a taken in an overdose or when a high TCA plasma level occurs as a result of slow metabolism (136). For that reason, most clinicians reserve TCAs for the child or adolescent who has at least a moderate depressive disorder unresponsive to a trial of one or more newer antidepressants. In such instances, TDM should be done at least once to ensure plasma concentrations greater than 450 ng/mL do not develop (137). Such levels are associated with an increased risk of the following:

- Delirium
- Seizures
- Slowing of intracardiac conduction, which can lead to heart blocks, arrhythmias, and sudden death (138)

Several cases of sudden death in children and adolescents taking desipramine for a variety of indications have been reported (139, 140). These cases have raised significant concern among child psychiatrists, even though the drug was barely detectable at autopsy, indicating that it was unlikely to have been a contributor to the sudden death. These events have led some clinicians to recommend frequent electrocardiographic (ECG) monitoring (e.g., baseline and at every dose increase) without evidence that such monitoring will achieve early detection of a problem and avoid an untoward outcome.

Treatment of Anxiety-Related Disorders in Children and Adolescents

The nosology of anxiety disorders has changed considerably over the past 40 years (141). Such disorders were not mentioned in the original DSM. In DSM-II, problems with anxiety were considered a subset of behavioral disorders and were restricted to "overanxious" and "withdrawing" reactions. The DSM-III defined three types of anxiety disorders in children and adolescents: overanxious, avoidant, and separation disorder. The DSM-III also acknowledged that children and adolescents could meet adult criteria for simple phobias, panic disorder, posttraumatic stress disorder, and obsessive-compulsive disorder (OCD). In DSM-IV (45), generalized anxiety disorder (GAD) and social phobia (or social anxiety disorder with childhood onset) replaced overanxious disorder and avoidant disorder, respectively. Selective mutism was considered to be a variant of social phobia or social anxiety disorder. In contrast, separation anxiety disorder was considered to be a unique developmental disorder of childhood often presenting as school refusal.

Perhaps because of these changes, few treatment studies have been conducted in this area (142–145). Of the studies reported, most have been open label and involved only a small number of patients. Of the various conditions subsumed under anxiety disorders, OCD is the best studied in children and adolescents, with five double-blind trials leading to formal FDA labeling of several medications for use in such patients. Four double-blind studies for school phobia or refusal and five for GAD or mixed diagnostic groups have also been conducted. None of these studies, however, has been sufficient to lead to formal labeling by the FDA as indicated for the treatment of these conditions in children or adolescents.

Obsessive-Compulsive Disorder

OCD typically begins in adolescence, but may also become apparent in childhood. Features are the same regardless of the age of onset, with the illness tending to run a chronic course. Until recently, patients were given a series of medications, as well as psychotherapy, frequently without substantial improvement.

That situation has changed with the development of clomipramine and the SSRIs, which appear to have unique efficacy in treating OCD when compared with other types of psychotropics (see Chapter 13, "Obsessive-Compulsive Disorder"). In addition, more effective behavioral approaches have been developed, which, in combination with medication, can substantially ameliorate this condition.

Clomipramine

The first agent proven to be effective in OCD was the TCA, clomipramine. Its efficacy in pediatric-age patients with OCD was demonstrated in two double-blind, placebo-controlled studies (146, 147). These findings were further supported by a double-blind crossover study with desipramine (148). This latter study provided support for serotonin uptake inhibition being the mechanism of action responsible for the efficacy of clomipramine in OCD. Despite this evidence, there are several limitations to the use of clomipramine because of its multiple mechanisms of action:

- Blockade of α_1-*adrenergic receptors*, which can cause orthostatic hypotension
- Blockade of *histamine* receptors, which can produce sedation and possibly weight gain
- Blockade of *cholinergic* receptors, which can result in a variety of peripheral anticholinergic adverse effects and memory impairment
- Inhibition of Na^+ *fast channels,* which can inhibit electrically excitable membranes and produce intracardiac conduction delays (137)

The latter action is responsible for the serious CNS and cardiac toxicity (e.g., delirium, seizures, cardiac arrhythmias, and cardiac arrest) that can occur at high plasma drug concentrations of clomipramine just as with any TCA. These effects are problematic with adults and may be of even greater concern with children and adolescents.

Other concerns of particular relevance to children and adolescents are due to pharmacokinetic differences between them and adults. Although clomipramine is the most potent TCA in terms of inhibiting the neuronal serotonin uptake pump, its major metabolite, desmethylclomipramine, is a potent inhibitor of the neuronal uptake of norepinephrine. Depending on the patient's hepatic metabolism profile, either desmethylclomipramine or clomipramine may be the predominant form of the circulating drug. Children tend to be extensive demethylators of TCAs. For this reason, desmethylclomipramine can account for 70% of the circulating drug in children on clomipramine. If serotonin uptake inhibition is critical to its effectiveness in treating OCD, then clomipramine may fail to work as a result of extensive conversion to desmethylclomipramine.

For these reasons, TDM can serve several roles when using clomipramine. First, it can be used to determine whether clomipramine or its demethylated metabolite constitutes the majority of the circulating drug. Second, TDM can be used to guide dose adjustment to ensure plasma concentrations equivalent to those seen in adults whose OCD is successfully treated. This approach also ensures that concentration levels do not approach or exceed the toxic threshold for TCAs (i.e., greater than 450 ng/mL). Like adults, children and adolescents demonstrate a wide variability in their capacity to metabolize TCAs. As mentioned earlier, children are usually faster metabolizers of these drugs than adults, so they typically need doses of approximately 2.5 to 3.5 mg/kg. Once puberty has been reached, the required doses can be reduced by as much as 50%.

Selective Serotonin Reuptake Inhibitors

Both fluvoxamine and sertraline are approved for the treatment of OCD in children and adolescents. Fluvoxamine was proven effective in a 10-week, double-blind, placebo-controlled trial in patients 8 to 17 years of age with OCD (149). Dosages in this study were adjusted to a total daily fluvoxamine dose of approximately 100 mg per day over the first 2 weeks using a balanced, twice-daily dosing schedule. After that, the dose was adjusted within a range of 50 to 200 mg per day based on clinical assessment of efficacy and tolerability. Fluvoxamine was superior to placebo on the Children's Yale-Brown Obsessive-Compulsive Scale (CY-BOCS) at weeks 1 to 6 and week 10. However, the effect was mainly in the 8- to 11-year-old versus the 12- to 17-year-old age group. The significance of this age difference is not known.

The effectiveness of sertraline in pediatric patients (ages 6 to 17 years) with OCD was demonstrated in a 12-week, double-blind, placebo-controlled study (150). Patients were initiated at a dose of either 25 mg per day (ages 6 to 12 years) or 50 mg per day (ages 13 to 17 years) and then adjusted over the next 4 weeks to a maximal dose of 200 mg per day as tolerated. The mean dose of completers was 178 mg per day. Dosing was once a day, either morning or evening. No differences in efficacy based on age or gender were observed.

As expected, children and adolescents were found to metabolize sertraline slightly more efficiently than adults. Relative to adults, the area under the plasma concentration-time curve and the peak plasma concentration of sertraline was on average 22% lower in children and adolescents compared with that in adults when the dose was adjusted based on body weight. The half-life did not differ between three groups: 26.2 hours for the 6- to 12-year-old age group, 27.8 hours for the 13- to 17-year-old age group, and 27.2 hours for the 18- to 45-year-old age group (from a separate study involving the same dose).

Finally, a small, double-blind, placebo-controlled, crossover trial of fluoxetine in 14 children and adolescents with OCD also showed a significant decrease in CY-BOCS total scores (151).

Other Anxiety Disorders

The medical management of other childhood anxiety disorders has included the use of BZDs, antihistamines, β-adrenergic blockers, and clonidine (152, 153). These medications are used by clinicians to treat a wide range of anxiety-related conditions, including separation anxiety, school phobia, and panic disorder. None of these agents, however, has been the subject of systematic, double-blind, placebo-controlled studies in children or adolescents, and opinions about their effectiveness depend primarily on anecdotal experience and reports.

Only a few studies have been done with BZDs in children and adolescents. The conclusions that can be drawn from these studies are limited by the small sample sizes, the short duration of the trials, the low doses used, and the high placebo response rate. Grae and colleagues (154) did not find *clonazepam* to be superior to placebo. Simeon and colleagues (155) did not find alprazolam at doses up to 0.04 mg per kg per day to be effective in children with either GAD or social phobia. There is only one small (n = 12) double-blind, placebo-controlled study showing clonazepam to be effective in pediatric panic disorder and none in posttraumatic stress disorder (156).

BZDs are, in general, more rapidly absorbed and metabolized in children than in adults (157). For this reason, the initial dose (in terms of milligrams per kilogram per day) of BZDs in children and adolescents are the same as in adults. The dose is then adjusted based on a clinical assessment of response rather than empirical data dictating the most appropriate doses, or how long the patient should remain on a given dose before

adjusting it or switching to another agent. The safety and tolerability of these medications do not appear to differ significantly whether used by children, adolescents, or adults. Unstudied issues in the pediatric population include the abuse and dependency potential of BZDs, as well as long-term effects on school performance and advancement.

The efficacy of TCAs, principally *imipramine*, has also been tested as treatment of separation anxiety and school phobia. Four placebo-controlled studies involving 140 children have been conducted (153, 158–160). Whereas early studies were positive, subsequent reports were not. Gittelman-Klein and Klein (161) demonstrated a significant benefit over placebo from 6 weeks of treatment with imipramine (mean dose = 159 mg per day) in 45 children with school phobia. A subsequent study using lower amounts of clomipramine (40 to 75 mg per day) was negative but the doses used make interpretation difficult. Also, because of its tolerability and safety profile, clomipramine is generally not used as an anxiolytic agent in children or adolescents.

Few trials have tested the potential efficacy of SSRIs to treat anxiety disorders other than OCD in children and adolescents. Black and colleagues (162) found a significant difference between *fluoxetine* and placebo in four of six children with selective mutism (believed to be a variant of social phobia) but only on the global rating of change and parent's rating of mutism change. In another small open-trial study, fluoxetine (10 to 60 mg per day) reduced anxiety and increased speech in 76% of children (age 5 to 14 years) with selective mutism (163).

No pharmacokinetic, dose-finding, controlled efficacy, or safety studies of *buspirone* in children or adolescents have been conducted. Although *β-blockers* have been used to treat anxiety and aggressive dyscontrol in children and adolescents, no controlled studies and no pharmacokinetic data exist.

Treatment of Psychotic Disorders in Children and Adolescents

Both typical (e.g., haloperidol) and atypical (e.g., clozapine) antipsychotics are used in children and adolescents, primarily to treat schizophrenia, psychotic mood disorder, and pervasive developmental disorders. These agents are also used on occasion to treat a range of other conditions including conduct disorder, impulsive and aggressive disorders, Tourette's disorder, and ADHD.

Younger patients with schizophrenia may be less responsive to pharmacotherapy than adult patients (164,165). Nonresponse to typical antipsychotics is as high as 40% to 50% in some reports. Thought disorder is the most drug-refractory of the classic psychotic symptoms in children and adolescents with schizophrenia. Thus, even when the more florid symptoms (e.g., hallucinations and delusions) abate following treatment with antipsychotics, these patients frequently continue to have substantial impairment in social functioning and scholastic performance.

Most studies in children and adolescents have been conducted with neuroleptics. A computerized literature search for the period 1974 to 1999 identified only five double-blind, placebo-controlled clinical trials that investigated the use of atypical antipsychotic medications in children and adolescents (166, 167). These studies involved a total of 105 patients. Numerous open-label and case series were also found.

Haloperidol is the best-studied antipsychotic medication in children and adolescents with schizophrenia. In a double-blind, placebo- and active-controlled study, haloperidol (2 to 16 mg per day) and loxapine (10 to 200 mg per day) were equally effective and superior to placebo (168). This finding was replicated in a placebo-controlled, crossover study of haloperidol (doses of 0.5 to 3.5 mg per day or 0.02 to 0.12 mg/kg per day) in children 5.5 to 12 years of age (169). In this study, haloperidol was more effective than placebo in reducing ideas of reference, persecutory ideas, hallucinations, and thought disorder.

The recommended dose range for haloperidol in children is 0.5 to 16.0 mg per day (0.02 to 0.2 mg/kg per day), but the initial dose should be low, with gradual increments upward as needed and tolerated. Dose should be increased no more than twice per week, except in unusual instances. Older adolescents with schizophrenia typically require doses in the adult range, and younger adolescents fall between the recommendations

for children and adults. As with adults, the final maintenance dose in children and adolescents must be empirically determined, based on both benefit and tolerability.

As in adults, the main acute untoward effects of high-potency, typical antipsychotics are extrapyramidal symptoms (EPS) syndromes, particularly acute dystonia, and sedation (167). Parkinsonism is rare in preschool-aged children but does occur in school-aged children and adolescents.

Adolescent boys may be more vulnerable to acute dystonia than adults. Although these adverse effects can be treated with anticholinergic agents, dose reduction should also be considered. For acute dystonia, diphenhydramine (25 to 50 mg) may be given orally or intramuscularly, as can equivalent doses of benztropine (1 to 2 mg/day). Diphenhydramine has both sedative and anticholinergic properties, with the former being helpful in calming the patient whereas the latter reverses the reaction itself.

The common adverse effects of low-potency antipsychotics (e.g., chlorpromazine, thioridazine) seen in adults also occur in children and adolescents and include sedation; peripheral anticholinergic effects (e.g., dry mouth, constipation); slowing of intracardiac conduction; and orthostatic blood pressure changes. **Children and adolescents are generally more tolerant of the blood pressure—lowering effects, so that they may develop greater changes before becoming clinically symptomatic. For that reason, it is important to monitor their blood pressure early during the dose adjustment phase.**

The term "behavioral toxicity" has been used in the child psychiatry literature to describe the following adverse effects of antipsychotics, particularly low-potency phenothiazines (e.g., chlorpromazine, thioridazine):

- Hypoactivity
- Apathy
- Social withdrawal
- Cognitive dulling
- Sedation

Although similar effects can occur in adults, they are particularly problematic in children and adolescents for three reasons:

- *Sedation is more likely to develop* in children and adolescents than in adults (165).
- Children and adolescents *may complain less about these effects,* so that the physician must monitor more closely to detect their development.
- These effects, if not promptly detected, *may have long-term adverse effects on the patient's development* by interfering at critical psychosocial stages and by compromising the ability to perform in school. These complications could offset any gains in psychosocial and school performance resulting from effective treatment of psychotic symptoms.

Clozapine

Among the atypical antipsychotics, clozapine has the most convincing evidence of efficacy in children and adolescents with schizophrenia (166, 167, 170). Kumar and colleagues (171) conducted a double-blind, randomized trial of clozapine versus haloperidol in 21 children and adolescents (mean age = 14 years) whose psychosis had been previously unresponsive to typical antipsychotics. Clozapine at a mean dose of 176 mg per day was superior to haloperidol for both positive and negative symptoms. These results are consistent with an open-label study by Remschmidt and colleagues (172). This group found that clozapine at a mean dose of 154 mg per day produced notable improvement in 27 of 36 (75%) adolescents with schizophrenia previously unresponsive to at least two trials of typical antipsychotics.

The adverse effects of clozapine in children and adolescents are generally comparable with those seen in adults, including decreased neutrophil counts and weight gain (i.e., up to 6.5 kg in 6 weeks) (166). As in adults, clozapine produces asymptomatic electroencephalographic (EEG) changes at doses that are otherwise therapeutic in 10% to 44% of children and adolescents (171, 173). Seizures can also occur in children and adolescents given clozapine without preexisting seizure histories (171).

In contrast to adults, children and adolescents may be more prone to development of acute EPS on clozapine, with two open-label studies reporting a 15% risk of acute EPS (172, 174).

Risperidone

No double-blind, controlled studies with risperidone in children and adolescents with schizophrenia have been conducted. One open trial and several case series, however, have been reported (167, 175). An open-label trial of risperidone (0.5 to 4 mg per day) for 2 to 12 months in 26 hospitalized young patients with mixed diagnoses and aggression reported this agent to be helpful (176). Because of the small sample size and uncontrolled nature of these reports, no firm conclusions can be drawn about either the efficacy or adverse effect profile of risperidone in this age group. Based on the available data, risperidone appears to cause the same adverse effects in children and adolescents as in adults; however, weight gain may be more problematic in this group. In the open-label trial by Lombroso and colleagues (177), all seven adolescents gained 3.6 to 6.3 kg in 6 weeks. Hepatotoxicity may result, and this concern has led to the recommendation that liver function be checked in patients who gain significant weight during treatment with risperidone (178). An open-label trial by Armenteros and colleagues (179) also found a rate of EPS comparable with that seen with typical antipsychotic medications in ten adolescents given risperidone. A few cases of dyskinesia have also been reported in children given risperidone (167).

Olanzapine

One open trial and several case series reports have examined the potential use of olanzapine in children and adolescents with schizophrenia (167, 180). Kumar and colleagues (180) have suggested that clozapine may be superior to olanzapine in the treatment of children and adolescents with schizophrenia unresponsive to typical antipsychotics. These investigators found a response rate of only 25% in their patients in an open-label trial of olanzapine (mean dose = 17.5 mg per day or 0.27 mg/kg per day) versus a 53% response rate in their double-blind trial of clozapine versus haloperidol (171). This conclusion is consistent with adult data indicating the superiority of clozapine over olanzapine in the patients with schizophrenia unresponsive to typical antipsychotics (see Chapter 5). Although the data are limited, olanzapine appears to be capable of producing the same adverse effects in children and adolescents as in adults. For example, Kumar and colleagues (180) reported an average weight gain of 3.4 kg in eight patients over the 6-week period of this open-label trial.

Long-Term Treatment with Antipsychotics

No formal, prospective, long-term efficacy or safety studies of either typical or atypical antipsychotics in children and adolescents with schizophrenia have been conducted (166, 167). However, reports of the long-term treatment of children and adolescents with conduct disorder (181, 182), autism (183), and Tourette's disorder (184) with either haloperidol or thioridazine suggest that the tolerability of these medications in children and adolescents is comparable with that in adults.

Tardive and withdrawal dyskinesias are the most common long-term, untoward effects of high-potency neuroleptics (e.g., haloperidol). As in adults, the incidence of tardive and withdrawal dyskinesia in children and adolescents given these medications varies widely (i.e., 8% to 51%) (185). The phenomenology of such dyskinesias in children and adolescents is similar to that seen in adults. Risk factors for the development of dyskinesias include the following:

* Greater cumulative *dose*
* Longer *exposure*
* *Mental retardation*
* *Autism*
* Female *gender* (186)

Some evidence based on MRI studies suggests that long-term treatment with *clozapine* may increase basal ganglia volume (187). The significance of this finding is unknown, including any relationship to the development of tardive dyskinesia.

To minimize the risk of development of dyskinesias, patients should be carefully examined for any baseline movement abnormalities before starting a neuroleptic. The use of one of the available scales (e.g., the Abnormal Involuntary Movements Scale) can help structure the examination and quantify symptoms.

Special Treatment Issues in Children and Adolescents

There are a variety of other conditions in this age range that are mentioned here only in overview. Further discussion of these topics may be found in various textbooks on child psychiatry or by reviewing the primary literature.

Conduct Disorder

Conduct disorder occurs in 2% to 10% of the general pediatric population and represents the largest diagnostic group referred to outpatient psychiatric clinics (146). Nevertheless, only a few double-blind, controlled treatment studies have been conducted of this condition. Although no studies show a single treatment to be more effective for conduct disorder, some data exist about the treatment of specific symptoms.

For example, several studies have reported that antisocial behavior, such as stealing and fighting, can be reduced with psychostimulants (188–190). Available data suggest that mood stabilizers are more effective than psychostimulants in reducing aggressive outburst (191–193). Lithium (600 to 1,800 mg per day, serum levels of 0.53 to 1.70 mEq/L) was found to be superior to placebo in reducing aggression in 50 hospitalized children with conduct disorder (192). Haloperidol (1 to 6 mg per day, mean 2.95 mg per day) was found to be superior to placebo and as effective as lithium for reducing aggressiveness and explosiveness in hospitalized children and adolescents with conduct disorder. Molindone and thioridazine were found to be equally effective in reducing aggression in a similar group of patients (194). One note of caution with antipsychotics, particularly neuroleptics, is that there is a risk of neurological adverse sequelae, including tardive dyskinesia. Although CBZ has been widely used for this indication, the one controlled study was negative (195). Although clonidine has also been widely used to reduce aggression, studies are limited to two small open trials (196). That fact, plus the concerns discussed earlier in this section about clonidine, suggests it should be used cautiously, if at all, for this indication.

Tourette's Disorder

Tourette's syndrome consists of tics (i.e., rapid, purposeless movements), noises (e.g., grunts, squeals, barks), and sometimes coarse speech, usually with an onset in childhood. It is inherited by an autosomal dominant mechanism. In some cases, drug treatment is not required, and simply explaining the neurological basis of the condition to the parent and child is often reassuring. In some cases, enduring the tics is less of a burden than suffering from the dysphoric adverse effects of antipsychotics.

Nevertheless, this condition is responsive to treatment with dopamine-2 receptor antagonists. Hence, this condition is one of the clearest childhood indications for treatment with these medications. In theory, any dopamine-2 blocking receptor antagonist could be used. *Haloperidol* has been the most extensively tested and used medication for this condition (167). The typical dose for children aged 3 to 12 years old is 0.2 mg/kg per day. More recently, in a double-blind study of 36 boys with Tourette's syndrome, *risperidone* was effective in reducing tics in 88% versus 60% for haloperidol (197), perhaps making risperidone a better option than a neuroleptic in terms of neurological adverse effects.

Pimozide is an alternative agent for refractory cases or those unable to tolerate haloperidol. In a double-blind, crossover study, pimozide was superior to both haloperidol and placebo (198), in part because of the higher rate of treatment-limiting adverse effects of haloperidol versus pimozide (41% versus 14%). Nevertheless, there is concern about pimozide because it may cause concentration-dependent prolongation of the QT interval. In addition, three patients died suddenly while taking pimozide (199, 200). In the first report, the dose of pimozide had been rapidly adjusted to 70 to 80 mg per day over a 2-week interval. In the second report, clarithromycin was added to a stable dose of pimozide, leading to a substantial reduction in pimozide clearance and increase in its levels. Thus, pimozide should not be administered with CYP 3A inhibitors (see Chapter 3) without careful TDM-driven dose adjustment.

Clonidine has also been useful in one controlled study and in a few case reports. Although this agent has the advantage of avoiding acute and chronic EPS associated with neuroleptics, its effects on blood pressure have appropriately constrained its use in this age population. There is also the concern regarding rebound hypertension if this agent is abruptly discontinued (e.g., noncompliance).

Autistic Disorder

Approximately 16 of every 10,000 babies are born with autism or one of its related disorders (201). Diagnosis requires that the patient display the following:

- Impairment in *social interactions*
- Impairment in *communication*
- Restricted and repetitive *interests* and *behavior*

Haloperidol has documented efficacy in both the short-term and the long-term treatment of such patients (167). Specifically, haloperidol can reduce

- *Stereotypic behavior*
- *Hyperactivity*
- *Aggressive behavior*, including self-abusive behavior
- Social *withdrawal*
- Temper *tantrums*

These patients, however, may be at increased risk for development of tardive dyskinesia. *Naltrexone* has also been used with reported positive effects, but hepatotoxicity in younger individuals is a concern (202). *Propranolol* can reduce rage outbursts, aggression, and severe agitation (152). An open-label study involving 11 subjects suggests that *risperidone* (1 to 4 mg per day) can also reduce repetitive and aggressive behavior in patients with autism (203). A double-blind trial found risperidone more effective than placebo in the short-term management of autistic symptoms in adults (204).

Bipolar Disorder

The differentiation between the emotional vicissitudes of adolescence and more subtle episodes of bipolar disorder can be difficult. Nonetheless, a sizable minority (30%) of adult patients with bipolar disorder report having their first symptoms during adolescence. Furthermore, classic manic (type I) episodes have been observed during adolescence, and the earlier the onset, the more likely the patient will have a psychotic form (14). Childhood-onset mania can be severe and is frequently co-morbid with ADHD and other psychiatric disorders (205).

There are few systematic data on the treatment of adolescence-onset bipolar disorder. Only one single double-blind, randomized clinical trial of a mood stabilizer in adolescents has been reported (206). In this study, Geller and colleagues found that lithium was significantly better than placebo with regard to reducing manic symptoms and secondary drug dependency. Despite these limited data, lithium has become popular among clinicians to treat a wide variety of adolescent behavior problems, reformulated as bipolar disorder, to rationalize the use of this drug. Because of its rapid renal clearance, higher lithium doses may be needed to achieve and maintain plasma concentrations in the range of 0.8 to 1.2 mEq/L. The adverse effects of lithium are similar to those seen in adults, including weight gain, decreased motor activity, excessive sedation, gastrointestinal complaints, pallor, headache, and polyuria. The most serious concerns in children and adolescents are the long-term consequences of lithium accumulation in bone, as well as its effects on thyroid and renal function.

When a patient responds to lithium, the inevitable question of duration of therapy arises. The period of highest risk for relapse is at least the first 6 months after remission, but this vulnerable interval may extend up to 18 months (207). Therefore, many clinicians recommend leaving the lithium-responsive patient on medication for at least 2 years after remission.

Like adults, some adolescents do not respond to lithium, and clinicians often try an anticonvulsant, such as valproate or carbamazepine. The use of these agents is based primarily on their antimanic activity in adults because only a limited number of case reports about the treatment of bipolar adolescents with CBZ are available (207). There are 29 reports in the world literature, however, examining the efficacy of CBZ in the treatment of behavioral dyscontrol or high activity level in children. Of these, three double-blind, placebo-controlled studies were done in the early 1970's and involved a total of 53 patients on CBZ and 53 on placebo (two studies had a crossover design). The majority of subjects had "abnormal EEGs." The overall response rate was 71% for CBZ versus 26% for placebo. The relevance of these results to the use of CBZ to treat mania in children and adolescents is uncertain.

In addition, an open-label study was conducted examining the efficacy of valproate in ten adolescents with chronic temper outbursts and mood lability (193). The authors report that valproate was associated with improvement in all subjects, that discontinuation led to relapse, and that there was subsequent improvement on rechallenge in five of six subjects. Although encouraging, these data are modest in terms of both the numbers and design and must be balanced against the risk of toxicity (e.g., hepatic and pancreatic) with valproate in children.

Because CBZ and valproate have been used for many years to treat seizure disorders in children and adolescents, more systematic knowledge about their clinical pharmacology in this age group is available than there is about lithium. However, pediatric patients with epilepsy are often on concomitant therapy with other anticonvulsants. That fact complicates attempts to extrapolate from this experience to the use of CBZ or valproate as monotherapy for childhood or adolescent bipolar disorder. For example, the risk of serious and potentially fatal hepatotoxicity with valproate occurs almost exclusively in children younger than age 10 years (usually 2 years or younger) who are on multiple anticonvulsants for congenital seizure disorders. How or whether this risk translates to children or adolescents who are on monotherapy with valproate for bipolar disorder is unknown. Nonetheless, clinicians need to be aware of this possible risk and take the following steps to increase the likelihood of early detection in case this problem arises:

- Appropriately warning the patient and the family of the *early symptoms of hepatotoxicity*
- *Monitoring the patient* appropriately during follow-up visits by inquiring about these early symptoms
- Performing *periodic liver function tests*

Other than the question of hepatotoxicity in children and adolescents, there are no other unique toxicity considerations when using anticonvulsants in this age range.

Finally, consistent with the impression that novel antipsychotics may have mood-regulating properties in adults, a recent retrospective chart review found risperidone helpful for manic and aggressive symptoms in 28 juvenile manic patients (208).

Enuresis

Nocturnal enuresis may be caused by the following:

- *Genetic* factors
- Reduced *bladder capacity*
- *Sleep disorders*
- Abnormal secretion of *antidiuretic hormone* (209)
- *Psychological* factors
- *Neurological* factors
- *Bacteria*
- *Diet*

Treatment approaches include pharmacotherapy, behavioral strategies, or a combination of these approaches (210).

Nonpharmacological management is preferable, with an alarm (e.g., bell, vibrator pad) conditioning paradigm considered to be most helpful (211). More recently, *desmopressin nasal spray* (1 to 2 puffs) has been found to be beneficial as a short-term solution and for those unresponsive to the conditioning paradigm. This agent may be used either as the sole therapy or as an adjunct to the alarm method (212). Treatment

with *imipramine* is decreasing because of associated adverse effects, concerns about the potential for a fatal overdose, and a very high relapse rate (212).

Conclusion

Whereas various childhood disorders have been reported to benefit from drug therapies, systematic data to support their use are usually minimal or lacking. An additional complication is the clinically significant pharmacokinetic (and perhaps pharmacodynamic) differences between the adult and younger age groups. Thus, the use of drugs in any treatment plan must be carefully considered and cautiously monitored to maintain the risk–benefit ratio in favor of the child or adolescent patient.

THE PERSONALITY-DISORDERED PATIENT

The DSM-IV currently groups personality disorders into three clusters:

- **Cluster A:** paranoid, schizotypal, schizoid
- **Cluster B:** borderline, antisocial, histrionic, narcissistic
- **Cluster C:** obsessive-compulsive, avoidant, dependent (see Appendix S)

Several studies have noted that some personality disorders may partially benefit from trials with psychotropic agents. Although the majority of trials have involved borderline personality (a Cluster B disorder), no clear specific drug therapy has emerged for this or any other personality disorder. Instead, most authors suggest that drug therapy should be symptom-oriented. Thus, these agents can be targeted to specific symptoms, regardless of the type of personality disorder (213).

With this approach, a variety of symptom presentations might benefit from the same agents indicated for the full diagnostic syndrome, including the following:

- *Antipsychotics*, usually in low doses for brief periods of time, for transient psychosis, paranoia, impulsivity, and cognitive disorders, particularly in Cluster A and borderline patients

- *Antidepressants* for panic attacks, phobias, compulsive symptoms, and depressive syndromes
- *Mood stabilizers* for dyscontrol, rage, violence, affective lability, and impulsivity
- *Anxiolytics* for panic symptoms, social phobia or agoraphobia, and acute conversion symptoms

Ayd (214) has summarized the critical issues to consider whenever considering drug therapy in these patients:

- Emphasize that drugs are *not a panacea.*
- Address *unrealistic expectations* for therapy.
- Always use *concurrent nonpharmacological therapies* in addition to medication.
- *Avoid polypharmacy:* Serial drug substitutions are preferable to concurrent multiple drug use.
- If possible, *avoid drugs that may cause tardive dyskinesia, paradoxical disinhibition,* or *lower the seizure threshold.*
- Continually review for *informed consent.*

Cluster A Disorders

Paranoid Personality Disorder

A few controlled studies and some anecdotal information indicate that low-dose antipsychotics may benefit some of these patients when used in conjunction with psychotherapy (215).

Schizotypal and Related Personality Disorders

In one single-blind study, 17 schizotypal patients were given a modest dose of haloperidol (i.e., 2 to 12 mg per day), which produced some benefit, although many were sensitive to the adverse effects of this drug (216). The study by Goldberg et al. (217) also found that thiothixene benefited both schizotypal disorder and borderline personality disorder (BPD). Similarly, low-dose antipsychotics had a modest effect in patients with both schizotypal and obsessive-compulsive personality disorders (218).

Although the term pseudoneurotic schizophrenia has been dropped from the nomenclature, Klein (219) made an interesting observation regarding the drug treatment of this condition. Specifically, in an investigation comparing the effects of chlorpromazine and imipramine in a wide variety of patients, imipramine was observed to be beneficial. Thus, in this controlled study, imipramine produced a positive outcome in 60% of subjects, in contrast to placebo, which produced only a 25% positive outcome.

Cluster B Disorders

Borderline Personality Disorder

BPD is characterized by a pervasive pattern of unstable affect, stormy interpersonal relationships, and behavioral dyscontrol. An estimated 1% to 2% of the general population manifest this syndrome. It is also a co-morbid condition with major mood disorders (i.e., different studies estimate from 25% to 75% of these patients have a major depression and 5% to 20% a bipolar disorder). Furthermore, as many as 25% of bulimics may also suffer from BPD, and approximately 70% of BPD patients abuse alcohol or drugs. Self-mutilation, suicide attempts, and completed suicides are all too frequent. **Indeed, it is estimated that 3% to 10% of these patients will take their own lives.**

There is a modest link to mood disorders, but it is weak in magnitude and somewhat inconsistent. For example, some studies suggest that BPD often exists in families with other members who have bipolar disorder (220).

The symptoms of BPD can be divided into three groups:

- *Impulsive,* consisting of both aggressive and self-damaging acts, eating disorders, and sensation seeking, which includes substance abuse
- *Affective,* which includes mood lability and depressive symptoms
- *Psychotic*

In this context, New et al. (221) have commented that no single drug treats all three groups of symptoms seen in this disorder.

Treatment of Borderline Personality Disorder

Impulsive Group. One of the problems that plague the investigation of BPD is that many patients fit multiple diagnostic criteria. For example, there is a significant overlap in criteria among hysteroid dysphoria, bipolar type II, and BPDs. It is also extraordinarily difficult to do well-controlled clinical trials with highly disturbed, manipulative patients such as those with acute mania or severe borderline features. Thus, although recognizing the heroic nature of doing such work, it must also be kept in mind that some of the borderline studies include very small sample sizes.

In the multiple crossover study of Gardner and Cowdry (222), which compared various agents with placebo over a 3-week drug trial, there were only six pairs for alprazolam versus placebo, eight pairs for CBZ versus placebo, five pairs for trifluoperazine versus placebo, and eight pairs for tranylcypromine versus placebo. Four of 16 patients on tranylcypromine had a moderate or marked improvement, whereas only 1 of 13 placebo patients showed similar improvement. Of note, those receiving alprazolam had significant increases in dyscontrol in comparison with those on placebo. In another study, Hedberg et al. (223) conducted a double-blind, crossover design in a sample of schizophrenic patients that included 28 characterized as "pseudo-neurotic," 14 of whom responded to tranylcypromine. Thus, these two small-sample studies provide some evidence that tranylcypromine may be beneficial for borderline personality and related disorders (224).

Soloff et al. (225) carried out a particularly important comparison of phenelzine versus haloperidol in BPD with depression. Although this study had reasonable sample sizes (i.e., 38 on phenelzine, 36 on haloperidol, and 34 on placebo), it failed to find a clear advantage for phenelzine over placebo. It did, however, find that phenelzine produced a significantly better improvement in hostility than placebo and a greater antidepressant response than haloperidol. The authors then maintained their patients on these same regimens for an additional 4 months, with little evidence that phenelzine had a continued greater beneficial effect than placebo.

A number of open trials with SSRIs (e.g., fluoxetine and sertraline) in BPD indicate that they may be most helpful for impulsive aggression and irritability (226–231). Salzman (232) has also reported a small, placebo-controlled, double-blind, random-assignment study of fluoxetine in patients with mild to moderately severe borderline personality disturbance. This was a 13-week trial with 13 patients on fluoxetine and nine on placebo. There was a striking reduction in measures of anxiety in those on fluoxetine (i.e., seven times as likely to show decrease in anger versus patients on placebo). Furthermore, this change was independent of the level of depression. Norden (230) investigated 12 patients with BPD without major depression and found that fluoxetine produced substantial improvement, which was maintained through a follow-up period of 6 months. Seventy-five percent of the patients were assessed as much or very much improved for a wide variety of symptoms, including rejection sensitivity, anger, mood lability, irritability, and impulsivity, including substance abuse and overeating. Of note, six patients who interrupted medicine at some point during this lengthy trial experienced an increase in symptoms, which remitted with the resumption of fluoxetine. Thus, this finding supports the Salzman study (232).

Coccaro and Kavoussi (233) conducted a randomized, placebo-controlled study of mixed personality disordered patients (approximately one third were borderline) with impulsive aggression and found fluoxetine decreased aggression to a significantly greater degree in comparison with placebo. At end point, 18 of 27 fluoxetine-treated patients improved in comparison with three of 13 placebo-treated patients. Clinical experience indicates that the effect of an SSRI on impulsivity often occurs early and disappears quickly upon drug discontinuation, which suggests a different mechanism of action than the antidepressant effect. These researchers have also reported on their clinical experience with valproate. In this study, six of eight borderline patients responded with decreases in both irritability and impulsive aggression (234). Pinto and Akiskal (235) also found that several treatment-resistant borderline patients (particularly those with a bipolar component to their illness) had a robust response to lamotrigine over a 1-year period and one had an excellent response to valproate.

Links et al. (236) reported a small, blind, crossover study in BPD patients treated with lithium, desipramine, and placebo. Whereas eight of 13 patients responded to desipramine, six of 12 also responded to placebo. Of those patients with high scores for anger and suicide symptoms, four of 11 responded to desipramine, in comparison with five of six with placebo. Finally, another trial also found CBZ to be beneficial (237).

Affective Group. Conventional TCAs have had a variable and sometimes lackluster effect on the depressive symptoms seen in BPD. Indeed, some studies indicate that these drugs may worsen symptoms, particularly by increasing irritability and agitation (238). By contrast, Cole et al. (239) did a retrospective evaluation of drug response in patients with BPD and major depression, noting that five of six who received TCAs responded, whereas BPD patients without depression treated with a TCA did not respond.

Klein and colleagues (240, 241) investigated the effects of antidepressants in patients with emotionally unstable personalities, a condition characterized by excitability and ineffectiveness when confronted with minor stress. This syndrome is primarily found in female adolescents whose moods consist of short periods of intense unhappiness, social withdrawal, depression and irritability, episodes of impulsivity, rejection of religious rules, and pleasure seeking. They found that imipramine produced improvement in 67% and chlorpromazine produced improvement in 81% of these cases, with both agents demonstrating statistically significantly greater improvement in comparison with placebo.

Rifkin (242) also investigated 21 patients with emotionally unstable character disorder whose core psychopathology consisted of depression or hypomanic mood swings lasting hours to days. Although they had a history of chronic maladaptive behavior patterns (e.g., truancy, poor work history), their symptoms seemed more consistent with bipolar disorder or cyclothymia. Although

there are certain similarities between emotionally unstable character disorder and BPD, the patients described in this double-blind study may have a variant of bipolar disorder. In this light, it is noteworthy that lithium produced a beneficial effect on mood swings. Furthermore, Cowdry and Gardner (224) reported that 10 of 11 similar patients also had a modest improvement in mood when given CBZ.

Although we have reviewed evidence that both MAOIs and SSRIs may benefit the impulsivity cluster of BPD as expected, some of these same studies also demonstrated that these antidepressants were effective in controlling mood. Because patients with BPD are prone to suicide attempts, it is important to remember that TCAs and MAOIs are lethal in overdose, whereas the SSRIs are very safe. Furthermore, this last group may have antidepressant as well as antiimpulsivity and aggression properties.

Psychotic Group. **Several placebo-controlled studies indicate that antipsychotics are efficacious in BPD.** For example, Goldberg et al. (217), in a double-blind, placebo-controlled study of 50 borderline or schizotypal personality-disordered patients, found that thiothixene (mean dose = 8.7 mg per day) was superior to placebo, with improvement most evident for illusions, ideas of reference, and psychoticism. Of note, there were seven patients with BPD only, six with schizotypal personality disorder only, and 11 with both, with meaningful improvement occurring only in the latter two patient groups. In Cowdry and Gardner's multiple crossover design (224), trifluoperazine was compared with tranylcypromine, CBZ, alprazolam, and placebo in 16 female patients with BPD. Although many in the neuroleptic group did not tolerate the drug or clinically deteriorated, the five who completed the trial experienced modest benefit.

Several open studies have also found antipsychotics useful in BPD (214, 243, 244). For example, Leone (244) found that both loxapine and chlorpromazine were effective and equal in most respects.

Soloff et al. (245) compared haloperidol, amitriptyline, and placebo in 61 patients and found the neuroleptic clearly superior to amitriptyline or placebo, particularly for psychotic symptoms. The study is particularly noteworthy in that the sample size is reasonably large, with approximately 28 in each group. Although haloperidol benefited psychotic symptoms (e.g., paranoid ideation, psychoticism), general severity, and depression, it also improved depressive symptoms, as did amitriptyline.

Serban and Siegal (246) investigated a population of borderline-schizotypal personalities and found thiothixene was more effective than haloperidol. This population, however, was less psychotic than those in the earlier studies. Cornelius et al. (247) investigated haloperidol, phenelzine, and placebo in a 4-month continuation study. Those on haloperidol deteriorated faster, with two thirds dropping out in the first 8 weeks in contrast to only one fourth on placebo. Furthermore, those receiving haloperidol showed more depression, particularly in comparison with those on phenelzine. Overall, there were no significant changes on a global assessment scale.

In an open trial of antipsychotics for outpatients with BPD, Teicher and colleagues (243) noted that sustained melancholic depression developed in three patients, necessitating removal from the trial and treatment with antidepressants. In this context, Gardner and Cowdry (248) also reported that melancholia developed in three patients on CBZ, necessitating drug discontinuance and treatment for depression. Hence, clinicians should anticipate that severe depression can develop in some patients with BPD and be prepared to treat with antidepressants.

In Cole's previously mentioned retrospective chart review of BPD, all nine patients falling into the schizophrenic group were given antipsychotics and improved. In addition, three of four patients with major depression who received antipsychotics alone also responded. By contrast, four patients with core BPD without psychosis or depression did not improve on antipsychotics.

Atypical Antipsychotics. Open studies of the atypical antipsychotics are beginning to appear in the literature. Several of these studies have used *clozapine* in chronically hospitalized patients at the very severe end of the borderline personality "spectrum." They report dramatic decreases in psychosis, self-mutilation, aggression, impulsivity, and affective related symptoms (249–251). Frankenburg and Zanarini (252) conducted an open study in 15 patients who met the criteria for BPD but also had a substantial degree of psychosis. Indeed, their highest rating on the Brief Psychiatric Rating Scale (BPRS) was on the suspiciousness, hallucinations, and unusual thought content items. Treatment with clozapine produced substantial improvement, as was evident from a systematic follow-up of these patients, and was effective despite a history of nonresponse to neuroleptics. Because these trials were in hospitalized patients, some with more severe schizophrenia, it may have been the comorbid psychosis that responded to clozapine rather than the BPD per se. By contrast, alprazolam was ineffective, and indeed, seven of 12 patients on this agent either attempted suicide or were assaultive.

In an open study of 11 patients with "typical" borderline personality, Schulz et al. (253) found substantial improvement with *olanzapine,* particularly in psychosis, but also in anergia, hostility, and interpersonal sensitivity. Szigethy and Schulz (254) reported improvement in one patient whose BPRS went from 46 to 28 with *risperidone.* Remission of self-mutilation has also been reported in one borderline patient undergoing treatment with risperidone, as well as an SSRI, for depression (255). This patient was then able to return to a full-time job. Although one should reserve judgment until more definitive studies are completed, the more favorable side effect profile of *risperidone* and olanzapine suggests that these drugs may be useful when psychotic or near psychotic symptoms are present.

BPD can be life-threatening with a stormy course, at times necessitating inpatient hospitalization, or it can be a milder disorder managed on an outpatient basis. Thus, because one sample of patients may be more severely disturbed or has more psychotic features than another, discrepancies in outcome among studies may be due to these differences. In addition, because several studies combine schizotypal and BPDs, it is

important to separate these patients when analyzing the results.

Antisocial Personality Disorder

Antisocial personality disorder is characterized
by a blatant disregard for or violation of other's
rights. Although the relationship between type II
alcoholism and antisocial personality is unclear,
there is excellent evidence that impulsive violence in type II alcoholics may be related to low
brain serotonin levels, as manifested by low cerebrospinal fluid (CSF) 5-HIAA. In this context,
although it has been asserted that the SSRIs may
precipitate suicidal ideation and violence, evidence also indicates that they typically do not induce and can even reduce such impulsivity (256).
This finding leads to the hope that elucidating the
biology of impulsivity may lead to effective drug
treatments.

Sheard (257) investigated men in a maximum
security prison who repeatedly committed aggressive acts but were not psychotic or brain-
damaged. In this blinded study of lithium, he
found that it reduced impulsivity and aggression. Without knowledge of an individual's psychopathology, however, it is difficult to know for
whom lithium may be most useful, but his observation warrants further study. By contrast, Schiff
(258) reported a case in which lithium exacerbated interictal aggression in patients with complex partial seizures.

Histrionic Personality Disorder

Histrionic personality disorder is similar to the
syndrome that Liebowitz and Klein (259) have
termed hysteroid dysphoria or atypical depression. MAOIs have proven to be very helpful in
this condition and these data are reviewed in
Chapter 7. As noted earlier, Rifkin et al. (242)
also investigated the effects of antidepressants
in patients with emotionally unstable personalities, a syndrome characterized by excitability
and ineffectiveness when confronted with minor stress. This syndrome is primarily found in
female adolescents whose moods consist of the
following:

- Short periods of *intense unhappiness*
- *Social withdrawal*
- Depression and *irritability*
- Episodes of *impulsivity*
- *Rejection of religious rules*
- *Pleasure* seeking

They found that imipramine produced improvement in 67% and chlorpromazine helped in
81% of these cases, with both agents demonstrating a statistically significant greater improvement over placebo.

Cluster C Disorders

Obsessive-Compulsive Personality Disorder

Obsessive-compulsive *disorder* is rare in
obsessive-compulsive *personalities*. One study
found that only 6% of these personality disorders
have OCD; thus, it is quite likely that the two
conditions are distinct (260). The implication
for treatment is that agents helpful for OCD
(e.g., clomipramine) may not benefit obsessive-
compulsive personality disorder. Definitive
studies to address this issue have not been
conducted, however.

Avoidant Personality Disorder

Patients with avoidant personality disorder manifest social inhibition, a sense of inadequacy, and
hypersensitivity to negative evaluation. Because
most patients with avoidant personality disorder also have social phobias, these conditions
overlap to a substantial degree. Indeed, some
investigators estimate that as many as 85% of
these patients also meet diagnostic criteria for social phobia (261, 262). Therefore, social phobias
should always be considered when the diagnosis
of avoidant personality is made.

Patients with social phobias feel anxious and
are subject to such peripheral symptoms as
anxiety-like heart palpitations, blushing, and
sweating, especially when they feel people are
looking at or evaluating them.

The prevalence of social phobias is about
2.8%, and they can be subdivided into discrete
and generalized types. Discrete social phobias
consist of anxiety regarding specific activities

such as speaking or performing in public. General social phobia is the fear of interacting with other people and the avoidance of groups, an observation that is confirmed by others. This is different from patients who are pathologically shy or fearful of certain social events, like a cocktail party, where they are concerned about embarrassing themselves or believe that people will be unduly critical. Here, the fear does not lead to physical symptoms such as tremor or rapid heartbeat, but is more like embarrassment and fear of being watched or judged.

Because patients with the formal diagnosis of avoidant personality respond to the same drugs (e.g., MAOIs and SSRIs) that patients with social phobias do, we believe avoidant personalities often include patients with social phobia and should undergo treatment with these drugs (263, 264). Given the present evidence and risk–benefit ratio, SSRIs would be our first-line therapy and MAOIs reserved as a second choice.

Conclusion

Until recently in the United States, a great variety of patients, including some who would now be classified as BPD, were diagnosed as schizophrenic or "borderline" schizophrenic. This is understandable because many patients have difficult psychological problems, often requiring aggressive inpatient intervention. In addition, proper diagnosis and optimal psychopharmacotherapy of all personality disorders are hampered as a result of the lack of a clear separation of co-morbid conditions. Thus, when a patient has two disorders (e.g., schizophrenia or depression plus BPD), treatment becomes more complicated, and simply managing the Axis I condition should not necessarily be construed as adequate treatment of the co-morbid personality disorder. Because SSRIs have a specific effect on obsessive-compulsive symptoms not mediated by their antidepressant effect, and because these agents (as well as MAOIs) benefit social phobia not associated with co-morbid depression, it may be possible to develop similar drug strategies to disentangle other personality disorders from Axis I co-morbid conditions.

It is also possible that there may not be a strict isomorphism between personality disorders and other diagnostic entities. Thus, a "personality disorder" may be a psychological condition that only exists in patients who have a major psychiatric disorder, such as schizophrenia, atypical depression, or social phobia. One example is mania, which can present with interpersonal behaviors such as attacking people's weaknesses, sensitivity to division, and manipulative behavior with staff. This syndrome disappears completely, however, when the patient undergoes treatment with a mood stabilizer.

In summary, major psychiatric disorders co-morbid with various personality disorders should be recognized and properly treated. Although this approach will not alter an underlying and separate personality disorder, it often brings about significant symptomatic improvement. **Implicit in this approach is a drug treatment strategy that targets symptom patterns and not specific personality disorders.**

THE ELDERLY PATIENT

Elderly patients are exquisitely susceptible to the effects of drugs, and there are many reasons for this. Aging affects the following:

- The *cardiovascular* system, with cardiac output and perfusion of other organs diminished
- *Kidney* function, which is slowed because of diminished renal blood flow and glomerular filtration rate
- *Liver* function, which is often compromised

Also associated with these bodily changes is the development of *CNS compromise* as a result of a variety of diseases.

For these reasons, before prescribing any psychoactive drug, clinicians should be familiar with the physical status of the elderly patient, and, equally important, the clinician should always take a comprehensive personal drug history. This includes describing all medicines prescribed for the patient in the prior 6 months, as well as all over-the-counter preparations that elderly patients often use to self-medicate, natural remedies, and the use of alcohol or other substances. A personal drug history may confirm the use of multiple drugs dispensed by several different physicians, most of whom are unaware that other doctors are also prescribing. A good drug history will help identify the following:

- *Noncompliance*
- Potential or actual *adverse drug interactions*
- Inappropriate drug *prescription* or *management*

Finally, a good personal drug history often reveals that iatrogenic polypharmacy contributes to ill health, both physical and psychiatric, in elderly patients.

Pharmacokinetic and Pharmacodynamic Issues

Bodily changes that accompany aging often produce alterations in the pharmacological actions of drugs. Thus, drug absorption and distribution are often modified because of altered blood flow, bodily composition, hepatic metabolism, protein binding, and renal excretion. In addition, there are also age-related effects in receptor sensitivity (i.e., pharmacodynamic changes) (see Chapter 3). Another factor that should not be overlooked in elderly patients is alcohol consumption because of its impact on the clearance of many drugs.

Mindful of the age-related pharmacokinetic changes for all drugs, prescribers of psychotropics should always

- Initiate therapy with a *low dose*
- *Gradually increase the dose* with low increments, days or weeks apart
- Prescribe as *few drugs* as possible
- *Regularly monitor* the patient for therapeutic and adverse drug effects
- Use *TDM* when warranted
- Enlist the patient's collaboration in *individualizing* and *simplifying the drug regimen* as much as possible (e.g., discontinuing all drugs not absolutely necessary)
- Work with the patient to *ensure compliance* by limiting the total number of drugs and by simplifying dosing schedules

Compliance Issues

Compliance with psychopharmacotherapy can be enhanced by fully informing the elderly patient about what can reasonably be expected from the prescribed drug and by enlisting relatives as informed, knowledgeable helpers. This can be achieved by explaining drug therapy to both patients and their relatives using the guidelines such as those recommended by Blackwell (265). Key to rational and effective treatment is the explanation of therapy made to the patient, thus influencing expectations, response, compliance, and the ability to tolerate adverse effects.

The ideal discussion covers the following:

- The *name* of the drug
- Its *appearance*
- *Regimen* and *dose*
- *Reason* for prescribing
- Anticipated *degree* and *rate of response*
- Common or troublesome *adverse effects*
- Likely *duration* of therapy

Adverse effects can be explained in a matter-of-fact way without arousing alarm. The precise nature of the explanation should be tempered to match the patient's clinical state, but it should never be entirely overlooked. An acutely disturbed schizophrenic may comprehend little, but will still cooperate more readily if some rapport is attained. Depressed, anxious, or obsessive patients may require reassurance that they will not become addicted to medication, and it may also be necessary to explain that, although therapeutic effect is somewhat delayed, adverse effects can be immediate.

For some schizophrenic or suicidal patients, explanations should also be given to relatives who may need to assume responsibility, but in other instances it may be important for the patient to assume complete control. The latter may be particularly true of patients who tend to place the onus for a "cure" entirely on the physician.

Finally, it is important to caution the patient about *possible drug interactions* and about *possible interference with activities* such as driving.

Prescribing Drugs for Elderly Patients

Rational psychopharmacotherapy for elderly patients first acknowledges that most of them need few medicines, as Stubbs (266) has emphasized:

> What the elderly needs is to be mentally active, socially active, and physically active–and in that order. Their greatest pleasure is to be independent and to be comfortable. The purpose of treatment is to secure these things for them. Too often, it does the reverse. Medication, which is not simple, may be taken wrongly or may need to be administered by others. Frequent dosage is time-consuming, disturbs social life, and tends in many cases to noncompliance. Ineffective or unnecessary medicines are, to say the least, wasteful. The moment we begin to think about our health, we endanger it, for hypochondriasis has begun. Overtreatment confirms to many people their fears of ill health. The doctor's greatest gift to his patient is courage. To take that away is a poor service indeed. All too often our patients' disabilities are worsened or even due to the very remedies we prescribe.
>
> It is usually possible to discuss with the patient steps proposed in treatment and the gains hoped for. Some will ask for treatment to be simplified. Many are heartened to find they do as well with less. In the case of those already forgetful or muddled, the doctor might well consider what real gain treatment might achieve.
>
> In the old, sedatives and hypnotics are best avoided. When mental capacity or reserve is already reduced, these medicines can only reduce it further. In some people memory is worsened and control of the limbs impaired by as little as half a tablet of nitrazepam at night. Its withdrawal may restore their liberty. Confusion, falls, fractures, fear, urinary incontinence, antisocial behavior, and aggression are all seen at times to be due to sedatives and hypnotics.

Although these points may seem obvious, too many elderly patients leave their physicians' offices without sufficient information about the drugs prescribed for them. Whenever possible, oral instructions should be accompanied by the same information in writing because elderly patients may seem to understand in the office but forget once they get home or when confronted with a particular situation such as a missed dose or a possible adverse effect. Providing the same information to relatives is also beneficial.

In summary, the presence of other medical disorders, other nonpsychotropic agents, expectable changes with aging, and a decreased functional reserve in certain organ systems (e.g., the brain or the kidney) make elderly patients a more difficult population for drug treatment.

Antipsychotics

As a general principle, psychotic disorders in the geriatric age group are the same as those experienced earlier in life. Indeed, manic or schizophrenic patients who are first symptomatic in their late teens often have the same disorder in their 70s and 80s. Although the overall treatment strategy is the same, there may be tactical differences. For example, as noted earlier, elderly patients often suffer from medical problems and, consequently, are receiving a variety of medications. Thus, drug–drug interactions between psychotropics and other general medical agents are a frequent complicating issue. The medical disease itself may also interfere with the use of a psychotropic. Patients with preexisting heart block, for example, may be particularly vulnerable to the conduction disturbances induced by certain psychotropics.

Some of the expected changes with age, such as the reduction in cholinergic neurons or the presence of Alzheimer's dementia, may accentuate the anticholinergic effects of many antipsychotics and antidepressants. **Thus, elderly patients have increased sensitivity to these properties, often resulting in a central anticholinergic syndrome** (267). This condition is characterized by the loss of immediate memory, confusion, disorientation, and florid visual hallucinations, at times superimposed on other psychoses, such as schizophrenia or psychotic depression.

Elderly patients who suffer from schizophrenia, as well as those who suffer from psychotic depression and mania, usually require antipsychotics. In general, however, for most elderly patients, the dosage requirements are substantially lower than for younger age groups. Because many patients may respond to a very small dose and experience excessive adverse effects to doses even lower than those needed when they were younger, the clinician should start with a lower dose (often the lowest dose possible) and adjust upward at a much more gradual rate. Some elderly patients, however, may require moderate or, rarely, high doses. In this patient population, recommended starting doses of novel antipsychotics are as follows:

- Risperidone, 0.25 to 0.5 mg per day (268)
- Olanzapine, 2.5 mg per day (269)
- Quetiapine, 25 mg per day (270)
- Clozapine, 6.25 to 12.5 mg per day (271)

Doses should be slowly increased with the lowest possible increment, and maximal doses are usually one third to one half those recommended for younger adult patients.

Management of Agitation

Agitation in both the demented and the nondemented elderly patient represents an important clinical problem that can occur in nursing homes, state hospitals, or in the patient's own home, as well as when he or she is living with adult children or grandchildren. This phenomenon should not be confused with schizophrenia, mania, psychotic depression, or simple generalized anxiety. Despite the large number of elderly and the importance of managing this common condition, it has received little scrutiny in either open or controlled clinical investigations.

Experienced geriatric psychiatrists generally recommend low doses of antipsychotics for the agitated elderly (272–276). Because these agents are often effective, some have hypothesized a common physiological basis between agitation in the elderly patient and other psychotic processes. Although we know empirically that antipsychotics are effective and anxiolytics are usually ineffective, we do not know whether these agents are uniquely indicated for agitation in those elderly individuals who have never previously experienced a psychotic episode. In part, this is because most studies have intermixed schizophrenia and psychotic depression, as well as other major disorders with agitation, with cases of patients who have no previous history of psychosis. Thus, generalizations about appropriate indications are not possible. A properly designed study should only include those who have a psychosis resulting from either aging or a known brain disorder.

At least two double-blind, controlled studies (277, 278) have found antipsychotics superior to placebo in treating agitation in elderly patients. There have also been five double-blind studies of organic psychosis in state hospital geriatric units (279–283) (Table 14-5). A limited number of studies have focused on psychosis resulting from a wide variety of organic brain disorders (284). This population undoubtedly includes some of the agitated, demented elderly, but differs from the nursing home population, at least in part, because psychosis predominates in these patients; in the nursing home setting, senility is the predominant problem.

More recently, 206 nursing home patients with moderate to severe Alzheimer's dementia with behavior disturbances or psychosis were randomly assigned to either placebo or a fixed dose of olanzapine at 5, 10, or 15 mg per day for up to 6 weeks of treatment (285). In this multicenter, double-blind, placebo-controlled study,

TABLE 14-5. *Drug treatment of organic psychosis*

Study	Number of subjects	Responders (%)		Difference (%)
		AP (%)	Placebo (%)	
Hamilton L, Bennett J (1962)	27	22	0	22
Sugerman A et al. (1964)	18	56	0	56
Rada R, Kellner R (1976)	42	45	20	25
Petrie W et al. (1982)	59	35	9	26
Stotsky B (1984)	363	79	43	36
Totals	**509**	**66%**	**35%**	**31%**

Chi square $= 64$; $df = 1$; $p = 1 \times 10^{-15}$.

olanzapine was significantly more efficacious than placebo in reducing psychosis and behavioral disturbances. The best result was obtained with the 5-mg dose in patients who did not have delusions or hallucinations. Although these patients were selected because of behavioral disturbance, hallucinations, or delusions, 75% did not have hallucinations at baseline, 43% did not have delusions at baseline, and 38% did not have psychosis at baseline. At end point, of those patients without hallucinations at baseline, hallucinations developed in 7.4% on olanzapine, compared with 21.9% on placebo ($p = 0.045$). For those without delusions, 17% of placebo patients and 4% of olanzapine patients experienced delusions. For those subjects without psychosis (i.e., neither hallucinations nor delusions), psychosis developed in 8% of olanzapine patients and 25% of placebo patients ($p = 0.006$). Thus, olanzapine also seemed to prevent the occurrence of psychotic symptoms as the disease progressed.

These limited data show that antipsychotics are clearly superior to placebo, when considering the studies individually or pooling them by a meta-analysis.

Therapeutic Calvinism in the Treatment of Nursing Home Agitation. Elderly patients who receive a variety of medications have a greater propensity for drug–drug, drug–disease, and drug–aging interactions. In a patient with an impaired brain, sedatives may disrupt what little cognitive reserve is left, resulting in a worsening of behavior. Similarly, because anticholinergics may differentially impair memory in a patient with preexisting memory loss, clinicians should avoid using drugs with these properties. For example, because diphenhydramine has substantial anticholinergic properties, it is not the antihistamine or sedative of choice in the elderly patient. Unfortunately, a therapeutic calvinism is developing, which suggests that many of these medications are unnecessary and, indeed, may be harmful. Some report that, with little expense and effort, one can reduce the number of medications prescribed in nursing homes with only a risk of minimal deterioration (286).

This position has resulted in federal agencies mandating the curtailment of psychopharmacological agents, especially antipsychotics, based on documentation of their inappropriate use. As a result, an empirical investigation found a 37% reduction in antipsychotic use 1 year after these regulations were implemented, as well as a 20% reduction in dose; however, there was also an increased mortality rate. This last issue was also noted in an empirical study, in which four deaths occurred in the placebo group (278). Thus, it is possible that untreated agitation may propel some elderly patients into a decompensation, ultimately leading to serious morbidity and even death.

We support the intelligent choice of medications based on rational reasons, but avoid the position that all medication is bad, serving only as a substitute for adequate staffing. In this context, there is a great deal of trial and error in dosage adjustment, and there is no substitute for close monitoring in conjunction with frequent feedback from nursing staff.

Antidepressants

Depressive symptoms occur in about 15% of community residents older than age 65 years (287). The prevalence of major depression in elderly patients is estimated to be about 3%. Notably, a depressive episode is predicted to develop in 13% of patients admitted to a nursing home within 1 year. Elderly patients are even more predisposed to depression than younger age groups because of the following:

- Concurrent *medical disorders*
- Chronic *pain* (288)
- *Increased use of drugs,* both prescribed and over-the-counter
- *Sadness* and *bereavement* as a result of life cycle issues
- Social *isolation*

Although depression may be the most common psychological symptom in old age, the appropriate diagnosis is often missed or mistaken for another condition (e.g., dementia) (289). For example, many older patients complain of cognitive impairment or vague somatic symptoms that are compatible with other commonly suspected or concurrent medical problems, but for which no firm physical basis can be established.

Depression in the elderly patient can be divided into early onset and late-onset types (i.e., first episode occurs at age 60 years or earlier, versus after age 60 years, respectively). The distinction has clinical utility, especially for the late-onset type, in that:

- It is usually *triggered by medical disorders.*
- There is a higher frequency of *cognitive impairment,* cerebral atrophy, white matter changes.
- Genetic and *developmental factors* may play a greater role.
- *Family history* of depression is less frequent.
- *Early insomnia, agitation, hypochondriasis, delusions,* and *atypical presentation* are more frequent with this type.
- There is a higher *mortality* rate.

For example, completed suicide rates in 80- to 84-year-olds are more than twice the ratio in the general population (i.e., 26.5 versus 12.4/100,000).

Several factors must be considered if antidepressant therapy is to be optimized in this age group. In addition to a thorough medical evaluation, as outlined earlier in this chapter as well as in Chapter 1, other potential contributing issues must be considered and dealt with if a satisfactory outcome is to be achieved. These may include the following:

- *Social* situation and *support system*
- Level of *independence*
- *Financial status*

For these, as well as other reasons (e.g., altered life roles, chronic medical disorders), psychosocial therapies must always be included as part of a comprehensive treatment strategy for depression in elderly patients.

Another major problem is that these patients are often either overtreated or undertreated. The former usually occurs when various age-related pharmacokinetic and pharmacodynamic factors are ignored. The latter is most often due to an overly conservative approach because of the patient's advanced age or concurrent medical problems. Finally, an important issue is the frequency of noncompliance (intentional or otherwise) in this group.

Choice of Antidepressant

In contrast to the controlled data available for younger adults, randomized clinical drug trials are limited in the depressed elderly. In general, the most important issues in choosing a drug for the elderly patient are similar to those outlined in Chapter 7. Additionally, increased emphasis should be given to the side effect profile of a drug and the value of TDM to ensure adequate versus toxic or subtherapeutic dosing. For example, in a patient with cardiac conduction delay, the TCAs would not be the ideal first choice. In a physically healthy elderly patient, however, the *cautious use of secondary amine TCAs,* such as nortriptyline or desipramine, may be appropriate because of their clearly defined therapeutic plasma levels, proven efficacy, and known side effect profile.

The *SSRIs* may avoid some of the more serious adverse effects seen with the TCAs. Thus, if expense is not a major concern, the SSRIs are increasingly considered an appropriate first choice (290, 291). *Trazodone* and *bupropion* are also appealing because of their milder anticholinergic and cardiovascular effects (292). With milder mood disturbances, a brief trial with *psychostimulants,* such as *methylphenidate,* can be attempted.

MAOIs are usually not recommended because of uncertainty about adherence to dietary restrictions and the very real problem of hypotension. When used in selected patients, however, phenelzine has been found to be safe and effective. As noted in Chapter 7, however, the eventual introduction of selective, reversible MAOIs, such as moclobemide, may lead to a greater use of this class of antidepressants in all age groups.

For more severe forms of depression, characterized by a rapidly deteriorating course or nonresponsiveness to drug intervention, or in patients with serious concurrent medical disorders, *ECT* may be the most appropriate alternative (see Chapter 8) (293).

Dose **Whatever agent is chosen, a general rule is to start at half the usual adult dose**

(and even lower if organicity is involved) and to increase the drug at a slower rate. Thus, for a drug such as desipramine or nortriptyline, 10 to 25 mg per day may be the best initial strategy. Fluoxetine can be initially given in doses of 5 mg per day, 10 mg per day, or 20 mg every second or third day. Sertraline (initiated at 25 mg per day) is also an appropriate alternative strategy (294). If sedation is required, an agent such as trazodone (e.g., starting dose 25 mg at bedtime) may be used as the primary antidepressant or cautiously in combination with one of the other compounds discussed.

Adequate length of treatment may be longer (e.g., 6 to 12 weeks) in this population as a result of age-related pharmacokinetic and pharmacodynamic changes. TDM may be helpful to ensure levels that are therapeutic and nontoxic. Maintenance doses comparable with acute levels for 6 to 12 months after remission are usually appropriate.

Psychotherapy

A recent review also finds that cognitive-behavioral therapy may be beneficial for older depressed patients either as the sole treatment or in combination with an antidepressant (295).

Mood Stabilizers

As with depression in late life, mania can be divided into early onset and late-onset types. It is estimated that 5% to 10% of elderly patients with affective disorders have manic symptoms (296). Presentation tends to be more atypical, with secondary mania being a much more common phenomenon in the elderly versus younger patient population. As with the younger cohort, mania may be recurrent and disabling in some older patients.

Whereas *lithium* has been the standard approach, increased complications in elderly patients, especially when there is compromise of the CNS, endocrine, or renal systems, makes this agent a less attractive choice. Lower doses (e.g., 150 to 300 mg) should be initiated, with many elderly patients achieving adequate response on total daily doses of lithium in the 450- to 600-mg range. If a more rapid response is necessary,

low-dose high-potency antipsychotics can also be used in the early phases. Alternatively, a BZD, such as clonazepam or lorazepam, may be indicated (297).

An alternate strategy to lithium may be an anticonvulsant. For example, an open trial in seven elderly patients found that *valproate* produced marked to moderate improvement in five previously refractory patients. Furthermore, the drug appeared safe in this group of patients who also suffered from several medical disorders (298). Clearly, controlled trials in this age group are necessary to clarify the relative risk—benefit ratio of the available mood stabilizers.

Benzodiazepines

As a symptom, *anxiety* appears to be common among elderly patients, and Table 14-6 lists frequent factors that underlie this symptom (299). Nevertheless, only limited data are available on the incidence and prevalence of anxiety disorders in this population (300). Simple phobia may be the only anxiety disorder with an onset after age 60 years (301). According to an Epidemiologic Catchment Area Survey, phobic disorders may be the most common anxiety-related condition among those older than age 65 years, followed by GAD. By contrast, panic disorder may be relatively rare (302, 303). As in younger adults, anxiety in elderly patients may be due to a variety of causes; however, recent onset of nonphobic anxiety suggests an organic or iatrogenic basis that merits thorough investigation before treatment is initiated (300).

Sleep disturbances are common among elderly patients. According to a National Institutes of Health (NIH) Consensus Development Conference, disrupted sleep afflicts more than half of Americans age 65 years or older who live at home and about two thirds of those who live in long-term care facilities (304). Although changes in sleep–wake patterns appear to accompany advancing age, disrupted sleep may also be secondary to a wide variety of factors (302). As with anxiety, careful diagnosis is important before any treatment is initiated. Factors that commonly contribute to disturbed sleep are listed in Table 14-7.

TABLE 14-6. *Factors that may cause anxiety in the elderly*

Physical illness
  Respiratory disease
  Cardiac disease
  Gastrointestinal syndromes
  Anemia
  Metabolic disorders
  Endocrine disorders
Psychiatric/neurological illness
  Major depressive disorder
  Alzheimer's disease
  Delirium
  Seizure disorders
  Encephalopathies
  Postconcussion syndrome
Other
  Withdrawal syndromes (alcohol, nicotine,
    caffeine, sedatives, hypnotics)
  Grief and mourning
  Hospitalization
  Institutionalization
  Insomnia
Drugs
  Caffeine
  Alcohol
  Bronchodilators
  Salicylates
  Sympathomimetics
  Antiparkinsonian agents
  Neuroleptics (akathisia)
  Hypotensive agents
  Steroids
  Anorectics
  Diuretics
  Digitalis toxicity
  Anticholinergic toxicity

Choice of Benzodiazepine

If BZDs are used in elderly patients, they should be prescribed at the lowest possible dose for the shortest possible time, and on an intermittent rather than a regular basis. The decision to use these agents should be made with considerable caution, and only after possible underlying causes of the patient's symptoms have been explored and treated appropriately. Although surveys indicate that BZDs are frequently prescribed for elderly patients, the NIH Consensus Development Conference stated that the efficacy and safety of sedatives and hypnotics have not been established for older people, nor has the extent to which they contribute to or alleviate sleep problems (302,

305, 306). Salzman (307) has pointed out that relatively few research studies, most of which are seriously flawed, have examined the therapeutic effect of these agents in elderly patients. **Thus, recommendations for the use of BZDs in elderly patients are derived almost exclusively from studies of young adult patients, studies of pharmacokinetics and toxicity in elderly patients, and clinical and anecdotal experience.**

TABLE 14-7. *Factors that may disturb sleep in the elderly*

Physical illness
  Respiratory disease
  Cardiac disease
  Arthritis, pain syndromes
  Prostate disease
  Endocrine disease
  Sleep apnea syndrome
  Restless legs syndrome
Psychiatric/neurological illness
  Major depressive disorder
  Anxiety disorders
  Alzheimer's disease
  Delirium
Environment
  Situational anxiety
  Hospitalization
  Poor sleep hygiene
  Extensive bed rest
  Lack of appropriate exercise
  Confinement to a nursing home
  Circadian rhythm disturbances
  Noise
  Nondiuretic nocturia
  Light
  Grief and mourning
Drugs
  Alcohol
  Nicotine
  Caffeine
  Long-term use of hypnotics (prescription and
    over-the-counter)
  Diuretics
  Bronchodilators
  Steroids
  Respiratory stimulants
  β-Blockers
  Corticosteroids
  Alerting antidepressants
  Monoamine oxidase inhibitors
  Immunosuppressants
  Methyldopa
  Phenytoin

Age can significantly alter the pharmacokinetics of BZDs metabolized by oxidation, tending to reduce their clearance (see also Chapters 3 and 12). This change may lead to drug accumulation and possible toxicity during chronic administration, particularly in elderly men (308). BZDs transformed by conjugation have relatively short half-lives and accumulate less during multiple dosing, in part because the conjugation (as opposed to the oxidation) process appears to be less influenced by age. Age also appears to enhance pharmacodynamic sensitivity to BZDs, so that at any given plasma or brain concentration, the elderly patient experiences an increased intensity of drug effect compared with the younger patient (308). In addition, physical or emotional illness (e.g., stroke, Parkinson's disease, dementia, and disorders that impair protein binding, hepatic metabolism, or renal clearance) may increase sensitivity. Finally, concomitant use of other drugs with CNS effects (e.g., antidepressants, stimulants, steroids, alcohol) may exacerbate BZD toxicity (307).

Adverse Effects

Use of both long and short half-life BZDs in elderly patients has been associated with a number of potentially serious unwanted effects, of which the most common are excessive sedation and cerebellar, psychomotor, and cognitive impairment (Table 14-8).

Although short half-life BZDs are usually recommended for the elderly patient because they are less likely to accumulate and are rapidly eliminated, few comparisons have been made of their effects on performance in the elderly population. In one study of nonanxious elderly volunteers, both diazepam (long half-life, oxidation) and oxazepam (short half-life, conjugation) produced comparable self-rated sedation and fatigue during long-term administration (303). These effects persisted in diazepam subjects during a 2-week washout period, but rapidly returned to baseline in the oxazepam subjects.

Long half-life BZDs may increase the risk of daytime sedation, lethargy, cognitive impairment, and delirium, as well as falls and hip fractures (309–311). Long-term use of flurazepam

TABLE 14-8. *Adverse effects of benzodiazepines in the elderly*

CNS depression
   Excessive sedation
   Drowsiness
   Fatigue
Cerebellar
   Ataxia
   Dysarthria
   Incoordination
   Unsteadiness
   Falls, hip fractures
Psychomotor
   Slowed reaction time
   Diminished motor accuracy
   Impaired eye-hand coordination
CNS stimulation
   Paradoxical excitement
   Nightmares
   Insomnia
   Agitation
   Hallucinations
   Belligerence
Cognitive
   Confusion
   Anterograde amnesia
   Impaired short-term recall
   Increased forgetfulness
   Decreased attention
   Delirium

(30 mg per day) has been associated with an increased incidence of ataxia and hallucinations (312). However, short half-life BZDs also may cause serious adverse effects. Ataxia, depression, confusion, amnestic syndromes, and oversedation have been reported in elderly lorazepam users, and there is some evidence that short-acting BZDs may also increase the risk of falls (313–317).

Triazolam. In 1983, the FDA approved triazolam, 0.5, 0.25, and 0.125 mg based on data suggesting these doses would be safe and effective. Five years later, the FDA withdrew the 0.5-mg dose from the United States market, but continued approval of the 0.125-mg dose and the 0.25-mg dose (currently the recommended starting dose for nonelderly insomniacs) without new studies to demonstrate its efficacy in such patients. These actions were in response to scientific data indicating the risk of adverse reactions to triazolam is dose-dependent, a fact not emphasized by either the manufacturer or by the FDA.

In the early 1990's, the Committee on Safety of Medicines of the United Kingdom concluded that the risks of treatment with triazolam at the licensed doses (0.25 and 0.125 mg) outweighed the benefits. The United Kingdom and a few other countries banned triazolam primarily because of persistent reports of adverse reactions. As of 1992, France, Spain, and New Zealand suspended the 0.25-mg dose of triazolam but allowed continued marketing of the 0.125-mg dose, whereas Canada and Japan lowered the recommended starting dose for nonelderly insomniacs to 0.125 mg.

Since 1992, the FDA approved labeling on triazolam recommending that prescriptions be written only for short-term (7 to 10 days) treatment of insomnia, that use for more than 2 to 3 weeks requires a complete reevaluation of the patient, and that for geriatric or debilitated patients, a dose of 0.25 mg should not be exceeded, with higher doses being reserved for exceptional cases.

Between 1980 and 1991, only a few published studies examined the safety and the hypnotic efficacy of the 0.125-mg dose of triazolam in elderly patients (318–324). These studies and case reports indicate that with continued use, the initial efficacy of the 0.125-mg dose of triazolam in elderly patients begins to wane after 1 week and progressively diminishes to ineffectiveness, usually by the sixth week of continuous administration. During the same period, the risk of potentially serious adverse reactions increases.

One study evaluated only the cognitive effects of single doses of 0.125-mg triazolam (324). Although the others assessed hypnotic efficacy, in all but one of these, study duration was 2 to 14 nights. In the remaining study, with a duration of 3 to 9 weeks, five of 22 elderly subjects (23%) were taken off triazolam between the third and fifth weeks because of serious adverse effects (323). The researchers reported, "At week 3 significantly more triazolam patients were rated as more restless during the day ($p < 0.05$) and they also appeared more hostile, less relaxed, more irritable, and more anxious. After withdrawal of triazolam, these adverse reports were reduced.... Our study suggests that the use of triazolam in

older patients, given in conservative doses, may have significant disadvantages."

The investigators who studied only the cognitive effects of triazolam (0.125 mg) stated, "Elderly persons may remain unaware of or fail to express on standard rating instruments, the sedative effects of triazolam seen by an observer and evident in the results of tests of psychomotor function and memory" (321).

Triazolam may cause sedation, learning and memory impairment, confusion, irritability, paranoid delusions, aggression and irrational behavior, reversible delirium, anterograde amnesia, and automatic movements (314, 325–329). In a placebo-controlled study of the pharmacokinetic and pharmacodynamic effects of single doses (0.125 and 0.25 mg) of triazolam in healthy young and elderly subjects, triazolam caused a greater degree of sedation and greater impairment of psychomotor performance in the elderly than in the young subjects (324). Triazolam also has a narrow therapeutic range in elderly patients, and overdosage may occur with as little as 2 mg, an amount only four to eight times the recommended dose (330). Three cases of fatal triazolam overdose have been reported in elderly patients who were debilitated or had taken other psychotropic drugs and alcohol (331).

BZD-induced amnesia, confusion, depression, and oversedation in elderly patients may be misdiagnosed as dementia (332).

Sedatives and hypnotics as a group, and BZDs in particular, are frequently implicated in drug-related hospital admissions in the elderly (333, 334). This group is at particular risk for abrupt drug discontinuation when hospitalized, with resulting withdrawal symptoms that may be unrecognized as such and attributed to other health problems (313, 335–337). BZD hypnotics should not be routinely prescribed in the hospital unless the patient has a demonstrated sleep disorder (338). Even then, reassurance that restless sleep is normal in such a situation may obviate the need for a hypnotic (330).

Patients with Breathing Disorders. Some evidence indicates that BZDs may exacerbate breathing difficulties in patients with chronic lung disorders (339, 340). Because flurazepam has been reported to exacerbate sleep apneas in middle-aged and elderly normal volunteers, the possibility of undiagnosed sleep apnea should always be considered before a BZD is prescribed (341).

Demented Patients. As mentioned earlier in the discussion on antipsychotics, although BZDs are commonly used to treat the severe agitation, anxiety, and restlessness that may accompany dementia, response is unpredictable (342). These drugs may exacerbate confusion and agitation, producing mild-to-severe amnestic syndromes resembling dementia of the Alzheimer's type (343–347). Demented elderly patients may also be at risk for BZD-caused oversedation (272, 346, 347). If long half-life BZDs are used, oversedation and aggravation of dementia may become chronic (272). Buspirone is often a useful alternative (348).

Although severe disruption in the sleep–wake cycle is a common feature of dementia, the use of BZDs in such cases may also produce significant behavioral toxicity. Alternative drug approaches include bedtime use of olanzapine in nondepressed patients or trazodone in depressed patients.

Benzodiazepine Discontinuation in Elderly Patients

Evidence indicates that abrupt discontinuation of long-term BZD use may be associated with severe withdrawal symptoms, including confusion, disorientation, and hallucinations in elderly patients (332, 336, 337). Gradual discontinuation, however, appears to be tolerated as well by the elderly patients as by the younger patients (349). The cognitive impairment associated with BZD administration is reversible with drug discontinuation, often improving memory and concentration (306, 307).

BZD hypnotics such as midazolam and triazolam are primarily metabolized via the P450 3A3/4 microenzyme system. Other BZDs often used as hypnotics, such as diazepam, can also be metabolized by CYP 33/4 and CYP 2C19. Any drugs that act as inhibitors or inducers of these isoenzymes could increase or decrease BZD levels, respectively (350). Thus, ketocona-

zole, macrolide antibiotics (e.g., erythromycin), SSRIs (e.g., fluoxetine-norfluoxetine and fluvoxamine), and other antidepressants (especially nefazodone) may decrease clearance and increase BZD levels to potentially toxic ranges. Conversely, rifampacin, CBZ, and dexamethasone may increase clearance and decrease BZD levels to potentially subtherapeutic ranges.

Alternative Therapies

Drug Therapy

Despite the serious drawbacks to the use of BZDs in elderly patients, there are few pharmacological alternatives. *Barbiturates* and *meprobamate* have a high incidence of adverse effects and toxicity and should not be used. Small doses of *sedating antidepressants*, although generally well tolerated as hypnotics in younger patients, may produce a higher incidence of anticholinergic effects in the elderly. *Antihistamines,* a common ingredient in over-the-counter sleeping aids, are less effective than BZDs and may cause delirium if dosage is not carefully adjusted. Although *chloral hydrate* is contraindicated in patients taking drugs that may interact adversely with it (e.g., warfarin, phenytoin), it is unlikely to cause habituation or delirium (330). Confusion and hallucinations, however, have been reported (351).

Buspirone may be an effective anxiolytic in the elderly patient and less likely than BZDs to produce excessive sedation (352–355). Dizziness, however, may be a problem. *Zolpidem* or *zaleplon,* particularly in lower doses (i.e., 2.5 to 5.0 mg at bedtime) may be viable alternatives (356). The elimination half-life of these two agents is approximately 3 hours in the elderly. Although it has sleep-enhancing properties similar to BZD hypnotics, it is less likely to alter sleep architecture. Whereas *antidepressants* and *β-blockers* may be useful alternatives in younger patients, no data document their effectiveness for anxiety in elderly patients (307). Although *antipsychotics* may be helpful in reducing severe agitation, their side effect profile makes them unsuitable for use in subjective anxiety states (300, 307).

Nondrug Therapies

Nondrug therapies include patient education regarding the following:

- Good *sleep hygiene* and what constitutes "normal" sleep
- *Avoidance of stimulating substances* (alcohol, caffeine)
- *Reduction of environmental stimuli* that may disturb sleep (noise, light)
- *Reducing worry* at bedtime
- *Regular exercise* (302) (see also Chapter 12)

Efforts directed toward helping patients understand and cope with specific problems (e.g., bereavement, finances, illness, reduced social interactions) should be considered whenever possible. Various psychotherapies may also be useful (300).

Whenever considering drug treatment of dyssomnia in an elderly patient, several issues should be carefully considered. The first is whether a sleep disorder can be explained by another psychiatric or medical condition, which should be addressed first (e.g., an antidepressant for sleep disruption prescribed after a major depressive episode or analgesics in a patient with disabling pain of arthritis). Next, consider whether any prescribed or nonprescribed drugs could explain the disorder. Over-the-counter agents and excessive caffeine ingestion may go unappreciated unless inquired about. Nonpharmacological interventions often suffice. In particular, a detailed review of sleep hygiene issues combined with instruction about stimulus control and sleep restriction may be most useful.

If a medication is judged appropriate, we suggest an initial trial with low doses of zolpidem or zaleplon (e.g., 2.5 to 5 mg at bedtime) or a short- to intermediate-acting BZD hypnotic (e.g., estazolam, 0.5 to 1 mg at bedtime). When drug therapy is initiated, it is extremely important to monitor older patients for cumulative effects, given their heightened organ system sensitivity (e.g., CNS) and decreased clearance rates (e.g., hepatic compromise). If sleep problems persist beyond 2 weeks, a careful reassessment of diagnosis should be undertaken before represcribing a sedative-hypnotic.

Conclusion

Like for the very young, the aging body and mind are in many respects uncharted territory when considering psychopharmacotherapeutic interventions. What is known is that drug management is often unnecessary, may do more harm than good, and when used may adversely interact with a host of other medications that elderly patients require. Although the judicious use of psychotropics may be warranted in certain situations, the clinician must remain especially vigilant when choosing this course of action.

THE DYING PATIENT

Perhaps no other area in medicine and psychiatry has been more neglected than the appropriate role of psychopharmacotherapy for the dying patient (357). The need for more careful attention to and, when ethically feasible, controlled studies in this area is supported by a report from the National Hospice Study, which found that a variety of psychotropic drugs were used to manage terminal cancer, including antidepressants in 3% of patients, antihistamines in 2%, barbiturates in 7%, BZDs in 16%, and antipsychotics in 7% (358). In this context, our intention is to review the role of these agents in the dying patient as part of an overall treatment strategy to effectively manage their symptoms, as well as to improve their quality of life.

Patients often undergo a protracted course [e.g., acquired immunodeficiency syndrome (AIDS), newly diagnosed cancer, primary degenerative dementia], whose ultimate outcome may be years away. This allows for numerous opportunities to intervene with a variety of therapeutic modalities including various psychotropics, depending on the particular phase or presenting symptoms. The eventual goal of all these therapeutic interventions is to provide the best circumstances possible to enhance the quality of life and ultimately for a peaceful death.

While we focus on medication management, Fawzy et al. (359) have emphasized the integral role of various psychiatric interventions, including the following:

- Health *education*
- *Behavioral training* and *stress management*
- Individual *psychotherapy*
- Short-term, structured, psychosocial *support groups*

Complicating the proper assessment and, by implication, the most appropriate therapy for many patients, is the very real possibility of neuropsychiatric syndromes that may mimic classic psychiatric disorders, exacerbate them, or coexist with such disorders as major depression, panic attacks, and brief reactive psychosis. Thus, the CNS may be affected by various primary malignancies or secondary metastases; cardiovascular disorders, leading to ischemic episodes or hemorrhagic events; and several HIV-related complications.

Analgesics

One of the primary goals is to control pain. Thus, pain must frequently be factored into both the assessment and treatment equations, because it is often an ongoing symptom for the terminally ill. Its management, as well as the amelioration of associated psychiatric disturbances, is a major focus. For example, the World Health Organization has summarized the basic pharmacological principles of cancer pain management in an "analgesic ladder" (360, 361), which incorporates the following recommendations:

- *Mild pain:* nonopioid analgesic with or without an adjuvant agent
- *Moderate pain:* weak opioid with or without a nonopioid or adjuvant agent
- *Severe pain:* strong opioid with or without a nonopioid or adjuvant agent

Adjuvant agents can include a variety of drugs, many of which are psychotropics (e.g., antidepressants, anticonvulsants, anxiolytics, antipsychotics, psychostimulants).

Although a common and severe problem in certain disorders, pain is frequently mismanaged (362). In part, this may be due to the incorrect use of analgesics, but it may also be complicated by a "cure-oriented" culture and concerns about

criticism for practicing euthanasia (363). In this context, the hospice movement has provided a means for terminally ill patients to be cared for in the intimate and comforting surroundings of their own homes, while affording the family or significant others the opportunity to serve as primary caregivers.

There are two major classes of pain medications, nonopioids and opioids. The *nonopioids* used to treat *mild pain* include agents such as acetaminophen, both steroid and nonsteroidal antiinflammatory drugs (NSAIDs), and acetylsalicylic acid. Anticonvulsants suppress neuronal firing and are also helpful in neuropathic pain. Antiinflammatory agents (e.g., NSAIDs or corticosteroids) may be particularly helpful when bony involvement occurs and are often used for low-intensity pain. Steroids decrease inflammatory edema and are useful in cases of nerve and spinal cord compression, lymphedema, visceral pain caused by organ enlargement, and bone pain. Finally, short-term corticosteroid therapy may also produce euphoria (thus ameliorating less severe depressions) as well as reverse anorexia.

Moderate pain can be treated by *nonopioid–weak opioid* combinations, such as acetaminophen with codeine, or acetaminophen with oxycodone. The *strong opioids,* such as morphine and hydromorphone, are the primary agents used to treat severe pain. Transdermal or oral transmucosal *fentanyl* (an anesthetic found to have analgesic properties) is another option and can be effective for up to 72 hours (364, 365). Opioid doses should be adjusted to the patient's report of discomfort, recognizing that those with chronic pain often do not display the usual objective signs such as moaning, grimacing, or decreased activity. "As-needed" dosing is not appropriate for continuous pain, and long-acting morphine can be given orally every 8 to 12 hours, with short-acting morphine as needed for breakthrough pain. Morphine has no ceiling effect, and the risk of respiratory depression and sedation is low as long as pain is present (366). Addiction should not be a concern, even though a patient becomes tolerant to drugs and requires higher doses, especially because pain often increases as the disease advances. Clonidine or bupivacaine combined with epidural narcotic analgesics have been used to control intractable pain, especially when neurogenic in origin (367). **Meperidine should *never* be used when caring for terminally ill patients because of its short half-life, toxic metabolites, and poor oral efficacy** (368).

Antipsychotics may be useful adjuncts, facilitating sedation, diminishing nausea and vomiting, and perhaps serving as coanalgesics. *Antidepressants* such as the SSRIs (e.g., fluoxetine, sertraline, paroxetine) or amitriptyline enhance CNS serotonin activity, a neurotransmitter that inhibits pain, with the usual analgesic dose of these agents often being lower than that required for an antidepressant effect (369). *Anticonvulsants* such as CBZ or clonazepam may improve neuropathic pain when used alone or in combination with antidepressants (370).

Although analgesics and adjuvant agents are the mainstay of effective pain management, nondrug approaches such as relaxation techniques, imagery, and hypnosis can also help to raise a patient's threshold for pain, allowing for lower doses or less frequent administration of such agents.

Anxiolytics and Sedative-Hypnotics

Anxiety is a universal phenomenon, occurring in myriad circumstances. Dying patients experience various degrees of apprehension, at times culminating in debilitating anxiety (e.g., GAD, panic attacks, phobic symptoms). Whereas a variety of anxiolytics, antidepressants, and narcotics may ease the anxiety of these patients, perhaps the most therapeutic intervention that can be offered is a person's time to lend support and empathy. Indeed, adequate contact or providing other allied specialists to offer support and the opportunity to express feelings may often diminish or even preclude the need for antianxiety medication. Thus, initial strategies to reduce stress and related symptoms, including supportive psychotherapy, deep breathing exercises, guided imagery, and hypnosis, can all be helpful in minimizing a patient's discomfort (371).

In more severe episodes, especially those complicated by panic, BZDs may be useful. In this context, we emphasize that patients should be actively discouraged from using over-the-counter sedatives, many of which possess significant anticholinergic properties. Clinicians also need to consider the cumulative effects of BZDs, because they are primarily metabolized through the liver, and hepatic function of these patients is often compromised. Thus, agents with longer half-lives (e.g., diazepam, flurazepam) may result in excessive daytime sleepiness, apathetic states, and confusion, with or without paradoxical agitation (which may already be present as part of the dying process), and should be avoided. Agents with the shortest half-life, such as triazolam, may not be well tolerated either because they often cause interdose withdrawal symptoms, amnesia, and worsening of neurocognitive functioning. *Thus, short- to intermediate-acting agents, such as oxazepam, lorazepam, and alprazolam, are preferable.* Lower initial doses (e.g., 0.5 to 1 mg lorazepam or 0.25 to 0.5 mg alprazolam given on an as-needed basis) are the preferred strategy. As a patient reaches an end-stage phase and is unable to swallow, lorazepam can be given sublingually or subcutaneously in much higher doses (up to 2 mg every 1 to 2 hours as needed).

Midazolam has also been used as an effective medication in palliative medicine when symptom management supersedes the problem of side effects (372, 373). It is used for a variety of indications, including for terminal agitation, for muscle relaxation, and as an anticonvulsant. Recommended therapy is a loading subcutaneous dose of 5 to 10 mg, depending on weight, age, and degree of debility, followed by a continuous infusion of 1.5 mg per hour. The rate is titrated by 0.5 to 1.0 mg per hour, with boluses of 3.0 mg.

An alternative strategy, particularly when considering a drug to alleviate sleep disturbances, may be a sedating antidepressant such as *trazodone* (25 to 50 mg at bedtime). A second strategy is the use of the nonbenzodiazepine anxiolytic *buspirone* (5 to 15 mg per day as a starting dose). Although this agent appears to avoid many of the complications associated with BZDs, its slower onset of action and lack of benefit in some patients have limited its use. A third approach may be the *opioids*, which when used to control pain can also alleviate anxiety. For example, morphine for those with advanced terminal illness has been particularly helpful in decreasing associated anxiety, especially in those experiencing significant dyspnea.

Antipsychotics

Often, toxic organic states that may be complicated by psychotic symptoms develop in terminally ill patients. Acute confusion has been reported in up to 85% of terminal cancer patients, with restlessness and agitation occurring in up to 42%. Unfortunately, the cause of delirium is determined in only 21% of these patients (373, 374). Common sources can include the following:

- Hyponatremia
- Hypoglycemia
- Hypercalcemia
- Medications (including steroids, nonprescription medication, digoxin, and anticholinergic drugs)

Whereas the development of classic disorders such as schizophrenia in a dying patient with no previous history is an unlikely occurrence, many symptoms, such as hallucinations, delusions, and disordered thinking, are commonly encountered. Some episodes may be reversible and, when the causative source is recognized, can be readily treated by the physician. For example, high-dose steroids are often used to manage metastatic brain lesions, but it is also well known that they can induce a psychotic state. Simply reducing the dose, when possible, may quickly abort a psychotic episode.

When medication is required to manage psychotic symptoms, low-dose, higher potency antipsychotics with less problematic adverse effect profiles are usually the drugs of choice. Thus, agents such as haloperidol or risperidone, lower in anticholinergic, antihistaminic, and α-adrenergic blocking properties, are better than antipsychotics possessing such properties (e.g., chlorpromazine, thioridazine). Doses required are often dramatically less than the typical starting amounts used in a healthy, young adult

schizophrenic patient. Patients experiencing a toxic organic psychosis can often be managed with as little as 0.5 to 1 mg haloperidol given i.m. or i.m. or risperidone given in liquid form in doses as low as 0.25 mg, with doses repeated on an as-needed basis. In the home, haloperidol can also be given orally or subcutaneously. Standard doses (e.g., 5 to 10 mg per day haloperidol, 3 to 6 mg per day risperidone) are not generally necessary and may worsen rather then improve a toxic psychotic state. The rule is to start with very low amounts and to proceed very slowly with small dose increments.

It is also important to remember that these agents are primarily metabolized by the liver, and because various medical disorders can compromise hepatic function (e.g., congestion secondary to heart failure, metastases, or cirrhotic states), the elimination half-lives of these drugs may be significantly prolonged. This may lead to excessive accumulation over several days to weeks of treatment, ultimately culminating in further deterioration. Thus, the judicious use of as-needed or short-term drug use is ideal.

Antidepressants and Mood Stabilizers

Depression

If depression occurs, it is usually a transitory phenomenon, requiring sensitivity and supportive interventions to help work through this phase of the dying process (375). Indeed, feelings of loss, loneliness, hopelessness, anxiety, grieving, and spiritual distress are at times more intense than the physical symptoms, and social withdrawal is a natural occurrence as the active phase of dying begins (375, 376).

More severe forms of depression with classic neurovegetative signs can pose a complicated management issue. For example, many of the classic depressive signs and symptoms (e.g., anorexia, weight loss, disrupted sleep, fatigue, psychomotor retardation) are not only typical of a major depression but also common in patients suffering from a terminal condition.

As noted earlier, because the possibility of an unrecognized neuropsychiatric phenomenon is always a danger, antidepressants with fewer adverse effects, particularly anticholinergic-related, are the preferred treatment. Little information is available on the use of more recent antidepressant classes (e.g., SSRIs, bupropion, venlafaxine, nefazodone, or mirtazapine) for the dying patient. If drug therapy is required and there is a significant agitated component (e.g., insomnia, anxiety) associated with the episode, a more sedating agent, such as trazodone, may be helpful, especially because it has anticholinergic and cardiotoxic properties (377). In patients in whom excessive fatigue or sedation is a problem, low doses of less sedating drugs, such as bupropion (e.g., 25 mg) or fluoxetine (e.g., 5 to 10 mg), may be more useful.

Suicide

In any terminally ill patient, the issue of suicide must be acknowledged and discussed, especially during periods of more severe depression. As a patient's physical and cognitive status begins to deteriorate, the risk may become even greater. For example, it is estimated that patients with Huntington's disease have a 25% suicide rate during the course of their illness (378, 379). In contrast, fewer patients suffering from terminal cancer commit suicide (380).

Developing good rapport early in the treatment relationship is critically important so that the individual can more comfortably talk about increasing thoughts or intentions of suicide. During the course of their decline, many terminally ill patients verbalize, "Is life worth living like this?" or "I wish this were over; how long can this go on?" Caregivers should listen supportively, validate these feelings as normal, and attempt to find ways to improve the quality of life.

In more emergent circumstances (e.g., mood is rapidly deteriorating), patients suffering from such conditions as Huntington's or AIDS may benefit from a course of ECT, which can often work quickly, perhaps avoiding an unnecessary tragic outcome. To achieve optimal efficacy and minimize cognitive complications, unilateral-nondominant electroconvulsive therapy with high electrical dose stimulus may be the preferable method of administration, if this modality is used (381, 382).

Mania

Manic syndromes are a possible complication in terminal patients, even in those who do not have a prior personal or family history of bipolar disorder. Gilmer and Busch (383), for example, reported on one AIDS patient in whom manic symptoms developed associated with zidovudine (AZT) therapy, which remitted when the drug was discontinued, only to return when reintroduced. They also reported on two other patients who were able to continue AZT when lithium was added to control their manic symptoms. Although not as common as depression, anxiety, and reactive psychosis, when mania occurs, it may pose a more serious hazard. Thus, given the often belligerent and explosive nature of the syndrome, an effective treatment must be quickly instituted. Again, very low doses of a more potent antipsychotic, such as haloperidol (0.5 to 5 mg i.v., repeated as necessary) may abort the development of a full manic syndrome. This may be a particularly useful strategy in HIV patients, because the intravenous route of administration is less likely to induce acute extrapyramidal reactions, in contrast to the more typical oral administration. Alternatively, olanzapine has been demonstrated to have antimanic, as well as antipsychotic effects (384, 385). Its anticholinergic properties, however, must be considered, dictating lower and perhaps less effective doses.

Conclusion

Traditional medical interventions seek a cure or attempt to prolong life. Many terminally ill patients no longer wish to prevent death, but rather want to die peacefully and pain-free at home. The treatment of such cases is often complicated by the frequent development of psychiatric symptoms, in addition to the terminal disease process. Effective strategies are needed to manage pain, anxiety, psychosis, depression, and mania. With increasing frequency, drug therapies are used in the context of the hospice movement, which developed out of the specialized needs of the dying patient, perhaps too long overlooked by the medical profession. **Thus, psychiatrists should anticipate increasing involvement in the hospice team, with a special reliance on their expertise in psychopharmacotherapy.**

THE ALCOHOLIC PATIENT

The World Health Organization defined alcoholism as a chronic behavior disorder manifested by repeated drinking of alcoholic beverages in excess of community norms for dietary and social purposes and to an extent that it interferes with one's health or social and economic functioning (386).

Subsequently, a committee composed of representatives from the National Council on Alcoholism and Drug Dependence and the American Society of Addiction Medicine have developed a definition that includes typical behavioral changes, as well as the concept of denial (387). They characterized alcoholism as the following:

• A *primary chronic disease* with genetic, psychosocial, and environmental factors influencing its development and manifestations
• Often *progressive* and *fatal*
• *Impaired control* over drinking
• *Preoccupation* with this drug
• *Use despite adverse consequence*
• Distortions in thinking, especially *denial*
• *Continuous* or *periodic*

After heart disease and cancer, alcohol-related disorders are considered the third most important health problem in the United States, estimated to account for at least one fourth of all hospitalizations in this country. Almost 50% of those who suffer from alcohol dependence also abuse other legal and illicit drugs (see Appendix D). Alcohol is involved in 25% to 35% of all *suicides* and 50% to 70% of all homicides; it also figures prominently in *accidental deaths* and *domestic violence* (388, 389). Furthermore, causes of death resulting from excessive alcohol use include the following:

• *Cirrhosis*
• *Cancers* of the *oropharynx*

• *Breast cancer* in women
• *Injuries* and other external causes in men (390)

In contrast, moderate alcohol consumption in the middle-aged and elderly slightly reduced overall mortality risk.

Of the approximately 100 million Americans who imbibe, about 10% suffer from alcoholism, while consuming about 50% of all alcoholic beverages in this country. There are also an estimated 10 to 12 million "problem drinkers," with men's risk for development of severe problems being three to four times higher than women's. Although the heaviest drinking occurs at an earlier age for men than for women, the abstinence rate for both sexes begins to increase after age 50 years (391). The "end-stage" drinker constitutes less than 3% of the alcoholic population and describes an individual who is, generally,

• *Unemployed*
• *Transient*
• A *daily* drinker
• Without *social* and *economic support*
• In a *deteriorated psychological* and *physical state*

Adolescents abuse alcohol more frequently than any other drug, with an incidence ranging from 15% to 25%. Traffic accidents involving teenagers often have alcohol as a contributing factor, and the number of traffic-related deaths increases or decreases concomitantly with the lowering or raising of the legal drinking age in various states.

The precise incidence of alcoholism in the *elderly* remains unknown, but retired and recently widowed men seem to be at higher risk (392). Physicians and family members often overlook the effects of alcohol on an elderly person's physical and psychological health and may mistake this problem for an organic mental disorder. In the elderly, preexisting organic mental disorders, a decreased volume of distribution, and the concurrent use of other medication may potentiate the effects of alcohol on cognition, affect, and behavior (see "The Elderly Patient" earlier in this chapter).

Strong evidence indicates at least a familial pattern and perhaps a hereditary basis for some types of alcoholism (393). More recent data show that genotype accounts for approximately 33% of the overall variance in liability (394). In addition, specific neurocircuitry and neurochemical systems appear to be important in the etiology of alcoholism (395). Thus, positive reinforcement may be mediated by activation of γ-aminobutyric acid (GABA)$_A$ receptors, release of opioid peptides and dopamine, inhibition of glutamate receptors, and interactions with the 5-HT system. Furthermore, neurobehavioral effects of alcohol and their association with these various neurotransmitters serve as potential targets for novel drug therapies.

Alcohol dependence requires intervention aimed at medical, psychological, and social complications. The goal is to reduce or eliminate the desire to drink, to produce a reduction or cessation in alcohol consumption, and to minimize its harmful consequences. Treatment involves detoxification and rehabilitation (396).

Alcohol-Related Psychiatric Complications

Alcohol abuse is associated with many psychiatric complications, starting with those involving acute consumption or withdrawal:

- *Intoxication* and its complications (e.g., disinhibition, aggressiveness, depression, and suicide)
- *Idiosyncratic* (or pathological) *intoxication*
- *Withdrawal syndrome,* which may include *tremors, hallucinosis, seizures,* and *delirium* (e.g., delirium tremens)

A patient who is intoxicated or undergoing alcohol withdrawal should be hospitalized for management if any of the following are present:

- History of *severe withdrawal symptoms*
- Recent *seizure* or history of withdrawal seizures
- Recent *head trauma*
- Serious *medical complications* (e.g., pancreatitis, gastrointestinal bleeding, hepatitis, cirrhosis, or pneumonia)
- *Delirium* or hallucinosis
- *Temperature* greater than 101° Fahrenheit
- Significant *malnutrition* or *dehydration*

- The *Wernicke-Korsakoff* syndrome
- Severe *depression* or *suicide risk* (397)

In regard to this last issue, the question of comorbid depression associated with alcohol dependence can represent a difficult clinical picture. Whereas antidepressants may be appropriate and useful, premature intervention may be unnecessary. Dackis and colleagues (398), for example, found that 80% of 49 severely depressed alcoholics remitted after 2 weeks of unmedicated sobriety. They concluded that many severe depressions are alcohol-induced organic mood syndromes and improve spontaneously with abstinence.

Most intoxicated individuals do not need hospitalization, display none of the previous medical problems, and experience minimal withdrawal symptoms. Observing and treating them in the emergency room or a nonmedical detoxification center (i.e., social intoxication) for 6 to 12 hours may be all that is required.

Acute Alcohol Intoxication

Alcohol is similar to other general anesthetics in that it depresses the CNS. Clinically, however, it may appear to be a stimulant because it first suppresses inhibitory control mechanisms, resulting in early disinhibition. In general, the effect of alcohol on the CNS is proportionate to its blood concentration, but the effects are more marked when the concentration is increasing.

In the alert intoxicated patient, general management is primarily supportive and protective. Thiamine 100 mg i.m. is given initially and repeated three times a day orally for the next several weeks. A multivitamin preparation should also be given orally each day. If the patient is restless, a short-acting BZD such as lorazepam (1 to 2 mg i.v., i.m., or orally) may be given and repeated as frequently as needed. If the patient is violent or severely agitated, an antipsychotic may be necessary with low-dose, high-potency agents, such as haloperidol (2 to 5 mg i.m. or i.v. as needed). If larger doses are necessary, one should reconsider the diagnosis.

Alcohol Idiosyncratic Intoxication

This syndrome has similarities to the paradoxical reaction seen with barbiturates or BZDs, as well as epileptoid syndromes, including temporal lobe seizures and intermittent explosive disorder. Brain injury from trauma or encephalitis may also predispose some to an abnormally excessive response to even small amounts of alcohol.

Clinical signs and symptoms include sudden onset of irrational, combative, or destructive behavior after ingesting relatively small amounts of alcohol. The behavior is atypical of the individual when not drinking, and usually begins within minutes to hours. After the acute outburst, the patient usually lapses into deep sleep and upon awakening has only fragmentary memory or total amnesia for the episode. Treatment should attempt to diminish stimulation as much as possible, and antipsychotics, such as haloperidol (2 to 5 mg orally, i.m., or i.v.) may reduce combative or destructive behavior.

Alcohol Withdrawal or Abstinence Syndrome

This condition may emerge after a period of relative or absolute abstinence, with the cause being unknown. The duration of drinking and quantity of alcohol required to produce noticeable symptoms vary widely. Abstinence may also result from intercurrent illness, hospitalization for an unrelated illness, or lack of money to buy alcohol. The full spectrum of this syndrome, which ranges from an early, mild withdrawal picture to delirium is frequently seen in large urban hospital emergency room settings.

Early withdrawal peaks at about 24 hours and rarely can emerge several days after cessation. Symptoms can clear in a few hours or last up to 2 weeks, and may include the following:

- *Tremulousness,* which is the earliest and most common sign. Associated symptoms may last for 10 to 14 days, and include nausea, vomiting, tension, and insomnia.
- *Alcoholic hallucinosis,* which usually consists of auditory hallucinations (but may also be visual) in the presence of a clear sensorium. They usually emerge within the first few days and may persist after all other withdrawal symptoms have resolved.
- *Seizures* ("rum fits"), which are generalized motor events that usually peak 12 to 48 hours after cessation of alcohol consumption. Partial seizures suggest a focal lesion and require careful neurological evaluation.
- *Withdrawal delirium* (delirium tremens), which usually appears 1 to 4 days after abstinence and peaks at about 72 to 96 hours. The mortality rate may be as high as 15% if serious complicating medical problems are also present. Clinical signs and symptoms include profound confusion, illusions, delusions, vivid hallucinations, agitation, insomnia, and autonomic hyperactivity. Death results from infection, cardiac arrhythmias, fluid and electrolyte abnormalities, or suicide (e.g., in response to hallucinations, illusions, or delusions).

Treatment

The treatment of alcohol withdrawal incorporates *general supportive measures,* as well as management of specific symptoms. Supportive measures include abstinence from alcohol, ample rest, adequate general nutrition, and reality orientation. It is important to treat the syndrome vigorously and, when appropriate, to prevent it by using sufficient doses of medication.

Typically, the *BZDs* are used on an as-needed basis to treat objective signs of withdrawal, such as tremor, tachycardia, or hypertension. The longer-acting BZDs, such as chlordiazepoxide and diazepam, have the advantage of less frequent dosing but the risk of drug accumulation. The intermediate-acting agents, such as lorazepam, are less likely to accumulate but need to be administered more frequently to prevent reemergence of signs and symptoms. One approach might be lorazepam, 2 mg orally every 2 hours as needed, for as long as needed. The acute dose is then tapered over a 1- to 2-week period, using a twice-daily or three-times-daily regimen. Total daily doses of more than 10 to 12 mg are rarely required. A fixed-dose regimen may not work because of the variability in duration and severity of symptoms. In the severely agitated patient, lorazepam i.m. (2 mg per hour) or diazepam i.v. (5 to 10 mg slowly) may be necessary. *β-Adrenergic blockers,* such as atenolol, have been tried as adjuncts to BZDs to treat autonomic hyperactivity. For example, atenolol (100 mg orally daily) has been given for moderate to severe tachycardia. Occasionally, *antipsychotics,* such as haloperidol (2 to 10 mg i.m. or orally), may be needed.

Treatment of withdrawal seizures depends on whether there is a prior history. For example, in one study of patients who had experienced a withdrawal seizure, lorazepam 2 mg i.v. was significantly more effective than normal saline placebo in reducing the risk of a recurrent seizure (399). If there is no history, prophylactic anticonvulsants will probably not help. Furthermore, BZDs used for sedation also have anticonvulsant properties, so adequate doses should minimize the risk of seizures. If an antipsychotic is required, one should avoid agents that can lower the seizure threshold and cause extrapyramidal symptoms and hypotension. Patients with a more complicated history of withdrawal or other seizure disorders are at greater risk and should be given an anticonvulsant. If the patient is currently receiving a maintenance dose, it should be continued. If the patient is not receiving medication or if it was discontinued 5 or more days previously, a loading dose of phenytoin, 15 mg/kg intravenously in saline, could be given at a rate not to exceed 50 mg per minute. Maintenance doses should be started 24 hours later. Some withdrawal seizures can be prevented by restoring serum magnesium levels with *magnesium sulfate* (2 mL of a 50% solution, up to three doses), given with intravenous fluids over 8 hours.

Treatment of delirium includes the following:

- *Reduce environmental stimulation.*
- Monitor *vital signs* frequently.
- *Restrain* combative or agitated patients.
- Monitor *fluid* and *electrolyte* balance, correcting any imbalance.
- Maintain *blood pressure* with intravenous saline and glucose.
- Give *thiamine,* 100 mg i.m. initially, then 100 mg orally three times a day.
- Replenish other *vitamin stores* with folate, B-complex, and multivitamin supplements.

- Give a *BZD,* such as diazepam, 5 to 10 mg orally every 1 to 2 hours, as needed for sedation, with a maximum of 80 to 100 mg per day. If the patient is severely agitated, give 5 to 10 mg diazepam intravenously slowly every 20 minutes, until the patient is sedated.
- If necessary, use low-dose high-potency *antipsychotic,* such as haloperidol (2 to 5 mg i.m. every 2 to 4 hours), to control acute symptoms on an as-needed basis.
- *Search for and treat complicating illnesses* such as pneumonia, gastrointestinal bleeding, hepatic decompensation, pancreatitis, subdural hematoma, and fractures.

Alternative adjunctive strategies with some evidence for efficacy include the following:

- Clonidine
- *β*-Blockers
- Other anticonvulsants (e.g., valproate)
- Calcium antagonists (400)

Complicating Medical Conditions in the Alcoholic Patient

Because several major diseases are commonly associated with alcoholism, treatment of alcohol-related psychiatric disorders may have to be modified if one of these conditions is present.

Cirrhosis

Ninety-five percent of all alcohol is metabolized in the liver; the remaining 5% is excreted via the kidneys and the lungs (see Chapter 3). The rate of metabolism increases with fasting and after protracted periods of drinking. Alcohol has a direct toxic effect on the liver, and whereas significant hepatic damage develops in only 10% to 20% of long-term heavy drinkers, BZDs must be used cautiously because they are primarily metabolized by this organ. If there is evidence of disease, oxazepam and lorazepam are the BZDs of choice because they are not metabolized by the liver. When oral drugs cannot be used, lorazepam (2 to 8 mg i.m. daily) is preferred.

As discussed in Chapter 3, the phases of alcohol consumption can have varying effects on the metabolism of concomitantly administered psychotropics. Thus, *acute alcohol ingestion* generally interferes with the metabolism of drugs, increasing plasma concentration. *Ingestion over several weeks* stimulates hepatic enzymes, accelerating the metabolism of many other drugs. Finally, cirrhosis induced by *long-term alcohol consumption* diminishes enzyme concentration and liver mass, again increasing plasma levels of various concurrently administered drugs metabolized by this system. Fluid and electrolyte therapy must take into account the development of ascites and the possibility of right-sided heart failure. Salt restriction to 500 mg per day and bed rest are the initial conservative treatments, with medical consultation usually required.

Other Medical Conditions

Because heavy cigarette smoking is typically associated with alcohol dependence and may lead to impaired *pulmonary function,* BZDs should be used more cautiously to reduce the risk of oversedation and respiratory depression. Hypoxia can cause agitation and is exacerbated by treatment with sedative drugs. Again, shorter half-life agents and those with fewer active metabolites should be used (e.g., oxazepam or lorazepam). Alcoholic patients also have an increased risk of aspiration of gastric contents or infected oropharyngeal material, with resulting aspiration pneumonia.

Erosive *gastritis* caused by recent excessive ingestion of alcohol is the most common cause of gastrointestinal bleeding in alcoholics. Bleeding usually subsides with cessation of drinking and administration of antacids. If the patient has cirrhosis, bleeding from esophageal varices must be suspected.

Alcohol-Related Neurological Disorders

The following chronic neuropsychiatric disorders may arise from nutritional deficiencies, gastric malabsorption, and hepatic dysfunction:

• The *Wernicke-Korsakoff* syndrome
• Cerebral *cortical atrophy* (alcohol-associated dementia)
• *Cerebellar degeneration*

• *Polyneuropathy*
• Alcohol *myopathy*
• *Pellagra* (401)

Deficiencies of thiamine and B vitamins arising from poor nutrition and malabsorption are usually the basis for these neurological sequelae.

The *Wernicke-Korsakoff* syndrome consists of both an acute (i.e., Wernicke's encephalopathy) and a chronic phase (i.e., Korsakoff's psychosis). The acute encephalopathy may be precipitated or worsened by carbohydrates (including intravenous glucose) unless thiamine is also replenished before or during administration. Wernicke's encephalopathy may first be manifested by the following:

• *Mental status abnormalities,* especially global confusion, inattentiveness, and a hypokinetic delirium
• *Ataxia*
• *Ocular findings,* including nystagmus (horizontal or vertical), weakness or paralysis of the lateral recti muscles, and weakness or paralysis of conjugate gaze

Korsakoff's psychosis is most characterized by the following:

• Anterograde and retrograde *amnesia*
• *Decreased insight*
• *Apathy*
• *Inability to learn*

Although *confabulation* (unconscious fabrication of facts because of memory impairment) is often considered a key symptom, it is not always present. Thiamine, initially given i.m. and then orally (100 to 300 mg per day), can improve many of these symptoms, assuming irreversible changes have not occurred.

Pellagra is often characterized by mental abnormalities such as anxiety, irritability, and depression. The classic symptoms of pellagra are known as the "4 Ds"–*dementia, diarrhea, dermatitis,* and *death.* Inflammation of mucosal surfaces, weakness, anorexia, and other gastrointestinal disturbances are also seen. Niacin (300 to 500 mg per day) is the definitive therapy.

Other neurological syndromes (e.g., cerebral cortical atrophy, myopathy, cerebellar degeneration) are also associated with alcoholism, but their pathogenesis is less certain than that of nutritional deficiency disorders. Abstinence from alcohol plus vitamin replacement and physical therapy comprise the standard treatment approach for these conditions.

Complicating Psychiatric Conditions in the Alcoholic Patient

Proper diagnosis, important with any illness, is even more crucial in treatment planning for patients with a dual diagnosis. Because psychoactive substance use can obfuscate the diagnosis, special care must be taken to preclude organically based syndromes. Thus, adequate periods of abstinence must first be achieved, and then the patient reexamined for residual symptoms compatible with a nonaddictive, non–substance-induced psychiatric disorder (402).

Important demographic information relevant to the pharmacotherapy of patients with a dual diagnosis can be gleaned from several studies. For example, in their report of chronic mentally ill patients, with or without addictions, Drake and Wallach (403) found that the dually diagnosed were

- Generally *younger*
- Usually *male*
- More frequently *hostile, suicidal,* and *disordered in their speech*
- *Less compliant* with medication
- *Less able to manage their lives* in the community in terms of maintaining regular meals, adequate finances, stable housing, and regular activities

Smith and Hucker (404) note the following characteristics in the population of schizophrenic addicts included in their review of the literature:

- More *violence*
- More *suicide*
- More *noncompliance*
- Earlier *psychotic breakdown*
- *Exacerbations* of psychosis
- Relative *antipsychotic refractoriness*

- Increased rates of *hospitalization*
- Increased *tardive dyskinesia*
- *Poor prognosis* overall

Additionally, Noordsy and colleagues (405) contribute data indicating that a family history of alcoholism in alcoholic schizophrenics is associated with a more severe course of illness, greater resistance to treatment, and more frequent abuse of other drugs.

Drug Therapy During Rehabilitation

Treatment is best approached by using a disease model in which alcoholism is considered a chronic medical disorder and not simply a psychological or social problem. As with any other chronic illness, relapse is a normal part of the recovery process. Because the etiology of alcoholism is unknown and it afflicts a heterogeneous population, therapeutic strategies must keep in mind that some will not respond to more accepted forms of management. In this context, agents that reduce one's desire to drink may be important adjuncts (406).

Disulfiram

Disulfiram (Antabuse) is an aversive drug that can be prescribed in conjunction with other forms of therapy such as Alcoholics Anonymous and individual counseling. Although controlled trials have not consistently demonstrated benefit with this agent in comparison with placebo, many clinicians believe it has a psychological effect that may attenuate impulsive drinking in selected patients (407). Furthermore, this strategy is recommended only for patients with good compliance and no serious physical condition (e.g., cardiovascular disease). After 6 to 12 months, disulfiram may be stopped if a patient has been able to remain sober; however, some patients may require the drug indefinitely to ensure sobriety. The usual loading dose is 250 to 500 mg per day for 3 to 5 days, although adverse effects may require a lower dose. Most patients are adequately maintained on 125 to 200 mg per day. A patient who drinks while taking this agent may experience facial flushing, sweating, headaches, nausea, vomiting, chest pain, dyspnea, weakness, dizziness, blurred vision, and confusion within minutes. Respiratory depression, shock, arrhythmias, seizures, and death are rare. Before disulfiram is prescribed, patients must be informed about these adverse effects and about the possibility of a serious disulfiram-ethanol reaction; patients must be aware that many foods and aftershave lotion contain alcohol, as well as some over-the-counter mouthwashes and cough syrups. Written informed consent should be obtained. Disulfiram may also interfere with the action of other commonly coprescribed drugs such as anticoagulants, phenytoin, and isoniazid.

Although disulfiram is sometimes helpful as an adjunct to nonpharmacological treatments for alcoholism, it has the potential to worsen psychosis. Kofoed (408, 409) notes, however, that these findings are based on untreated chronically affected patients given high doses. He and his colleagues used disulfiram with a small number of dually diagnosed psychotic and alcohol-dependent patients after they were stabilized on appropriate antipsychotic medications. They found that compliance with disulfiram therapy in their dual-diagnosis group was as good as in primary alcoholic outpatients. They also reported no particular problems, concluding that disulfiram seemed less of a risk than continued alcohol misuse (410, 411).

Opioid Antagonists

Several studies have indicated that the opioid system may be involved in the regulation of alcohol intake in various animals. *Naltrexone* has been shown to reduce alcohol consumption in alcohol-craving animals (412, 413). Two well-controlled studies using naltrexone in humans produced dramatically effective results (414, 415). Thus, the FDA has approved this agent (under the trade name Revia) as an adjunct to a comprehensive treatment plan. Typical starting doses are 25 to 50 mg per day by mouth. A large multicenter usage study reported that in 570 patients on naltrexone, the most common adverse effects were nausea (9.8%) and headache (6.6%), with 15% of patients dropping out because of nausea (416). Although no deaths occurred, a single case re-sport has raised the question of a possible association between naltrexone and rhabdomyolysis (417).

More recently, a double-blind, placebo-controlled trial with another opioid antagonist, *nalmefene* (20 or 80 mg per day), found that this agent had a significant benefit over placebo in preventing relapse to heavy drinking (418).

The promising findings of the trials already mentioned, as well as the possible benefits of opiate antagonists in treating symptoms of schizophrenia or bipolar disorder without alcohol dependence or co-morbid alcohol and cocaine dependence, however, warrant studies in these difficult-to-treat populations (419–422). Furthermore, some data support a synergistic therapeutic effect when naltrexone is combined with cognitive-behavioral therapy (423).

In summary, naltrexone and perhaps other opioid antagonists such as nalmefene are promising agents in the pharmacotherapy of alcohol dependence with or without coexisting psychiatric and addictive disorders (418).

Acamprosate

Acamprosate (calcium acetylhomotaurine) has a chemical structure similar to homotaurine and GABA and appears to normalize N-methyl-D-aspartate (NMDA) receptor tone in the glutamate system.

Results from animal studies indicating a decrease in voluntary alcohol intake led to a number of double-blind, placebo-controlled trials involving more than 4,500 patients with alcohol dependence (424). In a review of these data, Mason and Ownby (424) found that 14 of 16 studies demonstrated a significantly superior benefit from acamprosate versus placebo in terms of the following:

- Greater rate of *treatment completion*
- Time to *first drink*
- *Abstinence* rate
- Cumulative *abstinence duration*

Dose-response data indicate that 2 grams per day was optimal. In addition, this agent demonstrates an excellent safety profile, with loose stools or diarrhea being the only adverse effects reported more often than with placebo. Other data indicate that this agent can be safely administered concurrently with disulfiram or naltrexone.

Alcoholism and Mood Disorders

Ample evidence shows that although alcoholism and depression are often associated, they may also present as distinct entities and not different presentations of identical processes (425). In this context, Schuckit et al. (426) addressed the issue of induced versus independent MDD in 2,945 alcoholics. These authors concluded that it was possible to distinguish between substance-induced and independent episodes. However, common symptoms often overlap, at times making proper diagnosis more difficult.

Clinical studies of depressed alcoholics give some suggestions of the course of treatments. Brown et al. (427) demonstrated that those male patients in their sample with dual diagnoses of alcohol dependence and a mood disorder did not demonstrate more severe depressive symptoms or a slower recovery than their counterparts with either diagnosis alone. Evidence from another study shows that depression in schizophrenic alcoholics on acute inpatient admission resolves within the same time frame as does depression in non-dually diagnosed alcoholics (428). If supported and broadened by further investigation, this finding would simplify treatment strategies by including patients with a dual diagnosis in established trends for mainstream addiction treatment.

Tricyclic Antidepressants

The role of tricyclics for depressed alcoholics has usually been limited to the period of acute withdrawal and not for longer-term maintenance. Other methodological problems with studies in this area include the following:

- Relative inattention to *different subtypes* of depression
- Inadequate use of *TDM*
- Failure to monitor both *mood* and *drinking behavior* in response to treatment (429)

Despite these design flaws, many of the studies support the beneficial effects of tricyclic antidepressants in the treatment of depression associated with alcohol withdrawal. These benefits, however, do not exceed those of placebo after 3 weeks, and thus may have only limited application in actual clinical practice.

Of the antidepressants available, imipramine is the most extensively studied. A trial assessing this agent's effectiveness for alcoholism with comorbid depression had certain advantages over its predecessors, including the following:

- *Lifetime histories* to establish diagnoses of depression (thus avoiding transient depressive effects of alcohol)
- A *double-blind* design during the second phase of the study
- *Adequacy of dosing* as monitored by plasma levels (430)

Although criteria for response are incomplete, the investigators report that, of 60 alcoholics who had major depression and who completed an initial 12-week open-label trial of imipramine, 27 (45%) responded, showing improvement in both mood (posttreatment Hamilton Depression Rating Scale score = 3; SD = 3) and drinking behavior (30% achieving abstinence and another 15% at a "much reduced level"). These response rates were further enhanced after dose increases or treatment with disulfiram. Patients who improved with imipramine in the initial open trial were then randomized into a subsequent 6-month double-blind maintenance phase. During this phase, seven of 10 (70%) suffered a relapse on placebo, in contrast to only four of 13 (31%) on imipramine. Although the sample sizes were small, the investigators believed that this represented a significant improvement for those on medication in a common dual-diagnosis scenario.

Serotonergic Agents

New possibilities emerged with the introduction of the SSRIs. Basic studies using these agents in animals substantiated a decrease in alcohol preference and consumption, whereas nonspecific monoamine uptake blockers (e.g., amitriptyline, doxepin) did not (431). Using animal models of spontaneous alcohol consumption, Gorelick reported evidence that increased brain serotonin activity tended to decrease alcohol preference and consumption. Extrapolating these results from the laboratory to the clinical arena, Gorelick and Paredes (432) then studied the effect of fluoxetine on alcohol consumption in 20 men with chronic dependence. After a 28-day double-blind, placebo-controlled period, these investigators found that the fluoxetine group had a 14% lower alcohol intake, primarily during the first week. The beneficial effect was associated with a lower proportion of requests as well as less craving for alcohol. As in the imipramine outcomes, however, these investigators did not find a significant effect in later weeks (i.e., virtually no differences in scores on the Hamilton Depression and Anxiety Scales or the abridged Hopkins Symptom Checklist).

Although the mechanism of action of SSRIs in treating alcohol dependence remains unclear, Gorelick and Paredes (432) postulate that it is not due to motor inhibition or general sedation. Rather, they believe it may be "related to decreased appetite and food intake or a conditioned taste aversion mediated by increased brain serotonin activity." Other competing theories have been summarized by Thomas (433):

- *Antidepressant* and anxiolytic effects
- Decrease in *impulsivity*
- Extinction of *reward* contingencies

Several early outpatient studies of SSRIs used in early stage problem drinkers and chronic alcoholics also supported this trend by demonstrating reductions in various parameters used to measure drinking during variable time frames (434–437).

Garbutt and colleagues (407) reviewed the existing evidence for the usefulness of SSRIs in the management of alcoholic patients with and without significant depression or anxiety. The studies varied in design and outcome, but overall these investigators believed the data were limited and not promising (438–443). Furthermore, the results may have been confounded by high rates of co-morbid mood and anxiety symptoms.

Trials with buspirone and ondansetron have yielded similar mixed results (444–447).

Mood Stabilizers

In general, all mood-stabilizing agents used for the dually diagnosed population can at least facilitate treatment of the psychiatric and the addictive disorder by stabilizing patients, thus promoting more appropriate participation in treatment. Lithium, however, has not fulfilled its initial promise for the treatment of primary alcoholism with and without a concurrent affective disorder. Dorus and colleagues (448) studied 457 male alcoholics in a Veterans Administration collaborative study and found that lithium did not alter the use of alcohol in either depressed or nondepressed alcoholics. Specifically, they reported abstinence in 38% of lithium-treated nondepressed alcoholics (compared with 28% of placebo-controlled subjects) and 32% of lithium-treated depressed alcoholics (compared with 37% of their placebo-controlled subjects). Fawcett and colleagues (449) reported beneficial effects of lithium in 104 alcoholics studied in a double-blind, placebo-controlled design. They found, however, that 19 of 51 (37%) patients given lithium and 22 of 53 (42%) patients on placebo were abstinent at the 6-month follow-up, with the numbers being even more similar at 12-month follow-up.

Although lithium no longer appears promising to treat alcohol dependence itself, it may have a place in pharmacotherapy of the overall syndrome. A small pilot study (n = 12) by Nagel and colleagues (450) assessed lithium in a double-blind, placebo-controlled design focusing on recently (3 to 7 days before entry into study) detoxified alcoholics who manifested a syndrome resembling hypomania. Symptoms consisted of elevated psychomotor activity, grandiosity, irritability, a heightened desire for social contact, loquaciousness, and sexual preoccupation. The severity of symptoms was significantly decreased by treatment with low-dose lithium carbonate (serum levels 0.3 to 0.5 mEq/L), but was not affected by placebo treatment.

Anticonvulsants such as valproate and CBZ are effective mood-stabilizing agents and may be useful in withdrawal states from alcohol, BZDs, and cocaine (451, 452). Because lithium shows some utility in certain patients whose dual diagnosis includes bipolar disorder, and because the anticonvulsants attenuate several types of withdrawal syndromes, these agents may be useful and safe for selected alcoholic patients with bipolar and related disorders.

Alcoholism and Anxiety

Anxiety is a common complaint that invariably complicates addictive illnesses. Estimates of co-morbid anxiety and alcohol disorders range from 20% to 50%, with men more likely to self-medicate anxiety than women (453–455). Some investigators have also found increased rates of alcoholism in family members of patients with anxiety disorders (456, 457). Patients with alcohol or drug dependence show a tendency for development of panic disorder earlier, and it has been suggested that repeated alcohol withdrawal may be the trigger for panic attacks in susceptible individuals (458, 459). Finally, BZDs, the primary pharmacological treatment for these disorders, are themselves addictive and sometimes associated with anxiety syndromes, especially on their discontinuation (460).

Two studies have evaluated buspirone for alcoholism with coexisting depression and anxiety (445, 446). This non-BZD, partial serotonin agonist with anxiolytic properties may be particularly valuable in treating a dual diagnosis because it is nonaddicting. In this light, Kranzler and colleagues' placebo-controlled trial of buspirone in anxious alcoholics indicated that this agent led to the following:

- A greater likelihood of *completing treatment*
- Reduction of *anxiety* symptoms
- A slower rate of heavy alcohol *relapse*
- More days of *abstinence* during the follow-up period (445)

Conclusion

To paraphrase William Osler, "If you know alcoholism, you know all of medicine." This observation is particularly pertinent given alcohol's myriad neuropsychiatric manifestations, co-morbid mental disturbances, and complicating medical conditions. The interaction between alcohol and its related physical disturbances requires the careful use of various psychotropics to safely detoxify patients and to help prevent more serious medical or emotional complications. The use of BZDs should only be short-term, because many patients are likely to transfer their dependence from alcohol to these agents. Various drugs have the ability to decrease alcohol craving by different mechanisms and may benefit selected patients. Finally, those suffering from co-morbid medical or psychiatric disorders in addition to their alcohol disorder, require specialized management of these concurrent conditions to achieve a successful outcome.

THE HUMAN IMMUNODEFICIENCY VIRUS—INFECTED PATIENT

HIV-related psychological complications present a unique challenge to the clinician (460a). These patients not only have severe associated psychosocial stressors but also varied neuropsychiatric manifestations that complicate any

TABLE 14-9. *Etiology of neuropsychological disorders in patients with HIV-1 infection*

Direct CNS infection with HIV
Secondary malignancies of the CNS from immuno-compromise
    Primary CNS lymphoma
    Burkitt's lymphoma
    Disseminated Kaposi's sarcoma
    Other sarcomas
    Candidiasis
Secondary CNS infections from immunocom-promise
    Cerebral toxoplasmosis
    Herpes simplex encephalitis
    Cryptococcosis
    Mycobacterium tuberculosis (rare)
    Atypical mucobacterial infection (rare)
    Progressive multifocal leukoencephalopathy (papillomavirus)
Systemic complications of HIV infection or side effects of its treatment
    Nutritional deficiencies, especially vitamin B_{12} deficiency
    Drug-related neurotoxicities
    Metabolic encephalopathies
Psychological reactions of the patients to having disease

From Jobe TH. Neuropsychiatry of HIV disease. In: Flaherty J, Davis JM, Janicak, PG, eds. *Psychiatry: diagnosis and therapy.* 2nd ed. New York: Appleton and Lange, 1993, with permission.

potential intervention (Table 14-9) (461, 462). In this context, one study found that AIDS patients with concurrent psychiatric disorders who were hospitalized for medical reasons had significantly longer average lengths of stay than their counterparts without a diagnosable psychiatric disorder (463).

From another perspective, mentally ill patients who have tested positive can pose some difficult management issues, particularly when they require hospitalization (464). For example, simply testing for the AIDS antibody is fraught with controversy, including such ethical and legal questions as

- *Who* should be tested?
- When and to whom should the *results be disclosed?*
- What is the best way to balance a *patient's right to privacy* with a "duty to warn"? (465)

AIDS and AIDS-related complex (ARC) are distinguished by weight loss, chronic fatigue, fevers, night sweats, oral leukoplakia, oral candidiasis, and generalized lymphadenopathy. They also show evidence of neurotropic as well as their better-known lymphotropic features. **As many as 70% of these patients have clinically apparent mental changes during the course of their disease. Neuropsychological impairment may, in fact, be the first symptom of HIV-related disorders** (462, 466).

Early studies have found that, among HIV outpatients, 67% manifest adjustment disorder with mixed emotional features, and 80% of inpatients manifest an organic mental disorder. Indeed, a study by the World Health Organization suggested that the significance of the psychopathological complications of symptomatic HIV-1 infection may have been underestimated by earlier studies, which included more stable patient samples (467). Furthermore, postmortem studies on patients who suffered from AIDS have found that neuropathological abnormalities occur in approximately 90%. These abnormalities have included the following:

- *Toxoplasmosis*
- *Fungal* infections
- *Bacterial* infections
- *Viral* infections

- *Vascular* lesions
- *Neoplasms*

In the CNS, tumors include primary and secondary lymphomas and, rarely, Kaposi's sarcoma. It is also thought that the HIV retrovirus itself may be encephalopathic (468).

Because an increasing number of patients with a concurrent psychiatric disorder and HIV infection are requiring intervention, this poses an important challenge to the mental health field.

Unfortunately, relative to the general population, chronic psychiatric patients typically have inadequate information about HIV and AIDS. Furthermore, they are more likely to engage in lifestyles that substantially increase their risk of contracting this disease. Such factors include sexual impulsivity, transient and often dysfunctional social relationships, more frequent risk-taking behavior, and poor judgment (469). DiClemente and Ponton (470), for example, reported that adolescents in psychiatric facilities engaged in a very high rate of sexual and drug-related behaviors that increased the risk for contracting HIV-related disorders.

Psychiatric Diagnosis in HIV-Infected Patients

The most common diagnosis given to these patients is an *adjustment disorder with mixed emotional features;* however, one must always be cognizant of the potential for an underlying, but as yet unrecognized, organic process. The typical neuropsychiatric complications can be divided into four major categories:

- AIDS-related *dementia complex* and *delirium*
- *Psychosis*
- *Mood* disorders
- *Anxiety*

Oftentimes, these conditions coexist, making diagnosis and treatment planning exceedingly complicated.

General Management of the HIV-Infected Patient

General *nonpharmacological* therapeutic approaches consist of the following:

- Normalization of *nutritional deficiencies* and *supplementation* beyond normal levels (471)
- *Supportive psychotherapy*
- *Psychoeducation*
- *Family therapy*
- *Mobilization of social support systems*
- *Follow-up neuropsychological testing*

A related issue is the growing number of AIDS-phobic individuals, who often benefit from empathic, informed reassurance, thus avoiding HIV-antibody testing or the need for more intensive treatment.

When informed that they have tested HIV-positive, many patients initially react to this knowledge with anger, depression, and suicidal thoughts (461). This may be further complicated by the potential for impaired judgment as a result of cognitive disruption and drug-induced adverse drug reactions (e.g., delirium) when medicating these sensitized individuals.

An important related problem is the trend toward demedicalization of state mental health facilities. Given a host of clinical and economic realities, many HIV-infected patients can only be served by such institutions (472). Their complicated psychiatric and medical presentations, however, require a high level of clinical sophistication, particularly in recognizing and managing their physical co-morbidities (473, 474). Indeed, an increasing number of patients suffer from a "triple" diagnosis (i.e., a psychiatric disorder with co-morbid substance abuse and HIV-positive status) (475).

Drug Therapy

Because these patients may be exquisitely sensitive to the effects of medication, the general principle is always to start with the lowest dose and increase medication only if necessary and very slowly. The route of administration may also be problematic, because some patients have very poor absorption, and thus medications may not be adequately assimilated. Parenteral administration is also often complicated by decreased muscle mass, thrombocytopenia, and difficulty in finding veins.

Dementia and Delirium

Zidovudine (AZT) was the first agent approved for the treatment of HIV infection, and there is also some evidence that it may partially reverse the cognitive disruption associated with AIDS-dementia complex (476). This agent, however, may also cause CNS complications, such as headache, insomnia, and restlessness. Some authors have also reported dramatic responses with *methylphenidate,* whether depression was present or not (477). More recently, antiretroviral agents such as *protease inhibitors, nucleoside-analogue reverse transcriptase inhibitors* and *non-nucleoside analogue reverse inhibitors* have made it possible to suppress viral replication to undetectable levels and produce more sustained CD4 cell counts (478, 479, 479a), improving all aspects of this disease (e.g., cognitive disturbances). These agents, however, can produce significant adverse effects and drug interactions.

Psychosis

In cases of organic psychosis or delirium, pharmacotherapy with a moderately potent antipsychotic agent such as molindone, which also has limited anticholinergic adverse effects, is indicated. High-potency antipsychotics should be avoided because of their tendency to produce unusually severe extrapyramidal side effects or neuroleptic malignant syndrome (480, 481). This may be due to underlying damage in the basal ganglia resulting from HIV-induced changes. Alternatively, i.m. or i.v. "microdoses" of haloperidol (e.g., 0.5 mg twice daily) may be helpful, while minimizing the chances for an extrapyramidal side effect reaction.

The introduction of the novel antipsychotics such as risperidone and olanzapine may represent an important alternative treatment option for this population. These agents may be particularly helpful in managing psychotic symptoms while avoiding some of the more troublesome adverse experiences with neuroleptics on the one hand and clozapine on the other (482, 483). Because adverse effects such as hypotension can be a problem, however, lower doses should be given an adequate trial before attempting an escalation. In patients manifesting psychotic symptoms, who also have difficulty with the extrapyramidal side effects associated with the higher potency agents, olanzapine or quetiapine may be the better choice. These drugs may also be preferable in the seizure-prone patient. Each new agent, however, must be considered in terms of its potential for adverse events, especially cardiovascular and anticholinergic effects.

Some commonly used drugs may also induce organic mental syndromes in these patients. For example, medications with anticholinergic properties (e.g., antiparkinsonian agents, tricyclics, low-potency antipsychotics, certain antiemetics such as prochlorperazine, and antihistamines) may all induce a delirium characterized by visual or tactile hallucinations, confusion, and agitation. If an antiparkinsonian agent is needed to counteract neuroleptic-induced adverse effects, some recommend *amantadine* rather than benztropine. The dose is usually 50 mg twice a day, with a gradual increase to 100 mg twice daily, if necessary. The optimal treatment, however, is discontinuation of the offending agent and waiting for the symptoms to subside.

In situations characterized by agitation, Gilmer and Busch (484) have recommended lorazepam in small doses (0.5 mg) given intravenously by slow push or intramuscularly. The anticipated availability of acute parenteral (i.m.) novel antipsychotics (e.g., olanzapine, ziprasidone) may be reasonable alternatives.

Mood Disorders

Mood disorders often accompany, and can seriously complicate, the diagnosis and management of patients with HIV infections (484a).

Depression

Lyketsos and colleagues (485) have reported a dramatic, sustained increase in depressive symptoms as early as 18 months before the clinical diagnosis of AIDS. Mood disturbance, primarily depression, can range from mild adjustment phenomena to a major depressive episode with psychotic features. Depression in this group can be categorized as

- *Reactive* depressive syndromes, including adjustment disorders
- *Concomitant MDDs,* which were either preexisting or recently identified
- *Organic* depressive syndromes

One problem in making the diagnosis of depression in HIV- or AIDS-related disorders is the lack of specificity of the typical neurovegetative signs and symptoms. Thus, fatigue, insomnia, anorexia, and weight loss are common in both conditions. Again, if antidepressant therapy is contemplated, one should start with lower doses, increase more gradually, and preferably avoid agents with greater anticholinergic properties. Limited information is available, however, on the use of SSRIs, MAOIs, venlafaxine, nefazodone, mirtazapine, or bupropion in these patients.

Reactive depression that results from knowledge of seropositivity or the onset of serious physical symptoms is best managed by supportive therapy and, if necessary, by antidepressants. The drug of choice is an agent with low anticholinergic potency (e.g., sertraline, trazodone), started more slowly and maintained at a lower level than in non-AIDS patients.

The SSRIs, venlafaxine, or nefazodone may be reasonable alternatives to earlier generation antidepressants because of their less problematic side effect profiles (486). The propensity to increase activity, the lack of sedation, gastrointestinal symptoms, and alterations in blood pressure are potential complications, however. Given AIDS-induced altered metabolism, for many of these agents, TDM may be helpful in establishing an effective, nontoxic dose.

There is a clinical impression that psychostimulants may be helpful in HIV- or AIDS-related affective syndromes (487, 488). Thus, *methylphenidate* 10 to 20 mg per day (up to 40 mg per day) or *dextroamphetamine* 5 to 15 mg per day (up to 60 mg per day) has been helpful in patients with mild depression who also show symptoms of social withdrawal, fatigue, and apathy, as well as mild cognitive impairment. At times, the combination of low-dose antidepressant and psychostimulant may be more effective and less likely to induce adverse CNS effects.

Suicide is almost always an issue when a patient is severely depressed, and many with HIV disease will consider this option at one time or another during the course of their illness. The potential for suicide may increase rapidly as the physical symptoms accelerate, because of the patient's fear that he or she will not be able to act on these thoughts when their debilitation becomes severe. Developing a good rapport with the patient is very important if the patient's suicidal desire is to be diminished through counseling or psychotherapy. ECT may be the treatment of choice in more emergent situations.

Mania

Although mania in AIDS patients appears to be uncommon, such episodes can pose a serious hazard and require rapid control. Intravenous haloperidol or droperidol may be effective strategies, in part because this route of administration may be less likely than oral doses to induce acute extrapyramidal side effects (489, 490). Some concern, however, has been raised with the potential prolongation of the QT_c interval with droperidol, requiring caution in this regard.

Gilmer and Busch (485) reported on one patient in whom manic symptoms developed in association with AZT therapy and whose affective symptoms remitted when the drug was discontinued, only to return when it was reintroduced. Two other patients were able to continue AZT when lithium was added to control manic symptoms.

Halman et al. (491) conducted a retrospective chart review on 11 patients who were HIV-positive and presented with an acute manic episode. Whereas the six patients with abnormal MRI findings demonstrated intolerance to standard drug treatment (i.e., lithium, conventional neuroleptics), all benefited from a trial with an anticonvulsant (e.g., valproate, CBZ, clonazepam).

The introduction of novel antipsychotics such as risperidone and olanzapine has led to a series of case reports and controlled trials regarding their use for patients with mania, whether complicated by psychotic symptoms or not (384, 492, 493). Singh and Catalan (494), for example, found risperidone helpful in four male AIDS patients who were also experiencing a manic phase of their schizoaffective disorder. Notably, low doses (i.e., 1 or 2 mg twice daily) seemed sufficient.

Anxiety Disorders

During the initial, asymptomatic period of HIV disease, nearly all patients experience varying degrees of anxiety and bouts of dysphoria. Stress-reducing techniques and supportive psychotherapy may be effective in dealing with such symptoms. BZDs are indicated for those with severe episodic anxiety (often bordering on panic) that is not sufficiently responsive to these nondrug interventions. Patients should be counseled about and discouraged from using over-the-counter hypnotics that contain anticholinergic agents.

In the management of anxiety, the cumulative effects of longer half-life BZDs often result in excessive sleepiness, apathetic states, and confusion (with or without paradoxical agitation). Thus, short- and intermediate-acting agents such as oxazepam, lorazepam, and alprazolam are preferable. Lower doses (e.g., 0.5 to 1.0 mg of lorazepam; 0.25 to 0.5 mg of alprazolam) are preferable. Agents with very short half-lives, such as midazolam and triazolam, are not well tolerated, especially in those with more severe neurocognitive disruption. In this context, low-dose antipsychotics were found more effective than lorazepam in the treatment of AIDS-related delirium (495).

Because BZDs can cause excessive sedation and misuse, especially in drug-abusing HIV-infected patients, buspirone may be a useful alternative. Batki (496) reported on the use of this agent in 17 opiate abusers with AIDS or ARC who were also taking methadone. In the 14 patients who remained on the drug for at least 2 weeks, there was a reduction in several aberrant behaviors without any incidence of abuse.

Small doses of *trazodone* (25 to 50 mg) at bedtime may be useful as a sedative-hypnotic. More data are required on pain control and analgesia using *low-dose opioids* on a short-term basis, which may also benefit anxiety. For example, the use of morphine in patients with advanced disease has been found to be particularly helpful in decreasing their associated anxiety.

Conclusion

In addition to offering increasingly effective drug therapies, clinicians must offer the utmost sensitivity and constant support in the face of this devastating illness. Thus, intelligent application of both nondrug and drug therapies must always be complemented by hope and comfort. The aim should not be to simply prolong life, but whenever possible, to improve its quality. When psychotropics are used, drug-induced delirium is a real and ever-present complication. This is due to increased CNS sensitivity as well as AIDS-induced gastrointestinal and hepatic compromise, which can alter a drug's metabolism and disposition. Thus, low drug doses, increased very gradually with the smallest dose increments, should be the guiding principle.

THE EATING-DISORDERED PATIENT

Approximately 5 million Americans annually are affected by eating disorders. These conditions are characterized by

- Serious *disturbances in eating*
- Excessive concern about *body shape* or *weight*
- Potentially devastating *effects on health*
- A *mortality rate* in young women with anorexia nervosa that is 12 times that of their nonanorectic counterparts (497)

Although these disorders are more common in adolescent girls or young women, 5% to 15% of anorexia nervosa and bulimia nervosa and approximately 40% of binge-eating disorders occur in boys and men (498).

Thus, a comprehensive management strategy must address the medical, nutritional, and psychological aspects of these disorders.

The role of pharmacotherapy in eating-disordered patients has yet to be clearly defined. In those with concurrent disorders, such as dysthymia or psychosis, appropriate psychotropic agents may be beneficial. Furthermore, some promising, albeit preliminary, data indicate that

SSRIs may have at least short-term "antibulimic" properties. **In all situations, the clinician must keep in mind the potential for greater adverse effects because of the malnourished status or the binging- and purging-related complications.** Furthermore, the propensity toward substance abuse and self-destruction may find a fatal outlet when these patients are prescribed drugs such as the TCAs. Leach (499) has provided an excellent review of the literature on drug therapies for eating disorders, which can be divided into the following:

- Anorexia nervosa
- Bulimia nervosa
- Bulimia nervosa multisymptomatic

Anorexia Nervosa

Anorexia nervosa is a heterogeneous and multifactorial eating disorder that occurs most commonly in prepubertal, adolescent, and young adult females. It is most characterized by a relentless pursuit of thinness and a morbid fear of fat. The distortion of body image is considered central to the diagnosis by most experts. This disorder is also characterized by refusal to maintain a normal body weight and obsession with dieting to the point of inducing profound weight loss, with body weights at least 15% below that expected. Most of the weight loss is accomplished in secret.

The critical change between the DSM-IV and DSM-III-R nosologies is subtyping based on the presence or absence of binging or purging. This feature acknowledges significant clinical differences between anorectic *restrictors,* who lose weight through dieting, fasting, or excessive exercise, and anorectic bulimics, who regularly engage in binge eating and purging.

Anorectic patients often suffer from complications such as hypotension, hypothermia, and abnormal ECGs, all of which are consistent with starvation. In women, amenorrhea is common with this syndrome. Like patients with depression, they also have high cerebrospinal fluid concentrations of corticotropin-releasing hormone.

Drug Therapy of Anorexia Nervosa

Several psychotropics have been tried to manage this disorder, including the following:

- *Antidepressants* such as the tricyclics, SSRIs, and MAOIs
- *Antipsychotics* (e.g., chlorpromazine, pimozide, olanzapine)
- Appetite *stimulants* (e.g., cyproheptadine)
- *Lithium*

None of these has been found to be more than minimally or partially beneficial, and most have caused adverse effects that outweigh any therapeutic advantages. The only appetite stimulant shown in controlled double-blind trials to be of some benefit is *cyproheptadine,* but only in nonbulimic anorectic patients.

There are several reasons to anticipate that antidepressants might be effective in the treatment of anorexia nervosa. Malnutrition has been shown to produce a syndrome that is virtually indistinguishable from depression, with anhedonia, weight loss, motor retardation, anergia, and decreased ability to think or concentrate. In addition, the high association of comorbidity between anorexia nervosa and mood disturbances, as well as the preponderance of mood disorders in first-degree relatives of those with anorexia nervosa, have led some clinicians to consider and treat this condition as a depressive variant.

Halmi and colleagues (500) found that patients given *amitriptyline* doses averaging 160 mg per day reached weight goals almost 13 days quicker and had a greater decrease in depressive symptoms compared with those given placebo. By contrast, Biederman's group (501) randomly assigned 43 patients to placebo or amitriptyline in doses averaging 115 mg per day for 5 weeks, but found no relationship between serum levels and weight gain or psychiatric symptoms.

More recently, investigators have focused on the *SSRIs* for several reasons:

- Serotonin has been shown to be important in *regulating feeding behaviors in animals.*
- Anorectic patients have demonstrated *disturbances of serotonergic activity.*

- These agents have proven beneficial for *obsessive-compulsive symptoms.*

For example, Gwirtsman and colleagues (502) reported on six patients with chronic, refractory anorexia nervosa who were openly given fluoxetine. All patients had diminished depressive symptoms and associated weight gain. Kaye's group (503) administered fluoxetine to 31 anorectic patients for an average of 11 months, with 29 patients able to maintain themselves at or above 85% average body weight. Response was also categorized based on improvement in eating behaviors, mood, and obsessional symptoms, judged as good in 10, partial in 17, and poor in four patients. Restrictor anorectics fared significantly better than bulimic anorectics, because the authors had previously demonstrated that the restrictor subgroup has increased serotonin turnover compared with their bulimic counterparts.

Antidepressants should be used with caution in this medically compromised population. In particular, heterocyclic-induced side effects such as hypotension and arrhythmias may be fatal.

Antipsychotics also have been used in the treatment of anorexia nervosa. The apparent role of dopamine in feeding and satiety involves increased receptor activity, producing symptoms similar to those found in anorexia nervosa. Thus, it seems reasonable to use dopamine antagonists to alter these behaviors. It also seems appropriate to use the sedative side effects of these drugs to decrease anxiety associated with eating.

Chlorpromazine has been widely used in this context despite the lack of controlled studies demonstrating its efficacy. Two small crossover studies also examined the efficacy of other antipsychotics. In one, 4 to 6 mg per day of *pimozide* was marginally better than placebo, with patients demonstrating a small nonsignificant improvement in weight and in some attitudes toward eating (504). In another study, 400 to 600 mg per day of *sulpiride* was no more effective than placebo in terms of weight gain or characteristic behaviors or attitudes (505). The role of novel antipsychotics, such as risperidone and olanzapine, has yet to be explored in ment

controlled trials, but case reports have shown some benefit (506–509).

Similar to the heterocyclic antidepressants, antipsychotics must be used carefully and sparingly in this physiologically impaired population. In particular, low potency agents (most notably chlorpromazine) may cause extreme hypotension and hypothermia in these patients.

A meta-analysis of eating disorder programs suggests that medications alone fail to produce consistent weight gain in anorexia nervosa (510). Better results appear possible if medication is integrated into a comprehensive treatment approach, which includes the following:

- Nutritional counseling
- Behavior modification techniques
- Individual, group, and family therapy

Bulimia Nervosa

Bulimia nervosa has an unknown etiology, is more common in women, and is characterized by binging and purging, disturbances of mood, and neuroendocrine abnormalities. Binges range from 2 to 20 times per week, with 50% occurring daily and one third occurring several times a day. Up to one third of bulimics have a history of anorexia nervosa, and approximately one third also use laxatives. Each binge may be followed by a depressed episode, self-criticism, and self-induced vomiting. In addition, a subpopulation engages in regular binge eating without purging. Subtyping in the DSM-IV distinguishes between individuals who purge and those who use nonpurging behaviors. More significantly, the addition of a fifth criterion specifies that the disorder not occur exclusively during episodes of anorexia nervosa, thus preventing both diagnoses in the same patient.

Bulimic patients usually have a history of numerous strict or fad diets, punctuated by recurrent episodes of binging and persistent overconcern with body shape and weight (511, 512). MDD, as well as alcohol and drug abuse, often coexist in bulimia nervosa patients.

Drug Therapy of Bulimia Nervosa

Whereas attempts to treat anorexia nervosa pharmacologically have generally been disappointing, the role of medication in the treatment of bulimia nervosa is more promising. There are several positive studies published, many of which used larger sample sizes and were well controlled. Most have centered on the possible efficacy of the following:

- *Antidepressants*
- *Anticonvulsants*
- *Lithium*
- *Other agents* (e.g., opioid antagonists)

Antidepressants

Controlled trials have shown that antidepressants are more effective than placebo in reducing the frequency of overeating and the intensity of some of the symptoms of bulimia nervosa (513, 514). Furthermore, these agents have been effective whether or not the patient was depressed (515, 516), suggesting that the decrease in bulimic symptoms may be due to the direct effect of these drugs on brain mechanisms that control eating. There is no evidence, however, that they also have an impact on disturbed attitudes about body shape, weight, or extreme dieting (517, 518).

Pope and colleagues (519) published the first double-blind, placebo-controlled trial demonstrating the efficacy of antidepressants in bulimia nervosa. They found 200 mg per day of imipramine significantly superior to placebo in decreasing the following:

- The *frequency* of binges
- The *intensity* of binges
- The *preoccupation* with food

These results were replicated by Agras' group (520). Subsequently, Mitchell et al. (521) randomly assigned patients to 12 weeks of imipramine only, placebo only, imipramine plus group psychotherapy, or placebo plus group psychotherapy. The results suggested that the three active treatment cells were more efficacious than placebo in reducing bulimic behaviors and improving mood. Some bulimia nervosa subsets may not be as responsive to active treatment, however, with Rothschild's group (522) demonstrating that imipramine was no more effective than placebo in treating bulimia in atypical depressives.

Hughes et al. (515) demonstrated that desipramine serum levels were positively correlated with improvement of bulimic behaviors. Similar results were also obtained by Barlow and colleagues (523) using a crossover design.

Walsh and colleagues (524) examined the long-term effects of desipramine on bulimia nervosa outcome. After confirming the superiority of desipramine over placebo for short-term treatment in 78 bulimic patients, these researchers followed up 29 desipramine responders maintained on active drug for 1 week and found no further improvement during this time. Nine of these patients then underwent a 24-week, double-blind, placebo-controlled discontinuation phase. Four of five desipramine-treated bulimic patients completed the study without relapse, whereas two of four placebo-treated patients relapsed, only one completed the study, and another dropped out after 13 weeks. Although the sample size is too small to draw any definitive conclusions, this study suggests that it may be useful to treat bulimia with maintenance desipramine. In a subsequent study, Agras' group (525) followed up patients randomly assigned to 16 or 24 weeks of desipramine treatment for 1 year. The group treated with desipramine for 24 weeks maintained significantly higher rates of improvement and recovery.

Mitchell and Groat (526), by contrast, found active drug therapy only marginally effective in the treatment of bulimia nervosa. This may have been due in part to the relatively *low amitriptyline doses* used (maximum 150 mg per day), resulting in average blood levels of only 103 ng/mL.

The overlap between atypical depression and bulimia nervosa, particularly the hyperphagia common to both disorders, has led investigators to try *monoamine oxidase inhibitors* for bulimia nervosa. *Isocarboxazid* and *phenelzine* have both been found superior to placebo in controlled, double-blind studies (516, 527). In one study of atypical depressed bulimic patients, phenelzine was found to be significantly more effective than either placebo or imipramine in treating both the depressive and the bulimic symptoms (522). Of note, 11 of 18 patients receiving isocarboxazid and 24 of 27 patients receiving phenelzine in the aforementioned studies discontinued treatment as a result of side effects. Subsequently, the selective MAOI, *brofaromine,* was found to be superior to placebo in decreasing the frequency of vomiting in bulimia nervosa, but not in decreasing the frequency of binging, changing attitudes, or decreasing self-reports of depression or anxiety (528). Some clinicians justifiably question the safety of prescribing medications requiring dietary restrictions to a population whose symptoms include lack of control over food intake. As noted earlier in the discussion on anorexia nervosa, selective and reversible inhibitors of monoamine oxidase may prove to be safer, and thus more useful.

Two later-generation antidepressants, *bupropion* and *trazodone,* have demonstrated efficacy in bulimia nervosa, in well-controlled trials (529, 530). **Four of the patients given bupropion experienced grand mal seizures in this study, and this medication is contraindicated in patients with eating disorders.** Although *mianserin* is the only antidepressant other than amitriptyline not found to have an advantage over placebo in the treatment of bulimia nervosa, the 60-mg per day dose used was significantly less than the usual antidepressant dose of 150 mg per day (531). *Nomifensine,* which is no longer available because of its unacceptable adverse effects, was shown to be efficacious in two uncontrolled studies as well as in a small double-blind, placebo-controlled crossover design study (532–534).

The most promising results have come from studies with SSRIs in bulimia nervosa. The first controlled trial using fluoxetine was small, but showed a definite treatment advantage over placebo (513). Subsequently, a large multicenter study confirmed this finding (535). Almost 400 outpatients were randomly assigned to 20 or 60 mg per day of fluoxetine, or placebo for 8 weeks. Fluoxetine 60 mg per day was superior to both placebo and 20 mg of fluoxetine, in decreasing both vomiting and binging.

Fluoxetine 30 mg per day significantly decreased vomiting but not binging when compared with placebo. Both doses of fluoxetine were well tolerated by study participants. These findings conflict, however, with a double-blind trial of fluoxetine 60 mg per day versus placebo in 40 patients (536). In this study, both groups demonstrated improvement, with no significant difference between them. The authors posit the existence of a "ceiling effect" resulting from the intensive inpatient care and behavioral therapy. In essence, the effects of these factors is so great that they limit the ability to demonstrate any improvement gained by the addition of medication.

An open-label trial of fluvoxamine in 20 patients and a single case report with sertraline are also encouraging (537, 538).

Anticonvulsants

Studies using anticonvulsants to treat bulimia nervosa have had little success. Nineteen subjects underwent treatment for 12 weeks in a double-blind crossover study of unspecified doses of *phenytoin* and placebo (539). Although the mean number of binges on phenytoin decreased slightly, it was not significantly different from placebo. There are several problems with this study, however, including the fact that 7 of 19 patients had subtherapeutic phenytoin levels (including two patients whose levels indicated gross noncompliance). Furthermore, the study explicitly targeted binge eaters rather than bulimics. *CBZ* was administered to six patients in a double-blind crossover study, but the only patient who demonstrated marked improvement had a history consistent with bipolar disorder (540).

Lithium

A small controlled study of *lithium* was no more promising, with bulimia nervosa patients on active drug showing improvement similar to those on placebo (541). The relatively low lithium plasma levels (0.62 mEq/L) achieved may have been a factor.

Other Agents

Paralleling the anorexia nervosa story, animal studies implicating endogenous opioids in the regulation of stress-induced eating prompted a controlled trial of the *opioid antagonist* naltrexone. However, it failed to elicit a significant reduction in bulimic behaviors (542).

Other than antidepressants, the most encouraging research to date is in the area of serotonergic agonists, with fenfluramine being the best studied of these agents. Thus, two small trials found fenfluramine to have antibulimic potential, but a later study did not replicate these findings (543–545). In one study, 43 patients underwent treatment for 8 weeks with 45 mg per day of fenfluramine or placebo. Because abnormal eating behaviors improved in both groups, fenfluramine did not offer a significant advantage over placebo. The authors refer to the earlier hypothesized "ceiling effect" to explain this finding, because all patients also received cognitive-behavioral therapy. This agent has since been taken off the market because of potential cardiac complications (546).

Conclusion

The role of medication in the treatment of bulimia nervosa seems better established than its role in the treatment of anorexia nervosa. The American Psychiatric Association "Practice Guideline for Eating Disorders" (510) suggests that antidepressants may be useful in bulimia nervosa with or without depression. They may be particularly helpful, however, in those with depression, anxiety, obsessions, or who have failed psychosocial therapies.

Bulimia Nervosa Multisymptomatic

Patients with this disorder not only have a disturbed eating pattern but also problems with impulse control, often resulting in drug or alcohol abuse, self-mutilation, kleptomania, and sexual disinhibition. They also may have symptoms of obsessive-compulsive disorder or obsessive-compulsive personality disorder (498). In these individuals, manipulation of food is associated in varying degrees with alcohol and drug abuse. They are typically poor candidates for pharmacotherapy and, not surprisingly, have been unresponsive to a variety of psychotropics.

Summary

Eating disorders are well recognized psychiatric illnesses associated with significant morbidity and mortality rates. Attempts to treat anorexia nervosa with medications have proved disappointing; thus, psychotherapy using cognitive and behavioral interventions remains central to an effective strategy. Bulimia nervosa has been more responsive to pharmacotherapy. In particular, antidepressants appear to play an important role. Clearly, medications should never be the sole treatment of any eating disorder, but in selected patients may play a part in a comprehensive treatment strategy (510). Eating disorders are frequently accompanied by other Axis I conditions, which require pharmacotherapy.

CONCLUSION

Advances in psychopharmacotherapy are occurring at an ever-accelerating pace. These events demand an increasing sophistication on the part of all clinicians working in the mental health field. Whether they prescribe medications or not, clinicians must have knowledge about the role as well as potential benefits and risks of drug therapy as a prerequisite for providing the best care possible for patients. These issues are most evident when caring for the specialized needs of the patients considered in this final chapter. The aim of these discussions is to provide signposts and reasonable courses of action based on the present state of knowledge. The clinician must remain alert to such issues, as well as to the inevitable advances that will occur in the assessment and therapeutic management of these special populations.

REFERENCES

1. Coyle I, Wayner MJ, Singer G. Behavioral teratogenesis: a critical evaluation. *Pharmacol Biochem Behav* 1976;4:191–200.

2. Miller LJ. Clinical strategies for the use of psychotropic drugs during pregnancy. In: Janicak PG, Davis JM (guest eds). *Psychiatr Med* 1991;9:275–298.

3. Miller LJ. Psychiatric medication during pregnancy; understanding and minimizing risks. In: Janicak PG (guest ed). *Psychiatr Ann* 1994;24;69–75.

4. Koren G, Pastuszak A, Ito S. Drugs in pregnancy. *N Engl J Med* 1998;338:1128–1137.

5. Barki ZHK, Kravitz HM, Berki TM. Psychotropic medications in pregnancy. *Psychiatr Ann* 1998;28:486–500.

6. Gold LH. Use of psychotropic medication during pregnancy: risk management guidelines. *Psychiatr Ann* 2000;30:421–432.

7. Miller LJ. Pharmacotherapy during the perinatal period. *Dir Psychiatry* 1998;18:49–63.

8. Altshuler LL, Cohen L, Szuba MP, et al. Pharmacologic management of psychiatric illness during pregnancy: dilemmas and guidelines. *Am J Psychiatry* 1996;153:592–606.

9. Burr WA, Falek A, Strauss LT, et al. Fertility in psychiatric outpatients. *Hosp Community Psychiatry* 1979;30:527–531.

10. Kuny S, Binswanger U. Neuroleptic-induced extrapyramidal symptoms and serum calcium levels: results of a pilot study. *Pharmacopsychiatry* 1989;21:67–70.

11. Chambers CD, Johnson KA, Dick LM, et al. Birth outcomes in pregnant women taking fluoxetine. *N Engl J Med* 1996;335:1010–1015.

12. Cohen LS, Heller VL, Rosenbaum JF. Treatment guidelines for psychotropic drug use in pregnancy. *Psychosomatics* 1989;30:25–33.

13. Jacobsen SS, Jones K, Johnson K, et al. Prospective multicentered study of pregnancy outcome after lithium exposure during the first trimester. *Lancet* 1992;339:530–533.

14. Kaneko S. A rational antiepileptic drug therapy of epileptic women in child bearing age. *Jpn J Psychiatry Neurol* 1988;42:473–482.

15. Murasaki O, Yoshitake K, Tachiki H, et al. Reexamination of the teratological effect of antiepileptic drugs. *Jpn J Psychiatry Neurol* 1988;42:592–593.

16. Cohen LS. Psychotropic drug use in pregnancy. *Hosp Community Psychiatry* 1989;40:566–567.

17. McElhatton PR. The effects of benzodiazepine use during pregnancy and lactation. *Reprod Toxicol* 1994;8:461–475.

18. Saxen I. Cleft palate and maternal diphenhydramine intake. *Lancet* 1974;1:407–408.

19. Stahl MM, Saldeen P, Vinge E. Reversal of fetal benzodiazepine intoxication using flumazenil. *Br J Obstet Gynaecol* 1993;100:185–188.

20. American Psychiatric Association. *Diagnostic and statistical manual of mental disorders,* 4th ed. Washington, DC: American Psychiatric Press, 1994:711–718.

21. Yonkers KA, Brown WA. Pharmacologic treatments for premenstrual dysphoric disorder. *Psychiatr Ann* 1996;26:596–589.

22. Freeman EW, Rickels K, Sondheimer SJ, et al. A double-blind trial of oral progesterone, alprazolam, and placebo in treatment of severe premenstrual syndrome. *JAMA* 1995;274:51–57.

23. Harrison WM, Endicott J, Nee J. Treatment of premenstrual dysphoria with alprazolam. *Arch Gen Psychiatry* 1990;47:270–275.

24. Smith S, Rinehart JS, Ruddock VE, et al. Treatment of premenstrual syndrome with alprazolam: results of a double-blind, placebo-controlled, randomized crossover clinical trial. *Obstet Gynecol* 1987;70: 37–43.

25. Schmidt PJ, Grover GN, Rubinow DR. Alprazolam in the treatment of premenstrual syndrome. A double-blind, placebo-controlled trial. *Arch Gen Psychiatry* 1993;50:467–473.

26. Berger CP, Presser B. Alprazolam in the treatment of two subsamples of patients with late luteal phase dysphoric disorder: a double-blind, placebo-controlled crossover study. *Obstet Gynecol* 1994;84: 379–385.

27. Brown WA. PMS: a quiet breakthrough. *Psychiatr Ann* 1996;26:569–570.

28. Pearlstein T. Nonpharmacological treatment of premenstrual syndrome. *Psychiatr Ann* 1996;26:590–594.

29. Kauffman RE. Drug safety, testing and availability for children. *Children's Legal Rights J* 1998;18:178–185.

30. Tosyali MC, Greenhill LL. Child and adolescent psychopharmacology: important developmental issues. *Pediatr Clin North Am* 1998;45:1021–1035.

31. National Institute of Mental Health. Implementation of the national plan for research on child and adolescent mental disorders. PA-91-46. Washington, DC: US Dept of Health and Human Services, Public Health Service, Alcohol, Drug Abuse, and Mental Health Administration, 1991.

32. National Institute of Mental Health. Ethical and human subjects issues in mental health research with children and adolescents. Washington, DC: National Institute of Mental Health, 1993.

33. Kauffman RE, Banner W Jr, Berlin CM Jr, et al. Guidelines for the ethical conduct of studies to evaluate drugs in pediatric populations. *Pediatrics* 1995;95:169–177.

34. Preskorn SH, Bupp S, Weller E, et al. Plasma levels of imipramine and metabolites in 68 hospitalized children. *J Am Acad Child Adolesc Psychiatry* 1989;28: 373–375.

35. Magnus RD, Findling R, Preskorn SH, et al. An open-label pharmacokinetic trial of nefazodone in depressed children and adolescents [Abstract]. *Psychopharmacol Bull* 1997;33:550.

36. Derivan A, Aguiar L, Preskorn S, et al. A study of venlafaxine in children and adolescents with conduct disorder. Annual Meeting of the American Academy of Child and Adolescent Psychiatry, New Orleans, 1995.

37. Leeder JS, Kearns GL. Pharmacogenetics in pediatrics: implications for practice. *Pediatr Clin North Am* 1997;44:55–77.

38. Milavetz G, Vaughan LM, Weinberger E. Evaluation of a scheme for establishing and maintaining dosage of theophylline in ambulatory patients with chronic asthma. *J Pediatr* 1986;109:351–356.

39. Korinthenberg R, Haug C, Hannak D. The metabolism of carbamazepine to CBZ-10,11 epoxide in children from the newborn age to adolescence. *Neuropediatrics* 1994;25:214–224.

40. Carlson GA. Bipolar disorders in children and adolescents. In: Garfinkel B, Carlson GA, Weller E, eds. *Psychiatric disorders in children and adolescents.* Philadelphia: WB Saunders, 1990:21–36.

41. Goldman LS, Genel M, Bezman RJ, et al. Diagnosis and treatment of attention-deficit/hyperactivity disorder in children and adolescents. *JAMA* 1998;279:1100–1107.

42. Wilens TE. *Straight talk about psychiatric medications for kids.* New York: Guilford Press, 1999:7–106.

43. Greenhill LL, Abikoff HB, Arnold LE, et al. Medication treatment strategies in the MTA study: relevance to clinicians and researchers. *J Am Acad Child Adolesc Psychiatry* 1996;35:1304–1313.

44. Bradley C. The behavior of children receiving benzedrine. *Am J Psychiatry* 1937;94:577–588.

45. American Psychiatric Association. *Diagnostic and statistical manual of mental disorders,* 4th ed. Washington, DC: American Psychiatric Press, 1994.

46. Berry CA, Shaywitz BA. Girls with attention deficit disorder: a silent minority? A report on behavioral and cognitive characteristics. *Pediatrics* 1985;76:801–809.

47. Cantwell DP. Attention deficit disorder: a review of the past 10 years. *J Am Acad Child Adolesc Psychiatry* 1996;35:978–987.

48. Goodman R, Stevenson J. A twin study of hyperactivity, II: The etiologic role of genes, family relationships, and perinatal adversity. *J Child Psychol Psychiatry* 1989;30:691–709.

49. Gillis JJ, Gilger JW, Pennington BF. Attention deficit disorder in reading-disabled twins: evidence for a genetic etiology. *J Abnorm Child Psychol* 1992;20:303–315.

50. Barkley RA. *Attention deficit hyperactivity disorder: a handbook for diagnosis and treatment.* New York: Guilford Press, 1990.

51. Biederman J, Newcorn J, Sprich S. Comorbidity of attention deficit hyperactivity disorder with conduct, depressive, anxiety, and other disorders. *Am J Psychiatry* 1991;148:564–577.

52. Wilens TE. Update on attention deficit hyperactivity disorder. *Curr Affect Illness* 1996;15:5–12.

53. Shaywitz BE, Fletcher JM, Shaywitz SE. Defining and classifying learning disabilities and attention-deficit/hyperactivity disorder. *J Child Neurol* 1995;10:S50–S57.

54. Shaywitz BE, Fletcher JM, Shaywitz SE. Attention deficit hyperactivity disorder. *Adv Pediatr* 1997;44:331–367.

55. Hill JC, Schoener EP. Age-dependent decline of attention deficit hyperactivity disorder. *Am J Psychiatry* 1996;153:1143–1146.

56. Biederman J, Faraone S, Milberger S. Predictors of persistence and remission of ADHD: results from a four year prospective follow-up study of ADHD children. *J Am Acad Child Adolesc Psychiatry* 1995;35:343–351.

57. Cantwell DP. Hyperactive children have grown up: what have we learned about what happens to them. *Arch Gen Psychiatry* 1985;42:1026–1028.

58. Mannuzza S, Klein RG, Bessler A. Adult outcome of hyperactive boys. *Arch Gen Psychiatry* 1993;50:565–576.

59. Pelham WEJ, Wheeler T, Chronis A. Empirically supported psychosocial treatments for attention deficit-hyperactivity disorder. *J Clin Child Psychol* 1998;27:190–205.

60. Conners CK. Conners' Rating Scales–revised. Toronto: Multi-Health Systems, 1997.
61. Swanson JM. *School based assessments and intervention for ADD dtudents.* California: Irvine, KC Publishing, 1992.
62. Gaub M, Carlson CL. Behavioral characteristics of DSM-IV ADHD subtypes in a school based population. *J Abnorm Child Psychol* 1997;25:103–111.
63. Swanson JM, McBurnett K, Wigan T, et al. Effect of stimulant medication on children with attention deficit disorder: a review of reviews. *Except Child* 1993;60:154–162.
64. Dulcan MK. Using psychostimulants to treat behavioral disorders of children and adolescents. *J Child Adolesc Psychopharmacol* 1990;1:7–20.
65. Klein RG, Wender P. The role of methylphenidate in psychiatry. *Arch Gen Psychiatry* 1995;52:429–433.
66. Spencer T, Biederman J, Wilens T, et al. Pharmacotherapy of attention deficit hyperactivity disorder across the life cycle. *J Am Acad Child Adolesc Psychiatry* 1996;35:409–432.
67. Pelham WE, Midlam JK, Gnagy EM, et al. A comparison of Ritalin and Adderall: efficacy and time course in children with attention deficit hyperactivity disorder. *Pediatrics* 1999;103:343–353.
68. Swanson JM, Wigal S, Greenhill LL, et al. Analog classroom assessment of Adderall in children with ADHD. *J Am Acad Child Adolesc Psychiatry* 1998;37:519–526.
69. Coffey B, Shader RI, Greenblatt DJ. Pharmacokinetics of benzodiazepines and psychostimulants in children. *J Clin Psychopharmacol* 1983;3:217–225.
70. Elia J, Borcherding BG, Rapoport JL, et al. Methylphenidate and dextroamphetamine treatments of hyperactivity: are there true nonresponders? *Psychiatry Res* 1991;36:141–155.
71. Pelham WE, Bender ME, Caddell J, et al. Methylphenidate and children with attention deficit disorder: dose effects on classroom academic and social behavior. *Arch Gen Psychiatry* 1985;42:948–952.
72. Swanson L, Greenhill W, Pelham WE. Initiating Concerta (OROS methylphenidate HCl) qd in children with attention deficit hyperactivity disorder. *J Clin Res* 2000;3:59–76.
73. Conners CK, Taylor E. Pemoline methylphenidate, and placebo in children with minimal brain dysfunction. *Arch Gen Psychiatry* 1980;37:922–930.
74. Pelham WE, Swanson JM, Furman MB, et al. Pemoline effects on children with ADHD: a time response by dose response analysis on classroom measures. *J Am Acad Child Adolesc Psychiatry* 1995;34:1504–1513.
75. Jacobvitz D. Treatment of attentional and hyperactivity problems in children with sympathomimetic drugs: a comprehensive review. *J Am Acad Child Adolesc Psychiatry* 1990;29:677–688.
76. Whalen CK, Henker B, Swanson JM, et al. Natural social behaviors in hyperactive children: dose effects of methylphenidate. *J Consult Clin Psychol* 1987;55:187–193.
77. Barkley RA, Karlsson J, Strzelecki E, et al. Effects of age and Ritalin dosage on the mother-child interactions of hyperactive children. *J Consult Clin Psychol* 1984;52:750–758.
78. Barkley RA, Karlsson J, Pollard S, et al. Developmental changes in the mother-child interactions of hyperactive boys: effects of two dose levels of Ritalin. *J Child Psychol Psychiatry* 1985;26:705–715.
79. Gillberg C, Melander H, von Knorring AL, et al. Long term stimulant treatment of children with attention deficit hyperactivity disorder symptoms: a randomized double blind, placebo controlled trial. *Arch Gen Psychiatry* 1997;54:857–864.
80. Hechtman L, Abikoff H. Multimodal treatment plus stimulants vs stimulant treatment in ADHD children: results from a two year comparative treatment study. 42nd Annual Meeting of the American Academy of Child and Adolescent Psychiatry, New Orleans, 1995.
81. Arnold LE, Abikoff HB, Cantwell DP, et al. Design challenges and choices. *Arch Gen Psychiatry* 1997;54:865–870.
82. MTA Cooperative Group. 14 Month randomized clinical trial of treatment strategies for attention deficit/hyperactivy disorder: the MTA study. *Arch Gen Psychiatry* 1999;56:1073–1086.
83. Varley CK. Effects of methylphenidate in adolescents with attention deficit disorder. *J Am Acad Child Psychiatry* 1983;4:351–354.
84. Hechtman L, Weiss G, Perlman T. Young adult outcome of hyperactive children who received long term stimulant treatment. *J Am Acad Child Psychiatry* 1984;23:261–269.
85. Loney J, Kramer J, Milich RS. In: Gadow KD, Loney J, eds. *Psychosocial aspects of drug treatment for hyperactivity.* Boulder, CO: Westview Press, 1981:381–415.
86. Gittelman R, Mannuzza S, Shenker R, et al. Hyperactive boys almost grown up. I. Psychiatric status. *Arch Gen Psychiatry* 1985;42:937–947.
87. Hughes C, Preskorn SH, Weller E, et al. Follow-up of adolescents initially treated for prepubertal onset major depressive disorders with imipramine. *Psychopharmacol Bull* 1990;26:244–248.
88. Castellanos FX, Giedd JN, Elia J, et al. Controlled stimulant treatment of ADHD and comorbid Tourette's syndrome: effects of stimulant and dose. *J Am Acad Child Adolesc Psychiatry* 1997;36:589–596.
89. Gadow KD, Nolan EE, Sverd J. Methylphenidate in hyperactive boys with comorbid tic disorder: II. Short term behavioral effects in school settings. *J Am Acad Child Adolesc Psychiatry* 1992;31:462–471.
90. Jadad A, Atkins D. *The treatment of attention deficit/hyperactivity disorder: an evidence report.* Hamilton, Ontario: Ontario Agency for Health Care Policy and Research, 1998.
91. Biederman J, Baldessarini RJ, Wright V, et al. A double-blind placebo controlled study of desipramine in the treatment of ADD I: Efficacy. *J Am Acad Child Adolesc Psychiatry* 1989;28:777–784.
92. Biederman J, Thisted RA, Greenhill LL, et al. Estimation of the association between desipramine and the risk for sudden death in 5 to 14 year old children. *J Clin Psychiatry* 1995;56:87–93.
93. Popper CW, Ziminitzky B. Sudden death putatively related to desipramine treatment in youth: a fifth case and a review of speculative mechanisms. *J Child Adolesc Psychopharmacol* 1995;5:283–300.
94. Spencer T, Biederman J, Wilens T, et al. Nortriptyline treatment of children with attention deficit hyperactivity disorder and tic disorder or Tourette's syndrome.

J Am Acad Child Adolesc Psychiatry 1993;32:205–210.

95. Wilens TE, Biederman J, Geist DE, et al. Nortriptyline in the treatment of ADHD: a chart review of 58 cases. *J Am Acad Child Adolesc Psychiatry* 1993;32:343–349.

96. Wilens TE, Biederman J, Mick E, et al. A systematic assessment of tricyclic antidepressants in the treatment of adult attention deficit hyperactivity disorder. *J Nerv Ment Dis* 1995;183:48–50.

97. Daly JM, Wilens T. The use of tricyclics antidepressants in children and adolescents. *Pediatr Clin North Am* 1998;45:1123–1135.

98. Casat CD, Pleasants DZ, Van Wyck F. A double-blind trial of bupropion in children with attention deficit disorder. *Psychopharmacol Bull* 1987;23:120–122.

99. Barrickman LL, Perry PJ, Allen AJ, et al. Bupropion versus methylphenidate in the treatment of attention-deficit hyperactivity disorder. *J Am Acad Child Adolesc Psychiatry* 1995;34:649–657.

100. Conners CK, Casat CD, Gualtieri CT, et al. Bupropion hydrochloride in attention deficit disorder with hyperactivity. *J Am Acad Child Adolesc Psychiatry* 1996;35:1314–1321.

101. Hunt RD, Minderaa RB, Cohen DJ. Clonidine benefits children with attention deficit disorder and hyperactivity: report of a double blind placebo crossover therapeutic trial. *J Am Acad Child Psychiatry* 1985;24:617–629.

102. Leckman JF, Hardin MT, Riddle MA, et al. Clonidine treatment of Gilles de la Tourette's syndrome. *Arch Gen Psychiatry* 1991;48:324–328.

103. Singer HS, Quaskey S, Rosenberg LA, et al. The treatment of attention deficit hyperactivity disorder in Tourette's syndrome: a double blind placebo controlled study with clonidine and desipramine. *Pediatrics* 1995;95:74–81.

104. van der Meere J, Gunning B, Stemerdink N. The effect of methylphenidate and clonidine on response inhibition and state regulation in children with ADHD. *J Child Psychol Psychiatry* 1999;40:291–298.

105. Wilens TE, Spencer TJ. Combining methylphenidate and clonidine. *J Am Acad Child Adolesc Psychiatry* 1999;38:614–622.

106. Chappell PB, Riddle MA, Scahill L, et al. Guanfacine treatment of comorbid attention deficit hyperactivity disorder and Tourette's syndrome: preliminary clinical experience. *J Am Acad Child Psychiatry* 1995;34:1140–1146.

107. Horrigan JP, Barnhill LJ. Guanfacine for the treatment of attention deficit hyperactivity disorder in boys. *J Child Adolesc Psychopharmacol* 1995;5:215–223.

108. Hunt RD, Arnsten AFT, Asbell MD. An open trial of guanfacine in the treatment of attention deficit hyperactivity disorder. *J Am Acad Child Adolesc Psychiatry* 1995;34:50–54.

109. Scahill L, Chappell PB, Kim YS, et al. Guanfacine in attention deficit/hyperactivity disorder. 46th Annual Meeting of the American Academy of Child and Adolescent Psychiatry, Chicago, 1999.

110. Hughes CW, Preskorn SH, Weller E, et al. A descriptive profile of the depressed child. *Psychopharmacol Bull* 1989;25:232–237.

111. Brent DA, Holder D, Kolko D, et al. A clinical psychotherapy trial for adolescent depression comparing cognitive, family and supportive treatments. *Arch Gen Psychiatry* 1997;54:877–885.

112. Birmaher B. Should we use antidepressant medications for children and adolescents with depressive disorders? *Psychopharmacol Bull* 1998;34:35–39.

113. Hammen C, Rudolph K, Weiss J, et al. The context of depression in clinic-referred youth: neglected areas in treatment. *J Am Acad Child Adolesc Psychiatry* 1999;38:64–71.

114. Puig-Antich J, Perel J, Luptakin W, et al. Plasma levels of imipramine (IMI) and desmethylimipramine (DMI) and clinical response in prepubertal and major depressive disorder: a preliminary report. *J Am Acad Child Psychiatry* 1979;18:616–627.

115. Hughes C, Preskorn SH, Weller E, et al. The effect of concomitant disorders in childhood depression on predicting treatment response. *Psychopharmacol Bull* 1990;26:235–238.

116. Hoar W. Prozac Rx for children jumps 500%. *Ment Health News Alert* 1998;13.

117. Strober M, DeAntonio M, Schmidt-Lackner S, et al. The pharmacotherapy of depressive illness in adolescents: an open-label comparison of fluoxetine with imipramine-treated historical controls. *J Clin Psychiatry* 1999;60:164–169.

118. Simeon J, diNicola V, Ferguson HB, et al. Adolescent depression: a placebo-controlled fluoxetine treatment study and follow-up. *Prog Neuro-Psychopharmacol Biol Psychiatry* 1990;4:791–795.

119. Emslie GJ, Rush A, Weinberg WA, et al. A double-blind, randomized, placebo-controlled trial of fluoxetine in children and adolescents with depression. *Arch Gen Psychiatry* 1997;54:1031–1037.

120. Keller MB, Ryan NMD, Birmaher B, et al. Paroxetine and imipramine in the treatment of adolescent depression. New Research Program Abstracts, Annual Meeting of the American Psychiatric Association, Toronto, 1998.

121. Ambrosini PJ, Wagner KD, Biederman J, et al. Multicenter open label sertraline study in adolescent outpatients with major depression. *J Am Acad Child Adolesc Psychiatry* 1999;38:566–572.

122. Birmaher B, Ryan ND, Williamson DE, et al. Childhood and adolescent depression: a review of the past 10 years. Part I. *J Am Acad Child Adolesc Psychiatry* 1996;35:1427–1439.

123. Birmaher B, Ryan ND, Williamson DE, et al. Childhood and adolescent depression: a review of the past 10 years. Part II. *J Am Acad Child Adolesc Psychiatry* 1996;35:1575–1583.

124. Kashani JH, Shekim WO, Reid JC. Amitriptyline in children with major depressive disorder. A double blind crossover pilot study. *J Am Acad Child Psychiatry* 1984;23:348–351.

125. Preskorn SH, Weller E, Hughes C, et al. Depression in prepubertal children. Dexamethasone nonsuppression predicts differential response to imipramine vs. placebo. *Psychopharmacol Bull* 1987;23:128–133.

126. Preskorn SH, Weller E, Weller R. Depression in children: relationship between plasma imipramine levels and response. *J Clin Psychiatry* 1982;43:450–453.

127. Kramer A, Feiguine R. Clinical effects of amitriptyline in adolescent depression. *J Am Acad Child Psychiatry* 1981;20:636–644.

128. Geller B, Cooper TB, Graham DL, et al. Pharmacokinetically designed double-blind placebo-controlled study of nortriptyline in 6 to 12 year-olds with major depressive disorder. *J Am Acad Child Adolesc Psychiatry* 1992;31:34–44.

129. Kutcher S, Boulos C, Ward B, et al. Response to desipramine treatment in adolescent depression: a fixed-dose, placebo-controlled trial. *J Am Acad Child Adolesc Psychiatry* 1994;33:686–694.

130. Emslie GJ, Rush AJ, Weinberg WA, et al. Recurrence of major depressive disorder in hospitalized children and adolescents. *J Am Acad Child Adolesc Psychiatry* 1997;36:785–792.

131. McCauley E, Myers K, Mitchell J, et al. Depression in young people: initial presentation and clinical course. *J Am Acad Child Adolesc Psychiatry* 1993;32:714–722.

132. Rao U, Ryan ND, Birmaher B, et al. Unipolar depression in adolescents: clinical outcome in adulthood. *J Am Acad Child Adolesc Psychiatry* 1995;34:566–578.

133. Go FS, Malley EE, Birmaher B, et al. Manic behavior associated with fluoxetine in three 12–18 year olds with OCD. *J Child Adolesc Psychopharmacol* 1998;8:73–80.

134. Guiles JM. Sertraline induced behavior activation during the treatment of an adolescent with MDD. *J Child Adolesc Psychopharmacol* 1996;6:281–285.

135. Lake CR, Mikkelsen EJ, Rapoport JL. Effect of imipramine on norepinephrine and blood pressure in enuretic boys. *Clin Pharmacol Ther* 1979;39:647–647.

136. Preskorn SH. What happened to Tommy? *J Pract Psychiatry Behav Health* 1998;4:363–367.

137. Preskorn SH, Fast GA. Therapeutic drug monitoring for antidepressants: efficacy, safety and cost effectiveness. *J Clin Psychiatry* 1991;52[6, Suppl]:23–33.

138. Preskorn SH, Weller E, Jerkovich G, et al. Depression in children: concentration-dependent CNS toxicity of tricyclic antidepressants. *Psychopharmacol Bull* 1988;24:140–142.

139. Riddle MA, Nelson JC, Kleinman CS. Sudden death in children receiving norpramin: a review of three reported cases and commentary. *J Am Acad Child Adolesc Psychiatry* 1991;30:104–104.

140. Biederman J. Sudden death in children treated with a tricyclic antidepressant: a commentary. *Biol Ther Psychiatry* 1991;4:1–1.

141. Hughes CW, Emslie GA. Treatment of anxiety disorders in children and adolescents. In: Rush A, ed. *Current review of mood and anxiety disorders.* Baltimore: Williams & Wilkins, 1998;293–320.

142. Allen AJ, Leonard H, Swedo SE. Current knowledge of medications for the treatment of childhood anxiety disorders. *J Am Acad Child Adolesc Psychiatry* 1995;34:976–986.

143. Ambrosini PJ, Bianchi MD, Rabinovich H, et al. Antidepressant treatments in children and adolescents: II. Anxiety, physical, and behavioral disorders. *J Am Acad Child Adolesc Psychiatry* 1993;32:483–493.

144. Campbell M, Cueva J. Psychopharmacology in child and adolescent psychiatry: a review of the past seven years. Part I. *J Am Acad Child Adolesc Psychiatry* 1995;34:1124–1132.

145. Klein R, Slomkowski C. Treatment of psychiatric disorders in children and adolescents. *Psychopharmacol Bull* 1993;29:525–535.

146. De-Veaugh-Geiss J, Moroz G, Biederman J. Chlorimipramine hydrochloride in childhood and adolescent obsessive-compulsive disorder: a multicenter trial. *J Am Acad Child Adolesc Psychiatry* 1992;31:45–49.

147. Flament MF, Rapoport JL, Berg CJ. Clomipramine treatment of childhood obsessive-compulsive disorder. *Arch Gen Psychiatry* 1985;42:977–983.

148. Leonard HS, Swedo S, Rapoport JL. Treatment of obsessive-compulsive disorder with clomipramine and desmethylimipramine: a double-blind crossover comparison in children and adolescents. *Arch Gen Psychiatry* 1989;46:1088–1092.

149. McConville B, Minnery KL, Sorter MT, et al. An open study of the effects of sertraline on adolescent major depression. *J Child Adolesc Psychopharmacol* 1996;6:41–51.

150. Wolkow R, March J, Safferman A, et al. A placebo controlled trial of sertraline treatment for pediatric obsessive compulsive disorder. 6th World Congress of Biological Psychiatry 1997;42:213S–213S.

151. Riddle MA, Scahill L, King RA. Double blind trial of fluoxetine and placebo in children and adolescents with obsessive compulsive disorder. *J Am Acad Child Adolesc Psychiatry* 1992;31:1062–1069.

152. Coffey BJ. Anxiolytics for children and adolescents: traditional and new drugs. *J Child Adolesc Psychopharmacol* 1990;1:57–83.

153. Bernstein GA, Garfinkel BD, Borchart CM. Comparative studies of pharmacotherapy for school refusal. *J Am Acad Child Adolesc Psychiatry* 1990;29:773–781.

154. Grae F, Milner J, Rizzotto L, et al. Clonazepam in childhood anxiety disorders. *J Am Acad Child Adolesc Psychiatry* 1994;33:372–376.

155. Simeon JG, Ferguson HB, Knott V. Clinical, cognitive and neurophysiological effects of alprazolam in children and adolescents with overanxious and avoidant disorders. *J Am Acad Child Adolesc Psychiatry* 1992;31:29–33.

156. Kutcher SP, Reiter S, Gardner DM, et al. The pharmacotherapy of anxiety disorders in children and adolescents. *Psychiatr Clin North Am* 1992;15:41–67.

157. Simeon JG. Use of anxiolytics in children. *Encephale* 1993;19:71–74.

158. Gittelman-Klein R, Klein DF. Separation anxiety in school refusal and its treatment with drugs. In: Hersov L, Berg I, eds. *Out of school.* New York: Wiley, 1980;321–341.

159. Klein RG, Koplewicz HS, Kanner A. Imipramine treatment of children with separation anxiety. *J Am Acad Child Adolesc Psychiatry* 1992;31:21–28.

160. Berney T, Kolvin I, Bhate SR. School phobia: a therapeutic trial with clomipramine and short-term outcome. *Br J Psychiatry* 1981;138:110–118.

161. Gittelman-Klein R, Klein DF. School phobia: diagnostic consideration in the light of imipramine effects. *J Nerv Ment Dis* 1973;156:199–215.

162. Black B, Uhde TW, Tancer ME. Fluoxetine for the treatment of social phobia. *J Am Acad Child Adolesc Psychiatry* 1992;29:36–44.

163. Dummit ESI, Klein RG, Tancer NK, et al. Fluoxetine treatment of children with selective mutism: an open trial. *J Am Acad Child Adolesc Psychiatry* 1996;35:615–621.

164. Brenner HD, Dencker SJ, Goldstein MJ, et al. Defining treatment refractoriness in schizophrenia. *Schizophr Bull* 1990;16:551–561.

165. Realmuto GM, Erickson WD, Yellin AM. Clinical comparison of thiothixene and thioridazine in schizophrenic adolescents. *Am J Psychiatry* 1984;141:440–442.

166. Toren P, Laor N, Weizman A. Use of atypical neuroleptics in child and adolescent psychiatry. *J Clin Psychiatry* 1998;59:644–656.

167. Campbell M, Rapoport JL, Simpson GM. Antipsychotics in children and adolescents. *J Am Acad Child Adolesc Psychiatry* 1999;38:537–545.

168. Kowatch RA, Suppes T, Gilfillan SK, et al. Clozapine treatment of children and adolescents with bipolar disorder and schizophrenia: a clinical case series. *J Child Adolesc Psychopharmacol* 1995;5:241–253.

169. Pool D, Bloom W, Mielke DH. A controlled evaluation of Loxitane in seventy-five adolescent schizophrenia patients. *Curr Ther Res* 1976;19:99–104.

170. Spencer EK, Kafantaris V, Padron-Gayol MV, et al. Haloperidol in schizophrenic children: early findings from a study in progress. *Psychopharmacol Bull* 1992;28:183–186.

171. Kumar S, Frazier JA, Jacobsen LK, et al. Childhood onset schizophrenia: a double-blind clozapine haloperidol comparison. *Arch Gen Psychiatry* 1996;53:1090–1097.

172. Remschmidt H, Schulz E, Martin M. An open trial of clozapine in thirty-six adolescents with schizophrenia. *J Child Adolesc Psychopharmacol* 1994;4:31–41.

173. Frazier JA, Gordon CT, McKenna K, et al. An open trial of clozapine in 19 adolescents with childhood onset schizophrenia. *J Am Acad Child Adolesc Psychiatry* 1994;33:658–663.

174. Blanz B, Schmidt MH. Clozapine for schizophrenia [Letter, Comment]. *J Am Acad Child Adolesc Psychiatry* 1993;32:223–224.

175. Kumar S, Herion D, Jacobsen LK, et al. Case study: risperidone induced hepatoxicity in pediatric patients. *J Am Acad Child Adolesc Psychiatry* 1997;36:701–705.

176. Buitelaar JK. Open-label treatment with risperidone of 26 psychiatrically-hospitalized children and adolescents with mixed diagnoses and aggressive behavior. *J Child Adolesc Psychopharmacol* 2000;10:19–26.

177. Lombroso PJ, Scahill L, King RA, et al. Risperidone treatment of children and adolescents with chronic tic disorders: a preliminary report. *J Am Acad Child Adolesc Psychiatry* 1995;34:1147–1152.

178. Simeon JG. Pediatric psychopharmacology. *Can J Psychiatry* 1989;34:115.

179. Armenteros JL, Whitaker AH, Welikson M, et al. Risperidone in adolescents with schizophrenia: an open pilot study. *J Am Acad Child Adolesc Psychiatry* 1997;36:694–700.

180. Kumar S, Jacobson LK, Lenane M, et al. Childhood onset schizophrenia: an open label study of olanzapine in adolescents. *J Am Acad Child Adolesc Psychiatry* 1998;37:377–385.

181. Wong GH, Cock RJ. Long term effects of haloperidol on severely emotionally disturbed children. *Aust N Z J Psychiatry* 1971;5:296–300.

182. Gittelman-Klein R, Klein DF, Katz S, et al. Comparative effects of methylphenidate and thioridazine in hyperkinetic children, I: Clinical results. *Arch Gen Psychiatry* 1976;33:1217–1231.

183. Perry R, Campbell M, Adams P, et al. Long term efficacy of haloperidol in autistic children: continuous versus discontinuous drug administration. *J Am Acad Child Adolesc Psychiatry* 1989;28:87–92.

184. Shapiro AK, Shapiro E. Treatment of tic disorders with neuroleptic drugs. In: Richardson MA, Haugland G, eds. *Use of neuroleptics in children*. Washington, DC: American Psychiatric Press, 1996;137–198.

185. Campbell M, Grega DM, Green WH, et al. Neuroleptic induced dyskinesias in children. *Clin Neuropharmacol* 1983;6:207–222.

186. Campbell M, Armentereos JL, Malone RP, et al. Neuroleptic related dyskinesias in autistic children: a prospective, longitudinal study. *J Am Acad Child Adolesc Psychiatry* 1997;36:835–843.

187. Frazier JA, Giedd JN, Kaysen D, et al. Childhood onset schizophrenia: brain MRI rescan after 2 years of clozapine maintenance treatment. *Am J Psychiatry* 1996;153:564–566.

188. Hinshaw SP, Heller T, McHale JP. Covert antisocial behavior in boys with attention deficit hyperactivity disorder: external validation and effects of methylphenidate. *J Consult Clin Psychol* 1992;60:274–281.

189. Klein RG, Abikoff H, Klass E, et al. Clinical efficacy of methylphenidate in conduct disorder with and without attention deficit. *Arch Gen Psychiatry* 1997;54:1073–1080.

190. Murphy DA, Pelham WE, Lang AR. Aggression in boys with attention deficit hyperactivity disorder: methylphenidate effects on naturalistically observed aggression, response to provocation and social information processing. *J Abnorm Child Psychol* 1992;20:451–466.

191. Campbell M, Cueva J. Psychopharmacology in child and adolescent psychiatry: a review of the past seven years. Part II. *J Am Acad Child Adolesc Psychiatry* 1995;34:1262–1272.

192. Campbell M, Adams PB, Small AM. Lithium in hospitalized aggressive children with conduct disorder: a double blind placebo controlled study. *J Am Acad Child Adolesc Psychiatry* 1995;34:445–453.

193. Donovan SJ, Susser ES, Nunes EV, et al. Divalproex treatment of disruptive adolescents: a report of 10 cases. *J Clin Psychiatry* 1997;58:12–15.

194. Greenhill LL, Solomon M, Pleak R, et al. Molindone hydrochloride treatment of hospitalized children with conduct disorder. *J Clin Psychiatry* 1985;46:20–25.

195. Cueva JE, Overall JE, Small AM, et al. Carbamazepine in aggressive children with conduct disorder: a double blind and placebo controlled study. *J Am Acad Child Adolesc Psychiatry* 1996;35:480–490.

196. Kemph JP, DeVane CL, Levin GM, et al. Treatment of aggressive children with clonidine: results of an open pilot study. *J Am Acad Child Adolesc Psychiatry* 1993;32:577–581.

197. Nam M, Sook-Haeng J, Jung IW, et al. Comparative efficacy of risperidone and haloperidol in the treatment of Tourette's disorders. 44th Annual Meeting of the American Academy of Child and Adolescent Psychiatry, Toronto, 1997.

198. Sallee FR, Nesbitt L, Jackson C, et al. Relative efficacy of haloperidol and pimozide in children and adolescents with Tourette's disorder. *Am J Psychiatry* 1997;154:1057–1062.

199. Opler LA, Feinberg SS. The role of pimozide in clinical psychiatry: a review. *J Clin Psychiatry* 1991;52:221–233.

200. Flockhart DA, Richard E, Woosley RL, et al. A metabolic interaction between clarithromycin and pimozide may result in cardiac toxicity. *Clin Pharmacol Ther* 1996;59:189–189.

201. Rodier PM. The early origins of autism: new research into the causes of this baffling disorder is focusing on genes that control the development of the brain. *Sci Am* 2000;28(2):56–63.

202. Bernstein GA, Hughes JR, Mitchell JE, Thompson T. Effects of narcotic antagonists on self-injurious behavior: a single case study. *J Am Acad Child Adolesc Psychiatry* 1987;26:886–889.

203. McDougle CJ, Holmes JP, Bronson MR, et al. Risperidone treatment of children and onset bipolar adolescents with pervasive developmental disorders: a prospective, open label study. *J Am Acad Child Adolesc Psychiatry* 1997;36:685–693.

204. McDougle CJ, Holmes JP, Carlson DC, et al. A double-blind, placebo-controlled study of risperidone in adults with autistic disorder and other pervasive developmental disorders. *Arch Gen Psychiatry* 1998;55:633–641.

205. Wozniak J, Biederman J, Kiely K, et al. Mania-like symptoms suggestive of childhood-disorder in clinically referred children. *J Am Acad Child Adolesc Psychiatry* 1995;34:867–876.

206. Geller B, Cooper TB, Sun K, et al. Double blind and placebo controlled study of lithium for adolescent bipolar disorders with secondary substance dependency. *J Am Acad Child Adolesc Psychiatry* 1998;37:171–178.

207. Ryan ND, Bhatara VS, Perel JM. Mood stabilizers in children and adolescents. *J Am Acad Child Adolesc Psychiatry* 1999;38:529–536.

208. Frazier JA, Meyer MC, Biederman J, et al. Risperidone treatment for juvenile bipolar disorder: a retrospective chart review. *J Am Acad Child Adolesc Psychiatry* 1999;38:960–965.

209. Natochin YV, Kuznetsova AA. Nocturnal enuresis: correction of renal function by desmopressin and diclofenac. *Pediatr Nephrol* 2000;14:42–47.

210. Tietjen DN, Husmann DA. Nocturnal enuresis: a guide to evaluation and treatment. *Mayo Clin Proc* 1996;71:857–862.

211. Schulman SL, Colish Y, von Zuben FC, et al. Effectiveness of treatments for nocturnal enuresis in a heterogeneous population. *Clin Pediatr* 2000;39:359–364.

212. Harari MD, Moulden A. Nocturnal enuresis: what is happening? *J Paediatr Child Health* 2000;36:78–81.

213. Davis JM, Janicak PG, Ayd FJ, Jr. Psychopharmacotherapy of the personality disordered patient. *Psychiatr Ann* 1995;25:614–620.

214. Ayd FJ, Jr. Psychopharmacologic treatment of personality disorders. *Int Drug Ther Newsl* 1990;25:1–2.

215. Munro A. Monosymptomatic hypochondriacal psychosis. *Br J Hosp Med* 1980;24:34–38.

216. Hymowitz P, Frances A, Jacobsberg L, et al. Neuroleptic treatment of schizotypal personality disorder. *Compr Psychiatry* 1986;27:267–271.

217. Goldberg SC, Schulz SC, Schulz PM, et al. Borderline and schizotypal personality disorders treated with low-dose thiothixene vs placebo. *Arch Gen Psychiatry* 1986;43:680–686.

218. Schulz SC. The use of low dose neuroleptics in the treatment of "schizo-obsessive" patients. *Am J Psychiatry* 1986;143:1318–1319.

219. Klein DF. Importance of psychiatric diagnosis in the prediction of clinical drug effects. *Arch Gen Psychiatry* 1967;16:118–126.

220. Widiger TA, Frances AJ. Epidemiology, diagnosis, and comorbidity of borderline personality disorder. In: Tasman A, Hales RE, Frances AJ, eds. *Review of psychiatry,* Vol 8. Washington, DC: American Psychiatric Press, 1989:8.

221. New AS, Trestman RL, Seiver LJ. The pharmacotherapy of borderline personality disorder. *CNS Drugs* 1994;2:347–354.

222. Gardner DL, Cowdry RW. Alprazolam induced dyscontrol in borderline personality disorder. *Am J Psychiatry* 1985;142:98–100.

223. Hedberg DL, Houck JH, Glueck BC Jr. Tranylcypromine-trifluoperazine combination in the treatment of schizophrenia. *Am J Psychiatry* 1971;127:1141–1146.

224. Cowdry RW, Gardner DL. Pharmacotherapy of borderline personality disorder. Alprazolam, carbamazepine, trifluoperazine, and tranylcypromine. *Arch Gen Psychiatry* 1988;45:111–119.

225. Soloff PH, Cornelius J, George A, et al. Efficacy of phenelzine and haloperidol in borderline personality disorder. *Arch Gen Psychiatry* 1993;50:377–385.

226. Coccaro EF, Astill JL, Herbert JA, et al. Fluoxetine treatment of impulsive aggression in DSM-III-R personality disorder patients. *J Clin Psychopharmacol* 1990;10:373–375.

227. Cornelius JR, Soloff PH, Perel JM, et al. Fluoxetine trial in borderline personality disorder. *Psychopharmacol Bull* 1990;26:151–154.

228. Cornelius JR, Soloff PH, Perel JM, et al. A preliminary trial of fluoxetine in refractory borderline patients. *J Clin Psychopharmacol* 1991;11:116–120.

229. Markowitz PJ, Calabrese JR, Schulz SC, et al. Fluoxetine treatment of borderline and schizotypal personality disorder. *Am J Psychiatry* 1991;148:1064–1067.

230. Norden MJ. Fluoxetine in borderline personality disorder. *Prog Neuropsychopharmacol Biol Psychiatry* 1989;13:885–893.

231. Kavoussi RJ, Liv J, Coccaro EF. An open trial of sertraline in personality disorder patients with impulsive aggression. *J Clin Psychiatry* 1994;55:137–141.

232. Salzman C. Effect of fluoxetine on anger in borderline personality disorder [Abstract]. *Neuropsychopharmacology* 1994;10[Suppl 1]:826.

233. Coccaro EF, Kavoussi RJ. Fluoxetine and impulsive aggressive behavior in personality-disordered subjects. *Arch Gen Psychiatry* 1997;54:1081–1088.

234. Kavoussi RJ, Coccaro EF. Divalproex sodium for impulsive aggressive behavior in patients with personality disorder. *J Clin Psychiatry* 1998;59:676–680.

235. Pinto OC, Akiskal HS. Lamotrigine as a promising approach to borderline personality: an open case series without concurrent DSM-IV major mood disorder. *J Affect Disord* 1998;51:333–343.

236. Links PS, Steiner M, Boiageo BA, et al. Lithium therapy for borderline patients: preliminary findings. *J Pers Disord* 1990;4:173–181.

237. Gardner DL, Cowdry RW. Positive effects of carbamazepine on behavioral dyscontrol in borderline

personality disorder. *Am J Psychiatry* 1986;143:519–522.

238. Soloff PH, George A, Nathan RS, et al. Paradoxical effects of amitriptyline on borderline patients. *Am J Psychiatry* 1986;143:1603–1605.

239. Cole JO, Salomon M, Gunderson J. Drug therapy in borderline patients. *J Clin Psychiatry* 1984;25:249–254.

240. Klein DF. Chlorpromazine-procyclidine combination, imipramine and placebo in depressive disorders. *Can Psychiatr Assoc J* 1966;11[Suppl 1]:146–149.

241. Fink M, Klein DF, Kramer JC. Clinical efficacy of chlorpromazine-procyclidine combination, imipramine and placebo in depressive disorders. *Psychopharmacologia* 1965;7:27–36.

242. Rifkin A, Quitkin F, Carrillo C, et al. Lithium carbonate in emotionally unstable character disorder. *Arch Gen Psychiatry* 1972;27:519–523.

243. Teicher MH, Glod CA, Aaronson ST, et al. Open assessment of the safety and efficacy of thioridazine in the treatment of patients with borderline personality disorder. *Psychopharmacol Bull* 1989;25:535–549.

244. Leone NF. Response of borderline patients to loxapine and chlorpromazine. *J Clin Psychiatry* 1982;43:148–150.

245. Soloff PH, George A, Nathan S, et al. Amitriptyline versus haloperidol in borderlines: final outcomes and predictors of responses. *J Clin Psychopharmacol* 1989;9:238–246.

246. Serban G, Seigel S. Responses of borderline and schizotypal patients to small doses of thiothixene and haloperidol. *Am J Psychiatry* 1984;141:1455–1458.

247. Cornelius JR, Soloff PH, George A, et al. Haloperidol versus phenelzine in continuation therapy of borderline disorder. *Psychopharmacol Bull* 1993;29:333–337.

248. Gardner DL, Cowdry RW. Development of melancholia during carbamazepine treatment in borderline personality disorder. *J Clin Psychopharmacol* 1986;6:236–239.

249. Benedetti F, Sforzini L, Colombo C, et al. Low-dose clozapine in acute and continuation treatment of severe borderline personality disorder. *J Clin Psychiatry* 1998;59:103–107.

250. Chengappa KN, Ebeling T, Kang JS, et al. Clozapine reduces severe self-mutilation and aggression in psychotic patients with borderline personality disorder. *J Clin Psychiatry* 1999;60:477–484.

251. Frankenburg FR, Zanarini MC. Use of clozapine in nonschizophrenic patients. *Harvard Rev Psychiatry* 1994;2:142–150.

252. Frankenberg FR, Zanarini MC. Clozapine treatment of borderline patients: a preliminary study. *Compr Psychiatry* 1993;34:402–405.

253. Schulz CS, Camlin KL, Berry SA, et al. Olanzapine safety and efficacy in patients with borderline personality disorder and comorbid dysthymia. *Biol Psychiatry* 1999;46:1429–1435.

254. Szigethy EM, Schulz CS. Risperidone in comorbid borderline personality disorder and dysthymia. *J Clin Psychopharmacol* 1997;17:326–327.

255. Khouzam HR, Donnelly NJ. Remission of self-mutilation in a patient with borderline personality during risperidone therapy. *J Nerv Ment Dis* 1997;185:348–349.

256. Mann J, Kapur S. The emergence of suicidal ideation and behavior during antidepressant pharmacotherapy. *Arch Gen Psychiatry* 1991;48:1027–1033.

257. Sheard MH, Marini JL, Bridges CL, et al. The effect of lithium on impulsive aggressive behavior in man. *Am J Psychiatry* 1976;133:1409–1413.

258. Schiff HB, Sabin TD, Geller A, et al. Lithium in aggressive behavior. *Am J Psychiatry* 1982;139:1346–1348.

259. Liebowitz MR, Klein DF. Interrelationship of hysteroid dysphoria and borderline personality disorder. *Psychiatr Clin North Am* 1981;4:67–68.

260. Baer L, Jenike MA, Ricciardi JN, et al. Standardized assessment of personality disorders in obsessive-compulsive disorder. *Arch Gen Psychiatry* 1990;47:826–830.

261. Holt CS, Heimberg RG, Hope DA. Avoidant personality disorder and the generalized subtype of social phobia. *J Abnorm Psychol* 1992;101:318–325.

262. Schneier FR, Spitzer RL, Gibbon M, et al. The relationship of social phobia subtypes and avoidant personality disorder. *Compr Psychiatry* 1991;32:1–5.

263. Leibowitz MR. Pharmacotherapy of social phobia. *J Clin Psychiatry* 1993;54[Suppl 12]:31–35.

264. Tancer ME. Neurobiology of social phobia. *J Clin Psychiatry* 1993;54[Suppl 12]:26–30.

265. Blackwell B. Explaining psychoactive drug therapy to the patient. *Int Drug Ther Newsl* 1986;21:32.

266. Stubbs CM. Medication in the elderly. *Therapeutic Notes 186*. Wellington, Australia: Department of Health, April 14, 1982.

267. Sunderland T, Tariot PN, Cohen RM, et al. Anticholinergic sensitivity in patients with dementia of the Alzheimer type and age-matched controls. A dose-response study. *Arch Gen Psychiatry* 1987;44:418–426.

268. Madhusoodanan S, Brenner R, Cohen CI. Risperidone for elderly patients with schizophrenia or schizoaffective disorder. *Psychiatr Ann* 2000;30:175–180.

269. Street JS, Tollefson GD, Tohen M, et al. Olanzapine for psychotic conditions in the elderly. *Psychiatr Ann* 2000;30:191–196.

270. Yeung PP, Tariot PN, Schneider LS, et al. Quetiapine for elderly patients with psychotic disorders. *Psychiatr Ann* 2000;30:197–201.

271. Sajatovic M. Clozapine for elderly patients. *Psychiatr Ann* 2000;30:170–174.

272. Salzman C. Treatment of the agitated demented elderly patient. *Hosp Community Psychiatry* 1988;39:1143–1144.

273. Risse SC, Barnes R. Pharmacologic treatment of agitation associated with dementia. *J Am Geriatr Soc* 1986;34:368–376.

274. Sunderland T, Silver MA. Neuroleptics in the treatment of dementia. *Int J Geriatr Psychiatry* 1988;3:79–88.

275. Mintzer JE, Madhusoodanan S, Brenner R. Risperidone in dementia. *Psychiatr Ann* 2000;30:181–187.

276. Masand PS. Atypical antipsychotics for elderly patients with neurodegenerative disorders and medical conditions. *Psychiatr Ann* 2000;30:202–208.

277. Barnes R, Veith R, Okimoto J, et al. Efficacy of antipsychotic medications in behaviorally disturbed dementia patients. *Am J Psychiatry* 1982;139:1170–1174.

278. Finkel SI, Lyons SS, Anderson RL, et al. A randomized, placebo controlled trial of thiothixene missing

language?in agitated, demented nursing home patients. *Int J Geriatr Psychiatry* 1995;10:129–136.

279. Sugerman AA, Williams BH, Adlerstein AM. Haloperidol in the psychiatric disorders of old age. *Am J Psychiatry* 1964;120:1190–1192.

280. Hamilton LD, Bennett JL. The use of trifluoperazine in geriatric patients with chronic brain syndrome. *J Am Geriatr Soc* 1962;10:140–147.

281. Petrie WM, Ban TA, Berney S, et al. Loxapine in psychogeriatrics: a placebo- and standard-controlled clinical investigation. *J Clin Psychopharmacol* 1982;2:122–126.

282. Rada RT, Kellner R. Thiothixene in the treatment of geriatric patients with chronic organic brain syndrome. J Am Geriatr Soc 1976;24:105–107.

283. Stotsky B. Multicenter study comparing thioridazine with diazepam and placebo in elderly, nonpsychotic patients with emotional and behavioral disorders. *Clin Ther* 1984;6:564–559.

284. Devanand DP, Sackeim HA, Brown RP, et al. A pilot study of haloperidol treatment of psychosis and behavioral disturbance in Alzheimer's disease. *Arch Neurol* 1989;46:854–857.

285. Clark WS, Street JS, Sanger TM, et al. Olanzapine in the prevention of psychosis among nursing home patients with behavioral distrubances associated with Alzheimer's disease. Presented at the American College of Neuropsychopharmacology Annual Meeting, Acapulco, Mexico, December 12–16, 1999.

286. Avorn J, Soumerai SB, Everitt DE, et al. A randomized trial of a program to reduce the use of psychoactive drugs in nursing homes. *N Engl J Med* 1992;327:168–173.

287. NIH Consensus Development Panel on Depression in Late Life. Diagnosis and treatment of depression in late life. *JAMA* 1992;268:1018–1023.

288. Quinn C. Pharmacologic treatment of chronic pain in the elderly. *Pharm Ther* 2000;25:182–202.

289. Rothschild AJ. The diagnosis and treatment of late-life depression. *J Clin Psychiatry* 1996;57[Suppl 5]:5–11.

290. Newhouse PA. Use of serotonin selective reuptake inhibitors in geriatric depression. *J Clin Psychiatry* 1996;57[Suppl 5]:12–22.

291. Finkel SI. Efficacy and tolerability of antidepressant therapy in the old-old. *J Clin Psychiatry* 1996;57[Suppl 5]:23–28.

292. Wiehs KL, Settle EC Jr, Batey SR, et al. Buproprion sustained release versus paroxetine for the treatment of depression in the elderly. *J Clin Psychiatry* 2000;61:196–202.

293. Alexopoulos GS, Young RC, Abrams RC. ECT in the high-risk geriatric patient. *Convuls Ther* 1989;5:75–87.

294. Bondareff W, Alpert M, Friedhoff AJ, et al. Comparison of sertraline and nortriptyline in the treatment of major depressive disorder in late life. *Am J Psychiatry* 2000;157:729–736.

295. Thompson LW. Cognitive-behavioral therapy and treatment for late-life depression. *J Clin Psychiatry* 1996;57[Suppl 5]:29–37.

296. Shulman KI. Clinical aspects of mania in the elderly. *Therapeutic Strategies in the Older Adult* 1996:2(3):1–14.

297. Coppen A. Everyday management of affective disorders. *Lancet* 1987;i:886.

298. McFarland BH, Miller MR, Straumfjord AA. Valproate use in the older manic patients. *J Clin Psychiatry* 1990;51:479–481.

299. Gurian BS, Miner JH. Clinical presentation of anxiety in the elderly. In: Salzman C, Lebowitz BD, eds. *Anxiety in the elderly. Treatment and research.* New York: Springer, 1991.

300. Barbee JG, McLaulin B. Anxiety disorders: diagnosis and pharmacotherapy in the elderly. *Psychiatr Ann* 1990;20:439–445.

301. Thyer B, Parrish RJ, Curtis GC, et al. Ages of onset of DSM-III anxiety disorders. *Compr Psychiatry* 1985;23:113–122.

302. Prinz PN, Vitiello MV, Raskind MA, et al. Geriatrics: sleep disorders and aging. *N Engl J Med* 1990;323:520–526.

303. Salzman C, Shader RI, Greenblatt DJ, et al. Long vs. short half-life benzodiazepines in the elderly. *Arch Gen Psychiatry* 1983;40:293–297.

304. Monjan AA. Sleep disorders of older people: report of a consensus conference. *Hosp Community Psychiatry* 1990;41:743–744.

305. *National disease and therapeutic index (NDTI).* Ambler, PA: IMS, 1986.

306. Mellinger GD, Balter MB, Uhlenhuth EH. Prevalence and correlates of the long-term regular use of anxiolytics. *JAMA* 1984;251:375–379.

307. Salzman C. Pharmacologic treatment of the anxious elderly patient. In: Salzman C, Lebowitz BD, eds. *Anxiety in the elderly. Treatment and research.* New York: Springer, 1991.

308. Greenblatt DJ, Shader RI. Benzodiazepines in the elderly: pharmacokinetics and drug sensitivity. In: Salzman C, Lebowitz BD, eds. *Anxiety in the elderly. Treatment and research.* New York: Springer, 1991.

309. Ray WA, Griffin MR, Schaffner W, et al. Psychotropic drug use and the risk of hip fracture. *N Engl J Med* 1987;316:363–369.

310. Ray WA, Griffin MR, Downey M. Benzodiazepines of long and short elimination half-life and the risk of hip fracture. *JAMA* 1989;262:3303–3307.

311. Sorock GS, Shimkin EE. Benzodiazepine sedatives and the risk of falling in a community-dwelling elderly cohort. *Arch Intern Med* 1988;148:2441–2444.

312. Marttila JK, Hammel RJ, Alexander B, et al. Potential untoward effects of long-term use of flurazepam in geriatric patients. *J Am Pharmacol Assoc* 1977;17:692–695.

313. Ancill RJJ, Embury GD, MacEwan GW, et al. Lorazepam in the elderly–a retrospective study of the side-effects in 20 patients. *J Pharmacol* 1987;2:126–127.

314. Robin DW, Hasan SS, Lichtenstein MJ, et al. Dose-related effects of triazolam on postural sway. *Clin Pharmacol Ther* 1991;49:581–588.

315. Campbell AJ, Somerton DT. Benzodiazepine drug effect on body sway in elderly subjects. *J Clin Exp Gerontol* 1982;4:341–347.

316. Swift CG, Haythorne JM, Clarke P, et al. The effect of aging on measured responses to single doses of oral temazepam. *Br J Clin Pharmacol* 1981;11:414P–423P.

317. Doyle CJ. Halcion and bed-related falls. Loss control bulletin. Louisville, KY: Humana Inc., Insurance Department, 1987:5.
318. Lipani JA. Preference study of the hypnotic efficacy of triazolam 0.125 mg compared to placebo in geriatric patients with insomnia. *Curr Ther Res* 1978;24:397–402.
319. Day BH, Davis H, Parsons DW. An assessment of two hypnotics in the elderly. *Clin Trials J* 1981;273–286.
320. Roehrs T, Zorick F, Wittig R, et al. Efficacy of a reduced triazolam dose in elderly insomniacs. *Neurobiol Aging* 1985;6:292–296.
321. Bonnet MH, Dexter JR, Arand DL. The effect of triazolam on arousal and respiration in central sleep apnea patients. *Sleep* 1990;13:31–41.
322. Woo E, Proulx SM, Greenblatt DJ. Differential side effects profile of triazolam versus flurazepam in elderly patients undergoing rehabilitation therapy. *J Clin Pharmacol* 1991;31:168–173.
323. Bayer AJ, Bayer EM, Pathy MSJ, et al. A double-blind controlled study of chlormethiazole and triazolam as hypnotics in the elderly. *Acta Psychiatr Scand* 1986;73[Suppl 329]:104–111.
324. Greenblatt DJ, Harmatz JS, Shapiro L, et al. Sensitivity to triazolam in the elderly. *N Engl J Med* 1991;324:1691–1698.
325. Patterson F. Triazolam syndrome in the elderly. *South Med J* 1987;80:1425–1426.
326. Shader RI, Greenblatt DJ. Triazolam and anterograde amnesia: all is not well in the z-zone. *J Clin Psychopharmacol* 1983;3:273.
327. Schogt B, Conn D. Paranoid symptoms associated with triazolam. *Can J Psychiatry* 1985;30:462–463.
328. DeTullio PL, Kirking DM, Zacardelli DK, et al. Evaluation of long-term triazolam use in an ambulatory veterans administration medical center population. *Ann Pharmacother* 1989;23:290–293.
329. Thompson JF, Robinson CA. Triazolam in the elderly. *N Engl J Med* 1991;325:1743–1744.
330. Moran MG, Thompson TL, Nies AS. Sleep disorders in the elderly. *Am J Psychiatry* 1988;145:1369–1378.
331. Sunter JP, Bal TS, Cowan WK: Three cases of fatal triazolam poisoning. *BMJ* 1988;297:719.
332. Miller F, Whitcup S. Benzodiazepine use in psychiatrically hospitalized elderly patients. *J Clin Psychopharmacol* 1986;6:384–385.
333. Williamson J, Chopin JM. Adverse reactions to prescribed drugs in the elderly: a multicentre investigation. *Age Ageing* 1980;9:73–80.
334. Grymonpre RE, Mitenko PA, Sitar DS, et al. Drug-associated hospital admissions in older medical patients. *J Am Geriatr Soc* 1988;36:1092–1098.
335. Moss JH. Sedative and hypnotic withdrawal states in hospitalised patients [Letter]. *Lancet* 1991;338:575.
336. Foy A, Drinkwater V, March S, et al. Confusion after admission to hospital in elderly patients using benzodiazepines [Letter]. *BMJ* 1986;293:1072.
337. Speirs CJ, Navey FL, Brooks DJ, et al. Opisthotonos and benzodiazepine withdrawal in the elderly. *Lancet* 1986;2:1101.
338. Berlin RM. Management of insomnia in hospitalized patients. *Ann Intern Med* 1984;100:398–404.
339. Model DG, Berry DJ. Effect of chlordiazepoxide in respiratory failure due to chronic bronchitis. *Lancet* 1974;2:869–870.
340. Rudolf M, Geddes DM, Turner JA, et al. Depression of central respiratory drive by nitrazepam. *Thorax* 1978;33:97–100.
341. Guilleminault C, Silvestri R, Mondini S, et al. Aging and sleep apnea: action of benzodiazepines, acetazolamide, alcohol and sleep deprivation in a healthy elderly group. *J Gerontol* 1984;39:655–661.
342. Salzman C. Treatment of agitation, anxiety, and depression in dementia. *Psychopharmacol Bull* 1988;24:39–42.
343. Hale WE, Stewart RB, Marks RG. Antianxiety drugs and central nervous system symptoms in an ambulatory elderly population. *Drug Intell Clin Pharm* 1985;19:37–40.
344. Larson EB, Kukull WA, Buchner D, et al. Adverse drug reactions associated with global cognitive impairment in elderly persons. *Ann Intern Med* 1987;107:169–173.
345. Thompson TL, Moran MG, Nies AS. Psychotropic drug use in the elderly. *N Engl J Med* 1983;308:134–138.
346. Bartus RT, Dean RL, Beer B, et al. The cholinergic hypothesis of geriatric memory dysfunction. *Science* 1982;217:408–417.
347. Block RI, De Voe M, Stanley M, et al. Memory performance in individuals with primary degenerative dementia: its similarity to diazepam-induced impairments. *Exp Aging Res* 1985;11:151–155.
348. Colenda CC III. Buspirone in treatment of agitated demented patient [Letter]. *Lancet* 1988;1:1169.
349. Schweizer E, Case GW, Rickels K. Benzodiazepine dependence and withdrawal in elderly patients. *Am J Psychiatry* 1989;146:521–529.
350. Janicak PG, Davis JM. Pharmacokinetics and drug interactions. In: Sadock BS, Sadock V, eds. *Kaplan and Sadock's comprehensive textbook of psychiatry,* 7th ed, Vol 2. Philadelphia: Lippincott Williams & Wilkins, 2000:2250–2259.
351. Kramer C. Methaqualone and chloral hydrate: preliminary comparison in geriatric patients. *J Am Geriatr Soc* 1967;15:455–461.
352. Napoliello MJ. An interim multicentre report on 677 anxious geriatric outpatients treated with buspirone. *Br J Clin Pract* 1986;40:71–73.
353. Robinson D, Napoliello MJ. The safety and usefulness of buspirone as an anxiolytic in elderly versus young patients. *Clin Ther* 1988;10:740–746.
354. Singh AN, Beer M. A dose range finding study of buspirone in geriatric patients with symptoms of anxiety. *J Clin Psychopharmacol* 1988;8:67–68.
355. Levine S, Napoliello MJ, Domantay AG. Open study of buspirone in octogenarians with anxiety. *Hum Psychopharmacol* 1989;4:51–53.
356. Janicak PG, Ayd FA Jr. Sedative-hypnotics in the elderly population. In: Nelson JC, ed. *Geriatric psychopharmacology.* New York: Marcel Dekker, 1997.
357. Sheehan MK, Janicak PG, Dowd S. The role of psychopharmacotherapy in the dying patient. *Psychiatr Ann* 1994;24:98–103.
358. Greer DS, Mor V, Sherwood S, et al. National hospice study analysis plan. *J Chronic Dis* 1983;36:737–780.
359. Fawzy FI, Fawzy NW, Arndt LA, Pasnau RO. Critical review of psychosocial interventions in cancer care. *Arch Gen Psychiatry* 1995;52:100–113.

360. Marshall KA. Managing cancer pain: basic principles and invasive treatments. *Mayo Clin Proc* 1996;71:472–477.

361. World Health Organization. *Cancer Pain Relief.* Geneva: WHO, 1986.

362. Silverman HD, Croker NA. Pain management in terminally ill patients: how the primary care physician can help. *Postgrad Med* 1988;83:181–188.

363. Truog RD, Berde CV, Mitchell C, Grier HE. Barbiturates in the care of the terminally ill. *N Engl J Med* 1992;327:1678–1682.

364. Anonymous. Transdermal fentanyl: new preparation. An alternative to morphine. *Prescrire Int* 1998;7:137–140.

365. Reddy SK, Nguyen P. Breakthrough pain in cancer patients: new therapeutic approaches to an old challenge. *Curr Rev Pain* 2000;4:242–247.

366. Berry J. The use of analgesics in patients with pain from terminal disease. *Am J Hospice Care* 1988;5(5):26–42.

367. Erush SC. Clonidine for chronic cancer pain. *Pharm Ther* 1998:149–151.

368. Wener S. The pain of cancer. *Postgrad Med* 1988;84:79–92.

369. Schug SA, Dunlop R, Zech D. Treatment of cancer pain. *Drugs* 1992;43:44–53.

370. Levy MH. Pharmacologic treatment of cancer pain. *N Engl J Med* 1996;3351124–1132.

371. Kearney M. Management of the final 24 hours. *Ir Med J* 1992;85:93–95.

372. Johanson G. Midazolam in terminal care. *Am J Hospice Palliat Care* 1993;10(1):13–14.

373. Martin E. Confusion in the terminally ill: recognition and management. *Am J Hospice Palliat Care* 1990;7(3):20–24.

374. Enck R. The last few days. *Am J Hospice Palliat Care* 1992;9(14):11–13.

375. Kübler-Ross E. *On death and dying.* New York: Macmillan, 1969.

376. Lindley-Davis B. Process of dying: defining characteristics. *Cancer Nurs* 1991;14:328–333.

377. Walsh T. Symptom control in patients with advanced cancer. *Am J Hospice Palliat Care* 1992;9(6):32–40.

378. Huntington GW. On chorea. *Med Surg Rep* 1872;26:317.

379. Mayeux R. Emotional changes associated with basal ganglia disorders. In: Heilman KM, Satz P, eds. *Neuropsychology of human emotion.* New York: Guilford, 1983.

380. Hietanen P, Lonnqvist J. Cancer and suicide. *Ann Oncol* 1991;2:19–23.

381. Sackeim HA, Prudic J, Devanand DP, et al. Effects of stimulus intensity and electrode placement on the efficacy and cognitive effects of electroconvulsive therapy. *N Engl J Med* 1993;328:839–846.

382. Sackeim HA, Prudic J, Devanand DP, et al. A prospective, randomized, double-blind comparison of bilateral and right unilateral electroconvulsive therapy at different stimulus intensities. *Arch Gen Psychiatry* 2000;57:425–434.

383. Gilmer W, Busch K. Neuropsychiatric aspects of AIDS and psychopharmacologic management. In: Janicak PG, Davis JM, guest eds. *Psychiatr Med* 1991;9:313–329.

384. Tohen M, Sanger TM, McElroy SL, et al. Olanzapine versus placebo in the treatment of acute mania. *Am J Psychiatry* 1999;156:702–709.

385. Tohen M, Jacobs TG, Grundy SL, et al. A double-blind, placebo-controlled study of olanzapine in patients with acute bipolar mania. *Arch Gen Psychiatry* 2000;57:841–849.

386. DeLuca JR, ed. Fourth special report to the US Congress on alcohol. Washington, DC: U.S. Government Printing Office, 1981.

387. Morse RM, Flavin BK. The definition of alcoholism. *JAMA* 1992;268:1012–1014.

388. Schuckit MA. Alcohol-related disorders. In: Kaplan HI, Sadock BJ, eds. *Comprehensive textbook of psychiatry,* 6th ed, Vol. 1. Baltimore: Williams & Wilkins, 1995:775–791.

389. Black DW, Yates W, Petty F, et al. Suicidal behavior in alcoholic males. *Compr Psychiatry* 1986;27:227–233.

390. Thun MJ, Peto R, Lopez AD, et al. Alcohol consumption and mortality among middle-aged and elderly U.S. adults. *N Engl J Med* 1997;337:1705–1714.

391. Vaillant GE. *The natural history of alcoholism.* Cambridge, MA: Harvard University Press, 1983.

392. Atkinson RM. Alcohol and drug abuse in old age. Washington, DC: American Psychiatric Press, 1984.

393. O'Brien CP, Eckardt MJ, Linnoila MI. Pharmacotherapy of alcoholism. In: FE Bloom, DJ Kupfer, eds. Psychopharmacology: the fourth generation of progress. New York: Raven Press, 1995:1745–1755.

394. Goldman D, Bergen A. General and specific inheritance of substance abuse and alcoholism. *Arch Gen Psychiatry* 1998;55:964–965.

395. Koob GF, Roberts AJ. Brain reward circuits in alcoholism. *CNS Spect* 1999;4:23–37.

396. Swift RM. Drug therapy for alcohol dependence. *N Engl J Med* 1999;340:1482–1490.

397. Bean-Bayog M. Inpatient treatment of the psychiatric patient with alcoholism. *Gen Hosp Psychiatry* 1987;9:203–209.

398. Dackis CA, Gold MS, Pottash ALC, et al. Evaluating depression in alcoholics. *Psychiatry Res* 1986;17:105–109.

399. D'Onofrio G, Rathlev NK, Ulrich AS, et al. Lorazepam for the prevention of recurrent seizures related to alcohol. *N Engl J Med* 1999;340:915–919.

400. Mayo-Smith MF, American Society of Addiction Medicine Working Group on Pharmacological Management of Alcohol Withdrawal. Pharmacological management of alcohol withdrawal: a meta-analysis and evidence-based practice guideline. *JAMA* 1997;278:144–151.

401. Parsons AO, Butters N, Nathan PE, eds. Neuropsychology of alcoholism: implications for diagnosis and treatment. New York: Guilford Press, 1987.

402. Pechter B, Janicak P, Davis JM. Psychopharmacotherapy for the dually diagnosed. Novel approaches. In: Miller N, ed. *The principles and practice of addictions in psychiatry.* Philadelphia: WB Saunders, 1997:521–531.

403. Drake RE, Wallach MA. Substance abuse among the chronic mentally ill. *Hosp Community Psychiatry* 1989;40:1041–1045.

404. Smith J, Hucker S. Schizophrenia and substance abuse. *Br J Psychiatry* 1994;165:13–21.

405. Noordsy DL, Drake RE, Biesanz JC, et al. Family history of alcoholism in schizophrenia. *J Nerv Ment Dis* 1994;182:651–655.

406. Sellers EM, Naranjo CA, Peachey JE. Drug therapy: drugs to decrease alcohol consumption. *N Engl J Med* 1981;305:1255.

407. Garbutt JC, West SL, Carey TS, Lohr KN, et al. Pharmacological treatment of alcohol dependence: a review of the evidence. *JAMA* 1999;281:1318–1325.

408. Major LF, Lerner P, Ballenge JC, et al. Dopamine beta-hydroxylase in the cerebrospinal fluid: relationship to disulfiram-induced psychosis. *Biol Psychiatry* 1979;14:337–344.

409. Kofoed L. Outpatient vs. inpatient treatment for the chronically mentally ill with substance use disorders. *J Addict Dis* 1993;12:123–137.

410. Kofoed L, Kania J, Walsh T, et al. Outpatient treatment of patients with substance abuse and coexisting psychiatric disorders. *Am J Psychiatry* 1986;143:867–872.

411. Kofoed LL. Chemical monitoring of disulfiram compliance. A study of alcoholic outpatients. *Alcohol Clin Exp Res* 1987;11:481–485.

412. Myers RD, Borg S, Mossberg R. Antagonism by naltrexone of voluntary alcohol selection in the chronically drinking macaque monkey. *Alcohol* 1986;3:383–388.

413. Volpicelli JR, Davis MA, Olgin JE. Naltrexone blocks the post-shock increase of ethanol consumption. *Life Sci* 1986;38:841–847.

414. O'Malley SS, Jaffe A, Chang G, et al. Naltrexone and coping skills therapy for alcohol dependence: a controlled study. *Arch Gen Psychiatry* 1992;49:881–887.

415. Volpicelli JR, Alterman AI, Hayashida M, et al. Naltrexone in the treatment of alcohol dependence. *Arch Gen Psychiatry* 1992;49:876–880.

416. Croop RS, Faulkner EB, Labriola DF. The safety profile of naltrexone in the treatment of alcoholism. Results from a multicenter usage study. The Naltrexone Usage Study Group. *Arch Gen Psychiatry* 1997;54:1130–1135.

417. Zaim S, Wiley DB, Albano SA. Rhabdoymolysis associated with naltrexone. *Ann Pharmacother* 1999;33:312–313.

418. Mason BJ, Retno EC, Morgan RO, et al. A double-blind, placebo-controlled pilot study to evaluate the efficacy and safety of oral nalmefene HCl for alcohol dependence. *Alcohol Clin Exp Res* 1994;18:1162–1167.

419. Berger P, Watson S, Akil H, et al. The effects of naloxone in chronic schizophrenia. *Am J Psychiatry* 1981;138:913–915.

420. Watson SJ, Berger PA, Akil H, et al. Effects of naloxone in schizophrenia: reduction in hallucinations in a subpopulation of subjects. *Science* 1978;201:73–76.

421. Janowsky DS, Judd L, Huey L, et al. Naloxone effects on manic symptoms and growth-hormone levels. *Lancet* 1978;i:320.

422. Oslin DW, Pettinati HM, Volpicelli JR, et al. The effects of naltrexone on alcohol and cocaine use in dually addicted patients. *J Subst Abuse Treat* 1999;16:163–167.

423. Anton RF, Moak DH, Waid LR, et al. Naltrexone and cognitive behavioral therapy for the treatment of out patient alcoholics: results of a placebo-controlled trial. *Am J Psychiatry* 1999;156:1758–1764.

424. Mason BJ, Ownby RL. Acamprosate for the treatment of alcohol dependence: a review of double-blind, placebo-controlled trials. *CNS Spect* 2000;5:58–69.

425. Merikangas KR, Leckman JF, Pursoff BA, et al. Familial transmission of depression and alcoholism. *Arch Gen Psychiatry* 1985;42:367–372.

426. Schuckit MA, Tipp JE, Bergman M, et al. Comparison of induced and independent major depressive disorders in 2945 alcoholics. *Am J Psychiatry* 1997;154:948–957.

427. Brown SA, Inaba RK, Gillin JC, et al. Alcoholism and affective disorder: clinical course of depressive symptoms. *Am J Psychiatry* 1995;152:45–52.

428. Brady KT, Killeen T, Jarell P. Depression in alcoholic schizophrenic patients. *Am J Psychiatry* 1993;150:1255–1256.

429. Ciraulo DA, Jaffe JH. Tricyclic antidepressants in the treatment of depression associated with alcoholism. *J Clin Psychopharmacol* 1981;1:146–150.

430. Nunes EV, McGrath PJ, Quitkin FM, et al. Imipramine treatment of alcoholism with comorbid depression. *Am J Psychiatry* 1993;150:963–965.

431. Gorelick DA. Serotonin uptake blockers and the treatment of alcoholism. *Recent Dev Alcohol* 1989;7:267–281.

432. Gorelick DA, Paredes A. Effect of fluoxetine on alcohol consumption in male alcoholics. *Alcohol Clin Exp Res* 1992;16:261–265.

433. Thomas R. Fluvoxamine and alcoholism. *Int Clin Psychopharmacol* 1991;6:84–92.

434. Amit Z, Brown Z, Sutherland Z, et al. Reduction in alcohol intake in humans as a function of treatment with zimelidine: implications for treatment. In: Naranjo CA, Sellers EM, eds. *Research advances in new psychopharmacological treatments for alcoholism.* Amsterdam: Excerpta Medica, 1985:189–198.

435. Naranjo CA, Sellers EM, Jullivan JT, et al. The serotonin uptake inhibitor citalopram attenuates ethanol intake. *Clin Pharmacol Ther* 1987;41:266–274.

436. Naranjo CA, Sellers EM, Roach CA, et al. Zimelidine-induced variations in alcohol intake by non-depressed heavy drinkers. *Clin Pharmacol Ther* 1984;35:374–381.

437. Kranzler HR, Burleson JA, Korner P, et al. Placebo-controlled trial of fluoxetine as an adjunct to relapse prevention in alcoholics. *Am J Psychiatry* 1995;152:391–397.

438. Janiri L, Gobbi G, Mannelli P, et al. Effects of fluoxetine at antidepressant doses on short-term outcome of detoxified alcoholics. *Int Clin Psychopharmacol* 1996;11:109–117.

439. Kabel DI, Petty F. A placebo-controlled, double-blind study of fluoxetine in severe alcohol dependence. *Alcohol Clin Exp Res* 1996;20:780–784.

440. Kranzler HR, Burleson JA, Brown J, et al. Fluoxetine treatment seems to reduce the beneficial effects of cognitive-behavioral therapy in type B alcoholics. *Alcohol Clin Exp Res* 1996;20:1534–1541.

441. Tiihonen J, Ryynanen OP, Kauhanen J, et al. Citalopram in the treatment of alcoholism. *Pharmacopsychiatry* 1996;29:27–29.

442. Cornelius JR, Salloum IM, Ehler JG, et al. Fluoxetine in depressed alcoholics: a double-blind, placebo-

controlled trial. *Arch Gen Psychiatry* 1997;54:700–705.

443. Malec E, Malec T, Gagne MA, et al. Buspirone in the treatment of alcohol dependence. *Alcohol Clin Exp Res* 1996;20:307–312.

444. Malcolm R, Anton RF, Randall CL, et al. A placebo-controlled trial of buspirone in anxious inpatient alcoholics. *Alcohol Clin Exp Res* 1992;16:1007–1013.

445. Kranzler HR, Burleson JA, Del Boca FK, et al. Buspirone treatment of anxious alcoholics. *Arch Gen Psychiatry* 1994;51:720–731.

446. Sellers EM, Toneatto T, Romach MK, et al. Clinical efficacy of the 5-HT3 antagonist ondansetron in alcohol abuse and dependence. *Alcohol Clin Exp Res* 1994;18:879–885.

447. Naranjo C, Kadlic K, Sanhueza P, et al. Fluoxetine differentially alters alcohol intake and other consummatory behaviors in problem drinkers. *Clin Pharmacol Ther* 1990;47:490–498.

448. Dorus W, Ostrow DG, Anton R, et al. Lithium treatment of depressed and nondepressed alcoholics. *JAMA* 1989;262:1646–1652.

449. Fawcett J, Clark DC, Gibbons RD, et al. Evaluation of lithium therapy for alcoholism. *J Clin Psychiatry* 1984;45:494–499.

450. Nagel K, Adler LE, Bell L, et al. Lithium carbonate and mood disorder in recently detoxified alcoholics: a double-blind, placebo-controlled pilot study. *Alcohol Clin Exp Res* 1991;15:978–981.

451. Halikas J, Kuhn K, Carlsan G. The effect of carbamazepine on cocaine use. *Am J Addict* 1992;1:30–39.

452. Kosten TR, Gawin FH, Kosten TA, et al. Six-month follow-up of short-term pharmacotherapy for cocaine dependence. *Am J Addict* 1992;1:40–49.

453. Bowen RC, Cipywnyk D, D'Arcy C, et al. Alcoholism, anxiety disorders, and agoraphobia. *Alcohol Clin Exp Res* 1984;8:48–50.

454. Smail P, Stockwell T, Canter S, et al. Alcohol dependence and phobic anxiety states I. A prevalence study. *Br J Psychiatry* 1984;144:53–57.

455. Reich J, Chaudhry D. Personality of panic disorder alcohol abusers. *J Nerv Ment Dis* 1987;175:224–228.

456. Cloninger CR, Martin RL, Clayton P, Couze S. Follow-up and family study of anxiety neurosis. In: Klein DF, Rabkin J, eds. *Anxiety: New Research and Changing Concepts*. New York: Raven Press, 1981.

457. Crowe RR, Crowe RC, Pauls DL, et al. A family study of anxiety neurosis: morbidity risk in families of patients with and without mitral valve prolapse. *Arch Gen Psychiatry* 1980;37:77–79.

458. Starcevic V, Uhlenhuth EH, Kellner R, et al. Comorbidity in panic disorder: II. Chronology of appearance and pathogenic comorbidity. *Psychiatry Res* 1993;46:285–293.

459. George DT, Nutt DJ, Dwyer BA, et al. Alcoholism and panic disorder: is the comorbidity more than coincidence? *Acta Psychiatr Scand* 1990;81:97–107.

460. Ayd FJ Jr, Janicak PG, Davis JM, et al. Advances in the pharmacotherapy of anxiety and sleep disorders. In: Janicak PG, ed. *Principles and practice of psychopharmacotherapy update*, Vol 1, No. 4. Baltimore: Williams & Wilkins, 1996.

460a. Forstein M, McDaniel JS. Medical overview of HIV infection and AIDS. *Psych Annals* 2001;31(1):16.

461. Jobe TH. Neuropsychiatry of HIV disease. In: Flaherty J, Davis JM, Janicak PG, eds. *Psychiatry: diagnosis and therapy*, 2nd ed. New York: Appleton and Lange, 1993.

462. Janicak PG. Psychopharmacotherapy in the HIV-infected patient. *Psychiatr Ann* 1995;25:609–613.

463. Uldall KK, Koutsky LA, Bradshaw DH, et al. Psychiatric comorbidity and length of stay in hospitalized AIDS patients. *Am J Psychiatry* 1994;151:1475–1478.

464. American Psychiatric Association. AIDS policy: guidelines for inpatient psychiatric units. *Am J Psychiatry* 1992;149:722.

465. Binder RL. AIDS antibody tests on inpatient psychiatric units. *Am J Psychiatry* 1987;144:176–181.

466. Shapshak P, Fujimura RK, Srivastava A, et al. Dementia and the neurovirulence of HIV-1. *CNS Spect* 2000;5(4):31–42.

467. Maj M, Janssen R, Starace F, et al. WHO neuropsychiatric AIDS study, cross-sectional phase 1. *Arch Gen Psychiatry* 1994;51:39–49.

468. Concha M, Rabinstein A. Central nervous system opportunistic infections in HIV-1 infection. *CNS Spect* 2000;5(4):43–60.

469. Kalichman SC, Kellky JA, Johnson J, et al. Factors associated with risk for human immunodeficiency versus (HIV) infection among chronically mentally ill adults. *Am J Psychiatry* 1993;151:121–127.

470. DiClemente RJ, Ponton LE. HIV-related risk behaviors among psychiatrically hospitalized adolescents and school-based adolescents. *South J Psychiatry* 1993;150:324–325.

471. Baldewicz TT, Brouwers P, Goodkin K, et al. Nutritional contributions to the CNS pathophysiology of HIV-1 infection and implications for treatment. *CNS Spect* 2000;5(4):61–72.

472. Cournos F, Empfield M, Horwath E, et al. The management of HIV infection in state psychiatric hospitals. *Hosp Community Psychiatry* 1989;40:153–158.

473. Horwath E, Kramer M, Cournos F, et al. Clinical presentations of AIDS and HIV infection in state psychiatric facilities. *Hosp Community Psychiatry* 1989;40:502–514.

474. Jacobsberg LB, Perry S. Medical management of AIDS patients: psychiatric disturbances. *Med Clin North Am* 1992;76:99–106.

475. Batki SL. Drug abuse, psychoactive disorders and AIDS: dual and triple diagnosis. *West J Med* 1990;152:547–552.

476. Yarchoan R, Brouwers P, Spitzer AR, et al. Response of human-immunodeficiency associated neurological disease to 3'-azido-3'-deoxythymidine. *Lancet* 1987;1:132–135.

477. Fernandez F, Adams F, Levy JK, et al. Cognitive impairment due to AIDS-related complex and its response to psychostimulants. *Psychosomatics* 1988;29:38–46.

478. Carpenter CC, Fischl MA, Hammer SM, et al. Antiretroviral therapy for HIV infection in 1998: updated recommendations of the International AIDS Society-USA Panel. *JAMA* 1998;280:78–86.

479. Palella FJJ, Delaney KM, Moorman AC, et al. Declining morbidity and mortality among patients with advanced human immunodeficiency virus infection: HIV-1 Outpatient Study Investigators. *N Engl J Med* 1998;338:853–860.

479a. Gillenwater DR, McDaniel JS. Rational psychopharmacology for patients with HIV infection and AIDS. *Psych Annals* 2001;31(1):28–34.

480. Burch EA, Montoya J. NMS in an AIDS patient. *J Clin Psychiatry* 1989;9:228–229.

481. Ostrow D, Grant I, Atkinson H. Assessment and management of AIDS patients with neuropsychiatric disturbances. *J Clin Psychiatry* 1988;49[Suppl]:14–22.

482. Davis JM, Janicak PG, Preskorn SH, et al. Advances in the psychopharmacotherapy of psychotic disorders. In: Janicak PG, ed. *Principles and practice of psychopharmacotherapy update,* Vol 1, No 1. Baltimore: Williams & Wilkins, 1994.

483. Ayd FS Jr, Janicak PG, Davis JM. Advances in pharmacotherapy of psychotic disorders II. The novel antipsychotics. In: Janicak PG, ed. *Principles and practice of pychopharmacotherapy update,* Vol 1, No. 5. Baltimore: Williams & Wilkins, 1997.

484. Gilmer W, Busch K. Neuropsychiatric aspects of AIDS and psychopharmacologic management. *Psychiatr Med* 1991;9:313–329.

484a. Lyketsos CG, Treisman GJ. Mood disorders in HIV infection. *Psych Annals* 2001;31(1):45–49.

485. Lyketsos CG, Hoover DR, Guccione M, et al. Changes in depressive symptoms as AIDS develops. *Am J Psychiatry* 1996;153:1430–1437.

486. Preskorn S, Janicak PG, Davis JM, et al. Advances in the psychopharmacotherapy of depressive disorders. In: Janicak PG, ed. *Principles and practice of psychopharmacotherapy update,* Vol 1, No 3. Baltimore: Williams & Wilkins, 1995.

487. Sullivan MD. Treatment of depression at the end of life: clinical and ethical issues. *Semin Clin Neuropsychiatry* 1998;3:151–156.

488. Masand PS, Tesar GE. Use of stimulants in the medically ill. *Psychiatr Clin North Am* 1996;19:515–547.

489. Menza MA, Murray GB, Holmes VF, et al. Decreased extrapyramidal symptoms with intravenous haloperidol. *J Clin Psychiatry* 1987;48:278–280.

490. Chambers RA, Druss BG. Droperidol: efficacy and side effects in psychiatric emergencies. *J Clin Psychiatry* 1999;60:664–667.

491. Halman MH, Worth JL, Sanders KM, et al. Anticonvulsant use in the treatment of manic syndrome in patients with HIV-1 infection. *J Neuropsychiatry Clin Neurosci* 1993;5:430–434.

492. Lane HY, Chiu WC, Chang WH. Risperidone monotherapy for mania and depression. *Am J Psychiatry* 1999;156:1115.

493. Janicak PG, Keck PE Jr, Davis JM, et al. A double-blind, randomized, prospective evaluation of the efficacy and safety of risperidone versus haloperidol in the treatment of schizoaffective disorder. *J Clin Psychopharmacol* (in press).

494. Singh A, Catalan J. Risperidone in HIV-related manic psychosis [Letter]. *Lancet* 1994;344:1029–1030.

495. Breitbart W, Marotta R, Platt MM, et al. A double-blind trial of haloperidol, chlorpromazine, and lorazepam in the treatment of delirium in hospitalized AIDS patients. *Am J Psychiatry* 1996;153:231–237.

496. Batki SL. Buspirone in drug users with AIDS or AIDS related complex. *J Clin Psychopharmacol* 1990;10[Suppl 3]:111S–115S.

497. Becker AE, Grinspoon SK, Klibanski A, et al. Eating disorders. *N Engl J Med* 1999;340:1092–1098.

498. American Psychiatric Press. *Diagnostic and statistical manual of mental disorders,* 4th ed. Washington, DC: American Psychiatric Press, 1994;539–550, 729–731.

499. Leach A. The psychopharmacotherapy of eating disorders. *Psychiatr Ann* 1995;25:633–638.

500. Halmi KA, Eckert E, LaDu TJ, et al. Anorexia nervosa. Treatment efficacy of cyproheptadine and amitriptyline. *Arch Gen Psychiatry* 1986;43:177–181.

501. Biederman J, Herzog DB, Rivinus TM, et al. Amitriptyline in the treatment of anorexia nervosa: a double-blind, placebo-controlled study. *J Clin Psychopharmacol* 1985;5:10–16.

502. Gwirtsman HE, Guze BH, Vager J, et al. Fluoxetine treatment of anorexia nervosa: an open clinical trial. *J Clin Psychiatry* 1990;51:378–382.

503. Kaye WH, Weltzin TE, Hsu LKG, et al. An open trial of fluoxetine in patients with anorexia nervosa. *J Clin Psychiatry* 1991;52:464–471.

504. Vandereycken W, Pierloot R. Pimozide combined with behavior therapy in the short-term treatment of anorexia nervosa. *Acta Psychiatr Scand* 1982;66:445–450.

505. Vandereycken W. Neuroleptics in the short term treatment of anorexia nervosa: a double-blind, placebo-controlled study with sulpiride. *Br J Psychiatry* 1984;144:2788–2792.

506. La Via MC, Gray N, Kaye WH. Case reports of olanzapine treatment of anorexia nervosa. *Int J Eat Disord* 2000;27:363–366.

507. Hansen L. Olanzapine in the treatment of anorexia nervosa [Letter]. *Br J Psychiatry* 1999;175:592.

508. Jensen VS, Mejlhede A. Anorexia nervosa: treatment with olanzapine [Letter]. *Br J Psychiatry* 2000;177:87.

509. Newman-Toker J. Risperidone in anorexia nervosa [Letter]. *J Am Acad Child Adolesc Psychiatry* 2000;39:941–942.

510. American Psychiatric Association. Practice guideline for eating disorders. *Am J Psychiatry* 1993;150:212–228.

511. Mcgilley BM, Pryor TL. Assessment and treatment of bulimia nervosa. *Am Fam Physician* 1998;57:2743–2750.

512. Caruso D, Klein H. Diagnosis and treatment of bulimia nervosa. *Semin Gastrointest Dis* 1998;9:176–182.

513. Freeman CPL, Munro JKM. Drug and group treatments for bulimia/bulimia nervosa. *J Psychosom Res* 1988;32:647–660.

514. Agras WS, McCann U. The efficacy and role of antidepressants in the treatment of bulimia nervosa. *Ann Behav Med* 1987;9:18–22.

515. Hughes PL, Wells LA, Cunningham CJ, et al. Treating bulimia with desipramine: a double-blind, placebo-controlled study. *Arch Gen Psychiatry* 1986;43:182–186.

516. Walsh BT, Gladis M, Roose SP, et al. Phenelzine vs placebo in 50 patients with bulimia. *Arch Gen Psychiatry* 1988;45:471–475.

517. Rossiter EM, Agras WS, Losch M. Changes in self-reported food intake in bulimics as a consequence of anti-depressant treatment. *Int J Eat Disord* 1988;7:779–783.

518. Mitchell JE, Fletcher L, Pyle RL, et al. The impact of treatment on meal patterns in patients with bulimia nervosa. *Int J Eat Disord* 1989;8:167–172.

519. Pope HG, Hudson JI, Jonas JM, et al. Bulimia treated with imipramine: a placebo-controlled, double-blind study. *Am J Psychiatry* 1983;10:554–558.

520. Agras WS, Dorian B, Kirkley BG, et al. Imipramine in the treatment of bulimia: a double-blind controlled study. *Int J Eat Disord* 1987;6:29–38.

521. Mitchell JE, Pyle RL, Eckert ED, et al. A comparison study of antidepressants and structured intensive group psychotherapy in the treatment of bulimia nervosa. *Arch Gen Psychiatry* 1990;47:149–157.

522. Rothschild R, Quitkin HM, Quitkin FM, et al. A double blind placebo-controlled comparison of phenelzine and imipramine in the treatment of bulimia in atypical depressives. *Int J Eat Disord* 1994;9:1–9.

523. Barlow J, Blouin J, Blouin A, Perez E. Treatment of bulimia with desipramine: a double-blind crossover study. *Can J Psychiatry* 1988;33:129–133.

524. Walsh BT, Hadigan CM, Devlin MJ, et al. Long-term outcome of antidepressive treatment for bulimia nervosa. *Am J Psychiatry* 1991;148:1206–1212.

525. Agras WS, Rossiter EM, Arnow B, et al. One-year follow-up of psychosocial and pharmacological treatments for bulimia nervosa. *J Clin Psychiatry* 1994;55:179–183.

526. Mitchell JE, Groat RA. A placebo-controlled, double-blind trial of amitriptyline in bulimia. *J Clin Psychopharmacol* 1984;4:186–193.

527. Kennedy SH, Piran N, Warsh JJ, et al. A trial of isocarboxazid in the treatment of bulimia nervosa. *J Clin Psychopharmacol* 1988;8:391–396.

528. Kennedy SH, Goldbloom DS, Ralevski E, et al. Is there a role for selective monoamine oxidase inhibitor therapy in bulimia nervosa? A placebo-controlled trial of brofaromine. *J Clin Psychopharmacol* 1993;13:415–422.

529. Horne RL, Ferguson JM, Pope HG, et al. Treatment of bulimia with bupropion: a multi-center controlled trial. *J Clin Psychiatry* 1988;49:262–266.

530. Pope HG, Keck PE, McElroy S, et al. A placebo-controlled study of trazodone in bulimia nervosa. *J Clin Psychopharmacol* 1989;9:254–259.

531. Sabine E, Yonace A, Farrington AJ, et al. Bulimia nervosa: a placebo controlled, double-blind, therapeutic trial of mianserin. *Br J Pharmacol* 1983;15:195–202.

532. Nassr DG. Successful treatment of bulimia with nomifensine. *Am J Psychiatry* 1986;143:373–374.

533. Pope HG, Herridge PL, Hudson JI, et al. Treatment of bulimia with nomifensine. *Am J Psychiatry* 1986;143:371–372.

534. Price WA, Babai MR. Antidepressant drug therapy for bulimia: current status revisited. *J Clin Psychiatry* 1987;48:385.

535. Fluoxetine Bulimia Nervosa Collaborative Study Group. Fluoxetine in the treatment of bulimia nervosa: a multicenter, placebo-controlled, double-blind trial. *Arch Gen Psychiatry* 1992;49:139–147.

536. Fichter MM, Leibl K, Rief W, et al. Fluoxetine versus placebo: a double-blind study with bulimic in patients undergoing intensive psychotherapy. *Pharmacopsychiatry* 1991;24:1–7.

537. Aguso-Gutierrez JL, Palazo'n M, Ayusa-Mateos JL. Open trial of fluvoxamine in the treatment of bulimia nervosa. *Int J Eat Disord* 1994;15:245–249.

538. Roberts JM, Lydiard RB. Sertraline in the treatment of bulimia nervosa. *Am J Psychiatry* 1993;150:1753.

539. Wermuth BM, Davis KL, Hollister LE, et al. Phenytoin treatment of the binge-eating syndrome. *Am J Psychiatry* 1977;134:1249–1253.

540. Kaplan AS, Garfinkel PE, Darby PL, et al. Carbamazepine in the treatment of bulimia. *Am J Psychiatry* 1983;140:1225–1226.

541. Hsu LKG, Clement L, Santhouse R, et al. Treatment of bulimia nervosa with lithium carbonate: a controlled study. *J Nerv Ment Dis* 1991;179:351–355.

542. Mitchell JE, Christenson G, Jennings J, et al. A placebo-controlled, double-blind cross-over study of naltrexone hydrochloride in outpatients with normal weight bulimia. *J Clin Psychopharmacol* 1989;9:94–97.

543. Robinson PH, Checkley SA, Russell GFM. Suppression of eating by fenfluramine in patients with bulimia nervosa. *Br J Psychiatry* 1985;146:169–176.

544. Russell GFM, Checkley SA, Feldman J, et al. A controlled trial of d-fenfluramine in bulimia nervosa. *Clin Neuropharmacol* 1988;11:S146–S159.

545. Fahy TA, Eisler I, Russell GFM. A placebo-controlled trial of d-fenfluramine in bulimia nervosa. *Br J Psychiatry* 1993;162:597–603.

546. Connolly HM, Crary JL, McGoon MD, et al. Valvular heart disease associated with fenfluramine-phentermine. *N Engl J Med* 1997;337:581–588.

APPENDICES

INTRODUCTION

The third edition of the American Psychiatric Association's *Diagnostic and Statistical Manual of Mental Disorders* (DSM-III) marked the beginning of a new era in the classification of mental disorders in the United States (1). The emphasis on phenomenology in DSM-III and its revision, the DSM-III-R, was a significant departure from the impressionistic, theoretically based schema of its predecessors, the DSM-I (1952) and the DSM-II (1968) (2–4). The DSM-IV continues to emphasize the role of empirical findings as the basis for diagnosing psychiatric disorders, as well as strive for compatibility with the tenth revision of the International Classification of Diseases (ICD-10), whenever feasible (5, 6).

To effectively use this system, the clinician must carefully consider an extensive array of information before arriving at a diagnostic label. The myriad of possible diagnoses, as well as the exactness of the criteria within each category, can be a challenge to the most experienced clinician, and overwhelming to the novice. Thus, we have provided an overview highlighting the organization and critical criteria to facilitate assimilation of this information.

The general approach to diagnosis in the DSM-IV is multiaxial:

- Axes I and II, for mental disorders
- Axis III, to reflect any physical disorders substantively related to Axis I or II
- Axis IV, to provide data on any significant psychosocial stressors
- Axis V, to reflect the highest level of adaptational functioning in the previous year information should be provided, when possible, in all relevant areas.

To enhance the discussion in this text on indications for pharmacotherapy, we provide an overview of the critical criteria in DSM-IV pertinent to each diagnostic category on Axes I and II (7). Using a series of diagrams, we have designed a quick reference for the practitioner to more readily identify the salient criteria. These diagrams were adapted from Janicak PG, Andriukaitis SN. DSM-III: seeing the forest through the trees. *Psychiatr Ann* 1980;10(8): 6–30.

REFERENCES

1. American Psychiatric Association. *Diagnostic and statistical manual of mental disorders,* 3rd ed. Washington, DC: American Psychiatric Association, 1980.
2. American Psychiatric Association. *Diagnostic and statistical manual, mental disorders,* 1st ed. Washington, DC: American Psychiatric Association, 1952.
3. American Psychiatric Association. *Diagnostic and statistical manual of mental disorders,* 2nd ed. Washington, DC: 1968.

4. American Psychiatric Association. *Diagnostic and sta-tistical manual of mental disorders,* 3rd ed, revised. Washington DC: American Psychiatric Association, 1987.
5. American Psychiatric Association. *Diagnostic and statis-tical manual of mental disorders,* 4th ed. Washington DC: American Psychiatric Association, 1994.
6. American Psychiatric Association. *Diagnostic and statis-tical manual of mental disorders*, 4th ed. Washington DC: American Psychiatric Association, 2000.
7. Janicak PG, Andriukaitis SN. DSM-III: seeing the forest through the trees. *Psychiatr Ann* 1980;10(8):6–30.

Appendix A. An Overview of DSM-IV, Axes I and II.

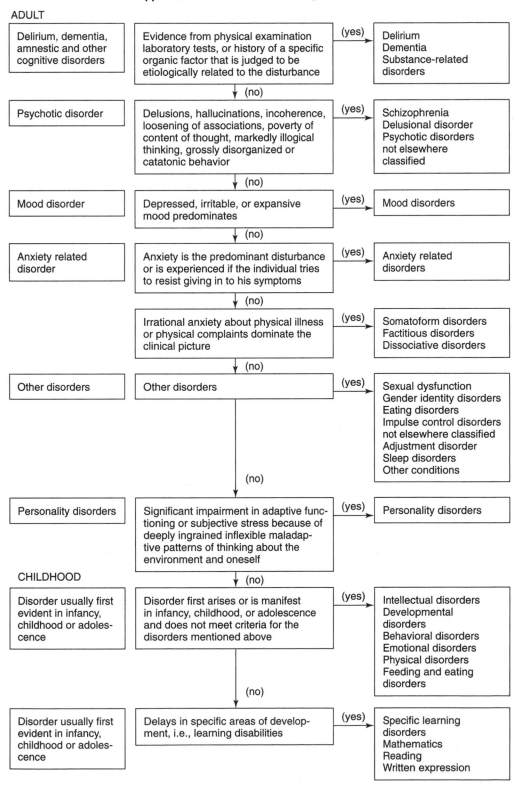

Appendix B. Disorders Usually First Diagnosed in Infancy, Childhood, or Adolescence.

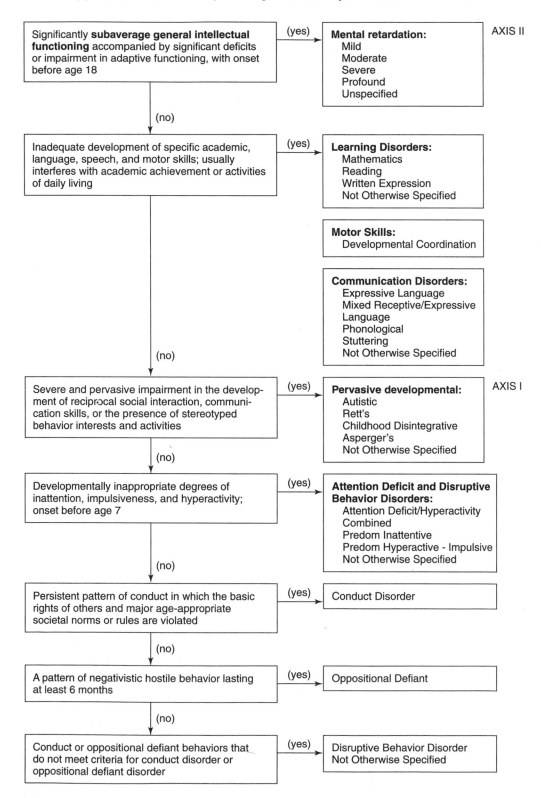

Appendix B. *continued*

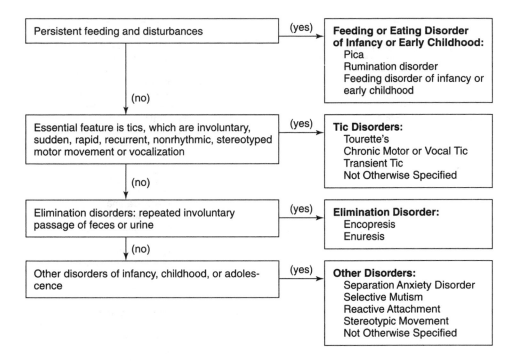

Appendix C. Delirium, Dementia, Amnestic, and Other Cognitive Disorders.

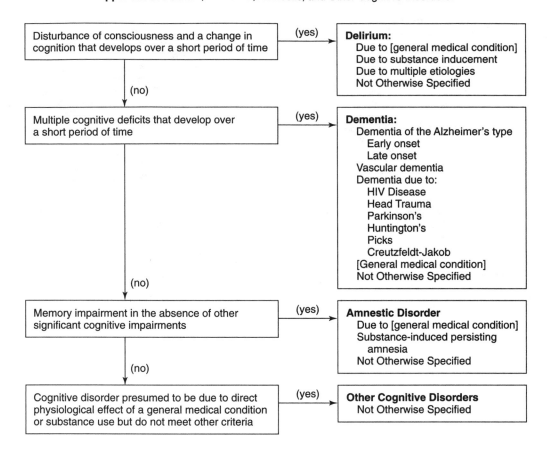

Appendix D. Substance-Related Disorders.

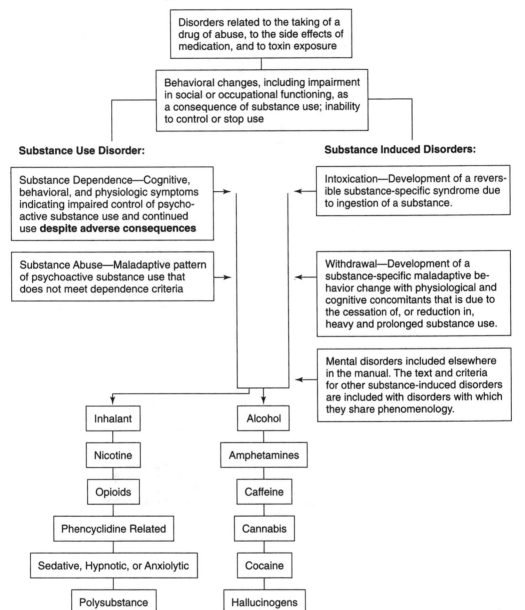

Appendix E. An Overview of Schizophrenic and Other Psychotic Disorders.

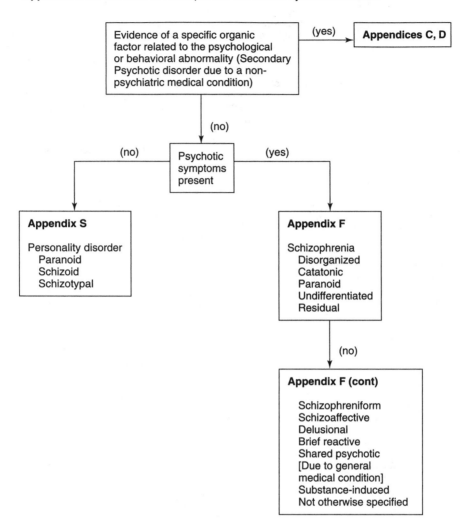

Appendix F. Schizophrenia and Other Psychotic Disorders.

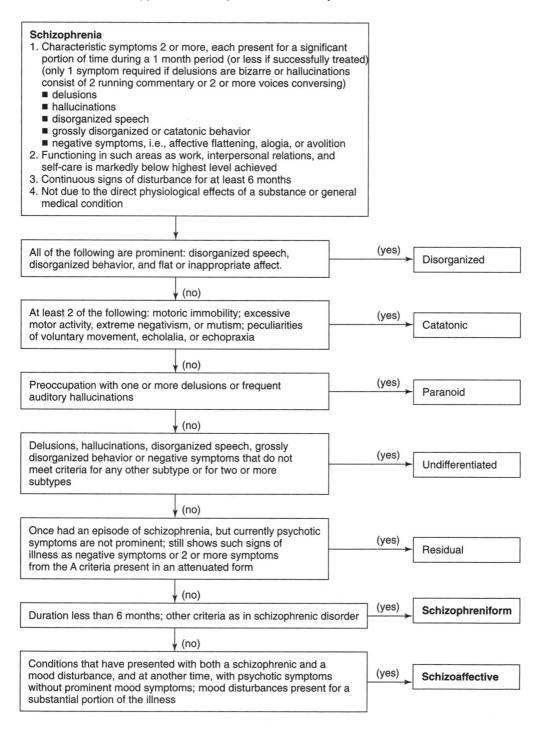

Appendix F. *continued*

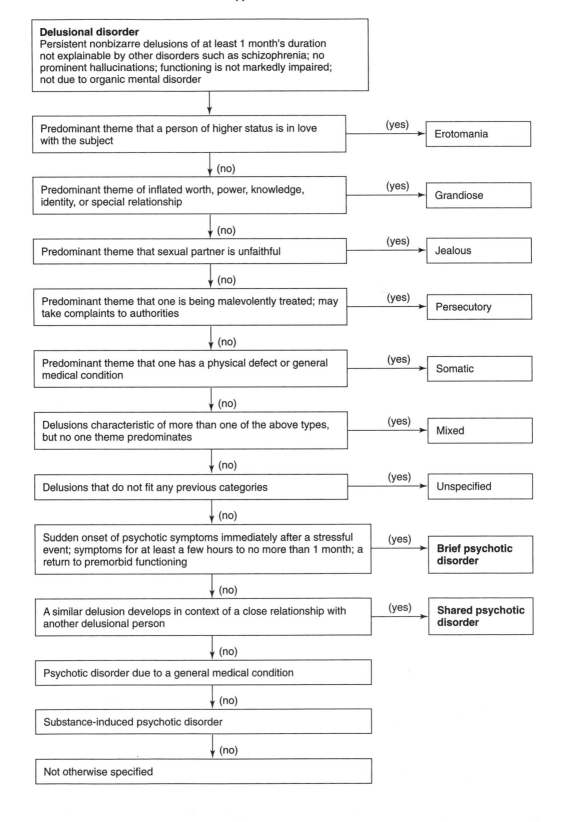

Appendix G. An Overview of Mood-Related Disorders.

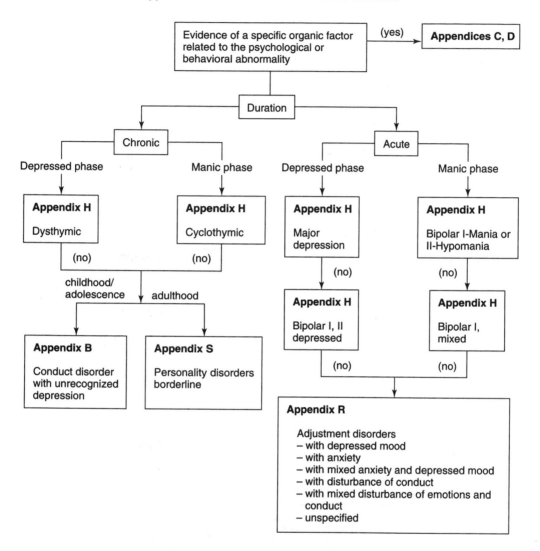

Appendix H. Mood Disorders.

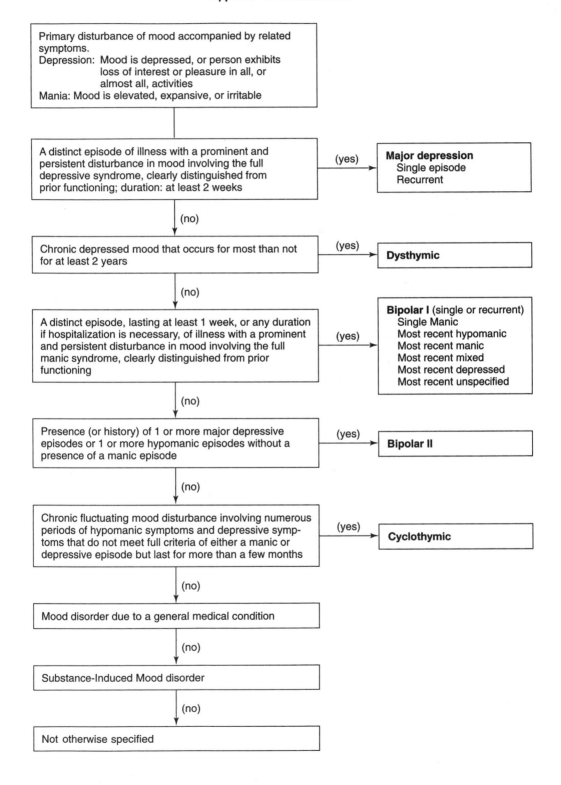

Appendix I. An Overview of Anxiety-Related Disorders.

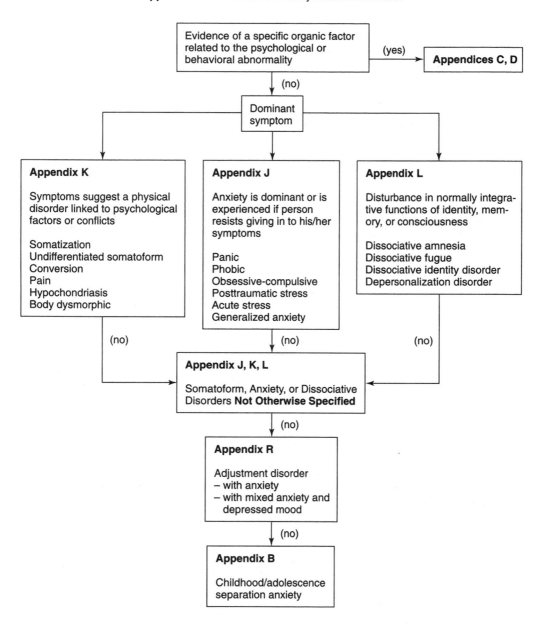

Appendix J. Anxiety Disorders.

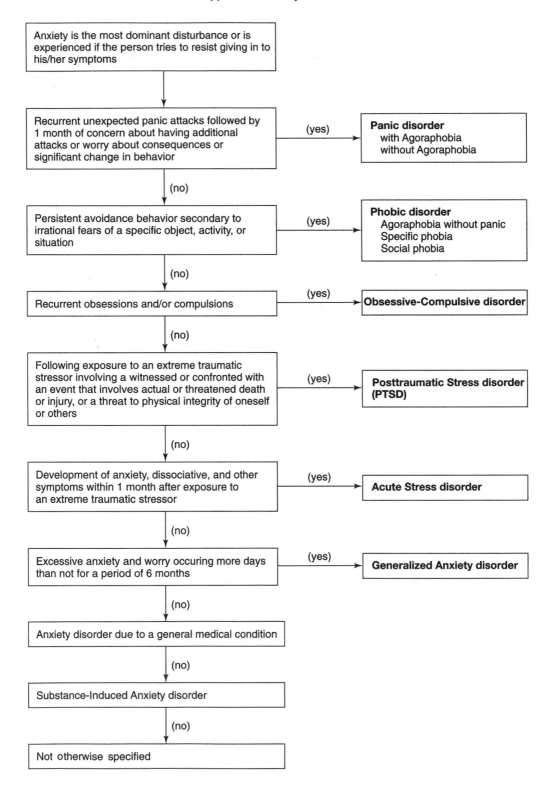

Anxiety is the most dominant disturbance or is experienced if the person tries to resist giving in to his/her symptoms

Recurrent unexpected panic attacks followed by 1 month of concern about having additional attacks or worry about consequences or significant change in behavior

(yes) →
Panic disorder
   with Agoraphobia
   without Agoraphobia

(no)

Persistent avoidance behavior secondary to irrational fears of a specific object, activity, or situation

(yes) →
Phobic disorder
   Agoraphobia without panic
   Specific phobia
   Social phobia

(no)

Recurrent obsessions and/or compulsions

(yes) →
Obsessive-Compulsive disorder

(no)

Following exposure to an extreme traumatic stressor involving a witnessed or confronted with an event that involves actual or threatened death or injury, or a threat to physical integrity of oneself or others

(yes) →
Posttraumatic Stress disorder (PTSD)

(no)

Development of anxiety, dissociative, and other symptoms within 1 month after exposure to an extreme traumatic stressor

(yes) →
Acute Stress disorder

(no)

Excessive anxiety and worry occuring more days than not for a period of 6 months

(yes) →
Generalized Anxiety disorder

(no)

Anxiety disorder due to a general medical condition

(no)

Substance-Induced Anxiety disorder

(no)

Not otherwise specified

Appendix K. Somatoform Disorders.

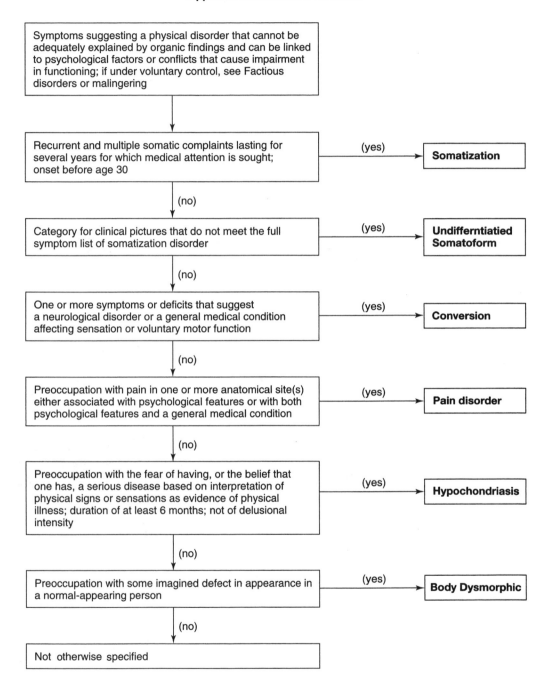

Appendix L. Dissociative Disorders.

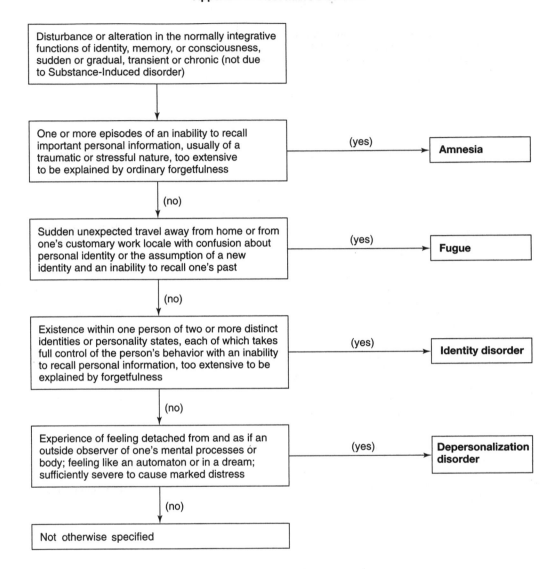

Appendix M. Factitious Disorders.

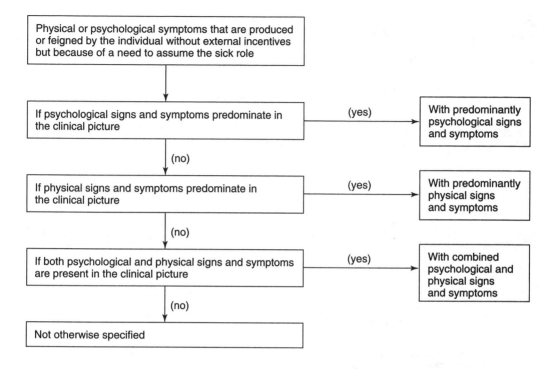

Appendix N. Sexual and Gender Identity Disorders.

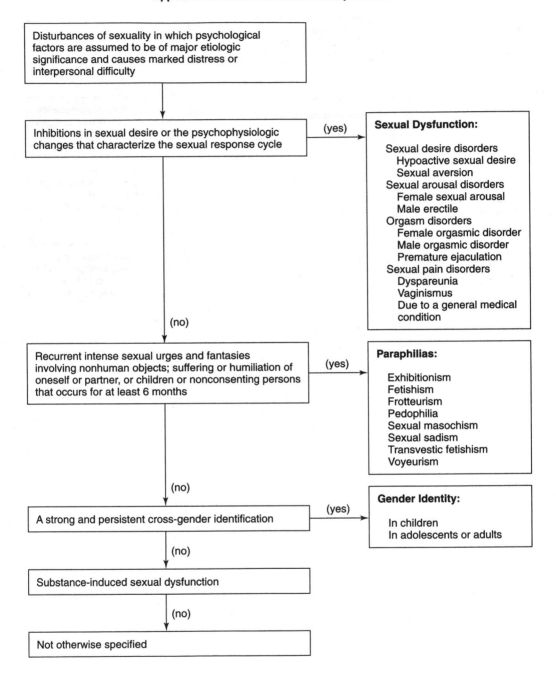

Appendix O. Eating Disorders.

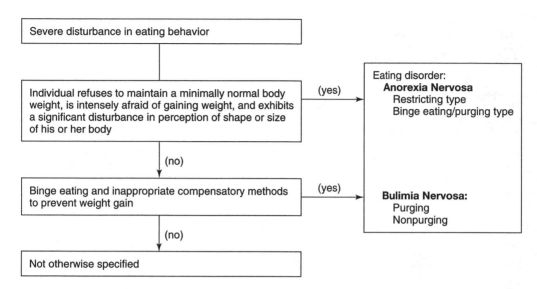

Appendix P. Sleep Disorders.

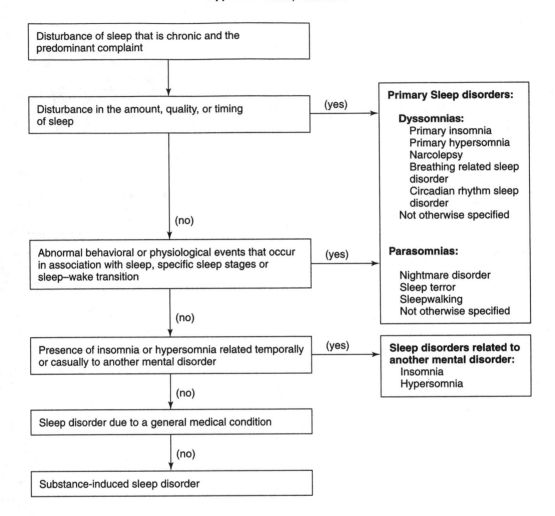

Appendix Q. Impulse Control Disorders Not Elsewhere Classified.

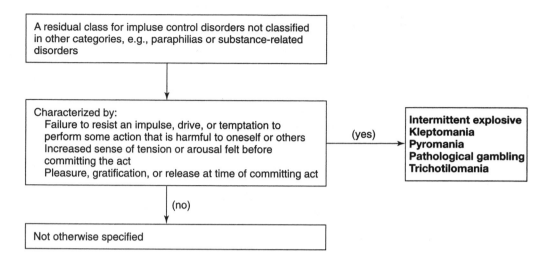

Appendix R. Adjustment Disorders.

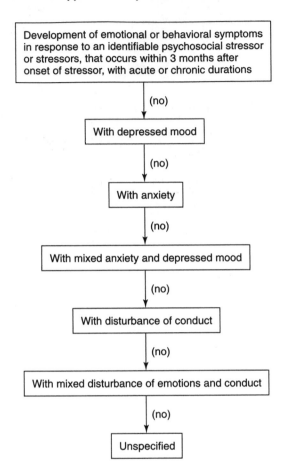

Development of emotional or behavioral symptoms
in response to an identifiable psychosocial stressor
or stressors, that occurs within 3 months after
onset of stressor, with acute or chronic durations

(no)

With depressed mood

(no)

With anxiety

(no)

With mixed anxiety and depressed mood

(no)

With disturbance of conduct

(no)

With mixed disturbance of emotions and conduct

(no)

Unspecified

Appendix S. Personality Disorders (Listed on Axis II).

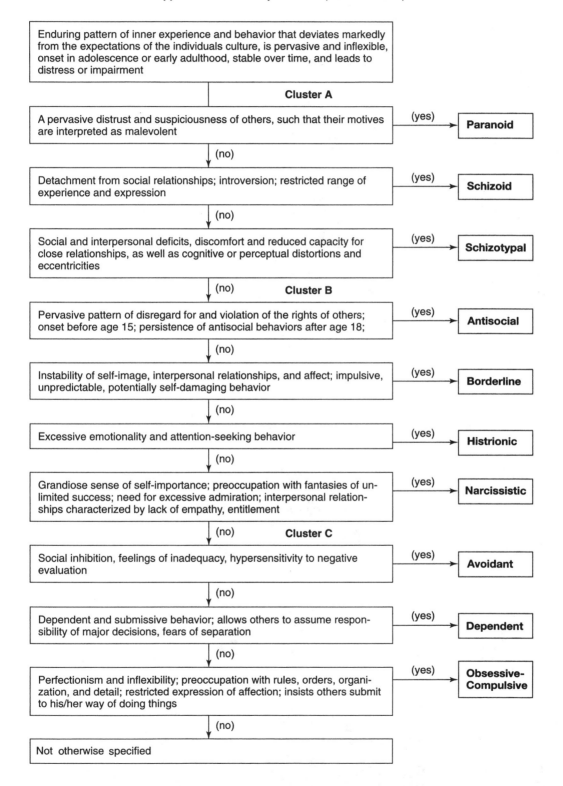

Appendix T. Other Conditions That May Be Focus of Clinical Attention.

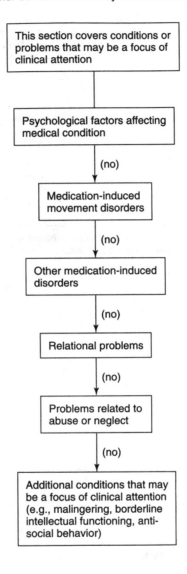

Subject Index

Page numbers followed by f refer to figures; page numbers followed by t refer to tables.